BLACK'S
MEDICAL
DICTIONARY

BLACK'S MEDICAL DICTIONARY

Edited by Gordon Macpherson, MB, BS

Thirty-seventh edition

A & C BLACK · LONDON

37th edition published by
A & C Black (Publishers) Limited
35 Bedford Row, London WC1R 4JH

ISBN 0-7136-3608-4

A CIP catalogue record for this book
is available from the British Library

In its earlier editions *Black's Medical Dictionary* was edited by:
J. D. Comrie, MD — first to seventeenth editions, 1906–42
H. A. Clegg, FRCP — eighteenth edition, 1944
W. A. R. Thomson, MD — nineteenth to thirty-fourth editions, 1948–84
C. W. H. Havard FRCP — thirty-fifth and thirty-sixth editions, 1987 and 1990

Typeset by Ace Filmsetting Ltd, Frome
Printed in Great Britain by The Bath Press

CONTENTS

PREFACE

Black's Medical Dictionary defines and explains over 5,000 terms relevant to medicine. Many aspects of anatomy, physiology, pathology, and therapeutics are explained, and the volume should prove helpful to anyone whose work or interests are part of or impinge on medical care.

For this, the 37th edition of a book first published in 1906, over 600 new entries have been prepared. In addition, around 350 existing entries have been revised, many with the help of nearly a score of distinguished experts. An appendix summarizing first-aid care has been added. While the dictionary gives an indication of the uses of various groups of drugs, it does not attempt to provide comprehensive lists or accounts of the many pharmaceutical products now available for treatment. Where specific drugs are mentioned the generic or official name is used as given in the *British Pharmacopoeia*.

I am very grateful to the following experts who have contributed to this edition: L. Beeley, FRCP; D. Blair-Fish, PhD; Professor A. W. Craft, FRCP; L. Dillner, FRCS; F. Eben, MRCOG; J. C. W. Edwards, MRCP; R. Goulding, FRCP; S. T. Green, MRCP; P. Groves, MRCPsych.; J. M. Harrington, FRCP; G. Jackson, FRCP; A. Owers, PhD; R. C. L. Page, MRCP; D. Parker, MRCP; C. G. A. Price, MRCP; P. J. Rees, FRCP; S. Rees, MB; H. M. Saxton, FRCR; and I. R. C. Swann, FRCS.

I am particularly indebted to Dr Stella Lowry and Dr Michael Weisz for their considerable and patient help in preparing new entries and revising existing ones.

Although extensively revised, the purpose of the dictionary remains the same: to provide a concise and understandable text on medicine's many aspects.

A

ABDOMEN is the lower part of the trunk. Above, and separated from it by the diaphragm or midriff, lies the thorax or chest, and below lies the pelvis, or basin, generally described as a separate cavity though directly continuous with that of the abdomen. Behind lie the spinal column and lower ribs which come within a few inches of the iliac or haunch bones; at the sides the protection afforded to the contained organs by the iliac bones and down-sloping ribs is still more effective; but in front the whole extent is protected only by soft tissues. The latter consist of the skin, a varying amount of fat, three layers of broad, flat muscle, another layer of fat, and finally the smooth, thin peritoneum which lines the whole cavity. The absence of rigidity allows the necessary distension when food is taken into the stomach, and the various important movements of the organs associated with digestion. The shape of the abdomen varies; in children it may protrude considerably, though if this is too marked it may indicate disease; in healthy young adults it should be either very slightly prominent or slightly indrawn, and should show the outline of the muscular layer,

especially of the pair of muscles running vertically (recti), which are divided into four or five sections by transverse lines; while with advance of age it is quite natural that a certain amount of fat should be deposited on and inside the abdomen.

Contents: The principal contents of the abdominal cavity are the digestive organs, i.e. the stomach and intestines, and the associated glands, the liver and pancreas. The position of the stomach is above and to the left when the individual is recumbent, but may be much lower in the erect position. The liver lies above and to the right, lying to a large extent under cover of the ribs, and occupying the hollow of the diaphragm, by which alone both it and the stomach are separated from the lungs and heart. Against the back wall on either side lie the kidneys, protected also to a great extent by the last two ribs; and from the kidneys run the ureters, or urinary ducts, down along the back wall to the bladder in the pelvis. The pancreas lies across the spine between the kidneys, and upon the upper end of each kidney lies a suprarenal gland. High up on the left and partly behind the stomach lies the spleen. The great blood-vessels and nerves, the absorbent vessels and the glands connected with them, lie on the

1 6th costal cartilage	7 9th costal cartilage	13 transverse colon
2 diaphragm	8 10th costal cartilage	14 left flexure of colon
3 7th costal cartilage	9 right flexure of colon	15 stomach
4 falciform ligament	10 caecum	16 liver
5 8th costal cartilage	11 small intestine	17 xiphoid process
6 gall bladder	12 position of umbilicus	

Contents of the abdomen in position.

back wall, and the remainder of the space is taken up by the intestines or bowels (see INTESTINE), the large intestine lying in the flanks on either side in front of the kidneys and crossing below the stomach from right to left, while the small intestine hangs from the back wall in coils which fill up the spaces between the other organs. Hanging down from the stomach in front of the bowels is the omentum, or apron, containing a considerable amount of fat, and helping to protect the bowels from cold and injury. In pregnancy the uterus, or womb, as it increases in size, rises up from the pelvis into the abdomen, lifting the coils of the small intestine above it.

The *pelvis* is that portion of the abdomen which lies within the bony pelvis (see BONE), and contains the rectum or end part of the intestine, the bladder, and, in the male the prostate, in the female the uterus, ovaries, and Fallopian tubes.

ABDOMEN, DISEASES OF: (See under STOMACH, DISEASES OF; INTESTINE, DISEASES OF; DIARRHOEA; LIVER DISEASES; PANCREAS, DISEASES OF; KIDNEYS, DISEASES OF; BLADDER, DISEASES OF; HERNIA; PERITONITIS; APPENDICITIS; TUMOUR.)

Symptoms: The symptoms of various diseases will be found under the above headings, and only some general symptoms of abdominal disease, or symptoms, the meaning of which is not plain, but which nevertheless point to trouble in definite organs, will be mentioned here.

PAIN: This is a most important symptom, because the internal organs being devoid of

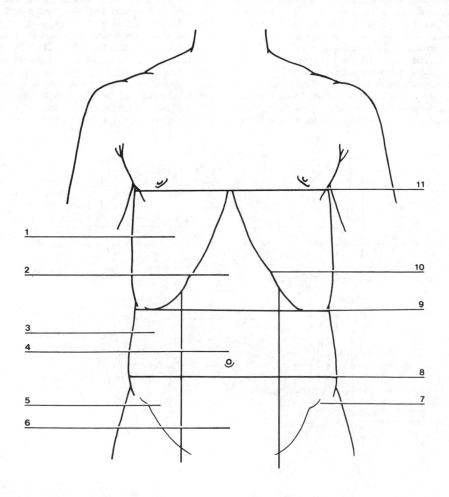

1 hypochondriac region	7 anterior superior iliac spine
2 epigastrium	8 intertubercular plane
3 lumbar region	9 subcostal plane
4 umbilical region	10 tip of 9th costal cartilage
5 iliac region	11 xiphisternal plane
6 hypogastric region	

Regions of the abdomen.

ordinary sensation, pain in them generally means a considerable interference with structure or function. The *site* of the pain may indicate the organ affected. Thus pain under the ribs on the left, or in the pit of the stomach, generally points to the stomach as being at fault. When it is felt on the right high up, and shoots through to the right shoulder, it indicates trouble connected with the liver or gallbladder. Pain situated on the right, and low down in the iliac region, may arise from a diseased appendix. On the left, and low down, or at the exit of the bowel, it means some rectal trouble. Finally, pain situated vaguely all over the front of the abdomen, especially round the navel, points to inflammation of the peritoneal lining of the abdomen, or to irregularity in movement of the small intestine.

The *character* of the pain is also important. A dull, aching pain is not generally serious, though, if persistent, it may indicate chronic peritonitis or obstruction. (See PERITONITIS; and INTESTINE, DISEASES OF.) A twisting, griping pain is generally, e.g. in babies, due to spasmodic movements of the small intestine, often produced by errors in diet, and called colic. A straining pain with frequent calls to stool indicates irritation low down in the large bowel. The pains of stomach trouble are of varied nature. (See DYSPEPSIA.) Sudden, colicky, agonizing pain is often due to the passage of a gallstone, if situated high up on the right, shooting through towards the back, or to the passage of a renal calculus, if shooting from the back down into the groin. Pain of a dull character slightly to the right of the pit of the stomach, especially when it is relieved by taking food, suggests some trouble in the duodenum.

TENDERNESS on pressure is generally a sign of inflammation either of an organ situated beneath the tender spot or of the peritoneum. (See APPENDICITIS; PERITONITIS.)

VOMITING is an important symptom. (See VOMITING.) When due to irritation of the stomach, it usually ceases as the contents of this organ are brought up. If it persists, it may be due to some obstruction in the bowels, or may be of nervous origin, e.g. in sea-sickness, or brain tumour, and have no direct connection with the abdomen.

DIARRHOEA is another important symptom, and may indicate serious trouble. (See DIARRHOEA.)

SWELLING of the abdomen may be so marked as to call the patient's attention to it. This may be due merely to excessive deposit of fat, especially in elderly people – for example, in women at the menopause. (See OBESITY; DIET.) Enlargement, of course, occurs in pregnancy. The abdomen in habitual constipation may become more distended, partly by accumulation of gas, or the enlargement may be due to chronic obstruction of the bowels. (See CONSTIPATION; and INTESTINE, DISEASES OF.) Finally, a collection of fluid may produce the swelling (see OEDEMA; LIVER DISEASES; HEART DISEASES; PERITONITIS), or it may be due to enlargement of a single organ.

INDRAWING of the abdomen occurs in wasting diseases, and also to a marked extent in meningitis. (See MENINGITIS.)

DISTENSION OF THE VEINS on the surface of the abdomen indicates some interference with the circulation in the portal vein or in the inferior vena cava.

VISIBLE MOVEMENTS are sometimes seen, due to the bowels or stomach being distended and contracting forcibly in the attempt to drive their contents onwards. They indicate (unless they are visible merely on account of extreme thinness of the abdominal wall) some obstruction in the bowel or stomach. (See PERISTALSIS.)

The differentiation of abdominal diseases is often one of the most difficult problems with which even an expert has to deal, and frequently it is only after a period of observation, lasting in difficult cases perhaps some weeks, that a diagnosis of approximate accuracy can be arrived at. This is partly due to the difficulty or impossibility of feeling the surface and dimensions of the contained organs, e.g. the kidneys, especially in stout people; partly to the vagueness of symptoms set up in organs which are very little sensitive to even extreme changes in their structure; and partly to the readiness with which the organs change their relative positions, and to the great changes in shape and position often brought about by previous disease.

Treatment: Details of treatment are given under the headings of the various diseases. On the whole, people are rather too much given to regarding abdominal symptoms as trivial and amenable to home treatment. In many cases incurable dyspepsia would have been got rid of in its early stages if its symptoms had not been neglected, and patients with acute obstruction of the bowels may die because a dose of castor oil was taken when a doctor should have been consulted. In this connection one may say that whenever the three symptoms of (a) abdominal pain, (b) vomiting or retching, and (c) stoppage of the bowels for a day or two, or stoppage followed by a little diarrhoea, have occurred together, the case demands skilled medical attention. If severe abdominal pain is directly traceable to some dietetic indiscretion, the offending material should be got rid of speedily by an emetic, if it is still in the stomach (see EMETICS); or by a purgative if the symptoms are referable to the bowels (see PURGATIVES). If the pain is griping in character, e.g. in babies, relief is often given by pressure; thus nurses often lay their charges stomach downwards across the arm, or adults get some relief by lying face downwards on a pillow. (See COLIC; LEAD-POISONING.) The application of heat, in the form of a hot-water bottle, may also give relief. When the pain is agonizing, stronger remedies are necessary. (See COLIC.)

ABDUCENT NERVE is the sixth nerve rising from the brain and controls the external rectus muscle of the eye, which turns the eye outwards. It is particularly liable to be paralysed in diseases of the nervous system, thus leading to an inward squint.

ABDUCT means to move a part of the body – for example, a limb – away from the mid line.

ABLATION means the removal of any part of the body by a surgical operation.

ABORTIFACIENT is a drug which causes artificial abortion.

ABORTION is defined as the expulsion of a fetus showing no signs of life before the 28th week of pregnancy.

SPONTANEOUS ABORTION, often called miscarriage, may occur at any time before 28 weeks, although it is commonest in the first 12 weeks of pregnancy. Of all diagnosed pregnancies 15–20 per cent end in spontaneous abortion.

The upper limit in the United Kingdom definition has recently been reduced to 24 weeks' gestation to take account of the fact that viability of a fetus is possible from 24 weeks' gestation onwards.

Spontaneous abortions occurring in early pregnancy (q.v.) are thought to be particularly associated with fetal defects such as chromosomal abnormalities. They have also been attributed to a lack of progesterone secretion during the developing pregnancy, abnormalities of the shape of the uterine cavity, and maternal disorders such as diabetes mellitus, thyroid disease and problems with the immune system. An incomplete response of the maternal immune system to pregnancy seems of particular importance in women who suffer recurrent miscarriages, defined as three or more spontaneous abortions.

Factors such as increased maternal age, a high number of previous pregnancies and smoking predispose to spontaneous abortion.

Ultrasound scans have altered the management of abortions. These make it possible to distinguish between threatened miscarriages, where the women have experienced some vaginal bleeding, but the fetus is alive; inevitable abortion, where the neck of the womb has started to open up; incomplete abortion, where part of the fetus or placenta is retained; and complete abortions. Whereas bed rest may be useful in treating threatened abortions, an inevitable or incomplete abortion will normally require the evacuation of the uterus and a complete miscarriage should require no treatment at all.

Evacuation of the uterus involves administering a general anaesthetic, gentle dilatation of the neck of the womb (cervix), and removal of the remaining products of the pregnancy.

Maternal factors are thought to account more often for late abortions. These include an inappropriately early opening of the neck of the womb (cervical incompetence), structural abnormalities and infections of the uterus.

Ultrasound scan is important to assess the condition of the intrauterine fetus. If the fetus appears normal uterine contractions may be suppressed with drugs.

In cases of cervical incompetence, it may be possible to close the cervical canal with a suture, which is removed at 38 weeks' gestation. THERAPEUTIC ABORTION Before this can take place, two doctors must agree that the continuation of the pregnancy would involve risk, greater than if the pregnancy were terminated, of injury to the physical or mental health of the mother or any existing child(ren). The new legislation introduced in 1990 states that at the time of abortion the pregnancy should not have exceeded the 24th week.

There is no time limit on therapeutic abortion where the termination is done to save the mother's life, there is substantial risk of serious fetal handicap, or of grave permanent injury to the health of the mother.

About 175,000 terminations are performed on residents in England and Wales, fewer than 500 were done over 20 weeks' gestation.

The mortality from therapeutic abortion is less than 1 per 100,000 women and, provided it is performed skilfully before 12 weeks of pregnancy, it is not associated with any reduction in fertility, increased rates of spontaneous abortion or preterm birth in subsequent pregnancies.

Methods of abortion: up to about 12 weeks into the pregnancy therapeutic abortion is performed by removing the contents of the uterus by suction under general anaesthetic after dilatation of the cervix.

In the future surgery may be avoided by using the drug mefepristone (RU 486), which causes abortion in about 85 per cent of cases.

Termination after 14 weeks usually requires induction of labourlike pains with PROSTAGLANDINS (q.v.).

ABO SYSTEM (see BLOOD GROUPS).

ABRASION means the rubbing off of the surface of the skin or of a mucous membrane due to some mechanical injury. Such injuries, though slight in themselves, are apt to allow entrance of dirt containing organisms and so to lead to an abscess or some severer form of inflammation.

Treatment: The most effective form of treatment consists in the thorough and immediate cleansing of the wound with soap and water. An antiseptic such as 1 per cent cetrimide can then be applied, and a sterile dry dressing.

DENTAL ABRASION is a form of trauma in which the teeth are worn away. This may be by bruxism or excessive use of the toothbrush, particularly if an abrasive toothpaste is used. It usually occurs at the junction of the crown and root of the tooth and is worst on the upper left teeth in a right-handed person.

ABREACTION: An emotional release caused by the recall of past unpleasant experiences. This is normally the result of psychoanalytical treatment in which psychotherapy, certain drugs, or hypnosis are used to effect the abreaction. The technique is used in the treatment of anxiety, hysteria, or other neurotic states.

ABRUPTIO PLACENTA Placental bleeding after the 28th week of pregnancy which may result in complete or partial detachment of the placenta from the wall of the womb.

ABSCESS is a localized collection of pus. A minute abscess is known as a pustule (see PUSTULE), a diffused production of pus is known as cellulitis or erysipelas (see ERYSIPELAS). An abscess may be acute or chronic. An acute abscess is one which develops rapidly within the course of a few days or hours. It is characterized by a definite set of symptoms.
Causes: The direct cause is various bacteria. In a few cases the presence of foreign bodies, such as bullets or splinters, or contact with poisonous plants, such as poison ivy, may produce abscesses, but these foreign bodies may remain for life buried in the tissues without causing any trouble provided they are not contaminated with bacteria or other micro-organisms.

The micro-organisms most frequently found are *staphylococci*, and next to these *streptococci*, though the latter cause more virulent abscesses. Other abscess-forming organisms are *Pseudomonas pyocyanea* and *Escherichia coli*, which lives always in the bowels, and under certain conditions wanders into the surrounding tissues and produces abscesses.

The presence of micro-organisms is not sufficient to produce suppuration (see IMMUNITY; and INFECTION); streptococci can often be found on the skin and in the skin glands of perfectly healthy individuals. Given the proper micro-organisms in the tissues, whether they will produce abscesses or not depends upon the virulence of the organism at the time, and the resisting power of the individual. They enter the body generally by a wound, but may also come through the mucous membrane of the intestine; they may also pass through the mucous membranes of the nose, mouth, respiratory and urinary passages, and cause local abscesses, or even through the skin's minute lubricating glands.

When bacteria have gained access, for example, to a wound, they rapidly multiply, and, by the formation of poisonous substances, irritate the surrounding tissues, and so produce local dilatation of the blood-vessels, slowing of the blood- stream, and exudation of blood corpuscles and fluid. The leucocytes, or white corpuscles of the blood, collect around the invaded area, apparently under some attracting influence of the bacteria (chemotaxis), and destroy the latter either by actually devouring and digesting them (see PHAGOCYTOSIS), or by forming some substances which cause their death. These white corpuscles undergo a granular fatty degeneration, and in turn die, and form the white constituent of the pus (pus corpuscles). Meanwhile, the area where these changes have been taking place has been cut off from communication with the rest of the body by plugging of the blood and lymphatic vessels around it. The tissues of the affected area die and are digested by the action of the white corpuscles, and the cavity so produced is distended by fluid and by the white corpuscles which flock to it in increasing numbers till all bacteria have disappeared. The abscess is shut off from healthy tissue by what is known as the abscess wall. The bacteria may find their way along a vessel to some little distance, where the same process takes place, and these secondary abscess cavities may coalesce with the original one.
Symptoms: The classic symptoms of inflammation are redness, warmth, swelling, pain and fever. When the cavity containing fluid has been formed, a sign, known as fluctuation, can be made out. The lymphatic glands in the neighbourhood may be swollen and tender in an attempt to stop the bacteria spreading to other parts of the body. Immediately the abscess is opened, or bursts, the pain disappears, the temperature falls rapidly to normal, the elasticity of the tissues around the cavity diminishes its bulk, and the healing of the small space left proceeds rapidly. If, however, the abscess discharges into an internal cavity, such as the bowel or bladder, it may heal very slowly, and the reabsorption of its poisonous products may cause general ill-health. When an abscess is deep-seated, an important sign for diagnosis is provided by examination of the blood. (See LEUCOCYTOSIS.)
Treatment: As soon as there is evidence that pus has formed, we can relieve pain, stop unnecessary destruction of tissue, and shorten the process by opening the abscess. Previous to this, an injection of penicillin, or some other antibiotic to which the causative micro-organism is sensitive, is given.

Abscesses can occur in any tissue in the body – for example, bones, brain, kidneys, lungs and appendix – but the principles of treatment are broadly the same: use of an antibiotic and, where appropriate, surgery.

A chronic abscess is one which takes weeks or months for its development. In some cases it is tuberculous, being caused by *Mycobacterium tuberculosis*, but other organisms such as the fungus actinomycosis or the staphyllococcus bacteria may be the cause.

ABSORPTION: Uptake by the body tissues of fluids or other substances. For example, food is absorbed from the digestive tract into the blood and lymph systems.

ABSTRACT: This is a dry powder produced by extracting the active principles from a crude drug with strong alcohol, mixing with sugar of milk, and drying. Abstracts are standardized so as to be twice the strength of the crude drug.

ACANTHOSIS NIGRICANS, is a darkly pigmented verrucous skin change, usually around the neck and axilla. It may be inherited but is most commonly acquired and is associated with adenocarcinoma, usually of the stomach (see CANCER), and certain hormonal disorders such as the polycystic ovary (q.v.), Addison's disease (q.v.) and Cushing's syndrome (q.v.).

ACARDIA: The congenital absence of the heart.

ACARUS: The group of animal parasites which includes *Sarcoptes scabiei*, the cause of the skin disease known as Itch, or Scabies. This parasite used to be known as *Acarus scabiei*. (See SCABIES.)

ACCIDENT PREVENTION IN THE HOME: Every year 5,500 people are killed in accidents in British homes, a further 2.2 million need hospital treatment and 900,000 consult their GPs. Domestic accidents in England and Wales cost the health service about £300 million a year. Many of these accidents happen to children or old people, and many of them are preventable.

Children's accidents can often be predicted by their stage of development. Small babies are most at risk of being dropped or having hot drinks spilled on them. As they learn to roll, crawl, and walk they are at risk of falls. As they become more inquisitive they are prone to poisoning from medicines and household chemicals. Older children are at risk from road traffic accidents. Boys are twice as likely to have accidents as girls, and children from deprived backgrounds are at particular risk. Sensible precautions will prevent many accidents. Small babies should not be left unattended on raised surfaces, and manufacturers' instructions should be followed when using all nursery equipment. Hot drinks should not be consumed anywhere near a baby or where a small child is running about. Heavy and dangerous objects should be moved out of children's reach, and parents should remember that children are quite capable of using toys as 'mounting blocks' to reach high shelves. All medicines and chemicals should be locked up. Bath water should be run from the cold tap first to ensure that a child does not get into a scalding running bath, and no child should be left unattended in a bath. Windows, especially on upper floors, should be fitted with locks that restrict the amount by which they can be opened, and stairgates can prevent many falls. By law all children's nightwear must be flameproof, but this does not remove the need for fireguards and care with naked flames and matches. Further information about preventing children's accidents can be obtained from the Child Accident Prevention Trust, 28 Portland Place, London W1N 4DE (071-636 2545).

Old people may be frail and have impaired eyesight, hearing, and mobility that increase their risk of an accident. Special precautions, similar to those for children, may be needed for people suffering from dementia, but more general rules include ensuring adequate lighting (especially on stairwells), removing unnecessary furniture and other obstacles from main thoroughfares in the home, removing loose mats from hard floors, and wearing well-fitting shoes. Specific help like walking aids, grab rails, and bath aids may help some people.

Many aspects of home safety apply to people of all ages. Domestic fires account for three-quarters of the deaths and injuries in fires in Britain. Wiring should be checked every five years, and electrical equipment should be installed and maintained according to the manufacturers' instructions. Architectural glass is a major health hazard. Toughened glass is best as it breaks into cuboid pieces. Such safety glass should be used for domestic glazing (at least at low levels). Further information about accidents at home can be obtained from the Royal Society for the Prevention of Accidents, Cannon House, The Priory, Queensway, Birmingham B4 6BS (021-200 2461).

Although many, if not all, accidents are potentially preventable, they continue to occur. Information on basic first aid can be found in APPENDIX: BASIC FIRST AID.

ACCOMMODATION: The process by which the refractive power of the lens of the eye is increased by constriction of the ciliary muscle, producing an increased thickness and curvature of the lens. Rays of light from an object further than 6 metres away are parallel on reaching the eye. These rays are brought to a focus on the retina mainly by the cornea. If the eye is now directed at an object closer than 6 metres away, the rays of light from this near object will be diverging by the time they reach the eye. In order to focus these diverging beams of light, the refracting power of the lens must increase. In other words the lens must accommodate.

With age the lens loses its elasticity and thus becomes less spherical when tension in the zonule relaxes. This results in an increased long

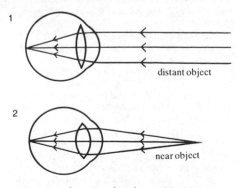

Diagram of eye in relaxed state (1) viewing a distant object and in an accommodated state; (2) with increased convexity of the lens for viewing a near object.

sightedness with age (*presbyopia*) requiring reading glasses for correction. (See AGE, NATURAL CHANGES IN).

ACEBUTOLOL (see ADRENERGIC RECEPTORS).

ACETABULUM is the cup-shaped socket on the pelvis in which rests the head of the femur or thigh-bone, the two forming the hip joint. (See HIP JOINT.)

ACETAZOLAMIDE is a drug which acts by inhibiting the enzyme carbonic anhydrase. This enzyme is of great importance in the production of acid and alkaline secretions in the body. Acetazolamide has proved of value in the treatment of glaucoma. There is some evidence that it is of value in the prevention of altitude sickness (q.v.).

ACETIC ACID, also called pyroligneous acid, is prepared by the distillation of wood and subsequent separation from tar. It is also synthesized from acetylene. In the pure form it is solid, being then known as glacial acetic acid. It is the active principle of vinegar, which is prepared from wine by the action of a particular ferment discovered by Pasteur. This grows on the surface of the vine, taking from the air oxygen which it gives up to the alcohol of the wine, so producing acetic acid. Weak acetic acid has all the actions of vinegar, and is less expensive. Strong acetic acid is a caustic and irritant poison.
Uses: In strong solution acetic acid is used to destroy warts or raise blisters. In cases of excessive sweating the weak acid is of value, because, sponged over the skin, it checks perspiration and produces a sense of coolness.

ACETONE is a chemical substance found in the urine in conditions of starvation, in diabetes mellitus, in prolonged vomiting, and in acute fevers – especially in children. With it occur in the urine beta-hydroxybutyric and acetoacetic acids, particularly in severe cases of diabetes. A large quantity of these acids and of acetone in the urine in diabetes indicates approaching coma. (See also ACIDOSIS.)

ACETYLCHOLINE is one of the substances which mediates the transmission of nerve impulses from one nerve to another, or from a nerve to the organ it acts on such as muscles. Its predominant role is in the parasympathetic nervous system (q.v.), but it also plays an important part in the transmission of nerve impulses in the brain. Acetylcholine is rapidly destroyed by cholinesterase, an enzyme present in the blood.

ACETYLCYSTEINE is a drug that is used in the treatment of fibrocystic disease of the pancreas (q.v.) and paracetamol poisoning (q.v.).

ACETYLSALICYLIC ACID (see ASPIRIN).

ACHALASIA is another term for spasm, but indicates not so much an active spasm of muscle as a failure to relax.

ACHALASIA OF THE CARDIA is a condition in which there is a failure to relax of the muscle fibres round the opening of the gullet, or oesophagus, into the stomach. (See OESOPHAGUS, DISEASES OF.)

ACHILLES TENDON: A thick tendon that joins the calf muscles to the heel bone (calcaneus) and pulls up that bone. Named after the mythical Greek hero Achilles, who was reputedly vulnerable to his enemies only in his heel, the tendon is prone to rupture in middle-aged people playing vigorous sports such as squash or tennis.

ACHLORHYDRIA means an absence of hydrochloric acid from the stomach juice; it occurs in about 4 per cent of healthy people and in several conditions, including pernicious anaemia, carcinoma of the stomach and gastritis.

ACHONDROPLASIA is a form of dwarfing in which the arms and legs are abnormally short. It is a dominant hereditary condition, and the commonest form of dwarfism. It affects both sexes and, whilst many are stillborn or die soon after birth, those who survive have normal intelligence and a normal expectation of life and good health.

ACHYLIA GASTRICA means the complete absence of ferments and of hydrochloric acid from the gastric juice; in this condition the food is passed from the stomach in a state of incomplete digestion.

ACID BASE BALANCE: The balance between the acid and alkaline elements present in the blood and body fluids. The normal hydrogen ion concentration of the plasma is a constant pH 7·4, and the lungs and kidneys have a crucial function in maintaining this figure. Changes in pH value will cause acidosis or alkalosis.

ACIDOSIS is a condition in which there is either (i) a production in the body of two abnormal acids – beta-hydroxybutyric and acetoacetic acids, or (ii) a diminution in the alkali reserve of the blood.
Causes: The condition is usually due to faulty metabolism of fat which results in the production of beta-hydroxybutyric and acetoacetic acids. It occurs in diabetes mellitus when this is either untreated or inadequately treated, starvation, persistent vomiting, and delayed anaesthetic vomiting. It also occurs in the terminal stages of glomerulonephritis when it is due to

failure of the kidneys. A milder form of it may occur in severe fevers, particularly in children. (See also ACETONE.)

Symptoms: General lassitude, vomiting, thirst, restlessness, and the presence of acetone in the urine form the earliest manifestations of the condition. In diabetes a state of coma may ensue and the disease end fatally.

Treatment: The underlying condition must always be treated: e.g. if the acidosis is due to diabetes mellitus insulin must be given. For the acidosis, alkalis should be given; e.g. bicarbonate of soda, either by mouth, or by injection if there is persistent vomiting or if the patient is unconscious. Glucose should also be given, and adequate fluids.

ACINUS is the name applied to each of the minute sacs of which secreting glands are composed, and which usually cluster round the branches of the gland-duct like grapes on their stem. (See GLANDS.)

ACNE: A skin complaint common in adolescence. It arises from sebaceous glands associated with hair follicles, especially on the face, chest, and neck. There is increased sebum production, with the development of blackheads. Proliferation of bacteria in the ducts of the sebaceous glands leads to inflammation. Adolescent acne usually clears with time. Topical treatment with benzoyl peroxide (q.v.) or salicylic acid may help. Vitamin A creams and ultraviolet light are sometimes useful, and severe cases may benefit from oral antibiotics such as oxytetracycline. Very severe acne may respond to a three-month course of 13-cis-retinoic acid, but this is teratogenic and can cause liver problems. It can only be prescribed in hospital.

ACNE ROSACEA (see ROSACEA).

ACOUSTIC NEUROMA: A slowly growing benign tumour in the auditory canal arising from the acoustic cranial nerve. The neuroma may cause facial numbness, hearing loss, unsteady balance, headache, and tinnitus. It can usually be removed surgically.

ACRIFLAVINE is an aniline derivative. It is an orange-red crystalline powder, readily soluble in water, which gives a rich yellow colour to substances brought into contact with it, and in a solution of 1 in 1000 of water, possesses strong antiseptic powers.

ACROCYANOSIS is a condition, occurring especially in young women, in which there is persistent blueness of hands, feet, nose and ears.

ACRODYNIA (see ERYTHROEDEMA).

ACROMEGALY is a disorder caused by the increased secretion of growth hormone by an adenoma of the anterior pituitary gland. It results in excessive body growth of both the skeletal and the soft tissues. If it occurs in adolescence before the bony epiphyses have fused the result is gigantism. If it occurs in adult life the skeletal overgrowth is confined to the hands, feet, cranial sinuses and jaw. Most of the features are due to overgrowth of the cartilage of the nose and ear and the soft tissues which increase the thickness of the skin and lips. Viscera such as the thyroid and liver are also affected. The overgrowth of the soft tissues occurs so gradually that the patient and spouse are often unaware of the change. It is only relatives who have not seen the patient for many months or years who are aware of the striking change in physical appearance.

The local effects of the tumour commonly cause headache and, less frequently, impairment of vision, particularly of the temporal field of vision, as a result of pressure on the nerves to the eye. The tumour may damage the other pituitary cells giving rise to gonadal, thyroid or adrenocortical insufficiency. The diagnosis is confirmed by measuring the level of growth hormone in the serum and by an X-ray of the skull which usually shows enlargement of the pituitary fossa. The treatment consists of removal or irradiation of the pituitary adenoma. This may have to be done via a craniotomy if the tumour is large but can often be done by an approach through the nose and sphenoid sinus. Deep X-ray therapy to the pituitary fossa is also effective treatment but it may take several years for irradiation to achieve its maximum effect. Drugs, such as bromocriptine, which are dopamine agonists, lower growth hormone levels in acromegaly and are particularly useful as an adjunct to radiotherapy.

ACROMION is the part of the scapula, or shoulder blade, forming the tip of the shoulder and giving its squareness to the latter. It projects forward from the scapula, and, with the clavicle or collar-bone in front, forms a protecting arch of bone over the shoulder joint.

ACROPARAESTHESIA is a disorder occurring predominantly in middle-aged women in which there is numbness and tingling of the fingers.

ACTH is the commonly used abbreviation for corticotrophin (q.v.).

ACTINOMYCIN D is an antibiotic isolated from *Streptomyces antibioticus* and *Streptomyces chrysomallus*; it has an inhibitory action on neoplastic cells (see CYTOTOXIC).

ACTINOMYCOSIS is an acute or chronic suppurative disease affecting cattle in which it is known as Woody Tongue, and sometimes found in man.

Causes: The direct cause is the ray-fungus or actinomyces known as *Actinomyces israeli*, which occurs as a commensal (q.v.) in the mouth. In certain circumstances still rather obscure, but one of which is undoubtedly trauma, such as a fractured jaw or extraction of a tooth, the *A. israeli* becomes active. It then causes hard swellings, abscesses and ulcers, in the pus of which the fungus is found in little yellow balls of a size which can just be made out by the naked eye. These little balls are found to consist of masses of thread-like material matted together, and of club-shaped bodies radiating from a common centre, hence the name of ray-fungus. It used to be thought that the human infection arose from the chewing of straw or grain, or was caught from cattle, but this is now known not to be the case. In over 50 per cent of cases the disease occurs in or about the mouth; in 20 per cent it occurs in the abdomen, and in 15 per cent in the thorax.

Symptoms: These are general bad health, the presence of hard fibrous masses about the mouth or tongue, or in other organs, and the development sooner or later in these masses of abscesses which after bursting form sinuses or ulcers that will not heal.

Treatment: The outlook has been changed completely since the introduction of the antibiotics. The best results are usually obtained with large doses of penicillin, but in some cases chlortetracycline is more effective. Surgical treatment may be required, as in the draining of abscesses.

ACUPUNCTURE is a traditional Chinese method of healing by inserting thin needles into certain areas beneath the skin and rotating them. Its rationale is that disease is a manifestation of a disturbance of Yin and Yang energy in the body, and that acupuncture brings this energy back into balance by what is described as 'the judicious stimulation or depression of the flow of energy in the various meridians'. What is still unclear to western doctors is why needling, which is the essence of acupuncture, should have the effect it is claimed to have. One theory is that the technique stimulates deep sensory nerves, promoting the production of pain-relieving endorphins (q.v.). Of its efficacy in skilled Chinese hands, however, there can be no question, and in China the technique is an alternative to anaesthesia for some operations.

ACUTE: An adjective to describe a disease of short duration that starts quickly and has severe symptons. It may also refer to a symptom, for example, severe pain. An ACUTE ABDOMEN is a serious disorder of the abdomen requiring urgent treatment, usually surgery. ACUTE HEART FAILURE is the sudden stopping or defect in the action of the heart. ACUTE LEUKAEMIA is a rapid growth in the numbers of white blood cells which is fatal if untreated.

ACYCLOVIR is an antiviral drug that is particularly useful in infections by herpes virus.

ADACTYLY: Absence of the digits.

ADDICTION: A vague term that may describe habitual cravings for tobacco or caffeine products to the physical and psychological dependence of a person on powerful substances such as morphine or heroin (see DRUG ADDICTION).

ADDISON'S DISEASE: The cause of Addison's disease is a deficiency of the adrenocortical hormones cortisol, aldosterone and androgens due to destruction of the adrenal cortex. It occurs in about 1:25,000 of the population. Although the destruction of the adrenal cortex in Addison's original description was due to tuberculosis, a much more common cause today is auto-immune damage. Rare causes of Addison's disease include metastases from carcinoma, usually of the bronchus, granulomata and haemochromatosis.

Symptoms: The clinical symptoms depend on the severity of the underlying disease process. The patient usually complains of anorexia, nausea and loss of weight. The skin becomes pigmentated due to the increased production of ACTH (q.v.). Faintness, especially on standing, is due to postural hypotension secondary to aldosterone deficiency. Women lose their axillary hair and both sexes are liable to develop mental symptoms such as depression.

Diagnosis depends on demonstrating impaired serum levels of cortisol and inability of these levels to rise after an injection of ACTH.

Treatment consists in replacement of the deficient hormones and this enable patients to lead a completely normal life and to enjoy a normal life expectancy.

ADENINE ARABINOSIDE is an anti-viral agent that is proving of value in the treatment of certain forms of herpes. (See HERPES SIMPLEX; and EYE, DISEASE AND INJURIES.)

ADENITIS means inflammation of a gland. (See LYMPHATICS.)

ADENO- is a prefix denoting relation to a gland or glands.

ADENOCARCINOMA: A malignant growth of glandular tissue. This tissue is widespread throughout the body's organs and the tumours may occur, for example, in the stomach, ovaries, and uterus. Adenocarcinomas may be subdivided into those that arise from mucous or serous secreting glandular tissue.

ADENOIDS (see NOSE, DISEASES OF).

ADENOMA means a benign tumour composed of glandular tissue. It may arise in any part of the body in which glandular tissue occurs: e.g. the thyroid gland. It must be differentiated from an adenocarcinoma, which is a malignant tumour composed of glandular tissue. (See TUMOUR.)

ADENOVIRUSES are a group of viruses which cause infections of the upper respiratory tract resembling the common cold, and often referred to as febrile catarrh.

ADHESION: This means the uniting together of structures which should normally be separate and freely movable. It is the result of acute or chronic inflammation. The medium by which the attachment takes place may at first be fibrin (q.v.) as a result of acute inflammation, but later is, in every case, fibrous tissue either in masses or in bands.
Causes: The most important adhesions are those taking place in serous and joint cavities. When one of these structures becomes inflamed there is a great exudation of fluid into the cavity. From this fluid a solid material separates and becomes deposited upon the smooth surface of the cavity. This solid 'fibrin' should, in the course of recovery, be reabsorbed; but, if the inflammation is very severe, or if there is repeated attacks of it, this absorption does not completely take place, the two layers of fibrin on the opposing surfaces of the cavity stick together, and the united mass is 'organized' into the less absorbable fibrous tissue (see FIBROUS TISSUE). As a result there is restricted movement in the parts concerned; thus in the case of a joint there is ankylosis (see JOINTS DISEASES OF); if the inflammation has been pleurisy the lung becomes adherent to the chest wall; if peritonitis, bands are formed between stomach, bowels, and other abdominal organs.
Symptoms: It is generally difficult to tell, except from the history of an inflammatory attack and from the presence of disordered function of internal organs, that adhesions are present (see PLEURISY; PERITONITIS). Sometimes adhesions between loops of bowels may be very serious and cause obstruction, if an old-standing and rigid fibrous band becomes twisted round a loop of bowel (see INTESTINE, DISEASES OF).
Treatment: While the adhesions are still *fibrinous* one expects complete absorption if the inflammation is speedily subdued. If the adhesions are *fibrous*, and show their presence by interference with the function of the organs concerned, one can seldom expect their complete absorption.

Sometimes, e.g. when obstruction of the bowels is due to an adhesion, an immediate operation is necessary, and the adhesion is then divided. Adhesions causing limitation of movement in joints can often be broken down by means of manipulation.

ADIPOSE TISSUE or FAT is a loose variety of fibrous tissue, in the meshes of which lie cells, each of which is distended by several small drops, or one large drop, of fat. This tissue replaces fibrous tissue when the amount of food taken is in excess of the bodily requirements. (See DIET; OBESITY.)

ADIPOSIS DOLOROSA, also known as Dercum's disease, is a condition in which painful masses of fat develop under the skin. It is commoner in women than in men.

ADOPTION (see CHILD ADOPTION).

ADRENAL GLANDS, also known as SUPRARENAL GLANDS, are two organs situated one upon the upper end of each kidney. Each measure about 5 cm (2 inches) in length from above downwards, rather less than that from side to side; and each is about 6 mm (¼ inch) thick. The two together weigh about 7 grams.
Structure: Each suprarenal gland has an enveloping layer of fibrous tissue. Within this the gland shows two distinct parts: an outer, firm, deep-yellow, *cortical* layer, and a central, soft, dark-brown, *medullary* portion. The cortical part consists of columns of cells running from the surface inwards, whilst in the medullary portion the cells are arranged irregularly and separated from one another by large capillary blood-vessels. Both the blood vessels and the nerves of the suprarenal glands are large and numerous, considering the small size of the organ.
Functions: It has long been known that removal of the suprarenal glands in animals is speedily followed by great muscular prostration and death in a few days. In human beings, disease of the suprarenal glands is apt to bring on Addison's disease, in which the chief symptoms are increasing weakness and bronzing of the skin. The medulla of the glands produces a substance – adrenaline – the effects of which closely resemble those brought about by activity of the sympathetic nervous system: dilated pupils, hair standing on end, quickening and strengthening of the heart-beat, immobilization of the gut, increased output of sugar from the liver into the blood-stream. From the cortex of the gland are produced a series of hormones which play a vital, though as yet incompletely elucidated, rôle in the metabolism of the body. Some (such as aldosterone) control the electrolyte balance of the body, others are concerned in carbohydrate metabolism, whilst others again are concerned with sex physiology. Cortisone is the most important hormone of the adrenal cortex and is essential for life. (See ADRENALINE; ADDISON'S DISEASE; CORTISONE.)

ADRENALINE is the secretion of the adrenal medulla. (See ADRENAL GLANDS.) In the United States Pharmocopoeia it is known as epinephrine. It is also prepared synthetically. When injected it produces the same effect as stimulation of the sympathetic nervous system (q.v.). Among its important effects are raising of the blood pressure, increasing the amount of glucose in the blood, and constricting the smaller blood- vessels.

It is applied directly to wounds on gauze or lint to check haemorrhage. Injected along with some local anaesthetic it permits painless, bloodless operations to be performed on the eye, nose, etc. It is injected hypodermically to relieve asthma, and to stimulate the heart in collapsed conditions. It is also injected as an antidote in the condition of hypoglycaemia, when too large a dose of insulin has been given.

ADRENERGIC RECEPTORS are the sites in the body on which adrenaline (q.v.) and comparable stimulants of the sympathetic system (q.v.) act. Drugs which have an adrenaline-like action are described as being adrenergic. There are four different types of adrenergic receptors, known as $alpha_1$, $alpha_2$, $beta_1$, and $beta_2$, respectively. Stimulation of alpha receptors leads to constriction of the bronchi, constriction of the blood vessels with consequent rise in blood-pressure, and dilatation of the pupils of the eyes. Stimulation of $beta_1$ receptors quickens the rate and output of the heart, whilst stimulation of $beta_2$ receptors dilates the bronchi.

For long it had been realized that in certain cases of asthma adrenaline had not the usual beneficial effect of dilating the bronchi during an attack; rather it made the asthma worse. This was due to its acting on both the alpha and beta adrenergic receptors. A derivative, isoprenaline, was therefore produced which acted only on the beta receptors. This had an excellent effect in dilating the bronchi, but unfortunately also affected the heart, speeding it up and increasing its output – an undesirable effect which meant that isoprenaline, still a valuable drug in the treatment of asthma, has to be used with great care. In due course drugs were produced, such as salbutamol, which act predominantly on the $beta_2$ adrenergic receptors in the bronchi and have relatively little effect on the heart.

The converse of this story was the search for what became known as beta-adrenoceptor-blocking drugs, or beta-adrenergic-blocking drugs. The theoretical argument was that if such drugs could be synthesized, they could be of value in taking the strain off the heart – for example: stress → stimulation of the output of adrenaline → stimulation of the heart → increased work for the heart. A drug that could prevent this train of events would be of value, for example, in the treatment of angina pectoris (q.v.). Now there is a series of beta-adrenergic-blocking drugs of use not only in angina pectoris, but also in various other heart conditions such as disorders of rhythm, as well as high blood- pressure. They are also proving of value in the treatment of anxiety states by preventing disturbing features such as palpitations. An unexpected dividend is that some of them at least appear to be of help in the treatment of migraine.

The first beta-blocker in therapeutic use and probably still the best known is propranolol. Many other beta-blockers are now available and in general they are all equally effective. There are, however, minor differences which may affect the choice in treating an individual patient. Some drugs have intrinsic sympathomimetic activity, a manifestation of the ability of these drugs to stimulate as well as to block adrenergic receptors. Oxprenolol, pindolol and acebutolol are members of this group and they therefore tend to cause less slowing of the pulse and less coldness of the extremities than the other beta-blockers. Some beta-blockers are lipid soluble and as a result pass the blood brain barrier with ease. They may therefore cause central effects such as sleep disturbances and nightmares. Water-soluble beta- blockers tend not to cross the blood brain barrier and are less likely to have these side-effects. Examples of the water soluble beta-blockers are atenolol, nadolol and sotalol. Being water soluble they are excreted by the kidneys and may therefore accumulate in patients with renal impairment.

Some beta-blockers tend to have less effect on the $beta_2$ or bronchial receptors and are therefore called cardio-selective. This is not completely true as if given in larger doses $beta_2$ effects will also occur. Nevertheless metoprolol, atenolol and acebutolol are relatively cardioselective and have less effect on airways resistance. Despite this, the precaution of avoiding beta-blockers in patients with obstructive airways disease also applies to the so-called selective drugs. Nevertheless the beta- adrenoceptor blocking drugs are most useful in the treatment of hypertension, angina pectoris, secondary prevention of myocardial infarction, migraine, anxiety states, essential tremor, thyrotoxicosis and glaucoma when used topically.

ADRENOCORTICOTROPHIC HORMONE (ACTH) A hormone which is released into the body during stress. Made and stored in the anterior pituitary gland, ACTH regulates the production of Corticosteroid hormones from the Adrenal Gland. ACTH is vital for the growth and maintenance of the adrenal cortical cells. Its production is in part controlled by the amount of hydrocortisone in the blood and also by the hypothalmus. The hormone is used to test adrenal function and treat conditions such as asthma.

ADRENOGENITAL SYNDROME: An inherited condition, the adrenogenital syndrome or congenital adrenal hyperplasia is an uncommon disorder affecting about one baby in 7,500. The condition is present from birth and the victim suffers from various enzyme defects as well as a block on the production of hydrocortisone and aldosterone by the adrenal gland. In girls the syndrome produces virilization of the genital tract, which may become enlarged. The metabolism of salt and water is disturbed causing dehydration, low blood pressure, and loss of weight. Enlargement of the adrenal glands occurs and the affected individual may also develop excessive pigmentation in the skin. Treatment requires replacement of the missing hormones and, if started early, may lead to normal sexual development.

ADULT RESPIRATORY DISTRESS SYNDROME (ARDS): A form of acute respiratory failure in which a variety of different disorders give rise to pulmonary injury by what is thought to be a common pathway. It has a high mortality (about 70 per cent).

The exact aetiology is unknown, but it is thought that, whatever the stimulus, activation of neutrophils (which may then be sequestered in the lungs) releases cytotoxic substances – substances that damage or kill cells – such as oxygen-free radicals and proteases which damage the alveolar capillary membranes. Once this is damaged protein-rich oedema fluid leaks into the alveoli and insterstitial spaces. Surfactant (q.v.) is also lost. This impairs gas exchange and gives rise to the clinical and pathological picture of acute respiratory failure.

The typical patient with ARDS has rapidly worsening hypoxaemia (lack of oxygen in the blood), often requiring mechanical ventilation, which contrasts with the relative lack of physical signs. There are all the signs of respiratory failure (see TACHYPNOEA, TACHYCARDIA, CYANOSIS, etc.), though the chest may be clear apart from a few crackles. Radiographs show bilateral, patchy, peripheral shadowing sparing the cardio and costophrenic angles. Blood gases will show a low PaO_2 (concentration of oxygen in pulmonary arterial blood) and usually a high $PaCO_2$ (concentration of carbon dioxide in pulmonary arterial blood). The lungs are 'stiff' – they are less effective because of the loss of surfactant and the non-cardiogenic pulmonary oedema. The causes of ARDS may be broadly divided into the following:

MICROBIOLOGICAL – pulmonary, distant, or generalized infection by bacteria, fungi, or viruses.
ACTIVATION OF HOST DEFENCE – massive transfusion, transfusion reaction, cardiopulmonary bypass, etc., may cause activation of neutrophils (q.v.) via complement pathways.
CHEMICAL – this includes drugs, inhaled toxic gases and smoke, and metabolic disorders like uraemia (q.v.) and pancreatitis (see pancreas, diseases of).
PHYSICAL – trauma to the lung, gastric aspiration, aspiration of water, etc. The principles of management are supportive, with treatment of the underlying condition if that is possible. Oxygenation is improved by increasing inspired oxygen concentration and mechanical ventilation of the lungs. Attempts are made to reduce the formation of pulmonary oedema by careful management of fluid balance. Secondary infections are treated if they arise, as are the possible complications of prolonged ventilation with low lung compliance (e.g., pneumothorax (q.v.)). There is some evidence that giving surfactant through a nebulizer or aerosol

may help to improve lung effectiveness and reduce oedema. There is little evidence that steroids are of use. Some experimental evidence supports the use of free radical scavengers and antioxidants, but these are not commonly used. In severe cases extracorporeal gas exchange has been advocated as a supportive measure until the lungs have healed enough for adequate gas exchange. (See also RESPIRATION DISTRESS SYNDROME AND HYALINE MEMBRANE DISEASE.)

ADVERSE REACTIONS TO DRUGS: There are a number of ways in which post-marketing studies permit the detection of adverse drug reactions. In the past techniques such as invididual case reports, the Committee on the Safety of Medicines' yellow card system, monitoring national mortality statistics and case control studies have successfully identified adverse drug reactions. The most useful method, when it is feasible, is the Cohort investigation. This requires that a cohort of patients starting treatment with a particular drug should be identified and the cohort should be sufficiently large to allow rarer adverse reactions to be detected. The system must look at adverse events and not merely suspected adverse reactions suffered by patients from the time of starting treatment to the end of the enquiry.

AEDES AEGYPTI is the scientific name of the mosquito which conveys to man (by biting) the viruses of yellow fever and of dengue or 'breakbone fever'. (See DENGUE; and YELLOW FEVER.)

AEGOPHONY is the bleating or punchinello tone given to the voice as heard by auscultation, when there is a small amount of fluid in the pleural cavity.

AERODONTALGIA is the relatively rare form of dental pain occasionally felt in restored or non-vital teeth by those who fly. It is thought that it is caused by expansion of gas entrapped in the pulp canal of the tooth, resulting from the change in altitude.

AEROPHAGY means air-swallowing, and is the name applied to a habit which some persons, especially when suffering from dyspepsia, contract of swallowing mouthfuls of air. This at first gives relief to the discomfort and pain of indigestion, but later prolongs and aggravates it. The resulting breathlessness can be relieved to some extent by taking peppermint water or chloroform water in doses of a tablespoonful, but the chief necessity is to overcome the habit of swallowing air.

AEROSOL (see INHALANTS).

AESTHESIOMETER is an instrument for measuring the sensation of touch in a person.

AETIOLOGY is the part of medical science dealing with the causes of disease.

AFFERENT An adjective to describe nerves, blood vessels, or lymphatic vessels that conduct their electrical charge or contents inwards to the brain, spinal cord or relevant organ.

AFIBRINOGENAEMIA is a condition in which the blood is incoagulable as a result of absence of fibrin (q.v.). It is characterized by haemorrhage. There are two forms: (a) a congenital form, and (b) an acquired form. The latter may be associated with advanced liver disease, or may occur as a complication of labour. Treatment consists of the intravenous injection of fibrinogen and blood transfusion.

AFTERBIRTH, or PLACENTA, is the name given to the thick, spongy disc-like cake of tissue which connects the embryo with the inner surface of the womb, the embryo otherwise lying free in the amniotic fluid. (See AMNION.) The placenta is mainly a new structure growing with the embryo, but, when it separates, a portion of the inner surface of the womb, called the maternal placenta, comes away with it. It is mainly composed of loops of veins belonging to the embryo, lying in blood-sinuses, in which circulates maternal blood. Thus, though no mixing of the blood of embryo and mother takes place, there is ample opportunity for the exchange of fluids, gases, and the nutriment brought by the mother's blood. The width of the full-sized placenta is about 20 cm (8 inches), its thickness 2·5 cm (1 inch). One surface is rough and studded with villi, which consist of the loops of foetal veins; the other is smooth, and has implanted in its centre the umbilical cord, or navel string, which is about as thick as a finger and 50 cm (20 inches) long. It contains two arteries and a vein, enters the foetus at the navel, and forms the sole connection between the bodies of mother and foetus. The name 'afterbirth' is given to the structure because it is expelled from the womb in the third stage of labour (see LABOUR).

AFTERPAINS are pains similar to but feebler than those of labour, occurring in the two or three days following childbirth.
Causes are generally the presence of a blood-clot or retained piece of placenta which the womb is attempting to expel.

AGAMMAGLOBULINAEMIA is a condition found in children, in which there is no gamma-globulin (q.v.) in the blood. These children are particularly susceptible to infections as they are unable to form antibodies to any infecting micro-organism.

AGAR, or AGAR-AGAR, is a gelatinous substance prepared from seaweed. It is used in preparing culture-media for use in bacteriologi-cal laboratories. It is sometimes given for relieving constipation.

AGE, NATURAL CHANGES IN: As age advances, the tissues become more rigid and less elastic. The bones become more brittle. The ligaments are stiffer, so that contortions of the body and limbs become impossible. Fat is deposited beneath the skin in middle life with accompanying increase in weight. It may be absorbed again in old age, leaving the skin wrinkled. Deposition of fat also occurs in internal organs, e.g. the heart, weakening their activity. The skin becomes thin, is less well lubricated, and its vessels do not react properly to heat and cold, so that cold is more acutely felt. The chief change is in the blood-vessels, the walls of which become first thicker, then more brittle. This means that obstruction (e.g. in the coronary arteries that supply the heart muscle with blood) or haemorrhage (e.g. into the brain, with apoplexy) more readily occurs. This change is hastened by alcoholic excesses and some diseases, and the extent to which it has occurred is the measure of the interference with the employments of active life. This thickening of the arteries in the brain and consequent narrowing of their calibre, causing a poorer blood-supply to the brain is one of the chief reasons of mental feebleness in old age. The menopause occurs in women between forty-five and fifty (see MENSTRUATION), and men sometimes about the age of sixty have some months' illness and feebleness, after which strength again returns. Sexual activity tends to diminish but seldom becomes dormant. Loss of elasticity in the lens of the eye brings about the need of spectacles for reading from forty upwards. Another eye change occurs after fifty in the appearance of a whitish ring (arcus senilis) round the cornea, near its edge: this is of no significance. Of more importance is the opacification of the lens known as cataract (q.v.) which tends to occur after fifty and may so interfere with sight that the lens has to be removed. After sixty the teeth, if still good, may begin to fall out and the hair whitens. (See also CLIMACTERIC; and EXPECTATION OF LIFE.)

AGENESIA, or AGENESIS, means incomplete development or the failure of any part or organ of the body to develop normally.

AGGLUTINATION is the adherence together of small bodies in a fluid. Thus, blood corpuscles agglutinate into heaps (rouleaux) when added to the serum of a person belonging to an incompatible blood-group. Bacteria agglutinate into clumps and die when exposed to the presence of antibodies in the blood. This is important in regard to diagnosis of certain diseases due to bacteria. In typhoid fever, for example, the blood of an animal is immunized against typhoid bacilli by repeated injections of these. The blood-serum of the animal, known now as anti-typhoid serum, is issued to laboratories for use when bacilli are found in the excretions of a patient who is possibly suffering from typhoid fever. The bacilli are exposed to the action of a drop of the serum; if the serum shows the power of agglutinating these bacteria, this forms evidence that the bacteria in question are typhoid bacilli. The reaction may also be carried out in the contrary manner: that is to say, the serum from the blood of a patient, who may be suffering from typhoid fever, but in regard to whom the diagnosis is still a matter of doubt, is added to a drop of fluid containing bacteria known to be typhoid bacilli; if these are agglutinated into clumps by the patient's serum, the patient is then known to be suffering from typhoid fever; if they do not agglutinate, his symptoms are due to some other condition. This reaction for typhoid fever is known as the Widal reaction. Comparable agglutination reactions, using an appropriate serum, are used in the diagnosis of a number of diseases, including glandular fever (when it is known as the Paul-Bunnell reaction), typhus fever (when it is known as the Weil-Felix reaction), undulant fever, and Weil's disease.

AGNOSIA is the condition in which, in certain diseases of the brain, the patient loses the ability to recognize the character of objects through the senses – touch, taste, sight, hearing.

AGONIST A muscle which contracts and causes a movement.

AGORAPHOBIA means a sense of fear experienced in large open spaces and public places, and is a symptom of psychological disorder (see MENTAL ILLNESS) . There are said to be 300,000 victims of it in the United Kingdom. Those who suffer from what can be a most distressing condition can obtain help and advice from the Phobics Society, 4 Cheltenham Road, Chorlton cum Hardy, Manchester M21 1QN. (061-881 1937.)

AGRANULOCYTOSIS is a condition in which the white corpuscles in the blood of the polynuclear or granular variety become greatly lessened in numbers or disappear altogether. It is usually caused by taking such drugs as amidopyrine, thiourea, sulphonamides, chloramphenicol and the immuno-suppressant drugs.

AGRAPHIA is the loss of power to express ideas by writing. (See APHASIA.)

AGUE (see MALARIA). The term is also sometimes applied to neuralgia (brow ague) and to a state of tremor of the muscles found in various diseases (such as brass founders' ague).

AIDS/HIV INFECTION: The first recognition of AIDS (acquired immune deficiency syndrome) was in 1981 in the USA when clusters of cases of a hitherto rare pneumonia, *Pneumocystis carinii* pneumonia (PCP), and an uncommon skin tumour, Kaposi's sarcoma (KS), were recognized. It has now been established beyond reasonable doubt that the cause of the syndrome is a ribonucleic acid (RNA (q.v.)) retrovirus, HIV (human immunodeficiency virus), and this agent is responsible for a whole constellation of clinical conditions with AIDS representing only the late clinical consequences of infection with HIV. The origins of HIV are not known, although it has several close relatives in the animal world.

Since clinical HIV infection was first recognized, cases have been reported from almost all countries in the world, and by 1991 the World Health Organization had estimated that worldwide there were at least 10 million infected (the majority in sub-Saharan Africa) and that 1 million of these had reached the stage known as AIDS. In the UK in 1991 there were at least 15,000 HIV-infected individuals. Retrospective studies have shown that the virus was in Africa at least as far back as the mid-1950s. HIV has now been subdivided into HIV-1 and HIV-2; both lead to profound immunodeficiency.

Africa	6 million
Asia	1 million
North America	1 million
South America	1 million
Europe	0·5 million
UK	15,000+

Estimated number of HIV-positive individuals worldwide in 1991 (WHO figures)

The ultimate target of HIV is the CD4+ ('T_4') lymphocyte, a cell essential for the proper functioning of the cell-mediated immunity arm of the immune system; once it has gained admission to the CD4+ cell the virus uses an enzyme, reverse transcriptase, to convert viral RNA into deoxyribonucleic acid (DNA (q.v.)), this DNA then being incorporated into the genome. This effectively converts the CD4+ lymphocyte into a 'virus factory'. In uninfected individuals the peripheral CD4+ cell count in the blood is more than 500/mm^3, but this begins to decline and most of the clinical consequences of HIV infection result from this process.

Initial impressions were that only individuals from certain 'high-risk groups' (e.g. homosexual men, injecting drug users and haemophiliacs) were susceptible to HIV infection. It is now abundantly clear that this is not so and that there are two principal modes of transmission of HIV: sexual (either heterosexual or homosexual); direct 'transplantation' of the virus from one individual's body to another (e.g. blood-product transfusion, organ transplant, sharing of needles by injecting drug users). Transmission does not occur through casual contact.

Individuals are regarded as being infected with HIV if they test positive for antibodies to

HIV-1 or HIV-2 (in either blood or saliva) and such individuals are said to be 'HIV-positive'. It is usual for a newly infected individual to commence producing specific antibodies around six to twelve weeks later. This period when antibodies cannot be detected is conventionally known as the 'window period'; thus HIV-testing before twelve weeks have elapsed since the high-risk incident occurred might not detect antibody, despite the individual's actually being infected.

The clinical picture can be regarded as a continuum, with patients moving from an asymptomatic phase to a symptomatic one. About three-quarters of cases show no initial evidence of clinical disease after acquiring the infection; the other 25 per cent develop a clinical syndrome resembling glandular fever six to twelve weeks after becoming infected (the 'seroconversion illness'); recovery is invariably complete. The asymptomatic phase may last for many years, but there is invariably progressive and systematic destruction of the cell-mediated arm of the immune system. As the plasma CD4+ cell count falls to less than 200/mm^3, the infected individual will begin to develop symptoms and possibly clinical signs showing progression. Early clinical indicators of progression include persistent generalized lymphadenopathy – enlargement of lymph glands – (PGL), thrombocytopenic purpura – spontaneous bruising and bleeding after injury as a result of the condition thrombocytopenia (q.v.), lethargy, fevers, night sweats, oral hairy leukoplakia (q.v.), seborrhoeic dermatitis (see SEBORRHOEA), weight loss and oral candidiasis (see CANDIDA). Ultimately, the CD4+ cell count falls so low that the individual becomes particularly susceptible to the development of certain viral, fungal, protozoal and mycobacterial infections and tumours, some characteristic, if not pathognomic, of HIV infection and rarely encountered in other clinical settings. Eventually antibody-mediated immune responses are also impaired and pyogenic bacterial infections occur more commonly than in immuno-competent individuals. The presence of certain infections and tumours places the HIV-infected individual into the category of 'AIDS'.

Among the more important clinical manifestations of advanced HIV disease are severe and recurrent herpes virus infections (e.g. Herpes simplex (q.v.), Herpes zoster (q.v.), gastrointestinal and invasive candidiasis, pneumonic illnesses (e.g. PCP, cytomegalovirus (CMV)), diarrhoeal illnesses (e.g. cryptosporidium, salmonella (q.v.)), meningitis (q.v.) (e.g. Cryptococcus neoformans), cerebral abscesses (e.g. Toxoplasma gondii), retinitis (see RETINA, DISORDERS OF) leading to blindness (e.g. CMV) and disseminated Mycobacterium avium-intracellulare. Specific chemotherapy exists for many (but not all) of these conditions and research and development continue.

Dementia (AIDS-dementia complex), cutaneous and gastrointestinal Kaposi's sarcoma and non-Hodgkin's lymphoma are other well recognized manifestations. All of these tend to

PROTOZOAL
Pneumocystis carinii*
Cryptosporidium*
Toxoplasma gondii*
Entamoeba histolytica
VIRAL
Cytomegalovirus*
JC virus (encephalopathy)*
Herpes simplex
Herpes varicella\zoster
FUNGAL
Candida (invasive)*
Cryptococcus neoformans*
Aspergillosis
Tinea
MYCOBACTERIAL
Mycobacterium avium-intracellulare*
Mycobacterium tuberculosis
BACTERIA
Salmonella
Staphylococci
Streptococci (inc. Strept. pneumoniae)
TUMOURS
Kaposi's sarcoma*
Non-Hodgkin's lymphoma*

* AIDS indicator condition

Important opportunistic pathogens and tumours in HIV infection

occur when the CD4+ count is less than 50/mm^3, and a recent revised definition of AIDS that regards HIV-infected individuals with a CD4+ cell count less than 200/mm^3 as having AIDS has been proposed.

Treatment: Most authorities accept that probably all HIV-infected individuals will ultimately develop serious life-threatening health problems, although these may take ten years or more to develop. Drugs such as zidovudine and dideoxyinosine, which inhibit HIV replication, can slow deterioration of the immune system, while the use of prophylactic drugs directed against PCP and other major opportunistic infections is also helping to maintain health and lengthen lives. Research continues and several new drugs and immunotherapies are under development.

Despite the therapeutic advances, the infection remains incurable. HIV dissemination continues and the World Health Organization estimates that by AD 2000 there will be 40 million infected people worldwide. At present an effective vaccine is a long way off. Accordingly continued monitoring and surveillance of the epidemic remain vital, as do measures directed towards the prevention of further spread. These include health promotion/educational initiatives targeted at sexual health and drug injecting (both among HIV-positive individuals and the general population), easy access to skilled counselling and HIV testing, improved condom availability, etc. The need for these measures will disappear only if and when an effective cure or a vaccine becomes available.

AIR: The general constituents of air are:

	per cent
Oxygen	20 94
Nitrogen	78 09
Argon	0 94
Carbonic acid	0 03

Besides these there are always ozone, minerals and organic matter in small and variable amounts, and more or less water vapour according to the weather. In the air of towns, sulphurous acid and sulphuretted hydrogen are important impurities derived from combustion. After air has been respired once, the oxygen falls by about 4 per cent and the carbonic acid rises to about 4 per cent, while organic matter and water vapour are greatly increased and the air rises in temperature. The cause of the discomfort felt in badly ventilated rooms and crowded halls is associated with the increase in the temperature and moisture of the air, but a high percentage of carbonic acid may be present without causing any noticeable discomfort or appreciable quickening of the respiration.

AIR-BEDS consist of stout rubber perforated in numerous places by rubber tubes which open on the upper and lower surfaces and add strength to the bed. The bed is pumped up from one end to the desired hardness. Such a bed is both easier for the nurse to manage and more comfortable to the patient than a water-bed. (See RIPPLE BEDS.)
Uses: In general an air-bed is placed under a bedridden person or one suffering from devitalizing disease of the nervous system, in order to prevent the formation of bed sores, by distributing pressure all over the patient's back. Apart from the tendency to bed sores, a patient who is long confined to bed, who is fevered, or who is emaciated, derives a sense of great coolness and comfort from an air-bed.

AIR EMBOLISM: A bubble of air in a blood vessel that affects the flow of blood from the heart. Air may enter the circulation after injury, infusions into the venous circulation, or surgery. The victim suffers breathlessness, chest discomfort, and acute heart failure.

AIR PASSAGES: These are the nose, pharynx or throat (the large cavity behind the nose and mouth), larynx, trachea or windpipe, and bronchi or bronchial tubes. The air, on entering the nose, passes through a high narrow passage on each side, the outer wall of which has three projections (the nasal conchae) which almost touch the dividing septum between the nostrils, thus making on each side three passages or meatuses, in which the air is warmed, moistened, and relieved of particles of dust. (See NOSE.) Mouth-breathing is, accordingly, a bad habit because the air is not prepared for entrance to the lungs. In the pharynx the food and air passages meet and cross. The larynx lies in front of the lower part of the pharynx and is the organ where the voice is produced (see VOICE AND SPEECH) by aid of the vocal cords. The opening between the cords is called the glottis, and shortly after passing this the air reaches the trachea or wind-pipe, a tube 10 to 12·5 cm (4 to 5 inches) long, and 2 cm (¾ inch) wide.

This leads into the chest and divides above the heart into two bronchi, one of which goes to each lung, in which it splits into finer and finer tubes (see LUNGS). The larynx is enclosed in two strong cartilages, the thyroid (of which the most projecting part, the Adam's apple, is a prominent point on the front of the neck) and the cricoid (which can be felt as a hard ring about an inch below). Beneath this, the trachea, which is stiffened by rings of cartilage, so that it is never closed in any position of the body, can be traced down till it disappears behind the breast-bone.

AIR-SICKNESS: The manifestations of this condition are very similar to those of sea-sickness. The most satisfactory remedy is hyoscine hydrobromide, (0·3 to 0·5 mg). (See MOTION SICKNESS.)

AKINESIA means loss, or impairment, of voluntary movement, or immobility. It is characteristically seen in Parkinsonism (q.v.).

ALASTRIM, or VARIOLA MINOR, is a form of smallpox which differs from ordinary smallpox in being milder and having a low mortality.

1 air	5 windpipe
2 tongue	6 gullet
3 epiglottis	7 eustachian tube
4 larynx	

Vertical section through the middle of the head and neck showing the upper air passages.

1 right bronchus
2 right apical bronchus
3 right subapical bronchus
4 right eparterial bronchus
5 right pectoral bronchus
6 right hyparterial bronchus
7 right middle lobe bronchus
8 right anterior basal bronchus
9 right axillary basal bronchus
10 right posterior basal bronchus
11 cardiac bronchus
12 right dorsal bronchus

13 left dorsal bronchus
14 left posterior basal bronchus
15 left axillary basal bronchus
16 left anterior basal bronchus
17 left lingular bronchus
18 left pectoral bronchus
19 left apical bronchus
20 left bronchus
21 trachea
22 cricoid cartilage
23 cricothyroid ligament
24 thyroid cartilage

The lower air passages.

ALBINISM: An inherited disorder in which there is an absence or decrease of melanin in the skin, hair and eyes. Those affected tend to have a very fair complexion and blonde or ginger hair. Many have nystagmus, poor visual acuity and a high incidence of squints. There is no treatment. Albinos tend to burn easily in sunlight, so barrier creams and dark glasses may be helpful.

ALBUMINS are proteins. They enter into the composition of all the tissues of the body. Their characters are that they are soluble in pure water; can be dried into a light, flaky, non-crystalline powder; are coagulated by heat, and precipitated by various agents like nitric acid, tannin, alcohol, or perchloride of mercury.
Varieties: Albumins are generally divided according to their source of origin, as muscle-albumin, milk-albumin, blood- or serum-albumin, egg-albumin, vegetable-albumin, etc. These differ both in chemical reactions and also physiologically, for though serum-albumin occurs in the blood, some albumins, e.g. egg-albumin, injected direct into the blood are highly poisonous.
Uses: When taken into the stomach they are all converted into a soluble form by the process of digestion (q.v.), and are then absorbed into the blood, whence they go to build up the tissues gradually worn out in the activity of the body. (See PROTEINURIA; GLOMERULONEPHRITIS.)

ALBUMINURIA (see PROTEINURIA).

ALCOHOL: A colourless liquid, also called ethanol or ethylalcohol, produced by the fermentation of carbohydrates by yeast. Medically, it is used as a solvent and an antiseptic. Recreationally, it is a widely used drug, taken in alcoholic drinks to give a pleasant taste and to relax, reduce inhibitions, and increase sociability. In moderate dose (see table) it seems to be safe and, indeed, research published in 1991 confirms that two standard drinks or units a day protect against high blood pressure and heart disease. In larger doses, however, alcohol causes a great deal of mental and physical harm.

1 standard drink	= 1 unit
	= 1/2 pint of beer
	= 1 measure of spirits
	= 1 glass of sherry or vermouth
	= 1 glass of wine

Safe limits within which alcohol causes no long-term health risks:

Women up to 2 units a day, 14 a week

(Pregnant women should avoid alcohol completely. If this is too difficult, 1 unit a day seems to be safe for the baby.)

Men up to 3 units a day, 21 a week

Women absorb alcohol more quickly than men.

Alcohol depresses the central nervous system and disturbs both mental and physical functioning. Drunkenness causes slurred speech, muddled thinking, amnesia, drowsiness, erectile impotence, poor co-ordination, and dulled reactions – thereby making driving or operating machinery dangerous. Disinhibition may lead to extreme euphoria, irritability, misery, or aggression, depending on the underlying mood at the start of drinking. Severe intoxication may lead to coma and respiratory failure.

Persistent alcohol misuse leads to physical, mental, social, and occupational problems. Misuse may follow several patterns – regular but controlled heavy intake, binge drinking, and dependence (alcoholism). The first pattern usually leads to mainly physical problems such as gastritis, peptic ulcer, liver disease, heart disease, and impotence. The second is commonest among young men and usually leads to mainly social and occupational problems – getting into fights, jeopardizing personal relationships, overspending on alcohol at weekends, and missing days off work because of hangovers. The third pattern – alcohol dependence – is the most serious, and can severely disrupt health and social stability.

Many researchers consider alcohol dependence to be an illness that runs in families, with a genetic component which is probably passed on as a vulnerable personality. But it is hard to disentangle genetic, environmental, and social factors in such families.

Alcohol causes tolerance and both physical and psychological dependence (see DRUG ADDICTION for definitions). Dependent drinkers classically drink early in the morning to relieve overnight withdrawal symptoms. These symptoms include anxiety, restlessness, nausea and vomiting, and tremor. Sudden withdrawal from regular heavy drinking can lead to life-threatening delirium tremens (DTs), with severe tremor, hallucinations (often visual – seeing spiders and monsters, rather than the pink elephants of romantic myth), and convulsions. This must be treated urgently with sedative drugs, preferably by intravenous drip. Similar symptoms, plus severe incoordination and double vision can occur in Wernicke's encephalopathy (q.v.), a serious neurological condition due to lack of the B vitamin thiamine (whose absorption from the stomach is markedly reduced by alcohol). If not treated urgently with injections of thiamine and other vitamins, this can lead to an irreversible form of brain damage called Korsakoff's psychosis, with severe amnesia. Finally, prolonged alcohol misuse can cause a form of dementia.

In addition to these severe neurological disorders, the wide range of life-threatening problems caused by heavy drinking includes hepatitis, liver cirrhosis, pancreatitis, gastrointestinal haemorrhage, fetal alcohol syndrome, and suicide. The social effects of alcohol misuse – such as marital breakdown, family violence, and severe debt – can be equally devastating.

Treatment of alcohol-related problems occurs largely in the NHS and is only moderately successful. First, many of the physical problems are treated in the short term by doctors who fail to spot or never ask about heavy drinking. Second, attempts at treating alcohol dependence by detoxification or drying out (substituting a tranquillizing drug for alcohol and withdrawing it gradually over about a week) are not always followed up by adequate support at home, and drinking starts again. Home support by community alcohol teams comprising doctors, nurses, social workers and, when appropriate, probation officers is a recent development that may have better results. Many drinkers find the voluntary organization Alcoholics Anonymous (AA) and its related groups for relatives (Al-Anon) and teenagers (Alateen) helpful because total abstinence from alcohol is encouraged by intensive psychological and social support from fellow ex-drinkers.

Useful addresses are Alcoholics Anonymous, PO Box 1, Stonebow House, Stonebow, York YO1 2NJ (0904-644026/7/8/9); Al-Anon Family Groups UK and Eire (including Alateen), 61 Great Dover Street, London SE1 4YF (071-403 0888); Alcohol Concern, 305 Gray's Inn Road, London WC1X 8QF (071-833 3471); Scottish Council on Alcohol, 137–145 Sauchiehall Street, Glasgow G2 3EW (041-333 9677, fax: 041-333 1606); Accept (community services for problem drinkers and tranquillizer misusers), 724 Fulham Road, London SW6 5SE (071-371 7477).

ALCURONIUM is a relaxant drug which is being used by anaesthetists in relatively short operations of around twenty minutes' duration.

ALDOSTERONE is a hormone secreted by the adrenal cortex. It plays an important part in maintaining the electrolyte balance of the body by promoting the reabsorption of sodium and the secretion of potassium by the renal tubules. It is thus of primary importance in controlling the volume of the body fluids.

ALEXIA is another name for word-blindness. (See APHASIA; DYSLEXIA.)

ALFACALCIDOL is a synthetic form (or analogue) of vitamin D. (See VITAMIN.)

ALGESIMETER is an instrument used in measuring the sensitiveness of areas of the skin.

ALIMENTARY CANAL is the passage along which the food passes, in which it is digested (see DIGESTION), and from which it is absorbed by lymphatics and blood-vessels into the circulation. The canal consists of the mouth, pharynx or throat, oesophagus or gullet, stomach, small intestine, and large intestine, in this order. For details see articles under these heads. The total length of the alimentary canal is about 9 metres in man.

1 mouth	11 appendix
2 hepatic ducts	12 rectum
3 gall-bladder	13 sigmoid flexure
4 common bile duct	14 descending colon
5 duodenum	15 jejunum
6 pancreatic duct	16 transverse colon
7 hepatic flexure	17 splenic flexure
8 ascending colon	18 stomach
9 ileum	19 oesophagus
10 caecum	

The alimentary canal.

ALKALI is a substance which neutralizes an acid to form a salt, and turns litmus and other vegetable dyes blue. Alkalis are generally oxides or carbonates of metals.

ALKALOIDS are substances found commonly in various plants. They are natural nitrogenous organic bases and combine with acids to form crystalline salts. Among alkaloids, morphine was discovered in 1805, strychnine in 1818, quinine and caffeine in 1820, nicotine in 1829, atropine in 1833. Only a few alkaloids occur in the animal kingdom, the outstanding example being adrenaline, which is formed in the medulla of the suprarenal, or adrenal, gland. Alkaloids are often used for medicinal purposes. The name of an alkaloid ends in 'ine' (in Latin ina).
NEUTRAL PRINCIPLES are crystalline substances with actions similar to those of alkaloids but having a neutral reaction. The name of a neutral principle ends in 'in', e.g. digitalin, aloin.

The following are the more important alkaloids, with their source plants:

Aconite, *from Monkshood*.
Atropine, *from Belladonna* (juice of Deadly Nightshade).
Cocaine, *from Coca leaves*.
Hyoscine, *from Henbane*.
Morphine, Codeine, *from Opium* (juice of Poppy).
Thebaine, Nicotine, *from Tobacco*.
Physostigmine, *from Calabar bean*.
Pilocarpine, *from Jaborandi leaves*.
Quinidine, *from Cinchona or Peruvian bark*.
Strychnine, *from Nux Vomica seeds*.

ALKALOSIS means an increase in the alkalinity of the blood, or, more accurately, a decrease in the concentration of hydrogen ions in the blood. It occurs, for example, in patients who have had large doses of alkalis for the treatment of gastric ulcer.

ALKAPTONURIA (see OCHRONOSIS).

ALKYLATING AGENTS are so named because they alkylate or react with certain biochemical entities, particularly those concerned with the synthesis of nucleic acid. Alkylation is the substitution of an organic grouping in place of another grouping in a molecule.

The importance of the alkylating agents in medicine is that by interfering with the growth of cells they have proved of value in the treatment of various forms of malignant disease. Unfortunately they interfere with the growth of normal cells as well as malignant cells, and this restricts their use to a considerable extent.

Nevertheless several of them, including mustine (q.v.) and thiotepa (q.v.) have proved of considerable value in the chemotherapy of malignant disease.

ALLANTOIN is a crystalline powder which occurs naturally in comfrey root, but is prepared synthetically. It is used in the treatment of skin ulcers to stimulate the formation of the surface epithelial layer of the skin.

ALLANTOIS is a vascular structure which, very early in the life of the embryo, grows out from its hind-gut. The end becomes attached to the wall of the womb. It spreads out at the end, becomes stalked, and develops later into the placenta and umbilical cord (see AFTERBIRTH), which forms the only connection between the mother and embryo.

ALLERGEN is the term applied to any substance, usually a protein, which, taken into the body, makes the body hypersensitive or 'allergic' to it. Thus in hay fever the allergen is pollen.

ALLERGY means special sensitiveness of an individual to certain foods, pollens or other products of plants, animal emanations, insect bites, etc., so that in such an individual conditions like asthma, dyspepsia, nettle-rash, hay fever, eczema and headache are produced. The term anaphylaxis (q.v.) is given to a similar serious reaction following the injection of serum. The substances that produce allergy, known as allergens, are generally of protein nature and include such ordinary foods as eggs, milk, flour and potatoes; also strawberries, tomatoes, cauliflower, walnuts, pork, shellfish, salmon, coffee, etc., as well as colouring agents and preservatives in food; it may also be caused by inhalation of dust from feathers (in pillows), of the hair of horses, dogs or cats, of face powder containing orris root, and of pollen, especially from grasses and certain flowers. What happens in allergic individuals is that allergens induce the formation of antibodies. When an allergen comes in contact with its antibody this leads to the release of those substances, such as bradykinin (q.v.) and histamine (q.v.), which are responsible for the actual allergic reaction, whether this be asthma, hay fever, eczema or the like.
Symptoms: The reaction in sensitive persons usually appears within a few minutes, but may be delayed for hours. One of the most common effects is nettle-rash or dropsical swellings in various parts; hay fever is another common result; sometimes there is swelling in a joint. Another type of reaction consists in spasmodic contractions of unstriped muscle so that the person affected may become urgently ill with asthma, or may develop spasms in the stomach with painful dyspepsia and vomiting, or in the intestine with symptoms resembling obstruction or severe diarrhoea, or may be troubled by irritability of the bladder. In other cases, neuralgia, headache or attacks of giddiness may come on.
Treatment: It is important to find out the food or other substance to which the individual is sensitive. Sometimes this has been discovered

by long personal experience. Skin testing may also be carried out by inoculating into a series of scratches extracts of various foods, etc., likely to cause allergy, and the substance responsible produces a weal (q.v.) surrounded by redness within a few minutes. When the substance is discovered, it should in future be carefully avoided, or, if it is an ordinary food, the sensitiveness can sometimes be abolished by taking this food constantly in small quantities, very gradually increased. In other cases, particularly of hay fever, it may be possible to desensitize the affected individual by a series of injections of a vaccine made from the substance (e.g. pollen) to which he or she is sensitive. Severe symptoms, as in asthma, may be relieved by inhalation or injection of sympathomimotic drugs. There is now available a range of antihistamine drugs (q.v.) which are of value in treating cases in which the cause of the condition cannot be avoided or is not known.

ALLOCHEIRIA is the name for a disorder of sensation in which sensations are referred to the wrong part of the body.

ALLOGRAFT is a piece of tissue or an organ, such as the kidney, transplanted from one to another of the same species: eg. from man to man. It is also known as a homograft.

ALLOPATHY is a term applied sometimes by homoeopathists to the methods used by regular practitioners of medicine and surgery. The term literally means curing by inducing a different kind of action in the body, and is an erroneous designation.

ALLOPURINOL is a drug of value in the treatment of gout. It acts by suppressing the formation of uric acid. It is also being used in treatment of uric acid stone in the kidney.

ALOPECIA is another name for baldness. (See BALDNESS.)

ALOPECIA AREATA is the term given to the disorder in which the hair comes out in patches, resulting in shiny, smooth, bald areas. (See BALDNESS.)

ALPHA FETOPROTEIN: A protein produced in the gut and liver of the fetus. Abnormality in the fetus, such as neural tube defect, may result in raised levels of alpha fetoprotein in the maternal blood. In Down's syndrome levels may be abnormally low. In either case screening of the pregnancy should be done, including amniocentesis to check the amount of alpha fetoprotein in the amniotic fluid. The protein may also be produced in some abnormal tissues in the adult, for example, in patients with liver cancer.

ALTERNATIVE MEDICINE: Systems of medical care that are based on methods of treatment or theories of disease that differ from those taught in recognized western-oriented medical schools. These systems include, for instance, herbal remedies, homeopathy, naturopathy, and faith healing. Acupuncture and osteopathy are examples of alternative medical techniques that are increasingly accepted by the medical establishment. Most alternative treatments, however, have not been proved by scientific testing and tend to be resorted to by patients unable to obtain relief or cure by orthodox medicine.

ALTITUDE SICKNESS This condition, also known as mountain sickness, occurs in mountain climbers or hikers who have climbed too quickly to heights above 3000 m, thus failing to allow their bodies to acclimatize to altitude. The lower atmospheric pressure and shortage of oxygen result in hyperventilation – deep, quick breathing – and this reduces the amount of carbon dioxide in the blood. Nausea, anxiety, and exhaustion are presenting symptoms and seriously affected individuals may be acutely breathless because of pulmonary oedema (excess fluid in the lungs). Gradual climbing over two or three days should prevent mountain sickness. In serious cases the individual must be brought down to hospital as a matter of urgency. Most attacks, however, are mild.

ALUM is either potash alum, potassium aluminium sulphate, or ammonia alum (ammonium aluminium sulphate). It is an astringent, and may be used as a powder to rub into abrasions when bleeding will not stop of itself. As an emetic, a teaspoonful of powdered alum may be given in water. A 1 to 4 per cent solution is used as a mouth-wash in stomatitis and pharyngitis, and a 2 per cent solution is useful when applied to the skin in cases of excessive perspiration.

ALVEOLITIS means inflammation of the alveoli (see ALVEOLUS) of the lungs caused by an allergic reaction. When the inflammation is caused by infection it is called pneumonia and when by a chemical or physical agent it is called pneumonitis. It may be associated with systemic sclerosis or rheumatoid arthritis.
EXTRINSIC ALLERGIC ALVEOLITIS is the condition induced by the lungs becoming allergic (see ALLERGY) to various factors or substances. It includes bagassosis (q.v.), farmer's lung (q.v.), mushroom-worker's lung (q.v.), budgerigar-fancier's lung (q.v.) and pigeon-breeders' lung. It is characterized by the onset of shortness of breath, tightness of the chest, cough and fever. The onset may be sudden or gradual. Treatment consists of removal of the affected individual from the offending material to which he has become allergic. Corticosteroids (q.v.) give temporary relief.

ALVEOLUS is a term applied to the sockets of the teeth in the jaw-bone. The term is also applied to the minute divisions of glands and the air sacs of the lungs.

ALZHEIMER'S DISEASE is a degenerative disorder of the cerebral cortex that produces a dementia (q.v.) in middle to late life. The commonest cause of dementia, the disease's onset is insidious and the first manifestation is usually failing memory. The cause is unknown, although various theories have been proposed, one being that the condition results from the deposition of aluminium in the brain cells. Heredity may play a part. There is no cure. Relatives can obtain help and advice from the Alzheimer's Disease Society, 158–160 Balham High Road, London SW12 9BN (081-675 6557).

AMANTADINE is a drug which is being used in the treatment of certain virus infections, and is proving of value in the prevention of certain forms of influenza. It is also used in the treatment of Parkinsonism (q.v.).

AMAUROSIS is the term applied to blindness in which there is no obvious lesion of the eye, the blindness being caused by disease of the optic nerve, retina or brain, or being due to hysteria.

AMAUROSIS FUGAX is the term given to sudden transitory impairment, or loss of, vision. It usually affects only one eye, and is commonly due to circulatory failure. In its simplest form it occurs in normal people on rising suddenly from the sitting or recumbent position, when it is due to the effects of gravity. It also occurs in migraine. A not uncommon cause, particularly in elderly people, is transient ocular ischaemia (see ISCHAEMIA), resulting from blockage of the circulation to the retina (see EYE) by emboli (see EMBOLISM) from the common carotid artery or the heart. Treatment in this last group of cases consists of control of the blood pressure if this is raised, as it often is in such cases; the administration of drugs that reduce the stickiness of blood platelets such as aspirin. In some instances removal of the part of the carotid artery from which the emboli are coming may be indicated.

AMBIVALENCE is the term applied to the psychological state in which a person concurrently hates and loves the same object or person.

AMBLYOPIA means defective vision for which no recognizable cause exists in any part of the eye. It may be due to such causes as defective development, hysteria, excessive use of tobacco or alcohol. The most important form is that associated with squinting (q.v.), or gross difference in refraction between the two eyes. It has

been estimated that in Britain 5·7 per cent of young adults have amblyopia due to this cause.

AMELIA: This is absence of the limbs, usually a congenital defect.

AMENORRHOEA is the absence of the menstrual flow during the time of life at which it should occur. (See MENSTRUATION.) If menstruation has never occurred the amenorrhoea is termed primary. If it ceases after having once become established it is known as secondary amenorrhoea. The only value of these terms is that some patients with either chromosome abnormalities or malformations of the genital tract fall into the primary category. Otherwise the age of onset of symptoms is more important.

The causes of amenorrhoea are numerous and treatment requires dealing with the primary cause. The commonest cause of amenorrhoea is pregnancy. Hypothalamic disorders such as psychological stress or anorexia nervosa also cause amenorrhoea. Poor nutrition or loss of weight by dieting may cause it and any serious underlying disease such as tuberculosis or malaria may also result in the cessation of periods. The excess secretion of prolactin, whether this is the result of a micro-adenoma (see ADENOMA) of the pituitary gland or whether it is drug induced will cause amenorrhoea and possibly galactorrhoea (q.v.) as well. Malfunction of the pituitary gland will result in a failure to produce the gonadotrophic hormones with consequent amenorrhea. Excessive production of cortisol, as in Cushing's syndrome, or of androgens, as in the adreno-genital syndrome or the polycystic ovary syndrome, will result in amenorrhoea. Amenorrhoea occasionally follows the use of the oral contraceptive pill and may be associated with both hypothyroidism and obesity. It is thus important to take a careful history with emphasis on psychological factors, weight fluctuations and the use of drugs that may stimulate the release of prolactin, and it is also important to look for evidence of virilization.

A gynaecological examination is necessary in primary amenorrhoea to exclude malformations of the genital tract. Estimations of the gonadotrophic hormone levels will reveal whether the amenorrhoea is primary ovarian failure or secondary to pituitary disease. In view of the frequent psychosomatic origins of amenorrhoea, reassurance of the patient is of great importance, in particular with reference to marriage and the ability to conceive. When weight loss is the cause of amenorrhoea restoration of body weight alone can result in spontaneous menstruation. Patients with raised concentrations of serum gonadotrophin hormones have primary ovarian failure. It is not amendable to treatment. Cyclical oestrogen/progestogen therapy will usually establish withdrawal bleeding. If the amenorrhoea is due to mild pituitary failure menstruation may return after treatment with clomiphene. Clomiphene is a non-steroidal agent which competes for oestrogen receptors in the hypothalamus. The patients who are most likely to respond to clomiphene are those who have some evidence of endogenous oestrogen and gonadotrophin production.

AMENT is an idiot or mentally deficient person – one having no mind.

AMENTIA is the state of being an ament; mental deficiency from failure of the mind to develop normally.

AMETHOCAINE is a powerful local anaesthetic which is used when a prolonged effect is required. It is also used as a spinal anaesthetic.

AMETROPIA (see REFRACTION).

AMIKACIN is a semi-synthetic derivative of kanamycin (q.v.) which is proving of value in the treatment of infections caused by micro-organisms resistant to gentamicin (q.v.) and tobramycin (q.v.).

AMILORIDE is a diuretic that acts without causing excessive loss of potassium (see DIURETICS).

AMINES are substances derived from ammonia or amino-acids (q.v.) which play an important part in the working of the body, including the brain and the circulatory system. They include adrenaline (q.v.), noradrenaline (q.v.) and histamine (q.v.). (See also MONOAMINE OXIDASE INHIBITORS.)

AMINO-ACID is the name given to the ultimate products of digestion of protein foods and from which the protein materials of the body are again built up. They are organic acids in which one or more hydrogen atoms have been replaced by the chemical group NH_2. (See PROTEIN.)

AMINOCAPROIC ACID is one of a group of drugs introduced for the the control of bleeding. These drugs act by inhibiting the fibrinolytic system. This is a complex system which helps to maintain the coagulation mechanism of the blood in such a state that clotting of the blood only occurs when it is necessary. Thus, if fibrinolysis is prevented then the blood will clot more easily and bleeding will stop.

AMINOGLUTETHIMIDE is a drug that inhibits the synthesis of adrenal corticorteroids. It is proving of value in the treatment of cancer of the breast in post-menopausal women.

AMINOGLYCOSIDES: These are a group of antibiotics that are usually kept for use in severe infections. They are effective against a wide range of bacteria but can cause side-effects that include damage to the kidneys and inner ear. Gentamycin, neomycin and streptomycin are important examples of this group of drugs.

AMINOPHYLLINE is the name given to a combination of theophylline and ethylenediamine. It is used in the treatment of bronchial asthma.

AMINOPTERIN is an antimetabolite (q.v.) which is proving of value in the treatment of acute leukaemia (q.v.).

AMITRIPTYLINE (see ANTIDEPRESSANTS).

AMMONIA is a pungent gas formcd by heating a mixture of sal ammoniac and quicklime. Dissolved in water it forms spirits of hartshorn, or liquor ammoniae. It is given off slowly from carbonate of ammonia, which is used as smelling salts. Carbonate of ammonia is the chief ingredient in aromatic spirits of ammonia or sal volatile. In chloride of ammonia or sal ammoniac it is fixed.
Uses: Externally, strong ammonia produces blistering. For bee stings, weak ammonia is applied locally to relieve the pain. (See ALKALI.) Internally it is a powerful stimulant, and therefore a teaspoonful of sal volatile in water is given, or smelling salts are applied to the nose, when fainting threatens. The chloride and the carbonate of ammonia are used as expectorants (q.v.), whilst the former is also a diuretic (q.v.).

AMNESIA means loss of memory.

AMNIOCENTESIS (see PRENATAL DIAGNOSIS).

AMNION is the tough fibrous membrane which lines the cavity of the womb during pregnancy, and contains from 0·5 to 1 litre (one to two pints) of fluid in which the embryo floats. It is formed from the ovum along with the embryo, and in labour the part of it at the mouth of the womb forms the 'bag of waters'. (See LABOUR.) When a child is 'born with a caul', the caul is a piece of amnion. (See CAUL.)

AMNIOSCOPY is the method whereby the fluid in the amniotic sac (see AMNION) can be assessed without interfering with the course of pregnancy. It is of value in determining whether the foetus is distressed and therefore whether or not labour should be induced, and also in finding out whether the fetus, or unborn child, is suffering from certain congenital diseases, such as mongolism. It is also possible to say what is the sex of the child.

AMNIOTIC FLUID The clear fluid contained within the amnion that surrounds the fetus in the womb and protects it from external pressure. The fluid, mainly water, is produced by the amnion and is regularly circulated, being swallowed by the fetus and excreted through the kidneys back into the amniotic sac. By the 35th week of pregnancy there is about one litre of fluid but this falls to half a litre at term. The amniotic sac normally ruptures in early labour releasing the fluid or 'waters'.

AMOEBA is a minute protozoan organism consisting of a single cell, in which a nucleus is surrounded by protoplasm that changes its shape as the protozoon progresses or absorbs nourishment. Several varieties are found under different conditions within the human body. One variety, *Entamoeba coli*, is found in the large intestine of man without any associated disease; another, *Entamoeba gingivalis*, is found in the sockets of the teeth associated with pyorrhoea; another, *Entamoeba histolytica*, is the causative organism of amoebic dysentery (see DYSENTERY). Two, *Acanthamoeba* and *Naegleria fowleri*, cause the infection of the brain known as meningoencephalitis (q.v.). *Entamoeba histolytica* may also cause meningoencephalitis. Other forms are found in the genital organs.

AMOEBIASIS (see DYSENTERY).

AMOXYCILLIN (see PENICILLIN, ANTIBIOTIC).

AMPHETAMINES are a group of drugs closely related to adrenaline and act by stimulating the sympathetic nervous system. When taken by mouth they have a profound stimulating effect on the brain, producing a sense of well-being and confidence and seemingly increasing the capacity for mental work. They are, however, drugs of dependence and their medical use is now strictly limited, for example, to the treatment of narcolepsy.

Because they inhibit appetite, they rapidly achieved a reputation for slimming purposes, but they should not be used for this purpose. The dangers of amphetamines far outweigh their advantages.

AMPHORIC is an adjective denoting the kind of breathing heard over a cavity in the lung. The sound is like that made by blowing over the mouth of a narrow-necked vase.

AMPHOTERICIN is a mixture of antifungal substances derived from *Streptomyces nodosus*, which is proving of value in the treatment of certain of the diseases classified under the heading of mycosis (q.v.). It is, however, a very toxic substance and is therefore only used in those infections in which the outlook is otherwise hopeless. It is also proving of value in the

treatment of certain cases of amoebic meningo-encephalitis. (See MENINGOENCEPHALITIS.)

AMPICILLIN (see PENICILLIN, ANTIBIOTIC).

AMPOULE is a small glass container having one end drawn out into a point capable of being sealed so as to preserve its contents sterile. It is used for containing solutions for hypodermic injection.

AMPUTATION means the severing of any limb or part completely from the body. In the case of organs other than limbs the word excision is generally used. An amputation through a joint without sawing of bone is called a disarticulation.

Objects of amputation: In the great majority of cases a limb is amputated because it has been damaged beyond the hope of recovery, though amputation of the lower limb may be performed because of chronically poor blood supply resulting from arterial disease. It is not always easy to say at once that a limb should, or should not, be removed after an injury, but the three chief points are, as to whether (1) extensive portions of muscle, skin, and bone are so crushed and torn as to make their death and separation inevitable; (2) the great nerves and blood-vessels are divided so as to destroy the viability of the limb; and (3) the laceration is so extensive, or involves joint cavities so as to render cleansing of the wound impossible and endanger the patient from blood-poisoning (q.v.) due to septic absorption. Often after gunshot wounds, crushes in machinery, or railway accidents, where a decision cannot be made at once, the injured limb is cleaned (blood-vessels tied, sinews stitched, etc.), and a careful watch maintained for some days to see if healing will take place. This is done especially

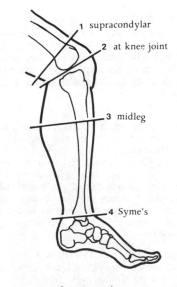

Sites for amputation.

in the case of the hand, where every fragment of tissue is valuable because of the delicate movements the upper limb executes, and where, fortunately, circulation by anastomosis (q.v.) is good. But in the lower limbs, the chief point is to have a small scar and a sound stump, so that the weight of the body can be borne. The more common sites of amputation in the lower limbs are shown in the illustration below. Site 4 is used for injuries in which the whole forefoot is mangled and for severe deformities of the foot. Site 3, or midleg amputation, is the site of selection for injuries around the ankle, while sites 2 and 1 are reserved for more extensive injuries. The planning of an amputation and choice of level must take into account the fitting of a prosthetic limb so as to ensure the minimum disability for the patient. (see PROSTHESES, PHANTOM LIMB.)

AMSACRINE (see CYTOTOXIC).

AMYLASE is an enzyme (q.v.) in pancreatic juice which facilitates the conversion of starch to maltose. (See PANCREAS.)

AMYL NITRITE is a volatile, oily liquid prepared by the action of nitric and nitrous acids upon amyl alcohol. It resembles other nitrites in its power of relieving spasms and dilating blood-vessels, and it acts with great rapidity when inhaled, producing its effects in a few seconds.

AMYLOIDOSIS, or WAXY DISEASE, is the condition in which deposits of complex protein, known as amyloid, are found in various parts of the body. It is a degenerative condition resulting from various causes such as chronic infection, including tuberculosis and rheumatoid arthritis.

AMYLOSE is the name applied to any carbohydrate of the starch group.

ANABOLIC STEROIDS: Nitrogen-retaining effect of androgen is responsible for the larger muscle mass of the male. This is called an anabolic effect. Attempts have been made to separate the anabolic effects of hormones from 'heir virilizing effects. This is only partially successful. Thus anabolic steroids have the property of protein building so that when taken they lead to an increase in muscle bulk and strength. All the anabolic steroids have some androgenic activity but they cause less virilization than androgens in women. Androgenic side-effects may result from any of these anabolic compounds, especially if they are given for prolonged periods. Norethandrolone, in addition to its anabolic effect, has a progestational action and so amenorrhoea (q.v.) or uterine bleeding may result from its withdrawal. All these compounds should therefore be used with caution in women, and are contra-indicted in

men with prostatic carcinoma. Jaundice due to stasis of bile in the intrahepatic canaliculi is a hazard, and the depression of pituitary gonadotrophin production is a possible complication. Norethandrolone and nandrolone phenylpropionate are the most important anabolic steroids.

Anabolic steroids have been used to stimulate protein anabolism in debilitating illness and to promote growth in children with pituitary dwarfism and other disorders associated with interference of growth. Stimulation of protein anabolism may also be of value in acute renal failure, and the retention of nitrogen and calcium is of probable benefit to patients with osteoporosis (q.v.) and to patients receiving corticosteroid therapy. Anabolic steroids may stimulate bone marrow function in hypoplastic anaemia.

Anabolic steroids have been widely abused by athletes aiming to improve their strength, stamina and speed. They should not be used for this purpose and athletes using them face bans from official competitions.

The anabolic steroids in therapeutic use, which can be given by mouth, include: ethyloestrenol, norethandrolone, oxymetholone and stanozolol. Those that require to be given by injection include: nandrolone decanoate, nandrolone phenylpropionate and norethandrolone.

ANAEMIA is the condition characterized by inadequate red blood cells and/or haemoglobin in the blood. It is considered to exist if haemoglobin levels are below 13 grams per 100 ml in males and below 12 grams per 100 ml in adult non-pregnant women. No simple classification of anaemia can be wholly accurate, but the most useful method is to divide anaemias into: (a) microcytic hypochromic anaemia, (b) megaloblastic hyperchromic anaemia, (c) aplastic anaemia, (d) haemolytic anaemia. In Britain, anaemia is much more common among women than in men. Thus, around 10 per cent of girls have anaemia at the age of 15, whilst in adult life the incidence is over 30 per cent between the ages of 30 and 40, around 20 per cent at 50, and around 30 per cent at 70. Among men the incidence is under 5 per cent until the age of 50, and it then rises to 20 per cent at the age of 70. Ninety per cent of all cases of anaemia in Britain are microcytic, 7 per cent are macrocytic, and 3 per cent are haemolytic or aplastic. (See also SICKLE-CELL ANAEMIA; and THALASSAEMIA.)

MICROCYTIC HYPOCHROMIC ANAEMIA: This corresponds to a large extent with what used to be known as 'secondary anaemia'. It takes its name from the characteristic changes in the blood.

Causes: (1) *Loss of blood.* (a) As a result of trauma. This is perhaps the simplest example of all, when, as a result of an accident involving a large artery, there is severe haemorrhage. (b) Menstruation. The regular monthly loss of blood which women sustain as a result of menstruation always puts a strain on the blood-forming organs. If this loss is excessive, then over a period of time it may lead to quite severe anaemia. (c) Child-birth. A considerable amount of blood is always lost at child-birth, and if this is severe, or if the woman was anaemic during pregnancy, a severe degree of anaemia may develop. (d) Bleeding from the gastro-intestinal tract. The best example here is anaemia due to 'bleeding piles' (see PILES). Such bleeding, even though slight, if maintained over a long period of time, is a common cause of anaemia in both men and women. The haemorrhage may be more acute and occur from a duodenal or gastric ulcer, when it is known as haematemesis (q.v.). (e) Certain blood diseases, such as purpura (q.v.) and haemophilia (q.v.), which are characterized by bleeding.

(2) *Defective blood formation*: (a) This is the main cause of anaemia in infections. The micro-organism responsible for the infection has a deleterious effect upon the blood-forming organs, just as it does upon other parts of the body. (b) Toxins. In conditions such as chronic glomerulonephritis and uraemia there is a severe anaemia due to the effect of the disease upon blood formation. (c) Drugs. Certain drugs, such as aspirin and the non- steroidal anti-inflammatory drugs, may cause occult gastro-intestinal **bleeding.**

(3) *Inadequate intake of iron*: The daily requirement of iron for an adult is 12 mg, and 15 to 20 mg during pregnancy. This is well covered by an ordinary diet, so that by itself it is not a common cause. But if there is a steady loss of blood, as a result of heavy menstrual loss or 'bleeding piles', the intake of iron in the diet may not be sufficient to maintain adequate formation of haemoglobin.

(4) *Inadequate absorption of iron*: This may occur in diseases of intestinal malabsorption.

In many cases the anaemia is found to be due to a combination of two or more of these causes. A severe form of this anaemia in women, known as chlorosis, used to be common, but it is seldom seen nowadays.

Symptoms: These depend upon whether the anaemia is sudden in onset, as in severe haemorrhage, or gradual. In all cases, however, the striking sign is pallor, the depth of which depends upon the severity of the anaemia. The colour of the skin may be misleading, except in cases due to severe haemorrhage, as the skin of many people is normally pale. The best guide is the colour of the internal lining of the eyelid. When the onset of the anaemia is sudden the patient complains of weakness and giddiness, and he loses consciousness if he tries to stand or sit up. The breathing is rapid and distressed, the pulse is rapid, and the blood-pressure is low. In chronic cases the tongue is often sore (glossitis), and the nails of the fingers may be brittle and concave instead of convex (koilonychia). In some cases, particularly in women, the Plummer-Vinson syndrome is present. This consists of difficulty in swallowing and may be accompanied by huskiness; in these cases glossitis is also present. There may

be slight enlargement of the spleen, and there is usually some diminution in gastric acidity.

Changes in the blood: The characteristic change is a diminution in both the haemoglobin and the red cell content of the blood. There is a relatively greater fall in the haemoglobin than in the red cell count. If the blood is examined under a microscope the red cells are seen to be paler and smaller than normal. These small red cells are known as microcytes.

Treatment consists primarily of giving sufficient iron by mouth to restore, and then maintain, a normal blood picture. The main iron preparation now used is ferrous sulphate, 200 mg, thrice daily after meals. When the blood picture has become normal, the dosage is gradually reduced. A preparation of iron is now available which can be given intravenously, but this is only used in cases which do not respond to iron given by mouth, or in cases in which it is essential to obtain a quick response.

If, of course, there is haemorrhage, this must be arrested, and if the loss of blood has been severe it may be necessary to give a blood transfusion. Care must be taken to ensure that the patient is having an adequate diet, and a period of rest in hospital, followed by a holiday, is often beneficial. If there is any underlying toxic or infective condition, this, of course, must be adequately treated.

MEGALOBLASTIC HYPERCHROMIC ANAEMIA: There are various forms of anaemia of this type, such as those due to nutritional but the most important is that known as PERNICIOUS ANAEMIA.

PERNICIOUS ANAEMIA: Up until about fifty years ago its cause was unknown and it was an invariably fatal disease. In 1926, two Americans, G. R. Minot and W. P. Murphy, reported that pernicious anaemia responded to treatment with liver. This discovery ranks in importance with that of insulin in the treatment of diabetes mellitus. This form of treatment is based upon the now well-proved fact that pernicious anaemia is due to lack of what is known as the *intrinsic factor*. For the formation of normal red blood corpuscles a substance known as the extrinsic factor is necessary. The efficient absorption of this factor into the body is dependent on the presence of intrinsic factor which is produced normally by the mucosa lining the distal part of the stomach. It is the inability of the patient to produce the intrinsic factor that leads to the onset of pernicious anaemia. In a normal person with adequate amounts of intrinsic factor, approximately 70 per cent of the extrinsic factor (which is vitamin B_{12} and is present in meat and other foods) in the daily diet is absorbed into the body. In patients with pernicious anaemia, however, less than 2 per cent is absorbed.

Symptoms: Pernicious anaemia is a disease of middle age, being rare under the age of 40 years. It affects both men and women. The onset is usually insidious, so that the anaemia is usually well developed before medical advice is sought. In addition to the general symptoms and signs already described in the section on microcytic anaemia, the important features of pernicious anaemia are as follows. The patient, who is often prematurely grey-haired, has a characteristic lemon-yellow complexion. The tongue is often sore and appears thinner, smoother, and redder than usual. There is often soreness and excoriation of the corners of the mouth – a condition known as cheilosis. There may be slight enlargement of the spleen. There is a complete absence of free hydrochloric acid in the stomach, even after the injection of histamine.

One of the most serious complications of pernicious anaemia is a disease with the cumbersome title of SUBACUTE COMBINED DEGENERATION OF THE CORD. This, as the name indicates, is a degenerative condition of the spinal cord, and the importance of recognizing its onset is that it can be cured by adequate treatment of the anaemia. Its early manifestations are a sensation of tingling or 'pins and needles' in the legs, accompanied by stiffness. Later, if untreated, the stiffness becomes progressively worse, finally leading to paralysis.

Changes in the blood: The red cells are larger than normal, i.e. macrocytes and they appear to be redder than normal. They also vary in shape (poikilocytosis) and in size (anisocytosis). Occasionally a few primitive red cells (normoblasts) may be found. The total white cell count is diminished: i.e. there is leucopenia. The final diagnosis depends upon an examination of the bone marrow, which is found to contain megaloblasts.

Treatment consists of the administration of vitamin B_{12} in the form of hydroxocobalamin. It is given by injection. It must always be remembered that a patient with pernicious anaemia requires to take vitamin B_{12} for the rest of his or her life.

APLASTIC ANAEMIA is a disease in which the red blood corpuscles are very greatly reduced and in which no attempt appears to be made in the bone marrow towards their regeneration. It is more accurately called hypoplastic anaemia as the degree of impairment of bone marrow function is rarely complete. The cause in many cases is not known, but in rather less than half the cases the condition is due to some toxic substance, such as benzol or certain drugs, or ionizing radiations. The patient becomes very pale, with a tendency to haemorrhages under the skin and mucous membranes, and the temperature may at times be raised. The red blood corpuscles diminish steadily in numbers. Treatment consists primarily of regular blood transfusions. Although the disease is often fatal, the outlook has improved in recent years. About 25 per cent of patients recover when adequately treated, and others survive for several years. In severe cases promising results are being reported from the use of bone marrow transplantation.

HAEMOLYTIC ANAEMIA results from the excessive destruction, or haemolysis (q.v.), of the red blood cells. This haemolysis may be due to undue fragility of the red blood cells, when the condition is known as congenital haemolytic anaemia, or acholuric jaundice.

ANAEROBE is the term applied to bacteria having the power to live without air. Such organisms are found growing freely, deep in the soil, as, for example, the tetanus bacillus.

ANAESTHESIA: The loss of sensation or feeling. It may be caused by a disease process, but its common usage describes a reversible process for abolishing sensation to allow painful procedures such as surgery to occur without pain or distress to the patient.

Anaesthesia is provided by a trained specialist who, in most countries, is a qualified medical practitioner. The anaesthetist will assess the patient's fitness for anaesthesia, choose and perform the appropriate type of anaesthetic, whilst monitoring and caring for the well-being of the patient, and, following reversal of the anaesthetic, supervise the recovery and postoperative analgesia for the patient. Anaesthesia can be broadly divided into general and local. GENERAL ANAESTHESIA: under general anaesthesia patients are given a combination of drugs to render them reversibly unconscious during a painful procedure. A so called 'balanced' anaesthetic provides unconsciousness, analgesia, and a greater or lesser degree of muscle relaxation. By using a combination of drugs the side-effects of any individual drug are minimized, while achieving the optimum anaesthetic effect.

A general anaesthetic may be divided into induction, maintenance, and recovery (or reversal). Historically anaesthesia has been divided into four stages (see below) but these are only seen clearly with a purely inhalational induction and maintenance.

Stage 1: onset of induction to unconsciousness.
Stage 2: stage of excitement.
Stage 3: plane 1 – deep regular breathing
        plane 2 – cessation of eye movement
        plane 3 – surgical anaesthesia
        plane 4 – diaphragmatic paralysis.
Stage 4: overdosage.

Induction merely means putting the patient to sleep. Most often this is performed by means of an intravenous injection, though an inhalation technique can be used instead. The most widely used agents are short-acting barbiturates, thiopentone, and methohexitone, whilst two newer agents etomidate and propofol are also used.

The maintenance of anaesthesia is usually by administration of oxygen and nitrous oxide containing a volatile anaesthetic agent. Anaesthetic machines and vaporizers provide a constant percentage of each constituent set by the anaesthetist. They are administered to the patient via a breathing circuit either through a mask or an endotracheal tube. For some operations the patient may be paralysed with a muscle relaxant, in which case their lungs will be artificially ventilated by a machine (see ARTIFICIAL VENTILATION OF THE LUNGS). Often opioids are given to supplement analgesia, as may a local anaesthetic block.

The most commonly used volatile agents in the UK are halothane (a halogenated hydrocarbon), isoflurane and enflurane (isomers of a halogenated ether). On a world-wide basis ether and chloroform are still often used. The mode of action of these agents is not fully understood, though there are several theories, but by whatever action they reversibly depress conduction of impulses in central nervous tissue and thereby produce unconsciousness.

Reversal of anaesthesia will occur when the patient is allowed to breathe oxygen or oxygen-enriched air and excrete via the lungs the volatile anaesthetic agent previously absorbed. Muscle relaxants and occasionally the effects of opioids are pharmacologically reversed.

Ketamine is an unusual anaesthetic sometimes used for general anaesthesia but more often for painful procedures such as burns dressings. It produces a dissociative anaesthesia under which patients may open their eyes and move but are unaware of what is happening. Though it is an excellent analgesic and depresses ventilation less than most other anaesthetics, it produces hallucinations and nightmares.

LOCAL ANAESTHETICS are drugs which reversibly block the conduction of impulses in nerves. They therefore abolish the motor and sensory function in the areas served by that particular nerve. Many drugs have local anaesthetic actions but all the ones used to produce local anaesthesia clinically are amide or ester derivatives of aromatic acids. If absorbed systemically in toxic amounts, they produce central-nervous-system and cardiovascular side-effects. Local anaesthesia may be used to supplement general anaesthesia, as the sole method if coexisting medical conditions make general anaesthesia unsuitable, or for the relief of chronic or acute pain. Several techniques are used as listed below.

Local infiltration – small quantities of local anaesthetic are infiltrated subcutaneously to produce a small area of anaesthetized skin. Similarly, deeper tissues may be infiltrated and anaesthetized. This technique is useful for removing small superficial lesions and suturing skin.

Nerve blocks – local anaesthetic is injected in the proximity of nerve plexuses or individual nerves. Once it has diffused into the nerve, surgical anaesthesia in the area subserved by the nerve is achieved. More than one nerve may need to be blocked.

Spinal – small volumes (2–4 ml) of local anaesthetic are injected into the cerebrospinal fluid (CSF) (q.v.) by means of a spinal needle inserted through the tissues of the back and the dura mater (q.v.). A dense symmetrical motor and sensory block is produced in the lower body. The height of the block is dependent on the volume of local anaesthetic injected, the position of the patient, and individual variation. If the block is too high, the respiratory muscles are paralysed and respiratory arrest occurs. Because the sympathetic nerves are also blocked, hypotension may occur as the blood vessels in the blocked area vasodilate. A spinal headache may occasionally complicate a spinal anaesthetic, possibly because of continuing leakage of CSF through the dural puncture.

Epidural – as with a spinal, anaesthesia is produced in the lower body. The spinal nerves are blocked in the epidural space by injection of local anaesthetic through a fine-bore plastic catheter inserted through a special needle (Tuohy needle). Because of the catheter the block can be augmented if necessary as it begins to wear off. This makes it ideal for the relief of labour pains as well as for operations below the waist. Potential complications are hypotension and headache (due to accidental dural puncture with the Tuohy needle – a rare occurrence). There is a risk of spinal-cord compression by clot or abscess because of the confined space within which it lies. For this reason both spinal and epidural anaesthesia are contraindicated in patients who are receiving anticoagulant drugs or who have generalized or local sepsis.

ANALEPTIC means a restorative medicine, or one which acts as a stimulant of the central nervous system: for example caffeine.

ANALGESIA means loss of the power to feel pain without loss of consciousness: e.g in some nervous diseases or due to some drugs. (See also AUDIOANALGESIA; CRYOANALGESIA.)

ANALGESICS are drugs that relieve pain. Unlike local anaesthetics they do not abolish other modalities of sensation. There are many drugs with different modes of action available, and the choice of analgesic will depend on the type and severity of the pain. Mild or moderate pain is usually treated with simple analgesics such as paracetamol, aspirin, or one of the wide range of drugs known collectively as non-steroidal anti-inflammatory drugs (q.v.) (NSAIDS).

Paracetamol acts within the central nervous system by inhibiting prostaglandin (q.v.) biosynthesis. It causes hepatic damage in overdosage.

The NSAIDS (including aspirin) have both central and peripheral action. They inhibit prostaglandin synthetase (cyclo-oxygenase) – an enzyme necessary for the production of certain prostaglandins implicated in the development of inflammation. A central, antipyretic, action also occurs. Side-effects include gastrointestinal bleeding from gastric erosions, inhibition of platelet (q.v.) aggregation, fluid retention, and a variable propensity for renal papillary damage.

Severe pain is often treated using opioid drugs. These mimic the action of naturally occurring analgesics (endorphins and enkephalins (qq.v.) at opioid receptors in the brain and spinal cord. They also produce euphoria, which helps in coping with pain. Respiratory depression, vomiting, constipation, and itching are possible side-effects. The older drugs are naturally occurring purified plant alkaloids (q.v.) (e.g. morphine and papaveretum). Semi-synthetic drugs such as diamorphine (heroin) are also useful and there is now a plethora of synthetic opioids which have various strengths and durations of action (e.g., pethidine, fentanyl, alfentanyl, and sufentanyl).

ANALYSIS means a separation into component parts by determination of the chemical constituents of a substance. The process of analysis is carried out by various means: e.g chromatographic analysis by means of the adsorption column; colorimetric analysis by means of various colour tests; densimetric analysis by estimation of the specific gravity; gasometric analysis by estimating the different gases given off in some process; polariscope analysis by means of the polariscope; volumetric analysis by measuring volumes of liquids. Analysis is also sometimes used as an abbreviation for psycho-analysis (q.v.).

ANAPHYLAXIS is a condition of excessive sensitiveness exhibited by certain persons or animals to the injection of foreign material into their tissues. A common example is the pain, swelling, eruption, feverishness and general prostration which occasionally follow the injection of serum containing diphtheria or tetanus antitoxin. An example of a slighter form of anaphylaxis is afforded by people who suffer from nettle-rash, asthma, and similar symptoms when they take some food of which their system is intolerant, or by other people who present similar symptoms when exposed to the emanations of certain animals, e.g horses, cats or fowls. There is an acute form, fortunately rare, known as anaphylactic shock which may occur within minutes of the injection of certain drugs or vaccines to which the injected individual is hypersensitive. It is characterized by severe shortness of breath, marked fall in blood-pressure and acute urticaria (q.v.). Treatment consists of the immediate intramuscular injection of 1 ml of adrenaline B.P. (See ADRENALINE; ALLERGY.)

ANAPLASIA means the state in which a body cell loses its distinctive characters and takes on a more primitive form; it occurs, for example, in cancer, when cells proliferate rapidly.

ANASTOMOSIS is a term describing the means by which the circulation is carried on when large vessels are narrowed or closed, as by pressure. In the limbs, especially around joints, and in internal organs, small arteries open freely into their neighbours to form a network from which the smallest vessels carry off the blood. By this means pressure from one side, or even the ligature of the main artery to a limb, is prevented from stopping the flow of blood to any part, because so soon as one artery is closed, the other arteries of the limb dilate, through relaxation of their muscle fibres, and the supply of blood passes on as before, but by new channels. Anastomosis is also a term describing the joining together (by operation) of any two parts of the alimentary tract or of blood-vessels.

ANATOMY is the science which deals with the structure of the bodies of men and animals. Brief descriptions of the anatomy of each important organ are given under the headings of the various organs. It is studied by dissection of bodies bequeathed for the purpose or of the bodies of those who die in hospitals and similar institutions, unclaimed by relatives.

ANCROD is an enzyme (q.v.) present in the venom of the Malayan pit viper which destroys the fibrinogen in blood and thereby prevents the blood clotting. In other words it is an anticoagulant (q.v.).

ANCYLOSTOMIASIS is the parasitic infestation caused by two nematodes, *Ancylostoma duodenale* and *Necator americanus*, perhaps better known as the hookworm. The former is also known as the tunnel-worm on account of the ravages it caused among the men at work on the St Gotthard tunnel. They produce great anaemia, debility, and cardiac weakness, sometimes leading to death. The disease is widespread in the tropics and subtropics, as well as certain mines in Europe. The estimated world prevalence is 700 million cases. *Ancylostoma duodenale* occurs in the Far East, the Mediterranean littoral and the Middle East, whilst *Necator americanus* is found in East, West and Central Africa, Central and South America and the Far East. In recent years these geographical demarcations have been largely broken down. The worms are about 12 mm) (½ inch) long, and inhabit the upper part of the small intestine, often in great numbers; here they embed themselves in the mucous membrane lining the bowel. In certain parts of India it is so common that about 75 per cent of the population are said to be affected; it is also very common in Egypt. The worms embedded in the small intestine produce an enormous number of eggs which pass from the body in the stools; the embryos, finding their way into water, mud, or damp earth, develop rapidly and can maintain their vitality for weeks or months, if moisture is present. In the insanitary conditions so widespread in the areas where the disease occurs, the embryos gain access to the human host through the skin – usually the feet. They may also gain access through the drinking of polluted water. Ultimately, through the blood-stream and the lungs, they gain access to the intestine, where they develop. The disease is a very serious one, partly in consequence of the numbers of people prevented from working by the debility it causes, and partly because death in such debilitated persons is not uncommon.

Treatment: The most effective remedies are tetrachloroethylene, bephenium hydroxynaphthoate, pyrantel embonate, and mebendazole. The anaemia which always accompanies chronic infestation with ancylostoma also needs intensive treatment.

ANDROGEN is the general term for any one of a group of hormones which govern the development of the sexual organs and the secondary sexual characteristics of the male. Testosterone, the androgenic hormone formed in the interstitial cells of the testis, controls the development and maintenance of the male sex organs and secondary sex characteristics. In small doses it increases the number of spermatozoa produced, but in large doses it inhibits the gonadotrophic activity of the anterior pituitary gland and suppresses the formation of the spermatozoa. It is both androgenic and anabolic in action. The anabolic effect includes the ability to stimulate protein synthesis and to diminish the catabolism of amino acids, and this is associated with retention of nitrogen, potassium, phosphorus and calcium. Doses in excess of 10 mg daily to the female may produce virilism.

Unconjugated testosterone is rarely used clinically because its derivatives have a more powerful and prolonged effect, and testosterone itself requires implantation into the subcutaneous fat, using a trocar and cannula for maximum therapeutic benefit. Testosterone propionate is prepared in an oily solution, as it is insoluble in water. It is effective for three days and is therefore administered intramuscularly twice weekly. Testosterone phenylpropionate is a long-acting micro-crystalline preparation, which, when given by intramuscular or subcutaneous injection, is effective for two weeks. Methyl-testosterone is only weakly active by mouth though it is absorbed sublingually. It does however produce a cholestatic jaundice in a significant proportion of patients and is therefore better avoided. Mesterolone is an effective oral androgen and is less hepatoxic. It does not inhibit pituitary gonadotrophic production and hence spermatogenesis is unimpaired. Testosterone undecanoate has recently been introduced and may well prove to be the oral androgen of choice.

The androgens in therapeutic use which can be given by mouth include: mesterolone, methyltestosterone, testosterone, testosterone undecanoate. Those that can be given by injection include: testosterone propionate, testosterone phenylpropionate, testosterone enanthate, testosterone esters and drostanolone.

ANENCEPHALY is the term given to the condition in which a child is born with a defect of the skull and absence of the brain. Anencephaly is the most common major malformation of the central nervous system. It has an incidence of 0·65 per 1,000 live births. There is complete absence of the cerebral hemispheres and overlying skull and the brain stem and cerebellum are atrophic. If the pregnancy goes to term the infants rapidly die but in 50 per cent of pregnancies associated with anencephaly spontaneous abortion occurs. It is possible to detect the presence of anencephaly in the fetus by measuring the level of alpha foeto protein in the mother's serum or in the amniotic fluid. (See SPINA BIFIDA.)

ANEUPLOIDY is the state in which there is an abnormal number of chromosomes (q.v.): e.g. Down's syndrome (q.v.) and Turner's syndrome (q.v.).

ANEURINE is an alternative name for vitamin B_1. (See THIAMINE.)

ANEURYSM means a dilatation upon an artery, due to yielding of the vessel-wall and gradual stretching by the pressure of the blood. They are called *dissecting* when the inner coat has given way somewhat suddenly and blood has passed between the coats and torn its way some distance along the vessel wall; *miliary* when the aneurysm is very small and looks like a millet seed on the side of the vessel, which is a form often found on the vessels in the brain. An *arteriovenous aneurysm* is one where there is a communication between an artery and a vein. **Causes**: The two main factors responsible for the formation of an aneurysm are (1) strain; (2) weakening of the wall of the artery. The latter is the more important. No amount of strain, whether due to a raised blood-pressure or to muscular effort, will lead to aneurysm formation unless there is some local weakening of the wall of the artery. The two most important causes of weakening of the arterial wall are atheroma (q.v.) and syphilis (q.v.). Most aneurysms of the thoracic aorta are due to syphilis. Atheroma is the more common cause of aneurysms in the abdominal aorta. Aneurysms may also be due to loss of the support provided by the surrounding tissues, e.g. in the lungs, where an aneurysm may form in one of the branches of the pulmonary artery as a result of destruction of the surrounding tissue by tuberculosis. Occasionally they may be due to congenital defects in the arterial wall: the most common site for such aneurysms is the circle of Willis (q.v.) at the base of the brain. More rarely they may arise as a result of repeated small trauma and strain in exposed arteries, such as the popliteal artery, which have not much support from the surrounding tissues; popliteal aneurysms were more common in the old coaching days among those who spent most of their working lives on horseback. Small aneurysms, known as *mycotic* aneurysms, may also arise in cases of severe sepsis, as a result of infection of the arterial wall. Aneurysms are more common in men than in women, and particularly among those who perform in hard physical labour. **Symptoms**: These vary greatly with the size and position of the aneurysm, but there are some which are characteristic of all forms. If the aneurysm is in a limb, a round *swelling* is noticed, perhaps as large as a walnut or Mandarin orange, which expands and diminishes with each heart-beat. The swelling is generally painless, and the skin over it is unchanged (unlike an abscess). Aneurysms rarely occur further from the trunk than the elbow or knee. If the aneurysm be internal it is situated upon a great vessel, and is often very large in size before it causes any definite symptoms, which are mainly due to interference with surrounding organs. *Pain* is felt only when the swelling presses upon nerves, upon the air passages, causing great breathlessness, or upon bone, wearing it gradually away. In the latter case pain may be agonizing, although in early cases it is not infrequently taken for mere rheumatic pain. *Breathlessness* or *difficulty in swallowing* may occur where there is a large thoracic aneurysm, from pressure on the windpipe or gullet, also *cough* of a barking, irritating nature, and changes in the voice, from irritation or paralysis of the left recurrent laryngeal nerve. In thoracic and abdominal aneurysm there may be a *bulging* in the upper part of chest or abdomen, as the case may be, which can be felt to throb when one hand is placed on it in front and the other on the back; in a later stage pulsation can also be seen. The *aneurysmal tippet* is the name given to a network of dilated veins which appears upon the chest and shoulders, owing to obstruction of the circulation through the great veins, by a thoracic aneurysm. *Swelling of the skin* or oedema is found with all aneurysms sooner or later from the same cause. Many other signs, such as inequality of the pupils, difference in the pulse on the two sides of the body, and murmurs heard over the swelling, are present in different aneurysms, but can be appreciated only by the trained observer. Congenital aneurysms of the circle of Willis usually cause no symptoms unless they rupture. This results in subarachnoid haemorrhage (q.v.) or sudden death. By rupturing they are a not uncommon cause of sudden death in apparently healthy young people after exercise.

Treatment: (*a*) MEDICAL: Although the aneurysm tends constantly to increase in size, another tendency is for the blood in contact with the unhealthy wall to clot. If this is encouraged, the aneurysm may become a solid mass, which practically may be looked on as a cure, because there is no more tendency to grow or to burst. If the aneurysm is syphilitic in origin, penicillin is given.

SURGICAL: Tremendous advances have been achieved in recent years in the surgical treatment of aneurysms. In many cases, as in aneurysms of arteries in the limbs, all that is required is to ligature the artery above and below the aneurysm, the circulation to the limb being maintained by anastomosis (q.v.) of the other arteries in the limb. In the case of other major arteries, such as the aorta, the aneurysm is replaced by a graft so that the circulation through the artery can be maintained. This graft may consist of a piece of an artery removed from a cadaver, or of synthetic material such as orlon.

ANGINA means literally choking, and is a term applied to swellings of the throat or other cause of difficulty in breathing, as *tonsillar angina* or quinsy, *laryngeal angina* or laryngitis, *membranous angina* or croup, *anginal scarlatina* or scarlet fever with abscesses round the throat.

ANGINA PECTORIS is a term applied to a painful sensation in the chest, arising for the most part in connection with disease of the coronary arteries.

Causes: Angina pectoris is generally held to be due to an inadequate blood-supply to the myocardium: i.e. the heart muscle. The myocardium receives its blood-supply through the coronary arteries. Thus angina pectoris may be due to spasm of the coronary arteries or to narrowing of the lumen of these arteries as a result of arteriosclerosis (see ARTERIES, DISEASES OF) or atheroma (q.v.). It is sometimes due to spasm alone. In the majority of cases it is due either to spasm plus arteriosclerosis (or atheroma) or to arteriosclerosis (or atheroma). Occasionally the defective blood-supply may be the result of disease of the first part of the aorta or of the aortic valve. Because of its association with coronary artery disease, angina pectoris is predominantly a disease of middle age and is more common in men than in women.

Symptoms: The characteristic feature of angina pectoris is the occurrence of pain behind the chest-bone, arising as a result of exertion and relieved by rest. This pain often spreads into the left arm. The amount of exertion necessary to induce the pain varies considerably, and to a certain extent gives some idea of the severity of the condition. Thus, it may only occur on hurrying, whilst in other cases the blood-supply to the myocardium may be so defective that the least exertion, e.g. turning over in bed, may be sufficient to induce a severe paroxysm of pain. Aggravating factors are exposure to cold, or exertion immediately following a meal. The paroxysm of pain seldom lasts for more than a few minutes, provided the affected individual remains at complete rest. In most instances the pain is so severe that the affected individual is unable to continue any exertion. Diagnostic tests include an *electrocardiogram* (ECG) and a cardiac-stress test – an ECG while exercising.

Treatment: The aim of treatment is to prevent the occurrence of pain by persuading the patient to restrict his activities. Thus, he should always rest for at least half an hour after a meal. He should always be warmly clad when he goes out of doors in cold weather. In more severe cases his bedroom should be on the ground floor and should be warmed in the winter. He should always allow himself plenty of time so that he never needs to hurry. If he is overweight he should restrict his diet so as to bring his weight down. Even with all these precautions, attacks of pain may still occur, and for the relief of these glyceryl trinitrate tablets B.P., or trinitrin tablets as they are also known, each containing 500 micrograms, are the most satisfactory. A tablet should be placed in the mouth, as soon as pain is felt, and allowed to melt in the mouth. Most patients with angina pectoris carry a small supply of these tablets about with them wherever they go, so that they are always available for immediate use. A preparation of glyceryl trinitrate is now available which is applied to the skin once a day and thereby maintains a steady absorption of the drug into the body. It is useful in more severe cases in which a steady supply of the drug is necessary to keep the pain under control. An alternative form of treatment is amyl nitrite, which is supplied in the form of small glass 'perles'. One of these, held in a handkerchief, is broken between the fingers and the contents then inhaled. Whilst usually as effective as trinitrin tablets, amyl nitrite is more liable to produce unpleasant side-effects such as headache and giddiness. The precise mode of action of these two preparations is still rather obscure, but all the evidence suggests that they act by reducing the demand of the heart muscle for oxygen. Other drugs used in the treatment of angina pectoris include propranolol (q.v.), perhexiline, and nifedipine. If the patient has high blood pressure, he or she should receive anti-hypertensive drugs.

If, despite drug treatment, attacks become more severe and there is angiographic evidence of narrowing of the coronary blood vessels, coronary-artery bypass surgery (*angioplasty*) may be performed.

ANGIOCARDIOGRAPHY means X-raying of the heart after injection into it of a radio-opaque substance.

ANGIOGRAPHY means rendering the blood-vessels visible on an X-ray film by injecting into them a radio-opaque substance. In the case of arteries this is know as *arteriography*; the corresponding term for veins being *venography* or *phlebography*. This procedure demonstrates whether there is any narrowing of the lumen of the vessel.

ANGIOMA is a tumour composed of blood-vessels. (See TUMOUR and NAEVUS.)

ANGIONEUROTIC OEDEMA is a painless swelling in the sub-cutaneous tissues or the sub-mucosa, usually occurring around the face and especially affecting the eyes, lips and tongue. It is similar in many ways to nettle rash (see URTICARIA). It is caused primarily by food allergy. There is also an hereditary form which is transmitted as an autosomal dominant trait and is due to an enzyme deficiency that inactivates one of the mediators of inflammation called Complement.

ANGIOPLASTY: A method of treating blockage or narrowing of a blood vessel or heart valve by inserting a balloon into the constriction to reopen it. The technique is used to treat a narrowed artery in the heart or a limb. About 65 per cent of patients treated benefit, but when symptoms persist or recur the procedure may be repeated. There is a small risk of damage to the vessel or valve.

ANGIOTENSIN is one of the factors responsible for hypertension, or high blood-pressure. (See ESSENTIAL HYPERTENSION; RENIN.)

ANGIOTENSIN-CONVERTING ENZYME INHIBITORS: The enzyme that converts angiotensin I to angiotensin II is called angiotensin-converting enzyme. Angiotensin II controls the blood pressure and is the most potent endogenous pressor substance produced in the body; angiotensin I has no such pressor activity. Inhibition of the enzyme that converts angiotensin I to angiotensin II will thus have marked effects on lowering the blood pressure. Captopril was the first angiotensin inhibitor to be synthesized. It lowers peripheral resistance by causing arteriolar dilatation and thus lowers blood pressure. Other drugs such as enalapril and lisinopril have since been developed. Some kidney disorders increase the production of angiotensin II and so cause hypertension.

ANGITIS, or ANGIITIS, means inflammation of a vessel such as a blood-vessel, lymph-vessel, or bile-duct.

ÅNGSTRÖM UNIT (called after the Swedish physicist) is a measurement of length and equals 1/10000 micrometre, or one-hundred-millionth of a centimetre. It is represented by the symbol Å and is used to give the length of electro-magnetic waves.

ANIDROSIS is the condition in which there is an abnormal diminution in the secretion of sweat.

ANISOCYTOSIS: This refers to a variation in the size of red blood cells.

ANKLE is the joint between the leg bones (tibia and fibula) above, and the talus (the Roman dice-bone) below. It is a very strong joint with powerful ligaments binding the bones together at either side, many sinews running over it, and bony projections from the leg bones, which form large bosses on either side, called the outer and inner malleoli, extending about 12 mm (half an inch) below the actual joint. Two common injuries near the ankle are a sprain, on the inner side, consisting of tearing of the internal ligament; and fracture of the fibula (Pott's fracture) on the outer side. (See also JOINTS, DISEASES OF.)

ANKYLOSING SPONDYLITIS (see SPINE AND SPINAL CORD, DISEASES AND INJURIES OF).

ANKYLOSIS is a term meaning the condition of a joint in which the movements are restricted by fibrous bands, or by malformation, or by actual union of the bones. (See JOINTS, DISEASES OF.)

ANKYLOSTOMA (see ANCYLOSTOMIASIS).

ANODYNES are curative measures which soothe pain. They act by removing the cause of pain, by soothing the irritated nerves of the painful part, or by paralysing the part of the brain by which the painful impression is received. Substances which destroy the power of feeling altogether are called anaesthetics (q.v.), those which destroy only the power of feeling pain are analgesics (q.v.).
Varieties: Alkaline applications are anodynes to bee-stings. Prolonged application of either cold or heat is an anodyne in inflammation. Chloroform, camphor and menthol are local anodynes, while internally various synthetic products like aspirin soothe pain in distant parts.
Uses: Opium is the oldest and most powerful anodyne, but can only be used in cases of excessive pain, because of its tendency to habit-formation. Barbiturates dull pain, but with it the mental faculties, so that they also interfere with the performance of everyday duties. Aspirin and paracetamol seem to have the power of dulling only that part of the brain which perceives the pain, and so are most suitable in slighter pains which do not incapacitate though they interfere with ordinary duties. (For further details, see NEURALGIA; HEADACHE; INFLAMMATION; and the various drugs named.)

ANOPHELES is the generic name of a widely distributed group of mosquitoes, certain species of which transmit to man the infecting agent of malaria. *Anopheles maculipennis* and *A. bifurcatus* are both found in England and can both transmit the malaria parasite.

ANOREXIA means loss of appetite. (See APPETITE.)

ANOREXIA NERVOSA (see EATING DISORDERS).

ANOSMIA means loss of sense of smell. (See NOSE, DISEASES OF.)

ANOVULAR: Absence of ovulation. Anovular menstruation occurs when a woman takes the contraceptive pill.

ANOXAEMIA means reduction of the oxygen content of the blood below normal limits.

ANOXIA is the term applied to that state in which the body tissues have an inadequate supply of oxygen. This may be because the blood in the lungs does not receive enough oxygen, or because there is not enough blood to receive the oxygen, or because the blood stagnates in the body. (See OXYGEN.)

ANTABUSE (see DISULFIRAM).

ANTACIDS are medicines which correct acidity, either general or stomachic. (See ALKALI; DYSPEPSIA.)

ANTAGONIST: (*a*) The action of one drug in opposing the action of another. (*b*) A muscle the contraction of which opposes that of another muscle called the *agonist* (q.v.). When the agonist contracts the antagonist relaxes.

ANTE- is a prefix meaning before or forwards.

ANTEFLEXION means the abnormal forward curvature of an organ in which the upper part is sharply bent forward. The term is especially applied to forward displacement of the uterus.

ANTENATAL is a term applied to conditions occurring before birth. It is used with reference both to mother and child. (For Antenatal Clinics, see MATERNITY AND CHILD WELFARE.)

ANTEPARTUM: An adjective describing an event before labour starts in pregnancy.

ANTERIOR: An adjective that describes or relates to the front part of the body, limbs, or organs.

ANTERIOR TIBIAL SYNDROME (see MUSCLE).

ANTEVERSION is the term applied to the forward tilting of an organ, especially of the uterus.

ANTHELMINTICS are substances which cause the death or expulsion of parasitic worms.

ANTHRACOSIS is the change which takes place in the lungs and bronchial glands of coal miners, and others, who inhale coal dust constantly. The lungs are amazingly efficient in coping with this problem. During a working lifetime a coalminer may inhale around 5000 grams of dust, but at post-mortem examination it is rare to find more than about 40 grams in his lungs. The affected tissues change in colour from greyish pink to jet black, owing to loading with minute carbon particles. This fine form of dust appears to be almost devoid of any harmful effect.

ANTHRAX is a very serious disease occurring in sheep and cattle, and in those who tend them or handle the bones, skins and fleeces, even long after removal of the latter from the animals. It is sometimes referred to as malignant pustule, wool-sorters' disease, splenic fever of animals or murrain. It is now a rare condition in the United Kingdom. The cause is a bacillus (*B. anthracis*) which grows in long chains and produces spores of great vitality. These spores retain their life for years, in dried skins and fleeces; they are not destroyed by boiling, freezing, 5 per cent carbolic lotion, or, like many bacilli, by the gastric juice. The disease is communicated from a diseased animal to a crack in the skin, e.g. of a shepherd or butcher, or from contact with contaminated skins or fleeces. Nowadays skins are handled wet, but if they are allowed to dry so that dust laden with spores is inhaled by the workers an internal form of the disease results. Instances have occurred of the disease being conveyed on shaving brushes made from bristles of diseased animals.

Symptoms: (*a*) EXTERNAL FORM: This is the 'malignant pustule'. After inoculation of some small wound, a few hours or days elapse, and then a red, inflamed swelling appears, which grows larger till it covers half the face or the breadth of the arm, as the case may be. Upon its summit appears a bleb of pus, which bursts and leaves a black scab, perhaps 12 mm (half an inch) wide. At the same time there is great prostration and fever. The inflammation may last ten days or so, when it slowly subsides and the patient recovers, if surviving the fever and prostration.

(*b*) INTERNAL FORM: This takes the form of pneumonia with haemorrhages, when the spores have been drawn into the lungs, or of ulcers of the stomach and intestines, with gangrene of the spleen, when they have been swallowed. It is usually fatal in two or three days.

Prevention is most important by disinfecting all hides, wool and hair coming from areas of the world. An efficient vaccine is now available. Treatment consists of the administration of large doses of penicillin or of one of the tetracyclines.

ANTI- is a prefix meaning against.

ANTIBIOTIC is the term used to describe any antibacterial agent derived from micro-organisms, such as penicillin, streptomycin, chloramphenicol and chlortetracycline.

The discovery and isolation of the penicillin nucleus, 6 amino penicillanic acid (6-APA) in 1958 provided the basis for the synthesis of a large number of new penicillins. These semi-synthetic penicillins now comprise the largest single group of antibiotics in clinical medicine (phenethicillin, ampicillin, propicillin, azidocillin, carbenicillin, ticarcillin, sulbenicillin, carindicillin, carfecillin, mezlocillin, piperacillin, apacillin, talampicillin, bacampicillin, amoxycillin, pivampicillin, methicillin, nafcillin,

oxacillin, cloxacillin, dicloxacillin, flucloxacillin, mecillinam, pivmecillinam). All these compounds are derivatives of 6 amino penicillin acid and at the present time there are nearly a score of different semi-synthetic penicillins in clinical use.

The cephalosporins are derived from the compound cephalosporin C which is obtained by fermentation of the mould cephalosporium. The cephalosporin nucleus 7 Amino cephalosporanic (7-ICA) acid has been the basis for the production of the semi-synthetic compounds of the cephalosporin nucleus. The first semi-synthetic cephalosporin, cephalothin, appeared in 1962; it was followed by cephaloridine in 1964. The original cephalosporins had to be given by injection but more recent preparations can be given by mouth. The newer preparations are less readily destroyed by beta lactamases and so they have a much broader spectrum of antibacterial activity. The newer cephalosporins include cephalexin, cefazolin, cephacetrile, cephapirin, cefamandole, cefuroxine, cephrodine, cefodroxil and cefotaxine. Inactivation of beta lactamase is the basis of bacterial resistance to both the penicillins and the cephalosporins so that attempts to prepare these antibiotics with resistance to beta lactamase is of great importance. A synthetic inhibitor of beta lactamase called clavulanic acid has recently been synthesized. This is used in combination with the penicillins and cephalosporins to prevent resistance. The cephamycins are a new addition to the beta lactam antibiotics. They are similar in structure to the cephalosporins but are produced, not by fungi, but by actinomycetes.

ANTIBODIES are substances in the blood which destroy or neutralize various toxins or 'bodies' (e.g. bacteria), known generally as antigens. The antibodies are formed, usually, as a result of the introduction into the body of the antigens to which they are antagonistic, as in all infectious diseases.

ANTICHOLINERGIC: An action or drug that inhibits the activity of acetylcholine (q.v.).

ANTICOAGULANTS are drugs which prevent coagulation of the blood. The main ones now in use are heparin (q.v.), phenindione (q.v.) and warfarin (q.v.). Patients who are on anticoagulants require to be under medical supervision, and it is now usual for them to receive from their doctors an Anticoagulant Card with instructions about the use of whatever anticoagulant drug they may be taking.

ANTICONVULSANT: A drug that reduced or prevents the severity of an epileptic convulsion or seizure. The nature of the fit and the patient's reaction influences the type of anticonvulsant used. Anticonvulsants inhibit the high level of electrical activity in the brain that causes the fit. Among regularly used anticonvulsants are carbamazepine, clonazopam, diazepam, phenobarbitone, phenytoin, primidone, and sodium valporate.

ANTIDEPRESSANTS are drugs which relieve depression and associated symptoms such as insomnia and poor appetite. They are not tranquillizers, although some cause sedation, and they do not seem to be addictive.

The antidepressant effect often takes two or three weeks to start, and at least three months of regular treatment may be needed to restore normal mood. Relapse may occur quickly, hence patients are usually advised to continue taking antidepressants for at least three months after recovery. The dose can then be reduced gradually and stopped. Alcohol should be avoided throughout the course of treatment.

There are three main types of antidepressant: tricyclics, serotonin reuptake inhibitors, and monoamine oxidase inhibitors. They probably work by restoring the balance of certain mood-regulating chemicals in the brain, such as noradrenaline and serotonin (also known as 5-hydroxytryptamine or 5HT). Two other drugs – lithium and carbamazepine – that can relieve depression are used mainly to regulate mood in manic depressive illnesses and are not discussed in detail here.

Tricyclic antidepressants, whose molecules usually contain three rings, have some sedative effects. Sedation may help patients who also feel anxious and agitated, but can be a nuisance. Other side-effects (often occurring only in the first week or two) may include dry mouth, blurred vision, tremor, constipation, weight increase, difficulty in urinating, and sexual difficulties. In elderly patients these drugs may cause dizziness, low blood pressure, and heart arrhythmias and should be introduced slowly. They should not be taken by patients with recent heart attacks or an arrhythmia called heart block and should be avoided in pregnancy. Commonly prescribed tricyclics and related drugs include amitriptyline, imipramine, trimipramine, clomipramine, lofepramine, and dothiepin.

Serotonin reuptake inhibitors or blockers are a fairly new group of antidepressants, used in Britain since the mid 1980s. They seem to work by increasing brain levels of the serotonin. They are as effective as the tricyclics and produce the same side-effects less often, so are increasingly prescribed for elderly patients. But some patients experience other side-effects with these drugs including agitation, nausea, and loss of appetite and weight. Examples of serotonin reuptake inhibitors include fluvoxamine, fluoexetine, paroxetine, and sertraline.

Monoamine oxidase inhibitors (MAOIs) are stimulants which may cause agitation and insomnia. They are rarely prescribed now because they can cause a dangerous increase in blood pressure when taken with foods containing the chemical tyramine (cheese, pickled herring, broad bean pods, meat and yeast extracts, game, and alcohol – particularly red wine). The same interaction can occur with other drugs (including treatments bought over the counter for coughs and colds), thus anyone taking MAOIs must check with a pharmacist before taking any other medicine. The MAOIs available in Britain are tranylcypromine, phenelzine, and isocarboxazid.

ANTIDIURETIC HORMONE (ADH) (see VASOPRESSIN).

ANTIDOTES are remedies which neutralize the effects of poisons. Thus acids have alkalis as antidote and vice versa.

ANTIEMETIC: A drug that counteracts nausea and sickness. Some antihistamines and anticholinergics have an antiemetic effect. They are used to combat motion sickness or nausea and vomiting brought on by other drugs.

ANTIGEN is the term applied to a substance which causes the formation of antibodies: it is usually a protein that is foreign to the body.

ANTIHISTAMINE DRUGS are drugs which antagonize the action of histamine (q.v.) and are therefore of value in the treatment of certain allergic conditions. They are also of some value in the treatment of vasomotor rhinitis. They reduce rhinorrhoea and sneezing but are usually less effective in relieving nasal congestion. All antihistamines are also useful in the treatment of urticaria and certain allergic skin rashes, insect bites and stings. They are also used in the treatment of drug allergies. Chlorpheniramine or promethazine injections are useful in the emergency treatment of angioneurotic oedema and anaphylaxis.

There is little evidence that any one antihistamine is superior to another and patients vary considerably in their response to them. The antihistamines differ in their duration of action and in the incidence of side-effects such as drowsiness. Most are short-acting, but some (such as promethazine) work for up to twelve hours. They all cause sedation but promethazine, trimeprazine and dimenhydrinate tend to be more sedating while chlorpheniramine and cyclizine are less so, as are astemizole, oxatomide and terfenadine. Patients should be warned that their ability to drive or operate machinery may be impaired and that the effects of alcohol may be increased.

ANTIHYPERTENSIVE DRUGS: A group of drugs which are used to treat high blood pressure (hypertension). Untreated hypertension leads to strokes, heart attacks and heart failure. The high incidence of hypertension in western countries has led to intensive research to discover antihypertensive drugs and many have been marketed. The drugs may work by reducing the power of the heart beat, by dilating the blood vessels or by increasing the excretion of salts and water in the urine (diuresis). (See ESSENTIAL HYPERTENSION; MALIGNANT HYPERTENSION.)

ANTIMETABOLITES are a group of drugs which have been introduced for the treatment of certain forms of malignant disease. Chemically, they closely resemble substances (or metabolites) which are essential for the life and growth of cells. When introduced into the body they are 'mistaken', so to speak, by the cell for the corresponding metabolite, thereby preventing the cell from making use of the metabolite, or substance, which is essential for its growth. By this means the life of the cell is affected and it ultimately dies.

ANTIMONY is the name applied to a metal and also to its sulphide, a black powder found in nature. The tartrate of potassium and antimony is commonly known as tartar emetic in reference to its chief property. The preparations of antimony, some of which are used in the treatment of tropical diseases such as kala-azar, are all irritants; hence in large doses they are poisons.

ANTIPERISTALSIS is a movement in the bowels and stomach by which the food and other contents are passed upwards, instead of in the proper direction. (See PERISTALSIS.)

ANTI-PSYCHOTIC DRUGS (see NEURO-LEPTICS).

ANTIPYRETICS are measures used to reduce temperature in fever.
Varieties: Cold-sponging, wet-pack, baths and diaphoretic drugs such as quinine, salicylate of soda, and aspirin.
Uses (see under above headings).

ANTISEPTICS prevent the growth of disease-causing micro-organisms without damaging living tissues.
     Among chemicals used are boric acid, carbolic acid, hydrogen peroxide and products based on coal tar, such as cresol. Chlorhexidines, iodine, formaldehyde, flavines, alcohol and hexachlorophane are also used. Antiseptics are applied to prevent infection – for example, in preparing the skin before operation. They are also used to treat infected wounds.

ANTISPASMODICS (see SPASMOLYTICS).

ANTITOXINS, ANTITOXIC SERUM (see IMMUNOLOGY: serum therapy).

ANTIVENINE, or ANTIVENOM, is the name given to SNAKE VENOM ANTISERUM, which is produced by the injection of venom from poisonous animals such as snakes, spiders or scorpions into animals in small but increasing doses. The animal becomes immune to the particular venom injected. Native tradition in countries in Africa and Asia has it that a comparable method provides protection against snake bites in the treatment given by traditional snake doctors who specialize in the treatment of snake bites. The antiserum prepared from the serum of such immunized animals is effective in neutralizing venom injected by the bite of a snake of the same species. No antiserum effective against all venoms is available. The custom is for each country to prepare antisera able to neutralize the venoms of indigenous snakes. The antivenom active against the venom of the adder is known as Zagreb antivenom. To be of any use, it must be administered as soon as possible after the snake bite. (See BITES AND STINGS.)

ANTROSTOMY is the operation in which an opening is made through the nose into the maxillary antrum. (See ANTRUM.)

ANTRUM means a natural hollow or cavity. The *maxillary antrum* is now known as the maxillary sinus (see SINUS). The *mastoid antrum* is situated in the mastoid process, the mass of bone felt behind the ear. It may become the seat of an abscess in cases of suppuration of the middle ear (see EAR, DISEASES OF). The *pyloric antrum* is the part of the stomach immediately preceding the pylorus (q.v.).

ANURIA is a condition in which no urine is voided. (See GLOMERULONEPHRITIS; URINE.)

ANUS is the opening at the lower end of the bowel. It is kept closed by two muscles, the external and internal sphincters. The latter is a muscular ring which extends about 25 mm (1 inch) up the bowel, is nearly 6 mm (¼ inch) thick, and is kept constantly contracted by the action of a nerve centre in the spinal cord. In disease of the spinal cord the muscle may be paralysed, and inability to retain the motions results.

ANUS, DISEASES OF (see RECTUM, DISEASES OF).

ANXIETY STATE (see NEUROSIS).

ANXIOLYTICS are drugs for the relief of anxiety. They will induce sleep when given in large doses at night and so are hypnotics as well. Conversely most hypnotics will sedate when given in divided doses during the day. Prescription of these drugs is widespread but physical and psychological dependence occurs as well as tolerance to their effects. This is particularly true of the barbiturates which are now limited in their use, but also applies to the benzodiazepines. Withdrawal syndromes may occur if drug treatment is stopped too abruptly. Hypnotic sedatives and anxiolytics should therefore not be prescribed indiscriminately, but reserved for short courses.

AORTA is the large vessel which opens out of the left ventricle of the heart and carries blood to all the body. It is about 45 cm (1½ feet) long and 2·5 cm (1 inch) wide. Like other arteries it possesses three coats, of which the middle one is much the thickest. This consists partly of muscle fibre, but is mainly composed of an elastic substance, called elastin. The aorta passes first to the right, and lies nearest the surface behind the end of the second right rib-cartilage; then it curves backwards and to the left, passes down behind the left lung close to the backbone, and through an opening in the diaphragm into the abdomen, where it divides, at the level of the navel, into the two common iliac arteries, which carry blood to the lower limbs. Its branches, in order, are: two coronary arteries to the heart wall; the brachiocephalic, left common carotid, and left subclavian arteries to the head, neck and upper limbs; several small branches to the oesophagus, bronchi, and other organs of the chest; nine pairs of intercostal arteries which run round the body between the ribs; one pair of subcostal arteries which is in series with the intercostal arteries; four (or five) lumbar arteries to the muscles of the loins; coeliac trunk to the stomach, liver and pancreas; two mesenteric arteries to the bowels; and suprarenal, renal and testicular arteries to the suprarenal body, kidney, and testicle on each side. From the termination of the aorta rises a small branch, the median sacral artery, which runs down into the pelvis. In the female the ovarian arteries replace the testicular.

The chief diseases of the aorta are atheroma and aneurysm. (See ARTERIES, DISEASES OF; ANEURYSM; and COARCTATION OF THE AORTA.)

AORTIC REGURGITATION: The back flow of blood through the aortic valve of the heart into the left ventricle caused by an incompetent valve. The failure to close may be caused by a congenital defect or by damage from disease. The defect may be cured by surgical replacement of the damaged valve with an artificial valve. (See HEART DISEASES.)

AORTIC STENOSIS: Narrowing of the aortic valve which obstructs the flow of blood through it with serious effects on the heart and the circulation. The muscle in the left ventricle works harder to compensate for the obstruction and thickens as a result. Stenosis is usually caused by the deposition of calcium on the valve and is commonly associated with atheroma. Untreated, the condition leads to heart failure, but nowadays the stenosis can be treated surgically.

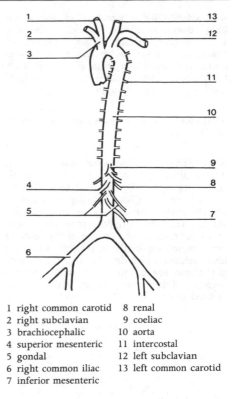

1 right common carotid	8 renal
2 right subclavian	9 coeliac
3 brachiocephalic	10 aorta
4 superior mesenteric	11 intercostal
5 gondal	12 left subclavian
6 right common iliac	13 left common carotid
7 inferior mesenteric	

Main branches of the aorta.

AORTIC VALVE: The valve that controls the flow of blood from the aorta to the left ventricle of the heart. (See HEART.)

AORTITIS means a degenerative condition of the lining of the aorta. It is usually produced by syphilis.

AORTOGRAPHY is the technique of rendering the aorta visible in an X-ray film by injecting a radio-opaque substance into it. (See also ANGIOGRAPHY.)

APACILLIN (see ANTIBIOTIC).

APERIENTS are medicines which produce a natural movement of the bowels. (See CONSTIPATION; PURGATIVES.)

APEX is the pointed portion of any organ which has a conical shape. The apex of each lung reaches about 3·5 to 5 cm (1½ or 2 inches) above the collar-bone into the neck. In health the apex of the heart can be felt below the fifth rib immediately inside the nipple.

APEX BEAT: This is the beat of the apex of the heart, which can be felt through the skin to the left of the breastbone between the fifth and sixth ribs.

APGAR SCORE is a method of assessing a baby's condition at birth, in which a value of 0, 1 or 2 is given to each of five signs: colour, heart-rate, muscle tone, respiratory (or breathing) effort, and the response to stimulation. A total score of 10 indicates that the newborn child is in excellent condition.

APHAKIA is a term which means absence of the lens of the eye.

APHASIA means a loss of the power of speech, due to injury to the centres which govern this act in the brain. The higher of these centres, which have to do with forming the ideas of speech, putting words together in sentences, and governing the movements of mouth, tongue and larynx, lie on the surface of the cerebral hemispheres, especially of the left; while the lower centres, which directly bring the muscles of the voice organs into action, under superintendence of the higher ones, are in the medulla or hind brain.

1 movements of tongue	6 memories of written
2 lateral	words
3 speech	7 sensation
4 hearing	8 central sulcus
5 sight	9 movement of leg
	10 movement of the
	trunk

Areas on the left surface of the cerebrum associated with definite functions.

Causes: The cause is destruction of a portion of the brain, including one of these higher centres, owing to rupture of a blood-vessel, and haemorrhage into the brain tissue; or owing to blocking of a blood-vessel by an embolus (see EMBOLISM), or by clotting of the blood on the diseased wall of a vessel (see THROMBOSIS), any one of which cuts off the supply of blood to the part concerned. The causes are thus the same as in a stroke, and aphasia may be one of the symptoms of a stroke especially when the right side of the body is paralysed, or may occur by itself, according to the extent of brain involved. Other diseases, such as tumours, may also be the cause, the important factor being interfer-

ence with the functions of certain definite areas of the brain.

Varieties: It was first pointed out by Broca that the inferior frontal gyrus on the left side of the brain in right-handed persons, and vice versa in left-handed persons, is, after death, found to be diseased in those who have, in life, suffered from inability to speak, although the intelligence and powers of silent reading and of writing may have remained. Such a condition is known as *motor aphasia*. But the state is generally more complicated. In addition to Broca's speech area, which governs the movements of the tongue, mouth and larynx that frame words to express ideas, there is a centre in the middle frontal gyrus of the left side, which regulates the power of writing intelligibly, and disease of this region produces loss of power to write rationally, even though the hand remains quite able to hold a pen, this condition being known as *agraphia*. These two forms involve loss of power of *production* of speech and writing, but there are corresponding losses of power of *perception* known as *word blindness* and *word deafness*, the two conditions being grouped together as *sensory aphasia*. In the former of these the afflicted person is unable to read correctly, though his vision is perfect, and he may be able to spell and even to write, though not to read what he writes. This condition is due to disease in the angular gyrus. In word deafness the disability consists in failure to understand what is said, and, though the sufferer hears perfectly, the sounds are to him like those of a foreign tongue which he does not understand; in this case the disease lies in the superior temporal gyrus. There are still more complicated forms in which the disease affects, not the surface of the brain, but the strands of nerve fibres, which run from one centre to another and reduce the working of the whole arrangement to a system.

Symptoms: The disorder generally follows a stroke and exists along with some paralysis on the right side of the body. *Aphasia* may come on suddenly and last only a few hours or days, being due then to a temporary circulatory disturbance in the brain. Generally it is permanent, and, naturally, a person with aphasia has always some mental impairment. Sometimes he is absolutely without the power of speech. When the condition is one of *sensory aphasia*, names of persons, of places, even of the commonest household articles.

Treatment: This is as in stroke, of which the condition often forms a part (see STROKE). The condition is seldom much improved if it has lasted more than a week without improvement. But in some patients improvement is achieved by teaching the afflicted person to read and speak just as one would teach a child, a new part of the brain apparently being educated.

APHONIA means loss of voice. It is caused by some disorder in the throat or in the nerves proceeding to the throat muscles, or by hysteria. (See VOICE AND SPEECH.)

APHTHAE (see THRUSH).

APHTHOUS ULCER: A small painful ulcer in the lining (mucosa) of the mouth. It is usually self limiting.

APICECTOMY is the minor operation carried out to try to save a tooth which has an abscess on it or which does not respond to root treatment. In this the abscess and the apex of the tooth are removed.

APLASIA: The complete or partial failure of tissue or an organ to develop.

APNOEA means stoppage of breathing, such as occurs when the blood is artificially supplied with too much oxygen; for example, by taking several deep breaths in quick succession. (See ASPHYXIA.)

APO- is a prefix implying separation or derivation from.

APODIA: Absence of the foot.

APOMORPHINE is a crystalline alkaloid closely related to morphine and having a powerful emetic action. Apomorphine hydrochloride is given hypodermically in doses of 2 to 8 mg in cases of poisoning in which the patient is unable to swallow or a very rapid emetic action is desired. It is also used in the treatment of alcoholism.

APONEUROSIS is the term applied to the white fibrous membrane which serves as an investment for the muscles and which covers the skull beneath the scalp.

APOPLEXY (see STROKE).

APPENDICECTOMY, or appendectomy, is the operation for the removal of the appendix vermiformis.

APPENDICITIS is an inflammatory disease starting in the vermiform appendix. It is the most common cause of abdominal sepsis in the western world and appendicectomy the most common surgical emergency. (See APPENDIX.)
Varieties: In the much less common form of grumbling or recurrent appendicitis the person affected is troubled by repeated slight attacks of pain or discomfort in the right iliac region. The *acute form* is usually known as an 'attack of appendicitis'. Unless adequately and properly treated, this form may proceed to *gangrenous appendicitis* in which the inflammation is so intense that the appendix sloughs away, and the bowels communicate, through the opening, with the peritoneal cavity. In *suppurative appen-*

dicitis, the appendix becomes the centre of an abscess. Both of these latter forms are extremely dangerous to life and are often very sudden in their development. This is why most patients with acute appendicitis are operated upon as soon as possible.

Acute appendicitis occurs at all ages, but is most common in the first twenty years of life, though rare under the age of two. It tends to be more common in males than in females. The precise cause is not known, but the condition is usually due to a combination of infection and obstruction. What probably happens in most cases is that the appendix becomes obstructed. This may be due to a small mass of faeces accumulating in the appendix or to kinking of the appendix. The contents of the obstructed appendix being infective, the whole appendix rapidly becomes infected, with the serious consequences already described, unless immediate skilled surgical treatment is available.

An attack of appendicitis comes on as a rule suddenly. The principal symptoms are: (*a*) sudden pain in the abdomen, often vague in situation at first, but usually settling in the right iliac region. (*b*) Disturbance of the digestive functions, consisting in loss of appetite, nausea, often vomiting, and constipation, which has usually been present for a day or two. (*c*) Tenderness to touch in the right iliac region, which in very many cases has its point of greatest intensity defined with curious exactitude at a point called Munro's or McBurney's point, situated about halfway between the spine of the iliac bone and the navel. (*d*) Fever of a moderate amount, generally about 39 °C (102 °F).
Treatment: A patient with acute appendicitis seen within thirty-six hours of the onset should be operated on forthwith, the mortality in the hands of good surgeons being very low: around 0·25 per cent. If the case is seen after forty-eight hours of the onset and improvement has set in, some surgeons recommend postponement of the operation until the inflammation has completely subsided; others hold that operation should be done at once. If the patient is suspected of having gangrenous appendicitis immediate operation is the only possible course; for the great danger of the disease consists in the production of a general peritonitis through the escape of bacteria and putrescent material from the interior of the appendix. (See PERITONITIS.)

APPENDIX is a term applied to appendages of several hollow organs. The epiploic appendices are a number of tags of fat hanging from the outer surface of the large intestine. The appendices of the larynx are two pouches, one on either side between the false and true vocal cords. The term appendix is most commonly applied to the vermiform appendix of the large intestine. It is a tubular prolongation of the large intestine with an average length of 9 or 10 cm and a width of 6 mm. It lies in the right lower corner of the abdomen and has peritoneal,

Part of the bowel in the right iliac region showing the relations of the appendix
to the ilium and the caecum.

muscular and mucous coats similar to those of the rest of the intestine.

APPETITE is the craving for the food necessary to maintain the body and to supply it with sufficient energy to carry on its functions. The ultimate cause of appetite is a question of supply and demand in the muscles and various organs, but the proximate cause is doubtful. Unlike hunger, it is probably an acquired, rather than an inborn, sensation. Thus, a newborn infant experiences hunger, but probably not appetite. Whatever other factors may be concerned, the tone of the stomach is of importance. This is supported by the fact that in conditions associated with poor appetite the tone of the stomach is poor, whilst in conditions such as duodenal ulcer which are characterized by a good, or even excessive appetite, the stomach is often hypertonic. Important factors in stimulating appetite are anticipation and the sight and smell of well-cooked food. Just as, conversely, the sight or smell of badly cooked food may remove all desire for food. Undoubtedly a good appetite is necessary to good digestion, and a perfectly healthy taste and appetite ought to be both a guide to the suitability of foods and a gauge of the amount required. Like every other bodily function, appetite may be out of order. It may be depraved, and may indicate quite unsuitable articles of diet, from toasted cheese in dyspeptics, who know by experience that such an article upsets their digestion, to cinders, hair, pebbles, etc., in the condition known as *pica*, which occurs sometimes during pregnancy, in children, in hysteria, and often in mental disorders. The two chief disorders, however, are excessive increase of appetite and diminution or loss of appetite.

Excessive appetite may be simply a bad habit, due to habitual over-indulgence in good food, and resulting in gout, obesity, etc., according to the other habits and constitution of the person.

It may also be a sign of diabetes mellitus or thyrotoxicosis. (See EATING DISORDERS.)

Diminished appetite is a sign common to almost all diseases causing general weakness, because the activity of the stomach and the secretion of gastric juice fail early when vital power is low. It is the most common sign of dyspepsia due to gastritis (see DYSPEPSIA) and of cancer of the stomach. In some cases it is a manifestation of stress or strain such as domestic worry or difficulties at work. Indeed, appetite seems to be particularly susceptible to emotional disturbances.

APPROVED NAMES is the term used for names devised or selected by the British Pharmacopoeia Commission for new drugs. The intention is that if any of the drugs to which these Approved Names are applied should eventually be included in the *British Pharmacopoeia* the Approved Name should be its official title. The issue of an Approved Name, however, does not imply that the substance will necessarily be included in the *British Pharmacopoeia* or that the Commission is prepared to recommend the use of the substance.

APRAXIA means loss of power to carry out regulated movements. Although there is no muscle weakness or incoordination, there is difficulty in formulating movement patterns.

APYREXIA means absence of fever.

ARACHIS OIL, also known as peanut oil, is the oil expressed from the seeds of *Arachis hypogoea*. It is sometimes used to replace olive oil when the latter is in short supply. It is commonly used as the vehicle for the intramuscular injection of drugs: e.g. penicillin.

ARACHNODACTYLY, or MARFAN'S SYN-DROME, is a congenital condition characterized by extreme length and slenderness of the fingers and toes and, to a lesser extent, of the limbs and trunk, laxity of the ligaments, and dislocation of the lens of the eye. The antero-posterior diameter of the skull is abnormally long, and the jaw is prominent. There may also be abnormalities of the heart.

ARACHNOID MEMBRANE is one of the membranes covering the brain and spinal cord (see BRAIN). Arachnoiditis is the name applied to inflammation of this membrane.

ARBOVIRUSES are a group of around 200 viruses, which are transmitted to man by arthropods. They include the viruses of dengue (q.v.) and yellow fever (q.v.) which are transmitted by mosquitoes.

ARC EYE (see EYE, DISEASE AND INJURIES).

ARCUS CORNEALIS (see EYE, DISEASE AND INJURIES).

ARENAVIRUSES are a group of viruses, so called because under the electron microscope they have a sand-sprinkled (Latin, *arenosus*) appearance. Among the diseases in man for which they are responsible are lassa fever (q.v.) in West Africa, Argentinian haemorrhagic fever (mortality rate 3 to 15 per cent), a similar disease in Bolivia (mortality rate 18 per cent), and lymphocytic choriomeningitis, in which deaths are uncommon.

AREOLA literally means a small space, and is the term applied to the red or dusky ring round the nipple, or round an inflamed part. Increase in the duskiness of the areola on the breast is an important early sign of pregnancy.

ARGYLL ROBERTSON PUPIL is a condition (described originally by Dr Argyll Robertson) in which the pupils contract when the eyes converge on a near object, but fail to contract when a bright light falls on the eye. It is found in several diseases, especially in locomotor ataxia and general paralysis of the insane.

ARGYRIA, or ARGYRIOSIS means the effect produced by taking silver salts over a long period, and consists of a deep duskiness of the skin, especially of the exposed parts.

ARM is the part of the upper limb between the shoulder and elbow, but is generally taken to include also the forearm and shoulder regions.

The upper limb is attached to the body by the strong pectoral muscles in front and by several powerful muscles springing from the spine and ribs behind. The great mobility of the shoulder is largely due to the fact that the only contact with the bones of the trunk takes place between the collar-bone and the upper end of the sternum or breast-bone, the shoulder-blade sliding freely between the muscles of the back as the arm is raised and lowered. The bones of the arm are the clavicle or collar-bone and the scapula or shoulder-blade lying at the upper part of the chest, the humerus, a single bone in the upper arm, and the radius and ulna lying side by side in the forearm. Eight small bones compose the wrist (or carpus) and connect the hand with the lower end of the radius.

The shoulder-joint is of the ball-and-socket variety, the head of the humerus resting against the glenoid cavity of the shoulder-blade. The elbow is a hinged joint formed at the lower end of the humerus above, while the ulna forms the chief part of the joint below, the radius resting lightly against the humerus. When the hand is rotated so as to lie palm up or back up, the radius in the first case lies alongside the ulna and in the latter crosses over it. The chief muscle which bends the elbow is the biceps in front of the upper arm, while the triceps lying behind straightens the limb. A group of muscles attached at the inner side of the elbow act to bend the wrist and fingers; another group of muscles attached to the outer side of the elbow have the general action of straightening and bending backwards the wrist and fingers.

One large artery (brachial artery) runs down the inner side of the upper arm corresponding to the seam of the coat sleeve in position. At the elbow this divides into two branches, the radial and ulnar arteries. The radial artery can be felt pulsating near the wrist and is generally known as the pulse. The ulnar artery lies to the inner side of the forearm, deeply imbedded in muscles. A large group of nerves lies at the inner side of the armpit, and these nerves run downwards to supply the muscles and skin of the arm. The ulnar nerve can readily be felt behind the inner side of the elbow, where it is exposed to bruising and is popularly known as the 'funny bone'. The large radial nerve runs down the back of the upper arm and the outer side of the forearm. At the back of the upper arm it is often damaged, leading then to the condition known as drop-wrist (q.v.), in which the hand hangs helpless and cannot be raised.

The collar-bone, by reason of its exposed position, is liable to fracture from falls on the shoulder, and the radius is often broken by falls on the palm of the hand. The shoulder-joint, on account of its great mobility, is prone to be dislocated in twists of the upper arm, but the elbow-joint is seldom injured. A small bursa or cavity lies between the skin and the end of the ulna at the point of the elbow, and this is often inflamed as the result of injury, and in the same way as the bursa in front of the knee is affected in the condition known as housemaid's knee. (See BURSITIS.)

ARMPIT, or AXILLA, is the pyramidal hollow between the upper arm and chest, bounded in front by the pectoral or breast muscles, behind by the shoulder-blade and its muscles, and running up to a point beneath the collar-bone. It contains the axillary vessels and nerves which run to the arm, also much fatty tissue, many sweat glands and lymphatic glands. The latter are important, because in poisoned wounds of the arm they may become inflamed, resulting in abscess; and still more, because in cancer of the breast they may become infected with cancer, and have to be removed with the breast. Wounds in the armpit are dangerous on the outer, front, and back walls, because large blood vessels run there.

ARRHYTHMIA means any variation from the normal regular rhythm of the heart-beat. The condition is produced by some affection interfering with the mechanism which controls the

beating of the heart, and includes the following disorders: sinus arrhythmia, atrial fibrillation, atrial flutter, heart block, extrasystole, pulsus alternans, and paroxysmal atrial tachycardia, ventricular tachycardia and ventricular fibrillation. (See HEART DISEASES.)

ARROWROOT is a West Indian plant (*Maranta arundinacea*). As sold, it is a white powder, consisting of almost pure starch, derived from the root of the plant. It is used as an invalid food, because it is easy to digest, but it must, of course, be combined with other forms of nourishment.

ARSENIC is a metal, but is better known by its oxide, white arsenic, by two arsenites of copper, Scheele's green and emerald green, and by two sulphides of arsenic, orpiment or king's yellow, and realgar. It is extensively used in dyeworks, in the manufacture of chemicals, in making

1 external iliac	13 arcuate	25 internal iliac
2 deep circumflex iliac artery	14 dorsalis pedis	26 superior gluteal
3 femoral artery	15 medial malleolar	27 inferior gluteal
4 lateral femoral artery	16 inferior medial genicular	28 perforating arteries 1-4
5 medial femoral circumflex	17 popliteal	29 popliteal
6 profunda femora	18 superior medical genicular	30 superior medial genicular
7 superior lateral genicular	19 supreme genu	31 superior lateral genicular
8 inferior lateral genicular	20 perforating arteries 1-4	32 anterior tibial
9 anterior tibial recurrent	21 profunda	33 fibular branch
10 anterior tibial	22 medial femoral circumflex	34 peroneal
11 lateral malleolar	23 obturator	35 posterior tibial
12 tarsal artery	24 inferior epigastric artery	36 medial malleolus

The arteries of the lower limb, anterior view (left) and the posterior view (right)

1 axillary	17 anterior interosseous
2 posterior humeral circumflex	18 common interosseus
3 anterior humeral circumflex	19 ulnar recurrent
4 profunda	20 superior ulnar collateral
5 brachial	21 subscapular
6 radial recurrent	22 lateral thoracic
7 radial	23 pectoral branch
8 palmar carpal	24 brachial artery
9 superficial palmar	25 inferior ulnar collateral artery
10 princeps pollicis	26 dorsal ulnar carpal artery
11 proper palmer digitals	27 first dorsal metacarpal artery
12 radiallis indicis	28 dorsal carpal radial artery
13 superficial palmer arch	29 posterior interosseous artery
14 deep palmar arch	30 profunda artery
15 deep palmar	31 posterior humeral circumflex artery
16 palmar carpal (ulnar)	

The arteries of the upper limb, anterior view (left) and posterior view (right).

enamel, in hardening shot and type, in fly-papers, sheep-dips, yellow and green paints, and is further given to horses to improve their coat. Applied pure, it is a strong germicide and caustic, and in large doses is a powerful irritant to stomach and intestines. When taken over long periods, larger and larger doses can be tolerated, till at last a quantity many times the poisonous dose has no apparent ill- effect. In some parts of the world, as among the mountaineers of Styria, its use has become a habit, and in these people it produces a sense of well-being and greater capacity for sustaining fatigue.

Most poisoning occurs through accidental ingestion, though arsenic has been used to murder people. Arsenic is a constituent of some pesticides and so may occur in rural communities, but industrial poisoning, once common, is now rare. Poisoning may be acute or chronic, the former causing inflammation of the stomach lining, resulting in nausea, vomiting, diarrhoea, and sweating. Chronic poisoning manifests as tiredness, weakness, loss of hair and dry and pigmented skin. Treatment includes the administration of dimercaprol.

ARTERIES are vessels which convey oxygenated blood away from the heart to the tissues of the body, limbs, and internal organs. In the case of most arteries, the blood has been purified by passing through the lungs, and is consequently bright red in colour, but in the pulmonary arteries which convey it to the lungs it is unoxygenated, dark, and like the blood in veins.

The arterial system begins at the left ventricle

1 internal cartoid
2 vertebral
3 right subclavian
4 brachiocephalic (innominate)
5 oesophageal
6 coeliac
7 middle suprarenal
8 renal
9 common iliac
10 internal iliac
11 external iliac
12 anterior tibial
13 peroneal
14 posterior tibial
15 nophiteal
16 femoral
17 ulnar
18 radial
19 middle sacral
20 spermatic
21 inferior mesenteric
22 brachial
23 superior mesenteric
24 inferior phrenic
25 superior phrenic
26 axillary
27 intercostals
28 left subclavian
29 internal mammery
30 thyrocervical trunk
31 costocervical trunk
32 common carotid
33 external carotid
34 superficial temperal

The chief arteries of the body.

The structure of an artery.

1 lumen

2 elastic membrane

3 muscular coat or media

4 adventitia

5 capillary supplying adventitia

of the heart with the aorta (see AORTA), which gives off branches that subdivide into smaller and smaller vessels, the final divisions, called arterioles, being microscopic, and ending in a network of capillaries, which perforate the tissues like the pores of a sponge, and bathe them in blood that is collected and brought back to the heart by veins. (See CIRCULATION OF THE BLOOD.)

The chief arteries after the *aorta* and its branches (see AORTA) are: (1) the *common carotid*, running up each side of the neck and dividing into *internal carotid* to the brain, and *external carotid* to the neck and face; (2) the *subclavian* to each arm, continued by the *axillary* in the armpit, and the *brachial* along the inner side of the arm, dividing at the elbow into the *radial* and the *ulnar*, which unite across the palm of the hand in arches that give branches to the fingers; (3) the two *common iliacs*, in which the aorta ends, each of which divides into the *internal iliac* to the organs in the pelvis, and the *external iliac* to the lower limb, continued by the *femoral* in the thigh, and the *popliteal* behind the knee, dividing into the *anterior* and *posterior tibial* arteries to the front and back of the leg. The latter passes behind the inner ankle to the sole of the foot, where it forms arches similar to those in the hand, and supplies the foot and toes by *plantar branches*.

Structure: The arteries are highly elastic, dilating at each heart-beat as blood is driven into them, and forcing it on by their resiliency (see PULSE). Every artery has *three coats*: (*a*) the outer or adventitia, consisting of ordinary strong fibrous tissue; (*b*) the middle or media, consisting of muscular fibres supported by elastic fibres, which in some of the larger arteries form distinct membranes; and (*c*) the inner or intima, consisting of a layer of yellow elastic tissue on whose inner surface rests a layer of smooth plate-like endothelial cells, over which flows the blood. In the larger arteries the muscle of the middle coat is largely replaced by elastic fibres, which render the artery still more expansile and elastic. When an artery is cut across, the muscular coat instantly shrinks, drawing the cut end within the fibrous sheath that surrounds the artery, and bunching

it up, so that a very small hole is left to be closed by blood-clot. (See HAEMORRHAGE.)

ARTERIES, DISEASES OF: ARTERIOSCLEROSIS, which is a condition of thickening and rigidity involving predominantly the inner and middle coat of medium-sized arteries, occurs as a natural change in old age. In some individuals, however, the change occurs earlier. The cause is still obscure, but certain facts are well established, even though they may only be predisposing factors. There is a hereditary tendency, and this is most marked in cases in which it develops at a relatively early age. There is a definite association with high blood-pressure in many cases, but arteriosclerosis can occur without a high blood-pressure. It is much more common in patients with diabetes mellitus than in individuals without this disease. It is also a common finding in gout. The distribution of arteriosclerosis throughout the arterial tree varies considerably. It may give rise to no symptoms, and only does so if it involves certain arteries. Thus, if it involves the arteries to the brain, the individual is liable to have a stroke; if it involves the coronary arteries which nourish the muscle of the heart, it may result in angina pectoris or a coronary thrombosis; if the arteries of the kidney are involved, a form of glomerulonephritis may develop; whilst if the arteries to the legs and feet are involved, gangrene may occur.

ATHEROSCLEROSIS is a condition characterized by the presence in the inner coat, or intima, of arteries of the degenerative condition known as atheroma. This manifests itself by nodes, or plaques, of yellowish material containing a high proportion of cholesterol (q.v.) and other lipids (q.v.). As these plaques enlarge, and the intima increases in thickness, the lumen of the artery becomes smaller and smaller. In due course the lumen of the artery may be so narrowed that it becomes blocked. If this occurs in the coronary arteries, which supply the heart muscle, the result is the all too common coronary thrombosis. If it occurs in the arteries in the brain it causes a stroke. The cause of atherosclerosis is not known, but one factor is the consumption of excessive saturated fats.

Following on atheroma, plates of lime may form in the arteries, or these vessels may, in extreme states, be changed into brittle calcareous tubes, very liable to tearing from slight injuries. When this condition occurs in older people, it is confined to the middle coat and is accompanied by marked calcification; it is known as *Mönckeberg's sclerosis*.

Syphilis and other inflammatory diseases may bring about an *obliterative inflammation*, in which the internal coat becomes greatly thickened (*endarteritis*) and in which the artery is more or less completely blocked. This leads to very serious effects, particularly in the case of arteries supplying the heart and brain. (See also THROMBOANGIITIS OBLITERANS; ANEURYSM.)

ARTERIOGRAPHY (see ANGIOGRAPHY).

ARTERIOLE is a small artery.

ARTERIO-VENOUS ANEURYSM is an abnormal communication between an artery and a vein. It is usually the result of an injury, such as a stab or a gunshot wound, which involves both a neighbouring artery and vein.

ARTERITIS means inflammation of an artery.

ARTHRALGIA: Pain in a joint in which there is no swelling or other indications of arthritis.

ARTHRITIS refers to any condition of joints of the limbs or spine associated with inflammatory or structural change. It is distinguished from arthralgia which simply implies joint pain with or without any inflammatory or structural change. The two main categories of arthritis are osteoarthritis, in which the primary change is thought of as mechanical failure of articular cartilage, and rheumatoid arthritis, in which the primary problem is a chronic inflammation of the synovial lining, of joints, tendon sheaths and bursae. Other less common forms of inflammatory arthritis include psoriatic arthritis, Reiter's syndrome, colitic arthritis and Behçet's syndrome. Spondarthritis refers to an inflammatory arthritis with involvement of the spine and is often associated with the HLA B27 tissue type. (See OSTEOARTHRITIS; RHEUMATOID ARTHRITIS; RHEUMATIC FEVER.)

ARTHRODESIS is the operation for fixing a joint in a given position, from which it cannot be moved. It results in a pain-free, stable, strong joint in certain cases of joint disease such as osteoarthrosis of the knee.

ARTHROPATHY is a term applied to any form of joint disease.

ARTHROPLASTY is the term applied to the operation for the making of a new joint as, for example, in advanced cases of osteoarthrosis of the hip, or the loosening of a fixed or stiff joint.

ARTHROPODS are segmented invertebrates with jointed legs. They include a wide range of organisms, such as scorpions, mites, ticks, spiders and centipedes.

ARTHROSCOPE: An instrument that enables the operator to see inside a joint cavity and, if necessary, take a biopsy or carry out an operation.

ARTICULAR means anything connected with a joint: e.g. articular rheumatism.

ARTICULATION is a term employed in two senses in medicine, either meaning the enunciation of words and sentences or meaning a joint.

ARTIFACT: A foreign body found in living tissue viewed under a microscope. It is usually caused by faulty preparation of a specimen with the result that disease or abnormality seems to be present.

ARTIFICIAL INSEMINATION: In this method of fertilization semen is collected either by the husband (AIH) or by a donor (AID) through masturbation and introduced into the upper vagina around the time of ovulation.

AIH is thought to be particularly useful for men with retrograde ejaculation or erectile impotence.

AID may be considered when the partner's sperm count is either very low or zero. Insemination can be made with fresh or frozen semen. Donors should be tested for sexually transmitted diseases and their identity remain unknown to the infertile couple. The pregnancy rate over six months is 50–60 per cent.

ARTIFICIAL KIDNEY (see KIDNEY, ARTIFICIAL).

ARTIFICIAL LIMBS AND OTHER PARTS: (see PROSTHESES).

ARTIFICIAL RESPIRATION (see APPENDIX: BASIC FIRST AID).

ARTIFICIAL VENTILATION OF THE LUNGS: Normally, on inspiration, air is drawn into the lungs by a subatmospheric pressure within the pleural space. This is achieved by expanding the lungs using the intercostal muscles and the diaphragm. Expiration is achieved by reversing the process and, when breathing heavily, contracting the abdominal muscles. To produce ventilation artificially this cycle of air flowing in and out of the lungs must be reproduced (see LUNGS). This may be achieved using intermittent positive or negative pressure as described below.

INTERMITTENT POSITIVE PRESSURE (ITP) – The simplest form of intermittent positive-pressure ventilation is mouth-to-mouth resuscitation (see APPENDIX: BASIC FIRST AID) where an individual blows his or her own expired gases into the lungs of an apnoeic person via the mouth or nose. Similarly gas may be blown into the lungs via a face mask (or down an endotracheal tube) and a self-inflating bag or an anaesthetic circuit containing a bag which is inflated by the flow of fresh gas from an anaesthetic machine, gas cylinder, or piped supply. In all these examples expiration is passive.

For more prolonged artificial ventilation it is usual to use a specially designed machine or ventilator to perform the task. The ventilators used in operating theatres when patients are anaesthetized and paralysed are relatively simple devices. Generally they consist of bellows which fill with fresh gas and which are then mechanically emptied (by means of a weight, piston, or compressed gas) via a circuit or tubes attached to an endotracheal tube into the patient's lungs. Adjustments can be made to the volume of fresh gas given with each breath and to the length of inspiration and expiration. Expiration is usually passive back to the atmosphere.

On the intensive-care unit, where patients are not usually paralysed, the ventilators are more complex. They have electronic controls which allow the user to programme a variety of pressure waveforms for inspiration and expiration. There are also programmes that allow the patient to breathe between ventilated breaths or to trigger ventilated breaths, or inhibit ventilation when the patient is breathing.

Indications for artificial ventilation are when the patient is unable to breathe adequately on his own. This may be due to injury or disease of the central nervous, cardiovascular, or respiratory systems or drug overdose. Artificial ventilation is performed to allow time for healing and recovery. Sometimes the patient is able to breathe but it is considered advisable to control ventilation – e.g. in severe head injury. Some operations require the patient to be paralysed for better or safer surgical access and this may require ventilation. With lung operations or very unwell patients ventilation is also indicated.

Artificial ventilation usually bypasses the physiological mechanisms for humidification of inspired air, so care must be taken to humidify inspired gases. It is important to monitor the efficacy of ventilation – e.g. by using blood gas measurement, pulse oximetry, and tidal carbon dioxide, and airways pressures.

Artificial ventilation is not without its hazards. The use of *positive pressure* raises the mean intrathoracic pressure. This can decrease venous return to the heart and cause a fall in cardiac output (q.v.) and blood pressure. Positive-pressure ventilation may also cause pneumothorax (q.v.), but this is rare. While patients are ventilated, they are unable to breath and so accidental disconnection from the ventilator may cause hypoxia and death.

NEGATIVE-PRESSURE VENTILATION is seldom used nowadays. The chest or whole body, apart from the head, is placed inside an airtight box. A vacuum lowers the pressure within the box causing the chest to expand. Air is drawn into the lungs through the mouth and nose. At the end of inspiration the vacuum is stopped, the pressure in the box returns to atmospheric, and the patient exhales passively. This is the principle of the 'iron lung' which saved many lives during the polio epidemics of the 1950s. These machines are cumbersome and make access to the patient difficult. In addition, complex manipulation of ventilation is impossible.

Jet ventilation is a relatively modern form of ventilation which utilizes very small tidal volumes (see LUNGS) from a high-pressure source at high frequencies (20–100/min). First developed by physiologists to produce low stable intrathoracic pressures whilst studying carotid-body reflexes (q.v.), it is sometimes now used in intensive therapy units for patients who do not achieve adequate gas exchanges with conventional ventilation. Its advantages are lower intrathoracic pressures (and therefore less risk of pneumothorax and impaired venous return) and better gas mixing within the lungs.

ARYTENOID is the name applied to two cartilages in the larynx.

ASBESTOSIS is a form of pneumoconiosis (q.v.), in which widespread fine scarring occurs in the lungs, leading to severe breathing disability. The main hazard, however, is the risk of cancer (mesothelioma) of the lung or pleura, or sometimes of the ovary. It is caused by the inhalation of mainly blue or brown asbestos dust, either during mining or quarrying, or in one of the many industries in which it is used: e.g. as an insulating material, in the making of paper, cardboard and brake linings. A person suffering from asbestosis is entitled to compensation as the disease is legally prescribed. About 900 people a year claim compensation, and 400 of these are for mesothelioma.

ASCARIASIS is the disease produced by infestation with the roundworm, *Ascaris lumbricoides*, also known as the maw-worm. Superficially it resembles a large earthworm. The male measures about 17 cm (7 inches) and the female 23 cm (9 inches) in length. It is a dirt disease, most prevalent where sanitation and cleanliness are lacking, particularly in the tropics and subtropics. Consumption of food contaminated by the ova (eggs), especially salad vegetables, is the commonest cause of infection. In children, infection is commonly acquired by crawling or playing on contaminated earth, and then sucking their fingers. After a complicated life-cycle in the body the adult worms end up in the intestines, whence they may be passed in the stools. A light infection may cause no symptoms. A heavy infection may lead to colic, or even obstruction of the gut. Occasionally a worm may wander into the stomach and be vomited up.

Treatment consists of the administration of levamisole, a piperazine derivative, pyrantel embonate, or mebendazole.

ASCITES is an accumulation of fluid in the abdomen. The causes include heart failure, cancer, cirrhosis of the liver and infections.

ASCORBIC ACID (VITAMIN) is a substance present in various natural sources such as fruits and vegetables, or synthetically prepared. (See VITAMIN.)

ASEPSIS is a term, used in distinction from 'antisepsis', to mean that principle in surgery by which, instead of strong germicides like corrosive sublimate or carbolic acid being applied to wounds, all the dressings, swabs, and instruments used are sterilized by steaming, boiling, or dry heat. Thin, sterilized, india-rubber gloves are worn by surgeons and prevent risk of infection from the hands. Aseptic surgery has the advantage that the germ-destroying activity of the tissues and their healing power after wounds are not lessened by antiseptics which decrease the vitality of the tissues. Healing is therefore surer and more rapid after an aseptic operation. (See also ANTISEPTICS.)

ASH stands for ACTION ON SMOKING AND HEALTH. It is a charity founded by the Royal College of Physicians in 1971 and supported by the DOH. Its aim is to alert and inform the public to the dangers of smoking and to try to prevent the disability and death which it causes. It gathers a wide range of information about smoking and disseminates it to the public to increase knowledge about the dangers of smoking and how to give up the habit. It commissions surveys on public attitudes to smoking and brings together working groups on such subjects as giving up smoking and how to prevent children from starting to smoke. It is largely due to the efforts of ASH that the majority of adults in the United Kingdom (more than six out of ten) are now non-smokers. ASH works on their behalf by pressing proprietors of public space to provide more smoke-free areas and advising them how to create and operate them. Hundreds of smokers who would like to give up smoking contact ASH for information every month. ASH has a small headquarters staff in London with other national and regional branches in Scotland, Wales, and Northern Ireland. More branches are opening every year. Further information can be obtained from ASH, 109 Gloucester Place, London W1H 3PH (071-935 3519, fax: 071-935 3463).

ASPARAGINASE is an enzyme that breaks down the amino-acid, asparagine. This is of no significance to most cells in the body as they can make asparagine from simpler constituents. Certain tumours, however, are unable to do this and therefore, if they cannot receive ready-made supplies of the amino-acid, they die. It is on this basis that asparaginase is proving of promise in the treatment of tumours which, by the administration of asparaginase, are deprived of an essential metabolite – and perish.

ASPARTANE is an artificial sweetener 200 times as sweet as sugar but without the bitter after-taste of saccharine.

ASPERGILLOSIS is a disease caused by invasion of the lung by the fungus, *Aspergillus fumigatus*. The infection is acquired by inhalation of air-borne spores of the fungus which settle and grow in damaged parts of the lung such as healed tuberculous cavities, abscesses, or the dilated bronchi of bronchiectasis (q.v.).

ASPERGILLUS is the name applied to a group of fungi including the common moulds. Several of these are capable of infecting the lungs and producing a disease resembling pulmonary tuberculosis.

ASPHYXIA means literally absence of pulse, but is the name given to the whole series of symptoms which follow stoppage of breathing and of the heart's action. Drowning is one cause but obstruction *of the air passages* may occur as the result of a foreign body or in some diseases, such as croup, diphtheria, swelling of the throat due to wounds or inflammation, asthma (to a partial extent), tumours in the chest (causing slow asphyxia), and the external conditions of suffocation and strangling. Placing the head in a plastic bag results in asphyxia and poisonous gases also cause asphyxia, for example, carbon monoxide gas, which may be given off by a stove or charcoal brazier in a badly ventilated room can kill people during sleep. (See CARBON MONOXIDE.) Several gases, such as sulphurous acid (from burning sulphur), ammonia, and chlorine (from bleaching-powder), cause involuntary closure of the entrance to the larynx, and thus prevent breathing. Other gases, such as nitrous oxide (or laughing-gas), chloroform, and ether, in poisonous quantity, stop the breathing by paralysing the respiration centre in the brain.

Symptoms: In most cases death from asphyxia is due to insufficiency of oxygen supplied to the blood. The first signs are rapid pulse and gasping for breath. Next comes a rise in the blood pressure, causing throbbing in the head, with lividity or blueness of the skin, due to failure of aeration of the blood, followed by still greater struggles for breath and by general convulsions. The heart becomes over-distended and gradually weaker, a paralytic stage sets in, and all struggling and breathing slowly cease.

When asphyxia is due to charcoal fumes, coal-gas, and other narcotic influences, there is no convulsive stage, and death ensues gently and may occur in the course of sleep.

Treatment: So long as the heart continues to beat, recovery may be looked for under prompt treatment. The one essential of treatment is to get the impure blood aerated by artificial respiration. Besides this, the feeble circulation can be helped by various methods. (See APPENDIX: BASIC FIRST AID, choking, cardiac/respiratory arrest.)

ASPIRATION means the withdrawal of fluid or gases from the natural cavities of the body or from cavities produced by disease. It may be performed either for curative purposes, or, very often, a small amount is drawn off for diagnosis of the nature or origin of the fluid.

Pleurisy with effusion is a condition requiring aspiration, and a litre or more of fluid may be drawn off by an aspirator or a large syringe and needle. *Chronic abscesses* and *tuberculous joints* may call for its use, the operation being done with a small syringe and hollow needle. *Pericarditis with effusion* is another condition in which aspiration is sometimes performed. The spinal canal is aspirated by the operation of lumbar puncture. (See LUMBAR PUNCTURE.) In children the ventricles of the brain are sometimes similarly relieved from excess of fluid by piercing the fontanelle (soft spot) on the infant's head. (See HYDROCEPHALUS.)

ASPIRIN, or ACETYLSALICYLIC ACID, is a white crystalline powder which is used like sodium salicylate as a remedy for reducing inflammation and fever. It has some action in relieving pain and producing sleep and is therefore often used for headache and slighter degrees of insomnia. Daily doses are now used in the prevention of coronary thrombosis. The dose is 300 mg to 1 g. Aspirin should be used with caution in children. (See ANALGESICS.)

ASPIRIN POISONING may not be common in relation to the vast amounts that are consumed every year, but nevertheless it is a worrying problem.

In ordinary doses it may induce bleeding from the stomach. This is usually quite mild, but it can be severe. In small doses it can produce a severe allergic reaction in individuals who are sensitive to it. This takes the form of asthma and angioneurotic oedema.

When an overdose is taken, there is marked over-breathing, sweating and vomiting. Later the individual becomes restless and irritable, and there may be convulsions before consciousness is finally lost.

Treatment: The stomach should be washed out, preferably with an alkaline solution, and a litre of 5-per-cent sodium bicarbonate should be left in the stomach. If there has been much loss of fluid by sweating and vomiting, fluids may need to be given intravenously. In severe cases oxygen may need to be administered.

ASSISTED CONCEPTION: There are two types of assisted conception: in vitro fertilization (IVF) and gamete intrafallopian transfer (GIFT).

IN VITRO FERTILIZATION: In this technique the female partner receives drugs to enhance ovulation. Just before ovulation several ripe eggs are collected under ultrasound guidance or through a laparoscope. The eggs are incubated with the prepared sperm. About 40 hours later, once the eggs have been fertilized, up to three embryos are transferred into the mother's uterus via the cervix. Pregnancy should then proceed normally. About one in five IFV pregnancies results in the birth of a child. The success rate falls rapidly if the female partner is aged 40 and over.

Indications: In women with severely damaged fallopian tubes IVF offers the only chance of pregnancy. The method is also used in couples with unexplained infertility, male-factor infertility where the sperm count is only slightly abnormal, and in women who have suffered an early or surgical menopause. In these cases donor eggs are used.

Almost one quarter of pregnancies are multiple. Twin or triplet pregnancies are associated with many more problems such as premature labour. As the likelihood of multiple pregnancy increases with the number of eggs replaced into the uterus, recent legislation in the United Kingdom has recommended that no more than three eggs are transferred in each IVF cycle.

It is also important to monitor the preovulation phase in the woman by ultrasound scan so that not too many eggs develop, as this may lead to hyperstimulation of the ovaries which can cause the development of ovarian cysts.

GAMETE INTRAFALLOPIAN TRANSFER: This method of fertilization may be used provided at least one fallopian tube is healthy and patent. As with IVF, ovulation is usually stimulated in the female partner. The woman then undergoes a laparoscopy just before ovulation during which the ripe eggs are picked up from the ovaries and injected into the fallopian tube together with prepared sperm from the husband. Fertilization then takes place as it does in natural conception.

GIFT is indicated in couples with unexplained infertility, minor male- or cervical-factor infertility. Associated problems are similar to IVF and are mainly related to an increased rate of multiple pregnancies.

The success rate for GIFT is about 17 per cent.

ASTEREOGNOSIS means the loss of the capacity to recognize the nature of an object by feeling it, and indicates a lesion (e.g. tumour) of the brain.

ASTHENIA means want of strength.

ASTHENOPIA means a sense of weakness in the eyes, coming on when they are used. As a rule it is due to long-sightedness, slight inflammation, or weakness of the muscles that move the eyes. (See VISION.)

ASTHMA is a disorder of breathing characterized by narrowing of airways within the lung. The main symptom is breathlessness. A major feature of asthma is the variability in the degree of airway narrowing. This reversibility of the obstruction may occur spontaneously or as a result of treatment.

Cause: Recent research has emphasized the importance of inflammation in the wall of the airways in asthma. This produces swelling in the airway wall which narrows the lumen and there is also contraction of the smooth muscle in the wall of the airway. The narrowing of the airways in the lung is responsible for the great difficulty in breathing which is the characteristic feature of asthma. The inflamed airway is irritable and further narrowing occurs in response to non-specific irritants and specific triggers. There is a large number of substances to which the asthmatic subject may be hypersensitive and contact with these may be responsible for an attack. These include pollens, skin scales of certain animals such as cats, dogs and horses, the house dust mite (*Dermatophagoides* species), certain industrial agents such as platinum salts (see OCCUPATIONAL DISEASES). In some asthmatic patients substances in the diet may be important, either colourings and additives or specific foodstuffs.

Asthmatic subjects have a genetic predisposition to form antibodies of the IgE class against allergens which they meet, particularly if these are inhaled. Skin tests may demonstrate this production of antibodies but there are often positive responses to many allergens and further investigation is usually necessary to accept that the particular allergen is important in the patient's asthma.

Asthma is often at its worst in the early hours of the morning causing disturbance of sleep. In some cases this may be related to specific allergens such as feathers in pillows, but usually it is just part of the pattern of daily variation in asthma. Non-specific factors such as dust, cold air, emotional disturbance and stress may exacerbate asthma and increase the sensitivity to other precipitants of asthma.

Asthma often runs in families and the genetic basis is under investigation. Asthmatic subjects often suffer from other allergic conditions such as hay fever and eczema as do other members of their family. Asthma most often begins in early childhood, by the age of 7. Asthma affects around 10 per cent of children, usually in a mild form. In this age group boys are affected twice as often as girls. Mildly affected children may grow out of their asthma and in adults the prevalence is nearer 5 per cent and males and females are equally affected. Asthma may come on at any age and, when it develops for the first time in adults, it is often more persistent with fewer identifiable precipitating factors. The death rate for asthma in the United Kingdom is around 2,000 per year and is steady or increasing slightly.

The prevalence of asthma varies around the world. In most developed countries rates are similar to the UK, although it is commoner in Australia and New Zealand. In less developed countries rates are lower but rise with increasing urbanization.

The term asthma is sometimes used in cardiac asthma. This describes the breathlessness associated with pulmonary oedema (q.v.) and left-sided heart failure. The term is used less than it was and should be abandoned.

Symptoms: The major symptoms of asthma are breathlessness and cough. Occasionally coughing may be the only symptom of asthma and this is more common in children when nighttime coughing attacks may be mistaken for bronchitis and treated inappropriately with antibiotics.

The amount of airway narrowing can be measured as the peak expiratory-flow rate by a simple meter. The hallmark of asthma is variability of airway narrowing; this may be intermittent mild breathlessness often precipitated by an obvious cause such as exercise or severe life-threatening attacks. Some asthma attacks have a sudden onset but routine recordings of peak expiratory-flow rate show that there is often a period of gradual decline for some days before the acute attack. A change in treatment during this decline will often prevent the severe attack and hospital admission.

The breathlessness of an acute attack of asthma produces distress in breathing out through the narrowed airways but the associated overinflation of the lungs results in difficulties in inspiration. The noise of turbulent air in narrowed airways produces wheezing noises, particularly on expiration. In a severe attack the breathing rate and the pulse rate increase and the patient may find it easier to breathe sitting up with the shoulders raised. In very severe attacks the patient may be too breathless to speak and reduced oxygen in the blood may result in the blueish colour of cyanosis. These features, together with lack of response to the usual inhaled treatment, indicate that the attack is very severe and urgent hospital treatment is necessary.

When asthma is poorly controlled for a long time in childhood, the chest may be left overexpanded. Chronic severe asthma may eventually result in airway narrowing which is no longer reversible in response to treatment but has become fixed.

Treatment: The first important consideration in the management of asthma is avoidance of precipitating factors. Sometimes this is possible where a specific animal, occupational exposure or foodstuff is involved. More often the problem is a widespread allergen such as pollen or house dust mite which is difficult or impossible to avoid. Exposure to specific allergens may produce prolonged reaction in the airways which remain more susceptible to other precipitants for days afterwards. Exercise should be considered differently. Although it may provoke asthma, it does not increase problems encountered with other substances and it is beneficial for asthmatics to stay fit. Exercise should continue with appropriate medication such as beta-agonist beforehand.

In some countries desensitization is commonly practised. This is done by taking an allergen to which the patient is sensitive and trying to produce tolerance by giving small injections of the substance and gradually increasing the dose. Antibodies which block the asthmatic response may develop. Severe reactions occur occasionally. There is a dispute about the effectiveness and desensitization is rarely used in the UK now.

There are two main forms of drug treatment. Bronchodilator drugs are used to dilate the airways and relieve breathlessness. They may also prevent problems when taken before exposure. The most useful group of bronchodilators are the beta adrenergic agonists. There are a range of these and the commonest-used drugs are salbutamol and terbutaline. These drugs should be used usually to control symptoms and not as regular therapy on their own. Other bronchodilators are anticholinergics such as ipratropium bromide and the theophylline group.

The second group of drugs are the suppressors or anti-inflammatory drugs. These are inhaled corticosteroids, sodium cromoglycate and nedocromil. When bronchodilators are used more than once a day regularly, then an anti-inflammatory agent should be considered. Sodium cromoglycate is often useful in children, inhaled corticosteroids are usually needed in adults. These prophylactic drugs must be taken regularly to be effective. This requires careful patient preparation and explanation.

All the drugs mentioned, apart from theophyllines, are best taken by inhalation into the respiratory tract. This means that only a small dose is necessary, little of the drug gets in to the rest of the body and few side-effects occur. Careful instruction is necessary to make sure the patient can use the inhalation device effectively. There are enough types of inhaler device currently available to suit almost anybody. Large doses of corticosteroids by inhalation can produce some systemic effects but are much less of a problem than steroid tablets. They can also produce local effects in the mouth such as candidiasis (thrush).

Newer drugs are being developed to deal with various aspects of the inflammatory process in asthma. At present inhaled corticosteroids are the most effective and are relatively free of adverse effects. They should be considered when a drug such as salbutamol (Ventolin) is being used more than once every day.

Asthmatic patients should stay fit using a warm-up period and a drug such as salbutamol or terbutaline prior to exercise.

Specific breathing exercises are of little use.

Every asthmatic should have a treatment plan to deal with exacerbations and a peak-flow meter available to measure the severity of the problem. Alternative therapies such as hypnosis have been used with some effect in selected patients.

Advice and support for research into asthma is provided by the National Asthma Campaign, Providence House, Providence Place, London N1 0NT (071-226 2260, fax: 071-704 0740).

ASTIGMATISM is an error of refraction in the eye due to the cornea (the clear membrane in front of the eye) being unequally curved in different directions, so that rays of light in different meridians cannot be brought to a focus together on the retina. The curvature, instead of being globular, is egg-shaped, longer in one axis than the other. The condition causes objects to seem distorted and out of place, a ball for instance looking like an egg, a circle like an ellipse. The condition is remedied by suitable spectacles of which one surface forms part of a cylinder. (See SPECTACLES.)

ASTROVIRUSES are small round viruses with no distinctive features, which have been isolated from the stools of infants with gastroenteritis (see DIARRHOEA).

ASYMPTOMATIC: The lack of any symptoms of disease whether or not a disease is present.

ASYNERGIA means the absence of harmonious and co-ordinated movements between muscles having opposite actions – e.g. the flexors and extensors of a joint – and is a sign of disease of the nervous system.

ASYSTOLE means arrest of the action of the heart.

ATARACTIC is the term used to describe drugs which induce peace of mind. For all practical purposes it is synonymous with tranquillizer (q.v.). It has never been widely adopted in Britain.

ATAVISM means the principle of inheritance of disease or bodily characters from grandparents or remoter ancestors, the parents not having been affected by these.

ATAXIA means loss of co-ordination, though the power necessary to make the movements is still present. Thus an ataxic person may have a good grip in each hand but be unable to do any fine movements with the fingers, or, if the ataxia be in the legs, he throws these about a great deal in walking, though he can lift the legs and take steps quite well. This is due to a sensory defect or to disease of the cerebellum. (See FRIEDREICH'S ATAXIA; LOCOMOTOR ATAXIA.)

ATELECTASIS means collapse of a part of the lung, or failure of the lung to expand at birth.

ATENOLOL is a drug that antagonizes beta adrenergic receptors (q.v.) and is of value in the treatment of high blood-pressure. One of its practical advantages is that only one dose a day need be taken. (See ADRENERGIC RECEPTORS.)

ATHEROMA is a degenerative change in the inner and middle coats of arteries. (See ARTERIES, DISEASES OF.)

ATHEROSCLEROSIS is a form of arteriosclerosis (q.v.), in which there is fatty degeneration of the middle coat of the arterial wall.

ATHETOID SPASMS are slow writhing movements affecting the distal parts of the limbs. They are due to disease of the extra-pyramidal system.

ATHETOSIS is the name for slow, involuntary, writhing, and repeated movements of the hands and feet, caused by disease of the brain.

ATHLETE'S FOOT is a somewhat loose term applied to a skin eruption on the foot, usually between the toes. It is commonly due to ringworm (q.v.), but may be due to other infections, or merely excessive sweating of the feet.

ATLAS is the name applied to the first cervical vertebra. (See SPINAL COLUMN.)

ATONY means want of tone or vigour in muscles and other organs.

ATOPY, meaning out of place, is a form of hypersensitivity characterized, amongst other features, by a familial tendency. It is due to the propensity of the affected individual to produce large amounts of reagin antibodies which stick to mast cells in the mucosa so that when the antigen is inhaled histamine is released from the mast cell. It is the condition responsible for asthma and hay fever. (See also ALLERGY.) It is estimated that 10 per cent of the human race are subject to atopy. (See also ECZEMA.)

ATRESIA means the absence of a natural opening, or closure of it by a membrane. Thus atresia may be found in new-born infants preventing the bowels from moving, and, in young girls after puberty, absence of the menstrual flow may be due to such a malformation.

ATRIAL NATRIURETIC PEPTIDE: The atria of the heart contain peptides with potent diuretic and vaso-dilating properties. It has been known since 1980 that extracts of human atria have potent diurectic and natriuretic effects in animals (see DIURETICS). In 1984 three polypeptide species were isolated from human atria and were called alpha, beta and gamma human atrial natriuretic peptides. Plasma concentration of immuno-reactive atrial natriuretic peptide can now be measured. The levels are low in healthy subjects and are increased in patients with congestive heart failure. Infusion of the peptides into human volunteers causes a natriuresis and diuresis. Atrial natriuretic peptide is thus the most recently isolated hormone.

ATRIAL SEPTAL DEFECT (see HEART DISEASES, Congenital heart disease).

ATRIUM is the name now given to the two upper cavities of the heart. These used to be known as the auricles of the heart. The term is also applied to the part of the ear immediately internal to the drum of the ear. (Plural: ATRIA.)

ATROPHY is a term used to describe a state of wasting due to some interference with the function of healthy nutrition. It is essential for the maintenance of health that a balance is maintained between the processes of waste and repair. When the appropriation of nutriment exceeds the waste, hypertrophy or increase in bulk of the tissues takes place. (See HYPERTROPHY.) When, on the other hand, the supply of nutritive matter is suspended or diminished, or when the power of assimilation is impaired, atrophy or wasting is the result. Thus the whole body becomes atrophied in many diseases; and in old age every part of the frame, with the exception of the heart, undergoes atrophic change. Atrophy may, however, affect single organs or parts of the body, irrespective of the general state of nutrition, and this may be brought about in a variety of ways. One of the most frequently observed of such instances is atrophy from disuse, or cessation of function.

Thus, when a limb is deprived of the natural power of motion, either by paralysis or by painful joint disease, atrophy of all its tissues sooner or later takes place. This form of atrophy is likewise well exemplified in the case of those organs and structures of the body which subserve important ends during fetal life, but which, ceasing to be necessary after birth, undergo a sort of natural atrophy, such as the thymus gland, and certain vessels specially concerned in the fetal circulation. The ovaries, after the child-bearing period, become shrunken.

Atrophy of a part may also be caused by interruption to its normal blood supply, as in the case of the ligature or obstruction of an artery. Again, long-standing disease, by affecting the nutrition of an organ and by inducing the deposit of morbid products, may result in atrophy, as frequently happens in affections of the liver and kidneys. Parts that are subjected to continuous pressure are liable to become atrophied, as is sometimes seen in internal organs which have been compressed by tumours or other morbid growths.

Atrophy may manifest itself simply by loss of substance; on the other hand, it is often found to co-exist with degenerative changes and the formation of fibrous or fatty growth, so that the part may not be reduced in bulk, although atrophied as regards its proper structure. Thus, in the case of the heart, when affected with fatty degeneration, there is atrophy of the proper muscular texture, but this, being largely replaced by fatty material, the organ may undergo no diminution in volume, but may, on the contrary, be increased in size. Atrophy is usually a gradual and slow process, but sometimes it proceeds rapidly. In the disease known by the name of *acute yellow atrophy of the liver*, that organ undergoes such rapidly destructive change as may result in its shrinking to half, or one-third, of its normal size in the course of a few days.

The term *progressive muscular atrophy* (*wasting* or *creeping palsy*) is applied to an affection of the muscular system, which is characterized by the atrophy and subsequent paralysis of certain muscles, or groups of muscles, and is associated with morbid changes in the anterior part of the grey matter in the spinal cord. This disease begins insidiously, and is often first observed to affect the muscles of one hand, generally the right. Gradually other muscles in the arms and legs become affected in a similar manner, their atrophy being attended with a corresponding diminution in power.

The term *idiopathic muscular atrophy* (also known as *muscular dystrophy*) is applied to a somewhat similar condition affecting young people in whom a progressive degeneration of the muscles occurs. In this condition no change is found in the nervous system after death, the cause apparently acting directly upon the muscles. (See MUSCLES, DISEASES OF.)

ATROPINE is the active principle of belladonna, the juice of the deadly nightshade. Because of its action in dilating the pupils it was at one time used as a cosmetic to give the eyes a full, lustrous appearance. It acts by antagonizing the action of the parasympathetic nervous system (q.v.). It temporarily impairs vision by paralysing accommodative power. (See ACCOMMODATION.) It has the effect of checking the activity of almost all the glands of the body, including the sweat glands of the skin and the salivary glands in the mouth. It relieves spasm by paralysing nerves in the muscle of the intestine, bile-ducts, bladder, stomach, etc. It has the power, in moderate doses, of markedly increasing the rate of the heart-beats, though by very large doses the heart, along with all other muscles, is paralysed and stopped.
Uses: Externally, liniment of belladonna is used in neuralgia, and other painful conditions. In eye troubles, atropine drops are used to dilate the pupil for more thorough examination of the interior of the eye, or to draw the iris away from wounds and ulcers on the centre of the eye; they also soothe the pain due to light falling on an inflamed eye, and are further used to paralyse the ciliary muscle and so prevent accommodative changes in the eye while the eye is being examined with the ophthalmoscope (q.v.). Belladonna is employed in cough-mixtures for bronchitis and whooping-cough to dry up the mucus and check spasmodic coughing. In renal colic, gall-stone colic, and other agonizing spasmodic conditions, atropine is given along with morphine by hypodermic injection. It is also used to decrease the amount of gastric secretion in peptic ulcer. It has been used as an antidote in opium poisoning and to muscarine, the poisonous principle of some toadstools.

ATROPINE or BELLADONNA POISONING: This may occur from children's eating the berries or leaves of the deadly nightshade. The appearance of a patient with atropine poisoning has been described as: 'hot as a hare, red as a beet, blind as a bat, dry as a bone, and mad as a wet hen'. The warning symptoms are: (1) great dryness of the mouth and throat, (2) wide dilatation of the pupils, (3) increased rate of the heart's action. There is sickness later, and the poisoned person has an excited delirium with, at the same time, bodily languor and weakness. If the dose has been very large, paralysis, unconsciousness, and gradual stoppage of heart and breathing ensue.
Treatment: The swallowed material should be got rid of by washing out the stomach followed by a saline purgative such as sodium sulphate, 30 grams in 250 millilitres of water. If breathing becomes feeble, artificial respiration must be performed. The patient should be given plenty to drink and be made to pass water frequently, as the poison is excreted by the kidneys, and may otherwise be reabsorbed. A sedative, such as diazepam or phenobarbitone, is given to control the excitement, as well as neostigmine which is a specific antidote.

AUDIOANALGESIA is a method of relieving the pains of childbirth. It is produced by the patient listening through headphones to a combination of white sound and music. The intensity of the sound is controlled by the woman herself according to the intensity of her pain. Experience suggests that the method is successful in women who are well adapted, like music and have some understanding of labour and delivery.

AUDIOMETRY is the testing of hearing.

AUDITORY NERVE (see VESTIBULOCOCHLEAR NERVE).

AURA is a peculiar feeling which persons, subject to epileptic seizures, have just before the onset of an attack. It may be a sensation of a cold breeze, a peculiar smell, a vision of some animal or person, an undefinable sense of disgust, or the like, but it is very important for persons who experience it, because it gives warning that a fit is coming and may enable a place of safety or seclusion to be reached.

AURAL: Relating to the ear.

AURICLE is a term applied both to the pinna or flap of the ear and also to the ear-shaped tip of the atrium of the heart.

AURISCOPE is an instrument for examining the ear. The source of illumination may be incorporated in the instrument, as in the electric auriscope, or it may be an independent light which is reflected into the ear by means of a forehead mirror.

AUSCULTATION is a term in medicine applied to the method employed by physicians for determining, by listening, the condition of certain internal organs. The ancient physicians appear to have practised a kind of auscultation, by which they were able to detect the presence of air or fluids in the cavities of the chest and abdomen.

In 1819, the French physician, Laennec, introduced the method of auscultation by means of the stethoscope. Initially a wooden cylinder, the stethoscope has evolved into a binaural instrument consisting of a small expanded chest-piece and two flexible tubes, the ends of which fit into the ears of the observer. Various modifications of the binaural stethoscope have been introduced.

The numerous conditions affecting the lungs can be recognized by means of auscultation and the stethoscope. The same is true for the heart, whose varied and often complex forms of disease can, by auscultation, be identified with striking accuracy. But auscultation is also helpful in the investigation of aneurysms and certain diseases of the oesophagus and stomach. The stethoscope is also a valuable aid in the detection of some forms of uterine tumours, especially in the diagnosis of pregnancy.

AUSTRALIAN ANTIGEN: An antigen associated with the hepatitis B virus (see HEPATITIS). The infection occurs in around 0·1 per cent of the population in Britain and the blood of people with it must not be used for transfusion. The name originated because the antigen was first discovered in an Australian aborigine.

AUTISM: The term autism was introduced by Kanner in 1943 to describe a disharmony of development in which children are unable to mature socially despite excellent motor skill. Thus, despite their manual dexterity they are unable to form emotional bonds, even with their parents. Because of their disregard of other people they are refractory to discipline. Although they may acquire some language, they communicate little.

Advice and information on autism may be obtained from The National Autistic Society,

276 Willesden Lane, London NW2 5RB (tel: 081-451 1114, fax: 081-451 5865).

AUTO- is a prefix meaning self.

AUTOANTIBODY: An antibody produced by a person's immune system that acts against the body's own tissues resulting in auto-immunity (q.v.).

AUTOCLAVE: This is one of the most effective ways of ensuring that material, e.g. surgical dressings, is completely sterilized and that even the most resistant bacteria with which it may be contaminated, are destroyed. Its use is based upon the fact that water boils when its vapour pressure is equal to the pressure of the surrounding atmosphere. This means that if the pressure inside a closed vessel be increased, the temperature at which water inside the vessel boils, will rise above 100 °C. By adjusting the pressure, almost any temperature for the boiling of the water will be obtained. This is now one of the most widely used methods of sterilization in hospitals and laboratories.

AUTOGENOUS means self-generated and is the term applied to products which arise within the body. It is applied to bacterial vaccines manufactured from the organisms found in discharges from the body and used for the treatment of the person from whom the bacteria were derived.

AUTO-IMMUNITY is the process whereby an individual develops antibodies which attack his own tissues. Normally an individual does not develop antibodies which attach his own tissues, but only to invaders of the body such as micro-organisms. The precise reason why some individuals develop this condition is still obscure but it is proving a fruitful line of investigation into the cause of some diseases. These include diabetes mellitus (q.v.), rheumatoid arthritis (q.v.) and systemic lupus erythematosus (see LUPUS).

AUTO-INTOXICATION means literally self-poisoning, and is any condition of poisoning brought about by substances formed in or by the body.

AUTOLYSIS means the disintegration and softening of dead cells brought about by enzymes in the cells themselves.

AUTOMATISM means the performance of acts without conscious will, as, for example, after an attack of epilepsy or concussion of the brain. In such conditions the person may perform acts of which he is neither conscious at the time nor has any memory afterwards. It is especially liable to occur when persons suffering from epilepsy, mental subnormality, or concussion consume alcoholic liquors. It may also occur following the taking of barbiturates or psychedelic drugs (q.v.). There are, however, other cases in which there are no such precipitatory factors. Thus it may occur following hypnosis, mental stress or strain, or conditions such as fugues (q.v.) or somnambulism (see SLEEP). The condition is of considerable importance from a legal point of view, because acts done in this state, and for which the person committing them is not responsible, may be of a criminal nature. According to English law, however, it entails complete loss of consciousness, and only then is it a defence to an action for negligence. A lesser impairment of consciousness is no defence.

AUTONOMIC NERVOUS SYSTEM is part of the nervous system which regulates the functions of some of the internal organs independently of the will power. It consists of two main divisions – the SYMPATHETIC and the PARASYMPATHETIC SYSTEMS (qq.v.).

AUTOPSY means a post-mortem examination, or the examination of the internal organs of a dead body. (See NECROPSY.)

AUTO-SUGGESTION is a peculiar mental state, which sometimes occurs after accidents, in which the will and judgement are partially perverted, so that slight or temporary injuries are greatly exaggerated in the imagination, and the person believes himself to be affected by some serious disability. Examples of this are found in paralysed and insensitive limbs following some minor bruise, for example in a railway accident, and the blindness, deafness, or inability to speak, which sometimes followed concussion in soldiers, especially when the injury was received in the dark. This state is also called 'traumatic suggestion'. The condition often approaches very near to, or is mingled with, the condition of malingering, in which the person consciously suggests to himself or produces some disability from an ulterior motive, as, for example, in some of the prolonged cases of disability following a trifling injury for which a person is in receipt of compensation. The term is also applied to the reverse process, by which, either as a result of suggestion by another person, or suggestion applied by the will-power of the person affected, a cure of such a condition is accomplished.

AVASCULAR: Without a blood supply. Avascular necrosis is the death of a tissue because the blood supply has been cut off.

AVERSION THERAPY is a form of psychological treatment in which such an unpleasant response is induced to his psychological aberration that the patient decides to give it up. Thus the victim of alcoholism is given a drug that makes the subsequent drinking of alcoholic liquors so unpleasant by inducing nausea and vomiting that he decides to give up drinking. (See ALCOHOL; and DISULFIRAM.) Another commonly used method of inducing aversion is an electric shock. Aversion therapy may help in the treatment of alcoholism, drug addiction, sexual deviations, such as transvestism, and compulsive gambling.

AVITAMINOSIS is the condition of a human being or an animal deprived of one or more vitamins.

AVOMINE is the trade name for promethazine theoclate, which is widely, and successfully, used as a remedy for travel sickness.

AVULSION: Forcible tearing away of one tissue from another. For example, a tendon may be avulsed from the bone to which it is attached or a nerve may be injured and torn away from the tissue in which it runs.

AXILLA is the anatomical name for the armpit. (See ARMPIT.)

AXIS is the name applied to the second cervical vertebra. (See SPINAL COLUMN.)

AXON: Nerve fibre: an elongated projection of a nerve cell or neurone that carries an electrical impulse to the tissue at the end of the axon. Large axons are covered by a sheath of insulating myelin which is interrupted at intervals by nodes of Lanvier, where other axons branch out.

AZATHIOPRINE is a cytotoxic and an immunosuppressive drug. In the first of these capacities it is proving of value in the treatment of acute leukaemia. As an immunosuppressive agent, by reducing the antibody response of the body it is proving of value in facilitating the success of transplant operations by reducing the chances of the transplanted organ, e.g. the kidney, being rejected by the body. It is also proving of value in the treatment of autoimmune diseases. (See CYTOTOXIC.)

AZOOSPERMIA is the condition characterized by lack of spermatozoa in the semen.

AZOTAEMIA means the presence of urea and other nitrogenous bodies in greater concentration than normal in the blood. The condition is generally associated with advanced types of kidney disease.

B

BABINSKI REFLEX is an abnormal response of the plantar reflex. When a sharp body is drawn along the sole of the foot, instead of the toes bending down towards the sole as usual, the great toe is turned upwards and the other toes tend to spread apart. This response may be obtained in normal infants, but after the age of about two years its presence indicates some severe disturbance in the upper part of the central nervous system.

BACAMPICILLIN (see ANTIBIOTIC).

BACILLI (See under MICROBIOLOGY.)

BACITRACIN is a polypeptide antibiotic derived from *Bacillus licheniformis*. It is active against the same range of bacteria as penicillin.

BACK: The back consists mainly of the spinal column and hinder parts of the ribs, and the wide-spreading iliac or haunch bones with the sacrum below. The bones are covered by thick and powerful muscles, which above support and move the head and which below pass round the flanks and downwards into the lower limbs. The skin covering the back is not very sensitive and is not greatly subject to painful conditions. The powerful muscles, of which the chief is the erector spinae, are much subject to minor injuries, the result of twists and strains, and also to rheumatic affections (see LUMBAGO). Diseases and injuries of the spinal column and spinal cord are of a very serious nature (see SPINAL COLUMN; SPINAL CORD).

BACKACHE is a symptom of many diseases. In addition to being the result of local causes, pain may be referred to the back from diseases in deep-seated organs. Medical causes which include inflammatory conditions, neoplasms and metabolic disorders are generally readily recognized but in total they are involved in only 1 or 2 per cent of all cases of chronic persistent backache. Similarly, sensations of pain experienced in the back but originating elsewhere in the body are usually identified by clinical history and laboratory investigations. A large majority of episodes of back pain stem from mechanical or structural disorders. Within this category diagnosis of a prolapsed intervertebral disc as the cause of suffering is relatively straightforward. In many other instances, however, the mechanical abnormalities giving rise to pain remain the subject of speculation. The main causes of back pain are:
(1) Mechanical and traumatic causes.
 (*a*) Musculo tenderness and ligament strain.
 (*b*) Fractures of the spine.
 (*c*) Prolapsed intravertebral disc.
 (*d*) Spondylosis.

(*e*) Congenital anomalies.
(2) Inflammatory causes.
 (*a*) Osteomyelitis.
 (*b*) Tuberculosis.
 (*c*) Brucellosis.
 (*d*) Paravertebral abcess.
 (*e*) Spondyloarthropathy.
 (*f*) Ankylosing spondylitis.
 (*g*) Reiter's syndrome.
 (*h*) Psoriatic arthropathy.
(3) Neoplastic causes.
 (*a*) Primary benign tumours.
 (*b*) Primary malignant tumours.
 (*c*) Metastatic disease.
(4) Metabolic bone disease.
 (*a*) Osteoporosis.
 (*b*) Osteomalacia.
 (*c*) Paget's disease.
(5) Referred pain.
 (*a*) Posterior duodenal ulcer.
 (*b*) Carcinoma of the pancreas.
 (*c*) Pelvic disease[d]prolapse of the womb. Ovarian inflammation and tumours.
(6) Psychogenic causes.
 (*a*) Anxiety.
 (*b*) Depression.
  People with backache can obtain advice from the National Back Pain Association, Grundy House, 31–33 Park Road, Teddington, Middlesex TW11 0AB (071–977 5474).

BACLOFEN is a muscle-relaxing drug that is proving of value in relieving the spasm of muscles in some cases of multiple sclerosis (q.v.).

BACTERAEMIA is the condition in which bacteria are present in the bloodstream.

BACTERIA is a term which, strictly speaking, means small micro-organisms of a simple primitive form, but the word is now vaguely used to cover a great variety of low microscopic forms of plant life. It is equivalent to terms such as 'germs', 'microbes', 'micro-organisms' (see MICROBIOLOGY).

BACTERICIDE strictly means anything which kills bacteria, but is usually applied to drugs and antiseptics which do this. Hence *bactericidal*.

BACTERIOLOGY (See MICROBIOLOGY).

BACTERIOPHAGE is the term given to a virus (q.v.) which has a bacterium (q.v.) as its host. Containing either single-stranded or double-stranded DNA or RNA (qq.v.), a particular phage generally may infect one or a limited number of bacterial strains or species. After infection, once phage nucleic acid has entered the host cell, a lytic or a lysogenic cycle may result, depending on the phage and host types. Some (virulent) phages always induce a lytic cycle, whereby the bacterial synthetic machinery is programmed to produce viral components, which are assembled into virus particles and released on bacterial lysis (disintegration). Other (temperate) phages induce a non-lytic, or lysogenic, state, in which phage nucleic acid integrates stably into and replicates with the bacterial chromosome. The relationship can revert to a lytic cycle and production of new phages. In the process the phage may carry small amounts of donor bacterial DNA which may be expressed in a new host individual during lysogeny: the production of diphtheria toxin by *Corynebacterium diphtheriae* and of erythrogenic toxin by *Streptococcus pyogenes* are well-known examples of the effects of lysogeny.

BACTERIOSTATIC: Preventing bacterial growth and cell division.

BACTERIURIA means the presence of bacteria in the urine, usually a sign of infection in the kidneys, bladder, or urethra.

BACUP stands for the British Association of Cancer United Patients and their families and friends. It was founded by Dr Vicky Clement-Jones after she was treated for ovarian cancer and it became fully operational on 31 October 1985. The aim of the association is to provide an information service to cancer patients who want to know more about their illness or who need practical advice on how to cope with it. It does not seek to replace the traditional relationship between the doctor and patient, nor does it recommend specific treatment for particular patients; but its aim is to help patients to understand more about their illness so that they can communicate more effectively and freely with their medical advisors and their families and friends.

The address of the Association is 121–123 Charterhouse Street, London EC1M 6AA and the telephone number of its Cancer Information Service is 071–608 1661.

BAGASSOSIS is an industrial lung disease occurring in those who work with bagasse, which is the name given to the broken sugar cane after sugar has been extracted from it. Bagasse, which contains 6 per cent silica, is used in board-making. The inhalation of dust causes an acute lung affection, and subsequently in some cases a chronic lung disease. (See ALVEOLITIS.)

BAL is the abbreviation for *British Anti-Lewisite*. (See DIMERCAPROL.)

BALANITIS means inflammation of the parts of the penis covered by the prepuce.

BALANTIDIASIS is a form of dysentery caused by a protozoon known as *Balantidium coli*, a common parasite in pigs, which are usually the source of infection. It responds to metronidazole.

BALDNESS is generally partial and slowly progressive, and is so universal that it may be looked on as a natural change in age. There is a gradual depletion in hair on the head with age: e.g. from an average of 615 per square centimetre at the age of 20 to 30 to 485 at 30 to 50 years of age. It is most common in Caucasoids, less so in Negroes and least common in Mongoloids. It may also occur rapidly in patches, or even every hair on the body may be lost, in the disease called alopecia areata.

Causes: Certain *serious diseases* are associated with partial loss of hair as one of their symptoms; but these diseases are of so much greater importance that the thinness of hair is not taken account of, and as a rule remedies itself as these diseases wear off. Such diseases are acute fevers, myxoedema, syphilis, influenza, anaemia, and great anxiety or nervous shock. Baldness is, to a considerable extent, hereditary, and it is generally preceded for some years by seborrhoeic eczema, a condition of dandruff on the scalp. If it first appears relatively early in life – the twenties or early thirties in men – it is likely to be rapidly progressive and total baldness can be expected within a few years. If it does not set in until later life it tends to progress much less rapidly. In women it seldom tends to be rapidly progressive even though it begins to appear relatively early and actual baldness seldom appears until late middle age, and not always then. Every day, in the healthy scalp, a certain number of hairs reach the end of their existence, and are combed out, being replaced in time by others growing up from below. Each hair-follicle in this way produces many hairs in the course of a person's life, but, if the change is too rapid, the hairs become gradually finer, then downy, until finally the hair-producing power of the follicle wears out. This rapid change is due to the eczematous condition of the scalp. Many skin diseases, like lupus, erysipelas, ringworm, which leave a hardened condition of the scalp behind them, cause baldness, and such cases are made worse by the various stimulating hair washes sold for baldness. Other causes include excessive exposure to ultra-violet light as in prolonged sun-bathing, and certain cosmetic procedures such as bleaching, permanent waving, and hair straightening. It can also result from certain hairstyles which impose a mechanical strain on the hair such as the 'ponytail', and by wearing of hair rollers, particularly in bed at night.

Treatment: There is little that can be done to prevent baldness in those predisposed to it. ALOPECIA AREATA, or patchy baldness, is common on the scalp, but may affect the hair all over the body. It occurs principally in adolescents and young adults. The cause is not known. It is doubtful whether treatment makes any difference. The hair regrows spontaneously in a majority of cases, though sometimes lighter in colour, or even white. Ultra-violet light is beneficial in some cases. The more extensive the areas of baldness, and the more often it recurs, the worse the outlook for regrowth of the hair.

BALLOTTEMENT: The technique of examining a fluid-filled part of the body for the presence of a floating object. For example, a fetus can be pushed away by a finger inside the mother's vagina. The fetus floats away from the examining finger and then bounces back on to it.

BALSAMS are substances which contain resins and benzoic acid. Balsam of Peru, balsam of tolu, and Friars' balsam (compound tincture of benzoin) are the chief. They are given internally for colds, and aid expectoration, while locally they are used to cover abrasions and stimulate ulcers. Friars' balsam, one teaspoonful, inhaled from a jug of boiling water, is of value in the alleviation of the common cold. Balsam of Peru is given internally in doses of 5 to 15 drops with beaten-up egg; balsam of tolu is similarly administered in doses of 300 mg to 1 g, or is given as the more familiar syrup of tolu in doses of one teaspoonful.

BANDAGES are pieces of material used to support injured parts or to retain dressings in position.
Types: *Triangular bandages* are made by taking a piece of calico 1 metre square and cutting it across cornerwise to form two triangles. The cut side of each is called the 'base', and the opposite right-hand corner is called the 'point'. *Crepe bandages*, which have a one-way stretch, consist of characteristic fabric of plain weave in which the warp threads are of cotton and wool and the weft threads are of cotton. They are used in the treatment of mild sprains and strains, and as compression bandages over paste bandages in the treatment of varicose ulcers. Much of the elasticity is lost during use, but can be restored by washing in soapy water. *Domette bandages* consist of union fabric of plain weave, in which the warp threads are of cotton or viscose, or of a combined cotton and viscose yarn, and the weft threads are of wool. It is used mainly for orthopaedic purposes, especially where a high degree of warmth, protection and support is needed. *Elastic bandages* provide firm support as in the treatment of varicose veins. *Plaster of Paris bandages* are impregnated with calcium sulphate and used as a form of splint. (See PLASTER OF PARIS.) *Netelast* is an elasticated tubular net of cellular cotton and elastic. It can be applied easily and quickly, can be washed and sterilized, and is available in different sizes. *Tubegauz* consists of seamless, circular cotton tubular material, which can be applied easily and quickly to any part of the body. *Tubifast* is a tubular bandage made from rayon with fine interwoven threads. It has a one way stretch which provides light pressure and so ensures that it holds itself in position.

For more detailed instruction in bandaging the reader is referred to *First Aid*, the authorized manual of the St John's Ambulance Association, St Andrew's Ambulance Association and British Red Cross Society (6th edition, 1991, London: Dorling Kindersley).

BARAGNOSIS means the inability on the part of a patient to recognize that an object placed in the hand has weight, a condition due to disease of the brain.

BARANY'S TEST is a test for gauging the efficiency of the balancing mechanism (the vestibular apparatus) by applying hot or cold air or water to the external ear.

BARBER'S ITCH (see SYCOSIS).

BARBITURATES: The barbiturate drugs are all derivatives of barbituric acid, so called because it was first prepared on St Barbara's Day (1899). They form a most extensive series of sedative, hypnotic, and anaesthetic drugs, but are being used to a decreasing extent in view of the ease with which they can be abused. They are being replaced largely by the tranquillizers (q.v.). (See also DRUG ADDICTION.)

BARIUM SULPHATE is a heavy white powder used in X-ray diagnosis. The mass of barium forms an opaque shadow and shows the outline of the cavity in which it lies. Thus the physician can see the size and position of the stomach in an X-ray photograph, or can trace a meal in its passage through the bowels.

BARORECEPTOR: Specialized nerve ending which acts as a stretch receptor in the carotid sinus, aortic arch, atria, pulmonary veins, and left ventricle. Increased pressure in these structures increases the rate of discharge of the baroreceptors. This information is relayed to the medulla and is important in the control of blood pressure.

BARRIER CREAMS are substances applied to the skin before work to prevent damage by irritants. They are also used in medicine: e.g. for the prevention of bedsores and napkin rashes.

There are three main types of barrier creams: a *dust barrier* to protect the skin against sensitizing dusts and against substances which, if absorbed, will produce systemic poisoning; a *water-repellent barrier* for those whose hands are constantly exposed to water, alkalis, and water-soluble oils; an *oil-repellent* or *water-miscible barrier*, which is a protective against oils, greases and solvents, and which facilitates their removal without the use of abrasives or oil solvents.

Silicones (q.v.), which are water repellent, are being used increasingly as barrier creams.

The hands should be clean and dry before applying a barrier cream. The cream should be applied sparingly to the whole of the hands. To get the full value from silicone creams, they should be applied twice daily for ten days before exposing the hands to irritants; after this a once-daily application should be sufficient.

The use of barrier creams must not be allowed to lead to any slackening in the attention paid to other more important protective measures, such as standards of cleanliness in workshops and the wearing of protective clothing.

BARRIER NURSING is the nursing of a patient suffering from an infectious disease in such a way that the risk of his passing on the disease to others is effectively reduced. Thus, precautions are taken to ensure that all infective matter, such as stools, urine, sputum, discharge from wounds, and anything that may be contaminated by such infective matter, such as nurses' uniforms, bedding and towels are so treated that they will not convey the infection. (See NURSING.)

BARTHOLIN'S GLANDS: Two small glands opening either side of the external vaginal orifice. Their secretions help to lubricate the vulva.

BASAL CELL CARCINOMA: Commonly called 'rodent ulcer' this tumour presents on the skin of the face as a shallow ulcer with a raised, rolled edge. If untreated it erodes slowly into the underlying structures of the face and head.

BASAL GANGLION: Grey matter near the base of the cerebral hemispheres, consisting of the corpus striatum (caudate nucleus and lenticular nucleus (globus pallidus and putamen)), claustrum, and amygdaloid nucleus. The basal ganglia are involved in the subconscious regulation of voluntary movement, and disorders in this region cause dyskinesias.

BASAL METABOLISM (see METABOLISM).

BASEDOW'S DISEASE is another name for exophthalmic goitre or Graves' disease. (See GOITRE.)

BASILIC VEIN is the prominent vein which runs from near the bend of the elbow upwards along the inner side of the upper arm. It is generally the vein opened in venesection for blood-letting.

BASOPHILIA is a term applied to the blueish appearance under the microscope of immature red blood corpuscles when stained by certain dyes. This appearance, with the blue areas collected in points, is seen in lead poisoning and the condition is called punctate basophilia. The term basophilia may also mean an increase in the numbers of basophil cells in the blood.

BAT EARS is the term commonly applied to prominent ears. The condition may be familial, but this is by no means the rule. Strapping the ears firmly back has no effect and is merely a waste of time and an embarrassment to the child. In cases in which the condition is proving a definite embarrassment to the child, it can be rectified by plastic surgery.

BATHER'S ITCH, also called SWIMMER'S ITCH, WATER ITCH, and SCHISTOSOME DERMATITIS, is the term given to a blotchy rash on the skin occurring in those bathing in water which is infested with the larvae of certain trematode worms known as *Schistosomes* (see SCHISTO-SOMIASIS). The worm is parasitic in snails. The skin rash is caused by penetration of the skin by the free-swimming larval cercaria. Bather's itch is common in many parts of the world, including USA, Canada, Central and South America, Australasia, Malaysia and Japan. It has also been found in Wales, France, and Germany.

BCG VACCINE: BCG (*Bacillus Calmette-Guérin*) vaccine, which was introduced in France in 1908, is the only vaccine that has produced significant immunity against the tubercle bacillus and at the same time has proved safe enough for use in human subjects. The original work of Calmette and Guérin has now been amply confirmed by investigators in many parts of the world. BCG vaccination is usually considered for five main groups of people. (1) Schoolchildren: the routine programme in schools usually covers children aged between 10 and 14. (2) Students, including those in teacher training colleges. (3) Children and new-born infants of Asian origin because of the high incidence of tuberculosis in this ethnic group. (4) Health workers, such as nurses, and others likely to be exposed to infection in their work. (5) Household contacts of people known to have active tuberculosis and new-born infants in households where there is a history of tuberculosis. A pre-vaccination tuberculin test is necessary in all age-groups except new-born infants, and only those with negative tuberculin reactions are vaccinated. Complications are few and far between. A local reaction at the site of vaccination usually occurs between two and six weeks after vaccination, beginning as a small papule that slowly increases in size. It may produce a small ulcer. This heals after around two months, leaving a small scar. (See IMMUNITY; TUBERCULIN.)

BEANS are widely used as a source of food. In the western world they include the kidney bean, or French bean (*Phaseolus vulgaris*) which is the now popular 'baked bean', the scarlet runner bean (*Phaseolus multiflorus*), haricot beans, navy beans and pea beans. In the East, and particularly in China, the most widely eaten bean is the soya bean (*Glycine hispida*) which has twice the protein content of most other beans. Modern methods have now been evolved whereby it can be converted into an acceptable imitation of meat. It is also a constituent of the vegetable milk substitutes being used in the developing countries of Africa, South America and Asia. (See PULSES; SOYA BEANS.)

BECHET'S SYNDROME: This is a syndrome of unknown aetiology. It is characterized by oral and genital ulceration, iridocyclitis and arthropathy. Thrombophlebitis is a common complication and involvement of the central nervous system may occur.

BECLOMETHASONE DIPROPIONATE is a corticosteroid that is proving of value as a cream or ointment in the treatment of certain skin diseases. It is also of value by inhalation in the treatment of asthma and hay fever, and by insertion into the nose in the treatment of perennial rhinitis. (See NOSE, DISEASES OF.)

BED BUG, or *Cimex lectularius*, is a wingless, blood-sucking insect, parasitic on man. It is a flat, rusty brown insect, 5 mm long and 3 mm wide, with an offensive, never forgotten smell, which cannot fly. The average life is 3 to 6 months, but it can live for a year without food. The bed bug remains hidden during the day in cracks in walls and floors, and in beds. It does not transmit any known disease. Eggs hatch out into larvae in 6 to 10 days, which become adult within about 12 weeks. A temperature of 44 °C kills the adult in an hour. Various agents have been used to disinfect premises, such as sulphur dioxide, ethylene oxide mixed with carbon dioxide, hydrogen cyanide and heavy naphtha, but insecticide is the most effective disinfecting agent.

BED SORES, or PRESSURE SORES, are areas of inflamed skin, tending to ulcerate, which appear on the body or limbs of people from confined to bed or to a wheelchair for long periods.
Causes: Sores are particularly likely to occur in people who are thin, elderly, or debilitated. People with neurological diseases are particularly at risk. The direct cause may be wrinkles left in the bed-clothes, discharges allowed to soil the invalid's back, and want of daily observation of the places where sores are likely to form.
Symptoms: Very often the invalid feels no pain. Sores commonly form where the bones show through the skin in the lower part of the back, on the heels, on the haunch, on the ankles, on the elbows, or on the shoulder blades. Redness of the skin over a prominence quickly turns blue and dusky. Then a black slough forms and comes away, leaving a raw surface which widens if not carefully treated.
Treatment: The best treatment is preventive, by keeping the patient's back scrupulously clean and dry; by examining night and morning for any sign of redness; and especially by changing the invalid's position so as to relieve the various

prominences from constant pressure. The twice-daily smearing of the skin with barrier creams (q.v.) containing silicone, such as dimethicone cream may help.

BED WETTING: Involuntary passage of urine at night. This usually stops as children grow older, but can persist into teenage, or even adult, life. Treatment is by positive reinforcement of bladder control, alarm systems such as the 'pad and bell', or occasionally by drugs.

BEER (see ALCOHOL).

BEE STINGS (see BITES AND STINGS).

BEHAVIOUR THERAPY: A form of psychiatric treatment based on learning theory. Symptoms are considered to be conditioned responses, and treatment is aimed at removing them, regardless of the underlying diagnosis. Desensitization, operant conditioning, and aversion therapy are examples of behaviour therapy.

BELCHING (see ERUCTATION).

BELLADONNA (see ATROPINE).

BELL'S PALSY is paralysis of the muscles of the face on one or both sides, causing inability to close the eye, to smile, to show the teeth, and the like, on the affected side. The paralysis is due to damage of the seventh cranial, or facial, nerve. When due to inflammation, it is often temporary, and complete recovery may ensue, but when due to a wound in front of the ear, to fracture of the base of the skull, or to a stroke or apoplexy, it is apt to be permanent, although apoplectic paralysis of the face is more favourable for recovery than that due to injury. (See PARALYSIS.)

B ENDORPHIN: A naturally occurring painkiller which is produced by the pituitary as part of a prohormone (pre-pro-opianomelanocortin). It is an agonist at opioid receptors, and its release is stimulated by pain and stress.

BENDS: (see CAISSON DISEASE).

BENIGN: Not harmful. Used especially to describe tumours that are not malignant.

BENNETT'S FRACTURE, so-called after an Irish surgeon, Edward Hallaran Bennett (1837–1907), is a longitudinal fracture of the first metacarpal bone, which also involves the carpometacarpal joint.

BENZEDRINE is a proprietary name for amphetamine sulphate (see AMPHETAMINES).

BENZENE HEXACHLORIDE is an insecticide which acts more rapidly than many insecticides but not for such a long time. When first sprayed it is very toxic to insects, but its action wears off in 3 to 4 months, whereas that of others will persist longer.

BENZHEXOL is a drug that is proving of value in the treatment of Parkinsonism (q.v.).

BENZOCAINE is a white powder with soothing properties used as a sedative for inflamed and painful surfaces.

BENZODIAZEPINES: A large family of drugs used as hypnotics, anxiolytics, tranquillizers, anticonvulsants, premedicants, and for intravenous sedation. They differ in their duration of action, metabolites, and lipid solubility. Short-acting ones are used as hypnotics (q.v.), longer acting ones as hypnotics and tranquillizers (q.v.), and those with high lipid solubility act rapidly if given intravenously. They act at a specific central- nervous-system receptor or by potentiating the action of inhibitory neuro-transmitters. They have advantages over other sedatives by having some selectivity for anxiety rather than general sedation. They do not induce hepatic enzymes and are safer in overdose. Unfortunately they may cause aggression, amnesia, excessive sedation, or confusion in the elderly. Those with long half lives or with metabolites having long half lives may produce a hangover effect, and dependence on these is now well recognized.

BENZOIC ACID is an antiseptic. It, or sodium benzoate, is still given internally in cases of infection along the urinary tract, especially in inflammation of the bladder with decomposition of the urine. Other acids are neutralized in the blood, but benzoic acid is excreted as hippuric acid and acidifies the urine. It is also used as a preservative in certain foodstuffs and beverages: e.g. fruit cordials, pickles.

BENZOIN is a balsamic resin, which is an ingredient of inhalations used in the treatment of bronchitis and common colds. The most widely used of these is Friars' balsam. (See BALSAMS.)

BENZOTHIADIAZINES, or THIAZIDES, are a group of diuretics (q.v.) which are effective when taken by mouth. They act by inhibiting the reabsorption of sodium and chloride in the renal tubules. They also have a blood-pressure-lowering effect. Chlorothiazide was the first member of this group to be introduced. Their main use is to relieve oedema in heart failure.

All thiazides are active by mouth with an onset of action within one to two hours, and a duration of twelve to twenty-four hours. Chlorthalidone is a thiazide-related compound that has a longer duration of action and only requires to be given on alternate days. The other thiazide drugs available include bendrofluazide, clopamide, cyclopenthiazide, hydrochlorothiazide, hydroflumethiazide, indapamide, mefruside, methyclothiazide, metolazone, polythiazide, and xipamide.

The loop diuretics are more potent than the thiazides. They are so called because they inhibit re-absorption from the ascending loop of Henle in the renal tubules. Frusemide, bumetanide, and ethacrynic acid are the three most important loop diuretics.

BENZOYL PEROXIDE is a bactericide (q.v.) used in the treatment of acne (q.v.). It is also used as a bleaching agent in the food industry.

BENZYL BENZOATE is widely used as a lotion in the treatment of scabies (q.v.).

BENZYLPENICILLIN (see PENICILLIN).

BERBERINE is an alkaloid (q.v.) derived from the roots and bark of the plant *Berberis aristata*, a deciduous evergreen shrub. It has a broad spectrum antibiotic activity against selective bacteria including vibrio cholera, shigella and pseudomonas, E Coli and proteus. It inhibits the action of the vibrio cholera toxin when administered before or with the enterotoxin in animals and it has been shown to be effective in the treatment of cholera and related diarrhoeas in man. (See CHOLERA.)

BEREAVEMENT: There is significantly increased psychiatric and physical morbidity following bereavement. Psychosomatic disorders, common neuroses, affective disorders, alcoholism and suicide may occur. The bereaved who are most at risk are those whose lives are complicated by crises other than bereavement and those who see their families as unsupportive. In the case of those who have been widowed, those whose marriage was ambivalent are particularly at risk and this is sometimes associated with an unrealistic idealization of the dead partner. Treatment should be directed towards encouragement of the expression of sorrow, anger, guilt, anxiety and helplessness and reassurance about the normality of the physiological accompaniments of grief.

BERIBERI is a disease found mainly in Japan, Malaysia, China, Manila, Fiji Islands, India, West Africa, Western Australia and round the Gulf of Mexico, and consists in inflammation of the nerves all over the body. (See NEURITIS.)

Causes: It is found among those living in certain parts of the tropics, whose diet consists mainly of highly milled rice. It also occurs in Newfoundland and Labrador, where the inhabitants' main item of diet is white wheaten flour. In both groups of population the removal of the husk of rice and of the wheat berry leaves the diet very deficient in vitamin B₁ (thiamine). It is the lack of this vitamin that causes the trouble.

Symptoms: The affected person becomes, first of all, for some days feverish and weak; then, though feeling better in general health, he gradually develops symptoms of paralysis, especially of the hands and feet, dropsy, palpitation of the heart and loss of sensation in large areas of the skin, especially about the legs. These pass off, in general, in the course of some weeks, and the sufferer gradually recovers health, or occasionally he gets worse and dies from heart failure.

Treatment: The treatment required is large doses of vitamin B₁ (thiamine) (q.v.), plenty of nourishing food, and complete rest.

BERKEFELD FILTER is a candle-shaped filter made of diatomaceous earth. It restrains ordinary bacteria but lets through viruses.

BERYLLIOSIS is a disease of the lungs caused by the inhalation of particles of beryllium oxide.

BETA BLOCKER: Competitive antagonist at beta adrenoreceptors. These antagonize the beta effects of the sympathetic nervous system, decreasing heart rate and blood pressure, for example. They may cause cardiac failure, hypotension, and bronchoconstriction. Large numbers of drugs are available, some of which are cardioselective. They are used to control hypertension, angina, myocardial reinfarction, tachydysrythmias, and ventricular outflow obstruction.

BETAMETHASONE is a corticosteroid (q.v.) which has an action comparable to that of prednisolone, but in much lower dosage. In the form of betamethasone valerate it is used as an application to the skin as an ointment, cream or lotion.

BETATRON (see RADIOTHERAPY).

BEZAFIBRATE (see HYPERLIPIDAEMIA).

BEZOAR: A mass of ingested foreign material found in the stomach, usually in children or people with psychiatric illnesses. It may cause gastric obstruction and require surgical removal. The commonest type consists of hair and is known as a trichobezoar.

BICARBONATE OF SODA, or BAKING SODA, is an alkali, sometimes used as a home remedy for indigestion or soothing insect bites.

BICEPS: A term used for a muscle that has two heads. The *biceps femoris* flexes the knee and extends the hip and the *biceps brachii* supinates the forearm and flexes the elbow and shoulder.

BICUSPID: Having two cusps. The premolars are bicuspid teeth, and the mitral valve is a bicuspid valve.

BIER'S BLOCK: A technique for producing anaesthesia of a limb, first described by Bier in 1908. The limb is exsanguinated and a tourniquet applied. A suitable volume of a local anaesthetic with low toxicity is then injected intravenously via a distally placed cannula. Anaesthesia and muscle relaxation in the limb develop rapidly and last until the tourniquet is released (not less than 20 minutes after injection to avoid systemic toxicity from the local anaesthetic). Suitable for short operations and manipulation of fractures. Although the technique is simple the potential complications necessitate that the practitioner is skilled in resuscitation.

BIFID: Split into two parts.

BIFOCAL LENS: A spectacle lens in which the upper part is shaped to assist distant vision and the lower part is for close work such as reading.

BIFURCATION: The point at which a structure (for example, a blood vessel) divides into two branches.

BIGUANIDES are a group of chemical substances which act as oral hypoglycaemic agents (that is, reduce the level of the blood sugar when given by mouth), and are proving of value in the treatment of diabetes mellitus. They include metformin (q.v.). They act by reducing the production of glucose in the liver. (See DIABETES MELLITUS.)

BILATERAL: Occurring on both sides of the body.

BILE is a thick, bitter, golden-brown or greenish-yellow fluid, secreted by the liver, and stored in the gall-bladder. It consists of water, mucus, pigments (bilirubin and biliverdin), salts of three complex acids (cholic, chenodeoxycholic and deoxycholic acids), cholesterol and some mineral salts, and it is discharged through the bile-ducts into the intestine, a few cms below the opening from the stomach. This discharge is constant, but is much increased shortly after food is taken, and again, some hours later, when the food is digested. Bile is partly an excretion of waste material thrown out by the liver, partly a secretion endowed with some functions in digestion, especially that of fats, and it further aids the absorption of nourishment from the food passing down the bowels, and prevents excessive decomposition by destroying various micro-organisms. About 0·5 to 1 litre (1 to 2 pints) is secreted daily in man, but the greater part of this is reabsorbed with the food, passes into the blood, and ultimately circulates back to the liver, to be again excreted, and so on.

JAUNDICE is a condition in which the flow of bile becomes obstructed, so that the bile is not poured into the intestine, but circulates in the blood. As a consequence, the bile pigments are deposited in the tissues, and the skin becomes yellow or olive-green, while, at the same time, the stools become grey or white and the urine dark. (See JAUNDICE.)

BILIOUS HEADACHE, or biliousness, is a vague term, applied either to migraine (see HEADACHE) or to the headache and vomiting which occur in acute catarrh of the stomach set up by errors in diet. (See DYSPEPSIA.)

VOMITING OF BILE occurs in the two last-named conditions, and is also a sign of obstruction of the bowels, but bile may be brought up in any case of persistent vomiting or retching.

BILHARZIASIS is another name for schisto-somiasis (q.v.).

BILIRUBIN is the chief pigment in human bile. It is derived from haemoglobin (q.v.) which is the red pigment of the red blood corpuscles. The site of manufacture of bilirubin is the reticulo-endothelial system (q.v.). When bile is passed into the intestine from the gall-bladder, part of the bilirubin is converted into stercobilin and excreted in the faeces. The remainder is reabsorbed into the blood-stream, and of this portion the bulk goes back to the liver to be re-excreted into the bile, whilst a small proportion is excreted in the urine as urobilinogen.

BILIVERDIN is the chief pigment of bile in herbivora and birds. It is a precursor of bilirubin in the production of the latter from haemo-globin, and there is a small amount in human bile.

BINAURAL: Relating to both ears.

BINOCULAR: Relating to both eyes. Binocular vision involves focusing on an object with both eyes simultaneously and is important in judging distance.

BINOVULAR TWINS are twins who result from the fertilization of two separate ova. (See MULTIPLE BIRTHS.)

BIO-AVAILABILITY is a term referring to that proportion of a drug which reaches the systemic circulation unchanged after a particular route of administration. The most important factor that determines how much of a drug reaches the circulation is the pre-systemic metabolism in either the intestine or the liver. This is called first pass metabolism. It limits the bio-availability of many lipid-soluble drugs such as the beta blockers, some tricyclic antidepressants and various opiate analgesics (qq.v.). Food can influence drug bio-availability. The first effect of food is to modify gastric emptying so that the rate of absorption of a drug is reduced. Also calcium in the food may chelate with drugs such as the tetracyclines and reduce their intestinal absorption.

BIOFEEDBACK is a technique whereby an auditory or visual stimulus follows on from a physiological response. Thus, a subject's electrocardiogram (q.v.) may be monitored, and a signal passed back to the subject indicating his heart rate: e.g. a red light if the rate is between fifty and sixty beats a minute; a green light if it is between sixty and seventy a minute. Once the subject has learned to discriminate between these two rates he can then learn to control his heart rate. How this is learned is not clear, but it is claimed that by this biofeedback it is possible to control the heart rate and blood-pressure, relax spastic muscles, and even bring migraine under control.

BIOPSY means the removal and examination of tissue from the living body for diagnostic purposes. For example, a piece of a tumour may be cut out and examined to determine whether it is cancerous.

BIOTIN is one of the dozen or so vitamins included in the vitamin B complex. It is found in liver, eggs, and meat, and it is also synthesized by bacteria in the gut. Absorption from the gut is prevented by avidin, a constituent of egg-white. The daily requirement is small: a fraction of a milligram daily. Gross deficiency results in disturbances of the skin, a smooth tongue and lassitude.

BIRD FANCIER'S LUNG, or PIGEON BREEDER'S LUNG as it is sometimes known, is a form of extrinsic allergic alveolitis resulting from sensitization to birds. In bird fanciers skin tests have revealed sensitization to birds' droppings, eggs, protein and serum, even through there has been no evidence of any illness. (See ALVEOLITIS).

BIRTH-MARKS are of various kinds. The most common are port-wine marks (see NAEVUS). Pigment spots are found, very often raised above the surface and more or less hairy, being then called moles (see MOLE).

BIRTH RATE: In 1989, the birth rate in England was 13·6 per 1000 population. The mean age at bearing the first child in marriage was 27. Around half of premaritally conceived births are to teenage mothers.

BISACODYL is a laxative which acts by stimulation of the nerve endings in the colon by direct contact with the mucous lining.

BISEXUAL: Having the qualities of both sexes. The term is used to describe people who are sexually attracted to both men and women.

BISMUTH is a metal, of which the carbonate, subnitrate, salicylate, subgallate and oxychloride are used in medicine.

Uses: In irritative and painful conditions of the stomach or of the bowels, e.g. when diarrhoea or vomiting is present, they have a sedative action. The salicylate of bismuth especially is used to check diarrhoea, the usual medicinal dose of it or of the subnitrate being about 1·2 g. Given internally, bismuth salts turn the stools black. The subgallate is used in the form of suppositories in the treatment of haemorrhoids.

Externally, as dusting powder, bismuth salts are used, both as a cosmetic and in eczema and other moist conditions of the skin, being commonly mixed, in equal proportions, with starch powder or oxide of zinc, or both.

BITES AND STINGS: Bites of animals are in general to be treated as punctured or lacerated wounds (see WOUNDS), but as animals' teeth are, in general, foul, suppuration is apt to arise if the bite be deep. The bite of some reptiles, scorpions, spiders, etc., causes definite symptoms of poisoning, while, after the bites of several animals, especially the wolf and the dog, there is often a risk of rabies. Wounds which are *septic*, i.e. poisoned by bacteria, are dealt with in the section on WOUNDS.

DOG BITES are treated by washing (not scrubbing) the bite with soap and water, and then applying hydrogen peroxide or cetrimide. The bite is then covered with a dressing. Penicillin is also given as a rule, and measures taken to prevent tetanus. More active treatment is required if there is possible risk of rabies (q.v.).

SNAKE BITES are not necessarily poisonous, for not only are many snakes harmless, but people can, like the snake-charmers of India, render themselves immune by the injection under the skin of gradually increasing doses of the poison. It is estimated that the annual death rate from snake bites, throughout the world, is 25,000 to 35,000, of which 20,000 to 25,000 occur in India. In Europe there are probably only 2 or 3 fatal cases every year. The last fatal case reported in England and Wales occurred in 1957, and in the previous fifty years only seven deaths due to snake bite had been reported. There was a fatal case in Scotland in 1975.

The principal poisonous snakes belong to the viper and cobra families, and all inject their poison through a pair of grooved or hollow teeth connected with poison glands. These include in Asia the cobra, the king cobra, the krait, the deboia and the phoorsa; in America the rattlesnake, the copperhead, and the moc-casin; in South America the fer-de-lance and the coral snake; in Africa cobras, vipers and the puff-adder; and in Australia the death-adder, tiger snake, copperhead, brown snake and black snake. The sea snakes of the Pacific and Indian Oceans are almost all poisonous. The only poisonous snake in Britain is the adder (*Vipera berus*). It is chiefly found in Scotland, Dartmoor and the New Forest. It is not found in Ireland. In a not inconsiderable number of cases of adder bite the victim is to blame as he has attempted to handle or torment the snake. Adders are not aggressive and usually try to get out of the way of humans.

The symptoms of snake-poisoning are swelling and paralysis of the bitten part, with general depression, palpitation, difficulty of breathing, faintness and later paralysis and convulsions, followed, in severe cases, by death. These symptoms appear within fifteen minutes to an hour after the bite. After the bite of a deboia or of one of the rattlesnakes very severe suppuration may occur in the neighbourhood of the bite in people who recover.

Treatment of an adder bite in Britain consists of immobilizing the limb by splinting, washing the wound with water, and giving an analgesic to relieve the pain. Medical advice should then be sought immediately, no matter how mild may appear to be the immediate effects of the bite. Victims of adder bites rarely need to be treated with *antivenine* (q.v.). Outside Britain, where the consequences can be much more serious, treatment consists of applying a tourniquet between the bite and the body, to prevent the poison being absorbed into the body. This should be released for a few seconds every fifteen minutes, in order to prevent gangrene. Bites should *not* be sucked as this will not help the victim and may harm the helper. The serum known as *antivenine* (q.v.), which is available as an antidote against many snake bites, should be injected intravenously in liberal amounts as soon as possible. Antivenoms are also becoming available which are active against the venoms of individual snakes, such as the carpet viper (*Echis carinatus*) which is widely distributed in Northern Africa, the Middle East, Pakistan, India and Sri Lanka. The individual should also be treated as for shock, i.e. resting quietly, kept warm, and given a blood transfusion and oxygen if necessary. The victim may be in shock and should not be given anything by mouth.

POISONOUS FISHES exist in most tropical waters, especially round the islands of the Pacific and Indian Oceans, and their venom may be conveyed to man either by poisonous stings or by their bite. The action of the poison is mostly a depressing one upon the heart, and in the case of some of the tropical fishes convulsions and even death may be produced.

Weever fish (known as bishop fish in Cornwall), which are found on Atlantic coasts, as well as on sandy Mediterranean coasts, have poisonous spines which can cause painful wounds – usually in the feet. As the poison is destroyed by heat, the affected foot should be repeatedly bathed in water as hot as the victim can tolerate. A wise precaution is to wear suitable footwear when paddling or bathing.

JELLY-FISH around British shores are fairly harmless, with the exception of the so-called Portuguese Man-of-War which occasionally invades our coasts. It has been described as looking 'rather like a pale blue Cornish pastie with a dark line down its back', and has tentacles up to 13 metres (40 feet) in length. The first thing to do in treatment is to withdraw the tentacle if it is still in the skin but this must not be done with the naked hand without the risk of being stung. A glove of wet sand, however, will usually give sufficient protection. The affected part should then be sprayed or gently washed with methylated spirit. Antihistamine preparations may also be helpful, either applied locally as a cream or, in more serious cases, given by mouth or by injection.

The stings of the much more dangerous jelly-fish found in North Australian and Pacific and Indian waters may prove fatal unless immediate medical attention is available.

SEA-URCHINS are a hazard, particularly to skin divers, because of their spines. The main culprit is *Paracentrobus lividus*, a sea urchin found on rocks in the Mediterranean, the Atlantic coasts of France and Spain, and the south coast of England. It has a black body, 2·5 to 5 cm (1 to 2 inches) in diameter, covered with sharp, purple articulated spines 2·5 cm (1 inch) long. The most severe injuries occur from treading on, or diving on to, collections of them on rocks. This produces a severe burning pain. Prevention consists of avoiding rocky shores when swimming or diving. First-aid treatment consists of removal of the spines as soon as possible. This may require the use of a local anaesthetic or anaesthetizing the skin with ethyl chloride (q.v.). Once removed, an antiseptic dressing should be applied to the affected area until the wound heals. If not removed, the spine may result in a small tender cyst and, if this is burst as a result of pressure on it, there may be a recurrence of severe burning pain.

TOADS AND SALAMANDERS secrete a milky fluid from the skin of the back which is irritating locally, and which, in small animals and weakly children, is said to kill if introduced by a wound.

CENTIPEDES, SCORPIONS AND TARANTULAS (large tropical spiders) kill their prey by poison, and can inflict a very painful, though probably seldom fatal, bite on human beings. The treatment is to apply a ligature as for snake bite at once, and to suck the wound or wash it well with a strong solution of permanganate of potassium. Some other substances have also a reputation as antidotes, such as ammonia, spirit of camphor, tobacco juice, turpentine, and camphor and chloral rubbed up together. An antitoxic serum has been prepared for use against scorpion bite in Egypt. If an abscess forms it is treated like an abscess from any other cause.

HARVEST-BUGS, FLEAS, TICKS, LICE AND MOSQUITOES often cause great irritation of the skin by their bite. Harvest-bugs may bury themselves in the skin and have to be picked out with a needle. Dimethyl phthalate applied to the skin or clothing is an effective repellent. Human beings vary much in their susceptibility to flea bites. The best preventive is dimethyl phthalate. Failing this, smearing the skin with oil of pennyroyal or oil of lavender is helpful, or dusting the underwear and socks with pyrethrum powder, menthol or camphor. Ticks are common parasites of household pets in Britain but seldom attack human beings. In Scotland, however, bites by sheep ticks are accepted as a natural minor hazard of life. The best preventive is dimethyl phthalate or diethyltoluamide. The ticks may be dislodged from the skin by applying the lighted end of a cigarette or the hot end of a match that has just been lit and blown out, or covering it with alcohol, petrol or petroleum jelly. Once bitten, calamine lotion relieves the itching. Lice may be got rid of, if in the hair, by the application of shampoos and lotions containing insecticides such as malathion or carbaryl used repeatedly over several days. The lice and nits can then be removed with a fine comb. They may be got rid of from the clothes by baking these in an oven or fumigating with burning sulphur for several hours, or by the use of an insecticide. (See also under INSECTS IN RELATION TO DISEASE.) Bites by mosquitoes or bugs are soothed by bathing with salt water, by painting with sal volatile or calamine lotion, or by applying an antihistamine cream or ointment. They may be prevented by smearing the skin with dimethyl phthalate (q.v.), or, if this is not available, camphor water, lime juice or one of the oils that are derived from lavender, cloves or cinnamon.

TROMBICULA AUTUMNALIS is the harvest mite. It is also known as red bug and chigger, and is found in fields, gardens and orchards in the autumn. It is the larva that attacks man by crawling up the legs. The adult, popularly known as the 'money spider', does not attack man. Measuring $1 \times 1·5$ mm, it can pass through ordinary clothing. It produces itchy red spots, known in Scotland as 'berry bugs' from their occurrence in those who have been picking raspberries and similar soft fruit. Similar trombiculid mites are found in the rest of Europe, America and Asia. In the Far East they are vectors (or carriers) of rickettsial diseases, such as mite-borne typhus (see TYPHUS FEVER.) Relief from the itching is obtained by bathing the affected part with weak ammonia or baking soda, or calamine lotion with or without the addition of 0·5 to 1 per cent phenol. Bites may be prevented by the use of an insect-repellent cream containing demethyl phthalate and diethyltoluamide, which is obtainable from chemists without a prescription. An alternative preventive measure in heavily infested areas is to wear a boiler suit previously soaked in gamma benzene hexachloride in water and then allowed to dry. When put on, the legs of the boiler suit are tucked into the top of Wellington boots.

ANTS, BEES, WASPS AND HORNETS cause great

irritation by their stings. Those of ants are allayed by eau-de-Cologne, vinegar or lemon juice. Bees sometimes leave a part of their sting as well as poison in the skin, and this should be looked for first of all and carefully wiped out. The sting of a wasp in the throat, the insect having been taken into the mouth in biting a fruit, has caused death owing to rapid swelling, which blocks the air passage. For bee stings the traditional treatment is the dabbing on of ammonia, bicarbonate of soda or washing blue. For wasp and hornet stings a weak acid, such as vinegar or lemon juice, is said to be better. But the experts claim that in both cases any benefit is psychological. A vaccine (Pharmalgen) is now available for those who are allergic to bee and wasp stings. It is estimated that one in every thousand people in Britain is potentially allergic to bee or wasp stings.

HAIRY-CATERPILLARS, by brittle, poisoned hairs, cause an itchy red rash after contact. It is relieved by vinegar or olive oil.

NETTLE STINGS are relieved by bruised dock leaves or raw onion juice.

BITOSCANATE is a drug that is proving of value in the treatment of hookworm infestations.

BITTERS are among the oldest drugs still prescribed. Wormwood is mentioned in the Papyrus Ebers from a tomb in Thebes (1500 BC), and bitters are referred to in the Hippocratic writings (*circa* 400 BC). They are alcoholic extracts of herbs used to stimulate the appetite and to a lesser extent as flavours for tonics and other remedies. Their precise action is not known.

BLACK CURRANTS, the fruit of *Ribes nigrum*, are a rich source of ascorbic acid (vitamin C). In the form of Black Currant Syrup BPC it is used as a dietary supplement, particularly for children, in a dosage of 5 to 10 millilitres. Ten millilitres contain 7·5 milligrams of ascorbic acid. It is also used as a flavouring agent in cough mixtures.

BLACK DEATH is an old name for plague. (See PLAGUE.)

BLACKHEADS (see ACNE).

BLACK MOTIONS are passed when there is great constipation, and when bismuth or iron is being taken; but the most important cause is blood changed by the digestive processes, and proceeding from ulceration somewhere in the stomach or bowels.

BLACK VOMIT is due to the presence of blood in the stomach. There may be dark masses, as in yellow fever, or a small amount of black sediment like coffee-grounds, as in ulcer of the stomach.

BLACKWATER FEVER is an acute illness characterized by haemoglobinuria ('black water'), jaundice, fever, vomiting, anaemia, and severe haemolysis. It is associated with malignant tertian malaria, and occurs in Central Africa, India and the Far East.

Although the precise cause is still obscure, it is known that the disease may be precipitated in malarial subjects by the taking of quinine or by exposure to cold, by fatigue, and by trauma. Predisposing factors include exposure by non-immune individuals to virulent strains of the malarial parasite and irregular and inadequate treatment of such infections. The mortality rate usually varies between 10 and 20 per cent, but may be as high as 40 per cent.

Symptoms: These are fever, rigor, nausea, bilious vomiting, epigastric discomfort, jaundice and the passage of pinkish, red or port-wine coloured urine – haemoglobinuria. The spleen and liver are enlarged and tender. After a few hours the temperature falls, there is profuse sweating, and the skin becomes jaundiced. Mild cases may recover in a day or two. Severe cases have a succession of attacks.

Treatment: This consists in (1) absolute rest in bed; (2) administration of plenty of alkaline fluids; (3) glucose given intravenously (and sodium bicarbonate if necessary); (4) blood transfusion, and subsequent remedies for anaemia.

BLADDER, DISEASES OF: For diseases of the gall-bladder see GALL-BLADDER, DISEASES OF. (See also URINE.)

The urinary bladder is subject to several diseases, but, partly owing to its inaccessibility, as it lies deep in the pelvis behind the pubic bones, partly owing to general ignorance as to its site and functions, symptoms set up in it are often attributed to the bowels and other organs. Diseased conditions in it are diagnosed in part by the symptoms they set up, in part by chemical and microscopical examination of the urine, and in the more obscure conditions by means of the cystoscope. The *cystoscope* consists of a narrow metal tube fitted up as a telescope, and bearing at its end a small electric lamp by which the cavity is lighted up. The instrument is introduced through the urethra, and shows any tumour or ulcer which may exist, and also whether blood in the urine comes from the bladder wall or runs out of the ureters from the kidneys. (See CYSTOSCOPE.) *Sounding* is another process, consisting in the introduction of a curved solid metal rod, when the presence of a stone is suspected, against which the sound can be felt or heard to strike. *Catheters* are narrow tubes, used to draw off the water when it is not possible to expel this voluntarily, or, when the bladder is to be washed out for some diseased condition. (See CATHETERS.) The following are some of the chief diseased conditions:

CYSTITIS, or INFLAMMATION OF THE BLADDER:
Causes: Bacteria live readily in the urine but they do not multiply in the healthy bladder. When some cause is present to weaken the bladder wall, or, when bacteria are introduced in large numbers, for example on a dirty catheter, they multiply inside this organ and set up inflammation.

There may be direct infection from neighbouring organs, as the urethra in gonorrhoea. Any cause that prevents the free voiding of the urine, such as stricture or narrowing of the urethra, or enlargement of the prostate gland at the outlet of the bladder, which is a common occurrence in elderly men, may produce a chronic form of cystitis. In women it is commonly associated with prolapse of the womb. A stone, if present, is apt by its irritation to do the same. One of the most frequent organisms found in the urine in cases of cystitis is *Escherichia coli*. Tuberculous cystitis may be found, due to the *Mycobacterium tuberculosis* which produces a chronic ulcer on the bladder wall. Another very chronic form is caused by the schistosome, a small parasitic worm which may settle in the minute blood-vessels of the bladder wall. This form is very common in Egypt and South Africa. (See SCHISTOSOMIASIS.)

Symptoms: Pain in the region of the bladder or in the small of the back, frequency of making water, and a condition of bad smell, turbidity and whitish sediment in the urine, are the chief facts noticed by the sufferer. In acute cases there may be high temperature and shivering fits. In the chronic form the very frequent desire to pass small quantities of urine is the most marked symptom.

Treatment: Rest in bed and hot applications, like rubber hot water bottles to the lower part of the abdomen, along with simple diet and large quantities of bland fluid, such as barley water, to drink, may be all that is necessary. Large doses of potassium citrate are also helpful, usually combined in a mixture with tincture of hyoscyamus. In the majority of cases, however, it is necessary to give drugs that will destroy the causative organism. In practice this means one of the sulphonamides or antibiotics. The choice is dependent upon which organism is responsible for the infection, and this is determined by submitting a specimen of urine to bacteriological investigation.

STONE, or CALCULUS, in the bladder may be of any size up to that of a hen's or goose's egg, or even larger. The largest one ever seen in England, in 1809, is said to have weighed 1·36 kg (2¾ lb.). An almost equally large one, weighing 1·13 kg (2½ lb.) was removed in a London hospital in 1975. There are three varieties of stone: (*a*) URATIC, associated with acidity or with the gouty constitution; (*b*) OXALIC, composed of oxalate of lime, and often associated with a nervous dyspeptic type of temperament; (*c*) PHOSPHATIC, which occur in long-standing cases of inflammation of the bladder, accompanied by constant decomposition of the urine. This is the most common type of stone found in the bladder.

Symptoms: The symptoms of inflammation of the bladder, together with discomfort on movement, and sudden pain immediately after the passing of water, are those generally found.

Treatment: Although control of the diet may reduce the tendency to the formation of stones in the bladder, the only method of treatment once they have formed is surgical removal. In spite of many vaunted claims, there is no drug known which can remove, or dissolve, stones in the bladder. In 1739 a secret remedy sold by Mrs Joanna Stephens was considered so effectual in stones that the secret was bought by the British Government for £5000. It was found to consist of calcined egg shells, soap and aromatic bitters – that is, its essentials were lime, phosphates and alkalis. Surgical removal of the stone (or stones) is carried out by either *litholapaxy* or *lithotomy*. Litholapaxy consists of passing into the bladder through the urethra an instrument known as a lithotrite which crushes the stone, after which the small pieces are removed through the urethra. The advantage of this method is that no incision is required and the patient is only laid up for one or two days. If the stone is larger than 5 cm (2 inches) in diameter, however, or if there are too many stones present, lithotomy has to be performed: i.e. the bladder is opened through an incision in the lower abdominal wall and the stone (or stones) are removed in this way.

CANCER: About 10,000 cases of cancer of the bladder are diagnosed every year in Britain, and it is responsible for about 5,000 deaths a year. How many of these cases are occupational in origin is not clear, but it has been stated that contact with benzidine, beta-naphthylamine and alpha-naphthylamine increases the over-all risk of dying from cancer of the bladder 30 times above that of the general population. It is over eighty years now since attention was first drawn to the fact that cancer of the bladder was frequent among workers in the chemical industry. There is new evidence that workers in the rubber and cable-making industries, rodent-control operators, laboratory workers using benzidine, as well as engineering workers using lubricant oils may develop it. Prevention of such industrial cases consists of regular six-monthly screening. In treatment, promising results are being obtained from the use of radioactive isotopes (see ISOTOPES) and doxorubicin (q.v.).

RUPTURE of the bladder may occur in old men who have long suffered from difficulty in passing water and cystitis, or in healthy people from a blow or crush.

BLADDERS are sacs formed of muscular and fibrous tissue and lined by a mucous membrane, which is united loosely to the muscular coat, so as freely to allow increase and decrease in the contained cavity. Bladders are designed to contain some secretion or excretion, and communicate with the exterior by a narrow opening through which their contents can be discharged. In man there are two, the *gall-*

kidney

pelvis

ureter

ureteral orifice

bladder

prostatic urethra

membranous urethra

spongy urethra

external urethral orifice

Diagram of the male urinary system.

bladder and the *urinary bladder*.

GALL-BLADDER: This is situated under the liver in the upper part of the abdomen, and its function is to store the bile, which it discharges into the intestine by the bile duct. For further details, see LIVER.

URINARY BLADDER: This is situated in the pelvis, in front of the last part of the bowel. The bladder, in the full state, rises up into the abdomen and holds about 570 ml (a pint) of urine. Two fine tubes, called the ureters, lead into the bladder, one from each kidney; and the urethra, a tube as wide as a lead pencil when distended, leads from it to the exterior, a distance of 4 cm (1½ inches) in the female and 20 cm (8 inches) in the male.

Structure: The wall of the bladder is similar in structure to that of the bowels, and consists of four coats. The inner surface is lined by a soft mucous membrane covered by epithelial cells of irregular shape. This is attached to the muscular coat by a loose, fibrous, sub-mucous coat, in which run numerous blood-vessels. In the muscular coat the muscle fibres are arranged in several layers, and run in various directions, thereby adding greatly to the strength of the wall. On its upper and back part, the bladder possesses a covering of serous membrane, formed by part of the general peritoneal lining of the abdominal cavity, but this outermost coat does not extend down to the base of the bladder, where the latter lies in close contact with the other pelvic organs. The bladder is suspended in position by numerous ligaments, four of which are fibrous bands, while the remaining

five are formed by thickened portions of the peritoneum. The base of the bladder is directed downwards and backwards, and in this part are the three openings of the ureters and urethra. The exit from the bladder is kept closed by a muscular ring, which is relaxed every time water is passed.

BLEEDER is a term applied to persons in whom it is difficult to stop bleeding when some small wound has been sustained. (See HAEMO-PHILIA.)

BLEEDING (see HAEMORRHAGE; and VENESECTION).

BLENORRHOEA means an excessive discharge of mucus or slimy material from a surface, such as that of the eye, nose, bowel, etc. The word catarrh is used with the same meaning, but also includes the idea of inflammation as the cause of such discharge.

BLEOMYCIN is an antibiotic, obtained from *Streptomyces verticillus*, that is being used with a certain amount of success in the treatment of cancer of the upper part of the gut, the genital tract and lymphomas. (See CYTOTOXIC.)

BLEPHARITIS means inflammation of the eyelids. (See EYE, DISEASE AND INJURIES.)

BLEPHAROSPASM (see EYE, DISEASE AND INJURIES.

BLIGHTED OVUM, or BLIGHTED FETUS, is the term used to describe a condition in which apparently normal development of the embryo and its surrounding membranes continues for a short time and then the embryo dies, leaving the membranes alive for a little longer. The causes are not clear but are assumed to be either defects (possibly hereditary) in the ovum or fertilizing sperm, or some fault in the mother's womb. (See ABORTION; FETUS.)

BLINDNESS: The statutory definition for the purposes of registration as a blind person under the National Assistance Act, 1948, is that the person is 'so blind as to be unable to perform any work for which eyesight is essential'. Generally this is vision worse than 6/60 in the better eye, or with better acuity than this but where 'the field of vision is markedly contracted in the greater part of its extent'. Partial sight has no statutory definition but there are Department of Health guidelines for registering a person partially sighted. Generally these are vision of 6/24 or worse with some contraction of the peripheral field, or better with gross field defects. The World Health Organization estimated that there were 28–42 million binocularly blind people in the world in 1979. The causes of blindness vary with age and degree of development of the country. In Western society the commonest causes are 'other retinal disease, glaucoma, diabetic retinopathy and senile cataract'. (See also VISION.)

Any blind person, or his or her relatives, can obtain help and advice from the Royal National Institute for the Blind, 224 Great Portland Street, London W1N 6AA (071–388 1266). NIGHT BLINDNESS (NYCTALOPIA): An inability to see in the dark. It can be associated with retinitis pigmentosa or Vitamin A deficiency.

BLIND SPOT (see VISION, FIELD OF).

BLISTERS AND COUNTER-IRRITANTS: These are employed in cases of both acute and chronic inflammation, on the principle that irritation of the skin causes congestion of the parts immediately below the skin, while it relieves congestion of deep-seated organs through an action upon the nerves that regulate the size of the minute blood-vessels.
Varieties: Substances so employed are spoken of generally as counter-irritants, and divided into *rubefacients*, or substances which merely redden the skin and cause it to peel off; and *vesicants*, or blistering applications, when, in addition, they produce a collection of fluid under the horny layer of the skin; but there is no sharp division between them, most rubefacients producing blisters if left on long enough. The chief *rubefacients* are: mustard, turpentine, cajuput oil, capsicum, tincture of iodine and liniments of ammonia, chloroform, etc., and of *vesicants* we have cantharides or Spanish fly, pure acetic acid, ammonia and chloroform.

BLOOD consists of cellular components suspended in plasma. It circulates through the blood vessels carrying oxygen and nutrients to the organs and removing carbon dioxide and other waste products for excretion. In addition, it is the vehicle by which hormones and other humoral transmitters reach their sites of action.
Composition: The cellular components are red cells or corpuscles (erythrocytes, q.v.), white cells (leucocytes and lymphocytes, qq.v.), and platelets.

The red cells are biconcave discs with a diameter of 7.5μm. They contain haemoglobin, which is an iron containing porphyrin compound, which takes up oxygen in the lungs and releases it to the tissues.

The white cells are of various types – nomenclature depending on their morphology. They can leave the circulation to wander through the tissues. They are involved in combating infection, wound healing, and rejection of foreign bodies. Pus consists of the bodies of dead white cells.

Platelets are the smallest cellular components and play an important role in blood coagulation.

Erythrocytes are produced by the bone marrow in adults and have a lifespan of about 120 days. White cells are produced by the bone marrow and lymphoid tissue. Plasma consists of water, electrolytes (q.v.), and plasma proteins. It comprises 48–58 per cent of blood volume. Plasma proteins are produced mainly by the liver and certain types of white cells. Blood volume and electrolyte composition are closely regulated by complex mechanisms involving the kidneys, adrenal glands, and hypothalamus (qq.v.).

Haemoglobin		
concentration:	men	14–18 g/dl
	women	12–16 g/dl
Erythrocyte count:	men	$4.5–6.0 \times 10^{12}/l$
	women	$3.5–5.0 \times 10^{12}/l$
Mean corpuscular volume		76–96 fl.
Mean corpuscular		
haemoglobin concentration		31–35 g/dl
Mean corpuscular haemoglobin		27–32 pg
White cell count:		$4–10 \times 10^9/l$
Neutrophils		40–75%
Eosinophils		1–6%
Basophils		0–1%
Monocytes		2–10%
Lymphocytes		20–50%
Platelet count:		$150–400 \times 10^9/l$
Packed cell volume:	men	42–52%
	women	37–47%

Range of normal blood count.

BLOOD BANK: A department in which blood products are prepared, stored, and tested prior to transfusion into patients.

BLOOD BRAIN BARRIER: A functional semi-permeable membrane separating the brain and cerebrospinal fluid from the blood. It allows small and lipid soluble molecules to pass freely but is impermeable to large or ionized molecules and cells.

BLOOD CLOT: A blood clot arises when blood comes into contact with a foreign surface, for example, damaged blood vessels, or when tissue factors are released from damaged tissue. An initial platelet plug is converted to a definitive clot by the deposition of fibrin, which is formed by the clotting cascade and erythrocytes.

BLOOD CORPUSCLE (see ERYTHROCYTE and LEUCOCYTE).

BLOOD COUNT: The number of each of the cellular components per litre of blood. It may be calculated using a microscope or by an automated process.

BLOOD, DISEASES OF: (see ANAEMIA; LEUKAEMIA).

BLOOD DONOR: An individual who donates his or her own blood for use in patients of compatible blood group who require transfusion.

BLOOD GASES: Specifically this describes the measurement of the tensions of oxygen and carbon dioxide in blood. However, it is usually used to describe the analysis of a sample of heparinized arterial blood not only for gases but for acid base assessment. This includes measurement of oxygen, carbon dioxide, oxygen saturation, pH, bicarbonate, and base excess (the amount of acid required to return a unit volume of the blood to normal pH).

BLOOD GROUPS: People are divided into four main groups in respect of a certain reaction of the blood. This depends upon the capacity of the serum of one person's blood to agglutinate the red blood corpuscles of another's in certain circumstances. The reaction depends on antigens, known as agglutinogens, in the red corpuscles and antibodies, known as agglutinins, in the serum. There are two of each, the agglutinogens being known as A and B. Anyone's blood corpuscles may have (1) no agglutinogens, (2) agglutinogen A, (3) agglutinogen B, (4) agglutinogens A and B: these are the four groups.

In blood transfusion, the person giving and the person receiving the blood must belong to the same blood group, or a dangerous reaction will take place from the agglutination that occurs when blood of a different group is present.

Group	Agglutinogens in the corpuscles	Agglutinins in the plasma	Frequency in Great Britain
AB	A and B	None	2 per cent
A	A	Anti-B	46 per cent
B	B	Anti-A	8 per cent
O	Neither A nor B	Anti-A and Anti-B	44 per cent

The four main blood groups

Rhesus factor: In addition to these A and B agglutinogens (or antigens) there is another one known as the Rhesus (or Rh) factor, so named because there is a similar antigen in the red blood corpuscles of the Rhesus monkey. About 84 per cent of the population have this Rh factor in their blood and are therefore known as 'Rh-positive'. The remaining 16 per cent who do not possess the factor are known as 'Rh-negative'.

The practical importance of the Rh factor is that, unlike the A and B agglutinogens, there are no naturally occurring Rh antibodies, but such antibodies may develop in an Rh-negative person if the Rh antigen is introduced into his or her circulation. This can occur (a) if an Rh-negative person is given a transfusion of Rh-positive blood, (b) if an Rh-negative mother married to an Rh-positive husband becomes pregnant and the fetus is Rh-positive. If this happens, the mother develops Rh antibodies which can pass into the fetal circulation, where they react with the baby's Rh antigen and cause haemolytic disease of the fetus and newborn. This means that the child may be stillborn or become jaundiced shortly after birth (see HAEMOLYTIC DISEASE OF THE NEW-BORN).

As about one in six expectant mothers is Rh-negative a blood-group examination is now considered an essential part of the antenatal examination of a pregnant woman. All such Rh-negative expectant mothers are now given a 'Rhesus card' showing that they belong to the rhesus-negative blood group. This card they should always carry with them. Rh-positive blood should never be transfused to an Rh-negative girl or woman.

BLOOD-LETTING (see VENESECTION).

BLOOD-POISONING or SEPTICAEMIA is a serious condition caused by the presence of micro-organisms in the blood stream. A very high temperature may be the only sign, but there is often associated shivering (rigor), profuse sweating and pains in the joints and muscles.

The introduction of aseptic surgery by Lister immensely reduced the frequency of blood-poisoning, and the problem was further improved by the introduction of antibiotics.

BLOOD-PRESSURE is the name given to the pressure that must be applied to an artery, say in the arm, in order to stop the pulse in the vessel beyond the point of pressure. It is generally assumed to be equivalent to the pressure to which the blood is subjected by the force of the heart and the elasticity of the vessels, but it is also dependent on the thickness and hardness of the vessel wall, and on the volume of blood thrown out of the heart at each beat.

The blood-pressure is greatest at each heart-beat (systolic pressure) and falls somewhat between the beats (diastolic pressure). The systolic pressure in children is equal to that of a mercury column about 100 mm high, in young adults about 120, and it tends to increase with advancing age as the arteries get thicker and harder, but this is by no means always the case.

The blood-pressure is raised temporarily by exposure to cold, and permanently by kidney disease, by some disorders of the ductless glands, and in the condition known as essential hypertension (q.v.). A blood-pressure of 180 is not uncommon, and it may be as high as 250 or occasionally even 300 mm. Mental worry combined with lack of sufficient exercise has also an important effect in producing raised blood-pressure. The pressure is below the normal as the result of warmth, e.g. after a hot bath, as well as in exhaustion, weakening diseases, fevers and generally in heart failure.

The blood-pressure may be estimated roughly by the pressure with which it is necessary to apply the finger at the wrist in order to obliterate the pulse. It is more exactly measured by means of an instrument known as the *sphygmomanometer*. This consists of a flat rubber bag which is strapped round the arm, and the interior of which communicates by two tubes with either a pressure gauge or a mercury manometer, and with a hand pump. The bag is pumped up so as to constrict the arm, and the systolic pressure is taken as that at which the pulse disappears as felt at the wrist or as heard in the artery at the bend of the elbow.

An abnormally high blood-pressure is often accompanied by disease of the arteries, so that people with greatly raised pressure are specially liable to a stroke. In cases associated with advanced disease of the kidneys, the heightened blood-pressure is to some extent a salutary matter, because the circulation of the blood through the diminished vessels of the kidneys is thereby increased. In such a case the general health of the patient is better while the pressure remains moderately high, and if it is reduced too much by drugs and other means the general health deteriorates.

BLOOD-SPITTING (see EXPECTORATION; HAEMOPTYSIS).

BLOOD TEST: Removal of venous, capillary, or arterial blood for haematological, microbiological, or biochemical laboratory investigations.

BLOOD TRANSFUSION (see TRANSFUSION OF BLOOD).

BLOOD VESSEL: Tubes through which blood is conducted from or to the heart. Blood from the heart is conducted via arteries and arterioles through capillaries and back to the heart via venules and then veins. (See ARTERIES and VEINS).

'BLOWING' OF CANS means the presence of gas in cans of food, the gas resulting from putrefaction or fermentation of the food, or from the action of fruit on the metal of the container, producing hydrogen. The ends of the can or tin bulge and give a tympanitic note on percussion. The food in such cans should not be eaten.

BOILS, or FURUNCLES, are small tender areas of inflamed skin containing pus. They often start in the roots of hairs and are usually caused by *Staphylococcus aureus* infection. A large number of boils close together is called a carbuncle. Boils usually heal quickly when the pus is released, but antibiotics are sometimes required. Anyone liable to recurrence of boils should be investigated to exclude diabetes mellitus.

BOLUS: A lump of food prepared for swallowing by chewing and mixing with saliva. The term is also used to describe the rapid intravenous injection of fluid or a drug, as opposed to a slower infusion.

BONDING: The formation of a close selective attachment, as in the relationship between a mother and her baby.

BONE forms the framework upon which the rest of the body is built up. The bones are generally called the skeleton, though this term also includes the cartilages which join the ribs to the breast- bone, protect the larynx, etc.
Structure of bone: Bone is composed partly of fibrous tissue, partly of bone matrix comprising phosphate and carbonate of lime, intimately mixed together. As the bones of a child are composed to the extent of about two-thirds of fibrous tissue, whilst those of the aged contain one-third, the toughness of the former and the brittleness of the latter are evident. The shafts of the limb bones are composed of *dense bone*, the bone being a hard tube surrounded by a membrane, the periosteum, and enclosing a fatty substance, the marrow; and of *cancellous bone*, which forms the short bones and the ends of long bones, in which a fine lace-work of bone fills up the whole interior, enclosing marrow in its meshes. The marrow (see BONE MARROW) of the smaller bones is of great importance. It is red in colour, and in it red blood corpuscles are formed. Even the densest bone is tunnelled by fine canals (Haversian canals) in which run small blood-vessels, nerves and lymphatics, for the maintenance and repair of the bone. Round these Haversian canals the bone is arranged in circular plates called lamellae, the lamellae being separated from one another by clefts, known as lacunae, in which single bone-cells are contained. Even the lamellae are pierced by fine tubes known as canaliculi lodging processes of these cells. Each lamella is composed of very fine interlacing fibres.
GROWTH OF BONES: Bones grow in thickness from the fibrous tissue and lime salts laid down by cells in their substance; while the long bones grow in length from a plate of cartilage (epiphyseal cartilage) which runs across the bone about 1·5 cm or more from its ends, and which on one surface is also constantly forming bone till the bone ceases to lengthen about the age of sixteen or eighteen. The existence of this cartilage is important to bear in mind, because in children an injury to it may lead to diminished growth of the limb.
REPAIR OF BONE is effected by cells of microscopic size: some called osteoblasts, elaborating the materials brought by the blood, and laying down strands of fibrous tissue, between which bone earth is later deposited; while other cells, known as osteoclasts, dissolve and break up dead or damaged bone. When a fracture has occurred, and the broken ends have been brought into contact, these are surrounded by a mass of blood at first; this is partly absorbed

skull

first and second thoracic vertebrae

cervical vertebrae

clavicle

scapular

sternum

humerous

eleventh and
thoracic vertebrae

lumbar vertebrae

hip bone

radius

sacrum

ulna

coccyx

carpus

metacarpals

phalanges

femur

patella

tibia

fibula

tarsus

metatarsals

phalanges

sesamoid

Human skeleton.

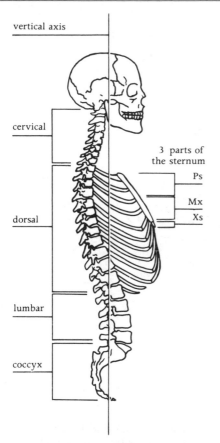

vertical axis

cervical

3 parts of
the sternum

Ps

Mx

Xs

dorsal

lumbar

coccyx

The spinal column.

1

2
3
4
5

6

7

1 body of vertebrae
2 articulas process for the head of corresponding
   rib
3 neural ring
4 notches by which nerves emege
5 articular process for the vertebrae above
6 transverse process
7 spinous process

Human dorsal vertebra seen from above.

and partly organized by these cells, first into fibrous tissue and later into bone. The mass surrounding the fractured ends is called the callus, and for some months it forms a distinct thickening, which is gradually smoothed away, leaving the bone as before the fracture. If the ends have not been brought accurately in contact a permanent thickening results.

VARIETIES OF BONES: Apart from the structural varieties, bones fall into four classes: (a) long bones like those of the limbs; (b) short bones composed of cancellous tissue like those of the wrist and the ankle; (c) flat bones like those of the skull; (d) irregular bones like those of the face or the vertebrae of the spinal column (or backbone).

THE SKELETON consists of over 200 bones. It is divided into an AXIAL part, consisting of the skull, the vertebral column, the ribs with their cartilages, and the breast-bone; and an APPENDICULAR portion consisting of the four limbs. The hyoid bone in the neck, together with the cartilages protecting the larynx and windpipe, may be described as the VISCERAL skeleton.

AXIAL SKELETON: The *skull* consists of the cranium, which has eight bones, viz. occipital, two parietal, two temporal, one frontal, ethmoid, and sphenoid; and of the face, which has fourteen bones, viz. two maxillae or upper jaw-bones, one mandible or lower jaw-bone, two malar or cheek bones, two nasal, two lacrimal, two turbinal, two palate bones, and one vomer bone. (For further details, see SKULL.) The *vertebral column* consists of seven vertebrae in the cervical or neck region, twelve dorsal vertebrae, five vertebrae in the lumbar or loin region, the sacrum or sacral bone (a mass formed of five vertebrae fused together and forming the back part of the *pelvis*, which is closed at the sides by the haunch-bones), and finally the coccyx (four small vertebrae representing the tail of lower animals). The vertebral column has four curves: the first forwards in the neck, the second backwards in the dorsal region, the third forward in the loins, and the lowest, involving the sacrum and coccyx, backwards. These are associated with the erect attitude, develop after a child learns to walk, and have the effect of diminishing jars and shocks before these reach internal organs. This is still further aided by discs of cartilage placed between each pair of vertebrae. Each vertebra has a solid part, the body in front, and behind this a ring of bone, the series of rings one above another forming a bony canal, up which runs the spinal cord to pass through an opening in the skull at the upper end of the canal and there join the brain. (For further details, see *spinal column*.) The *ribs*, twelve in number, on each side, are attached behind to the twelve dorsal vertebrae, while in front they end a few inches away from the breast-bone, but are continued forwards by cartilages. Of these the upper seven reach the breast-bone, these ribs being called true ribs, the next three are joined each to the cartilage above it, while the last two have their ends free and are called floating ribs. The

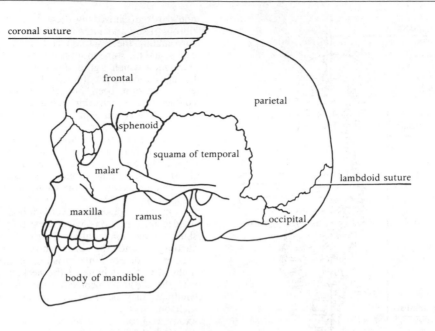

coronal suture

frontal

parietal

sphenoid

squama of temporal

malar

lambdoid suture

maxilla

ramus

occipital

body of mandible

Side view of skull.

breast-bone, or sternum, is shaped something like a short sword, about 15 cm (6 inches) long, and rather over 2·5 cm (1 inch) wide.

APPENDICULAR SKELETON: The *upper limb* consists of the shoulder region and three segments – the upper arm, the forearm, and the wrist with the hand, separated from each other by joints. In the shoulder lie the clavicle or collar-bone (which is immediately beneath the skin, and forms a prominent object on the front of the neck), and the scapula or shoulder-blade behind the chest. In the upper arm is a single bone, the humerus. In the forearm are two bones, the radius and ulna; the radius, in the movements of alternately turning the hand palm up and back up (called, respectively, supination and pronation), rotating round the ulna, which remains fixed. In the carpus or wrist are eight small bones – the scaphoid, lunate, triquetral, pisiform, trapezium, trapezoid, capitate, and hamate. In the hand proper are five bones called metacarpals, upon which are set the four fingers, each containing the three bones known as phalanges, and the thumb with two phalanges.

The *lower limb* consists similarly of the region of the haunch and three segments – the thigh, the leg, and the foot. The haunch-bone is a large flat bone made up of three – the ilium, the ischium, and the pubis, fused together, and forms the side of the pelvis or basin which encloses some of the abdominal organs. The thigh contains the femur, and the leg contains two bones – the tibia and fibula. In the tarsus are seven bones: the talus (which forms part of

the ankle joint), the calcaneus or heel-bone, the navicular, the lateral, intermediate, and medial cuneiforms, and the cuboid. These bones are so shaped as to form a distinct arch in the foot both from before back and from side to side. Finally, as in the hand, there are five metatarsals and fourteen phalanges, of which the great toe has two, the other toes three each.

Besides these named bones there are others sometimes found in sinews, called sesamoid bones, while the numbers of the regular bones may be increased by extra ribs or diminished by the fusion together of two or more bones.

BONE, DISEASES OF: Bone is made up of material called osteoid, which is heavily infiltrated with calcium and phosphate. The outer layer of bone is called periosteum.

ACUTE INFECTION in a bone is called osteomyelitis. It is usually caused by *Staphylococcus aureus* or a streptococcus and infection usually follows a skin graze or sore throat. It occurs mostly in children. The organism enters the bloodstream and settles towards the ends of the longer bones like the femur (thigh bone).

Symptoms: A few days after a minor injury the child becomes feverish and complains of severe limb pain. The limb is red, swollen and tender. In babies the diagnosis is often harder to make. The diagnosis is confirmed by taking blood cultures and growing the bacteria. Plain X-rays are only helpful after a week.

Treatment: At least two antibiotics are usually

needed for a minimum of six weeks, as well as pain relief.

CHRONIC INFECTION can follow acute infection, trauma or operations or it can develop on its own.

Following acute osteomyelitis: the infection may leave behind bits of dead bone (sequestra) which act as irritants and may cause flare-up of the disease or a chronically discharging sinus. Treatment is usually with antibiotics.

Following trauma or operation bacteria can enter and infect bone. An example of this is after a hip replacement where, if the implant becomes infected, it has to be removed before healing can occur. In chronic infections such as tuberculosis or syphilis bone is destroyed as part of a generalized disease.

ACHONDROPLASIA is a hereditary condition often known as dwarfism. It is due to a failure of the growing part of the bone to mature which means growth is arrested.

AVASCULAR NECROSIS occurs when bone dies after its blood supply has been interrupted. It may be seen on X-ray often before it causes pain and restriction of movement, as an area of increased density. It typically affects the femur at the hip. High doses of steroids, alcohol, fractures and infections are all major causes.

OSTEOCHONDRITIS is a condition mainly affecting young men in which a small piece of bone and its adjacent cartilage die and fall off. The knee is often involved, causing recurrent pain, swelling and locking. Repeated minor trauma is thought to be responsible. Sometimes surgical pinning or removal of the fragment is needed.

PAGET'S DISEASE OF BONE (OSTEITIS DEFORMANS) affects 3 per cent of people over 40 in the western world. It is rare in Africa. The turnover of bone becomes abnormally high, making the bone thick but brittle so that fractures occur. Many people have no symptoms.

For the following diseases see separate articles: RICKETS; ACROMEGALY; OSTEOMALACIA; OSTEOPOROSIS; OSTEOGENESIS IMPERFECTA.

Tumours of bone can be benign (non-cancerous) or malignant (cancerous). Most malignant tumours found in bone have spread there from another organ, such as the breast, lung or gut.

Osteoid osteoma is a harmless small growth which can occur in any bone. Its pain is typically removed by aspirin.

Ewing's tumour is a malignant growth affecting long bones, particularly the tibia (calf bone). The presenting symptoms are a throbbing pain in the limb and a high temperature. Treatment is combined surgery, radiotherapy and chemotherapy.

Osteosarcoma is a malignant tumour of bone with a peak incidence between the ages of 10 and 20. It typically involves the knees, causing a warm tender swelling. Removal of the growth with bone conservation techniques can often replace amputation as the definitive treatment. Chemotherapy can improve long-term survival.

Myeloma is a generalized malignant disease of blood cells which produces tumours in bones

which have red bone marrow such as the skull and trunk bones. These tumours can cause pathological fractures.

BONE MARROW means the softer substance enclosed in the interior of bones. It is of two kinds: *yellow marrow*, which occupies the large tubular space in the shaft of a long bone, such as a limb bone, and *red marrow*, which fills up the spaces in the interior of the ribs, sternum, and vertebral bodies, as well as the ends of the shafts of the long bones such as the femur and humerus. There is no essential difference between the two, although yellow marrow owes its colour to the large amount of fat contained in it, whilst red marrow is of a highly cellular structure. The marrow is the site of formation of red blood corpuscles, platelets, and granular white blood cells.

BONE TRANSPLANT: The insertion of a piece of bone from another site or from another person to fill a defect, provide supporting tissue, or encourage the growth of new bone.

BORAX, or BIBORATE OF SODA, acts in much the same ways as boric acid, but without its acid reaction.

Uses: Its chief use is in the form of a lotion (about 1 part to 30 of water) in all forms of itching and chapping of the skin. In thrush (q.v.) and other forms of irritation about the mouth in children the honey of borax, smeared on several times a day, is very soothing. To clean the mouth as well as soothe it, borax in honey wiped over the gums and tongue is very efficient. As in the case of boric acid, it should not be used in infants and young children.

BORBORYGMUS means flatulence in the bowels.

BORNHOLM DISEASE, also known as devil's grip, and epidemic myalgia, is an acute infective disease due to Coxsackie viruses (q.v.), and characterized by the abrupt onset of pain around the lower margin of the ribs, headache, and fever. It occurs in epidemics, usually during warm weather, and it is more common in young people than the old. The illness usually lasts seven to ten days. It is practically never fatal. The disease is named after the island of Bornholm in the Baltic, where several epidemics have been described.

BOTULISM: A rare type of food poisoning with a mortality greater than 50 per cent, caused by the presence of the exotoxin of the anaerobic bacterium *Clostridium botulinum*, usually in contaminated tinned or bottled food. Symptoms develop a few hours after ingestion.

The toxin has two components, one having haemaglutinin activity and the other neurotoxic activity which produces most of the symptoms. It has a lethal dose of as little as 1 mg/kg and is highly selective for cholinergic nerves. Thus the symptoms are those of autonomic parasympathetic blockade (dry mouth, constipation, urinary retention, mydriasis, blurred vision) and progress to blockade of somatic cholinergic transmission (muscle weakness). Death results from respiratory muscle paralysis. Treatment consists of supportive measures and 4 aminopyridine and 3, 4 di-aminopyridine, which may antagonize the effect of the toxin.

BOUGIES are solid instruments for introduction into natural passages in the body either in order to apply medicaments which they contain or with which they are coated, or, more usually, in order to dilate a narrow part or stricture of the passage. Thus we have, for example, urethral bougies, oesophageal bougies, rectal bougies, made usually of flexible rubber or, in the case of the urethra, of steel.

BOUILLON is a broth or soup prepared from meat. It is much used in various food preparations and also as a medium for cultivating organisms in bacteriological laboratories.

BOVINE SPONGIFORM ENCEPHALO-PATHY: A fatal disease of cattle, equivalent to scrapie in sheep and similar to human Creutzfeldt-Jakob disease or kuru. It has recently reached epidemic proportions, generating public concern that it may be transmissible to humans. The disease is probably transmitted by ingestion of infected animal products and has a long incubation period – up to five years. The causative agent has not yet been identified but may be a slow-acting virus.

BOWELS (see INTESTINE).

BOWEN'S DISEASE: This is a form of carcinoma *in situ* in the skin. It presents as an isolated scaling plaque. Round papules appear on the chest and back. It is due to abnormal keratin in the hair follicles and is a genetically determined disease.

BOW LEGS, or GENU VARUM: A deformity of the legs which comprises outward curvature between knee and ankle. It may be normal in infancy and occurs in osteoarthrosis, rickets, and other metabolic bone disease. In early childhood it may correct with growth, but in other cases surgical correction by *osteotomy* or ephiphyseal stapling is possible.

BOXING INJURIES rank eighth in frequency among sports injuries. A recent survey of causes of head injuries requiring admission to hospital in Scotland showed golf ranking well ahead of boxing.

According to the 'Report on the Medical Aspects of Boxing' issued by the Committee on Boxing of the Royal College of Physicians of London in October 1969, of 224 ex-professional boxers examined, 37 showed evidence of brain damage which was disabling in thirteen. Commenting on this, the report says: 'This prevalence rate of 17 per cent indicates that one in six of the boxers studied showed evidence of some damage to their nervous systems attributable to boxing but probably only a third of these were affected severely enough to be recognized as "punch drunk".' The report also notes that 'the Committee has had discussions with members, including medical officers, of the British Boxing Board of Control and appreciate that professional boxing under their auspices is, today, closely and carefully controlled. It is therefore difficult to draw conclusions about the risk of brain damage in professional boxing today'.

In 1984 a report of a working party of the British Medical Association was published. It concludes that there are two main ways in which boxing may lead to structural damage to the brain. The first type of damage occurs as an acute episode in which one or more severe blows leads to loss of consciousness and occasionally to death. Death in the acute phase is usually due to intracranial haemorrhage and this carries a mortality of 45 per cent even with the sophisticated surgical techniques currently available. The second type of damage develops over a much longer period and is cumulative, leading to the atrophy of the cerebral cortex and brain stem. The repair processes of the brain are very limited and even after mild concussion it may suffer a small amount of permanent structural damage. Brain scanning techniques now enable brain damage to be detected during life. Brain damage of the type previously associated with the punch-drunk syndrome is now being detected before obvious clinical signs have developed. Evidence of cerebral atrophy has been found in relatively young boxers including amateurs and those whose careers have been considered successful. The tragedy is that brain damage can only be detected after it has occurred.

BRACHIAL means 'belonging to the upper arm'. There are, for example, a brachial artery, and a brachial plexus of nerves through which run all the nerves to the arm. The brachial plexus lies along the outer side of the armpit, and is liable to be damaged in dislocation at the shoulder.

BRACHYCEPHALIC means short-headed and is a term applied to skulls the breadth of which is at least four-fifths of the length. Brachycephaly is a characteristic of the Alpine race.

BRACHYDACTYLY is a term applied to the conditions in which the fingers or toes are abnormally short.

BRADYCARDIA means slowness of the beating of the heart with corresponding slowness of the pulse (below 60 per minute). (See HEART DISEASES.)

BRADYKINESIA is a term used to describe the condition in which the movements of the body and limbs are abnormally slow.

BRADYKININ is a substance derived from plasma proteins, which plays an important role in many of the reactions of the body, including inflammation (q.v.). Its prime action is in producing dilatation of arteries and veins. It has also been described as 'the most powerful pain-producing agent known'.

BRAIDISM, after James Braid, who introduced it into medicine, is another name for hypnotism. (See HYPNOTISM.)

BRAILLE: A system of printing or writing for the blind using tangible dots or points to represent the characters.

BRAIN: The brain and spinal cord together form the central nervous sytem, the twelve nerves passing on each side from the brain, and the thirty-one from the cord being called the peripheral nervous system, while the complex chains of nerves and ganglia lying within the chest and abdomen, and acting to a large extent independently of the other two systems, though closely connected with them, make up the autonomic system, and govern the activity of the viscera.

Divisions: The brain in its simplest form in lowly vertebrate animals is a thickened part at the front end of the spinal cord, developed in order to govern the organs of special sense, viz. smell, sight, hearing, and taste, lodged near at hand. Higher in the scale, in fishes for example, there are marked bulgings of nervous matter forming the fore-brain, the mid-brain, and the hind-brain, and that part connected with the nerves of the eyes appears to be the highest governing part. In man, however, the part in front of this is specially developed, and not only forms the great bulk of the entire brain, but governs the activities of the rest. This part is called the cerebrum.

The CEREBRUM forms the great bulk of the brain in amount and consists of two cerebral hemispheres which occupy the entire vault of the cranium and are incompletely separated from one another by a deep median cleft, the longitudinal cerebral fissure. At the bottom of this cleft the two hemispheres are united by a thick band of some 200 million transverse nerve fibres: the corpus callosum. Other clefts or fissures, or sulci as they are known, make deep impressions, dividing the cerebrum into lobes. Of these the chief are the lateral sulcus and the central sulcus. The lobes of the cerebrum are the frontal lobe in the forehead region, the parietal lobe on the side and upper part of the brain, the occipital lobe to the back, and the

temporal lobe lying just above the region of the ear.

Numbers of shallower infoldings of the surface called furrows or sulci separate raised areas called convolutions or gyri. The outer 3 mm or thereabouts of the cerebral hemispheres consists of grey matter largely made up of ganglion cells, while in the deeper part the white matter consists of medullated nerve fibres connecting different parts of the surface and passing down to the lower parts of the brain. Among the white matter lie several rounded masses of grey matter, the lentiform and caudate nuclei. In the centre of each cerebral hemisphere is an irregular cavity, the lateral ventricle, each of which communicates with that on the other side and behind with the 3rd ventricle through a small opening, the interventricular foramen, or foramen of Monro.

The BASAL NUCLEI consist of two large masses of grey matter imbedded in the base of the cerebral hemispheres in man, but forming the chief part of the brain in many animals. Between these masses lies the 3rd ventricle, from which the infundibulum, a funnel-shaped process, projects downwards into the pituitary body, and above lies the pineal gland. This region includes the important *hypothalamus*.

The MID-BRAIN, or *mesencephalon*, is a stalk about 20 mm long connecting the cerebrum with the hind-brain. Down its centre lies a tube, the cerebral aqueduct, or aqueduct of Sylvius, connecting the 3rd and 4th ventricles. Above this aqueduct lie the corpora quadrigemina, and beneath it are the crura cerebri, strong bands of white matter in which important nerve fibres pass downwards from the cerebrum.

The PONS is a mass of nerve fibres, some of which run crosswise and others are the continuation of the crura cerebri downwards.

The CEREBELLUM lies towards the back, underneath the occipital lobes of the cerebrum.

The MEDULLA OBLONGATA is the lowest part of the brain, in structure resembling the spinal cord, with white matter on the surface and grey matter in its interior. This is continuous through the large opening in the skull, the foramen magnum, with the spinal cord. Between the medulla, pons, and cerebellum lies the 4th ventricle of the brain.

Structure: The brain is made up of grey and white matter. In the cerebrum and cerebellum the grey matter is arranged mainly in a layer on the surface, though both have certain grey masses imbedded in the white matter. In the other parts the grey matter is found in definite masses called nuclei, from which the nerves spring. The grey matter consists mainly of cells in which all the activities of the brain begin. These cells vary considerably in size and shape in different parts of the brain, though all give off a number of processes, some of which form nerve fibres. The cells on the surface of the cerebral hemispheres, for example, are very numerous, being set in layers five or six deep. In shape these cells are pyramidal, giving off processes from the apex, from the centre of the base, and from various projections elsewhere on the cell. The grey matter is everywhere penetrated by a rich supply of blood-vessels, and the nerve cells and blood- vessels are supported in a fine network of fibres, known as neuroglia. The white matter consists of nerve fibres, each of which is attached, at one end, to a cell in the grey matter, while, at the other end, it splits up into a tree-like structure round another cell in another part of the grey matter in the brain or spinal cord. The fibres have insulating sheaths of a fatty material, which, in the mass, gives the white matter its colour, and they convey messages from one part of the brain to the other (association fibres), or, grouped into bundles, leave the brain as nerves, or pass down into the spinal cord, where they end near, and exert a control upon, cells from which in turn spring the nerves to the body. Both grey and white matter are bound together by a felt-work called neuroglia. The general arrangement of fibres can be best understood by describing the course of a motor nerve fibre. Arising in a cell on the surface in front of the central sulcus, such a fibre passes inwards towards the centre of the cerebral hemisphere, the collected mass of fibres as they lie between the lentiform nucleus and optic thalamus being known as the internal capsule. Hence the fibre passes down through the crus cerebri, giving off various small connecting fibres as it passes downwards. After passing through the pons it reaches the medulla, and at this point crosses to the opposite side (decussation of the pyramids). Entering the spinal cord, it passes downwards to end finally in a series of branches (arborization) which meet and touch (synapse) similar branches from one or more of the cells in the grey matter of the cord (see SPINAL CORD).

Size: The weight of the average male brain is 1·4 kg, ranging from 1·24 to 1·68 kg, of the female brain 1·25 kg, ranging from 1·13 to 1·51 kg, but brains have been found as heavy as 1·8 kg, or, in exceptional cases, even more. The maximum mass of brain tissue is reached at the age of 20, and then decreases steadily.

Functions: The cerebrum is associated with the intellectual faculties in man, and also exerts a guiding influence over the rest of the nervous system. It is not, however, necessary to actual life. If the cerebrum of a frog is destroyed it still breathes and its heart beats, it can hop if pinched, and swim if put in water, but when left alone it sits still till it perishes. If the same happens to a pigeon it can fly when thrown in the air, and can alight, but it does not fly away when threatened, nor will it take food, having lost even the instinct to preserve life. If, on the other hand, the cerebellum of a pigeon is destroyed, the bird cannot maintain its balance, the cerebellum being concerned in the regulation of muscular movements and in preserving the equilibrium of the body.

1 frontal lobe	6 temporal lobe	11 parietal lobe
2 frontal pole	7 preoccipital notch	12 postcentral gyrus
3 lateral (sylvian) sulcus	8 occipital lobe	13 central sulcus
4 temporal pole	9 angular gyrus	14 precentral gyrus
5 superior temporal sulcus	10 supramarginal gyrus	

Side view of the brain.

Plato recognized three mental faculties, which he placed, respectively, in the liver, heart, and brain, these organs being supposed to secrete the 'animal spirits' appropriate to each faculty; and this view was accepted by the medical writers of antiquity. In the Middle Ages the Arabian physicians, however, following Galen's opinion, placed the different mental faculties in the several ventricles of the brain, this theory being adopted by Duns Scotus, Thomas of Aquino, and referred to by Burton in his *Anatomy of Melancholy*.

Descartes (1596–1650) had the fanciful idea that the pineal body was the seat of the mind. After his time it was thought that the whole brain must act together in every process, from the fact that, in cases of severe injury to the head, much substance can be lost from some parts of the brain without impairment of any one definite function or memory.

But it is now known that definite areas of the surface are associated with definite functions. The earliest systematic attempt to localize the functions of the brain to certain areas was made by Gall and Spurzheim, who founded the system of phrenology in the first quarter of the nineteenth century. Although this system was proved to be wrong both as regards the functions of the brain and the philosophic analysis of mental processes, the criticism it called forth gave a great impetus to the attempt to localize the functions of the brain in definite spots. Between 1820 and 1840 it became established that, in people who have lost the power of speech during life, the brain shows some disease in the left frontal lobe after death, and in 1861 Broca made the first definite discovery in cerebral localization by proving that the faculty of speech is governed by a centre in the region of the inferior frontal gyrus, named (after him) Broca's convolution. His discovery was followed later by the important observation of Hughlings Jackson that certain forms of epilepsy, associated with movements beginning in a definite limb, are caused by disease affecting the part of the brain that borders on the central sulcus, and this discovery was confirmed and extended by many experimenters and physicians. Fritsch, Hitzig, Ferrier, Sherrington, Grünbaum and others have shown that definite areas near the central sulcus are associated with the movement of definite parts. Further, the occipital lobes are associated with the sense of sight, the temporal lobe with hearing, and the inner surface of the same lobe with taste and smell. The purely intellectual faculties are probably associated with the frontal lobes, which seem to govern nothing else. The cerebellum has to do with the powers of balancing and of regulating movements. The medulla and pons have important functions, governing many of the processes most essential to life, e.g. those of respiration, rate of the heart, swallowing, vomiting, and giving off all the nerves which arise from the brain, except the first four.

MEMBRANES: The brain is separated from the skull by three membranes: the dura mater, a thick fibrous membrane; the arachnoid mater, a more delicate structure; and the pia mater, adhering to the surface of the brain, and containing the blood- vessels which nourish it. Between each pair is a space containing fluid on which the brain floats as on a water-bed. The fluid beneath the arachnoid membrane mixes

1 sulcus of corpus callosum	4 lingual gyrus	7 precuneus
2 uncus	5 calcarine sulcus	8 subparietal sulcus
3 hippocampal sulcus	6 cuneus	9 paracentral lobule

Vertical section through the middle of the brain.

with that inside the ventricles through a small opening in the 4th ventricle, called the median aperture, or foramen of Magendie.

These fluid arrangements have a great influence in preserving the brain from injury.

NERVES: Twelve nerves come off the brain:

I.	Olfactory, to the nose (smell).	
II.	Optic, to the eye (sight).	
III.	Oculomotor	
IV.	Trochlear	to eye-muscles.
V.	Abducent	
VI.	Trigeminal, to skin of face.	
VII.	Facial, to muscles of face.	
VIII.	Vestibulocochlear, to hear (hearing and balancing).	
IX.	Glossopharyngeal, to tongue (taste).	
X.	Vagus, to heart, larynx, lungs, and stomach.	
XI.	Spinal accessory, to muscles in neck.	
XII.	Hypoglossal, to muscles of tongue.	

BLOOD-VESSELS: Four vessels carry blood to the brain: two internal carotid arteries in front, and two vertebral arteries behind. These communicate to form a circle (circle of Willis) inside the skull, so that if one is blocked the others, by dilating, take its place. The chief branch of the internal carotid artery on each side is the middle cerebral, and this gives off a small but very important branch which pierces the base of the brain and supplies the region of the internal capsule with blood. The chief importance of this vessel lies in the fact that the blood in it is under specially high pressure, owing to its close connection with the carotid artery, so that haemorrhage from it is liable to occur and thus give rise to apoplexy. Two veins, the internal cerebral veins, bring the blood away from the interior of the brain, but most of the small veins come to the surface and open into large venous sinuses, which run in grooves in the skull, and finally pour their blood into the internal jugular vein that accompanies the carotid artery on each side of the neck.

BRAIN, DISEASES AND INJURIES OF: The signs of brain disease are in general indirect, being manifested by some defect in sensation or in the power of action, or by some peculiarity of conduct. (See APHASIA; ENCEPHALITIS; EPILEPSY; HEADACHE; HYDROCEPHALUS; MENINGITIS; MENTAL ILLNESS; PARALYSIS; STROKE.) The following are some of the conditions more exclusively connected with the brain.

ABSCESS is a very serious condition. It results from wounds of the scalp which suppurate and in which the inflammatory matter does not get free exit, or from suppurating ear disease, in which the discharge from the ear has been stopped. The symptoms are rather vague, but sooner or later there are severe headache and vomiting, with rise of temperature, and often some interference with vision. When the abscess lies in the temporal lobe the temperature is often below normal. The treatment should be prevention, by keeping every scalp wound clean, and by having every case of discharging ear disease under medical supervision (see EAR, DISEASES OF). When it is recognized that an abscess has occurred in the brain, it is customary to trephine the skull and evacuate the abscess, after which recovery often takes place.

ANAEMIA OF THE BRAIN is the cause of fainting when suddenly brought on by weakness of the heart's action. Anaemia of a more chronic type is a cause of sleeplessness in elderly persons, accompanied by weakness of mental power and drowsiness during working hours. It also causes headache, giddiness, and ringing in the ears.

COMPRESSION OF THE BRAIN may be caused by the growth of a tumour in the brain, a collection of blood between the brain and skull from injury of the membranes, or suppuration in the same locality from a neglected scalp wound or fracture of the skull. Unconsciousness coming on some hours after a blow on the side of the head is generally due to a fracture tearing one of the arteries in the membranes and producing a large clot between the skull and brain. The symptoms are vague, but, in addition to unconsciousness, there are generally difficulty of breathing, feeble pulse, and paralysis down one side of the body. The treatment is trephining of the skull (see TREPHINING).

CONCUSSION is a bruising of part of the brain as the result of a blow on the head (generally at the back) or a severe shake of the body. Cases vary in severity from mere giddiness and headache for an hour or two, to complete loss of consciousness lasting for weeks, and include those curious instances of lost memory for facts or even for personal identity which have been much used by novelists. The person lies unconscious and can be roused with difficulty. If he answers questions at all he does so irrelevantly, and shows great irritability of temper, going off to sleep again at once. He lies turned away from the light, with his knees drawn up on the body. Consciousness and convalescence come on very gradually, and for months there may be loss of memory, bad temper, and great susceptibility to the effects of alcohol. Recovery is generally good, but a tendency to epilepsy may remain. The treatment is complete rest in a darkened room, with careful nursing to ensure that no complications develop in the lungs and to prevent the development of bed sores. The urine may need to be drawn off. Once consciousness is regained, there should be a prolonged period of rest in order to prevent persisting or recurring headaches. Even the mildest form of concussion should be followed by a few days' rest. Otherwise there is a tendency to a persisting troublesome headache.

BRAIN FEVER is a popular name for several conditions. One is a state of prostration following some severe mental strain. This is not very serious and passes off in the course of a few weeks of rest. Another condition known under this name is encephalitis lethargica, also known popularly as 'sleepy sickness', in which inflammatory changes accompanied by oedema and haemorrhages take place in parts of the brain, causing a serious and often fatal disorder. (See

ENCEPHALITIS.) Another condition often called by this name is inflammation of the membranes of the brain, or meningitis, which occurs most commonly in children and which may be a dangerous disease (see MENINGITIS).

HAEMORRHAGE into the brain causes apoplexy. (See STROKE.)

LACERATION of the brain may occur in fracture of the skull. When the injury affects the upper part of the cerebrum, it is not of so great importance as the fact of whether the wound is kept clean and free from suppuration, although near the central sulcus damage to the brain may result in paralysis of a limb. When it occurs at the base of the skull serious injury of the brain is apt to result, often ending in death (see FRACTURES).

SOFTENING of the brain is a term used in a strictly scientific sense and in a popular sense. In the former case an actual area of brain tissue softens owing to its blood supply being cut off by plugging of its blood-vessels, or in consequence of some long-standing inflammatory process. The symptoms are then those of apoplexy, though not so sudden as if the cause were haemorrhage. In the popular sense, when people, who have been the subjects of gout, alcoholism, or syphilis, especially elderly people, become gradually dull in intellect, drowsy, absent-minded, emotional, and finally demented, because of their diseased blood-vessels diminishing the blood supply to, and causing deterioration of, the brain, these symptoms are also attributed to 'softening of the brain'.

TUMOURS of the brain produce very insidious and very complex symptoms, depending on the region they affect. Among the general symptoms are headache, giddiness, vomiting independent of food, and tenderness of the head on pressure. Blindness and mental symptoms come on later, owing to rise of pressure inside the skull. Sometimes these tumours are tuberculous or syphilitic in origin, when the general treatment for these diseases is of help. Occasionally a tumour produces definite 'localizing' symptoms indicating its position in the brain. In such cases an operation may be performed for the complete and successful removal of the tumour, or it may be treated with radio-isotopes (see isotopes). As a result of advances in neurosurgery and in nuclear medicine, it is becoming possible to deal successfully with an increasing number of tumours of the brain.

People who have had brain injuries, and their relatives, can obtain help and advice from Headway National Head Injuries Association, 7 King Edward Court, King Edward Street, Nottingham NG1 1EW (0602-240800).

BRAIN-STEM DEATH: When brain damage results in the irreversible loss of brain function, including brain-stem function, the individual is incapable of life without the aid of a ventilator. Criteria have been developed to recognize that 'death' has occurred and allow cessation of ventilation. The British criteria require that the patient is deeply unconscious and unable to breathe spontaneously.

All reversible pharmacological, metabolic, endocrine, and physiological causes must be excluded, and there should be no doubt that irreversible brain damage has occurred. Diagnostic tests are performed by two senior doctors which confirm that brain-stem reflexes are absent. These tests must be repeated after a suitable interval before death can be declared. The tests for brain death are:

(1) Fixed, dilated pupils
(2) Absent corneal reflex
(3) Absent vestibulo-ocular reflex
(4) No cranial motor response to somatic stimulation
(5) Absent gag and cough reflexes
(6) No respiratory effort in response to apnoea and adequate arterial CO_2.

BRAN is the meal derived from the outer covering of a cereal grain. It contains little or no carbohydrate, and is mainly used to provide roughage (q.v.) in the control of bowel function and the prevention of constipation.

BRANCHIAL CYST: A cyst arising in the neck from remnants of the embryological branchial clefts. They are usually fluid filled and will therefore transilluminate.

BRANDY (see ALCOHOL).

BREAD is one of the cheapest of foods and contains a reasonable amount of protein. In Britain it is made almost exclusively from wheat flour. Wholemeal flour may be refined by milling processes, in the course of which much of the roughage is removed.

Gluten is the mixture of proteins that constitutes the nitrogenous content of flour. COELIAC DISEASE (q.v.), or gluten enteropathy, is caused by sensitivity to gluten.

BREAK-BONE FEVER is another name for dengue (q.v.).

BREASTS, or MAMMARY GLANDS, are found in the most highly developed class of animals, called the Mammalia, for the purpose of suckling the young. As a rule they are confined to the female sex, though the male has rudimentary nipples, and, even in man, individuals occur in the male sex who have well-developed glands and have been known to produce milk. These glands are developed in the front of the chest, and, in the full-grown female, extend from the second to the sixth or seventh rib, being at the centre about 5 cm (2 inches) thick. There is usually one on each side, but small supplementary breasts are occasionally found in the armpit or low down on the abdomen. In the centre is a dark patch, called the areola, which surrounds the nipple. This areola darkens during pregnancy. This, together with enlargement of the whole breast and dilatation of its veins, forms an important and early sign of this condition. In structure each breast consists of from twelve to twenty compartments, each of which contains a system of branching tubes lined by cells that form the fatty and fluid materials composing the milk. In each section the tubes open on the surface of the nipple by a single small tube, or duct, of which therefore there are twelve to twenty in all. Between these gland tubes lie muscle fibres (which give the breasts their firmness), fibrous tissue, and fat (which is specially plentiful in elderly women).

BREASTS, DISEASES OF: These glands go through great changes during the course of life, becoming considerably enlarged about the age of puberty, afterwards congested at each monthly period, then undergoing great development during pregnancy, so as to be double the usual size during the time of suckling, and finally, with advancing years, undergoing gradual absorption, though, in stout persons, their actual size increases from deposit of fat.

ACUTE INFLAMMATION, or MASTITIS, and ABSCESS: **Causes**: This is most common during the period of suckling a child, and particularly during the first two months. The infection usually reaches the breast from the nipple, as a result of cracks of the nipple and lack of cleanliness. Another common cause is an indrawn nipple. Passing congestion, producing swelling and tenderness, sometimes appears in boys or girls at the time of puberty, but rarely goes on to abscess formation.

Symptoms: Discomfort in some part of the breast, with increased hardness and fullness, usually towards the lower edge, is first noticed, and, if treatment be then begun, the majority of cases do not go on to an abscess. If the condition remains untreated, definite pain next comes on, especially when the infant sucks, along with redness, swelling, and heat, the general signs of abscess. Finally, the skin over one spot, usually about 6 cms from the nipple, turns purple, and here the abscess bursts.

Treatment: It is essential that every care should be taken to prevent infection of the breast, by scrupulous attention to cleansing of the breast during the later stages of pregnancy and during suckling. This is best done by careful washing with soap and water; scrubbing with a brush is usually unnecessary. If the nipples are retracted during pregnancy, they should be drawn out every day. During suckling, the nipples should be carefully cleaned with sterile (i.e. boiled) water each time the baby is put to the breast.

If, in spite of these precautions, the breast becomes hard, tender, or congested, the breast should be firmly bandaged over by a large pad of cotton-wool. The affected breast should be emptied by gentle expression, or this may be done by a breast pump. The common practice today is to start using an antibiotic, usually penicillin, at a very early stage as this reduces the risk of abscess formation. If an abscess forms, it is opened and drained. In severe cases in which it is necessary to wean the baby, the secretion of milk is stopped by taking one of the oestrogenic hormones: e.g. stilboestrol (q.v.). The secretion of milk ceases in about half the women who develop a breast abscess.

CHRONIC INFLAMMATION, or mastitis, may take the form of a chronic abscess, but, more commonly, it consists of simple swelling and pain in one part of the breast, often erroneously believed by the affected person to be cancer. **Symptoms**: This condition is not due to infection, but to some disturbance of the normal control of the breast exerted by the ovaries and the pituitary gland. It occurs with increasing frequency after the age of 30 years, and is more liable to occur in women who have borne children. Pain is the principal symptom. This is worse just before the monthly period or during the early days of the period. It may be confined to one part of the breast or may involve the whole breast. Both breasts may be involved. One or more swellings may be seen or felt in the breast.

Treatment: The condition is made much worse by the patient allowing her mind to dwell on it and by constant handling of the swelling, so that when the breast is completely covered up and supported by a well-fitting brassière, complete recovery may speedily take place. The first essential, however, is that medical advice is sought, to decide whether or not the pain and swelling are due to cancer of the breast.

NEURALGIA may be very painful during pregnancy, in pelvic disorders, or in general troubles like anaemia and rheumatism. It is treated like neuralgia elsewhere.

CRACKED NIPPLES are sometimes very troublesome. For their treatment see under acute INFLAMMATION. When there is a chronic eczematous condition, a nipple-shield should be applied and fixed with plaster or tapes.

TUMOURS: In consequence of the fact that the breast is one of the organs most frequently attacked by cancer, many women render themselves unnecessarily unhappy over some swelling in the breast, taking for cancer what is often simply chronic inflammation, or a cyst or adenoma, the two latter being common non-malignant growths. In every case, immediately a woman discovers a small nodule in her breast she should consult a doctor. If the swelling is not cancer – and usually it is not – her mind will be relieved, and the treatment, whether by operation or not, will not in general necessitate the removal of the breast. If cancer is present, then the earlier an operation is done the more chance there is of a complete cure. A further advantage of early operation for cancer is that it may be possible to remove the growth without removing the whole breast. Such an operation, known colloquially among surgeons as 'lumpectomy', is followed by a course of radiotherapy (q.v.). (See MASTECTOMY.)

BREAST SCREENING: A set of investigations aimed at the early detection of breast cancer. It includes self-screening by monthly examination of the breasts and formal programmes of screening by palpation and mammography in special clinics. In Britain the Forrest report* recommended triennial mammographic screening by invitation of all women aged 50–64 and screening of older women on demand, but whether this is the most cost-effective system is currently under debate.

BREATH, DISORDERS OF: The manner in which breathing is affected is described under RESPIRATION. (See also BREATHLESSNESS; CHEST DISEASES; LUNGS, DISEASES OF.)

BAD BREATH, or halitosis, is sometimes extremely unpleasant to those around the subject of the trouble, although the smell may be extremely foul without the person himself being conscious of it.

Causes: Frequent causes are bad teeth, infections of the gums (e.g. Vincent's angina), chronic tonsillitis, and indigestion. Besides these, an excessively foetid condition is caused by bronchiectasis (q.v.), by ulceration about the bones of the nose, and by disease of the nose, in which crusts constantly form there (see NOSE, DISEASES OF.) A 'mousey' odour of the breath is often detectable during menstruation or premenstrually. In certain diseases there may be a characteristic odour of the breath: e.g. a sweet odour in cases of diabetes mellitus verging on coma; a musty odour (foetor hepaticum) in severe acute liver failure; a urine-like odour in uraemia (q.v.). Certain drugs, notably paraldehyde and disulfiram, also give a characteristic odour to the breath, as do certain foodstuffs, notably garlic.

Treatment: Careful attention to the hygiene of the mouth is the first essential (see TEETH), or the dental treatment of any defective teeth or infection of the gums. Tonsillectomy may be required if the tonsils are chronically inflamed. In one form of tonsillitis, small cheesy pellets of secretion collect in the hollows of the tonsils and putrefy; the tendency to this is lessened by gargling daily (see GARGLES). Indigestion with furred tongue is also credited with being a frequent cause of bad breath (see DYSPEPSIA). The smell may be temporarily relieved by placing a small drop of some essential oil, such as cloves, occasionally on the tongue, or by various scented sweets, or by means of a mouth wash containing one teaspoonful of concentrated peppermint water BP, and one teaspoonful of salt in 200 millilitres of water.

BREATH-HOLDING: Breath-holding attacks are not uncommon in infants and toddlers. They are characterized by the child's suddenly stopping breathing in the midst of a bout of crying evoked by pain, some emotional upset, or loss of temper. The breath may be held so long that the child goes blue in the face. The attack is never fatal and the condition disappears spontaneously after the age of 3 to 5 years, but once a child has acquired the habit it may recur quite often.

The attacks require no treatment as recovery is spontaneous and rapid. In no circumstances should the parents dramatize the situation by slapping, pinching, or drenching the child with water.

BREATHING (see RESPIRATION).

BREATHLESSNESS may be due to any condition which renders the blood impure or deficient in oxygen, and which therefore produces excessive involuntary efforts to gain more air.

Causes: Many diseased *conditions of the lungs* diminish the area available for breathing: e.g. pneumonia, tuberculosis, emphysema, bronchitis, collections of fluid in the pleural cavities, and pressure by a tumour or aneurysm.

Pleurisy causes short, rapid breathing to avoid the pain of deep inspiration.

Narrowing of the air passages may produce sudden and alarming attacks of difficult breathing, especially among children: e.g. in croup, asthma, and diphtheria (see these headings).

Almost all *affections of the heart* cause breathlessness when the person undergoes any special exertion.

Anaemia is a frequent cause.

Obesity is often associated with shortness of breath.

Among the *general diseases* which may interfere with breathing, uraemia (q.v.) and the coma which may occur in diabetes mellitus must be noted.

Treatment: In young girls who become breathless on very slight exertion the treatment is generally that for anaemia (q.v.). For the treatment of breathlessness in stout people, see OBESITY. In all conditions of breathlessness due to disease of a lung, the patient finds most ease in breathing when he lies upon the affected side. In many inflammatory conditions of the air passages much relief is gained from steam inhalations. The subjects of heart disease, if able to go about, should not unduly exert themselves, and are benefited by one of the forms of treatment mentioned under HEART DISEASES. Persons confined to bed by a heart affection are often unable to lie down, and must be provided with a comfortable bed-rest. Their difficulty of breathing is often due to bronchitis (see BRONCHITIS), or to collection of fluid in the chest (see OEDEMA), which requires special and energetic treatment. For breathlessness with lividity, oxygen inhalation is often usefully employed.

(*Forrest P. *Breast Screening: Report to the Health Ministers of England, Wales, Scotland and Northern Ireland by a Working Group Chaired by P. Forrest.* London: HMSO, 1986.)

BREATH SOUNDS: The transmitted sounds of breathing, heard when a stethoscope is applied to the chest. Normal breath sounds are described as *vesicular*. Abnormal sounds may be heard when there is increased fluid in the lungs or fibrosis (crepitation or crackles), when there is bronchospasm (rhonchi or wheezes), or when the lung is consolidated (bronchial breathing). Absent breath sounds occur with pleural effusion, pneumothorax, or after pneumonectomy.

BREECH PRESENTATION: Buttock presentation. The baby lies within the uterus so that it would be delivered buttocks first. This mode of delivery carries an increased risk of damage to baby and mother.

BRIGHT'S DISEASE (see GLOMERULO-NEPHRITIS).

BRITISH NATIONAL FORMULARY is a pocket book for those concerned with the prescribing, dispensing and administration of medicines in Britain. It is produced jointly by the Royal Pharmaceutical Society and the British Medical Association and is revised twice yearly.

BRITTLE BONE DISEASE is another name for osteogenesis imperfecta (q.v.).

BROMIDES are salts of bromine. The bromides of potassium, sodium, strontium, and ammonium are used in medicine. They act chiefly by depressing activity, and dulling sensibility of the brain.
Uses: Introduced to clinical medicine just over a hundred years ago, the bromides were for long the standard treatment of epilepsy. For this purpose they have now been largely replaced by the barbiturates, or more recent anticonvulsant drugs, but they are still of value in occasional cases of epilepsy which do not respond satisfactorily to the newer drugs. Their other use is as an occasional sedative in mild cases of insomnia: either alone (0·6 to 1·2 g), or in combination with chloral hydrate. They have the disadvantage of tending to produce an eruption, especially about the face. (See BROMISM.) As a result of taking bromides for a long time some people may show symptoms of a disturbed balance of mind, which pass off when the drug is omitted.

BROMIDROSIS means the excretion of evil-smelling perspiration. (See PERSPIRATION.)

BROMISM is the name given to a group of symptoms consisting of acne on the face, mental dullness, sleepiness, weakness, unsteady gait, and bad breath, which shows that too much bromide is being taken.

BROMOCRIPTINE is an ergot (q.v.) alkaloid which is being successfully used in the treatment of acromegaly (q.v.). It is also proving of value in the treatment of Parkinsonism (q.v.),

the suppression of lactation (q.v.), and the pain in the breast that sometimes precedes menstruation.

BROMPTON MIXTURE is a prescription of somewhat variable constituents, but consisting basically of morphine, cocaine and whisky (or rum) which was used as an effective pain-reliever, particularly in the terminal stages of painful diseases such as cancer.

BRONCHIAL TUBES (see AIR PASSAGES; BRONCHUS; LUNGS).

BRONCHIECTASIS is a condition characterized by dilatation of the bronchi. This is the result as a rule of infection of the bronchial tree leading to obstruction of the bronchi. As a result of the obstruction the affected individual cannot get rid of the secretions in the bronchi beyond the obstruction. This accumulates and becomes infected and gradually weakens the wall of the bronchi which dilate and become an increasingly large deposit of infected material. The initial infection may be due to bacterial or viral pneumonia or the infection of the lungs complicating measles or whooping-cough. Other causes are obstruction of the bronchi by tuberculosis, cancer of the lung or the inhalation into the lungs of a foreign body, such as a tooth during dental extraction. It usually starts in childhood but may not manifest itself until adult life. It manifests itself by the coughing up of large amounts of putrid, foul- tasting, foul-smelling expectoration, which may contain blood. The condition is not immediately dangerous to life, but as a rule it results in a gradual deterioration of health, with night sweats, clubbing of the fingers and toes (see CLUBBING), and an aggravated form of chronic bronchitis.
Treatment consists of getting rid of the accumulated secretion in the dilated bronchi by means of what is known as postural drainage. This consists of the patient lying on the affected side over the edge of the bed with a pillow under him, and the head well down, so as to drain the affected area. This allows the infected secretion to drain to the trachea (or windpipe) whence it is coughed up. This should be carried out for a quarter of an hour night and morning. It helps to increase the amount of secretion got rid of if someone percusses, or firmly taps, on the chest over the affected area. At the same time the patient should take deep breaths and cough firmly to dislodge the secretion and get rid of it. Should there be a flare-up of the condition, as there often is, this postural drainage should be done four times a day. If the odour is particularly unpleasant, this may be kept in check by inhalations of creosote, or by vaporizing creosote and other aromatic substances in steam near the bed. If there should be a flare-up of the condition due to infection, this is controlled by antibiotics. If the condition is localized to one lobe of the lung, an operation (lobectomy) may be performed to remove the affected lung.

Patients with bronchiectasis should be immunized against influenza every autumn, should not smoke, and should ensure that they have a well-balanced diet and as much fresh air as possible.

BRONCHIOLES is the term applied to the finest divisions of the bronchial tubes.

BRONCHIOLITIS is the name sometimes applied to bronchitis affecting the finest bronchial tubes, also known as capillary bronchitis.

BRONCHITIS means inflammation of the mucous membrane of the bronchial tubes. Well known as one of the most common hazards of the climate of Great Britain, bronchitis exists in either an *acute* or a *chronic* form.
(a) ACUTE BRONCHITIS, like other inflammatory affections of the chest, often develops following exposure to cold, particularly if accompanied with damp, or sudden change from a heated to a cool atmosphere. It may also arise as the result of inhaling irritating dust or vapours. The exciting cause is infection of the bronchial tree with one or more of the catarrh- producing organisms, and great numbers of these bacteria are commonly found in the expectoration.
Symptoms: The symptoms vary according to the severity of the attack, and more especially according to the extent to which the inflammatory action spreads in the bronchial tubes. The disease usually manifests itself at first in the form of catarrh, or the common cold; but the accompanying feverishness and general constitutional disturbance proclaim the attack to be something more severe, and symptoms denoting the onset of bronchitis soon present themselves. A short, painful, dry cough, accompanied with rapid and wheezing respiration, a feeling of rawness and pain in the throat and behind the breast-bone, and of oppression or tightness throughout the chest, mark the early stages of the disease.

After a few days, expectoration begins to come with the cough, at first scanty and viscid or frothy, but soon becoming copious and of purulent character. In general, after free expectoration has been established the more urgent and distressing symptoms abate; and, while the cough may persist for a length of time, often extending to three or four weeks, in the majority of instances convalescence advances, and the patient is ultimately restored to health, although not infrequently a tendency is left to a recurrence of the disease on exposure to its exciting causes.

When the ear or the stethoscope is applied to the chest of a person suffering from such an attack, there are heard in the earlier stages snoring or cooing sounds, mixed up with others of wheezing or fine whistling quality, accompanying respiration. These are named dry sounds or rhonchi, and they are occasionally so abundant and distinct as to convey their vibrations to the hand applied to the chest, as well as to be audible to a bystander at some distance. As the disease progresses these sounds become to a large extent replaced by others of crackling or bubbling character, which are termed moist sounds or crackles. Both these kinds of abnormal sounds are readily explained by a reference to the pathological condition of the parts. One of the first effects of inflammation upon the bronchial mucous membrane is to cause some degree of swelling, which, together with the presence of a tough secretion closely adhering to it, tends to narrow the tubes. The respired air as it passes through the narrowed tubes gives rise to the dry or sonorous breath sounds, the coarser being generated in the large, and the finer or wheezing sounds in the small divisions of the bronchi. Before long, however, the discharge from the bronchial mucous membrane becomes more abundant and less glutinous, and accumulates in the tubes till dislodged by coughing. The respired air, as it passes through this fluid, causes the moist crackles, above described. In most instances both moist and dry sounds are heard abundantly in the same case, since different portions of the bronchial tubes are affected at different times in the course of the disease.

Such are briefly the main characteristics presented by an ordinary attack of acute bronchitis running a favourable course.

The case, however, is very different when the inflammation spreads into, or when it primarily affects, the minute ramifications of the bronchial tubes which are in immediate relation to the air-cells of the lungs, giving rise to that form of the disease known as *bronchiolitis*. When this takes place all the symptoms already detailed become greatly intensified, and the outlook becomes much more serious in consequence of the interrruption to the entrance of air into the lungs, and thus to the due aeration of the blood. Indeed the condition may become indistinguishable from broncho-pneumonia. The feverishness and restlessness increase, the cough becomes incessant, the breathing extremely rapid and laboured, the nostrils dilating with each effort, and evidence of impending suffocation appears. The surface of the body is pale or dusky, the lips are livid, while breathing becomes increasingly difficult and is attended with suffocative paroxysms which render the recumbent posture impossible. Unless speedy relief is obtained by coughing and expectoration, the patient's strength gives way, somnolence and delirium set in, and death ensues. All this may be brought about in a few days, and such cases, particularly among the very young or the aged, sometimes prove fatal within forty-eight hours.

In addition to the auscultatory signs present in ordinary bronchitis, there generally exist in this form of the disease abundant fine crackles at the bases of both lungs; and the appearance of these organs after death shows the minute bronchi and many of the air-cells to be filled with matter similar to that which had been expectorated, and which has thus acted as a mechanical hindrance to the entrance of the air and caused death by asphyxia.

Acute bronchitis is pre-eminently dangerous at the extremes of life, and mortality statistics show it to be one of the most fatal of the diseases of those periods.

Bronchitis is also apt to be very severe when it occurs in alcoholics. Again, in those who suffer from any disease affecting directly or indirectly the respiratory functions, such as tuberculosis or heart disease, the supervention of an attack of acute bronchitis is an alarming complication, increasing, as it necessarily does, the embarrassment of breathing. The same remark is applicable to those numerous instances of its occurrence in children who are, or have been, suffering from such diseases as have always associated with them a certain degree of bronchial irritation, such as measles and whooping-cough.

One other source of danger of a special character in bronchitis remains to be mentioned: collapse of the lung. Occasionally a branch of a bronchial tube becomes plugged up with secretion, so that the area of the lung to which this branch brings air ceases to be inflated on inspiration. The small quantity of air imprisoned in the portion of lung gradually escapes, but no fresh air enters, and the part collapses and becomes of solid consistence. Increased difficulty of breathing is the result, and when a large portion of lung is affected by the plugging up of a large bronchus, a fatal result may rapidly follow, the danger being specially great in the case of children. Fortunately, the obstruction may sometimes be removed by vigorous coughing, and relief is then obtained.

Treatment: In those mild cases which are more of the nature of a simple catarrh little else will be found necessary than confinement in a warm room, or in bed, for a few days, and the use of light diet, together with warm diluent drinks, warm milk being specially beneficial. Additional measures are called for when the disease is more markedly developed. An antibiotic should be given. In the early stages of the disease, when the cough is harsh and unproductive, linctuses give considerable relief. Sedatives are also usually required at night. Opium or morphine must never be given to a patient with bronchitis, because of their depressant effect upon the respiratory centre. In the later stages of the disease, as the cough becomes looser, expectorants (q.v.) are of value. From the outset of the attack the employment of warm applications to the chest, in the form of an electric pad, medicated wool, or a rubber hot-water bottle, affords great relief. In children, rubbing the chest with some stimulating liniment such as camphorated oil has a similar effect.

In the earlier stages few remedial measures are of greater value than the frequent inhalation of steam. This is accomplished readily enough in the case of adults by the use of an inhaler or simply by breathing over an open-mouthed vessel containing boiling water. In children, in whom this plan cannot be carried out in the same manner, there is in general no difficulty in surrounding them with an atmosphere of steam by erecting over the bed or cot a tent, formed by a screen and blanket, under which can be led the orifice of a tin kettle heated by a spirit lamp or electric heater, and provided with a long spout. Various drugs of soothing or expectorant qualities, such as tincture of benzoin and menthol, can also be added to the water in the kettle, or poured upon a sponge which is placed in the end of the spout, and so inhaled in the steam (see INHALATION).

(*b*) CHRONIC BRONCHITIS: **Causes**: This form of the disease may arise as the result of repeated attacks of the acute form, or it may exist altogether independently. It occurs more often among persons advanced in life than among the young, although no age is exempt from it.

It is a common cause of death in this country and is much more common than in any other country. Hence its international reputation as the 'English disease'. Whilst there is probably a constitutional predisposition to the disease, there are in addition six important contributory factors:

(1) Exposure to irritant dust, smoke or fumes either as an occupational hazard or as part of the atmospheric pollution prevalent in industrial areas.

(2) Excessive cigarette smoking

(3) Bad housing

(4) A cold, damp, foggy climate

(5) Obesity

(6) Recurring respiratory infections.

The usual history of this form of bronchitis is that of a cough recurring during the colder seasons of the year, and in its earlier stages, departing entirely in summer, so that it is often called 'winter cough'. In many persons subject to it, however, attacks are apt to be excited at any time by very slight causes, such as changes in the weather; and in advanced cases of the disease the cough is seldom altogether absent.

Chronic bronchitis may arise secondarily to some other ailment. This is especially the case in heart disease, in which it often proves a serious complication.

Symptoms: The symptoms and auscultatory signs of chronic bronchitis are on the whole similar to those pertaining to the acute form, except that the febrile disturbance and pain are much less marked. The cough is usually more troublesome in the morning than during the day. There is usually free and copious expectoration of a thin frothy fluid, and occasionally this is so abundant as to constitute what is termed *bronchorrhoea*.

Chronic bronchitis leads to alterations of structure in the affected bronchial tubes, their mucous membrane becoming thickened or even ulcerated, while occasionally permanent dilatation of the bronchi takes place, often accompanied with profuse foetid expectoration. In long-standing cases of chronic bronchitis, the nutrition of the lungs becomes impaired, and dilatation of the air-sacs (*emphysema*) and other complications result, giving rise to more or less constant breathlessness and leading to deformity of the chest (*barrel-shaped chest*).

Chronic bronchitis does not often prove directly fatal, nor is it necessarily inconsistent with long life. Its chief danger lies in the tendency to intercurrent acute attacks, particularly in the aged; and in this manner it is a disturbingly common cause of death.

Treatment: The treatment to be adopted in chronic bronchitis depends upon the severity of the case, the age of the patient, and the presence or absence of complications. Attention to the general health is a matter of prime importance in all cases, more particularly among persons whose work entails exposure. As severe bronchitis is seldom found in one who has never smoked, smoking – certainly of cigarettes – should be given up. If the victim is overweight, he should take steps to get his weight down.

The value of antibiotics in chronic bronchitis is still undecided. Some recommend their routine use every winter, whilst others contend that this is unnecessary and not without its drawbacks. In many cases infection plays a relatively unimportant part, and for such patients antibiotics are obviously of little value, and treatment must consist of the general measures outlined above. In the presence of infection, as exemplified by a purulent sputum and/or the finding of antibiotic-sensitive organisms in the sputum, antibiotics may be of great value. Those who are subject to chronic bronchitis should be vaccinated against influenza every autumn.

Acute attacks of the disease, which are so apt to arise in the chronic form, must be dealt with on the principles already indicated in treating of acute bronchitis.

BRONCHODILATOR: These drugs reduce the tone of smooth muscle in the bronchioles and therefore increase their diameter. They are used in the treatment of asthma and other causes of bronchoconstriction. As bronchiolar tone is a balance between sympathetic and parasympathetic activity, most bronchodilators are either B2 receptor agonists or cholinergic receptor antagonists, although theophyllines are also useful.

BRONCHOGRAPHY means rendering the outline of the bronchial tree visible on an X-ray film by means of the injection of a radio-opaque substance through the larynx. This is a simple procedure carried out under general anaesthesia and allows the accurate location of, for example, a lung abscess, bronchiectasis (q.v.), or a tumour in the lung.

BRONCHOPHONY means the resonance of the voice as heard by auscultation over the site of the large bronchial tubes, and, in diseased conditions, conveyed beyond these by cavities or solidification of parts of the lung.

BRONCHOPLEURAL FISTULA: An abnormal communication between the tracheo-bronchial tree and the pleural cavity (see LUNGS). Most commonly occurring from breakdown of the bronchial stump following *pneumonectomy*, it may also be caused by trauma, neoplasia, or inflammation.

BRONCHO-PNEUMONIA (see PNEUMONIA).

BRONCHOSCOPE is an instrument constructed on the principle of the telescope, which on introduction into the mouth is passed down through the larynx and windpipe and enables the observer to see the interior of the larger bronchial tubes.

BRONCHUS, or bronchial tube, is the name applied to tubes into which the windpipe divides, one going to either lung. The name is also applied to the divisions of these tubes distributed throughout the lungs, the smallest being called bronchioles.

BROW AGUE is a term used to denote both frontal neuralgia or tic douloureux (see NEURALGIA) and migraine or megrim (see MIGRAINE).

BRUCELLOSIS, also known as UNDULANT FEVER, MALTA FEVER, MEDITERRANEAN FEVER.

Causes: In Malta and the Mediterranean littoral the causative organism is the *Brucella melitensis* which is conveyed in goat's milk. In Great Britain, the USA, and South Africa, the causative organism is the *Brucella abortus*, which is conveyed in cow's milk. This is the organism which is responsible for contagious abortion in cattle. In Great Britain brucellosis is largely an occupational disease and is now prescribed as an industrial disease (see OCCUPATIONAL DISEASES), and insured persons who contract the disease at work can claim industrial injuries benefit.

Year	England and Wales
1967	221
1970	324
1971	221
1973	217
1974	162
1977	58
1978	39
1979	33
1980	17
1984	21
1985	20
1986	30
1987	17
1988	30
1989	17

No. of cases of brucellosis in England and Wales, 1967–89

Symptoms: The characteristic features of the disease are undulating fever, drenching sweats, pains in the joints and back, and headache. There are, however, many atypical cases, and the diagnosis may be difficult. The liver and spleen may be enlarged. The diagnosis is confirmed by the finding of *Br. abortus*, or antibodies to it, in the blood. Recovery and convalescence tend to be slow.

Treatment: Treatment is directed towards relieving the symptoms. The condition responds well to one of the tetracycline antibiotics, and also to gentamicin and co-trimoxazole, but relapse is all too common. In chronic cases a combination of streptomycin and one of the tetracyclines is often more effective.

Prevention: It can be prevented by boiling or pasteurizing all milk used for human consumption. In Scandinavia, the Netherlands, Switzerland and Canada the disease has disappeared following its eradication in animals. Brucellosis has been eradicated from farm animals in the United Kingdom.

BRUISES, or CONTUSIONS, are injuries of the deeper parts of the skin and underlying tissues, accompanied by bleeding from damaged vessels, but unattended by corresponding open wounds.

The simplest type consists of a slight bluish discoloration due to the tearing of minute vessels and the escape of blood into the cellular spaces of the skin. The effusion of blood resulting from a more severe injury may cause a large swelling. In some diseases, like haemophilia and scurvy, extensive bruises are produced by little or no violence.

The colour of a bruise is at first black or bluish, later becoming brown, and finally changing to yellow, which fades away as alterations take place in, and absorption occurs of, the blood pigment. The time taken for a bruise to disappear depends largely upon the amount of blood effused.

Treatment of slight bruises consists chiefly in preventing the effusion of blood after an injury. This is done by firm pressure over the site for three to five minutes. This may be followed by cold compresses firmly fixed in position by suitable bandages. Ice may also be applied with good results.

BRUIT and **MURMUR** are words used to describe abnormal sounds heard in connection with the heart, arteries, and veins on auscultation.

BRUXISM or TOOTH GRINDING is the habit of grinding the teeth, usually while asleep and without being aware of it. The teeth may feel uncomfortable on wakening. It is very common in children and is of no significance, although more severe forms, even during the waking period, may occur in the mentally retarded. In adults it may be associated with stress or a malpositioned tooth or an overfilled tooth. It is also found in some patients taking drugs, such as fenfluramine and levodopa, which cause

minor tremors and reduced muscle control. If the bruxism persists, then excessive wear may result in the loss of enamel and cause pain. Treatment is not very successful unless a cause can be found and removed. A plastic splint fitted over the teeth may help.

BUBO means a swelling of a lymphatic gland in the groin in venereal disease or in plague. (See PLAGUE.)

BUCCAL: Relating to the mouth or inside of the cheek.

BUCHU is a remedy derived from the leaves of *Agathosma betulina* and similar plants. It contains volatile oil and mucilage and is administered in inflammatory conditions of the bladder.

BUDGERIGAR-FANCIER'S LUNG is a form of extrinsic allergic alveolitis, resulting from sensitization to budgerigars, or parakeets as they are known in North America. Skin tests have revealed sensitization to the birds' droppings and/or serum. As it is estimated that budgerigars are kept in 5–6 million homes in Britain, current figures suggest that anything up to 900 per 100,000 of the population are exposed to the risk of developing this condition. (See ALVEOLITIS.)

BUERGER'S DISEASE (see THROMBOANGIITIS OBLITERANS).

BULBAR PARALYSIS (see PARALYSIS).

BULIMIA means insatiable appetite of psychological origin.

BULIMIA NERVOSA is a variant of anorexia nervosa. It is characterized by overpowering urges to eat large amounts of food followed by induced vomiting or abuse of laxatives to avoid any gain in weight. Most of the cases are prone to being overweight and all have a morbid fear of obesity. They indulge in bouts of gross overeating, or 'binge rounds' as they describe them, to 'fill the empty space inside'. By their bizarre behaviour, most of them manage to maintain a normal weight. The condition is accompanied by irregular menstruation, often amounting to amenorrhoea. It is most common in women in their 20s. Although there are many similarities to anorexia nervosa, it differs in that there is no attempt at deceit, and it is freely admitted that there is an eating disorder and there is distress about the symptoms it produces. In spite of this, the response to treatment, which is as in anorexia nervosa, is far from satisfactory. (See EATING DISORDERS.)

BULLA is another word for blister.

BUMETANIDE is a diuretic (q.v.) which is active when taken by mouth. It acts quickly – within half-an-hour – and its action is over in a few hours. (See BENZOTHIADIAZINES, DIURETICS.)

BUNDLE BRANCH BLOCK: An abnormality of the conduction of electrical impulses through the ventricles of the heart, resulting in delayed depolarization of the ventricular muscle. The electrocardiograph (see ELECTROCARDIOGRAM) shows characteristic widening of the QRS complexes. Abnormalities of the right and left bundle branches cause delayed contraction of the right and left ventricles respectively.

BUNDLE OF HIS, or atrioventricular bundle, is a bundle of special muscle fibres which pass from the atria to the ventricles of the heart and which form the pathway for the impulse which makes the ventricles contract, the impulse originating in the part of the atria known as the sinuatrial node.

BUNIONS (see CORNS AND BUNIONS).

BUPIVACAINE is a local anaesthetic. It is four times as potent as lignocaine (q.v.).

BURKITT'S LYMPHOMA: Malignant lymphoma in children previously infected with Epstein Barr virus (q.v.). It occurs mainly in the jaw and abdominal organs. It is common in parts of Africa where malaria is endemic.

BURNING FEET is a syndrome (q.v.) characterized by a burning sensation in the soles of the feet. It is rare in temperate climes but widespread in India and the Far East. The precise cause is not known, but it is undoubtedly associated with malnutrition, and lack of one or more components of the vitamin B complex is the likeliest cause.

BURNING MOUTH is a common complaint. It is most commonly associated with faulty dentures. (See TEETH, DISEASES OF.) Other causes include infections of the mouth. (See MOUTH, DISEASES OF.) It is a not uncommon complaint at the time of the menopause and diabetic subjects are liable to complain of it, especially if their diabetes is not under control. Vitamin deficiency, particularly of certain members of the vitamin B complex, may be responsible. It may be due to a fungal infection following the administration of antibiotics.

BURNS AND SCALDS: Burns are injuries caused by dry heat, scalds by moist heat, but the two are similar in symptoms and treatment. Severe burns are also caused by contact with electric wires, and by the action of acids and other chemicals. The burn caused by chemicals differs from a burn by fire only in the fact that

the outcome is more favourable, because the chemical destroys the bacteria on the part, so that less suppuration follows.

Severe and extensive burns are most frequently produced by the clothes, for example, of a child, catching fire. This applies especially to cotton garments, which blaze up quickly. It should be remembered that such a flame can immediately be extinguished by making the individual lie on the floor so that the flames are uppermost, and wrapping him in a rug, mat, or blanket. As prevention is always better than cure, particular care should always be exercised with electric fires and kettles or pots of boiling water in houses where there are young children or old people. Equally important is it that children's night-clothes and frocks be made of non-inflammable material. Pyjamas are also much safer than nightdresses. Severe scalds are usually produced by escape of steam in boiler explosions.

Degrees of burns: The French surgeon Dupuytren divided burns into six degrees, according to their depth. In practice, however, today burns are referred to as either *superficial* (or partial thickness) burns when there is sufficient skin tissue left to ensure regrowth of skin over the burned site; and *deep* (or full thickness) when the skin is totally destroyed and grafting will be necessary.

Symptoms: Whilst many domestic burns are minor and insignificant, more severe burns and scalds can prove to be very dangerous to life. The main danger is due to shock (q.v.). This arises as a result of loss of fluid from the circulating blood at the site of the burn. This loss of fluid leads to a fall in the volume of the circulating blood. As the maintenance of an adequate blood volume is essential to life, the body attempts to compensate for this loss by withdrawing fluid from the uninjured areas of the body into the circulation. This, however, in turn, if carried too far begins to affect the viability of the body cells. As a sequel, essential body cells, such as those of the liver and kidneys, begin to suffer, and the liver and kidneys cease to function properly. This will show itself by the development of jaundice (q.v.) and the appearance of albumin in the urine. (See PROTEINURIA.) In addition, the circulation begins to fail with a resultant lack of oxygen (see ANOXIA) in the tissues, and the victim becomes cyanosed (see CYANOSIS), restless and collapsed and, in some cases, death ensues. In addition, there is a strong risk of infection occurring. Particularly is this the case with severe burns which leave a large raw surface exposed and very vulnerable to any micro-organisms. The combination of shock and infection can all too often be life-threatening unless expert treatment is immediately available.

The immediate outcome of a burn is largely determined by its extent. This is of more significance than the depth of the burn. To assess the extent of a burn in relation to the surface of the body, what is known as the Rule of Nine has been evolved. From the figure below it will be seen that the head and each arm cover 9 per cent of the body surface, whilst the front of the body, the back of the body, and each leg each cover 18 per cent, with the perineum (or crutch) accounting for the remaining 1 per cent. The greater the extent of the burn, the more seriously ill will the victim become from loss of fluid from his circulation, and therefore the more prompt should be his removal to hospital for expert treatment. The depth of the burn, unless this is very great and reaches the 5th or 6th degree, is mainly of import when the question arises as to how much surgical treatment, including skin grafting, will be required.

Treatment: This depends upon the severity of the burn. In the case of quite minor burns or scalds, all that may be necessary if they are seen immediately is to hold the part under cold running water until the pain is relieved. Cooling is one of the most effective ways of relieving the pain of a burn. If the burn involves the distal part of a limb, e.g. the hand and forearm, one of the most effective ways of relieving pain is to immerse the burned part in lukewarm water and add cold water until the pain disappears. As the water warms and pain returns more cold water is added. After some three to four hours, pain will not reappear on warming, and the burn may be dressed in the usual way. Thereafter a simple dressing – e.g. a piece of sterile gauze covered by cotton-wool, and on top of this a bandage or a piece of Elastoplast – should be applied. The part should be kept at rest and the dressing kept quite dry until healing takes place. Blisters should be pierced with a sterile needle, but the skin should not be cut away. No ointment or oil should be applied, and an antiseptic is not usually necessary.

In slightly more severe burns or scalds, it is probably advisable to use some antiseptic dressing. These are the cases which should be taken to a doctor – whether a general practitioner, a factory doctor, or a casualty officer in hospital. There is still no general consensus of expert opinion as to the best 'antiseptic' to use. Among those recommended are chlorhexidine, and antibiotics such as bacitracin, neomycin and polymixin. An alternative is to use a Tulle Gras dressing which has been impregnated with a suitable antibiotic. One of the many methods recommended is to apply a cream containing chlorhexidine and lignocaine (which has the double advantage of being both antiseptic and pain-relieving), covering this with a Tulle Gras dressing, covered in turn by cotton-wool and a crêpe bandage. To ensure that the burn is completely sealed off the ends of the dressing are completely sealed with zinc oxide plaster. The dressing is left on for four or five days before being changed unless the burn becomes painful or there is any evidence of infection (such as redness, swelling and pain), when it is changed immediately.

In the case of severe burns and scalds, the only sound rule is immediate removal to hospital. Unless there is any need for immediate resuscitation, such as artificial respiration, or attention to other injuries there may be, such as fractures or haemorrhage, nothing should be done on the spot to the patient except to make sure that he is as comfortable as possible and to keep him warm, and to cover the burn with a sterile (or clean) cloth such as a sheet, pillowcases, or towels wrung out in cold water. If pain is severe, morphine should be given – usually intravenously. Once the victim is in hospital, the primary decision is as to the extent of the burn, and whether or not a transfusion is necessary. If the burn is more than 9 per cent of the body surface in extent, a transfusion is called for. The precise treatment of the burn varies from hospital to hospital, but the essential is to prevent infection if this has not already

1 Epidermis   2 Dermis
3–4 Full-thickness burn requiring grafting.
5 Partial-thickness burn which will usually heal within 3 weeks.
6 Partial-thickness burn which will heal in 7–10 days.

The structure of the skin in relation to the depth
of a burn.

occurred, or, if it has, to bring it under control as quickly as possible. A high-protein diet, with ample fluids, is also necessary to compensate for all the protein that has been lost along with the fluid from the circulation. The process of healing is slow and tedious in the case of extensive burns, and involves careful nursing, the maintenance of morale, physiotherapy and occupational therapy. A vital decision is as to whether skin grafting is required, and when this should be initiated.

So far as the ultimate outcome is concerned, the main factor, as has already been noted, is the extent of the burn. The greater this is, the worse the outlook. The outlook is also poor in infants and old people.

Chemical Burns: Phenol or lysol can be washed off promptly before they do much damage. Acid or alkali burns should be neutralized by washing them repeatedly with sodium bicarbonate or 1 per cent acetic acid, respectively. Alternatively, the following buffer solution may be used for either acid or alkali burns: monobasic potassium phosphate (70 grams), dibasic sodium phosphate (70 grams) in 850 millilitres of water. (See also PHOSPHORUS BURNS.)

BURSAE are natural hollows in the fibrous tissues, lined by smooth cells and containing a little fluid. They are situated at points where there is much pressure or friction, and their purpose is to allow free movement without stretching or straining the tissues: for example, on the knee-cap or the point of the elbow, and, generally speaking, where one muscle rubs against another or against a bone. They develop also beneath corns and bunions, or where a bone comes to press in an unwonted manner on the skin.

BURSITIS means inflammation within a bursa. Acute bursitis is of the nature of an abscess, being produced by injury of a bursa, especially on the knee or elbow, when the prominent part of the joint becomes swollen, hot, painful, and red. It is treated as an abscess. (See ABSCESS.)

Chronic bursitis is due to too much movement of, or pressure on, a bursa. For example, the condition of housemaid's knee is a chronic inflammation of the patellar bursa in front of the knee, due to too much kneeling. This condition may consist of either a collection of fluid in the bursa, or, less frequently, in thickening of its walls, producing in either case an elastic swelling over the joint, with pain. In the former case, resting the limb, with counter-irritation (see BLISTERS AND COUNTER-IRRITANTS) over the swelling, or injection of some irritant substance into its interior, forms the treatment; in the latter case, removal by operation.

Chronic bursitis about the sinews round the wrist and ankle is generally called a ganglion. (See GANGLION.)

BUSULPHAN is a preparation allied to the nitrogen mustard group of compounds (q.v.), with an action on dividing cells similar to that of irradiation. It is proving of value in the treatment of chronic myeloid leukaemia. (See CYTOTOXIC.)

BUTYROPHENONES are a group of drugs, including haloperidol, which are proving to be effective in the treatment of psychotic illness.

BYSSINOSIS is a pneumoconiosis (q.v.), or chronic inflammatory thickening of the lung tissue, due to the inhalation of dust in textile factories. It is found chiefly among cotton and flax workers and, to a lesser extent, among workers in soft hemp. It is rare or absent in workers in jute and the hard fibres of hemp and sisal.

C

CACHET means an oval capsule, generally made of rice paper, for enclosing a dose of unpleasant medicine. Cachets are softened by moistening with water prior to swallowing.

CACHEXIA is the feeble state produced by serious disease, such as cancer.

CADAVERIC RIGIDITY is the stiffness which comes on after death. (See DEATH, SIGNS OF.)

CADMIUM POISONING is a recognized hazard in certain industrial processes, such as the manufacture of alloys, cadmium plating and glass blowing (see OCCUPATIONAL DISEASES). It is also now known that sewage sludge, which is used as fertilizer, may be contaminated by cadmium from industrial sources. Such cadmium could be taken up into vegetable crops. Cadmium levels in sewage are carefully monitored; surveys performed of people eating their own vegetables, grown in gardens fertilized with contaminated sludge, have shown no adverse health effects. Cadmium in the form of the sulphide occurs with zinc minerals, and investigations of an old zinc mining area near Shipham in Somerset have revealed a high level of cadmium in the soil and in vegetables grown in it. So far no adverse effect has been detected in those living in the region and eating vegetables grown there. Where an excess of cadmium is consumed it causes gastroenteritis, resulting in diarrhoea and vomiting. The most important source of cadmium is food, particularly some vegetables (cabbage, spinach, lettuce, kale, rhubarb and celery) when grown on soils fertilized with large amounts of contaminated sewage sludge, shellfish and kidneys. Smoking of cigarettes is the second major source of intake. The EEC Directive on the Quality of Water for

Human Consumption lays down 5 milligrams per litre as the upper safe level.

CAECUM is the dilated commencement of the large intestine lying in the right lower corner of the abdomen. Into it the small intestine and the appendix vermiformis open, and it is continued upwards through the right flank as the ascending colon.

CAESAREAN SECTION means the delivery of a child by opening the abdomen and womb from in front. It is supposed to get its name from the traditional, but unproven, story that Julius Caesar was so delivered. The more probable explanation is that it was named after Caesarean Law which forbade the burying of a pregnant mother until her baby had first been removed. According to Ovid, Aesculapius, the God of Physic, was born by caesarean section. The first caesarean section in the British Isles is said to have been performed in 1738 by an Irish midwife, Mary Donnally. Her patient, who had been in labour for twelve days, successfully survived the operation. It is performed when delivery by the natural passage is undesirable because of the risk to mother and child: for example, because of bony deformity of the pelvis; also when the mother has died just before labour, so as to save the child.

CAESIUM-137: An artificially produced radioactive element that is used in radiotherapy treatment (q.v.).

CAFFEINE is a white crystalline substance obtained from coffee, of which it is the active principle. Its main actions are as a cerebral stimulant, a cardiac stimulant, and as a diuretic. It is also of value in some cases of asthma. It is a constituent of many tablets for the relief of headache, usually combined with aspirin and paracetamol. Granular effervescent citrate of caffeine forms a useful, non-intoxicating stimulant in headache due to tiredness.

CAISSON DISEASE, or COMPRESSED AIR ILLNESS, affects workers in compressed air, such as underwater divers and workers in caissons. Its chief symptoms are pains in the joints and limbs (bends), pain in the stomach, headache and dizziness, and paralysis. Sudden death may occur. The condition is caused by the accumulation of bubbles of nitrogen in different parts of the body.

CALAMINE, or CARBONATE OF ZINC, is a mild astringent used, as calamine lotion, to soothe and protect the skin in many conditions such as eczema and urticaria.

CALCANEUS is the heelbone or os calcis.

CALCICOSIS is the term applied to disease of the lung caused by the inhalation of marble dust by marble-cutters.

CALCIFEROL, or VITAMIN D_2, is a crystalline substance extracted from irradiated ergosterol, and has the same action as vitamin D. Man attains vitamin D in two ways: from food naturally containing or fortified with vitamin D, or from its production in the skin by the action of ultraviolet light on the precursor 7-dehydrocholesterol. The vitamin D produced in the skin and occurring naturally in food products is cholecalciferol or vitamin D_3 while the product used for food fortification or prescribed as calciferol is the synthetic compound ergocalciferol or vitamin D_2. The biological activity of both ergocalciferol and cholecalciferol is the same and both are metabolized in identical manner. Cholecalciferol itself has little, if any, biological activity and it is metabolized in the liver and subsequently in the kidney to produce the active metabolite one alpha 25-dihydroxy vitamin D and this is known as calcitriol. One alpha cholecalciferol (alfacalcidol) is a synthetic analogue which is rapidly converted to the active metabolite.

The action of vitamin D is to increase the absorption of calcium from the gut and to increase the calcium release from bone. If there is a deficiency of vitamin D from the diet, or if vitamin D is not absorbed adequately, or if renal disease prevents the hydroxylation of cholecalciferol to dihydroxycholecalciferol, the bone disease of osteomalacia (q.v.) will result. This is a particularly common condition in the Asian immigrant population in Britain who tend to take a diet low in vitamin D and also tend to avoid sunlight on the skin so that the production of ergocalciferol is impaired.

The treatment of osteomalacia is to provide vitamin D. For low-dose treatment the most widely used preparation is Calcium with vitamin D (B.P.C.).

CALCIFICATION is the process of deposit of lime salts.

CALCITONIN is a hormone produced by the thyroid gland (q.v.) which lowers the concentration of calcium in the blood.

CALCIUM is the metallic element present in chalk and other forms of lime. The chief preparations used in medicine are calcium carbonate (chalk), calcium chloride, calcium gluconate, calcium hydroxide (slaked lime), liquor of calcium hydroxide (lime-water), calcium lactate, and calcium phosphate (see LIME). Although still commonly used in the treatment of chilblains, there is little evidence that calcium is of any real value in this condition. Calcium gluconate is freely soluble in water and is used in conditions in which calcium should be given by injection. Calcium chloride is sometimes used in the resuscitation of patients with cardiopulmonary collapse.

Calcium is a most important element in diet; the chief sources of it are milk and cheese. Calcium is especially needed by the growing child and the pregnant and nursing mother.

The recommended daily intakes of calcium are: 500 mg for children, 700 mg for adolescents, 500–900 mg for adults and 1200 mg for pregnant or nursing mothers.

CALCIUM CARBIMIDE is a drug used in the treatment of alcoholism that has the same action as disulfiram (q.v.) but produces a milder reaction.

CALCIUM-CHANNEL BLOCKERS (OR CAL-CIUM ANTAGONISTS): The influx of calcium is particularly important in the contraction of cardiac and smooth muscle cells. In cardiac muscle it occurs through specialized slow channels during the plateau of the action potential. Analagous channels are important in arterial smooth muscle. The calcium antagonists or calcium-channel blockers inhibit the movement of calcium across the cell membrane. Because they relax smooth muscle they have important applications in the treatment of hypertension and angina of effort. Four calcium antagonists are currently available in the United Kingdom. Verapamil has been available since 1967, nifedipine since 1977, while diltiazem and lidoflazine were introduced in 1984 and Nicardipine in 1986. All these drugs are rapidly and completely absorbed but undergo extensive first-pass metabolism in the liver so that bio-availability is only around 20 per cent. The calcium antagonists are effective in the treatment of angina, both by their action in dilating coronary arteries and also by dilating peripheral arterioles and so reducing cardiac work. They are also effective in the treatment of hypertension by virtue of their effect in dilating arterioles. Their hypotensive effect is additive with that of a beta-blocker. Only verapamil is effective in cardiac arrhythmias and is the drug of choice in terminating supra ventricular tachycardia. These drugs are particularly useful in patients in whom a beta-blocker is contraindicated.

CALCULI is the general name given to concretions in, for example, the bladder, kidneys, gallbladder.

CALIBRE is a talking book service which is available to all blind and handicapped people who can supply a doctor's certificate certifying that they are unable to read printed books in the normal way. Its catalogue contains over 370 books for adults and over 250 for children, and additions are being made at the rate of around three a week. Full details can be obtained from Calibre, Aylesbury, Bucks HP22 5XQ (0296 432339, 81211).

CALLIPER is a two-pronged instrument with pointed ends, for the measurement of diameters, such as that of the pelvis in obstetrics.

CALLIPER SPLINT is one that is applied to the broken leg in such a way that in walking the weight of the body is taken by the hip bone and not by the foot.

CALLOSITIES are thickenings of the outer skin or epidermis. (See CORNS AND BUNIONS.)

CALLUS is the new tissue formed round the ends of a broken bone. (See FRACTURES.)

CALORIE is the name applied to a unit of energy. Two units are called by this name. The small calorie, or gram calorie, is the amount of heat required to raise one gram of water one degree centigrade in temperature. The large Calorie or kilocalorie, which is used in the study of dietetics and physiological processes, is the amount of heat required to raise one kilogram of water one degree centigrade in temperature. The number of Calories required to carry on the processes necessary for life and body warmth, such as the beating of the heart, the movements of the chest in breathing, and the chemical activities of the secreting glands, is, for an adult person of ordinary weight, somewhere in the neighbourhood of 1600 Calories. For ordinary sedentary occupations an individual requires about 2500 Calories, for light muscular work slightly over 3000 Calories, and for hard continuous labour about 4000 Calories daily.

Under the International System of Units (SI) (see WEIGHTS AND MEASURES) the kilocalorie has been replaced by the joule, the abbreviation for which is J (1 kilocalorie=4186·8 J). As the term calorie, however, is so well established in medical writing, it has been retained in this edition. Conversion from Calories (or kilocalories) is made by multiplying by 4·186, but a factor of 4·2 is simpler and accurate enough for all practical purposes.

CALVARIA is another name for the skull cap or vault of the head.

CALYX means a cup-shaped cavity, the term being especially applied to the recesses of the pelvis of the kidney.

CAMPHOR is a solid, crystalline, oily substance distilled from the wood of a species of laurel grown in Japan and Formosa, or made synthetically. Liniment of camphor and camphorated oil (28·5 g of camphor in 228 ml of olive oil) are useful as a mild counter-irritant to produce a warm glow when rubbed into the chest in bronchitis and similar conditions.

CAMPYLOBACTER is a species of microorganism found in farm and pet animals, and there is increasing evidence of its transmission from such sources to man. Outbreaks of infection with it have occurred following the drinking of unpasteurized milk from infected cows and eating undercooked meat and poultry. It causes diarrhoea, and it is considered that it may be responsible for 8 per cent of sporadic cases of infective diarrhoea as a result of the inflammation of the small intestine (enteritis) that it produces. During 1989 over 32,000 cases were reported in England, a reflection of the continuing increase in the diagnosis and reporting of the disease since its implication in gastrointestinal disease was recognized in the mid-1970s.

CANALICULUS means a small channel, and is applied to (*a*) the minute passage leading from the lacrimal pore on each eyelid to the lacrimal sac on the side of the nose; (*b*) any one of the minute canals in bone.

CANCELLOUS is a term applied to loose bony tissues as found in the ends of the long bones.

CANCER is the general term used to refer to a malignant tumour, irrespective of the tissue of origin. 'Malignancy' indicates that (i) the tumour is capable of progressive growth, unrestrained by the capsule of the parent organ and/or (ii) capable of distant spread via lymphatics or the blood stream resulting in development of secondary deposits of tumour known as 'metastases'. Microscopically, cancer cells appear different from the equivalent normal cells in the affected tissue. In particular they may show a lesser degree of differentiation (i.e. they are more 'primitive'), features indicative of a faster proliferative rate and disorganized alignment in relationship to other cells or blood vessels. The diagnosis of cancer usually depends upon the observation of these microscopic features in biopsies, i.e. tissue removed surgically for such examination.

Cancers are classified according to the type of cell from which they are derived as well as the organ of origin. Hence cancers arising within the bronchi, often collectively referred to as 'lung cancer', include both adenocarcinomas (derived from glandular epithelium) and squamous carcinomas (derived from squamous epithelium). Sarcomas are cancers of connective tissue, including bone and cartilage. The behaviour of cancers and their response to therapy vary widely depending on this classification as well as on numerous other factors such as growth rate, differentiation in cell and characteristics and size at the time of presentation. It is entirely wrong to see cancer as a single disease entity with a universally poor prognosis.

Incidence: In most western countries cancer is the second most important cause of death after heart disease and accounts for 20–5 per cent of all deaths. There is wide international variation in the most frequently encountered types of cancer, reflecting the importance of environmental factors in the development of cancer. In the UK as well as the USA, carcinoma of the bronchus (q.v.) is the most common. Since it is usually inoperable at the time of diagnosis, it is even more strikingly the leading cause of cancer deaths. In women, breast cancer is most common, accounting for a quarter of all cancers; nevertheless, fewer than a half of women in whom breast cancer is discovered will die from the disease. Other common sites are as follows: males – colon and rectum, prostate and bladder; females – colon and rectum, uterus, ovary and pancreas.

In England and Wales in 1986 over 205,000 people were registered as suffering from cancers of all types. Over 25,000 of them had lung cancer, over 25,000 had large bowel cancer, nearly 23,000 breast cancer and more than 7,500 uterine cancer. The incidence of cancer varies with age, the older a person is the more likely is he or she to develop the disease: the over 85s have an incidence about nine times greater than those in the 25–44 age group.

Causes of cancer: In most cases the causes of cancer remain unknown. Rapid advances have, however, been made in the past two decades in understanding the differences between cancer cells and normal cells at the genetic level. It is now widely accepted that cancer results from acquired changes in the genetic make-up of a particular cell or group of cells which ultimately lead to a failure of the normal mechanisms regulating their growth. It appears that in most cases a cascade of changes is required for cells to behave in a truly malignant fashion; the critical changes affect specific key genes (q.v.), known as oncogenes, which are involved in growth regulation.

Since small genetic errors occur within cells at all times, most but not all of which are repaired, it follows that some cancers may develop as a result of an accumulation of random changes which cannot be attributed to environmental or other causes. The environmental factors known to cause cancer such as radiation and chemicals (including tar from tobacco, asbestos, etc.) do so by increasing the overall rate of acquired genetic damage. Certain viral infections can induce specific cancers (e.g. Hepatitis B virus and hepatoma, Epstein Barr virus and lymphoma (qq.v.)) probably by inducing alterations in specific genes. Hormones may also be a factor in the development of certain cancers such as those of the prostate and breast. Where there is a particular family tendency to certain types of cancer, it now appears that one or more of the critical genetic abnormalities required for development of that cancer may have been inherited. Where environmental factors such as tobacco smoking or asbestos are known to cause cancer, then health education and preventive measures can reduce the incidence of the relevant cancer.

Treatment: Many cancers can be cured by surgical removal if they are detected early, before there has been spread of significant numbers of tumour cells to distant sites. Important within this group are breast, colon and skin cancer (melanoma). The probability of early detection of certain cancers can be increased by screening programmes in which (ideally) all people at particular risk of development of such cancers are examined at regular intervals. Routine screening for cervical cancer and breast cancer is currently practised in the UK.

If complete surgical removal of the tumour is not possible because of its location or because spread from the primary site has occurred, an operation may nevertheless be helpful to relieve symptoms (e.g. pain) and to reduce the bulk of the tumour remaining to be dealt with by alternative means such as radiotherapy or chemotherapy. In some cases radiotherapy is preferable to surgery and may be curative, for example, in the management of tumours of the larynx or of the uterine cervix. Certain tumours are highly sensitive to chemotherapy and may be cured by the use of chemotherapeutic drugs alone. These include testicular tumours, leukaemias (q.v.), lymphomas (q.v.) and a variety of tumours occurring in childhood. These tend to be rapidly growing tumours composed of primitive cells which are much more vulnerable to the toxic effects of the chemotherapeutic agents than the normal cells within the body.

Unfortunately neither radiotherapy nor currently available chemotherapy provides a curative option for the majority of common cancers if surgical excision is not feasible. New effective treatments in these conditions are urgently needed. Nevertheless the rapidly increasing knowledge of cancer biology will almost certainly lead to novel therapeutic approaches – including probably genetic techniques – at least by the early twenty-first century. Where cure is not possible, there often remains much that can be done for the cancer-sufferer in terms of control of unpleasant symptoms such as pain. Many of the most important recent advances in cancer care relate to such 'palliative' treatment, and include the establishment in the UK of palliative care hospices.

Families and patients can obtain valuable help and advice from Marie Curie Cancer Care, 28 Belgrave Square, London SW1X 8QG (071-235 3325), Cancer Relief Macmillan Fund, Anchor House, 15/19 Britten Street, London SW3 3TZ (071-351 7811), or the British Association of Cancer United Patients, 121–123 Charterhouse Street, London EC1M 6AA (071-608 1661 for information).

CANCRUM ORIS, also called WATER CANKER or NOMA, is a gangrenous ulcer about the mouth which affects weakly children, especially after some severe disease, such as measles. It is due to the growth of bacteria in the tissues.

CANDIDA: CANDIDIASIS or MONILIASIS is an infection due to the fungus *Candida albicans*. It is the most common fungal infection. When it infects the mouth it is called thrush and appears as white patches on the throat and tongue. Although it can occur in any debilitated patient, it is particularly common in individuals on prolonged antibiotic treatment. It is cured by the anti-fungal agent Nystatin given as lozenges so that it is retained in the mouth. Candida infections are also common in skin folds and the vulva. Candida is also a common cause of vaginal infection which presents as a vaginal discharge and responds to Nystatin pessaries. Generalized fungal infection may occur in individuals in whom the immune system is compromised, as in patients with AIDS or patients on immunosuppressive drugs. Such more generalized infections require systemic treatment with the anti-fungal drug ketoconazole given by mouth or amphotericin by intravenous injection.

CANINE TEETH, or EYE-TEETH, (see TEETH).

CANKER is the name applied to small ulcers which form about the mouth and lips as the result of some local irritation, e.g. a jagged tooth, or in a condition of dyspepsia and deteriorated general health. (See MOUTH, DISEASES OF.)

CANNABIS is one of the oldest euphoriants. Cannabis does not cause physical dependence but its abuse leads to passivity, apathy and inertia. Acute adverse effects of cannabis include transient panic reactions and toxic psychoses. The panic reactions are characterized by anxiety, helplessness and loss of control and may be accompanied by florid paranoid thoughts and hallucinations. The toxic psychoses are characterized by the sudden onset of confusion and visual hallucinations. Even at lower doses cannabis can precipitate functional psychoses in vulnerable individuals. The acute physical manifestations of short-term cannabis abuse are conjunctival suffusion and tachycardia.

CANNABIS INDICA consists of the flowering tops of *Cannabis sativa*.

CANNED FOOD, originally popularized in the United States of America, had to overcome considerable prejudice in Great Britain. Such prejudice still persists to a certain extent but, irrespective of the merits of the controversy of fresh versus preserved food, it must be recognized that the advantages of canned food far outweigh the disadvantages. Modern methods of canning are so efficient that not only is the purity of the food preserved but its nutritional value is retained. There is, of course, some loss of vitamin content but this has been much reduced of recent years. Indeed there is probably less loss of vitamins in canning than in average domestic cooking. The further great advantage of canning is that it makes available to many people foodstuffs which otherwise they either would never be able to obtain or could only obtain at certain seasons of the year.

Methods of canning vary according to the foodstuff, but the two essentials of all canning processes are (1) heat treatment of the food and (2) expulsion of all air, after which the can is hermetically sealed. One of the major problems in canning is achieving the optimum temperature that will kill all bacteria but will not affect the nutritive value of the food or spoil its taste. A step to cope with this problem is the introduction of aseptic canning, in which the food is sterilized before it is sealed in sterilized cans. Many canned foods will keep for long periods: e.g. canned fish, meat preparations and soups will keep for two years. These, however, are safer figures. Cans of up to 20 years of age have been found to be in good condition, and the contents quite edible.

DANGERS OF CANNED FOOD: Outbreaks of food poisoning caused by canned food are relatively rare unless the food is contaminated after the container is opened, though, as Aberdeen learned to its cost, outbreaks of typhoid fever can occur as a result of the contamination of the contents of cans cooled in contaminated water. And, in 1979, there were several outbreaks of staphylococcal food poisoning in England due to the consumption of faultily canned corned beef from Brazil. In 1960–63 (inclusive), in England and Wales, 63 of the 749 outbreaks of food poisoning, for which information was available, were due to canned food: canned meat on 44 occasions, canned fish on 13 occasions, and canned vegetables on six occasions. The organism most commonly responsible was the staphylococcus. In other cases decomposition of canned fish or meat may occur due to faulty cans, whilst the acid in fruits or vegetables may lead to erosion of faulty tinplate or soldering, with contamination of the foodstuff with tin or lead.

EXAMINATION OF CANNED FOOD: Most cases of poisoning with canned food could be avoided if cans were examined before use. Canned food is carefully inspected either in the canning factory, if made in this country, or at the port of entry, if imported. About 1·5 per cent of canned meat is rejected in this country. It is a sound rule never to buy a canned food which does not bear a manufacturer's name. Another sound rule is that good cans usually contain good food. Any can which is leaking should be immediately discarded, and much rusting should be regarded with suspicion. 'Blowing', or bulging of the ends of the can, is the most important sign of a faulty can, but this must be differentiated from the bulging of one side of a can due to an indentation in the opposite side. Tapping of a sound can should produce a dull note; if the note is drum-like, this suggests gas-formation in the can due to decomposition. Shaking should produce no sound in a can of meat, but this test, of course, is of no value in the case of canned fruit, which contains syrup. If on opening the can an unpleasant or a stale odour is noted, or if, in the case of meat, there is a loss of firmness of the contents or a fading of the colour, the contents should be discarded.

CANNULA is a tube for insertion into the body, designed to fit tightly round a trocar, a sharp pointed instrument which is withdrawn from the cannula after insertion, so that fluid may run out through the latter.

CANTHARIDES, or SPANISH FLY, is a powder made of the body and wings of a dried beetle, *Cantharis vesicatoria*, which inhabits Spain, Italy, Sicily and Southern Russia.
Action: It is an irritant, first, to the part with which it is brought in contact, and, secondly, to the genital and urinary organs by which it is discharged from the body.
Uses: Its only use is for blistering (see BLISTERS AND COUNTER-IRRITANTS), and it may be applied as a plaster, in a paste, or painted on in ethereal solution called liquor epispasticus but it is seldom used now.

CANTHUS is the name applied to the angle at either end of the aperture between the eyelids.

CAPILLARIES are the minute vessels which join the ends of the arteries to the commencement of the veins. Their walls consist of a single layer of fine, flat transparent cells, bound together at the edges, and the vessels form a meshwork all through the tissues of the body, bathing the latter in blood with only the thin capillary wall interposed, through which gases and fluids readily pass. These vessels are less than 0·025 mm in width. (See CIRCULATION OF THE BLOOD.)

CAPSULE is a term used in several senses in medicine. The term is applied to a soluble case, usually of gelatine, for enclosing small doses of unpleasant medicine. *Enteric-coated capsules*, which have been largely superseded by enteric-coated tablets, are capsules treated in such a manner that the ingredients do not come in contact with the acid stomach contents but are only released when the capsule disintegrates in the alkaline contents of the intestine.

The term is also applied to the fibrous or membranous envelope of various organs, as of the spleen, liver or kidney. It is also applied to the ligamentous bag surrounding various joints and attached by its edge to the bones on either side.

CAPTOPRIL is a drug that has been introduced for the treatment of patients with severe hypertension (q.v.) resistant to other hypertensive agents. It acts by lowering the concentration in the blood of angiotensin II which is one of the factors responsible for high blood-pressure. (See ANGIOTENSIN; RENIN.)

CAPUT MEDUSAE is the term describing the abnormally dilated veins that form round the umbilicus in cirrhosis of the liver.

CAPUT SUCCEDANEUM is the temporary swelling which is sometimes found on the head of the new-born infant. It is due to oedema in and around the scalp, caused by pressure on the head as the child is born. It is of no significance and quickly disappears spontaneously.

CARBACHOL is a drug which stimulates the parasympathetic nervous system. It is given, for example, for paralysis of the gut and for retention of urine due to atony.

CARBAMAZEPINE is a drug which is proving of value in the treatment of trigeminal neuralgia (see TRIGEMINAL NEURALGIA). It is also of value in the treatment of certain cases of epilepsy. Because of its occasional action in causing aplastic anaemia and jaundice it must only be used under careful medical supervision.

CARBARYL is a broad-spectrum insecticide effective against lice. It was introduced because lice began to show resistance to DDT and gamma benzene hexachloride. It is particularly effective against head lice. (See INSECTS IN RELATION TO DISEASE.)

CARBENOXOLONE is a derivative of glycyrrhizinic acid, the active principle of liquorice, which is proving of value in the treatment of gastric ulcer.

CARBIMAZOLE is at present one of the most widely used drugs in the treatment of hyperthyroidism. It acts by interferring with the synthesis of thyroid hormone in the thyroid gland.

CARBOHYDRATE is the term applied to an organic substance in which the hydrogen and oxygen are usually in the proportion to form water. Carbohydrates are all, chemically considered, derivatives of simple forms of sugar and are classified as monosaccharides (e.g. glucose), disaccharides (e.g. cane sugar), polysaccharides (e.g. starch). Many of the cheaper and most important foods are included in this group, which comprises sugars, starches, celluloses and gums. When one of these foods is digested, it is converted into a simple kind of sugar and absorbed in this form. In the disease known as diabetes mellitus (q.v.), the most marked feature consists of an inability on the part of the tissues to assimilate and utilize the carbohydrate material. Each gram of carbohydrate is capable of furnishing slightly over 4 Calories of energy. (See DIET.)

CARBOLIC ACID, or PHENOL, precursor of all antiseptics, is a coal-tar preparation that was first introduced into medicine by Lord Lister.

Carbolic acid first paralyses and then destroys all forms of life, having a specially destructive action upon lowly organisms like bacteria. It has a softening action upon tissues, pus, etc., and it also vaporizes readily, so that it has much greater penetrating power than alcohol and other powerful antiseptics. It has been superseded by less harmful antiseptics, though it is used in calamine lotion for its anaesthetic effect.

CARBON DIOXIDE, or CARBONIC ACID, is the gas formed by the tissues and exhaled by the lungs (see AIR and VENTILATION). It effervesces from aerated waters and sparkling wines, and is used in baths for stimulation to the skin. Carbon dioxide in cylinders, combined with oxygen, is used to control breathing in anaesthesia and in cases of carbon monoxide poisoning.

CARBON DIOXIDE SNOW is formed when carbon dioxide (CO_2), stored under pressure in a cylinder, is allowed to escape through a small nozzle. This sudden expansion lowers its temperature to about $-70\ ^\circ$C and the CO_2 is obtained as a white powder or 'snow', which is then compressed into a cake or tube for application to the skin. It is a most effective method of freezing a localized area, and is commonly used in the treatment of warts (q.v.).

CARBON MONOXIDE is a colourless and odourless gas, the presence of which in a room is undetectable by the occupants. Hence its danger because it has 300 times the affinity for oxygen that haemoglobin (q.v.) has. It converts haemoglobin into carboxyhaemoglobin, and thereby deprives the tissues of the body of oxygen, as there is no haemoglobin left to pick up oxygen in the lungs and carry it throughout the body. As the gas is odourless, the occupants of the room – or garage – have no idea that they are breathing it. The result is that they become unconscious in the contaminated atmosphere and, all too often, by the time they are found, they are dead. Carbon monoxide has a special action on the ganglia at the base of the brain, and, if sufficient amounts are inhaled, permanent destructive changes occur in this vital part of the nervous system. What makes carbon monoxide poisoning all the more dangerous is its insidious onset. One of the commonest causes of carbon monoxide poisoning used to be coal gas but this risk has been brought under control in Britain since natural gas was introduced; this contains no carbon monoxide. Natural gas is not absolutely safe, however, because when burned in the absence of sufficient oxygen, or, whenever, for any reason, combustion is incomplete, carbon monoxide is formed. The risk is particularly high with water heaters in inadequately ventilated bathrooms. Care about maintaining adequate ventilation must be observed with all forms of heating derived from carbon-containing fuel. Perhaps the greatest risk in this respect today is from the use of oil heaters in rooms in which all sources of ventilation, such as windows and ventilators, have, in effect, been hermetically sealed. This is one of the major reasons why deaths in the home from carbon monoxide poisoning, other than piped gas, have increased. The exhaust gas of petrol vehicles is also dangerous. This is why the engine of a car must *never* be switched on in a garage unless the garage doors are open. The main manifestations of carbon monoxide poisoning are shown in the table below. One of the most striking signs of carbon monoxide poisoning is the cherry-red appearance of the victim's face. This is due to the large amount of carboxyhaemoglobin in the blood.

Carbon monoxide, which has a deleterious effect on arteries, aggravating the arterial disease which occurs in high blood-pressure (see ESSENTIAL HYPERTENSION) and coronary thrombosis (q.v.), is present in cigarette smoke.

Degree of saturation of haemoglobin with carbon monoxide per cent	Signs and symptoms
0 to 10	No symptoms
10 to 20	Tightness across the forehead
	Possibly headache
	Flushed skin
	Yawning
20 to 30	Headache
	Dizziness
	Palpitations on exercise
30 to 40	Severe headache
	Weakness
	Dizziness
	Nausea
	Collapse (possibly)
40 to 50	As above, with increased respiratory rate and pulse rate, and more possibility of collapse
50 to 60	Syncope
	Coma
	Cheyne-Stokes' respiration
60 to 70	Coma
	Weakened action of the heart and breathing
	Death imminent or actually takes place
70 to 80	Respiratory failure
	Death
90	Immediate arrest of the heart

The manifestations of carbon monoxide poisoning, according to the amount of carbon monoxide in the blood. The limit of safety is 18 to 20 per cent

Treatment of carbon monoxide poisoning consists of the immediate removal of the victim into the open air, followed by, and if available, the inhalation of oxygen and carbon dioxide. In this context 'immediate' means 'instant'.

CARBOXYHAEMOGLOBINAEMIA is the term applied to the state of the blood in carbon monoxide poisoning, in which this gas combines with the haemoglobin, displacing oxygen from it. (See CARBON MONOXIDE.)

CARBUNCLE like a boil, is an infection of a hair follicle and sebaceous gland or of a sweat gland, but unlike a boil it does not remain localized but spreads more deeply. The infecting organism is usually a staphylococcus. (See BOILS; KIDNEYS, DISEASES OF.)

CARCINOGENESIS is the means or method whereby the changes responsible for the induction of cancer are brought about.

CARCINOMA is a type of cancer (q.v.).

CARCINOMATOSIS: The spread of cancer cells from their original site of growth to other tissues in the body. Such a spread of cancer, which takes place mainly via blood and lymph vessels, is usually fatal.

CARDIA is a term applied to the upper opening of the stomach which lies immediately behind the heart.

CARDIAC ARREST occurs when the pumping action of the heart stops. This may be because the heart stops beating (see ASYSTOLE) or because the heart muscle starts contracting too fast to pump effectively (ventricular systole, the period when the heart contracts). Coronary thrombosis is the most frequent cause of arrest. Irreversible brain damage and death result without prompt treatment. Heart massage, defibrillation and artificial respiration, are customary treatment. Other causes of cardiac arrest are respiratory arrest, anaphylactic shock, and electrocution. (See APPENDIX: BASIC FIRST AID: cardiac/respiratory arrest.)

CARDIAC CATHETERIZATION: A diagnostic procedure in which a tube is inserted into a blood vessel and threaded through to the chambers of the heart to monitor blood flow, blood pressure, blood chemistry, and the output of the heart, and to take a sample of heart tissue. It is only performed for life-threatening conditions.

CARDIAC CYCLE: The various sequential movements of the heart that comprise the rhythmic relaxation and expansion of the heart muscles as first the atria contract and force the blood into the ventricles (diastole) which then contract (systole) to pump the blood round the body.

CARDIAC DISEASE (see HEART DISEASES).

CARDIAC MASSAGE is the procedure used to restart the action of the heart if it is suddenly arrested. For long the only recognized method of doing this was by opening the chest wall and massaging the heart directly by hand. This is perfectly feasible if the heart stops beating during an operation. Elsewhere, however, it is seldom a practicable proposition.

Recently it has been shown that in many cases the arrested heart can be made to start beating again by rhythmic compression of the chest wall.

This is done by placing the patient on a hard surface – a table or the floor – and then placing the heel of the hand over the lower part of the sternum and compressing the chest wall firmly, but not too forcibly, at the rate of 60 to 80 times a minute. At the same time artificial respiration must be started by the mouth-to-mouth method. (See APPENDIX: BASIC FIRST AID.)

CARDIAC MUSCLE: The muscle, unique to the heart, which comprises the walls of the atria and ventricles. It consists of long broadening cells (fibres) with special physiological characteristics which enable them to keep contracting and expanding indefinitely.

CARDIAC OUTPUT: The volume of blood pumped out by the ventricles during each cardiac cycle.

CARDIAC PACEMAKER: The rate and rhythm of the heart are controlled by a small collection of specialized nervous tissue known as the sinuatrial node, situated at the base of the heart (see HEART). This is the natural pacemaker of the heart – or cardiac pacemaker. When the impulse sent out by this pacemaker cannot reach all parts of the heart (a condition known as heart-block), the heart either stops or contracts in an irregular manner. (See HEART DISEASES.)

In these cases the natural pacemaker can be replaced by an artificial pacemaker, which, for all practical purposes, is a battery which stimulates the heart and allows it to beat at normal speeds. Most pacemakers are powered by mercury cells. Batteries powered by lithium-iodide batteries are also available, as well as an isotope-powered one, the potential longevity of which is 20 to 30 years, compared with two years for mercury batteries and 10 years for lithium batteries. The majority of cardiac pacemaker units are normally adjusted to deliver 65 to 75 impulses a minute. The pacemaker is either fixed to the outside of the chest or implanted in the armpit, and connnected to an electrode catheter which is passed through the main vein in the neck, into the heart. Approximately one person in every 2000 of the population in the United Kingdom has a pacemaker.

Under the Motor Vehicles (Driving Licences) Amendment Regulations 1973, which came into force on January 1, 1974, patients with heart disease whose condition has been brought under control by the fitting of a pacemaker can be given a licence to drive provided they satisfy the following conditions: (a) that their driving vehicle is not likely to be a source of danger to the public; (b) that the applicant has made adequate arrangements to receive regular medical supervision by a cardiologist throughout the currency of the licence and is complying with these arrangements.

There are many possible sources of electrical interference with pacemakers. These include the anti-theft devices in shops and libraries, and airport weapon detectors. Surgical diathermy is a common source of interference. Short-wave heat treatment of the type used in physiotherapy departments should not be applied to pacemaker patients. Inhibition of what is known as a demand pacemaker by low frequency acupuncture has been reported, and some dental apparatus, including the ultrasonic cleaner, is a potential danger. Over-all, however, the risks from interference are very slight. Their efficacy is demonstrated by the report from Guy's Hospital of pacemaker patients who have achieved county standard at athletics, competitive swimmers and scuba divers as well as many golfers.

CARDIAC TAMPONADE: Compression of the heart due to abnormal accumulation of fluid within the fibrous covering of the heart (pericardium). The result is irregular rhythm and death if the fluid is not removed.

CARDIOANGIOGRAPHY means rendering the outline of the heart visible on an X-ray film by injecting a radio-opaque substance into it.

CARDIOLOGY is the term applied to that branch of medical science devoted to the study of the diseases of the heart.

CARDIOMYOPATHIES are diseases of heart muscle of unknown cause. There are three distinct varieties: (1) *Hypertrophic cardiomyopathy* is characterized by massive ventricular hypertrophy. This hypertrophied muscle is not efficient and cannot relax adequately so that the ventricles do not fill properly during diastole. (2) *Congestive cardiomyopathy* is characterized by dilatation of both ventricles causing severe impairment of contraction. (3) *Restrictive cardiomyopathy* – organic material collects around the endocardium and myocardium which restricts the inflow of blood to the ventricles.

The disorder usually presents with congestive cardiac failure for which there does not appear to be a known cause.

CARDIOPLEGIA: A procedure whereby the heart is stopped by reducing its temperature (hypothermia), by injecting the muscle with a solution of salts or by electrostimulation. This enables surgeons to operate safely on the heart.

CARDIOPULMONARY BYPASS: A procedure in which the body's circulation of blood is kept going when the heart is intentionally stopped to enable heart surgery to be carried out. A heart-lung machine substitutes for the heart's pumping action and the blood is oxygenated at the same time.

CARDIOSPASM means the spasmodic contraction of the muscle surrounding the opening of the oesophagus into the stomach: also termed *achalasia of the cardia*. (See OESOPHAGUS, DISEASES OF.)

CARDIOVASCULAR SYSTEM: This refers to the whole circulatory system: the heart, the systemic circulation (the arteries and veins of the body) and the pulmonary circulation (the arteries and veins of the lungs). Blood circulates throughout the cardiovascular system bringing oxygen and nutrients to the tissues and removing carbon dioxide and other waste products.

CARDIOVERSION: A way of reinstating the heart's normal rhythm in patients with an abnormally fast or irregular beat. A carefully timed direct-current shock is administered to the chest wall of a patient under general anaesthetic.

CARIES, dental decay, is the material remaining after the calcified structure of the tooth has been removed in dental disease. This is probably initiated by bacteria. As the decay is removed a hole develops and the tooth may collapse.

CARMINATIVES are preparations to relieve flatulence, and any resulting griping, by the bringing up of wind, or eructation (q.v.). Their essential constituent is an aromatic volatile oil, usually of vegetable extraction. As in the case of bitters, their precise mode of action is not known, but in practice, when swallowed, they induce a pleasant taste which may be accompanied by an increased flow of saliva. This is followed by a sensation of warmth as they are swallowed, and sooner or later there ensues the bringing up of wind. There is a large variety of carminatives, some of which are referred to elsewhere, such as caraway, cardamon, chamomile, cinnamon, cloves, dill, ginger, nutmeg and peppermint. Most of them are now used more for their flavouring effects either in medicine or in the kitchen, but, again as in the case of bitters, if used in moderation in correct dosage, they can undoubtedly help the individual to renew his or her interest in food, and thereby increase, or at least restore, his interest in life. Whether this is accompanied by the bringing up of wind is incidental.

CARNEOUS MOLE is an ovum which has died in the early months of pregnancy. It usually requires no treatment and evacuates itself.

CAROTENE is a colouring matter of carrots, other plants, butter and yolk of egg, and is the precursor of vitamin A, which is formed from carotene in the liver. (See VITAMIN.)

CAROTID BODY is a small reddish-brown structure measuring 5 to 7 × 2·5 to 4 millimetres, situated one on each side of the neck, where the carotid artery divides into the internal and external carotid arteries. Its main function is in controlling breathing so that an adequate supply of oxygen is maintained to the tissues of the body. Oxygen levels are controlled by a reflex operating between the carotid body and the respiratory centre in the brain.

CARPAL TUNNEL SYNDROME is a condition characterized by attacks of pain and tingling in the first three or four fingers of one or both hands, which usually occur at night. It is caused by pressure on the median nerve as it passes under the strong ligament that lies across the front of the wrist. It often responds to rest induced by fixing the wrist in a plaster splint. If it does not respond to this treatment, the pressure is relieved by surgical division of the compressing ligament.

CARPUS is the Latin term for the wrist, composed of eight small bones firmly joined together with ligaments, but capable of a certain amount of sliding movement over one another. (See WRIST.)

CARRIERS OF DISEASE (see INFECTION).

CARTILAGE is a hard but pliant substance forming parts of the skeleton, e.g. the cartilages of the ribs, of the larynx and of the ears. Microscopically, cartilage is found to consist of cells arranged in twos or in rows, and embedded in a ground-glass-like material devoid of blood-vessels and nerves. The end of every long bone has a smooth layer of cartilage on it where it forms a joint with other bones (articular cartilage), and in young persons up to about the age of sixteen there is a plate of cartilage (epiphyseal cartilage) running right across the bone about 12 mm (half an inch) from each end. The latter, by constantly thickening and changing into bone, causes the increase in length of the bone. (See BONE.) In some situations there is found a combination of cartilage and fibrous tissue, as in the discs between the vertebrae of the spine. This fibro-cartilage, as it is known, combines the pliability of fibrous tissue with the elasticity of cartilage. (For cartilages of the knee, see KNEE.)

CARUNCLE is the name applied to any small fleshy eminence, whether normal or abnormal.

CASEATION is a process which takes place in the tissues in tuberculosis and some other chronic diseases. The central part of a diseased area, instead of changing into pus and so forming an abscess, changes to a firm cheese-like mass which may next be absorbed or may be converted into a calcareous deposit and fibrous tissue, and so healing results with the formation of a scar.

CASEIN is that part of milk which forms cheese or curds. It is produced by the union of a substance, caseinogen, dissolved in the milk, with lime salts also dissolved in the milk, the union being produced by the action of rennin, a ferment from the stomach of the calf. The same change occurs in the human stomach as the first step in the digestion of milk, and therefore when milk is vomited curdled it merely shows that digestion has begun.

CASTRATION is the operation for removal of the testicles or ovaries.

CASTS of hollow organs are found in various diseases. Membranous casts of the air passages are found in diphtheria and in one form of bronchitis, and are sometimes coughed up entire. Casts of the interior of the bowels are passed in cases of mucous colitis associated with constipation, and casts of the microscopic tubules in the kidneys passed in the urine form one of the surest signs of glomerulonephritis.

CATALEPSY is a term applied to a nervous affection characterized by the sudden suspension of sensation and volition, accompanied by a peculiar rigidity of the whole, or of certain muscles, of the body. The exciting cause of an attack is usually mental emotion operating either suddenly, as in the case of a fright, or more gradually in the way of prolonged depression. Sometimes the typical features of the disease are exhibited in a state of complete insensibility, together with a statue-like appearance of the body, which will retain any attitude it may be made to assume during the continuance of the attack. In this condition the whole organic and vital functions appear to be reduced to the lowest possible limit consistent with life, and to such a degree as to simulate actual death. The attack may be of short duration, passing off within a few minutes. It may, however, last for many hours, and in rare instances persist for several days; and it is conceivable that in such cases the appearances presented might be mistaken for real death, as is alleged to have happened occasionally. Catalepsy is sometimes associated with epilepsy and with serious mental disease such as schizophrenia. From what has been stated it follows that the successful treatment of such a disease as catalepsy must depend upon the due recognition of both its corporeal and mental relations. (See ECSTASY; HYSTERIA; SLEEP.)

CATAPLEXY is a condition in which the patient has a sudden attack of muscular weakness affecting the whole body. (See also NARCOLEPSY.)

CATARACT: An opacity of the lens.
Classification: One method is by the cause of cataract formation:
AGE RELATED (senile): With age, changes occur within the lens which render it gradually opaque. These changes begin at about the age of fifty years and are progressive at a variable rate during later life. Changes include lens protein aggregation, increased amounts of insoluble lens protein and increased pigmentation of the lens nucleus. These changes occur in eyes that are otherwise perfectly healthy (see AGE, NATURAL CHANGES IN).
TRAUMA (see EYE, DISEASE AND INJURIES): This is the commonest cause of monocular cataract in the young. Cataract may be the result of penetrating or blunt injury, infra-red energy, electric shock or ionizing radiation (the commonest cause is following irradiation of an ocular tumour).
METABOLIC DISORDERS: *Diabetes* can produce two types of cataract. The commoner is the 'age related' cataract which develops at an earlier age and is more rapidly progressive in diabetics than in non-diabetics. True diabetic cataracts can occur at any age. Other metabolic conditions associated with cataracts include galactosaemia, Fabry's Disease, Wilson's Disease and hypoparathyroidism.
DRUGS can cause cataracts, in particular steroids.
ASSOCIATED WITH OTHER EYE CONDITIONS, e.g. uveitis, acute glaucoma, retinitis pigmentosa.
CONGENITAL CATARACTS: These may be *hereditary*, i.e. passed on genetically from one generation to the next. They may be present due to infection of the patient's mother during pregnancy. Typically *rubella* can cause cataracts in this way. Certain congenital syndromes are associated with cataracts, e.g. Down's syndrome.

The acquired form of cataracts results in a progressive deterioration in vision. In senile cataracts this occurs fairly slowly over months or years. Traumatic cataracts can develop over a few hours with subsequent rapid loss of vision. Congenital cataracts are usually detected in routine examination of a child, or because there is a family history. Treatment of a cataract is undertaken for a variety of reasons: (*a*) in order to improve vision; (*b*) where the cataract is causing or is likely to cause complications that may damage the eye with consequent permanent loss of vision; (*c*) where the presence of a cataract may hinder treatment of other eye disorders because the doctor cannot see well enough through the cataract. Cataracts do not need to be removed just because they are there.
TYPES OF CATARACT SURGERY: The two common forms of cataract extraction are (i) *intracapsular extraction*: the zonule is first dissolved with chymotripsin (an enzyme) and the whole lens (capsule, cortex and nucleus) is removed in its

entirely by means of a cryoprobe (a device whose tip can be frozen so that it sticks to the lens). This method was the more common until a few years ago. (ii) *extracapsular extraction*: a small hole is made in the anterior lens capsule; the cortex and the nucleus are then removed through this small hole, leaving the posterior part of the lens capsule in place. This is now the commoner method of surgery. Modern surgery requires the use of an operating microscope. Surgery can be performed under local or general anaesthetic and the length of stay in hospital varies from 24 hours to a few days in uncomplicated cases. An estimated 500,000 cataract operations are performed in the USA each year. Having had a cataract removed the eye is made long sighted. An alternative means of focusing light on the retina must be found. The three usual alternatives are cataract glasses, contact lenses or a perspex intra-ocular lens (or implant). Implants by and large give the best results, but are not suitable for all patients.

CATARRH is a state of irritation of the mucous membranes, particularly those of the air passages, associated with a copious secretion of mucus. This complaint, so prevalent in damp and cold weather, usually begins as a nasal catarrh or coryza, with a feeling of weight about the forehead and some difficulty in breathing through the nose, increased on lying down. Fits of sneezing, accompanied with a profuse watery discharge from the nostrils and eyes, soon follow, while the sense of smell and to some extent that of taste become considerably impaired. Sore throat, fever and bronchial irritation may occur, causing hoarseness and cough. Sometimes the vocal apparatus becomes so much inflamed (laryngeal catarrh) that temporary loss of voice results. After two or three days the symptoms begin to abate, though sometimes infection spreads to the lungs. (See BRONCHITIS; CHILLS AND COLDS.)

CATATONIA is a symptom of mental disease in which the patient remains rigidly in the same position, behaving very much like a statue. Catatonia minor is a term applied to the group of symptoms occurring in the mental disease, schizophrenia, in which the patient shows peculiar mannerisms, continuing to repeat the same words or actions. (See MENTAL ILLNESS.)

CATECHOLAMINES are substances produced in the body from the dietary amino-acids (q.v.), phenylalanine and tyrosine. They include adrenaline (q.v.) and noradrenaline (q.v.).

CATGUT is used in surgery for tying cut arteries and stitching wounds. It is made from the fibrous coat of the intestines of animals, especially of the sheep, requires very careful purification, and in the tissues is gradually absorbed – in about five to ten days – as it is itself an animal substance. Hardened catgut is catgut which has been treated with a suitable hardening agent to prolong the time taken for it to be absorbed; catgut hardened by treatment with chromium compounds is known as chromicized catgut.

CATHARTICS are substances which produce an evacuation of the bowels. (See PURGATIVES.)

CATHETERS are hollow tubes used for passing into various organs of the body, either for investigational purposes or to give some form of treatment.
Varieties: *Cardiac catheters* are introduced through a vein in the arm and passed into the heart in order to diagnose some of the more obscure forms of congenital heart disease, and often as a preliminary to operating on the heart. *Endotracheal catheters* are used to pass down the trachea into the lungs, usually in the course of administering anaesthetics (q.v.). *Eustachian catheters* are small catheters that are passed along the floor of the nose into the Eustachian tube (q.v.) in order to inflate the ear. *Nasal catheters* are tubes passed through the nose into the stomach to feed a patient who cannot swallow: so-called nasal feeding. *Rectal catheters* are catheters passed into the rectum in order to give injections. *Suprapubic catheters* are catheters passed into the bladder through an incision in the lower abdominal wall just above the pubis, either to allow urine to drain away from the bladder, or to wash out an infected bladder. *Ureteric catheters* are small catheters that are passed up the ureter into the pelvis of the kidney, usually to determine the state of the kidney, either by obtaining a sample of urine direct from the kidney or to inject a radio-opaque substance preliminary to X-raying the kidney. (See PYELOGRAPHY.) *Urethral catheters* are catheters that are passed along the urethra into the bladder, either to draw off urine or to wash out the bladder. It is these last three types of catheters that are most extensively used.
Sterilization: The cleaning and sterilization of catheters is of paramount importance. After use, catheters must be carefully cleaned at once. This is done by rinsing them through with running water, and then syringing through with cetrimide. The outside is then well washed with soap and water. Rubber, silver and glass catheters are sterilized by being placed in boiling water. Once the water has again come to the boil, the catheter is boiled for ten minutes. Plastic (vinyl) catheters can be sterilized by boiling, or by autoclaving at 120 °C at 15 pounds pressure for fifteen minutes, after which they must be removed at once from the autoclave. The introduction of disposable catheters, which are only used once and then discarded, has led to their being used to an increasing extent. They are sterilized by gamma radiation.
Uses: The use of any form of catheterization of the bladder, whether urethral, ureteric or suprapubic, must be made under the strictest possible sterile conditions. Not only must the catheter be sterilized, but the hands of those

passing the catheter must be prepared with the same care as for a surgical operation, and the opening of the urethra must be sterilized with the utmost care so as to avoid passing any infection into the bladder. The greatest gentleness must be exercised in introducing the catheter. This applies particularly in passing a urethral catheter in men, in whom the urethra is so much longer than in women.

'CAT SCANNER' (see CT SCANNER).

CAT-SCRATCH FEVER is a disease, probably due to a virus, which is characterized by enlargement of the glands. In spite of the name, there is a history of a cat scratch in only about half the cases; in others the infection is acquired through a puncture of the skin by a splinter or thorn. The glandular swelling is usually slight and of short duration, but in some cases may go on to abscess formation which requires aspiration. The infection is not controlled by penicillin.

CAUDA: A tail or a tail-like structure. For example, the cauda equina is a collection of nerve roots from the lumbar sacral and coccygeal spinal nerves that runs down inside the spinal column until it leaves it through their respective openings.

CAUL is the piece of amnion which sometimes covers a child when he or she is born.

CAULIFLOWER EAR is the term applied to the distortion of the external ear produced by repeated injury in sport. Initially it is due to a haematoma (q.v.) in the auricle (see EAR). To prevent deformity the blood should be drawn off from this haematoma as soon as possible, and a firm pressure bandage then applied. Subsequent protection can be given to the ear by covering it with a few layers of two-way stretch strapping wound round the head.

CAUSALGIA: A severe burning pain in a limb in which the sympathetic and somatic nerves have been damaged.

CAUSTICS AND CAUTERIES are used to destroy tissues, the former by chemical action, the latter by their high temperature.

CAVERNOUS BREATHING indicates a peculiar quality of the respiratory sounds heard on auscultation over a cavity in the lung.

CAVERNOUS SINUS: A channel for venous blood placed either side of the sphenoid bone at the base of the skull behind the eye sockets. Blood drains into it from the eye, the nose, the brain and part of the cheek and leaves via the internal jugular and facial veins.

CEFOXITIN is a semi-synthetic antibiotic, given by injection, which is proving of value in the treatment of infections due to Gram-negative micro-organisms such as *Proteus* which are resistant to many other antibiotics.

CELLS are the microscopic particles which build up the tissues, of which they are the smallest structural divisions. There are around 10 billion in the human body.

Every cell consists essentially of a cell-body of soft albuminous material called cytoplasm, in which lies a kernel or nucleus which seems to direct all the activities of the cell. Within the nucleus may be seen a minute body, the nucleolus; and there may or may not be a cell-envelope around all. (See also MITOCHONDRIA.)

Cells vary much in size, ranging in the human body from 0·0025 mm to about 0·025 mm.

All animals and plants consist at first of a single cell (the egg-cell, or *ovum*), which begins to develop when fertilized by the sperm-cell derived from the opposite sex. Development begins by a division into two new cells, then into four, and so on till a large mass is formed. These cells then arrange themselves into layers, and form various tubes, rods, and masses which represent in the embryo the organs of the fully developed animal. (See FETUS.)

When the individual organs have been laid down on a scaffolding of cells, these gradually change in shape and in chemical composition. The cells in the nervous system send out long processes to form the nerves, those in the

1	mitochondria	golgi apparatus	8
2	nucleus	centrosphere	7
3	inclusion bodies	nucleolus	6
		caryosome	5
		vacuole	4

A semi-diagrammatic representation of a cell.

muscles become long and striped in appearance, and those which form fat become filled with fat droplets which distend the cells. Further, they begin to produce, between one another, the substances which give the various tissues their special character. Thus, in the future bones, some cells deposit lime salts, and others form cartilage; while, in tendons, they produce long white fibres of a gelatinous substance. In some organs the cells change little: thus the liver consists of columns of large cells packed together, while many cells, like the white blood corpuscles, retain their primitive characters almost entire.

Thus cells are the active agents in forming the body, and they have a similar function in repairing its wear and tear. Tumours (q.v.), and especially malignant tumours, have a highly cellular structure, the cells being of an embryonic type, or, at best, forming poor imitations of the tissues in which they grow.

CELLULITIS means an inflammation taking place in cellular tissue and usually refers to infection in the subcutaneous tissue. The word is erroneously used in the slimming business to refer to excess fatty tissue in the arms, buttocks and thighs. (See ABSCESS; ERYSIPELAS.)

CELLULOSE is a carbohydrate substance forming the skeleton of most plant structures. It is colourless, transparent, insoluble in water and is practically unaffected by digestion. In vegetable foods it therefore adds to the bulk, but it is of no value as a food-stuff. It is found in practically a pure state in cotton-wool.

CEMENT (see TEETH).

CEMENT BURNS arise as a result of prolonged contact of the skin with builders' cement. They are due to quicklime which constitutes 65 per cent of cement. As they are chemical, and not thermal, burns, the victim feels no immediate pain and therefore allows the contact to persist. The precautions that should be taken include adequate protection of the hands and feet, and avoidance of prolonged contact of the skin with cement.

CENSOR is a term applied to the mental influence which prevents certain subconscious thoughts and wishes from coming into consciousness unless they are disguised so as to be unrecognizable.

CENTENARIANS (see EXPECTATION OF LIFE).

CENTRAL NERVOUS SYSTEM: This comprises the nervous tissue of the brain and spinal cord but does *not* include the cranial and spinal nerves and the autonomic nervous system. This latter group makes up the peripheral nervous system.

CENTRAL VENOUS PRESSURE: The pressure of blood within the right atrium of the heart as measured by a catheter and manometer.

CENTRE is a term applied to a collection of nerve cells which give off nerve fibres and control some particular function: e.g. the speech centre and the vision centre in the brain.

CEPHALOSPORINS have been described as 'a valuable and versatile group of broad-spectrum, non-toxic antibiotics'. Most of them available at the moment are semi-synthetic derivatives of cephalosporin C, an antibiotic originally derived from a sewage outfall in Sardinia. They include cephaloridine, cephalothin, cephalexin, cephradine, and cephalozin. The term is sometimes used to include a group of semi-synthetic antibiotics with a comparable range of antibacterial action, but derived from a species of streptomyces. Strictly speaking this group, which includes cefoxitin, should be described as cephamycins. The indications for the use of individual members of the group vary. Some are active when given by mouth. Some have to be given by injection. One of their valuable features is that they are sometimes active against micro-organisms that have become resistant to penicillin, such as the gonococcus.

CERATE is a medicinal preparation, intended for external application, made with a basis consisting of wax in whole or in part which can be spread on the skin without melting: e.g. camphor cerate, compound menthol cerate.

CEREAL is the term applied to any plant of the nature of grass bearing an edible seed. The important cereals are wheat, oats, barley, maize, rice and millet. Along with these are usually included tapioca (derived from the cassava plant), sago (derived from the pith of the sago palm) and arrowroot (derived from the root of a West Indian plant), all of which consist almost entirely of starch. Semolina, farola and macaroni are preparations of wheat.

	per cent
Water	10 to 12
Protein	10 to 12
Carbohydrate	65 to 75
Fat	0·5 to 8
Mineral matter	2

Composition of cereals

Cereals consist predominantly of carbohydrate. They are therefore an excellent source of energy. On the other hand, their deficiency in protein and fat means that to provide a balanced diet, they must be supplemented by other foods rich in protein and fat, such as meat, milk and eggs.

	Water	Protein	Fat	Carbo-hydrate	Cellu-lose	Ash
Wheat	12·0	11·0	1·7	71·2	2·2	1·9
Oatmeal	7·2	14·2	7·3	65·9	3·5	1·9
Barley	12·3	10·1	1·9	69·5	3·8	2·4
Rye	11·0	10·2	2·3	72·3	2·1	2·1
Maize	12·5	9·7	5·4	68·9	2·0	1·5
Rice (polished)	12·4	6·9	0·4	79·4	0·4	0·5
Millet	12·3	10·4	3·9	68·3	2·9	2·2
Buck-wheat	13·0	10·2	2·2	61·3	11·1	2·2

Composition of certain cereals.

CEREBELLUM AND CEREBRUM (see BRAIN).

CEREBRAL PALSY is the term used to describe a group of conditions characterized by varying degrees of paralysis and occurring in infancy or early childhood. In some 80 per cent of cases this takes the form of spastic paralysis: hence the lay description of them as 'spastics'. The incidence is believed to be around 2 or 2·5 per 1000 of the childhood community. In the majority of cases the abnormality dates from before birth or occurs during birth. Among the pre-natal factors are some genetic malformation of the brain, a congenital defect of the brain, or some adverse effect on the fetal brain as by infection during pregnancy. Among the factors during birth that may be responsible are trauma to the child or prolonged lack of oxygen such as can occur during a difficult labour. This last factor is considered by some to be the most important single factor. In some 10 to 15 per cent of cases the condition is acquired after birth, when it may be due to kernicterus (q.v.), infection of the brain, cerebral thrombosis or embolism, or trauma. The congenital form is commoner in boys than girls, and a high proportion of the cases are first-born children.

The disease manifests itself in many ways. The victim may be spastic or flaccid, or the slow, writhing involuntary movements, known as athetosis, may be the predominant feature. These involuntary movements often disappear during sleep and may be controlled, or even abolished, in some cases by training the child to relax. The paralysis varies tremendously. It may involve the limbs on one side of the body (hemiplegia), both lower limbs (paraplegia), or all four limbs (tetraplegia). Mental subnormality is not uncommon.

The outlook for life is good, only the more severely affected cases dying in infancy. Although there is no cure, much can be done to help these unfortunate children, particularly if the condition is detected at an early stage. Little can be done to help those who have severe mental subnormality, but much can be done for those with normal intelligence by team work, giving attention to education, physiotherapy, occupational therapy and speech training. In this way many of these handicapped children are now reaching adult life as useful members of the community. Much help in dealing with these children can be obtained from the Spastics Society, 12 Park Crescent, London W1N 4EQ (071-636 5020); and the Scottish Council for Spastics, 22 Corstorphine Road, Edinburgh EH12 6HP (031-337 9876).

CEREBROSPINAL FEVER is another name for cerebrospinal meningitis. (See under MENINGITIS.)

CEREBROSPINAL FLUID is the fluid within the ventricles of the brain and bathing its surface and that of the spinal cord. It is normally under a pressure of 60 to 150 mm of water and contains 0 to 5 lymphocytes per cm^3. In each 100 millilitres of cerebrospinal fluid there are normally between 10 to 20 mg of protein (mostly albumin), 50 to 80 mg of glucose, and 725 to 750 mg of chlorides.

CEREBROVASCULAR ACCIDENT (see STROKE.)

CERUMEN is the name for the wax-like secretion found in the external ear.

CERVICAL means anything pertaining to the neck, or to the neck of the womb.

CERVICAL CANCER: Cancer of the cervix, the neck of the womb, is one of the most common cancers affecting women throughout the world. In some areas its incidence is increasing. This cancer has clearly identifiable precancerous stages with abnormal changes occurring in the cells on the surface of the cervix. These changes can be detected by a cervical smear test. Early cancer can be cured by diathermy, laser treatment, electrocoagulation or cryosurgery. If the disease has spread into the body of the cervix or beyond, more extensive surgery and possibly radiotherapy may be needed. The cure rate is 95 per cent if treated in the early stages but may fall as low as 10 per cent in some severe cases. About 4500 patients are diagnosed as having cervical cancer every year in the United Kingdom and about 2500 die from it. The sexual behaviour of a woman and her male partners influences the chances of getting this cancer. The earlier a woman has sexual intercourse and the more partners she has, the greater is the risk of developing the disease.

CERVICAL SMEAR: This test detects abnormal changes in the cells of the cervix and this enables an affected woman to have early treatment. The National Health Service has arrangements to check women regularly. A woman's first test should be within six months of her first experience of intercourse and thereafter at three-yearly intervals for the rest of her life. The test is simple, with some cells being scraped off the cervix with a spatula and the tissue then being examined microscopically.

CERVICAL VERTEBRAE: The seven bones of the top end of the backbone that form the neck. The first cervical vertebra is the atlas and this articulates with the base of the skull. The axis is the second vertebra, which contains a shaft of bone that allows the atlas to rotate on it, thus permitting the head to turn.

CERVICITIS means inflammation of the cervix uteri or neck of the womb.

CERVIX UTERI is the neck of the womb or uterus and is placed partly above and partly within the vagina. (See UTERUS.)

CETRIMIDE (also known as CETAVLON) is the official name for a mixture of alkyl ammonium bromides. It is a potent antiseptic, and as a 1-per-cent solution is used for cleaning and disinfecting wounds, and in the first-aid treatment of burns. As it is also a detergent, it is particularly useful for cleaning the skin, and also for cleansing and disinfecting greasy and infected bowls and baths.

CHAFING OF THE SKIN occurs in infants at the natural folds, e.g. groins, armpits, elbows, where two moist surfaces constantly rub one another; in stout elderly people at similar positions; and generally where the clothes cause friction or pressure, as in the armpits or on the feet of those who walk great distances.

To prevent chafing the folds of the skin should be kept specially clean by washing with warm water and super-fatted soap, carefully dried, and then dusted with fuller's earth or any dusting-powder, such as a mixture of starch, zinc oxide and subnitrate of bismuth in equal parts.

CHAGAS' DISEASE, or American trypanosomiasis, is a disease widespread in Central and South America, and caused by the *Trypanosoma cruzi*. The disease is transmitted by the biting bugs, *Panstrongylus megistus* and *Triatoma infestans*. It occurs in an acute and a chronic form. The former, which is most common in children, practically always affects the heart, and the prognosis is poor. The chronic form is commonest in adolescents and young adults and the outcome depends upon the extent to which the heart is involved. There is no effective drug treatment. It has been suggested that Charles Darwin acquired the disease during his historic voyage on *The Beagle* and that it was the chronic form that turned him into an invalid for 40 years of his life after his return home and ultimately was responsible for his death in 1882. (See also SLEEPING SICKNESS.)

CHALAZION (see EYE, DISEASE AND INJURIES).

CHALICOSIS is a disorder of the lungs found among stonecutters, and due to the inhalation of fine particles of stone.

CHALK is calcium carbonate.

CHALK-STONES (see GOUT).

CHALYBEATE tonics or waters are those containing salts of iron. (See IRON.)

CHAMOMILE TEA is a bitter made by infusing chamomile flowers in boiling water for fifteen minutes and then straining. It is used cold in wineglassful doses.

CHANCRE means the primary lesion of syphilis.

CHANCROID means a soft or non-syphilitic venereal sore. It is caused by a micro-organism known as *Haemophilus ducreyi*. It is usually acquired by sexual contact, and responds well to treatment with sulphadimidine (q.v.). Fewer than 100 cases are diagnosed in Britain annually.

CHANGE OF LIFE (see CLIMACTERIC; MENSTRUATION).

CHAPPED HANDS occur in cold weather, when the activity of the sweat and sebaceous glands is reduced and there is therefore less natural protection of the skin. If the hands are then degreased by prolonged immersion in soapy water, and afterwards exposed to cold air, the skin becomes inelastic and cracks.
Prevention: A mop should be used for washing up, and household rubber gloves worn when using strong bleaching solutions, ammonia or degreasing compounds for cleaning ovens. A barrier cream (q.v.), such as petroleum jelly or lanolin, may be used, but most housewives find these too greasy. A more effective, and less greasy barrier cream is the *British Pharmacopoeia* Oily Cream. Adequate drying of the hands is essential, and the hands should be protected from cold weather so far as possible.
Treatment: Once chapping has occurred, a cream, such as the Oily Cream just mentioned or another *British Pharmacopoeia* preparation, Aqueous Cream, should be applied every night at bedtime. After it has been applied, the hands should be covered with thin cotton gloves. The painful cracks which are so liable to form at the fingertips are best treated with a paint consisting of equal parts of tincture of benzoin and collodion.

CHAPPED LIPS (see LIPS).

CHAPPED NIPPLES (see BREASTS, DISEASES OF).

CHARCOAL as used in medicine is a black powder prepared from vegetable matter such as sawdust, peat, cellulose residues and coconut shells by carbonization and activation. Its medicinal value is a result of its ability to absorb both gases and chemicals. It is available in the form of a powder, granules, tablets or biscuits.
Uses: Its traditional use is in the treatment of flatulence in a dose of 4 grams, on the principle that it absorbs the intestinal gases, but its value in this role is doubtful. It is also used in the treatment of poisoning with many drugs such as aspirin, paracetamol, barbiturates and morphine, all of which it absorbs. Here the dosage is much higher – up to 50 grams in water. A strawberry-flavoured preparation is now available which makes it more palatable and easier to administer to children. This is supplied as a powder containing 20 grams in a 200-millilitre bottle. The powder is stable for several years. When needed, the bottle is filled with water and the suspension swallowed. Another traditional use is as a deodorizing application to foul ulcers.

CHARCOT-LEYDEN CRYSTALS are sharp crystals found in the sputum of those suffering from asthma, and of those affected by some blood diseases.

CHARCOT'S JOINTS is the name applied to a painless swelling and disorganization of the joints which is the result of damage to the pain fibres that occurs in diabetic neuropathy and tabes dorsalis. (See TABES.)

CHEILOSIS is an eczematous condition of the lips, especially at the angles of the mouth, and believed to be due to deficiency in the diet of one of the vitamins in the vitamin B complex – riboflavin. ANGULAR STOMATITIS and PERLÈCHE are other terms used to describe the condition, which may be associated with a red, sore tongue; fine desquamation at the junction of nose and lip, just inside the nose, and in the ears; eczema of the scrotum and perineum.

CHEIROPOMPHOLYX is the term applied to a disease of the skin in which little blisters filled with clear fluid suddenly appear on the hands and fingers. (See also POMPHOLYX.)

CHELATING AGENTS are compounds that will render an ion (usually a metal) biologically inactive by incorporating it into an inner ring structure in the molecule. (Hence the name from the Greek *chele*=claw.) When the complex formed in this way is harmless to the body and is excreted in the urine, such an agent is an effective way of ridding the body of toxic metals such as mercury. The main chelating agents are dimercaprol (q.v.), penicillamine (q.v.) and sodium calciumedetate.

CHEMOSIS: Swelling of the conjunctiva. (See EYE, DISEASE AND INJURIES.)

CHEMOTAXIS means the property possessed by certain cells of attracting or repelling other cells.

CHEMOTHERAPY is the treatment of disease by chemical substances. In the modern sense it dates from the discovery by Paul Ehrlich, in 1910, of the action of Salvarsan ('606') in destroying the spirochaete of syphilis. This organic arsenical preparation revolutionized the treatment of syphilis. The next great advance in chemotherapy was the introduction of the sulphonamides in 1935. Just as Salvarsan had revolutionized the treatment of syphilis so did the sulphonamides revolutionize the treatment of infections with the streptococcus, pneumococcus, gonococcus and similar organisms. They remained supreme in the treatment of such infections as septicaemia, pneumonia, and certain forms of meningitis, until the introduction of penicillin during the 1939–45 War. Subsequently a series of new antibiotics (q.v.) have been discovered, including streptomycin, chloramphenicol, the tetracyclines and the cephalosporins.
Chemotherapy has also played an important rôle in tropical medicine: e.g. mepacrine and proguanil for the treatment of malaria; the amidines in the treatment of sleeping sickness in man, and the sulphones in the treatment of leprosy.
In recent years it has played an increasing part in the treatment of cancer (q.v.).

CHENODEOXYCHOLIC ACID is one of the bile acids (see BILE), which is used in the treatment of cholesterol gall-stones (see GALL-BLADDER, DISEASES OF).

CHEST, or THORAX, is the upper part of the trunk. It is enclosed by the breast-bone(sternum) and the twelve ribs which join the sternum by way of cartilages and are attached to the spine behind. At the top of the thorax the opening in between the first ribs admits the windpipe (trachea), the gullet (oesophagus (q.v.)) and the large blood vessels. The bottom of the thorax is separated from the abdomen below by the muscular diaphragm (q.v.) which is the main muscle of breathing. Other muscles of respiration, the intercostal muscles, lie in between the ribs. Overlying the ribs are layers of muscle and soft tissue including the breast tissue.
Contents: The trachea divides into right and left main bronchi which go to the two lungs (q.v.). The left lung is slightly smaller than the right. The right has three lobes (upper, middle and lower) and the left lung has two lobes (upper and lower). Each lung is covered by two thin

membranes lubricated by a thin layer of fluid. These are the pleura and similar structures cover the heart (pericardium). The heart lies in the middle, displaced slightly to the left. The oesophagus passes right through the chest to enter the stomach just below the diaphragm. Various nerves, blood vessels and lymph channels run through the thorax. The thoracic duct is the main lymphatic drainage channel emptying into a vein on the left side of the root of the neck.

CHEST, DEFORMITIES OF

CHEST, DEFORMITIES OF: The healthy chest is gently rounded all over, its contour being more rounded in women by the breast tissue. In cross section it is oval shaped with a longer dimension from side to side than back to front.

BARREL CHEST is found in long-standing asthma or chronic bronchitis and emphysema when the lungs are chronically enlarged. The anterio-posterior dimension of the chest is increased and the ribs are near horizontal. In this position they can produce little further expansion of the chest and breathing often relies on accessory muscles in the neck lifting up the whole thoracic cage on inspiration.

PIGEON CHEST is one in which the cross-section of the chest becomes triangular with the sternum forming a sort of keel in front. It may be related to breathing problems in early life.

RICKETY CHEST is uncommon now and is caused by rickets in early life (see RICKETS). There is a hollow down each side caused by the pull of muscles on the softer ribs in childhood. The line of knobs produced on each side where the ribs join their costal cartilages is known as the rickety rosary.

PECTUS EXCAVATUM is quite a common abnormality where the central tendon of the diaphragm seems to be too short so that the lower part of the sternum is displaced inwards and the lower ribs are prominent. When severe it may displace the heart further to the left side.

LOCAL ABNORMALITIES in the shape of the chest occur when there is a deformity in the spine such as scoliosis which alters the angles of the ribs. The chest wall may be locally flattened when the underlying lung is reduced in size locally over a prolonged period. (See SPINE AND SPINAL CORD, DISEASES AND INJURIES OF.) This may be seen over a scarred area of lung such as that seen in pulmonary tuberculosis (q.v.).

CHEST DEVELOPMENT

CHEST DEVELOPMENT is affected by underlying disorders in the lungs. Local disease in the lungs may reduce the volume of all or part of one lung and lead to a local deformity in the overlying ribs. Long-standing narrowing of the airways such as that seen in asthma (q.v.) or emphysema (q.v.) may lead to a general expansion of the chest wall.

The muscles of respiration can be developed to some extent by training, either general fitness training or specific respiratory muscle work such as playing an instrument which involves blowing against a high resistance.

CHEST DISEASES

CHEST DISEASES: The lungs and the heart are within the chest but the term chest disease usually refers to abnormalities of the lungs. However, lung problems are often intimately associated with heart disorders. The lungs are the site of gas exchange in the body where oxygen is brought into the blood and the waste product, carbon dioxide, removed. Smoking is a very important cause of lung disease and is responsible for most cases of lung cancer, chronic bronchitis and emphysema.

Symptoms: *Breathlessness* is a common complaint in lung disease. Abnormalities in other systems such as the heart and the blood may cause breathlessness but lung problems are the most common cause. Shortness of breath limits exercise in many lung conditions. These are particularly diseases such as asthma, chronic bronchitis and emphysema which narrow the airways into the lungs (obstructive lung disorders) and those conditions which limit the expansion of the lungs (restrictive disorders) such as lung fibrosis, pneumonia, lung collapse or fluid around the lung (pleural effusion). Breathlessness also occurs when the muscles of the chest wall and diaphragm are weak or the chest wall is deformed. *Cough* is another common sympton and is caused by irritation at some site in the lungs or the airways to the lungs. Cough may be dry or produce sputum or phlegm. The colour of the sputum is yellow or green when infection is present. *Haemoptysis* is the production of sputum containing blood and is a symptom which should always be taken seriously and investigated. The lungs themselves do not produce painful sensations but inflammation of the lining around the lung (the pleura) leads to a pain which is worse on breathing, coughing and sometimes on movement (pleuritic pain).

Signs: signs of lung disease may be seen outside the chest, for example, the blue coloration of the lips and skin (cyanosis) which occurs when the lungs are unable to bring enough oxygen into the blood.

Treatment: Oxygen is useful in many lung diseases. In some patients with chronic lung disease the amount of oxygen needs to be carefully controlled. Antibiotics (q.v.) are used for pneumonia and other chest infections, with special antibiotics used over many months for tuberculosis. In asthma drugs can be used by inhalation directly into the airways. They can widen the airways and relieve breathlessness and also reduce the inflammation in the walls of the airways in the lungs. In cancer of the lung surgery may cure the disease but often it is not possible to remove the tumour and alternative treatments such as radiotherapy and chemotherapy may be used.

CHEYNE-STOKES BREATHING

CHEYNE-STOKES BREATHING is a type of breathing seen in some serious nervous affections, such as brain tumours and stroke, and also in the case of persons with advanced disease of the heart or kidneys. When well marked it is a sign that death is impending, though milder degrees of it do not carry such a serious implication in elderly patients. The breathing gets very faint for a short time, then gradually deepens till full expirations are taken for a few seconds, and then gradually dies away to another quiet period, again increasing in depth after a few seconds and so on in cycles.

CHIASMA: This is an X-shaped crossing. The optic chiasma is where the nerve fibres from the nasal half of each retina cross over the mid line to join the optic tract from the other side.

CHICKENPOX, or VARICELLA, is an acute contagious disease predominantly of children, though it may occur at any age, characterized by feverishness and an eruption on the skin. The name, chickenpox, is said to be derived from the resemblance of the eruption to boiled chick-peas.
Causes: The disease occurs in epidemics affecting especially children under the age of ten years. It has no connection with smallpox, to which it bears a superficial resemblance. It is due to the varicella zoster virus, and the condition is an extremely infectious one from child to child. Although an attack confers life-long immunity, the virus may lie dormant and manifest itself in adult life as *herpes zoster* or shingles (see HERPES ZOSTER).
Symptoms: There is an incubation period of fourteen to twenty-one days after infection, and then the child becomes feverish or has a slight shivering, or may feel more severely ill with vomiting and pains in the back and legs. Almost at the same time, an eruption consisting of red pimples which quickly change into vesicles filled with clear fluid appears on the back and chest, sometimes about the forehead, and less frequently on the limbs. These vesicles appear over several days and during the second day may show a change of their contents to turbid, purulent fluid and within a day or two they burst, or, at all events, shrivel up and become covered with brownish crusts. The small crusts have all dried up and fallen off in little more than a week and recovery is almost always complete.
Treatment: The child must be isolated from susceptible children for a week from the appearance of the rash or until all the vesicles are dry, but there is no need to wait until the scabs have separated. Calamine lotion or a simple dusting powder relieves the itchiness. No other treatment beyond isolation is required.

CHIGGER is another name for *Trombicula autumnalis*, popularly known as the harvest mite (see BITES AND STINGS).

CHILBLAIN, or ERYTHEMA PERNIO, is an inflamed condition of the skin of the hands or feet, or even of the ears, occurring in persons of defective circulation and in those of poor health.
Causes: Chilblains are found especially in child-hood and adolescence. Under-feeding, poor clothing and a defective circulation favour their appearance. People who suffer from them have habitually cold and numb hands and feet, and are subject to chills and colds in the head. In these people tight footwear is often sufficient to bring on chilblains of the feet, and warming the hands at the fire when they are cold produces chilblains on the fingers, the skin becoming engorged with blood in consequence of the irritation or warmth, and later losing its vitality.

True chilblains should not be confused with a cracked or chapped condition of the hands, feet, lips, or ears brought on by cold wind, or washing with hot water during cold weather in people of robust constitution but delicate skin.

Preventive treatment is the best. Good food and warm clothing improve the general condition upon which chilblains depend. Regular exercise improves the circulation.

CHILD ABUSE: The physical or emotional mistreatment of a child. Neglect, physical injury, and sexual abuse are all forms of child abuse and they may be caused by parents, relatives, or carers. Greater awareness of the problem has led to an increase of reported incidents, but whether the incidence of abuse is actually rising is uncertain. Physical abuse or non-accidental injury is the most easily recognized form. Victims of sexual abuse may not reveal their experiences until adulthood and often not at all. Where child abuse is suspected, full investigation of the circumstances is necessary, and this may mean admitting a child to hospital or to local authority care. Abuse may be the result of impulsive action by adults or it may be premeditated, for example, the continued sexual exploitation of a child over several years. Premeditated physical assault is rare but is liable to cause serious injury to a child and requires urgent action when identified. Adults will go to some lengths to cover up persistent abuse. The child's interests are paramount but the parents may well be under severe stress and also require sympathetic handling.

CHILD ADOPTION: Adoption was relatively uncommon until the Second World War with only 6,000 adoption orders annually. This peaked at nearly 25,000 in 1968 as adoption became more socially acceptable and the numbers of babies born to lone mothers rose in a climate hostile to single parenthood.

Adoption declined as the availability of babies fell with the introduction of the Abortion Act, 1968, improving contraceptive services and increasing acceptability of single parenthood.

However, with 10 per cent of couples suffering infertility, the demand continued, leading to the adoption of those previously perceived as difficult to place, i.e. physically, intellectually and/or emotionally disabled children and adolescents, those with terminal illness and children of ethnic-minority groups.

Recent controversies regarding homosexual couples as adoptive parents, adoption of children with or at high risk of HIV/AIDS, transcultural adoption and the increasing use of intercountry adoption to fulfil the needs of childless couples have provoked urgent consideration of the ethical dilemmas of adoption and its consequences for the children, their adoptive and birth families and society generally.

Detailed statistics have been unavailable since 1984 but in general there has been a downward trend with relatively more older children being placed. In 1989 7,044 adoption orders were granted (with an approximately equal ratio of boys to girls); 16 per cent were under 1 year, 26 per cent 1–4 years, 32 per cent 5–9 years, 19 per cent 10–14 years and 7 per cent 15–17 years old. Detailed reasons for adoption (i.e. interfamily, step-parent, intercountry, etc.) are not available but approximately one-third were adopted from local-authority care.

In the UK *all* adoptions (including interfamily and step-parent adoption) *must* take place through a registered adoption agency which may be local-authority based or provided by a registered voluntary agency. All local authorities must act as agencies, the voluntary agencies often providing specialist services to promote and support the adoption of more difficult-to-place children. Occasionally an adoption allowance will be awarded.

Adoption orders cannot be granted until a child has resided with its proposed adopters for 13 weeks. In the case of new-born infants the mother cannot give formal consent to placement until the baby is 6 weeks old, although informal arrangements can be made before this time.

In the UK the concept of responsibility of birth parents to their children and their rights to continued involvement after adoption are acknowledged by the Children Act, 1989. However, in all discussions the child's interests remain paramount. The Act also recognizes adopted children's need to have information regarding their origins. At present (1991) the adoption law is under review.

BAAF – British Agencies for Adoption and Fostering – is the national organization of adoptive agencies, both local authority and voluntary sector. The organization promotes and provides training service, development and research, has several specialist professional subgroups (i.e. medical, legal, etc.) and produces a quarterly journal. Its address is 11 Southwark Street, London SE1 1RQ (071-407 8800, fax: 071-403 6970).

PPIAS – Parent to Parent Information Service on Adoptive Services – is an effective national support network of adoptive parents who offer free information, a 'listening ear' and, to members, a quarterly newsletter: Lower Boddington, Daventry, Northamptonshire, NN11 6YB.

National Organization for Counselling Adoptees and their parents (NORCAP), 3 New High Street, Headington, Oxford OX3 7AJ, is concerned with adopted children and birth parents who wish to make contact.

The Registrar General operates an Adoption Contact Register for adopted persons and anyone related to that person by blood, half blood or marriage. Information can be obtained from the Office of Population Censuses and Surveys, The General Register Office, Adoptions Section, Smedley Hydro, Trafalgar Road, Birkdale, Southport PR8 2HH.

CHILD-CROWING (see CROUP).

CHILD DEVELOPMENT: Children develop new skills in predictable patterns which can be observed as series of milestones along the road to maturity. Up to the age of 3 years milestones are traditionally charted in four areas: (1) *motor* – a reflection of physical strength; (2) *social interaction* with parents and strangers; (3) *language* – including hearing – and (4) *fine co-ordination* – including vision. Health-care professionals use these milestones to assess overall developmental progress and as an aid to pinpoint specific problems. Whilst the sequence is generally similar, the age at which a child reaches a given milestone is variable, even within one family, and reflects the child's physical health, environment and personality. If a child has a limited disability, one area of development may lag behind the others. A deaf child will have delayed language but will smile, walk and build towers at the expected time. A mild delay in all areas may reflect personality, chronic hospitalization or poor environmental stimulation, but a severe generalized delay suggests major brain dysfunction.

A child should at 6 months (1) roll over from front to back, (2) reach for and shake a rattle, (3) look round to see where noises are coming from and (4) transfer a cube from one hand to the other; at 1 year (1) walk holding on to furniture, (2) hold and drink from a cup, (3) use four words with meaning and (4) pick up a small object between thumb and forefinger; at 18 months (1) climb on to furniture, (2) pull socks off, (3) attempt to join in rhymes and (4) build a tower of three bricks; at 2 years (1) kick a ball, (2) tell about experiences, (3) name five toys and (4) copy vertical and horizontal lines; at 3 years (1) hop on one foot, (2) wash hands, (3) know first name and (4) copy a circle.

After the age of 3 the discovery of major developmental problems is unlikely. However, deafness and learning disabilities may go unappreciated until the child is much older.

CHILLS AND COLDS: Although in general trivial ailments, on occasion they can be the prelude to serious diseases.
Causes: The so-called 'common cold' may follow some chill to the surface, such as exposure to a draught of cold air, breathing in a foggy atmosphere, wetting of the feet on a cold day, sudden immersion in water, some persons being specially liable after one of these to develop a catarrh of the respiratory passages

and feverish state. These, however, are only predisposing factors, and the primary cause is a virus. Often a 'cold in the head' runs through all the members of a family or school or a group of persons employed together, and such an 'infectious cold' is due to the causative virus passed from one person to another by sneezing or coughing.

Varieties and symptoms: A cold in the head with catarrh of the nose is known to every one; the catarrh sometimes extending up into the frontal sinuses and causing a severe browache, or involving the maxillary sinuses (see SINUS) and causing face-ache, or even spreading up the Eustachian tubes and causing inflammation of the middle ear with painful earache. Generally, these secondary affections disappear as the cold gets well, but suppuration may result in these various cavities, most commonly in the middle ear, though seldom in the frontal sinus. When the throat is the part affected, inflammation of the tonsils may result. (See TONSILLITIS.) In persons who use the voice much, or in those who take too much in alcohol, the larynx is a weak point, and laryngitis, with huskiness or even temporary loss of voice, is the common result of a chill. The cold may affect the respiratory passages further down and bronchitis then results, or if the surfaces of the air spaces in the lungs be inflamed, pneumonia is the condition produced. When the air passages from the larynx downwards contain mucus, coughing results, this being a series of involuntary explosive expirations designed to force the irritating substance up into the mouth, from which it is spat out. Some persons have a liability, as the result of a chill, to catarrh not of the respiratory, but of the alimentary system, as shown by ensuing dyspepsia or diarrhoea. It should be remembered that a so-called 'cold' is the commencement of several infectious and serious diseases, such as measles, whooping-cough, influenza, and tuberculosis. Medical advice should therefore be sought whenever this apparently trivial malady lasts more than a few weeks.

Treatment: There is little one can do in the treatment of a cold. Most people have their pet remedies, and most of these are harmless. On 'catching a cold', with a temperature above normal, the best thing to do is to go to bed and stay there at least 24 hours, if not two days. In this way the course of the cold will be cut short, and at the same time the sufferer will not be exposing other people to his infection. The best way to prevent colds is to isolate the infected person. Equally important is it that those suffering from a cold should not cough or sneeze indiscriminantly as their secretions are loaded with the causative organism, which is why health, and not merely politeness, demands coughing or sneezing into a handkerchief. On the other hand, this means that the handkerchief becomes loaded with micro-organisms. It has been reported that 15,000 organisms can be removed from a used handkerchief during thirty seconds of gentle manipulation, which is why disposable paper handkerchiefs should be used when one has a cold, sore throat or the like. Vaccines seem to be ineffectual in the prevention of colds.

CHIMERA is an organism, whether plant, animal or human being, in which there are at least two kinds of tissue differing in their genetic constitution. In recent years it has become possible to combine together two embryos (q.v.) at a very early stage of development so that they develop as a single individual. Such an animal, which thus can have four parents, instead of two, is an example of a chimera.

CHIROPODY is that part of medical science which is concerned with the health of the feet. The modern chiropodist is a specialist capable of providing a fully comprehensive foot-health service. This includes the palliation of established deformities and dysfunction both as short-term treatment for immediate relief of painful symptoms and long-term management to secure optimum results. This requires the backing of effective appliances and footwear services. It also involves curative footcare, including the use of various therapeutic techniques, including minor surgery and the prescription and provision of specialized and individual appliances. Chiropody also has a preventative role which includes inspection of children's feet and the detection of foot conditions requiring treatment and advice and also foot-health education. The chiropodist is trained to recognize medical conditions which manifest themselves in the feet, such as circulatory disorders, diabetes mellitus and diseases causing ulceration.

The scope of practice of chiropodists is defined by the Society of Chiropodists as comprising the maintenance of the feet in healthy condition and the treatment of their disabilities by methods covered by the syllabus of training hitherto approved by the Department of Health. A chiropodist should confine his practice to this field of work and to such forms of advice and treatment as his training and experience qualify him to give. The only course of training in the United Kingdom recognized for the purpose of state registration by the Chiropodists Board of the Council for Professions Supplementary to Medicine is the Society of Chiropodists 3-year full-time course. The course includes instruction and examination in the relevant aspects of anatomy and physiology, local analgesia, medicine and surgery, as well as in podology and therapeutics. The registered address of the Society of Chiropodists is 53 Welbeck Street, London W1M 7HE (071-486 3381, fax: 071-935 6359).

CHIROPRACTOR is a term applied to a person who practises chiropractic. This is a system of adjustment by hand of supposed minor displacements of the spinal column. These minor displacements, or subluxations (q.v.) of the spine, chiropractors contend, affect the associated or neighbouring nerves. By manipulating the affected part of the spinal column the patient's complaint, whatever it may be – for example, backache – is relieved. Information can be obtained from the Chiropractor Advancement Association, 56 Barnes Crescent, Wimborne, Dorset BH21 2AZ.

CHLAMYDIA is a genus of micro-organisms which include those responsible for non-specific urethritis (q.v.), ornithosis (q.v.), psittacosis (q.v.), and trachoma (q.v.). They are also widespread in birds and animals. Chlamydia can be sexually transmitted and 36,000 cases were reported in England in 1988.

CHLOASMA: This is an increase in the melanin pigment of the skin as a result of hormonal stimulation. It is commonly seen in pregnancy and sometimes in women on the contraceptive pill. It mainly affects the face.

CHLORAL HYDRATE is a substance which, when taken internally in moderate doses, produces sound, dreamless, refreshing sleep, like natural sleep. Particularly useful for old people, it acts rapidly, within about half-an-hour, and its effect lasts for about eight hours. It is, however, dangerous in large doses, and people taking it frequently may become habituated. It should not be taken in conjunction with alcohol.

CHLORAMBUCIL is a derivative of nitrogen mustard (q.v.), which is proving of value in the treatment of chronic lymphatic leukaemia (see LEUKAEMIA and Hodgkin's disease (q.v.)). It is given by mouth. (See CYTOTOXIC.)

CHLORAMPHENICOL is an antibiotic derived from a soil organism, *Streptomyces venezuelae*. It is also prepared synthetically. It is active against a wide range of organisms, but its most striking feature is its activity against certain rickettsias (q.v.). It has proved effective in the treatment of typhus, scrub typhus, Rocky Mountain spotted fever, typhoid and paratyphoid fevers. Its activity against certain organisms not susceptible to the sulphonamides and penicillin is proving of value. Particularly is this true of its use in the treatment of meningitis due to *H. influenzae*. It is given by mouth.

It is an antibiotic, however, that must be administered with discrimination because in certain individuals it may cause aplastic anaemia (see ANAEMIA), particularly if given for too long a period or in repeated courses.

CHLORDANE is an insecticide which has been used sucessfully against flies and mosquitoes resistant to DDT, and for the control of ticks and mites. It requires special handling as it is toxic to man when applied to the skin.

CHLORDIAZEPOXIDE is a widely used antianxiety drug. (See TRANQUILLIZERS, BENZODIAZEPINES.)

CHLORHEXIDINE, also known as HIBITANE, is an antiseptic which has a bacteriostatic action against many bacteria.

CHLORINATED LIME, also known as CHLORIDE OF LIME, is a white powder made by passing chlorine gas over slaked lime. Chlorine is a greenish gas, heavier than air, with a pungent, choking smell, and highly poisonous to all forms of bacterial life. By virtue of its power to give off chlorine, chlorinated lime is a powerful bleaching agent and disinfectant, especially when mixed with an acid. To disinfect rooms, chlorinated lime may be mixed with an equal bulk of water acidulated with sulphuric acid, and exposed on flat dishes for some hours. To disinfect water-closets and drains, 450 g (1 pound) of the chlorinated lime may be mixed with 4·5 l (1 gallon) of water and poured down the drain.

To disinfect swimming baths it should be added in such an amount that the free chlorine, after combining with any organic matter in the water, is left in a concentration of 0·25 to 1 part per million parts of water. It is an efficient disinfectant for drinking water when added in the proportion of 28·3 g to 9000 l (1 ounce to 2000 gallons). The residual taste of chlorine can be removed by adding a small crystal of sodium thiosulphate, about the size of a grain of rice, to a quart jug of water.

CHLORINE (see CHLORINATED LIME, and SODIUM HYPOCHLORITE).

CHLORMETHIAZOLE is a useful hypnotic particularly for elderly patients because of its freedom from hang-over effect. It is particularly useful in the acute withdrawal symptoms of alcoholism. Dependence may occur occasionally and therefore the length of period for which the drug is used should be limited. Sideeffects include sneezing, conjunctival irritation and occasional headache.

CHLOROFORM is a colourless, volatile liquid, half as heavy again as water, and, unlike ether, non-inflammable. It was discovered by Liebig in 1831, and is a compound of carbon, hydrogen, and chlorine ($CHCl_3$). It does not dissolve to a large amount in water, but mixes readily with alcohol or ether. It dissolves sulphur, phosphorus, fats, resins, and most substances which contain a large proportion of carbon; it is therefore very useful as a cleansing agent. It was introduced into medicine in 1847 by Sir J. Y. Simpson, who was then in search of a substance which could produce unconsciousness for operative purposes more conveniently than ether, introduced a short time previously by Morton in America. (See ANAESTHESIA.)

Uses: Chloroform is used as a solvent of fats, resins, etc., in many chemical processes. It is now rarely used in medicine.

CHLOROMA, or GREEN CANCER, is the name of a disease in which greenish growths appear under the skin, and in which a change takes place in the blood resembling that in leukaemia.

CHLOROPHYLL is the name of the green colouring matter of plants. Its main use is as a colouring agent, principally for soaps, oils and fats. It is also being found of value as a deodorant dressing to remove, or diminish, the unpleasant odour of heavily infected sores and wounds.

CHLOROQUINE, which is a 4-aminoquinoline, was introduced during the 1939–45 War for the treatment of malaria. It has also been found of value in the treatment of the skin condition known as chronic discoid lupus erythematosus, and of rheumatoid arthritis.

CHLOROTHIAZIDE is a potent benzothiadiazine (q.v.) diuretic which is active when taken by mouth. It has also a blood-pressure-lowering effect when used in conjunction with other hypotensive drugs.

CHLOROTRIANISENE is a synthetic oestrogen (q.v.) which is active when taken by mouth. (See OESTROGEN.)

CHLOROXYLENOL is an antiseptic which is used for treating cuts, abrasions and wounds. It is also widely used in obstetric practice. It is only slightly soluble in water (1 in 3000).

CHLORPROMAZINE is chemically related to the antihistamine drug, promethazine. One of the first antipsychotic drugs to be marketed, it is used extensively in psychiatry on account of its action in calming psychotic activity without producing undue general depression or clouding of consciousness. The drug is used particularly in schizophrenia and mania.

CHLORPROPAMIDE is one of the oral hypoglycaemic agents. It is a sulphonamide derivative and acts by stimulating the release of insulin from the pancreas. As it has a prolonged action, it need only be given once a day. Those taking chlorpropamide should bear in mind that in around 10 per cent of people it causes undue sensitivity to alcohol, resulting in severe flushing of the face, headache and a feeling of intoxication. (See also DIABETES MELLITUS, SULPHONYLUREAS.)

CHLORTETRACYCLINE (See TETRA-CYCLINES.)

CHOKING is the process which results from an obstruction to breathing situated in the larynx (see AIR PASSAGES). It may occur as the result of disease causing swelling round the glottis (the entrance to the larynx), or of some nervous disorders that interfere with the regulation of the muscles which open and shut the larynx, but generally it is due to the irritation of a piece of food or other substance introduced by the mouth, which provokes coughing but only partly interferes with breathing. As the mucous membrane lining the upper part of the latter is specially sensitive, coughing results in order to expel the cause of irritation. At the same time, if the foreign body is of any size, lividity of the face appears, due to partial suffocation (see ASPHYXIA).

Treatment: The choking person should take slow, deep inspirations, which do not force the particle further in (as sudden catchings of the breath between the coughs do), and which produce more powerful coughs. If the coughing is weak, one or two strong blows with the palm of the hand over either shoulder blade, timed to coincide with coughs aid the effect of the coughing. In the case of a child the patient may be held up by the legs, when the substance causing the obstruction is more readily dislodged.

If this fails to dislodge the foreign body, what is known as the Heimlich manoeuvre should be tried. If the victim is standing or sitting, stand behind him and wrap your arms round his waist. Grasp the closed fist of the bottom hand with the other hand, and place the thumb side of the first against the abdomen slightly above the navel and below the ribs. Then press your fist against the abdomen with a quick upward thrust. Repeat several times if necessary. If the victim is lying down, whether semi-conscious or unconscious, kneel astride his hips facing him. With one hand on top of the other, place the heel of the bottom hand on the abdomen slightly above the navel and below the ribs. Press into the abdomen with a quick upward thrust. Repeat several times if necessary. Should the victim vomit, turn him quickly on his side and wipe out his mouth to prevent him inhaling the vomited material. Another method in adults is to draw the thighs up towards the body with the knees bent. The thighs are then pressed suddenly and violently into the abdomen. If this fails, call the doctor.

CHOLAGOGUES are substances which increase the flow of bile by stimulating evacuation of the gall-bladder. The great majority of these act only by increasing the activity of the digestive organs, and so producing a flow of bile already stored up in the gall-bladder. Substances which stimulate the liver to secrete more bile are known as CHOLERETIC.

CHOLANGIOGRAPHY is the process whereby the bile ducts and the gall-bladder are rendered radio-opaque and therefore visible on an X-ray film. (See SODIUM DIATRIZOATE.)

CHOLANGITIS is the term applied to inflammation of the bile ducts.

CHOLECYSTECTOMY means the removal of the gall-bladder by operation.

CHOLECYSTITIS means inflammation of the gall-bladder (q.v.).

CHOLECYSTOGRAPHY is the term applied to the process whereby the gall-bladder is rendered radio-opaque and therefore visisble on an X-ray film. (See SODIUM DIATRIZOATE.)

CHOLECYSTOKIN is the hormone (q.v.) released from the lining membrane of the duodenum (q.v.) when food is taken, and which initiates emptying of the gall-bladder.

CHOLELITHIASIS means the presence of gall-stones in the bile- ducts and/or in the gall-bladder. (See GALL-BLADDER, DISEASES OF.)

CHOLELITHOTOMY: The removal of gall-stones by cholecystomy, an operation to open the gall-bladder which is done when cholecystectomy (q.v.) is not possible.

CHOLERA belongs originally to Asia, more particularly to India and Bangladesh, where epidemics are known to have occurred at various times for several centuries. It was not, however, till 1817 that the attention of European physicians was specially directed to the disease by the outbreak of a violent epidemic of cholera at Jessore in Bengal. This was followed by its rapid spread over a large portion of British India, where it caused immense destruction of life among both natives and Europeans. By 1823 it had extended into Asia Minor and Russia in Asia, and it continued to advance steadily though slowly westwards, and spread onwards to England, appearing in Sunderland in October 1831, and in London in January 1832. The disease subsequently spread through North and Central America, reaching even to the military posts on the upper Mississippi. In 1835 it was general throughout North Africa, after which this epidemic disappeared.

About the year 1841 another great epidemic of cholera appeared in India and China, and soon began to extend in the direction traversed by the former, but involving a still wider area. This epidemic appears to have been even more deadly than the former, especially in Great Britain and France.

A third great outbreak of cholera took place in the East in 1850, entering Europe in 1853. It was specially severe throughout both North and South America.

A fourth epidemic visited Europe again in 1865–66, but was on the whole less extensive and destructive than its predecessors. In 1884, and again in 1892 and 1893, there were outbreaks in the middle of Europe, the last one being specially severe in Hamburg and some other cities, but, apart from occasional cases brought by ship, there has been no epidemic in Britain or in the United States for many years.

In 1977, a world total of 60,000 cases of cholera was notified, affecting thirty-four countries, including several around the Eastern Mediterranean. In 1980, four imported cases were notified in England.

In 1971 what is known as the el tor bio-type of *Vibrio cholerae* entered Europe from the Far East. Between 1970 and 1978 twenty imported cases of this type of cholera were reported in England and Wales, but there was no spread of infection. Neither were there any deaths. In view of the high standard of sanitation in Britain, the possibility of such imported cases leading to an epidemic is most remote. Only a small number of cases of cholera occur in the United Kingdom each year. In 1991 a cholera epidemic affected some South American countries.

Causes: The cause of the disease is the *Vibrio cholerae*, or comma-bacillus, discovered by Koch. This organism is constantly found in the discharges from the bowels of those suffering from the disease. The most important mode of transmission is by means of contaminated water, but the infection is also conveyed by flies, which contaminate food with infected faeces. The crowding which occurs under conditions of war and famine also favours epidemics.

Symptoms: The incubation period is a few hours to five days. The disease varies in severity from mild cases which do not feel ill enough to take to bed, to cases which are fatal within twenty- four hours. Over 90 per cent of cases, however, are of the so-called *Cholera gravis* type, in which three stages are recognized.

The *first stage*, which lasts for three to twelve hours, is of sudden onset with painless diarrhoea and vomiting. The stools rapidly become frequent and copious, resembling rice-water and containing flakes of fibrin. This is soon followed by agonizing cramps, first in the limbs and then in the abdomen. The patient complains bitterly of thirst and becomes restless and exhausted, with cold bluish skin, sunken eyeballs, and husky voice. The pulse is weak and the temperature taken in the rectum is 38·3 to 40 °C) (101 to 104 °F).

The *second stage* is termed the stage of collapse, or algid stage. The symptoms now advance with rapidity. The signs of collapse increase. The surface of the body becomes colder and assumes a dusky blue or purple hue, the skin is dry and wrinkled, indicating the intense draining away, in the evacuations, of the fluids of the body. The features are pinched and the eyes more deeply sunken, the pulse at the wrist is imperceptible, and the voice is reduced to a hoarse whisper (the 'vox cholerica'). There may be complete suppression of the urine.

In this condition, death often takes place in less than one day, but, in epidemics, cases are sometimes observed in which the collapse is so sudden and complete as to prove fatal in one or two hours without any great amount of previous purging or vomiting. In most instances the mental faculties are comparatively unaffected, although in the later stages there is generally more or less apathy.

Reaction may, however, take place, and this constitutes the *third stage*. It consists in the arrest of the alarming symptoms of the second stage, and the gradual but evident improvement in the patient's condition. The pulse returns, the surface assumes a natural hue, and the bodily heat is restored. Before long, the vomiting ceases, and, though diarrhoea may continue for a time, it is not of a severe character and soon subsides, as do also the cramps. The urine may remain suppressed for some time, and on returning is often found to be albuminous.

Even in this stage, however, the danger is not past, for relapses sometimes occur which speedily prove fatal; while, again, the reaction may be of imperfect character, and there may succeed an exhausting fever (the so-called *typhoid stage* of cholera), which may greatly retard recovery, and under which the patient may sink at a period even as late as two or three weeks from the start of the illness.

The death-rate varies tremendously: from over 50 per cent in epidemics to around 5 per cent among patients who have received adequate treatment. The outcome is worst in children and old people. Many mild cases are probably never detected in countries where the disease is epidemic.

The bodies of persons dying of cholera are found to remain long warm, and the temperature may even rise after death. Muscular contractions have been observed to take place after death, so that the position of the limbs may become altered.

Treatment: PREVENTIVE TREATMENT: When cholera threatens to invade any place, however favourably circumstanced as to its hygienic condition, increased vigilance will be requisite on the part of those entrusted with the care of the public health. Cholera may be introduced into a community by one or more individuals who have themselves only suffered from the first or milder stage of the disease (cholera diarrhoea), since the discharges from the bowels abound in the infective organisms, and, where sanitary arrangements are deficient, may readily contaminate the water of a locality.

Where suspicion attaches to the water, it should be boiled or chlorinated before being used; milk should also be boiled. Water and food should be protected against pollution with flies, and houses should be fly-proofed. Instructions should be issued by the authorities warning all persons against the use of unwholesome food, unripe fruit, and excesses of every kind, and recommending early application for medical advice where there is any tendency to diarrhoea. The discharges from cholera patients should be treated, as soon as passed, with strong disinfectants (see DISINFECTION), and special care should be taken that they are not disposed of in places where they can contaminate drinking-water. In 1893 Haffkine introduced a vaccine for preventive inoculation against cholera, and this seems to afford a certain amount of protection over a period of some six months. It is recommended for all those going to subtropical or tropical Africa or Asia and wherever there is an outbreak. A genetically engineered vaccine is under trial in America.

Curative treatment: Strict rest in bed is essential. All but a small percentage of cases can now be treated successfully by the administration by mouth of electrolyte solutions. This can be accomplished effectively and economically by the distribution of packets containing pre-weighed amounts of glucose, sodium chloride, potassium chloride and sodium bicarbonate to be added to measured volumes of boiled water in hospital, local treatment centres and, most importantly, in the home, even in the most rural and underdeveloped areas. In severe cases an intravenous infusion is necessary. The infusion fluid consists of two volumes of isotonic sodium chloride (0·9 per cent) plus one volume of sodium lactate (1·75 per cent) or sodium bicarbonate (1·4 per cent). An alternative is the so-called Dacca solution:

Sodium chloride	5 grams
Sodium bicarbonate	4 grams
Potassium chloride	1 gram
Water	to 1 litre

A blood-pressure below 70 mm of mercury, especially if there is associated cyanosis, restlessness, cramps, and cold extremities, is an indication for immediate transfusion with isotonic saline solution.

Chemotherapy is useful only in reducing the period during which the vibrio remains in the stool. For this purpose, chlortetracycline, or one of the insoluble sulphonamides (e.g. sulphaguanidine) should be used.

CHOLERETIC is the term applied to a drug that stimulates the flow of bile (q.v.).

CHOLESTASIS: A reduction or stoppage in the flow of bile (q.v.) into the intestine caused either by a blockage such as a stone in the bile duct or by liver disease disturbing the production of bile. The first type is called extrahepatic biliary obstruction and the second intrahepatic cholestasis. The patient develops jaundice and itching and passes dark urine and pale faeces.

CHOLESTEROL is a sterol, which is one of a class of solid alcohols; these are waxy materials derived from animal and vegetable tissues. It is widely distributed throughout the body, being especially abundant in the brain, nervous tissue, adrenal glands and skin. It is also found in egg yolk and gall-stones. It plays an important role in the body, being essential for the production of the sex hormones, as well as the repair of membranes. It is also the source from which bile acids are manufactured. The total amount in the body of a man weighing 70 kilograms (10 stones) is around 140 grams, and the amount present in the blood is 3·6 to 7·8 m.mol per litre or 150 to 250 milligrams per 100 millilitres.

A high blood-cholesterol level – that is, one over 6 m.mol per litre or 238 mg per 100 ml – is undesirable as there appears to be a correlation between a high blood cholesterol and atheroma (q.v.), the form of arterial degenerative disease associated with coronary thrombosis and high blood-pressure. This is well exemplified in diabetes mellitus (q.v.) and myxoedema (q.v.), two diseases in which there is a high blood cholesterol, sometimes going as high as 20 m.mol per litre; patients with these diseases are known to be particularly prone to arterial disease. There is also a familial disease known as hypercholesterolaemia, in which members of affected families have a blood cholesterol of around 18 m.mol per litre, or more, and are particularly liable to premature degenerative disease of the arteries.

The rising incidence of arterial disease in western countries in recent years has drawn attention to this relationship between high levels of cholesterol in the blood and arterial disease. The available evidence indicates that there is a relationship between blood-cholesterol levels and the amount of fat consumed. Thus, in Cape Town it has been shown that in men aged 45 the mean blood- cholesterol level was 234 mg per 100 ml in the European community and 166 mg per 100 ml in the Bantu community, and this was correlated with the basic difference between the diets of the two communities: 40 per cent of the calories in the European's diet was fat, compared with 20 per cent or less in the Bantu's diet. The suggestion was therefore made that the rising incidence of coronary heart disease, and other manifestations of arterial disease, such as high blood-pressure and strokes, might be arrested by persuading those living in western communities, such as Western Europe and USA, to eat less fat. One of the troubles is that the blood-cholesterol level bears little relationship with the amount of cholesterol consumed, most of the cholesterol in the body being produced by the body itself. Thus, it has been reported that even eating ten eggs, and eggs are the only rich source of cholesterol in the diet, does not usually raise the level of cholesterol in the blood.

On the other hand, it has been shown that diets containing fats with a high proportion of what are known as saturated fatty acids raise the blood-cholesterol level, whereas those with fats containing a high proportion of unsaturated fatty acids lower it. Fats with a high proportion of saturated fatty acids include animal fats such as butter, dripping and the like, whereas the fats with a high proportion of unsaturated fatty acids are predominantly vegetable oils such as olive oil, corn oil, and sunflower oil. The recommendation therefore is that people should reduce their consumption of 'saturated' fats and concentrate on 'unsaturated' fats. There is little doubt that there is a tendency to eat too much animal fat today. It is also generally admitted that, if an individual's blood cholesterol is on the high side, even if he is not suffering from diseases such as diabetes mellitus, then it is wise for him to curtail his intake of saturated fats, just as he should aim at avoiding obesity. The same probably applies to a man who has had a coronary thrombosis.

CHOLESTYRAMINE is a drug that is proving of value in the treatment of the pruritus, or itching (q.v.), which occurs in association with jaundice. This it does by 'binding' the bile salts in the gut and so preventing their being reabsorbed into the bloodstream, where their excess in jaundice is responsible for the itching. It is also proving useful in reducing the level of cholesterol and triglycerides in the blood and thereby, like clofibrate (q.v.), helping to reduce the incidence of coronary artery heart disease. (See CORONARY THROMBOSIS; HYPERLIPIDAEMIA.)

CHOLINE is one of the many constituents of the vitamin B complex. Lack of it in the experimental animal produces a fatty liver. It is found in egg-yolk, liver, and meat. The probable daily human requirement is 500 mg, an amount amply covered by the ordinary diet.

CHOLINERGIC: A description of nerve fibres that release acetylcholine (q.v.) as a neurotransmitter (q.v.).

CHONDROMA is a tumour composed in part of cartilage. (See TUMOUR.)

CHORDA: A nerve fibre, tendon or cord.

CHOREA, or ST VITUS'S DANCE, is a disorder of the nervous system occurring for the most part in children, and characterized mainly by involuntary jerking movements of the muscles. The name, St Vitus's dance, was originally applied to those remarkable epidemic outbursts of combined mental and physical excitement which for a time prevailed among the inhabitants of some parts of Germany in the Middle Ages. It is stated that sufferers from this dancing mania were wont to resort to the chapels of St Vitus, the saint believed to possess the power of curing them. The name was transferred to chorea, though the conditions are unconnected. The term, SYDENHAM'S CHOREA, is also applied to this disorder to distinguish it from Huntington's chorea (q.v.), a disease of hereditary nature which appears late in life and is accompanied by mental defects.

Causes: Chorea is a condition resulting from involvement of the central nervous system by the same factor (or factors) as are responsible for acute rheumatism (see RHEUMATIC FEVER). It is more common in girls than in boys, in the proportion of 3:1. Like acute rheumatism it is rare under the age of 3 years and uncommon under the age of 5 years. There is no definite evidence that it is hereditary, but it is more likely to occur in excitable, intelligent, ambitious children than in the phlegmatic child. There may be a history of some precipitating factor such as a fright or worry over an impending examination. It forms an occasional but rare complication of pregnancy.

Although chorea is the manifestation of acute rheumatism which is most likely to occur without manifestations of rheumatism elsewhere, the main importance of chorea is that about one-third of children who develop it show evidence of rheumatism elsewhere in the body, and usually in the heart. Recurrences occur in about one-third of the cases, usually within a year of the first attack. Such recurrences are more common in girls than in boys. If the heart is not involved in the first attack, it is unlikely to be affected in recurrent attacks.

Symptoms: The characteristic features are: (1) involuntary, purposeless, incoordinated movements; (2) weakness of voluntary movements; (3) loss of precision of movement; (4) psychological disturbances. The symptoms are usually preceded by changes in the temper and disposition, the child becoming sad, irritable and emotional, while at the same time the general health is impaired. The convulsive muscular movements usually show themselves first in one part, such as an arm or a leg, and in most instances they may remain localized to that limited extent, whilst in all cases there is a tendency for the disorderly symptoms to be more marked on one side than on the other. The symptoms are aggravated when purposive movements are attempted, or when the child is watched. Speech is affected, and eating becomes difficult. The heart may be affected as in acute rheumatism, and this may lay the foundation of permanent heart disease (see HEART DISEASES). Usually, there is a remission of the symptoms during sleep.

Rarely this disease assumes a very acute and aggravated form, in which the disorderly movements are so violent as to injure the patient and to necessitate forcible control. In the great majority of cases, however, complete recovery occurs after one to two months, or even longer.

Treatment: The first step in treatment is to provide the patient with complete rest, and under suitable conditions the disease tends to recover of itself. Sodium salicylate and aspirin are helpful, especially the latter.

CHORIOCARCINOMA is a form of cancer affecting the chorion (q.v.), in the treatment of which particularly impressive results are being obtained from the use of methotrexate.

CHORION is the more external of the two fetal membranes. (See AFTERBIRTH.)

CHORIONIC GONADOTROPHIC HORMONE: A hormone produced by the placenta (see AFTERBIRTH) during pregnancy. It is similar to the pituitary gonadotrophins, which are blocked during pregnancy. Large amounts appear in a woman's urine when she is pregnant and are used as the basis for pregnancy tests. Human gonadotrophins are used to treat delayed puberty and premenstrual tension.

CHOROID (see EYE).

CHOROIDITIS (see UVEITIS).

CHOROID PLEXUS: An extensive web of blood vessels occurring in the ventricles of the brain and producing the cerebrospinal fluid. (See BRAIN.)

CHRISTMAS DISEASE is a hereditary disorder of blood coagulation which can only be distinguished from haemophilia (q.v.) by laboratory tests. It is so called after the surname of the first case reported in this country. About one out of every ten patients clinically diagnosed as haemophiliac has in fact Christmas disease. It is due to lack in the blood of Factor IX.

CHROMAFFIN is a term applied to certain cells and organs in the body, such as part of the adrenal glands, which have a peculiar affinity for chrome salts. These cells and tissues generally are supposed to secrete substances which have an important action in maintaining the tone and elasticity of the blood-vessels and muscles.

CHROMIC ACID is used in several industries, particularly in chromium plating. Unless precautions are taken it may lead to dermatitis of the hands, arms, chest and face. It may also cause deep ulcers, especially of the nasal septum and knuckles.

Uses: The chief medicinal use of chromic acid is as a caustic for the treatment of warts and indolent ulcers. It is also sometimes used in a 2 or 3 per cent solution for the treatment of sweating feet.

CHROMOSOMES are the rod-shaped bodies to be found in the nucleus of every cell in the body. They contain the genes, or hereditary elements, which establish the characteristics of an individual. They occur in pairs, and human beings possess forty-six, made up of twenty-three pairs. The number of chromosomes is specific for each species of animal. (See GENETIC CODE; GENETICS; HEREDITY; MEIOSIS; SEX CHROMOSOMES.)

CHRONIC: A persistent or recurring condition. The disease, which may or may not be severe, often starts gradually and changes will be slow. Opposite of ACUTE.

CHYLE is the milky fluid which is absorbed by the lymphatic vessels of the intestine. The absorbed portion consists of fats in very fine emulsion, like milk, so that these vessels receive the name of lacteals (L. *lac*, milk). This absorbed chyle mixes with the lymph and is discharged into the thoracic duct, a vessel as large as a quill, which passes up through the chest to open into the jugular vein on the left side of the neck, where the chyle mixes with the blood.

CHYLURIA means the passage of chyle (q.v.) in the urine. This results in the passing of a milky-looking urine. It is one of the manifestations of filariasis (q.v.), where it is due to obstruction of the lymphatics (q.v.) by the causative parasite.

CHYME is the name given to the partly digested food as it issues from the stomach into the intestine. It is very acid and grey in colour, containing salts and sugars in solution, and the animal food softened into a semi-liquid mass. It is next converted into chyle.

CHYMOPAPAIN is an enzyme (q.v.) obtained from the paw-paw, which is being used in the treatment of prolapsed intervertebral discs (q.v.). When injected into the disc it dissolves it.

CHYMOTRYPSIN is an enzyme (q.v.) produced by the pancreas (q.v.) which digests protein. It is used as an aid in operations for removal of a cataract (see ZONULOLYSIS), and also by inhalation to loosen and liquefy secretions in the windpipe and bronchi.

CICATRIX is another word for scar.

CILIA is a term applied to minute, lash-like processes which are seen with the aid of the microscope upon the cells covering certain mucous membranes: e.g. the trachea (or windpipe) and nose and which maintain movement in the fluid passing over these membranes. They are also found on certain bacteria which have the power of rapid movement.

CILIARY BODY: That part of the eye that connects the iris and the choroid. The ciliary ring is next to the choroid, the ciliary processes comprise many ridges behind the iris, to which the lens's suspensory ligament is attached, and the ciliary muscle, which contracts to change the curvature of the lens and so adjust the accommodation of the eye. (See EYE.)

CIMETIDINE is a drug (known as an H_2 antagonist (q.v.)) that is proving of value in the treatment of peptic ulcer (q.v.). It acts by reducing the hyperacidity of the gastric juice by antagonizing histamine receptors in the stomach.

CIMEX LECTULARIUS (see BED BUG).

CINCHONA is the general name for several trees in the bark of which quinine is found. This bark is also known as Jesuit's bark, having been brought first to notice by Spanish priests in South America and brought to Europe first by the Countess of Cinchon, wife of the Viceroy of Peru, in 1640. The red cinchona bark is that which contains most quinine, and from which it is usually prepared. (See QUININE.) Various extracts and tinctures are made direct from cinchona bark, and used in place of quinine.

CINNAMON is the bark of *Cinnamomum zeylanicum*, a species of laurel grown in Sri Lanka (Ceylon). It has a stimulating action upon the stomach, and assists digestion; hence its use as a condiment. It is also an antispasmodic.

CIRCLE OF WILLIS, or CIRCULUS ARTERIOSUS, is a circle of arteries at the base of the brain, which is formed by the junction of the basilar, posterior cerebral, internal carotid and anterior cerebral arteries. Congenital defects may occur in these arteries and lead to the formation of aneurysms (q.v.).

CIRCULATION OF THE BLOOD: This principle was demonstrated for the first time by William Harvey in 1628. Harvey proved, first of all, mainly by the examination of living animals, that the arteries contain only blood. Secondly, he showed by three main propositions that this blood must go round from arteries to veins in a continuous circuit. (1) The quantity of blood passing from the veins into the heart in the course of a whole day is so great that it is quite impossible it could all be manufactured from the food. (2) The blood in the arteries passes in a constant stream to all the members of the body, and does not return by the same route. (3) The blood in the veins flows incessantly to the heart, and does not ebb and flow, as is shown by the valves in veins and in the heart, and by the fact that veins when pressed on do not fill from above. Having proved these points, he assumed there must be 'pores in the flesh' through which the blood 'percolated' from the ends of the arteries to the commencements of the veins. The last link in the evidence was supplied some thirty years later by Malpighi, an Italian scientist, who with

Diagram of the capillary bed. The direction of the blood flow is shown by the arrows.

1 superior vena cava	10 intestines
2 pulmonary	11 kidney
3 right atrium	12 left ventricle
4 right ventricle	13 left atrium
5 inferior vena cava	14 aorta
6 hepatic vein	15 pulmonary vein
7 liver	16 lungs
8 portal vein	17 head
9 limbs	

General plan of the circulation

the help of the microscope showed these 'pores' to be the minute vessels now called capillaries.

The course of the circulation is as follows: The veins pour their blood, coming from the head, trunk, limbs and abdominal organs, into the right atrium of the heart. This contracts and drives the blood into the right ventricle, which then forces the blood into the lungs by way of the pulmonary artery. Here it is contained in thin-walled capillaries, over which the air plays freely, and through which gases pass readily out and in. The blood gives off carbon dioxide (CO_2) and takes up oxygen (see RESPIRATION), and passes on by the pulmonary veins to the left atrium of the heart. The left atrium expels it into the left ventricle, which forces it on into the aorta, by which it is distributed all over the body. Passing through capillaries in the various tissues, it enters the veins, which ultimately unite into two great veins, the superior and the inferior vena cava, these emptying into the right atrium. This complete circle is accomplished by any particular drop of blood in about half a minute.

In one part of the body there is a further complication. The veins coming from the bowels, charged with food material and other products, split up, and their blood undergoes a

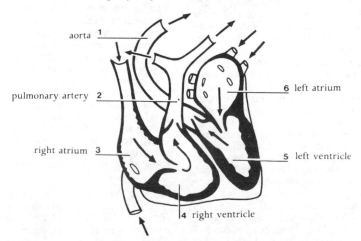

Diagram of the heart opened from in front to show the action of the valves

second capillary circulation through the liver. Here it is relieved of some food material and purified, and then passes into the inferior vena cava, and so to the right atrium. This is known as the portal circulation.

The circle is maintained always in one direction by four valves, situated one at the outlet from each cavity of the heart. (See HEART.)

The blood in the arteries going to the body generally is bright red, that in the veins dull red in colour, owing to the former being charged with oxygen, the latter with carbon dioxide (see RESPIRATION). For the same reason the blood in the pulmonary artery is dark, that in the pulmonary veins bright. There is no direct communication between the right and left sides of the heart, the blood passing from the right ventricle to the left atrium through the lungs.

In the embryo, before birth, the course of circulation is somewhat different, owing to the fact that no nourishment comes from the bowels nor air into the lungs. Accordingly, two large arteries pass out of the navel, and convey blood to be changed by contact with maternal blood (see AFTER-BIRTH), while a large vein brings this blood back again. There are also communications between the right and left atria, and between pulmonary artery and aorta. The latter is known as the ductus arteriosus. At birth all these extra vessels and connections close and rapidly shrivel up.

CIRCULATION, DISORDERS OF: The steady maintenance of the circulation depends upon two factors: (1) the power and regularity of the heart; and (2) the condition of the walls of the vessels, especially of the small arteries. The arteries are not rigid tubes, nor are they merely elastic tubes of a definite size, for each vessel has the power of dilating and contracting within wide limits, so as to let a larger or smaller stream of blood pass through. These motions are controlled by constricting and dilating nerves governed by the nervous system, and upon the action of these, more than upon the heart, depends the state of circulation in various parts. For example, when cold strikes the skin the constrictor nerves are stimulated, the vessels contract, and the blood is driven from the skin, which becomes pallid. On the other hand, blushing is due to loss of control by these nerves over the vessels, or, when the redness is extreme, to stimulation of the dilating nerves by some emotion powerfully affecting the nervous system. Similar changes occur, under other conditions, in all the organs.

Causes and symptoms: *Inflammation* in its early stages is associated with great redness and swelling, due to excessive inflow of blood to the inflamed part through widely dilated arteries. *Congestion* is a condition sometimes due to inflammation, sometimes to an obstruction to the veins which should carry off the blood, or very often to the feebleness of the heart, which cannot drive the blood upwards from dependent parts like the feet, or like the back portions of the lungs in bed-ridden persons. In old persons with diseased vessels, in which blood-clots are liable to form, congestion of the brain readily takes place from such obstructions. In weak persons, or those exhausted by illness, lying constantly on the back, congestion of the lungs is very apt to come on. Congestion of the lungs with bronchitis, and congestion of the liver and stomach with various disorders of digestion, are common results of valvular disease of the heart (see HEART DISEASES). *Oedema* and *varicose veins* are similar disorders often due to obstruction to veins. Oedema is also a usual result of heart disease and of kidney disease (see OEDEMA; VEINS, DISEASES OF). *Bloodlessness* of parts is a disorder in the opposite direction, due to spasm and extreme narrowing of arteries (see RAYNAUD'S DISEASE). A local blanching often precedes *chilblains*, which occur in people of sluggish circulation. *Cold feet and hands*, especially at night, form a milder variety of the same condition. *Insomnia* in elderly people is sometimes due to disordered circulation in the brain, because the vessels are extremely narrowed by disease.

Treatment: Where any failure of the heart is present, the case is treated by various cardiac drugs, by rest, and by graduated exercises. Some cases of disordered circulation depending on the vessels are benefited by cold baths and daily vigorous exercises, while good diet, warm clothing and tonics are of importance for their cure. (See also CHILBLAIN.)

CIRCUMCISION: A surgical procedure to remove the prepuce of the penis in males and a part or all of the external genitalia in females. Circumcision is mainly done for religious or ethnic reasons. There is virtually no medical or surgical reason for circumcision in the male new-born infant. The prepuce is not normally retractable in infancy so this is not an indication for circumcision. By the age of one the prepuce is retractable in most boys. The Americans are more enthusiastic about circumcision. And the reason offered is that cancer of the penis occurs only when a foreskin is present. This is however a rare disease. In the uncircumcised adult there is an increased transmission of herpes and cytomegalo viruses during the reproductive years but this can be reduced by adequate cleansing. Phimosis is an indication for circumcision. Haemorrhage infection and meatal stenosis are rare complications of circumcision. Circumcision in women is a damaging procedure, the results of which can cause psychological and sexual problems and complications in child-birth, and which has no known benefit to the woman's health, though cultural pressures have resulted in its continuation in some Muslim and African countries.

CIRRHOSIS, or FIBROSIS, is a diseased condition, in which the proper tissue is replaced by fibrous tissue similar to scar tissue. The name cirrhosis was originally given by Laennec to the disease as occurring in the liver, because of its yellow colour. (See LIVER DISEASES.)

CIRSOID ANEURYSM is the term applied to the condition in which a group of arteries become abnormally dilated and tortuous.

CISPLATIN (see CYTOTOXIC).

CITRIC ACID is the acid which gives their sharp taste to lemons, limes, unripe oranges, currants and raspberries. It is practically identical in action and appearance with tartaric acid, which is obtained from grapes and other fruits, although the two differ in chemical composition. It is similar also to malic acid, found in apples, pears and the berries of the mountain ash.
Uses: These vegetable acids and their salts (citrates and tartrates) are changed, on absorption into the blood, into alkaline substances, and act therefore to correct acidity. The acids themselves have the power of allaying thirst by stimulating the flow of saliva, and also of creating a feeling of coolness. For both these reasons they are much used for cooling drinks in fever. When, in addition, the stomach is irritable, they are best taken in the form of effervescing drinks, which soothe this organ.

CLAUDICATION: A cramplike pain that occurs in the legs on walking. It may cause the sufferer to limp or, if severe, stop him or her from walking. The usual cause is narrowing or blockage of the arteries in the legs due to atherosclerosis. Intermittent claudication occurs when a person has to stop every so often to let the pain, caused by the build-up of waste products in the muscles, to subside.

CLAUSTROPHOBIA means the fear of being in a confined space, or the fear experienced while in it.

CLAVICLE is the bone which runs from the upper end of the breast- bone towards the tip of the shoulder across the root of the neck. It supports the upper limb, keeps it out from the side, and gives breadth to the shoulders. The bone is shaped like an 'ƒ' with two curves, which give it increased strength. It is, however, liable to be broken by falls on the hand or on the shoulder, and is the most frequently fractured bone in the body. (See FRACTURES.)

CLAVUS is a form of neuralgia about the head, often found in hysterical people and others, compared by them to the pain of driving in a nail (see NEURALGIA). The term is also applied to a corn, or thickening of the horny epithelium upon the foot (see CORNS).

CLAW-FOOT, or PES CAVUS, is a familial deformity of the foot characterized by an abnormally high arch of the foot accompanied by shortening of the foot, clawing of the toes and inversion, or turning inwards, of the foot and heel. Its main effect is to impair the resilience of the foot resulting in a stiff gait and aching pain. Milder cases are treated with special shoes fitted with a sponge rubber insole. More severe cases may require surgical treatment.

CLAW-HAND is a condition of bending and wasting of the hand and fingers, especially of the ring and little fingers. The condition is generally due to paralysis of the ulnar nerve. A somewhat similar condition is produced by contraction of the fibrous tissues in the palm of the hand, partly due to rheumatic changes and partly to injury caused by the constant pressure of a tool against the palm of the hand. (See DUPUYTREN'S CONTRACTURE.)

CLAW-TOES (see CLAW-FOOT).

CLEFT FOOT is a rare congenital abnormality characterized by the absence of one or more toes and a deep central cleft that divides the foot into two. It is sometimes known as lobster foot or lobster claw. It may be accompanied by other congenital defects, such as cleft hand, absent permanent teeth, cleft lip and palate, absence of the nails, and defects of the eye.

CLEFT HAND is a rare congenital abnormality characterized by the absence of one or more fingers and a deep central cleft that divides the hand into two. It is sometimes known as lobster hand. It may be accompanied by other congenital defects, such as cleft foot, absent permanent teeth, cleft lip and palate, absence of the nails and defects of the eye.

The right clavicle, superior aspect.

CLEFT PALATE is the term applied to a fissure in the roof of the mouth (palate) and/or the lip which is present at birth. It is found in varying degrees of severity in about 1 in 700 children. Modern plastic surgery can greatly improve the appearance of the baby and often further cosmetic surgery later will not be necessary. The parent of the child who has cleft lip and/or palate will be given detailed advice specific to his case. In general the team of specialists involved are the paediatrician, plastic surgeon, dentist or orthodontic specialist, and speech therapist. (See PALATE, MALFORMATIONS OF.)

CLICKING FINGER is a condition in middle-aged people in which the victim finds on wakening in the morning that he or she cannot straighten the ring or middle finger spontaneously, but only by a special effort, when it suddenly straightens with a painful click. Hence the name. In due course the finger remains bent at all times unless a special effort is made to straighten it with the other hand. The condition is due to a swelling developing in one of the tendons of the affected finger. If the tendon sheath is slit open surgically, the condition is relieved. Many cases recover spontaneously if the patient is prepared to wait.

CLICKING THUMB is a comparable condition sometimes found in the new-born baby, and occasionally in adults. In the baby, surgery should not be resorted to, as the condition practically always clears up spontaneously. In the adult it can be such a nuisance that it should probably be operated on at a fairly early stage.

CLIMACTERIC was a word originally applied to the end of certain epochs or stages in the life of an individual, at which some great change was supposed to take place. (See also MENOPAUSE.)

CLIMATE IN RELATION TO DISEASE: Climate is of great medical importance, both because various diseases are found in one part of the world and not in others, so that it becomes necessary to know the reasons for this difference, and because removal of a diseased person to new conditions of air, warmth, moisture and the like, is often a valuable means of cure.

The broad division of climates is into hot, temperate and cold climates.

(*a*) **Hot climates** are generally considered as extending to about 35° from the equator, and possessing an average temperature throughout the year of about 29 °C (84 °F). In the Southern Hemisphere, Montevideo, Cape Town and Sydney lie just at the edge of this band, while north of the equator the limit divides the northern from the southern states of North America, skirts the south of Algeria, the north of India, and excludes Japan from the hot region. Generally speaking, there are, in this region, a wet and a dry season, but near the equator, two wet and two dry seasons.

(*b*) **Temperate climates** are those from about 35 to 55° of latitude, and have a mean temperature of about 3·3 °C (38 °F) in winter and 31 °C (68 °F) in summer. These regions include the northern states of USA, the south of Canada, Central and Southern Europe, and, in the East, Japan.

(*c*) **Cold climates** are those from 55° latitude to the poles. The cold is much modified, however, in some localities by ocean currents, so that Scotland, at the same latitude as Labrador, enjoys a temperate though moist climate, the surrounding seas and air being warmed by the Gulf Stream.

But, in estimating the effect of climate, far more than mere distance from the equator has to be considered. The degree of moisture in the air and presence of the sea near at hand, the rarefaction of the air in consequence of altitude, the difference between night and day temperatures, and the presence or absence of dust and bacteria are all of vital importance. For these reasons climates are classed into four sub-varieties: (1) seaboard and ocean climates; (2) inland low climates; (3) mountain climates; (4) dry climates.

SEABOARD AND OCEAN CLIMATES: The important features of these climates are the large amount of moisture in the air, the relatively high content of oxygen compared with mountain air, and the presence of salt and iodine. The air of the high seas is also free from dust and bacteria. Further, large expanses of water warm and cool more slowly than the earth, so that a seaboard climate tends to be more uniform than inland climates. The cases for which seaside air is most suitable are those convalescent from acute diseases, and those worn out by business or social worries.

INLAND LOW CLIMATES include most of the health resorts to which people go in order to drink mineral waters. The general character of inland climates is the great variation between the summer and winter temperature, but, as most of these places are resorted to only in the open part of the year, the climate goes often by the vague name of 'relaxing', in contradistinction to the 'bracing' climate of mountains. Diseases of the heart and other parts of the circulatory system are treated at some of the less relaxing of these resorts, such as Nauheim, where graduated exercises aid the restful action of the climate.

MOUNTAIN CLIMATES have, as their chief character, the rarity of the air, by reason of which the breathing and heart-beats are increased in rate, and a feeling of buoyancy and increased strength given to the whole system. Further, the air is drier and less laden with dust and bacteria, and there is greater difference between the day and night and between the sun and shade temperatures than at lower levels.

DRY CLIMATES or DESERT CLIMATES combine warmth and dryness. In addition, the air is relatively clear of bacteria, though apt to be dusty, and the nights are cold. Such climates are found in Egypt, Australia, some of the Western States of the USA, and, in a milder degree, on the Pampas of South America and the table-lands of Cape Province in South Africa. These are suited especially for chronic rheumatism and chest diseases.

CLINDAMYCIN is an antibiotic which is used in the treatment of serious infections. This restriction is imposed because it is liable to cause severe colitis. It is active against a wide range of micro-organisms.

CLINICAL means literally 'belonging to a bed', but the word is used to denote anything associated with the practical study or observation of sick people as clinical medicine, clinical thermometers.

CLINICAL PSYCHOLOGY: Psychology is the scientific study of behaviour. It may be applied in various settings including education, industry and health care. Clinical psychology is concerned with the practical application of research findings in the fields of physical and mental health. Training in clinical psychology involves a degree in Psychology followed by postgraduate training. Clinical psychologists are specifically skilled in applying theoretical models and objective methods of observation and measurement and in therapeutic interventions aimed at changing patient's dysfunctional behaviour, including thoughts and feelings as well as actions. Dysfunctional behaviour is explained in terms of normal processes and modified by applying principles of normal learning, adaption and social interaction.

Clinical psychologists are involved in health care in the following ways: (1) Assessment of thoughts, emotions and behaviour using standardized methods. (2) Treatment based on theoretical models and scientific evidence about behaviour change. Behaviour change is considered when it contributes to physical, psychological or social functioning. (3) Consultation with other health-care professionals about problems concerning emotions, thinking and behaviour. (4) Research on a wide variety of topics including the relationship between stress, psychological functioning and disease, the aetiology of problem behaviours, methods and theories of behaviour change. (5) Teaching other professionals about normal and dysfunctional behaviour, emotions and functioning.

Clinical psychologists may specialize in work in particular branches of patient care, including surgery, psychiatry, geriatrics, paediatrics, mental handicap, obstetrics and gynaecology, cardiology, neurology, general practice and physical rehabilitation. Whilst the focus of their work is frequently the patient, at times it may encompass the behaviour of the health-care professionals.

CLINICAL TRIALS: Voltaire defined medical treatment as the act of pouring drugs, of which one knew nothing, into a patient, of whom one knew less. This derisive appraisal of the therapeutics of his time was nearly true as there were virtually no drugs of significant therapeutic value and any benefit the patient received was usually a placebo effect.

The development of effective medical treatment only dates back 50 years or so. When useful drugs did become available in the 1940s and the 1950s doctors realized the importance of evaluating their effectiveness. This lead to the introduction of the so-called clinical trials. Systematic measures were introduced to assess the efficacy initially of new medicines and, later, of surgical operations. This is now done by controlled, randomized clinical trials which compare the new treatment under evaluation either with a placebo or the previous standard treatment. If possible this is done on a double blind basis when neither the patient nor the doctor knows at the time whether the test treatment or the control is being administered: this enables bias to be removed. Such trials have to be done to recognized ethical standards with the procedure properly explained to the participating subjects.

CLINICS (see MATERNITY AND CHILD WELFARE).

CLINIFEED (see ENTERAL FEEDING).

CLITORIS: A small sensitive organ comprising erectile tissue at the top of the female genitalia where the labial folds meet below the pubic bone. During sexual excitement the clitoris enlarges and hardens and may be the focus of orgasm.

CLOBAZAM (see BENZODIAZEPINES).

CLOFAZIMINE is a drug used in the treatment of leprosy.

CLOFIBRATE (see HYPERLIPIDAEMIA).

CLOMIPHENE is a drug that stimulates ovulation, or the production of ova, through the medium of the pituitary gland. It is thus being used in the treatment of female infertility. One of its hazards is that, if given in too big doses, it may produce multiple births.

CLOMIPRAMINE is an antidepressant drug. (See ANTIDEPRESSANTS.)

CLONAZEPAM is a drug that is proving of value in some cases of epilepsy, and in the restless-legs syndrome (q.v.). (See TRANQUILIZER.)

CLONE: A group of cells genetically identical to each other that have arisen from one cell by asexual reproduction (see CLONING).

CLONIC is a word applied to short spasmodic movements.

CLONIDINE is a drug originally introduced for the treatment of high blood-pressure. It is an alpha$_2$ adrenoreceptor agonist. It is also proving of value in the prevention of attacks of migraine. If it is used in the treatment of high blood-pressure, its use must not be stopped abruptly as this may result in a sudden rise of blood-pressure within a matter of hours to a dangerously high level. This is not likely to arise with the smaller doses used in the treatment of migraine.

CLONING, from the Greek *klon* meaning a cutting such as is used to propagate plants, is essentially a form of asexual reproduction. The initial stages have been successfully achieved in rabbits. In essence the technique consists of destroying the nucleus of the egg and replacing it with the nucleus from a body cell of the same species – either a male or a female. This provides the egg with a full complement of chromosomes (q.v.) and it starts to divide and grow just at it would if it had retained its nucleus and been fertilized with a spermatozoon. The vital difference is that the embryo resulting from this cloning process owes nothing genetically to the female egg. It is identical in every respect with the animal from which the introduced nucleus was obtained.

CLONUS: A succession of intermittent muscular relaxations and contractions usually resulting from a sustained stretching stimulus. An example is the clonus stimulated in the calf muscle by maintaining sustained upward pressure on the sole of the foot. The condition is often a sign of disease in the brain or spinal cord.

CLOPAMIDE is a diuretic of value in the treatment of oedema due to heart disease, cirrhosis of the liver and nephrosis. (See BENZOTHIADIAZINES.)

CLOSTRIDIUM is the genus, or variety, of micro-organisms that produce spores which enable them to survive under adverse conditions. They normally grow in soil, water and decomposing plant and animal matter, where they play an important part in the process of putrefaction (q.v.). Among the important members of the group, or genus, are *Clostridium welchii*, *Cl. septicum* and *Cl. oedematiens*, the causes of gas gangrene (see GANGRENE); *Cl. tetani*, the cause of tetanus (q.v.); and *Cl. botulinum*, the cause of botulism (q.v.).

CLOT is the term applied to any semi-solid mass of blood, lymph or other body fluid. Clotting in the blood is due to the formation of strings of fibrin produced by the action of a ferment. Milk clots in a similar manner in the stomach when exposed to the action of the ferment rennin. Clotting occurs naturally when blood is shed and comes in contact with tissues outside the blood-vessels. It occurs also at times in diseased vessels (*thrombosis*), producing serious effects upon the organs supplied by these vessels. Clots also form sometimes in the heart when the circulation is feeble and irregular. (See COAGULATION; EMBOLISM; THROMBOSIS.)

CLOTRIMAZOLE is a drug that is proving of value in the treatment of certain fungal or yeast infections, such as aspergillosis (q.v.) and cryptococcosis (q.v.).

CLOTTING TIME (see COAGULATION).

CLOVES are the unexpanded flower-buds of a species of myrtle, *Eugenia caryophyllus*, from the Indian Archipelago. Oil of cloves is an antiseptic, checks griping, and masks bad breath. It may be taken in doses of 2 or 3 drops on a lump of sugar, or one tablespoonful of infusion of cloves may be similarly used. Cotton-wool dipped in clove oil and put in a hollow tooth relieves toothache temporarily.

CLOXACILLIN (see PENICILLIN, ANTIBIOTIC).

CLUBBING is the term applied to the thickening and broadening of the finger tips and, less commonly, the tips of the toes, that occurs in certain chronic diseases of the lungs and heart. It is due to interstitial oedema especially at the nail bed leading to a loss of the acute angle between the nail and the skin of the finger. It is associated with lung cancer, empyema, bronchietasis and congenital cyanotic heart disease.

CLUB-FOOT, or TALIPES, is a deformity in which the foot is permanently twisted at the ankle-joint, so that the sole no longer rests on the ground in standing.
Varieties: The foot can be twisted in four directions. The heel may be pulled up so that the person walks on his toes (*talipes equinus*), or the toes may be bent up so that he walks on his heel only (*talipes calcaneus*), or the sole may look inwards so that he walks on the outer edge of the foot (*talipes varus*), or outwards so that he walks on the inside of the foot (*talipes valgus*). These are usually combined, the heel being drawn up and the sole turned inwards (*equino-varus*) or the heel resting on the ground and the sole looking outwards (*talipes calcaneo-valgus*). A more important division is into those cases in which the deformity exists at birth, which are generally at first fairly easily rectified; and into those cases which are acquired later in life as the result of some disease, which do not yield to such simple treatment.
Causes: The cases found at birth are due to some arrest of development resulting in a congenital deformity (talipes equino- varus), or

some faulty position of the fetus in the womb (talipes calcaneo-valgus). *Talipes equino-varus* occurs in about 1 per 1000 live births, is twice as common in boys as in girls, and in half the cases involves both feet. Children of affected parents are more likely to have club-foot than those of non- affected parents. Those which are acquired later may be caused by some spasm in the muscles of the one side of the leg (cerebral palsy), or by paralysis of the muscles on the side of the leg away from the deformity (poliomyelitis), or by rigidity due to the scar following a burn or inflammation.

Treatment: *Talipes calcaneo-valgus*, which is almost always due to a faulty position of the foot in the womb, and often involves both feet, responds well as a rule to manipulation. All that is required in most cases is that the affected part should be moulded into the *equino-varus* position each time mother attends to the babe. It is only in the more severe cases that the foot may need to be strapped into the correct position, or fixed in this position in plaster of Paris for a few weeks. The ultimate result is excellent, but there may be a tendency for the condition to relapse when the child starts walking. This is controlled by a wedge on the heel of the shoe. *Talipes equino-varus* is the most important of all forms of club-foot, and treatment depends upon the cause. If it is due to a congenital deformity, the baby must be referred to a specialist as soon as possible. The sooner treatment is begun the better. This consists of stretching and strapping under medical supervision, the baby being seen regularly by the doctor who does the re-strapping as the foot comes into the normal situation, and the mother being taught to stretch the foot regularly between visits to the clinic. In the more severe cases an operation may be needed if the condition has not responded to non-surgical treatment by the age of 2 or 3 months. In the cases which develop as a result of disease or injury after birth, treatment consists of splinting, strengthening the weakened muscles by massage and electrical stimulation. In the more severe cases operation for transplanting tendons may be necessary.

CLUSTER HEADACHES: This is a distinct entity separate from migraine, although it is sometimes referred to as migrainous neuralgia. The name derives from the fact that the headaches cluster in periods of six to twelve weeks at certain times of the year. The headache is usually on one side and often around the eye. Lacrimation and running of the nose are frequently associated. A chronic form in which attacks persist for more than six months exists. Prophylactic treatment with Lithium carbonate is usually effective.

COAGULATION of the blood is the process whereby bleeding (or haemorrhage) is normally arrested in the body. The process is summarized in the following diagram:

prothrombin + calcium + thromboplastin
|
thrombin + fibrinogen
|
fibrin

Prothrombin and calcium are normally present in the blood. Thromboplastin is an enzyme which is normally found in the blood platelets and in tissue cells. When bleeding occurs from a blood-vessel there is always some damage to tissue cells and to the blood platelets. As a result of this damage, thromboplastin is released and comes in contact with the prothrombin and calcium in the blood. In the presence of thromboplastin and calcium prothrombin is converted into thrombin, which in turn interacts with fibrinogen, a protein always present in the blood, to form fibrin. Fibrin consists of needle-shaped crystals, which, with the assistance of the blood platelets, form a fine network in which the blood corpuscles become enmeshed. This meshwork, or clot as it is known, gradually retracts until it forms a tight mass which prevents any further bleeding. It will thus be seen that clotting, or coagulation, does not occur in the healthy blood-vessel because there is no thromboplastin present. There is now evidence suggesting that there is an anti-thrombin substance present in the blood in small amounts, and that this substance antagonizes any small amounts of thrombin that may be formed as a result of small amounts of thromboplastin being released. The clotting or coagulation time is the time taken for blood to clot and can be measured under controlled conditions to ensure that it is normal (three to eight minutes). In certain diseases – haemophilia, for example – clotting time is greatly extended.

COAGULUM is the Latin term for a clot.

COAL-MINER'S LUNG (see ANTHRACOSIS).

COARCTATION OF THE AORTA is a narrowing of the aorta in the vicinity of the insertion of the ductus arteriosus. It is a congenital abnormality. Satisfactory results are now obtained from surgical treatment.

COBALAMINS are a group of substances which have an enzyme action (see ENZYME) and are essential for normal growth and nutrition. (See also CYANOCOBALAMIN; HYDROXOCOBALAMIN.)

COBALT-60 is a radioactive isotope which is being used as a substitute for radium and high-voltage X-rays in the treatment of malignant disease. (See RADIOTHERAPY.)

COBALT EDETATE is an antidote for cyanide poisoning (q.v.).

COCAINE: Coca leaves are obtained from two South American plants, *Erythroxylum coca* and *Erythroxylum truxillense*, and contain an alkaloid, cocaine, which has marked effects as a stimulant, and, locally applied, as an anaesthetic by paralysing nerves of sensation. The dried leaves have been used from time immemorial by the South American Indians, who chew them mixed with a little lime. Their effect is to dull the mucous surfaces of mouth and stomach, with which the saliva, produced by chewing them, comes into contact, thus blunting, for long periods, all feeling of hunger. The cocaine, being absorbed, produces on the central nervous system a stimulating effect, so that all sense of fatigue and breathlessness vanishes for the time. It was by the use of coca that the Indian post-runners of South America were able to achieve their extraordinary feats of endurance. The continued use of the drug, however, results in emaciation, loss of memory, sleeplessness and general breakdown. Addiction to cocaine or a derivative, 'crack', is now a serious social problem in many countries. (See DRUG ADDICTION.)

Uses: Before the serious effects that result from its habitual use were realized, the drug was sometimes used by hunters, travellers and others to relieve exhaustion and breathlessness in climbing mountains, to steady the nerves, and to dull hunger. The chief use in medicine is by local application to dull pain. Internally it is prescribed along with morphine or heroin for the relief of pain in advanced cancer. (See BROMPTON MIXTURE.) Here the risk of addiction is a secondary consideration. Otherwise it is practically only used in the treatment of diseases of the eye, and diseases of the ear, nose and throat. In the eye it is used as an anaesthetic in the form of eye-drops. It is also used in the form of lamellae to induce anaesthesia of the eye. A 5-per-cent spray solution is used to anaesthetize the throat and nose, whilst pastilles and lozenges containing 1·5 to 10 mg are used to reduce irritation of the throat and hoarseness. Artificial chemical compounds closely allied to cocaine are injected hypodermically in order to render painless small operations, such as amputation of the fingers, and by injection into the spinal canal to enable major operations to be done on the lower limbs without pain. (See PROCAINE.)

COCCUS is the name applied to a rounded form of bacterium. (See MICROBIOLOGY.)

COCCYDYNIA, or COCCYGODYNIA, means the sensation of severe pain in the coccyx.

COCCYX is the lower end of the spinal column, resembling a bird's beak and consisting of four nodules of bone, which represent vertebrae, and correspond to the tail in lower animals. They are deeply buried in the muscles in man, but in occasional cases they project backwards, and are surrounded by a fold of skin, so as to form an actual tail.

COCHLEA is the part of the inner ear concerned with hearing. (See EAR.)

CODEINE is one of the active principles of opium (q.v.). In the form of codeine phosphate it is widely prescribed for the relief of a useless, irritative cough, and also along with aspirin for the relief of headaches and rheumatic pains. It tends to be somewhat constipating.

COD-LIVER OIL is made by purification of the oil pressed from the fresh liver of the cod (*Gadus callarius*). Its principal value in medicine arises out of its high content of vitamin D, the vitamin used in the prevention and treatment of rickets. The official cod-liver oil of the *British Pharmacopoeia* contains not less than 85 international units of vitamin D per gram. Cod-liver oil is also a rich source of vitamin A, the official cod-liver oil of the *British Pharmacopoeia* containing not less than 600 units of vitamin-A activity per gram. The protective dose of vitamin D for infants and children is around 400 international units daily.

Human milk contains enough vitamins for the breast-fed baby provided the mother has enough vitamins in her diet and enough vitamin D from the action of sunlight on her skin, or by taking vitamin tablets during pregnancy and lactation when prescribed by her medical adviser. Cow's milk contains less vitamin D than human milk, but in Britain all baby foods contain added vitamin D (as well as vitamins A and C). There is therefore no need to give the bottle-fed baby vitamins as long as he or she is receiving vitamin-supplemented baby milks. Neither is there any need to give the breast-fed baby vitamin supplements as long as the mother has had sufficient of a mixed diet during pregnancy, has been out in the sunshine, and taken any prescribed vitamin tablets. When, however, the weaning process is begun, and the baby starts taking cow's milk, vitamin supplements are necessary.

COELIAC DISEASE is a wasting disease of childhood in which there is inability to absorb fat from the intestines; there is therefore an excess of fat in the stools. It is the result of a constitutional intolerance of gluten (a constituent of wheat flour) which damages the lining membrane of the small intestine. This in turn interferes with the absorption of fat. Treatment is by means of a gluten-free diet. People with coeliac disease, or parents or guardians of coeliac children can obtain help and guidance from the Coeliac Society of the United Kingdom, PO Box 220, High Wycombe, Bucks HP11 2HY (0494-437278). (See also GLUTEN; MALABSORPTION SYNDROME; SPRUE.)

COELIOSCOPY is a method of viewing the interior of the abdomen in patients in whom a tumour or some other condition requiring operation may be present but cannot with certainty be diagnosed. The examination is carried out by making a minute opening under local anaesthesia, and inserting an endoscope, a long flexible instrument bearing an electric lamp and telescopic lenses like that for examining the bladder (cystoscope), into the abdominal cavity. Certain of the abdominal organs can then be directly inspected in turn.

COITUS is sexual intercourse.
COITUS INTERRUPTUS (see CONTRACEPTION).

COLCHICUM, the bulb of *Colchicum autumnale*, or meadow-saffron, has long been used as a remedy for gout. How it acts is not quite certain.
Uses: Its main use is in gout, for which colchicine, the active principle of colchicum, in doses of 0·5 mg every one or two hours until the pain is relieved, followed by 0·5 mg thrice daily for about a week, is the form generally employed. Demecolcine, a derivative of colchicine, is sometimes of value in the treatment of chronic myelogenous leukaemia.

COLD, INJURIES FROM (see CHILBLAIN; FROSTBITE; HYPOTHERMIA; also CHILLS AND COLDS).

COLD SORES (see HERPES SIMPLEX).

COLD, USES OF: The application of cold to the surface of the body is capable of influencing the progress of disease in deep- seated parts to a considerable extent by acting on the blood at the surface, or through the nerves which end in the skin. Cold is applied for five chief purposes:
(a) *To subdue pain*: In headache, a wet cloth to the forehead, or sponging with an evaporating mixture of vinegar and water, or eau-de-Cologne and water, is a well-known remedy. Sprains, if treated by holding the injured joint at once under running water, are much relieved. Later on, however, cold applications do harm, rather than good, by preventing the absorption of the effused blood. The pain of pleurisy may also be relieved by the application of an ice-bag to the side. Small operations may be done painlessly after freezing the skin of the part by spraying ethyl chloride over it.
(b) *To lessen inflammation*: Ice-bags are used in inflammatory conditions to prevent the formation of an abscess. In meningitis, or inflammation of the membranes of the brain, they often give some relief when applied to the head.
(c) *To reduce high temperature*: In any fever, sponging the arms and legs, one by one, with tepid water, is harmless and often very soothing. When the temperature runs very high, e.g. to 40·5 to 41·8 °C (105 or 107 °F), wrapping the patient in a wet sheet and rubbing it with ice, or by putting him in a cold bath may be life-

saving. (See also under ENTERIC FEVERS; WET PACK.)
(d) *To stop haemorrhage*: In cases of increasing haemorrhage under the skin, for example, a bruised and blackening eye or a sprain, the amount of bleeding, and consequent discoloration, are lessened by applying compresses containing ice or some cooling lotion.
(e) *As a general stimulant*: Some diseases are systematically treated in certain countries by cold bathing: for example, typhoid fever. Others are benefited by an alternation of hot and cold bathing: for example, chronic rheumatism. (See also HYPOTHERMIA; CRYOANALGESIA; CRYOSURGERY.)

COLD WEATHER ITCH is a common form of itchiness that occurs in cold weather. It is characterized by slight dryness of the skin, and is particularly troublesome in the legs of old people. The dryness may be accompanied by some mild inflammation of the skin. It may be exacerbated by excessive central heating. Overwashing with soap should be avoided. A non-alkaline substitute for soap such as Aqueous Cream BP is often beneficial. Relief is obtained from the use of emollients such as E45, applied regularly and always after a bath. Rough winter clothing should not be worn next to the skin.

COLDS (see CHILLS AND COLDS).

COLECTOMY is the operation for removing the colon.

COLESTIPOL (see HYPERLIPIDAEMIA).

COLIC: By this term is generally understood an attack of spasmodic pain in the abdomen. SIMPLE COLIC commonly arises from the presence in the alimentary canal of some indigestible matter, which excites spasmodic contraction of the muscular coats of the intestines. The pain of colic is relieved by pressure over the abdomen, and there is no attendant fever – points which are of importance in distinguishing it from inflammation.
Attacks of this form of colic may occur in connection with a variety of causes other than that above mentioned: e.g. from accumulations of faeculent matter in the intestines in the case of those who suffer from habitual constipation; as an accompaniment of nervous ailments and not infrequently as the result of exposure to cold and damp, particularly where the feet become chilled, as in walking through snow. Similar attacks of colic are apt to occur in infants, especially those who are fed artificially; and in such cases it will generally be found that a temporary change of diet will be necessary. The duration of an attack of simple colic is seldom long, and in general no ill consequences follow from it. It is, however, not free from risk, especially that of sudden obstruction of the bowel from twisting, or invagination of one

part within another (intussusception) during the spasmodic seizure, giving rise to a very grave condition. Colic is also a serious symptom when due to obstruction of the bowel by a tumour or similar condition. (See INTESTINE, DISEASES OF; INTUSSUSCEPTION.)

LEAD COLIC (*Syn.* painter's colic, *colica Pictonum*, Devonshire colic, dry belly-ache) is due to the absorption of lead into the system. This disease had been observed and described long before its cause was discovered. Its occurrence in an epidemic form among the inhabitants of Poitou was recorded by Francis Citois, in 1617, and the disease was thereafter termed *colica Pictonum*. It was supposed to be due to the acidity of the native wines, but it was afterwards found to depend on lead contained in them. (See LEAD POISONING.)

BILIARY COLIC and RENAL COLIC are the terms applied to that violent pain which is produced, in the one case where a biliary calculus or gall-stone passes down from the gall-bladder into the intestine, and in the other where a renal calculus descends from the kidney along the ureter into the bladder. (See GALL-STONES; and KIDNEYS, DISEASES OF.)

Treatment: The treatment of colic consists in means to relieve the spasmodic pain, and in the removal, where possible, of the cause upon which it depends. When the attack appears to depend on accumulations of irritating matter in the alimentary canal, a brisk purgative, such as castor oil, will, in addition, be called for. It must be borne in mind that abdominal pain may indicate the onset of acute appendicitis or be a sign of, say, perforation of a peptic ulcer: in such cases purgatives must on no account be given.

Pressure upon the abdomen may relieve the pain partially if not completely. This may be effected, in the case of a baby, by laying him face downwards across the nurse's arm, and in the case of older people by laying a hot-water bottle upon the abdomen, or by lying face downward upon a folded-up pillow. The various substances known as carminatives (q.v.) or anti-spasmodics (see SPASMOLYTICS) also aid in giving relief.

COLIFORM: Description of a gram negative bacterium found in the faeces. It covers the bacterial groups *Enterobacter*, *Escherichia*, and *Klebsiella*.

COLISTIN is an antibiotic isolated from the soil organism, *Bacillus polymyxa* var. *colistinus*. It is active against many Gram-negative organisms, and is proving of value in the treatment of gastro-intestinal and genito-urinary infections.

COLITIS means inflammation of the colon, the first part of the large intestine. *Mucous colitis*, once a fashionable disease, is now recognized not to be a form of colitis and has been named *mucomembranous colic*, or *spastic*

or *irritable colon*. It is caused by painful spasms of the colon and occurs in nervous types of individuals. Treatment consists of dealing with the underlying nervous condition, the avoidance of all aperients, and a full diet without an excess of roughage. *Acute catarrhal colitis* occurs as part of an acute gastro-enteritis, usually due to food poisoning. The treatment is as for acute diarrhoea (q.v.). *Chronic catarrhal colitis* is usually due to the abuse of aperients and purgatives.

ULCERATIVE COLITIS is the most important form of colitis. It is an acute condition, the cause of which is not known. Although apparently precipitated at times by exposure to cold or damp or by dietetic indiscretions, these are not the primary cause. It is predominantly a disease of young adults. Once an individual has had the disease, it is very liable to relapses.

Symptoms: The onset may be sudden or insidious. In the acute form there is severe diarrhoea and the patient may pass up to twenty stools a day. The stools, which may be small in quantity, are fluid and contain blood, pus and mucus. There is always fever, which runs an irregular course. In other cases the patient first notices some irregularity of the movement of the bowels, with the passage of blood. This becomes gradually more marked. There is seldom actual pain except immediately prior to the passage of a stool, but there is always a varying amount of abdominal discomfort. The constant diarrhoea leads to emaciation and weakness, and there is always a well-marked anaemia. The acute form may be rapidly fatal, but as a rule the acute phase passes into a chronic stage. The chronic form is liable to run a prolonged course, and the majority of cases are subject to relapses for many years.

Treatment: Rest in bed is essential during the acute stage and as long as there is fever. The diarrhoea is controlled by corticosteroids which may be given either by mouth or by enema. The diet should be bland and nourishing and should contain a minimum of roughage: i.e. a low-residue diet (see DIET). The anaemia which is always present is treated by means of iron preparations. In some cases it may be necessary to use surgical measures to control the condition: e.g. by removing more or less of the affected colon. Corticosteroids, along with sulphasalazine (q.v.), have become the basic treatment. Another drug proving useful in this condition is azathioprine (q.v.). Once a patient has recovered and is back to work again, it is essential for him to remain on a low-residue diet, and to be particularly careful in avoiding unnecessary exposure to cold and damp; otherwise the condition is liable to recur. In the prevention of recurrences, sulphasalazine is proving most effective.

Patients and their relatives can obtain help and advice from the National Association for Colitis and Crohn's Disease, 98A London Road, St Albans, Herts AL1 1NX (0727–44296).

COLLAGEN is the most abundant protein in the body. It is the major structural component of many parts of the body and occurs in many different forms. Thus it exists as thick fibres in skin and tendons. It is also an important constituent of the heart and blood vessels. With calcium salts it provides the rigid structure of bone. It also occurs as a delicate structure in the cornea of the eye, and in what is known as the basement membrane of many tissues including the glomeruli of the kidneys and the capsule of the lens of the eye. It plays a part in many diseases, hereditary and otherwise. Among the inherited abnormalities of collagen are those responsible for aneurysms of the circle of Willis (q.v.) and for osteogenesis imperfecta (q.v.). On boiling it is converted into gelatin.

COLLAGEN DISEASES is a term used to describe a group of diseases, including acute rheumatism and rheumatoid arthritis, which are characterized by changes in the collagen of the tissues. The precise cause of these changes is not known, but they are probably a sensitization reaction to an unknown toxin, and they respond to cortisone and corticotrophin.

COLLAPSE is a condition of extreme weakness of all the bodily powers, and especially of the nervous system. It forms the termination of many severe diseases, such as cholera, typhoid fever, irritant poisoning. It is closely allied to the condition of surgical shock, but, whilst in collapse from the conditions mentioned the chief feature is feebleness of the heart's action, in shock there are numerous other prominent symptoms. (See SHOCK.)
Symptoms: The face is pale and drawn, the forehead sometimes covered with cold sweat, the eyes sunken and glassy. The voice is weak, the breathing shallow, and the pulse rapid and feeble or imperceptible. The temperature is usually reduced to 35·6 or 36·1 °C (96 or 97 °F). Generally the patient lies on his back, paying no attention to what is proceeding around him.
Treatment: The patient should be allowed to lie quietly on his back in a darkened room, well covered, and surrounded by hot bottles to maintain the body heat. Stimulants are also necessary.

COLLAPSE THERAPY is the term applied to the method of treating diseases of the lung by bringing about collapse of the diseased part through removing the supporting ribs (thoracoplasty), or introducing air into the pleural cavity (artificial pneumothorax).

COLLAR-BONE (see CLAVICLE).

COLLARGOL is a form of colloidal silver which mixes readily with water and any albuminous fluids, and has an antiseptic action. It is used especially for application to the eyes in inflammatory conditions.

COLLES'S FRACTURE is a fracture of the lower end of the radius close to the wrist, caused usually by a fall forwards on the palm of the hand, in which the lower fragment is displaced backwards. (See FRACTURES.)

COLLODIONS consist basically of a thick, colourless, syrupy liquid, made by dissolving gun-cotton (pyroxylin) in a mixture of ether and alcohol or with acetone. When painted on the skin the solvent evaporates, leaving a tough protective film behind that is useful for covering wounds. *Flexible collodion*, or collodion as it is often referred to, contains 1·6 per cent of pyroxylin, with colophony, castor oil and alcohol (90 per cent) in solvent ether. It should be kept in a well-sealed container. Being relatively elastic, it does not crack through the movements of the skin.

COLLOID is the name given to a type of cancer of internal organs, in which a glue-like substance collects in the interior of the tumour. The term is also applied to substances existing in a colloidal solution, and to the viscid iodine-containing material in the spaces of the thyroid gland.

COLLOIDAL SOLUTIONS are solutions in which a substance very finely divided into particles is suspended in another substance, as, for example, metals like silver and iron suspended in the form of minute particles in water or glycerin. The two constituents of the colloidal solution are called phases – the particles being known as the internal phase, and the medium in which they are suspended, the continuous or external phase. The term, suspensoid, is applied to colloids in which the particles consist of pure solid, and the term, emulsoid, is applied to those in which the particles absorb some of the liquid in which they are suspended.

COLOBOMA simply means a defect, but its use is usually restricted to congenital defects of the eye. These may involve, the lens, the iris, the retina or the eyelid.

COLON is the first part of the large intestine. (See INTESTINE.)

COLONIC IRRIGATION: Washing out the large bowel with an enema of water or other medication.

COLONOSCOPE is an instrument for viewing the interior of the colon. It is made of fibre glass which ensures flexibility, and incorporates a system of lenses for magnification and a lighting system.

COLOSTOMY is the operation for the establishment of an artificial opening into the colon. This acts as an artificial anus. The operation is carried out when there is an obstruction in the colon or rectum that cannot be overcome, or in cases, such as cancer of the rectum in which the rectum and part of the colon have to be removed. Such a colostomy opening can be trained to function in such a way that the patient can carry on a normal life, eating a more or less normal diet. Anyone wishing help or advice in the practical management of a colostomy should get in touch with the British Colostomy Association, 15 Station Road, Reading, Berkshire RG1 1LG (0734-391537, fax: 0734-569095). (See STOMA.)

COLOSTRUM is the first fluid secreted by the mammary glands for two or three days after childbirth. It contains less casein and more albumin than ordinary milk.

COLOUR BLINDNESS (see VISION, Defective colour vision).

COLPORRHAPHY is an operation designed to strengthen the pelvic floor in cases of prolapse of the uterus.

COLPOSCOPY is the method of examining the vagina and cervix by means of the binocular instrument known as the colposcope. It is proving of particular value in the early detection of cancer of the cervix.

COMA is a state of profound unconsciousness, in which not only can the sufferer not be roused, but there are not even reflex movements when the skin is pinched, the eyeball touched, etc. The breathing is generally stertorous, but deep, and the heart's action is strong. The cause of coma is usually apoplexy, but it may also be due to high fever, diabetes mellitus, glomerulonephritis, alcohol, epilepsy, cerebral tumour, meningitis, injury to the head, overdose of insulin, carbon monoxide poisoning, poisoning from opium and other narcotic drugs. Though usually of relatively short duration, and terminating in death, unless yielding to treatment, it may occasionally be long-lasting. The longest recorded case is that of the woman who died in the USA in 1978 at the age of 43, after having been in a coma for thirty-seven years following an operation for removal of her appendix. (See UNCONSCIOUSNESS.)

COMEDONES (see ACNE).

COMMENSAL is the term applied to microorganisms which live in or on the body (e.g. in the gut or respiratory tract, or on the skin) without doing any harm to the individual.

COMMINUTED FRACTURE: A break in a bone in which the broken ends splinter into pieces. It is usually the result of a crushing force which also damages surrounding tissues such as nerves, blood vessels and muscles. Such a fracture is harder to set than a simple (clean) break. (See FRACTURES.)

COMMISSURE means a joining, and is a term applied to strands of nerve fibres which join one side of the brain to the other, to the band joining one optic nerve to the other, to the junctions of the lips at the corners of the mouth, etc.

COMMITTEE ON SAFETY OF MEDICINES (CSM): The Committee for Safety of Drugs was set up in 1963 in response to the thalidomide disaster. When the Medicines Act became law in 1971 this Committee was replaced by the Committee on Safety of Medicines. The CSM is an advisory committee which scrutinizes drugs at three stages: before clinical trials (clinical trial certificate stage), before a drug is advertised or marketed (product licence stage), or after marketing, the stage at which most doctors first have a direct interest in its work. Until 1981 the first stage in the assessment of new products required the granting to the company concerned of a clinical trial certificate, without which the product could not be tested in man. The issue of a trial certificate requires detailed animal evidence of toxicology and of teratogenic effects. A product licence is normally valid for five years, after which it has to be renewed. Before such a licence is granted efficacy must be shown for each of the proposed indications and appropriate warnings about side effects, contra-indications and interactions given.

COMMON COLD (see CHILLS AND COLDS).

COMMOTIO CEREBRI is another term for concussion of the brain.

COMMUNICABLE DISEASE: This is an infectious or contagious disease, which can be passed from one person to another. Direct physical contact, the handling of an infected object or the transfer by droplets coughed or breathed out are all ways in which microorganisms can be transmitted. The government produces a list of notifiable diseases (q.v.), which includes all the dangerous communicable diseases.

COMMUNITY HEALTH COUNCIL (see NATIONAL HEALTH SERVICE).

COMMUNITY PHYSICIAN A doctor who works in the specialty that encompasses preventive medicine (q.v.), epidemiology (q.v.) and public health (q.v.).

COMPATIBILITY: The extent to which a person's defence systems will accept invading foreign substances, for example, an injection of a drug, a blood transfusion or an organ transplant. When incompatibility occurs there is usually a rapid antibody attack on the invading antigen with a severe local or system reaction in the individual receiving the antigenic substance.

COMPENSATION is a term applied to the counterbalancing of some defect of structure or function by some other special bodily development. The body possesses a remarkable power of adapting itself to even serious defects, so that disability due to these passes off after a time. The term is most often applied to the ability possessed by the heart to increase in size, and therefore in power, when the need for greater pumping action arises in consequence of a defective valve or some other abnormality in the circulation. A heart in this condition is, however, more liable to be prejudicially affected by strains and diseased processes, and the term 'failure of compensation' is applied to the symptoms that result when this power becomes temporarily insufficient.

COMPLEMENT is a normal constituent of blood serum which plays an important part in the antibody-antigen reaction which is the basis of many immunity processes. (See IMMUNITY.)

COMPLEMENTARY MEDICINE (see ALTERNATIVE MEDICINE).

COMPLEX is the term applied to a combination of various actions or symptoms. The term is particularly applied to a set of symptoms occurring together in mental disease with such regularity as to receive a special name.

COMPLEXION (see ACNE; SKIN DISEASES; SUNBURN).

COMPLIANCE: The extent to which a patient follows a doctor's advice. Compliance is better if the doctor explains the treatment to the patient.

COMPRESS is the name given to a pad of linen or flannel wrung out of water and bound to the body. It is generally wrung out of cold water, and may be covered with a piece of waterproof material. It is used to subdue pain or inflammation. (See COLD, USES OF.) A hot compress is generally called a fomentation. (See FOMENTATION.)

COMPRESSED AIR ILLNESS (see CAISSON DISEASE).

COMPRESSION SYNDROME (see MUSCLES, DISEASES OF).

COMPUTED TOMOGRAPHY: Tomography is an X-ray examination technique in which only structures in a particular plane produce clearly focused images. Whole-body computed tomography was introduced in 1977 and has already made a major impact in the investigation and management of medical and surgical disease. The technique is particularly valuable where a mass distorts the contour of an organ, e.g. a pancreatic tumour, or a lesion which has a density different from that of surrounding tissue, e.g. a metastasis in the liver. Computed tomography can distinguish soft tissues from cysts or fat, but in general soft tissue masses have similar appearances, so that distinguishing an inflammatory mass from a malignant process may be impossible. Computed tomography is particularly useful in patients with suspected malignancy. It can also define the extent of the cancer by detecting enlarged lymph nodes, indicating lymphatic spread. The main indications for computed tomography of the body are: mediastinal masses, suspected pulmonary metastases, adrenal disease, pancreatic masses, retroperitoneal lymph nodes, intra- abdominal abscesses, orbital tumours and the staging of cancer.

CONCEPTION signifies the complex set of changes which occur in the ovum and in the body of the mother at the beginning of pregnancy. The precise moment of conception is that at which the male element, or spermatozoon, and the female element, or ovum, fuse together. Only one-third of these conceptions survive to birth, whilst 15 per cent are cut short by spontaneous abortion or stillbirth. The remainder – over one half – are lost very early during pregnancy without trace. (See FETUS.)

CONCRETIONS are masses of various sizes and substances which form in many of the tissues and smaller cavities of the body in certain circumstances.
Varieties and causes: There is a special liability to the deposit of lime salts in damaged or degenerating tissues. The reason for this is probably much the same as that for the similar deposit from hard water inside kettles and boilers. The tissues in question being inactive do not produce sufficient carbon dioxide to keep dissolved the lime salts in the fluids circulating past and through them. Accordingly, healed-up areas in the lungs, which have been the seat of tuberculosis, the remains of dead parasites and other foreign bodies, degenerated blood-vessels, tumours and scars generally, are apt to have lime deposited in and around them till masses of considerable size are formed. The tartar on the teeth, some stones in the bladder, and the calculi sometimes found in the ducts of salivary glands in the cheek or beneath the tongue, are examples of a similar deposit of lime and phosphates, due to the action of bacteria.

Hair-balls, which are common in the stomachs of lower animals that lick themselves, occur sometimes in mentally deranged patients who have a habit of chewing their hair, and may reach the size of walnuts or larger. (See also BEZOAR.)

Various glands produce secretions, which, by a gradual process of sedimentation build up solid masses in the ducts of these glands. Examples of this are found in the gall-stones, formed of cholesterin separated from the bile, in the uratic stones found in the kidney or bladder of persons suffering from acidity, in the plugs of hardened wax which often give trouble in the ear, and in the cheese-like masses which accumulate in the tonsils and give rise to foetor of the breath.

Gout is a disease in which the pain is due to sharp uratic crystals which are deposited on the surfaces of joints, the same crystals being deposited in other tissues also, at a later stage of the disease, so that large solid masses called 'chalk-stones' are ultimately formed. (See GOUT.)

CONCUSSION OF THE BRAIN (see BRAIN).

CONDIMENTS (see DIET).

CONDITIONED REFLEX: The development of a specific response by an individual to a specific stimulus. The best-known conditioned reflex is the one described by Ivan Pavlov in which dogs that became accustomed to being fed when a bell was sounded salivated on hearing the bell even if no food was given. The conditioned reflex is an important part of behavioural theory.

CONDOM: A thin rubber or plastic sheath placed over the erect penis before sexual intercourse. It is the most effective type of barrier contraception and is also valuable in preventing the transfer between sexual partners of pathogenic organisms such as gonococci, which cause gonorrhoea, and human immunodeficiency virus, which may lead to AIDS.

CONDYLE is the name given to a rounded prominence at the end of a bone: for example, the prominences at the outer and inner sides of the knee on the thigh-bone (or femur). The projecting part of a condyle is sometimes known as an *epicondyle*, as in the case of the condyle at the lower end of the humerus (q.v.) where the epicondyles form the prominences on the outer and inner side of the elbow.

CONDYLOMA means a localized, rounded swelling of mucous membrane about the opening of the bowel, and the genital organs, sometimes known as 'genital warts' or 'anogenital warts'. There are two main forms of them: *Condyloma latum*, which is syphilitic in origin, and *Condyloma acuminatum*, which often occurs in association with venereal disease, but is only indirectly due to it, being primarily a virus infection.

CONDY'S FLUID is a powerful disinfectant containing permanganates.

CONE: (1) A light-sensitive cell in the retina of the eye that can also distinguish colours. The other type of light-sensitive cell is called a rod. There are around six million cones in the human retina and these are thought to comprise three types that are sensitive to the three primary colours of red, blue, and green. (2) A cone biopsy is a surgical technique in which a conical or cylindrical section of the lower part of the neck of the womb is excised.

CONGENITAL deformities, diseases, etc., are those which are either present at birth, or which, being transmitted direct from the parents, show themselves some time after birth.

CONGESTION means the accumulation of blood in a part due to over-filling of its blood-vessels. The condition may be due to some weakness of the circulation (see CIRCULATION, DISORDERS OF), but as a rule is one of the early signs of inflammation (see ABSCESS; INFLAMMATION).

CONJUGATE DEVIATION is the term for describing the persistent and involuntary turning of both eyes in any one direction, and is a sign of a lesion in the brain.

CONJUNCTIVA (see EYE).

CONJUNCTIVITIS (see EYE, DISEASE AND INJURIES).

CONNECTIVE TISSUE: This tissue holds together the different structures in the body. It comprises a matrix of substances called mucopolysaccharides in which are embedded a variety of specialist tissues and cells. These include elastic (yellow), collagenous (white) and reticular fibres as well as fibroblasts, macrophages and mast cells (q.v.). This variety is assembled in differing proportions to provide structures with varying functions: bone, cartilage, tendons and ligaments as well as fatty and elastic tissues.

CONSANGUINOUS: A relationship by blood: siblings are closely consanguinous, cousins, and grandparents and grandchildren less so.

CONSERVATIVE TREATMENT: Medical treatment which involves the minimum of active interference by the practitioner. For example, a disc lesion in the back might be treated by bed rest in contrast to surgical intervention to remove the damaged disc.

CONSOLIDATION is a term applied to solidification of an organ, especially of a lung. The consolidation may be of a permanent nature due to formation of fibrous tissue, or may be temporary, as in acute pneumonia.

CONSTIPATION, or COSTIVENESS, means a condition in which the bowels are opened too seldom or incompletely, the motions as a consequence being dry and hard. It should, however, be borne in mind that, though most persons have in health one daily movement of the bowels, some perform this act twice, while in others a motion once in two or more days is perfectly natural. Constipation is a chronic condition, and must be carefully distinguished from acute obstruction of the bowels, a much more serious condition. (See INTESTINE, DISEASES OF.) Great variations, however, take place in colour (see STOOLS), in amount, and in consistency, according to the nature and quantity of the food and drink taken.

Causes: The uncommon causes of constipation are mechanical – that is, obstruction by stricture of the bowel, by tumour, by adhesive bands. The common causes are (1) habit, (2) 'a greedy colon', which absorbs water too quickly, (3) a spastic colon, the muscle of which remains in a state of spasm, (4) lack of tone of the colon muscle, sometimes because of too little vitamin B_1 in the diet, (5) a diet which has not enough 'roughage' in it to stimulate the intestine to activity. Of these, habit is probably most important. Constant neglect to respond to the sensation in the rectum which indicates that it is full and needs emptying leads to retention of faeces, which become dry and hard. The condition is aggravated by the use of purgatives.

Symptoms and effects: The stools are dark, hard, and passed with difficulty, and in small amount. In severe, persistent cases there may be swelling of the abdomen, from the retention of large masses of the remnants from digestion. Colic may occur in long-standing cases, in which the accumulation in the lower part of the bowel is beginning to affect the rest of the gut. Piles, which are a cause of increasing constipation, are often brought on by inattention to the bowels to begin with. Headache and lassitude may be present, but this is largely due to the pressure of the accumulated faeces in the rectum, not to any so-called toxic effect.

Treatment: Assuming that there is no organic cause, such as tumour or other source of mechanical obstruction, the most important matter is the regulation of the daily habits. The person concerned should take a certain amount of exercise daily. Above all things, a habit of opening the bowels, at the same time every day, should be cultivated. The diet is of importance. On the whole, in cases of constipation this errs in being too concentrated and too unirritating. As a rule, the diet should be changed to include plenty of foods containing fibre, for instance, brown bread, green vegetables, and fruit, especially fruit like prunes, which have a large indigestible residue. A considerable amount of fluid should be taken, and the juice of an orange or grapefruit, or a glass of water, first thing in

the morning may help. There is much to be said for adding a dessertspoonful of wheat bran (in the form known as miller's bran) to the breakfast cereal, or lunch or dinner sweet.

The use of aperients and purgatives has usually exaggerated the condition, and as a general rule should be given up.

CONSTITUTION, or DIATHESIS, means the general condition of the body, especially with reference to its liability to certain diseases.

CONSULTANT: In Britain's National Health Service a consultant is the senior career post for a fully qualified specialist. He normally sees patients referred to him by general practitioners – hence the historical term 'consultant' – or emergency cases admitted direct to hospital. NHS consultants are also allowed to do a certain amount of private practice. A consultant has to undergo several years of specialist training in hospital as a 'junior' doctor and pass stiff, higher examinations. There were nearly 18,000 consultants in the United Kingdom in 1989 and over 33,000 general practitioners for a population of more than 57 million.

CONSUMPTION (see TUBERCULOSIS).

CONTACT LENSES are lenses worn in contact with the eye, behind the eyelids and in front of the cornea. They may be worn for cosmetic, optical or therapeutic reasons. The commonest reason for wear is cosmetic, many short-sighted people preferring to wear contact lenses instead of glasses. Optical reasons for contact-lens wear include cataract surgery (usually unilateral extraction) and the considerable improvement in overall standard of vision experienced by very short-sighted people by wearing contact lenses instead of glasses. Therapeutic lenses are those used in the treatment of eye disease, 'bandage lenses' are used in certain corneal diseases: contact lenses can be soaked in a particular drug and then put on the eye so that

	Hard lens	Soft lens
Cost	Cheap	Expensive
Fitting	Straightforward	Simpler
Adaptation time	Can be considerable	Much shorter
Wearing time	Limited	Longer
Comfort	May cause discomfort	Very comfortable
Visual acuity	Good	Poorer; may be unstable
Stability	May be displaced, or ejected from eye	Rarely displaced or ejected
Durability	Resistant to mishandling	More easily damaged
Length of service	Usually long	Limited
Care	Simple	More difficult

Relative advantages and disadvantages of hard and soft contact lenses.

the drug slowly leaks out on to the eye. Contact lenses may be hard, soft or gas permeable. Hard lenses are more optically accurate (because they are rigid), cheaper and more durable than soft. The main advantage of soft lenses is that they are more comfortable to wear. Gas-permeable lenses are so called because they are more permeable to oxygen than other lenses, thus allowing more oxygen to reach the cornea.

CONTAGION means the principle of spread of disease by direct contact with the body of an affected person.

CONTINUED FEVERS are typhus, typhoid and relapsing fevers, so called because of their continuing over a more or less definite space of time.

CONTINUOUS POSITIVE AIRWAYS PRESSURE: A method for treating babies who suffer from alveolar collapse in the lung as a result of hyaline membrane disease (respiratory distress syndrome) (q.v.).

CONTRACEPTION: A means of avoiding pregnancy despite sexual activity. There is no ideal contraceptive, and the choice of method depends on balancing considerations of safety, effectiveness, and acceptability. The best choice for any couple will depend on their ages and personal circumstances and may well vary with time. Contraceptive techniques can be classified in various ways, but one of the most useful is into 'barrier' and 'non-barrier' methods.
BARRIER METHODS: these involve a physical barrier which prevents sperm from reaching the cervix. Barrier methods reduce the risk of spreading sexually transmitted diseases, and the sheath is the best protection against HIV infection (q.v.) for sexually active people. The efficiency of barrier methods is improved if they are used in conjunction with a spermicidal foam or jelly, but care is needed to ensure that the preparation chosen does not damage the rubber barrier.
Condom (sheath): this is the most commonly used barrier contraceptive. It consists of a rubber sheath which is placed over the erect penis before intromission and removed after ejaculation. The failure rate, if properly used, is about 4 per cent.
Diaphragm or *cap*: a rubber dome that is inserted into the vagina before intercourse and fits snugly over the cervix. It should be used with an appropriate spermicide and is removed six hours after intercourse. A woman must be measured to ensure that she is supplied with the correct size of diaphragm, and the fit should be checked annually or after more than about 7 lbs. change in weight. The failure rate, if properly used, is about 2 per cent.
NON-BARRIER METHODS: these do not provide a physical barrier between sperm and cervix and so do not protect against sexually transmitted diseases, including HIV.

Coitus interruptus: this involves the man's withdrawing his penis from the vagina before ejaculation. Because some sperm may leak before full ejaculation, the method is not very reliable.
Safe period: this involves avoiding intercourse around the time when the woman ovulates and is at risk of pregnancy. The safe times can be predicted using temperature charts to identify the rise in temperature before ovulation or by careful assessment of the quality of the cervical mucus. This method works best if the woman has regular menstrual cycles. If used carefully it can be very effective and is free from side-effects, but it requires a highly motivated couple to succeed. It is approved by the Catholic church.
Spermicidal gels, creams, pessaries, etc.: these are supposed to prevent pregnancy by killing sperm before they reach the cervix, but they are unreliable and should be used only in conjunction with a barrier method.
Intrauterine contraceptive device (coil): this is a small metal or plastic shape placed inside the uterus that prevents pregnancy by disrupting implantation. Some people regard it as a form of abortion, so it is not acceptable to all religious groups. There is a significantly increased risk of pelvic infection and eventual infertility in women who have used coils, and in many countries their use has declined substantially. They must be inserted by a specially trained health worker, but once in place they permit intercourse at any time with no prior planning. Increased pain and bleeding may be caused during menstruation, but, if severe, these may indicate that the coil is incorrectly sited, and that its position should be checked.
Hormonal methods: these include the combined oestrogen and progesterone and progesterone-only contraceptive pills, as well as longer-acting depot preparations. They modify the woman's hormonal environment and prevent pregnancy by disrupting various stages of the menstrual cycle, especially ovulation. The combined oestrogen and progesterone pills are very effective and are the most popular form of contraception. A wide range of preparations is available and the *British National Formulary* contains details of the commonly used varieties.

The main side-effects are an increased risk of cardiovascular disease. The lowest possible dose of oestrogen should be used, and many preparations use phasic preparations in which the dose of oestrogen varies with the time of the cycle. The progesterone- only or 'mini' pill does not contain any oestrogen and must be taken at the same time every day. It is not as effective as the combined pill, but failure rates of less than 1-per-100 woman years can be achieved. It has few serious side-effects, but may cause menstrual irregularities. It is suitable for use by mothers who are breast feeding. Depot preparations include intramuscular injections, subcutaneous implants, and intravaginal rings. They are useful in cases where the woman cannot be relied on to take a pill regularly but needs effective contraception. Their main side-effect is their prolonged action, which means that users cannot suddenly decide that they would like to become pregnant.

Sterilization: permanent contraception can be achieved by sterilizing either the male or female partner. The operation on men is easier and safer. Although sterilization can sometimes be reversed, this cannot be guaranteed and couples should be counselled in advance that the method is irreversible. There is a small but definite failure rate with sterilization, and this should also be made clear before the operation is performed.

Post-coital contraception: this is, in effect, a high dose of the combined oral contraceptive given within 72 hours of unprotected intercourse. It can cause nausea and vomiting. It is useful in an emergency, e.g. if a sheath splits during intercourse or after rape, but, if a woman requests it repeatedly because she is forgetting to use her usual method of contraception, further counselling and a change of regular method is indicated.

CONTRACTURE means the permanent shortening of a muscle or of fibrous tissue. Contraction is the name given to the temporary shortening of a muscle.

CONTRAST MEDIUM: A material that is used to increase the visibility of the body's tissues and organs during radiography. A common example is the use of barium which is given by mouth or as an enema to show up the alimentary tract.

CONTRE-COUP means an injury in which a bone, generally the skull, is fractured, not at the spot where the violence is applied, but at the exactly opposite point.

CONTROLLED DRUGS: In the United Kingdom controlled drugs are those preparations referred to under the Misuse of Drugs Act, 1971. The act prohibits activities related to the manufacture, supply and possession of these drugs and they are classified into three groups which determine the penalties for offences involving their misuse. For example, class A includes cocaine, diamorphine, morphine, LSD and pethidine (qq.v.). Class B includes amphetamines, barbiturates, cannabis, codeine and pentazocine (qq.v.). Class C includes drugs related to amphetamines such as diethylpropion and chlorphentermine, meprobamate (q.v.) and most benzodiazepines (q.v.).

The Misuse of Drugs Regulations, 1985, define the classes of person authorized to supply and possess controlled drugs and lay down the conditions under which these activities may be carried out. In the Regulations drugs are divided into five schedules specifying the requirements for supply, possession, prescribing and record-keeping. Schedule 1 contains drugs, such as cannabis, which are not used as medicines. Schedules 2 and 3 contain drugs which are subject to the prescription requirements of the Act (see below). They are distinguished in the *British National Formulary* (BNF) (q.v.) by the symbol CD and they include morphine, diamorphine (heroin), other opioid analgesics, barbiturates, amphetamines, cocaine and diethylpropion. Schedules 4 and 5 contain drugs such as the benzodiazepines which are subject to minimal control. A full list of the drugs in each schedule can be found in the BNF.

Prescriptions for drugs in schedules 2 and 3 must be signed and dated by the prescriber, who must give his address. The prescription must be in the prescriber's own handwriting and provide the name and address of the patient and the total quantity of the preparation in both words and figures. The pharmacist is not allowed to dispense a controlled drug unless all the information required by law is given on the prescription.

The Misuse of Drugs (Notification and Supply of Addicts) Regulations, 1973, govern the notification of addicts. This is required in respect of the following commonly used drugs: cocaine, dextromoramide, diamorphine, dipipanone, hydrocodeine, hydromorphone, levorphanol, methadone, morphine, opium, oxycodone, pethidine, phenazocine and piritranide.

Any doctor who suspects that his patient may be addicted to one of these drugs must notify the Chief Medical Officer at the Home Office in writing within seven days. Notification in writing must be confirmed annually if the patient is still being treated by the doctor. The Home Office maintains an Index of Addicts which is available to doctors on a confidential basis.

CONTUSION (see BRUISES).

CONVALESCENCE means the condition through which a person passes after having suffered from some acute disease, and before complete health and strength are regained.

CONVERGENCE: (1) Inward turning of the eyes to focus on a near point with the result that a single image is registered by both retinas. (2) The coming together of various nerve fibres to form a nerve tract that provides a single pathway from different parts of the brain.

CONVOLUTIONS (see BRAIN).

CONVULSIONS are rapidly alternating contractions and relaxations of the muscles, causing irregular movements of the limbs or body generally, and usually accompanied by unconsciousness. They form really only a symptom of some other trouble, often, in children, of a trifling nature, but, on account of the alarm they cause and their occasional seriousness, they are treated often as a disease by themselves.

Causes: The most common cause of convulsions in adults is epilepsy (q.v.). As the vast majority of convulsive seizures occur in children, however, only these will be dealt with here. The relative frequency of convulsions in infants and young children is probably due to an instability of the immature nervous system. An American investigation showed that in a group of 8823 otherwise normal children, some 6 per cent had had one or more convulsions. Some children are more liable to develop convulsions than others, and this is probably due to a neurotic inheritance.

In young infants convulsions may be due to *birth injuries*, usually the result of a difficult labour. The convulsions in these cases are due to damage of the brain, either by bleeding from torn blood-vessels or concussion of the brain. In older infants convulsions may be due to the irritability of the brain often associated with *rickets*. This is the condition known as tetany, and before the introduction of the routine administration of vitamin D to infants and children, it was one of the most common causes of convulsions in older infants and young children. Other metabolic causes include hypoglycaemia and hypokalaemia.

A sudden *rise of temperature*, such as may occur in any infection, may induce convulsions in an infant and young child. This is most likely in pneumonia, and it would appear as if in the child a convulsion was the equivalent of the chill or rigor which occurs in adults. *Irritation* elsewhere in the body may cause convulsions in the predisposed child. This is most likely to occur with irritation in the bowels, e.g. the eating of unripe or indigestible food, colic, worms or even constipation. Infection of the kidneys or bladder may also be responsible, as may be earache, particularly if of sudden onset. The role of teething as a cause of convulsions has been exaggerated, but there is no doubt that, if painful, the teething process may occasionally produce convulsions.

Diseases of the brain, such as meningitis, encephalitis and tumours, or any disturbance of the brain due to bleeding, blockage of a blood-vessel, or irritation of the brain by a fracture of the skull, may also be responsible for convulsions.

Asphyxia, such as may occur in a young child during a paroxysm of whooping-cough, may also bring on convulsions. Breath-holding (q.v.), a not uncommon condition in infants and young children, may also persist long enough to bring on convulsions. These breath-holding attacks follow a severe bout of crying, at the end of which the infant holds his breath. As a rule, the worst that happens is that the infant holds his breath until he is blue in the face, and then starts breathing again. Occasionally, however, the breath-holding persists until there is a convulsion. An occasional breath-holding attack need not be taken too seriously but, if it is repeated, medical advice should be sought.

Finally, it must never be forgotten that *epilepsy* can occur in infants and young children.

Treatment: Convulsions are rarely dangerous to life unless they occur as part of a dangerous condition which is already threatening the child's life. The time-honoured custom is to put the child in a hot bath, but this is seldom necessary. On the other hand, tepid sponging may help if there is fever. If there is any possibility of the child biting his tongue, a spoon or a spatula should be put between the teeth. There is seldom any need to restrain the movements unless they are severe enough to throw the child off the bed or couch. If the convulsions persist, it may be necessary to give parenteral benzodiazepines. As a rule a sedative, or an injection of one of the barbiturates, controls the convulsions. Once these are under control, the cause of the convulsions must be sought and the necessary treatment given.

COOLEY'S ANAEMIA, or THALASSAEMIA, is a condition in which there is an inherited defect in the production of normal haemoglobin, resulting in a severe degree of anaemia.

COOMB'S TEST: A sensitive test that detects antibodies (q.v.) to the body's red cells (see ERYTHROCYTE). There are two methods: one, the direct, identifies those antibodies that are bound to the cells; the other, indirect, method identifies those circulating unattached in the serum.

CO-ORDINATION means the governing power exercised by the brain as a whole, or by certain centres in the nervous system, to make various muscles contract in harmony, and so produce definite actions, instead of meaningless movements. It is bound up intimately with the complex sense of localization, which enables a person with his eyes shut to tell, by sensations received from the bones, joints and muscles, the position of the various parts of his body. The power is impaired in various diseases, such as locomotor ataxia. It is tested by making the patient shut his eyes, moving his hand in various directions, and then telling him to bring the point of the forefinger steadily to the tip of the nose, or by other simple movements.

COPPER is an essential nutrient for man, and all tissues in the human body contain traces of it. The total amount in the adult body is 100 to 150 mg. Many essential enzyme systems are dependent on traces of copper. On the other hand, there is no evidence that dietary deficiency of copper ever occurs in man. Infants are born with an ample store, and the normal diet for an adult contains around 2 mg of copper a day. It is used in medicine as the two salts, sulphate of copper (blue stone) and nitrate of copper. The former is, in small doses, a powerful astringent, and in larger doses an irritant. Both are caustics when applied externally. Externally, either is used to rub on unhealthy ulcers and growths to stimulate the granulation tissue to more rapid healing.

COPROLALIA is the condition in which insane people give utterance to filthy and obscene words.

COPULATION: The act of coitus or sexual intercourse when the man inserts his erect penis into the woman's vagina and after a succession of thrusting movements ejaculates his semen.

CORDOTOMY, or CHORDOTOMY, is the surgical operation of cutting the antero-lateral tracts of the spinal cord to relieve otherwise intractable pain. It is also sometimes known as tractotomy.

CORNEA (see EYE).

CORNEAL GRAFT (KERATOPLASTY): If the cornea becomes damaged or diseased and vision is impaired, it can be removed and replaced by a corneal graft. The graft is taken from the cornea of a human donor. Some of the indication for corneal grafting include keratoconus, corneal dystrophies, severe corneal scarring following herpes simplex, alkali burns or injury. Because the graft is a foreign protein, there is a danger that the recipient's immune system may set up a reaction causing rejection of the graft. Rejection results in oedema of the graft with subsequent poor vision. Once a corneal graft has been taken from a donor, it should be used as quickly as possible. Corneas can be stored for a short while in tissue-culture medium at low temperature.

The Department of Health has drawn up a list of suitable eye-banks to which people can apply to bequeath their eyes, and an official form is now available for the bequest of eyes. (See also DONORS; TRANSPLANTATION.)

CORNS AND BUNIONS: A corn is a localized thickening of the cuticle or epidermis, of a conical shape, the point of the cone being directed inwards and being known as the 'eye' of the corn. A general thickening over a wider area is called a callosity. Bunion is a condition found over the joint at the base of the great toe, in which not only is there thickening of the skin, but the head of the metatarsal bone, in consequence of bending outwards of the toe by pointed or too short boots, becomes unduly prominent beneath thickened skin. Hammer-toe is a condition of the second toe, often caused by short boots, in which the toe becomes bent at its two joints in such a way as to resemble a hammer.
Causes: The cause of bunions is ill-fitting footwear. Corns are due similarly to the pressure of tight or badly fitting footwear, or, when on the under-surface of the foot, to unevenness in the sole. The skin grows more rapidly in consequence of the irritation, and becomes

changed by the pressure into a species of horn. Where the corns are between the toes, they become moist and sodden, and are called soft corns.

To prevent corns sufficiently large and properly shaped shoes should be worn. Relief from the pain of a corn may be obtained by wearing a ring of felt (corn plaster) round the corn, so as to free it from pressure. To remove the corn, the foot should be soaked in hot soapy water, and the corn then cut or scraped away with a clean knife or pair of scissors. After drying, the site of the corn should be covered with a small piece of soap plaster, or painted inside the felt ring with salicylic acid collodion to soften and break up the corn, which may be picked away gradually or rubbed down with pumice-stone.

Individuals who are liable to corns and bunions should attend a qualified chiropodist.

CORONARY is a term applied to several structures in the body encircling an organ in the manner of a crown. The coronary arteries are the arteries of supply to the heart which arise from the aorta, just beyond the aortic valve, and through which the blood is delivered to the muscle of the heart. Disease of the coronary arteries is a very serious condition producing various abnormal forms of heart action and the disease, angina pectoris.

CORONARY ARTERIES: The right coronary artery arises from the right sinus of the valsalva and passes into the right atrio-ventricular groove to supply the right ventricle, part of the intraventricular septum and the inferior part of the left ventricle. The left coronary artery arises from the left sinus and divides into an anterior descending branch which supplies the septum and the anterior and apical parts of the heart, and the circumflex branch which passes into the left antrio-ventricular groove and supplies the lateral posterior surfaces of the heart. Small anastomoses exist between the coronary arteries and they have the potential of enlarging if the blood flow through a neighbouring coronary artery is compromised. Coronary artery disease is damage to the heart caused by the narrowing or blockage of these arteries. It commonly presents as angina pectoris (q.v.) or acute myocardial infarction (see CORONARY THROMBOSIS).

CORONARY BYPASS GRAFT: When coronary arteries, narrowed by disease, cannot supply the heart muscle with sufficient blood the cardiac circulation may be improved by grafting a section of vein from the leg to bypass the obstruction. Around 10,000 people in the United Kingdom have this operation annually and the results are usually good. It is a major procedure that lasts several hours and is done by two surgeons.

CORONARY THROMBOSIS is the acute, dramatic manifestation of ischaemic heart disease, one of the major killing diseases of western civilization. In 1989, ischaemic heart disease was responsible for about 151,000 deaths in England and Wales, compared with an annual average of over 109,000 in England and Wales in the period 1958 to 1960, but between 1980 and 1989 the figures fell by over 20 per cent. The alternative name for ischaemic heart disease is coronary artery disease. The underlying cause is disease of the coronary arteries, which carry the blood supply to the heart muscle (or myocardium). This results in narrowing of the arteries until finally they are unable to transport sufficient blood for the myocardium to function efficiently. One of three things may happen. If the narrowing of the coronary arteries occurs gradually, then either the individual concerned will develop angina pectoris (q.v.) or he will develop signs of a failing heart. (See HEART DISEASES.)

If the narrowing occurs suddenly or leads to complete blockage, or occlusion, of a major branch of one of the coronary arteries, then the victim collapses with acute pain and distress. This is the condition commonly referred to as a coronary thrombosis because it is usually due to the affected artery suddenly becoming completely blocked by thrombosis (q.v.). More correctly, it should be described as coronary occlusion, because the final occluding factor need not necessarily be thrombosis. Alternatively, it is sometimes referred to as myocardial infarction, this describing the destructive changes produced in the myocardium by lack of its blood supply. (See INFARCTION.)

Causes: The precise cause is not known, but there is a wide range of factors which play a part in inducing coronary artery disease. Heredity is an important factor. It is commoner in men than in women. It is more common in those in sedentary occupations than in those who lead a more physically active life and the disease is more likely to occur in those with high blood-pressure than in those with normal blood-pressure. It is more common among smokers than non-smokers. The Royal College of Physicians in its report 'Smoking and Health' (1983) stated that 30 per cent of heart disease deaths are attributable to smoking. It is often associated with a high level of cholesterol (q.v.) in the blood. This in turn has been linked with an excessive consumption of animal, as opposed to vegetable, fats. In this connection the important factors seem to be the saturated fatty acids of animal fats which would appear to be more likely to lead to a high level of cholesterol in the blood than the unsaturated fatty acids of vegetable fats. As more research on the subject is carried out the arguments continue about the relative influence of the different factors.

Symptoms: The presenting symptom is the sudden onset, often at rest, of acute, agonizing pain in the front of the chest. This rapidly radiates all over the front of the chest and often down over the abdomen. It is often accompanied by nausea and vomiting, so that suspicion may be aroused of some acute abdominal condition such as gall-stone colic or a perforated peptic ulcer. The victim soon becomes collapsed, with a pale, cold sweating skin, rapid pulse and difficulty in breathing. There is usually some rise in temperature.

Treatment is immediate relief of the pain by injections of morphine. Thrombolytic drugs should be given as soon as possible and continued. Subsequent treatment includes the continued administration of drugs to relieve the pain, the administration of drugs that may be necessary to deal with the heart failure that commonly develops and the irregular action of the heart that quite often develops, and the administration of oxygen. Patients are usually admitted to coronary care units, where they receive constant supervision. Such units maintain an emergency, skilled, round-the-clock staff of doctors and nurses, as well as all the necessary resuscitation facilities that may be required.

The outcome varies considerably. The first few days are critical ones and, if survived, the outlook is quite good with a first coronary thrombosis, provided the patient does not have a high blood-pressure and is not overweight. Following recovery, there should be a gradual return to work, care being taken to avoid any increase in weight, unnecessary stress and strain, and to observe moderation in all things. Smoking should be stopped. At one time, patients who had had a coronary thrombosis were kept in bed for prolonged periods. Today, however, in uncomplicated cases the aim is to get them up and about as soon as possible. Most patients are in hospital for a week to ten days and back at work in three months or sooner.

CORONAVIRUSES, so called because in electron micrographs the spikes projecting from the virus resemble a crown, are a group of viruses which have been isolated from people with common colds, and have also been shown to produce common colds under experimental conditions. Their precise significance in the causation of the common cold is still undetermined.

CORONER: An independent legal officer of the Crown who is responsible for deciding whether to hold a postmortem and an inquest in cases of sudden or unexpected or unnatural death. He presides over an inquest, if held, sometimes with the help of a jury. Coroners are usually lawyers or doctors who have been qualified for at least five years. In Scotland the coroner is known as the procurator fiscal.

CORPORA QUADRIGEMINA form part of the mid-brain. (See BRAIN.)

CORPULENCE (see OBESITY).

COR PULMONALE is another name for pulmonary heart disease, which is characterized by hypertrophy and failure of the right ventricle of the heart as a result of disease of the lungs or disorder of the pulmonary circulation.

CORPUSCLE means a small body. (See BLOOD.)

CORPUS LUTEUM is the mass of cells formed in the ruptured Graafian follicle in the ovary from which the ovum is discharged about fifteen days before the onset of the next menstrual period. When the ovum escapes the follicle fills up with blood. This is soon replaced by cells which contain a yellow fatty material. The follicle and its luteal cells constitute the corpus luteum. The corpus luteum begins to disappear after ten days, unless the discharged ovum is fertilized and pregnancy ensues. In pregnancy the corpus luteum persists and grows and secretes the hormone, progesterone (q.v.).

CORRIGAN'S PULSE is the name applied to the collapsing pulse found with incompetence of the aortic valve. It is so called after Sir Dominic John Corrigan (1802–80), the famous Dublin physician, who first described it.

CORROSIVES are poisonous substances which corrode or eat away the mucous surfaces of mouth, gullet and stomach with which they come in contact. Examples are strong mineral acids like sulphuric, nitric and hydrochloric acids, caustic alkalis, and some salts like chlorides of mercury and zinc. (See POISONS.)

CORROSIVE SUBLIMATE, or PERCHLORIDE OF MERCURY, is a powerful antiseptic and an irritant poison. It is not to be confounded with subchloride of mercury or calomel. (See ANTISEPTICS; MERCURY.)

CORTEX: The tissues that form the outer part of an organ and which are positioned just below the capsule or outer membrane. Examples are the cerebal cortex of the brain and the renal cortex of the kidney.

CORTICOSTEROIDS is the generic term for the group of hormones with a cortisone-like action. Many chemical modifications of the cortisone molecule have been prepared in an attempt to dissociate therapeutic action from side effects. Analogues are already available with no mineralo-corticoid effects and steroids with a gluco-corticoid activity and no inflammatory action have been synthesized. The main corticosteroid hormones currently available are cortisone, hydrocortisone, prednisone, prednisolone, methyl prednisolone, triamcinolone, dexamethasone, beta-methasone and paramethasone. They are used clinically in three quite distinct circumstances. First they constitute replacement therapy in states of adrenocortical insufficiency or hypopituitarism. In this situation the dose is physiological, namely the equivalent of the normal adrenal

output under similar circumstances, and it is not associated with any side effects. Secondly, steroids are used to depress secretory activity of the adrenal cortex in conditions where this is abnormally high or where the adrenal cortex is producing abnormal hormones, as occurs in some hirsute women. The third application for corticosteroids is in suppressing the manifestations of disease in a wide variety of inflammatory and allergic conditions and in reducing antibody production in a number of auto-immune diseases. The inflammatory reaction is normally part of the body's defence mechanism and is to be encouraged rather than inhibited. However, in the case of those diseases in which the body's reaction is disproportionate to the offending agent, the steroid hormones can inhibit this undesirable response and although the underlying condition is not cured as a result it may resolve spontaneously. When such compounds are used for anti-inflammatory properties, the dose must be pharmacological; that is it must exceed the normal physiological requirement. Indeed, the necessary dose may exceed the normal maximum output of the healthy adrenal gland, which is about 250 to 300 mg cortisol per day. When doses of this order are used there are inevitable risks and side effects. A drug-induced Cushing's syndrome will result.

Corticosteroid treatment of short duration, as in angioneurotic oedema of the larynx or other allergic crises, may at the same time be life-saving and without significant risk. Prolonged therapy of such connective-tissue disorders, such as polyarteritis with its attendant hazards, is generally accepted because there are no other agents of therapeutic value. Similarly the absence of alternative medical treatment for such conditions as auto-immune haemolytic anaemia and auto-immune thrombocytopenia purpura establishes steroid therapy as the treatment of choice, which few would dispute. The place of steroids in such chronic conditions as rheumatoid athritis, asthma and eczema, is more debatable.

Although one must be aware of the side-effects, it is possible to become so obsessed with the risks of therapy as to underestimate the misery and danger of unrelieved chronic asthma or the incapacity, frustration and psychological trauma of rheumatoid arthritis. On the other hand, a form of treatment with the hazards of steroid therapy should never be undertaken lightly or until other established remedies have failed.

The incidence and severity of side-effects are related to the dose and duration of treatment. Prolonged daily treatment with 15 mg of prednisolone, or more, will cause hypercortisonism. Less than 10 mg prednisolone a day may be tolerated by most patients indefinitely. When used in pharmacological doses, steroid therapy is associated with certain side-effects which are so common as to be almost invariable but are not usually of serious consequence. These include gain in weight, fat distribution of the cushingoid type, acne and hirsutism, amenorrhoea, striae and increased bruising tendency. The more serious complications which fortunately occur much less frequently include infection, dyspepsia and peptic ulceration, gastrointestinal haemorrhage, adrenal suppression, osteoporosis, psychosis, diabetes mellitus, myopathy and potassium depletion.

CORTICOTROPHIN is the *British Pharmacopoeia* name for the adrenocorticotrophic hormone of the pituitary gland, also known as ACTH. It is so called because it stimulates the functions of the cortex of the suprarenal glands. This results, among other things, in an increased output of cortisone, Although first isolated from the pituitary gland in 1933, it was not until the discovery, in 1949, of the effect of cortisone and corticotrophin in rheumatoid arthritis that it came into general use. No means of synthesis has yet been discovered, and the only available sources are the pituitary glands of animals. It is only active when given by intravenous or intramuscular injection, but there are preparations available, which give a more prolonged action and which are given subcutaneously. As its action is predominantly the same as that of cortisone, the action of the two is discussed together in the section on cortisone (q.v.).

CORTISOL is another name for hydrocortisone (q.v.).

CORTISONE, originally known as Compound E, was isolated from beef adrenal glands in 1936 by workers at the Mayo Clinic. Its chemical name is 11-dehydro-17-hydroxycorticosterone. Mainly because of difficulties in obtaining adequate amounts, little interest was taken in it until, in 1949, Hench and Kendall and their colleagues demonstrated its dramatic, if transitory, effect in rheumatoid arthritis. The precise mode of action of cortisone is still not known. Among other things, it prevents (or delays) the proliferative changes in the tissues which are the normal response to infection and in allergic conditions. Among the conditions which have been shown to benefit from cortisone are rheumatoid arthritis, rheumatic fever, gout, certain eye conditions, certain skin conditions and Addison's disease.

Cortisone has two disadvantages which will always tend to restrict its use. One is that in chronic conditions such as rheumatoid arthritis the effect of cortisone is merely temporary, and tends to stop when administration is stopped. The other is that cortisone has certain toxic effects, and therefore it must only be used under medical supervision.

For all practical purposes corticotrophin (q.v.) and cortisone have the same action. (See also BETAMETHASONE; DEXAMETHASONE; HYDROCORTISONE; PREDNISOLONE; PREDNISONE; AND TRIAMCINOLONE.)

CORYZA is the technical name of a 'cold in the head'.

COSTAL means anything pertaining to the ribs.

COSTALGIA means pain in the ribs.

COSTIVENESS (see CONSTIPATION).

COT DEATH (see SUDDEN INFANT DEATH SYNDROME).

CO-TRIMOXAZOLE is an antibacterial agent which is proving of value in a wide range of infections. It is a combination of two antibacterial agents: trimethoprim and sulphamethoxazole.

COTTON WOOL, or ABSORBENT COTTON as it is now technically named by the *British Pharmacopoeia*, is a downy material made from the hairs on cotton plant seeds (GOSSYPIUM HERBACEUM). It is used in medicine for a great variety of purposes.

COUGH is a sudden indrawing of air with the glottis (q.v.) wide open. This is followed by a blowing out of air against a closed glottis. The glottis then suddenly opens and the air in the lungs is expelled under high pressure – up to 300 millimetres of mercury and at a speed of 960 kilometres (600 miles) an hour. Its purpose is to rid the air passages and windpipe of what are colloquially known as foreign bodies, including the excessive mucus and other secretions produced in infections of the lungs and upper air passages, such as bronchitis and sore throat. As such secretions contain many micro-organisms, it is clear what an important part coughing plays in spreading the common cold and other infections of the nose, throat and lungs. It is a reflex action (q.v.) produced by stimulation of nerve endings in the air passages and may therefore be induced by irritation of these nerve endings by inflammation without any secretion. This results in the dry irritable cough which can be such a troublesome feature of the early and late stages of acute bronchitis, tracheitis (q.v.) and laryngitis (q.v.). Conversely the inability to cough in inflammatory conditions of the lungs, such as bronchitis and bronchopneumonia, especially in old folk, is an ominous sign, and every effort must be made to stimulate coughing so far as this is possible.

COUGH SYNCOPE is the loss of consciousness that may be induced by a severe spasm of coughing. This is the result of the high pressure that may be induced in the chest – over 200 millimetres of mercury – by such a spasm. This prevents the return of blood to the heart, the veins in the neck begin to bulge and the blood-pressure falls. This may so reduce the blood flow to the brain that the individual feels giddy and may then lose consciousness. (See FAINT-ING.)

COWPOX is a disease affecting the udders of cows, on which it produces vesicles. It is communicable to man, and there has for centuries been a tradition that persons who have caught this cowpox from cows do not suffer afterwards from smallpox. This formed the basis for Jenner's experiments on vaccination. (See VACCINATION.)

COXALGIA means pain in the hip-joint.

COXA VARA is a condition in which the neck of the thigh-bone is bent so that the lower limbs are turned very much outwards and lameness results.

COXSACKIE VIRUSES are a group of viruses so-called because they were first isolated from two patients with a disease resembling paralytic poliomyelitis, in the village of Coxsackie in New York State. Thirty distinct types have now been identified. They constitute one of the three groups of viruses included in the family of enteroviruses (q.v.). They are divided into two groups: A and B. Despite the large number of types of group A virus (24) in existence, evidence of their role in causing human disease is limited. Some, however, cause aseptic meningitis, and others cause a condition known as herpangina (q.v.). Hand, foot and mouth disease (q.v.) is another disease caused by the A group. All 6 types of group B virus have been associated with outbreaks of aseptic meningitis, and they are also the cause of Bornholm disease (q.v.). Epidemics of type B$_2$ infections tend to occur in alternate years.

CRAB-LOUSE is another name for *Pediculus pubis*, a louse that infests the pubic region. (See PEDICULOSIS.)

CRACKED-POT SOUND is a peculiar resonance heard sometimes on percussion of the chest over a cavity in the lung, resembling the jarring sound heard on striking a cracked pot or bell. It is also heard on percussion over the skull in patients with diseases of the brain such as haemorrhages and tumours, and in certain cases of fracture of the skull.

CRADLE is the name applied to the cage which is placed over the legs of a patient in bed, in order to take the weight of the bed-clothes off the legs.

CRADLE CAP, or CRUSTA LACTEA as it is technically known, is the form of seborrhoea of the scalp which is not uncommon in nursing infants. It usually responds to an ointment containing equal parts of Salicylic Acid Oint-

ment of the *British National Formulary*, Sulphur Ointment BP, and White Soft Paraffin BP.

CRAMP is a painful spasmodic contraction of muscles, most commonly occurring in the limbs, but also apt to affect certain internal organs. This disorder belongs to the class of diseases known as local spasms, of which other varieties exist in such affections as tetany and colic. The cause of these painful seizures resides in the nervous system, and operates either directly from the great nerve centres, or, as is generally the case, indirectly by reflex action, as, for example, when attacks are brought on by some derangement of the digestive organs.

NIGHT CRAMP is most common in the elderly, during pregnancy, in diabetics and in those with peripheral vascular disease. It comes on suddenly, often during sleep, the patient being aroused by an agonizing feeling of pain in the calf of the leg or back of the thigh. During the paroxysm the muscular fibres affected can often be felt gathered up into a hard knot. The attack in general lasts but a few seconds and then suddenly departs, the spasmodic contraction of the muscles ceasing entirely; or, on the other hand, relief may come more gradually during a period of minutes or even hours. Even after the sharp pain has gone there is often a persisting ache. The cause is not known. It is more common in older people, but has been reported in soldiers during their preliminary period of training. It is also common in pregnancy.

Treatment: This painful disorder can be greatly relieved and often entirely removed by firmly grasping or briskly rubbing the affected part with the hand, or by anything which makes an impression on the nerves, such as the application of some cold substance to the part, or occasionally by warmth. Even a sudden and vigorous movement of the limb, in such a direction as to stretch the affected muscle, will often succeed in terminating the attack, though this may also exacerbate the condition. If troublesome during pregnancy, the mother should restrict her milk intake to 0·5 litre (1 pint) a day and take calcium gluconate tablets with or without vitamin D. In men and non-pregnant women, in whom the condition is irritatingly recurrent, 60 to 300 mg of quinine bisulphate, or 600 mg of calcium lactate the last thing before going to bed, have a high reputation as a preventive.

SWIMMER'S CRAMP includes usually spasm of the arteries as well as of the muscles, due to cold and exertion, so that death is apt to occur from stoppage of the heart. If treatment can be applied, friction of the limbs, warmth, and hot drinks are essential.

CRAMP OF THE STOMACH, or GASTRALGIA, is usually a symptom in connection with some form of gastric disorder (see STOMACH, DISEASES OF). For cramp affecting the muscular wall of the bowels, see COLIC.

HABIT SPASMS, or FUNCTIONAL SPASMS, are liable

to occur in individuals of almost any handicraft, and are often extremely troublesome.

SPASMODIC WRY-NECK is one of the most frequent forms which the disease takes. This comes on in shoemakers, tailors, and people generally whose employment necessitates their following, with the head, movements which the hands are making. The result is that the muscles of the neck assume the unpleasant habit of drawing the head to one side whenever the slightest attempt is made to turn and look at anything. Indeed, although actually a rare disease, no muscle or group of muscles which is specially called into action in any particular occupation is exempt from liability to this functional spasm, which is therefore ascribed to over-use of the parts concerned.

Treatment: In the treatment of habit spasms, the only effectual remedy is absolute cessation for a time (it may be a month or longer) from the work with which the attack is associated. It is sometimes recommended that the opposite hand or limb be used, so as to afford the affected part entire rest, but this may be followed by the extension of the disorder to that locality also. Special forms of penholder and other mechanical contrivances have been suggested so as to enable the occupation to be carried on, but they do not afford any relief to the disease, for the cure of which entire rest is important. There is often a strong psychological element in such cases, and psychotherapy is indicated. Where the spasmodically acting muscles are not of great importance to the bodily economy, their action can be controlled by division of their nerves of supply. For example, spasmodic wry-neck can be checked by division of the spinal accessory nerve on one side of the neck. Such a procedure is out of the question in the case of the hand.

HEAT CRAMPS are painful contractions of muscles occurring in men (e.g. stokers) working in high temperatures. The cramps are due to excessive loss of salt in the sweat, and can be cured, and prevented, by giving salt water to drink. (See also HEAT STROKE.)

CRANIAL NERVES are those arising from the brain. (See BRAIN.)

CRANIUM is the part of the skull enclosing the brain as distinguished from the face.

CREAM is the oily or fatty part of milk from which butter is prepared. Various medicinal preparations are known also as cream, e.g. *cold cream*, which is a simple ointment containing rose-water, beeswax, borax, and almond oil scented with oil of rose.

CREATINE is a nitrogenous substance, methyl-guanidine-acetic acid. In the adult human body there are about 120 grams of it, and 98 per cent of this is present in the muscles. Much of the creatine in muscle is combined with phosphoric acid as phosphocreatine, which plays an important part in the chemistry of muscular contraction.

CREATINE KINASE is an enzyme (q.v.) which is proving of value in the investigation and diagnosis of muscular dystrophy (see MYOPATHY), in which it is found in the blood in greatly increased amounts.

CREATININE is the anhydride of creatine and is derived from it. It is purely a waste product.

CREATININE CLEARANCE: A method of assessing the function of the kidney by comparing the amount of creatinine – a product of body metabolism which is normally excreted by the kidneys – in the blood with the amount appearing in the urine.

CREEPING ERUPTION is a skin condition caused by the invasion of the skin by the larvae of various species of nematode worms. It owes its name to the fact that as the larva moves through and along the skin it leaves behind it a long creeping thin red line. (See STRONGYLOIDIASIS.)

CREMATION (see DEAD, DISPOSAL OF THE).

CREOSOTE is a clear, yellow liquid, of aromatic smell and burning taste, prepared by distillation from pine-wood or from beech-wood. It mixes readily with alcohol, ether, chloroform, glycerin, and oils.

It is a powerful antiseptic and disinfectant. Creosote is an ingredient of some disinfectant fluids.

CREPITATIONS is the name applied to certain sounds which occur along with the breath sounds, as heard by auscultation, in various diseases of the lungs. They are signs of the presence of moist exudations in the lungs or in the bronchial tubes, are classified as fine, medium, and coarse crepitations, and resemble the sound made by bursting bubbles of various sizes.

CREPITUS means a grating sound. It is found in cases of fractured bones when the ends rub together; also in cases of severe chronic arthritis by the rubbing together of the dried internal surfaces of the joints.

CRESOL is an oily liquid obtained from coal tar. It is a powerful antiseptic and disinfectant. Uses: It is used combined with soap to form a clear saponaceous fluid known as lysol, which can be mixed with water in any proportions. For the disinfection of drains it is used at a dilution of 1 in 20; for heavily infected linen 1 in 40; for floors and walls 1 in 100.

CRETINISM is a disease which is due to defective thyroid function in fetal life or early in infancy. The clinical recognition of hypothyroidism (q.v.) during the first week or months of life is difficult. However if the infant has feeding problems, is constipated and fails to thrive, and is excessively sleepy, hypothyroidism should be considered. The physical signs include a typical facies, a hoarse voice, coarse or thin hair and a large tongue, umbilical hernia and large anterior fontanelle. If the diagnosis is delayed numerous neurological abnormalities occur with abnormal gait, speech difficulties and poor co-ordination. If the disorder is not treated early mental retardation will be permanent. In a population in North London screened for congenital hypothyroidism in 1980 only 40 per cent of the cases were clinically recognized before the age of three months. Experience in Switzerland and North America is similar. An early diagnosis, therefore, necessitates biochemical screening if the benefits of early treatment are to be utilized. A recent review showed that 55 per cent of infants treated in the first six weeks of life had an I.Q. of 90 or more but only 36 per cent of those starting treatment from 7 to 12 weeks of age achieved this level. Without early diagnosis one third of patients with cretinism will require special schooling and one quarter will have an I.Q. of less than 70.

Screening programmes for congenital hypothyroidism have thus been established in North America, some European countries and the United Kingdom. The incidence of primary hypothyroidism detected by such programmes is about 1:4400 live births. The screening programmes utilize cord blood serum, or capillary serum taken by a heel prick on day 5; the blood is used to assay the level of Serum Thyroxine and Serum TSH.

Treatment consists in giving thyroxine (q.v.) regularly.

CREUTZFELDT-JAKOB DISEASE is a rapidly progressive dementia occurring between the ages of forty and sixty-five. It is an uncommon disease in which dementia develops rapidly so that a normal healthy individual can be totally helpless within a year. The disease can be transmitted to animals by the innoculation of brain tissue from patients with the disease, after an incubation period of 11 to 71 months. The transmissible agent is thought to be a slow virus.

CRISIS is a word used with several distinct meanings. (1) The usual meaning is that of a rapid loss of fever and return to comparative health in certain acute diseases. For example, pneumonia, if allowed to run its natural course, ends by a crisis, usually on the eighth day, the temperature falling in twenty-four hours to normal, the pulse and breathing becoming slow and regular, and the patient passing from a partly delirious state into natural sleep. The opposite mode of ending to crisis is by lysis: for example, in typhoid fever, where the patient

slowly improves during a period of a week or more, without any sudden change. (2) A popular use of the word crisis, and still more frequently of critical, is to signify a dangerous state of illness in which it is uncertain whether the sufferer will recover or not. (3) The word crisis is also used to signify a paroxysm of pain in the larynx, stomach, or bowels occurring during the course of the tertiary stage of syphilis (q.v.).

CROHN'S DISEASE (see ILEITIS).

CROUP is a household term for a group of diseases characterized by swelling and partial blockage of the entrance to the larynx, occurring in children and characterized by crowing inspiration. There are various causes including diphtheritic laryngitis (see DIPHTHERIA) and acute laryngitis. It is an account of this last condition which will be given here. (See also LARYNGO-TRACHEO-BRONCHITIS.)

The important thing to remember about any form of croup is that it is always potentially dangerous – particularly in the case of an infant – because of the narrowness of the entrance to the larynx and therefore the comparative ease with which it may be blocked, thereby leading to suffocation of the infant.

Symptoms: The attack usually comes on at night, when the child is in bed, and follows a chill caught during the day, or an ordinary cold that has lasted perhaps for some days. The breathing is hoarse and croaking (hence the name of the disease), the voice thin, the cough paroxysmal and metallic in tone, and the air passes in with a harsh, loud noise. The child is frightened and excited at first, but later becomes feeble and livid. Still later, pallor, sweating, and great struggling for breath come on, and may last half-an-hour or several hours. After this the symptoms begin to abate, gradually pass away, and the child falls asleep, but there is always a danger that the larynx may become completely blocked, in which case death ensues in a few minutes. A fatal termination is rare if the child receives proper treatment, and the alarming symptoms usually abate on the day following the attack, to return, it may be, on the succeeding night. A child who has once had croup is liable to have future attacks, and so should be specially guarded against cold and damp till he has outgrown the tendency.

Treatment: The child should be put into a hot bath to which a tablespoonful of mustard has been added, and a tent should be made with a blanket over the bath, so that he may inhale the steam. When he is put back into bed the tent should be put over the bed and the nozzle of a steam kettle brought within it. To the water in the kettle may be added a teaspoonful of compound tincture of benzoin, of creosote inhalation (see CREOSOTE), or of other soothing substance (see INHALATION). At the beginning, an attack may be checked by the administration of a teaspoonful of ipecacuanha wine every ten minutes till vomiting takes place. Sometimes, when the spasm of the laryngeal muscles seems very great, inhalation of chloroform is resorted to.

CRUCIATE LIGAMENTS are two strong ligaments in the interior of the knee-joint, which cross one another like the limbs of the letter X. They are so attached as to become taut when the lower limb is straightened, and they prevent over-extension or bending forwards at the knee.

CRURAL means something connected with the leg.

CRUSH SYNDROME is the term given to a condition in which kidney failure occurs in patients who have been the victims of severe crushing accidents. The fundamental injury is damage to muscle. The limb swells. The blood volume falls. Blood urea rises; there is also a rise in the potassium content of the blood. The patient may survive; or he dies with renal failure. Post-mortem examination shows degeneration of the tubules of the kidney, and the presence in them of pigment casts.

CRUTCH-PALSY (see DROP-WRIST).

CRYOANALGESIA is the induction of analgesia (q.v.) by the use of cold produced by means of a special probe. The use of cold for the relief of pain dates back to the early days of man. Two millennia ago, Hippocrates was recommending snow and ice packs as a preoperative analgesic. The modern probe allows a precise temperature to be induced in a prescribed area. Among its uses is in the relief of chronic pain which will not respond to any other form of treatment. This applies particularly to chronic facial pain.

CRYOPRECIPITATE: When frozen plasma is allowed to thaw slowly at 4 °C, a proportion of the plasma protein remains undissolved in the cold thawed plasma and stays in this state until the plasma is warmed. It is this cold insoluble precipitate that is known as cryoprecipitate. It can be recovered quite easily by centrifuging. Its value is that it is a rich source of Factor VIII, which is used in the treatment of haemophilia (q.v.).

CRYOSCOPY means the method of finding the concentration of blood, urine, etc., by observing their freezing-point.

CRYOSURGERY is the use of cold in surgery. Its advantages include little associated pain, little or no bleeding, and excellent healing with little or no scar formation. Hence its relatively wide use in eye surgery. The coolants used include liquid nitrogen with which tempera-

tures as low as –196 °C can be obtained, carbon dioxide (–78 °C) and nitrous oxide (–88 °C).

CRYOTHERAPY is the term applied to the treatment of disease by refrigeration. The two main forms in which it is now used are HYPOTHERMIA (q.v.) and refrigeration anaesthesia. Perhaps the best example of the latter is when a gangrenous leg in chronic diabetes mellitus or arteriosclerosis is kept by means of ice bags at a temperature of 5 °C for from 1 to 5 hours. This form of anaesthesia much reduces the risks of shock and infection.

CRYPTOCOCCOSIS is a rare disease due to infection with a yeast known as *Cryptococcus neoformans*. Around 5 to 10 cases are diagnosed annually in the United Kingdom. It usually involves the lungs in the first instance, but may spread to the meninges and other parts of the body; including the skin. It responds well as a rule to treatment with amphotericin B, clotrimazole, and flucytosine.

CRYPTOCOCCUS is a genus of yeasts. *Cryptococcus neoformans* is widespread in nature and present in particularly large numbers in the faeces of pigeons. It occasionally infects man, as a result of the inhalation of dust contaminated by the faeces of pigeons, causing the disease known as cryptococcosis.

CRYPTORCHIDISM means an undescended testis. The testes normally descend into the scrotum during the seventh month of gestation. Until then the testis is an abdominal organ. If the testes do not descend before the first year of life they usually remain undescended until puberty and even then descent is not achieved in some instances. Fertility is impaired when one testis is affected and is usually absent in the bilateral cases. The incidence of undescended testis in full-term children at birth is 3·5 per cent, falling to less than 2 per cent at one month and 0·7 per cent at one year. Because of the high risk of infertility undescended testes should be brought down as early as possible and at the latest by the age of two. Sometimes medical treatment with human chorionic gonadotrophin is helpful but frequently surgical interference is necessary. This is the operation of orchidopexy.

CT SCANNER: The machine which combines the use of a computer and X-rays to produce cross-sectional images of the body (see COMPUTED TOMOGRAPHY).

CULDOSCOPY is a method of examining the pelvic organs in women by means of an instrument comparable to a cystoscope (q.v.) inserted into the pelvic cavity through the vagina. The instrument used for this purpose is known as a culdoscope.

CUPPING is a traditional practice, now rarely used, for treating cases of deep-seated congestion by drawing blood to the surface. It causes sudden dilatation of the superficial blood-vessels, and so probably contracts those of underlying organs. But whatever the explanation, it gives relief in difficulty of breathing due to asthma, bronchitis and pleurisy and brings relief in lumbago and various forms of rheumatic pain.

CUPRUM is the Latin word for copper.

CURARE, known also as CURARA, WOORALI, WOURARI, URARI, and TICUNAS, is a dark-coloured extract from some trees of the *Strychnos* family. It is used by the South American Indians as an arrow poison, and is extremely potent, its action depending upon a crystalline alkaloid: *d*-tubocurarine chloride. This alkaloid paralyses the nerve endings in muscle. For many years it was considered to be much too dangerous for use in man, but research has shown that the pure alkaloid can be used with safety. Its main use is in anaesthesia, where the muscular relaxation it produces is of invaluable assistance to the surgeon. With the aid of tubocurarine adequate muscular relaxation can be obtained with a lesser degree of anaesthesia than would be required were the drug not being used. It is a drug, however, that should only be used by a skilled anaesthetist. Its action is antagonized by neostigmine. It has also been used in the treatment of spastic conditions.

CURDLED MILK (see CASEIN).

CURETTE is a spoon-shaped instrument used in surgery for scooping out the contents of any cavity of the body: e.g. the uterine cavity.

CUSHING'S SYNDROME was described in 1932 by Harvey Cushing, the American neurosurgeon. It is due to the excess production of cortisol. It can thus result from an adrenal tumour secreting cortisol or from a pituitary tumour secreting ACTH and stimulating both adrenal cortexes to hypertrophy and secrete excess cortisol. It is sometimes the result of ectopic production of ACTH from non-endocrine tumours in the lung and pancreas. The patient gains weight and the obesity tends to have a characteristic distribution over the face, neck and shoulder and pelvic girdles. Purple striae develop over the abdomen and there is often increased hairiness or hirsutism. The blood pressure is commonly raised and the bone softens as a result of osteoporosis. The best test to establish the diagnosis is to measure the amount of cortisol in a 24-hourly specimen of urine. Once the diagnosis has been established it is then necessary to undertake further tests to determine the cause.

CUTANEOUS means belonging to the skin. (See SKIN; SKIN DISEASES.)

CUTICLE (see SKIN).

CUTS (see WOUNDS).

CYANIDE POISONING: Prussic, or hydrocyanic, acid is a very deadly poison with a sweet smell and pleasant taste, paralysing every part of the nervous system with which it comes in contact. In its dilute state it was once widely used as a remedy for irritable conditions of internal mucous membranes, such as that of the stomach, and for irritable skin diseases.

As a poison it acts with great rapidity, and, since potassium cyanide is much used in the processes of electroplating and photography, and is almost as deadly in its effects as the acid, those using the cyanide should be acquainted with the treatment which may save life in a case of poisoning.

Symptoms: After a large dose, the poison is very rapidly diffused through the body, and only a few minutes or seconds elapse before the symptoms appear. These are slowness of breathing, slowness and irregularity of the heart's action, and blueness of the face and lips. In a few minutes, insensibility with gradual stoppage of breathing and of the heart's action comes on, preceded in some cases by convulsions.

The suddenness and character of the symptoms and the sweet smell of prussic acid on the breath make the cause evident.

Treatment: Urgent hospital admission is required. Treatment is based upon the administration of nitrites, which convert cyanide in the blood into the harmless cyanmethaemoglobin. Amyl nitrite is given by inhalation for 30 seconds every two minutes and also, if the victim can still swallow, 0·5 gram of sodium nitrite in 10 millilitres of water, by mouth. Oxygen is administered. Injections of sodium nitrite and sodium thiosulphate are then given, as well as analeptics. An 'Ampin' Cyanide Emergency Kit is available which allows these injections to be given quickly. The victim must be watched carefully for forty-eight hours. Another antidote is cobalt edetate.

CYANIDES are salts of hydrocyanic or prussic acid. They are highly poisonous, and are also powerful antiseptics. (See CYANIDE POISONING; WOUNDS.)

CYANOCOBALAMIN is the name given by the British Pharmacopoeia Commission to vitamin B_{12}. It is a red cobalt-containing substance, and it owes its name to the fact that it contains cyanide and cobalt. Vitamin B_{12} was first isolated in 1948 and was found to be an effective substitute for liver in the treatment of pernicious anaemia. (See ANAEMIA.) It has now been replaced by hydroxocobalamin (q.v.) as the standard treatment for this condition. (See COBALAMINS.)

CYANOSIS is a condition of blueness seen particularly about the face and extremities, accompanying states in which the blood is not properly oxygenated in the lungs. It appears earliest through the nails, on the lips, and the tips of the ears, and over the cheeks. It may be due to blockage of the air passages, or to disease in the lungs, or to a feeble circulation, as in heart disease. (See METHAEMOGLOBINAEMIA.)

CYBERNETICS is the science of communication and control in the animal and in the machine.

CYCLAMATES are artificial sweetening agents which are about 30 times as sweet as cane sugar. After being in use since 1965, they were banned by Government decree in 1969 because of adverse reports received from the USA.

CYCLICAL OEDEMA: This is a syndrome in women characterized by irregular intermittent bouts of generalized swelling. Sometimes the fluid retention is more pronounced before the menstrual period. The eye lids are puffy and the face and fingers feel stiff and bloated. The breasts may feel swollen and the abdomen distended and ankles may swell. The diurnal weight gain may exceed 4 kg. The underlying disturbance is due to increased loss of fluid from the vascular compartment, probably from leakage of protein from the capillaries increasing the tissue osmotic pressure. Recent evidence suggests a decrease in the urinary excretion of dopamine may contribute as this catecholamine has a natriuretic action. This may explain why drugs that are dopamine antagonists, such as chlorpromazine, may precipitate or aggravate cyclical oedema. Conversely bromocriptine, a dopamine agonist, may improve the oedema.

CYCLIZINE HYDROCHLORIDE is an antihistamine drug (q.v.) which is mainly used for the prevention of sickness, including sea-sickness.

CYCLOPHOSPHAMIDE is a nitrogen mustard derivative (q.v.) which is proving of value in the treatment of various forms of malignant disease, including Hodgkin's disease and chronic lymphatic leukaemia. (See BENZOTHIADIAZINES.)

CYCLOPLEGIA denotes paralysis of the ciliary muscle of the eye, which results in the loss of the power of accommodation in the eye. (See ACCOMMODATION.)

CYCLOPROPANE is one of the most potent of the anaesthetics given by inhalation. Its advantages are that it acts quickly, causes little irritation to the lungs, and its effects pass off quickly.

CYCLOSERINE is an antibiotic derived from an actinomycete, which is of value in the treatment of certain infections of the genitourinary tract, and of limited value in the treatment of tuberculosis.

CYCLOSPORIN A is a drug that is proving of value in preventing the rejection of transplanted organs such as the heart and kidneys. (See TRANSPLANTATION.)

CYCLOTHYMIA is the state characterized by extreme swings of mood from elation to depression, and vice versa.

CYCLOTRON is a machine in which positively charged particles are so accelerated that they acquire energies equivalent to those produced by millions of volts. From the medical point of view its interest is that it is a source of neutrons. (See RADIOTHERAPY.)

CYESIS is another term for pregnancy.

CYPROHEPTADINE is a drug originally introduced as an antihistamine drug (q.v.), but is now known to be effective in stimulating appetite and allowing underweight children and adults to gain weight.

CYPROTERONE ACETATE is an anti-androgen. It inhibits the effects of androgens at receptor level and is therefore useful in the treatment of hirsutism in women and in the treatment of severe hypersexuality and sexual deviation in men. (See OESTROGEN.)

CYSTEAMINE is a drug used in the prevention and treatment of radiation sickness (q.v.), and the treatment of paracetamol poisoning (q.v.).

CYSTECTOMY: The surgical excision of the bladder. When this is done, usually to treat cancer of the bladder, an alternative means of collecting urine from the kidneys must be arranged. The ureters of the kidney are usually transplanted into a loop of bowel which is brought to the surface of the abdomen to form a stoma (q.v.) that exits into an externally worn pouch.

CYSTIC DUCT: The tube that runs from the gall bladder and joins up with the hepatic duct (formed from the bile ducts) to form the common bile duct. The bile produced by the liver cells is drained through this system and enters the small intestine to help in the digestion of food.

CYSTIC FIBROSIS is the commonest serious genetic disease in Caucasian children, with an incidence of about 1 per 2000 births. It is a disorder of the mucus-secreting glands of the lungs, the pancreas, the mouth, and the gastrointestinal tract, as well as the sweat glands of the skin. It is characterized by failure to gain weight in spite of a good appetite, by repeated attacks of bronchitis, and the passage of loose, foul-smelling and slimy stools. A simple, cheap, reliable test for detecting the disease by examination of the stools has now been evolved, which permits the early diagnosis of the disease. As yet there is no reliable method of detecting carriers of the disease or of detecting affected children before birth by antenatal tests. Treatment consists basically of regular physiotherapy and postural drainage, and the taking of pancreatic enzyme tablets and vitamins. The earlier treatment is started, the better the results. Whereas two decades ago, only 12 per cent of affected children survived beyond adolescence, today 75 per cent survive into adult life, and an increasing number are surviving into their 40's. Parents of children with cystic fibrosis, seeking help and advice, can obtain this from the Cystic Fibrosis Research Trust, Alexandra House, 5 Blyth Road, Bromley, Kent BR1 3RS (081-464 7211, fax: 081-313 0472).

CYSTITIS means inflammation of the bladder. The presenting symptom is usually dysuria; that is, a feeling of discomfort when urine is passed and frequently a stinging or burning pain in the urethra. There is also a feeling of wanting to pass water much more often than usual and yet there is very little urine present when the act is performed. Cystitis may be associated with a dragging ache in the lower abdomen. The urine usually looks dark or stronger than normal. It is frequently associated with haematuria, which means blood in the urine and is the result of the inflammation. It is a common problem; over half the women in Britain suffer from it at some time in their life. The cause of the disease is a bacterial infection of the bladder, the germs having entered the urethra and ascended into the bladder. The most common organism responsible is called E. coli. This organism normally lives in the bowel where it causes no harm. It is therefore likely to be present on the skin around the anus so that there is always a potential for infection. The disease is much more common in women because the urethra, vagina and anus are very close together and the urethra is much shorter in the female than it is in the male. It also explains why women commonly suffer cystitis after sexual intercourse and honeymoon cystitis is a very common presentation of bladder inflammation. In most cases the inflammation is more of a nuisance than a danger but the infection can spread up to the kidneys and cause pyelitis (q.v.) which is a much more serious disorder.

In cases of cystitis the urine should be cultured to grow the responsible organism. The relevant antibiotic can then be prescribed. Fluids should be taken freely not only for an acute attack of cystitis but also to prevent further attacks, because if the urine is dilute the organism is less likely to grow. Bicarbonate of soda is also helpful as this reduces the acidity of the urine and helps to relieve the burning pain, and inhibits the growth of the bacteria. Careful hygiene, in order to keep clean down below, is also important. (See BLADDER, DISEASES OF.)

CYSTOGRAM is an X-ray picture of the urinary bladder.

CYSTOMETER is an instrument for measuring the pressure in the urinary bladder.

CYSTOSCOPE is an instrument for viewing the interior of the bladder. It consists of a narrow tube carrying a small electric lamp at its end, a small mirror set obliquely opposite an opening near the end of the tube, and a telescope which is passed down the tube and by which the reflection of the brightly illuminated bladder wall in the mirror is examined. It is of great value in the diagnosis of conditions like ulcers and small tumours of the bladder.

Fine catheters can be passed along the cystoscope, and by the aid of vision can be inserted into each ureter and pushed up to the kidney, so that the urine from each kidney may be obtained and examined separately in order to diagnose which of these organs is diseased.

CYSTS are hollow tumours, containing fluid or soft material. They are almost always simple in nature.

Varieties: RETENTION CYSTS: In these, in consequence of irritation or other cause, some cavity which ought naturally to contain a little fluid becomes distended or the natural outlet from the cavity becomes blocked. Wens are caused by the blockage of the outlet from sebaceous glands in the skin, so that an accumulation of fatty matter takes place. Ranula (q.v.) is a clear swelling under the tongue, due to a collection of saliva in consequence of an obstruction to a salivary duct. Cysts in the breasts are, in many cases, the result of blockage in milk ducts, due to inflammation. Cysts also form in the kidney as a result of obstruction to the free outflow of the urine.

DEVELOPMENTAL CYSTS: Of these, the most important are the huge cysts that originate in the ovaries. The cause is doubtful, but the cyst probably begins at a very early period of life, gradually enlarges, and buds off smaller cysts from its wall. The contents are usually a clear gelatinous fluid. Very often both ovaries are affected, and the cysts may slowly reach a great size, often, however, taking a lifetime to do so.

A similar condition sometimes occurs in the kidney, and the tumour may have reached a great size in an infant even before birth (congenital cystic kidney).

Dermoid cysts are small cavities, which also originate probably early in life, but do not reach any great size till fairly late in life. They appear about parts of the body where clefts occur in the embryo and close up before birth, such as the corner of the eyes, the side of the neck, the middle line of the body. They contain hair, fatty matter, fragments of bone, scraps of skin, even numerous teeth.

HYDATID CYSTS are produced in many organs, particularly in the liver, by a parasite which is the larval stage of a tapeworm found in dogs. They occur in people who keep dogs and allow them to contaminate their food. (See TAENIASIS.)

CYTARABABINE (see CYTOTOXIC).

CYTO- is a prefix meaning something connected with a cell or cells.

CYTOGENETICS is the study of the structure and functions of the cells of the body, with particular reference to the chromosomes (q.v.).

CYTOLOGY is the study of cells.

CYTOMEGALOVIRUSES are a group of viruses belonging to the herpesvirus group. They are so-called from the swollen appearance of infected cells (*cytomegalo* = large cell). Their importance is that they are responsible for the condition of cytomegalic disease of the newborn. The virus is transmitted from the mother either to her unborn baby while still in the uterus or to the baby during birth. In some cases the baby may show no evidence of infection, but in others it may cause a fatal disease characterized by jaundice and an enlarged liver and spleen. In those who recover from this severe form of the disease, there may be permanent mental retardation. In England and Wales, around 400 babies a year are born mentally retarded because the mother was infected with the virus in pregnancy.

CYTOMETER is an instrument for counting and measuring cells.

CYTOPLASM is the name given to the protoplasm (q.v.) of the cell body. (See CELLS.)

CYTOTOXIC means being destructive to cells. Many cytotoxic drugs are now available for the treatment of cancer and to suppress the immune system to prevent rejection of organ transplants. In some patients with cancer the treatment with cytotoxic drugs, or chemotherapy (q.v.), is given with the aim of curing the disease. Under these circumstances some degree of drug-related toxicity is acceptable. Patients with acute leukaemia and lymphomas as well as some carcinomas can be be cured with cytotoxic drugs. They are frequently used in combination because of the enhanced response achieved when given in this way.

The cytotoxic drugs include: (1) the alkylating agents which act by damaging DNA, thus interfering with cell reproduction. Cyclophosphamide, ifosfamide, chlorambucil, kelphalan, busulphan, thiotepa and mustine are examples of alkylating agents.

(2) There are a number of cytotoxic antibiotics used in the treatment of cancer – doxorubicin, bleomycin, actinomycin D, mithramycin and amsacrine are examples. They are used primarily in the treatment of acute leukaemia and lymphomas.

(3) Antimetabolites – these drugs combine irreversibly with vital enzymes systems of the cell and hence prevent normal cell division. Methotrexate, cytarabine, fluorouracil, mercaptopurine and azathioprine are examples.

(4) Another group of cytotoxic drugs are the vinca alkaloids such as vincristine and vinblastine.

(5) Some newer cytotoxic drugs have been introduced, such as cisplatin. This cytotoxic agent is particularly useful in the treatment of carcinoma of the ovary and teratomas of the testis.

D

DACRYOCYSTITIS (see EYE, DISEASE AND INJURIES).

DACTYLITIS means inflammation of a finger or toe.

DANAZOL inhibits pituitary gonadotrophin secretion and is used in the treatment of endometriosis, menorrhagia and gynaecomastia. The dose is usually of the order of 100 mg twice daily and side-effects may include nausea, dizziness, flushing and skeletal muscle pain. It is mildly androgenic.

D and C (DILATATION AND CURETTAGE): Scraping the lining of the uterus using a curette after opening up the cervix using a series of dilators. Incomplete abortions (q.v.) and uterine polyps (q.v.) may be treated by this procedure, but it is usually used to obtain tissue samples to assist in diagnosis.

DANDRUFF, or SCURF, is the white scales cast off from the scalp. (See SEBORRHOEA.)

DANGEROUS DRUGS (see CONTROLLED DRUGS).

DANTROLENE is a muscle-relaxing drug that is proving of value in relieving the muscular spasm in some cases of multiple sclerosis (q.v.).

DAPSONE is one of the most effective drugs in the treatment of leprosy. An antibacterial drug, its use may cause nausea, vomiting and, occasionally, it may harm nerves, the liver and red blood cells. During treatment blood tests are done to check on liver function and the number of red cells in the blood.

The drug is also used to treat dermatitis herpetiformis, a rare skin disorder.

DARTOS is the thin muscle just under the skin of the scrotum which enables the scrotum to alter its shape.

DAY BLINDNESS is a condition in which the patient sees better in a dim light or by night than in daylight. It is only found in conditions in which the light is very glaring, as in the desert and on snow, and is relieved by resting the retina, for example by wearing coloured glasses for a time.

DDT is the generally used abbreviation for the compound which has been given the official name of dicophane. It was first synthesized in 1874, but it was not until 1940 that, as a result of research work in Switzerland, its remarkable toxic action on insects was discovered. This work was taken up and rapidly expanded in Great Britain and the USA, and one of its first practical applications was in controlling the spread of typhus. This disease is transmitted by the louse, one of the insects for which DDT is most toxic. Its toxic action against the mosquito has also been amply proved, and it thus rapidly became one of the most effective measures in controlling malaria. DDT is toxic to a large range of insects in addition to the louse and the mosquito; these include house-flies, bed-bugs, clothes-moths, fleas, cockroaches, and ants. It is also active against many agricultural and horticultural pests, including weevils, flour beetles, pine sawfly, and most varieties of scale insect.

DDT has thus had a wide use in medicine, public health, veterinary medicine, horticulture, and agriculture. Unfortunately, the indiscriminate use of DDT is potentially hazardous, and its use is now restricted or banned in several countries, including the United Kingdom.

The danger of DDT is that it enters the biological food chain with the result that animals at the end of the food chain such as birds or predators may build up lethal concentrations of the substance in their tissues.

In any case an increasing number of species of insects were becoming resistant to DDT. Fortunately, to date newer insecticides have been introduced which are toxic to DDT-resistant insects, but there is a certain amount of anxiety as to whether this supply of new insecticides can be maintained.

DEAD, DISPOSAL OF THE: Practically, only three methods have been used from the earliest times: burial; embalming; cremation.

BURIAL is perhaps the earliest and most primitive method. It was customary to bury the bodies of the dead in consecrated ground around the churches till the earlier half of the nineteenth century, when the utterly insanitary state of churchyards led to legislation for their better control, and now that cemeteries are supposed to be situated outside towns and in proper sites, the interment of the dead should seldom be a menace to the health of the living. Burials in Britain take place usually upon production of a certificate from a registrar of deaths, to whom notice of the death, accompanied by a medical certificate, must be given without delay by the nearest relatives.

EMBALMING is still used to a certain extent, particularly in the USA. The process consists in removing the internal organs by small openings and filling the body cavities with various aromatics of antiseptic power, the skin being swathed in bandages or otherwise protected from the action of the air. Bodies are also preserved by injecting the blood-vessels with strong antiseptics like perchloride of mercury. In certain circumstances bodies become naturally changed to a non-putrefying substance known as adipocere. (See PUTREFACTION.)

CREMATION provides a much speedier reduction of the body to its simple components than does burial, and one devoid of any harmful tendencies to the living. Not the least of its advantages is the amount of space that is saved. It is being used to an increasing extent.

In order to prevent any abuse, special certificates are required, and the necessary forms for these are obtained from the cremating authority. The law does not distinguish in England or the USA between cremation and burial, but special formalities are insisted upon by the crematorium authorities. The process of incineration takes between one and two hours. About 2·3 to 3·2 kg (5 to 7 pounds) of ash result from the combustion of the body, and there is no admixture with that from the fuel.

DEAD FINGERS (see RAYNAUD'S DISEASE).

DEADLY NIGHTSHADE is the popular name of *Atropa belladonna*, from which atropine is procured. Its poisonous black berries are sometimes eaten by children. (See ATROPINE.)

DEAD SPACE: Gas exchange only occurs in the terminal parts of the pulmonary airways. That portion of each breath that is taken into the lungs but does not take part in gas exchange is known as dead space. Anatomical dead space describes air in the airways up to the terminal bronchioles. Physiological dead space also includes gas in alveoli which are unable to take part in gas exchange because of structural abnormalities or disease.

DEAFNESS is the term commonly used for hearing impairment. The Medical Research Council Institute of Hearing Research National Study of Hearing conducted between 1980 and 1982 showed that some 16 per cent of the adult British population have a mild hearing impairment (25 dB HL loss for the speech frequencies), while 4 per cent have a moderate loss (45 dB HL) and 1 per cent a severe loss (65 dB HL).

In most people, this is a sensorineural hearing impairment, commonly known as *nerve deafness*. This means that the abnormality is located in the inner ear (the cochlea), the auditory nerve or in the brain itself. The prevalence of this type of hearing impairment rises greatly in elderly people to the extent that over 50 per cent of the over-70s have a moderate hearing impairment. In most cases, no definite cause can be found, but some are due to excessive exposure to noise, either at work (e.g. shipyards and steelworks) or from gunfire and explosions.

Conductive hearing impairment is the other main classification. Here there is an abnormality of the external or middle ear preventing the normal transmission of sound waves to the inner ear. This is most commonly due to chronic otitis media where there is inflammation of the middle ear with a perforation of the ear drum. It is thought that in the majority of cases this is a sequela of childhood middle-ear disease. Wax is an uncommon cause of hearing impairment. It is normal for ear canals to contain wax. Wax does not interfere with hearing unless it totally obstructs the ear canal or is impacted against the tympanic membrane, often due to injudicious use of cotton buds.

Conductive hearing impairment can be treated by an operation on the middle ear or by the use of a hearing aid. Sensorineural hearing impairments can be treated only with a hearing aid. In the UK hearing aids are available free on the NHS. Most NHS hearing aids are ear-level hearing aids, that is, they fit behind the ear with the sound transmitted to the ear via a mould in the external ear. The older body-worn hearing aids are now prescribed only for particular cases where an ear-level aid is unsuitable. Increasingly, however, smaller hearing aids are becoming available which fit within the ear itself and it is becoming much more common for people to wear hearing aids in both ears. Even though it is estimated that over 10 per cent of the adult population in the UK might benefit from the use of a hearing aid, fewer than 4 per cent have ever tried one. Those people with a hearing impairment which is so profound ('stone deaf') that they cannot be helped by a hearing aid can sometimes now be fitted with an electrical implant in their inner ear (a cochlear implant).

Congenital hearing loss accounts for a very small proportion of the hearing-impaired population. It is important to detect at an early stage as, if undetected and unaided, it may lead to delayed or absent ('deaf mute') development of speech. The commonest cause of hearing difficulties in childhood is otitis media with effusion (glue ear). This usually resolves spontaneously, though it may require surgical management by adenoidectomy (see NOSE, DISEASES OF) or insertion of ventilation tubes (see GROMMET) in the ear drum.

Advice and information on deafness and hearing aids may be obtained from the Royal National Institute for the Deaf, 105 Gower Street, London WC1E 6AH (071-387 8033, fax: 071-388 2346, Minicom: 071-383 3154).

DEAMINATION is the process of removal of the amino group, NH_2, from amino-acids not required for building up body protein. This is carried out mainly in the liver by means of an enzyme, deaminase. The fatty acid residue is either burnt up to yield energy, or is converted into glucose.

DEATH, CAUSES OF: Although the final cause of death is usually failure of the vital centres which govern the beating of the heart and the act of breathing, the practical question is the disease or injury which leads to this failure.

The principal causes of death in England in 1989 were ischaemic heart disease, which accounted for 30 per cent of all male deaths and 23 per cent of all female deaths, cerebral vascular disease, which accounted for 9 per cent of all male deaths and 14 per cent of all female deaths. Cancer of the respiratory organs accounted for 9 per cent of all male deaths and cancer of the digestive organs for 8 per cent of all male deaths, whereas cancer of the digestive organs accounted for 7 per cent of all female deaths.

DEATH CERTIFICATE: A certificate required by law to be signed by a medical practitioner stating the main and any contributary causes of a person's death.

DEATH RATE: In 1989, the death rate in England was 11·4 per thousand.

DEATH, SIGNS OF: There are some minor signs, such as relaxation of the facial muscles, which produces the staring eye and gaping mouth of the *Hippocratic countenance*, as well as a loss of the curves of the back, which becomes flat by contact with the bed or table; *discoloration of the skin*, which becomes of a wax-yellow hue, and loses its pink transparency at the finger-webs; *absence of blistering and redness* if the skin is burned (Christison's sign); and *failure of a ligature* tied round the finger to produce, after its removal, the usual change of a white ring, which, after a few seconds, becomes redder than the surrounding skin in a living person.

The only certain sign of death, however, is *stoppage of the heart*, and to ensure that this is permanent it is necessary to listen over the heart, that is, over the chest at the inner side of the nipple, for five minutes. This can be done by means of a stethoscope or by listening directly with the ear on the chest. *Stoppage of breathing* should also be noted, and this can be confirmed by observing that a mirror held before the mouth shows no haze, that a feather placed on the upper lip does not flutter, or that the reflection on the ceiling from a cup of water placed on the chest of the dead person shows no movement. An important sign is that if a cut is made in the skin or a vessel is opened no bleeding takes place after death.

In the vast majority of cases there is no difficulty in ensuring that death has occurred. The introduction of organ transplantation, however, and of more effective mechanical means of resuscitation, such as respirators, whereby an individual's heart can be kept beating almost indefinitely, has raised difficulties in a minority of cases. To solve the problem in these cases the concept of '*brain death*' has been introduced. In this context it has to be borne in mind that there is no legal definition of death. Death has traditionally been diagnosed by the irreversible cessation of respiration and heart-beat. In the Code of Practice drawn up in 1983 by a Working Party of the Health Departments of Great Britain and Northern Ireland, however, it is stated that 'death can also be diagnosed by the irreversible cessation of brain-stem function'. This is described as 'brain death'. The brain-stem consists of the mid-brain, pons and medulla oblongata which contain the centres controlling the vital processes of the body such as consciousness, breathing and the beating of the heart (see BRAIN). This new concept of death, which has been widely accepted in medical and legal circles throughout the world, means that it is now legitimate to equate brain death with death, that the essential component of brain death is death of the brain-stem, and that a dead brain-stem can be reliably diagnosed at the bedside.

Four points are important in determining the time that has elapsed since death. *Hypostasis*, or congestion, begins to appear as livid spots on the back, often mistaken for bruises, three hours or more after death. It is due to the blood running into the vessels in the lowest parts. *Loss of heat* begins at once after death, and the body has become as cold as the surrounding air after 12 hours, though this is delayed by hot weather, death from asphyxia, and some other causes. *Rigidity*, or rigor mortis, begins in six hours, takes another six to become fully established, remains for twelve hours and passes off during the succeeding twelve hours. It comes on quickly when extreme exertion has been indulged in immediately before death. Conversely it is slow in onset and slight in death from wasting diseases. It is slight or absent in children. It

begins in the small muscles of the eyelid and jaw and then spreads over the body. *Putrefaction* is variable in time of onset, but usually begins in 2 or 3 days, as a greenish tint over the abdomen. (See PUTREFACTION.)

DEBILITY means a state of weakness.

DEBRIDEMENT: The surgical removal of foreign material and damaged tissue from a wound.

DECIBEL is the unit of hearing. One decibel is the least intensity of sound at which a given note can be heard. The usual abbreviation for decibel is dB.

DECIDUA is the name of the soft coat which lines the interior of the womb during pregnancy and which is cast off at birth.

DECOCTION is a preparation made by boiling various plants in water and straining the fluid.

DECOMPENSATION means a failing condition of the heart in a case of valvular disease.

DECONGESTANTS: Drugs which relieve nasal congestion and stuffiness. They may be given orally or by nasal spray, and most are sympathomimetics which cause vasoconstriction in the nasal mucosa.

DECUBITUS is the name applied to the peculiar positions taken up in bed by patients suffering from various conditions. For example, patients with pleurisy or pneumonia prefer to lie upon the affected side; patients suffering from peritonitis, on the back; much exhausted people, far down in the bed.

The bed sores (q.v.) which such patients are liable to develop are known as decubitus ulcers.

DECUSSATION is a term applied to any point in the nervous system at which nerve fibres cross from one side to the other: e.g. the decussation of the pyramidal tracts in the medulla, where the motor fibres from one side of the brain cross to the other side of the spinal cord.

DEFAECATION means the act of opening the bowels. (See CONSTIPATION; DIARRHOEA.)

DEFIBRILLATION: If a heart is fibrillating (see VENTRICULAR FIBRILLATION) the application of a large electric shock via paddles applied to the chest wall causes simultaneous electrical depolarization of all the cardiac cells and may allow the pacemaker to re-establish sinus rhythm. One paddle is placed below the right clavicle and the other over the cardiac apex. Care must be taken that no one is in contact with the patient or the bed when the shock is given, to avoid electrocution.

DEFICIENCY DISEASE is the term applied to any disease resulting from the absence from the diet of any substance essential to good health: e.g. one of the vitamins.

DEFORMITIES may be present at birth, or they may be the result of injuries, or disease, or simply produced by bad habits, like the curved spine occasionally found in children. (See BURNS; CHEST, DEFORMITIES OF; CLUB-FOOT; FINGERS; FLAT-FOOT; KNOCK-KNEE; LEPROSY; PALATE, MAL-FORMATIONS OF; PARALYSIS; RICKETS; SCAR; SKULL; SPINE AND SPINAL CORD, DISEASES AND INJURIES OF; JOINTS, DISEASES OF.)

DEGENERATION means a change in structure or in chemical composition of a tissue or organ by which its vitality is lowered or its function interfered with. Degeneration is of various kinds, the chief being fatty, fibroid (see CIRRHOSIS), calcareous (see CONCRETIONS), waxy, colloid, and mucoid.

Causes of degeneration are, in many cases, very obscure. In some cases heredity plays a part, particular organs, for example the kidneys, tending to show fibroid changes in successive generations. Fatty, fibroid, and calcareous degenerations are part of the natural change in old age. Defective nutrition may bring them on prematurely, as may excessive and long-continued strain upon an organ like the heart. Various poisons, like alcohol, play a special part in producing the changes, and so do the poisons produced by various diseases, particularly syphilis and tuberculosis.

DEGLUTITION means the act of swallowing. (See CHOKING.)

DEHYDRATION: Removal of water. A reduction in the water content of the body. It may be caused by an inadequate intake or abnormal losses through sweating, vomiting, diarrhoea, or diuresis. The initial symptom is thirst which progresses to confusion and exhaustion. Rehydration may be produced by drinking, but in severe cases intravenous treatment may be necessary.

DELHI BOIL is a form of chronic sore occurring in Eastern countries, caused by a protozoan parasite, *Leishmania tropica*. (See LEISHMANIASIS.)

DELIRIUM is a condition of altered consciousness in which there is disorientation (as in a confusional state), incoherent talk and restlessness but with hallucination, illusions or delusions also present.

DELIRIUM (CONFUSION) The *milieu intérieur* of some old people is so fragile that acute confusion or acute brain syndrome is a common effect of physical illness. Elderly people are often referred to as being 'confused'; unfortunately this term is often inappropriately applied to a wide range of eccentricities of speech and behaviour as if it were a diagnosis. It can be applied to a patient with the early memory loss of dementia (q.v.), forgetful, disorientated and wandering; to the dejected old person with depression, often termed Pseudo-Dementia (Arie); to the patient whose consciousness is clouded in the delirium of acute illness; to the apranoid deluded sufferer of late-onset schizophrenia or even to the patient presenting with the acute dysphasia and incoherence of a stroke.

DELIRIUM TREMENS is the form of delirium most commonly due to withdrawal from alcohol, if dependent on it. There is restlessness, fear or even terror accompanied by vivid, usually visual, hallucinations or illusions. The level of consciousness is impaired and the patient may be disorientated for time, place and person.

Treatment is, as a rule, the treatment of causes. (See also ALCOHOL.) As the delirium in fevers is due partly to high temperature this should be lowered by tepid sponging (see COLD, USES OF). Careful nursing is one of the keystones of successful treatment, which includes ensuring that ample fluids are taken and nutrition is maintained. As for any withdrawal from alcohol dependence, sedation will be needed for delirium tremens, as an in-patient with medication such as benzodiazepines or chlormethiazole, on a gradually reducing basis. Care must be taken to exclude gross medical problems such as Wernicke's encephalopathy and it may be wise to give vitamin supplements by mouth or intramuscularly.

DELIVERY means the final expulsion of the child in the act of birth. (See LABOUR.)

DELTA WAVES is the term given to abnormal electrical waves observed in the electro-encephalogram. (See ELECTRO-ENCEPHALOGRAPHY.) The frequency of the normal alpha waves is ten per second. That of the delta waves is seven or less per second. They occur in the region of tumours of the brain, and in the brains of epileptics.

DELTOID is the powerful triangular muscle attached above to the collar-bone and shoulder-blade, and below, by its point, to the humerus, nearly half-way down the outer side of the upper arm. Its action is to raise the arm from the side, and it covers and gives roundness to the shoulder.

DELUSIONS are errors in judgment, regarding simple facts, which interfere with the ordinary conduct of life. Thus a man may have the delusion that he has no stomach and refuse to take food. No amount of argument or demonstration will convince the subject of a delusion as to the error of his belief. The existence of a delusion, of such a nature as to influence conduct seriously is one of the most important signs in reaching a decision to arrange for the compulsory admission of the patient to hospital for observation. (See MENTAL ILLNESS.)

DEMENTIA: Severe dementia occurs in 5 per cent of individuals aged over 65; mild intellectual impairment is present in an additional 10–15 per cent (benign senile forgetfulness); the incidence of significant dementia rises to 20 per cent in those aged over 80. The predominant causes of dementia are Senile Dementia of the Alzheimer Type (SDAT) and Multi-Infarct Dementia (MID), occurring in a ratio of 70:30, and both types must be distinguished from the reversible Dementia Syndrome which develops over a few months. SDAT is characterized by defects in orientation, memory, intellectual function, judgement and activity; it is an acquired persistent loss of intellectual function with impairments in at least three of the following spheres of mental activity; language, memory, visio-spatial skills, personality and cognition (e.g. abstraction, judgement, mathematics). These defects in function tend to be preceded by memory loss, specifically, short term, occurring in the two to three years prior to presentation.

DEMOGRAPHY: The study of populations and factors affecting their health.

DE MORGAN SPOTS, so called after the English physician who first described them, are small haemangiomas (q.v.) which occur in the skin of middle-aged people. They seldom exceed 3 millimetres in diameter. There are usually only one or two in any one individual, though occasionally they may be more widespread. They are of no significance.

DEMYELINATION: Destruction of the MYELIN SHEATH (see MYELIN) around NERVE FIBRES (see NERVES) which interferes with the nerve function. It can occur after injury to the nerve, but is particularly associated with multiple sclerosis.

DENDRITIC ULCER: A branching ulcer on the surface of the cornea caused by herpes simplex infection.

DENGUE, also called BREAK-BONE FEVER, DANDY-FEVER, and THREE-DAY FEVER, is a disease of tropical and sub-tropical regions caused by an arbovirus (q.v.) transmitted to man by the mosquito, *Aëdes aegypti*. It is a sudden and short infectious fever, with an incubation period (see INCUBATION) of a few days, characterized mainly by swelling and pains in the joints, and by skin eruptions.

Symptoms: It usually begins suddenly with pain in a joint and fever. Next appears redness of the face, spreading later over the body, very much like the rash of measles. This itches intensely. There are also sore throat and running of the eyes, and the muscles and joints generally become very painful. These symptoms endure for about three days, and then gradually pass off, leaving the person very weak. After two or three days a relapse generally takes place, very similar to the first attack. There may be a third or even a fourth relapse, and recovery from the weakness and pains in the joints is often slow, sometimes lasting over months. Death hardly ever occurs.

Treatment: Aspirin, with or without codeine, usually relieves the pains and reduces the temperature though in more severe cases pethidine may be needed to bring relief. Calamine lotion eases the itching of the rash.

DENGUE HAEMORRHAGIC FEVER is a more acute form of the disease which occurs predominantly in young children and seems to be confined largely to the indigenous population of South-east Asia.

DENERVATION: Interruption of the nerve supply to an organ or other structure.

DENTINE (see TEETH).

DENTIST is a person who diagnoses disease in the mouth, treats it and prevents its recurrence. There are a number of different groups. There is the *general dental practitioner* who is concerned with primary dental care. The *community dental practitioner* is part of the public-health team and is largely concerned with monitoring dental health and treating the young and the handicapped. In the *hospitals and dental schools* are those who are involved in only one of the specialities. The *restorative dentist* is concerned with the repair of teeth damaged by trauma and caries, and the replacement of missing teeth. The *orthodontist* is involved in the correction of jaws and teeth which are misaligned or irregular. This is done with appliances which may be removable or fixed to the teeth which are then moved with springs or elastics. *Oral and maxillofacial surgeons* are those who carry out surgery to the mouth and face. This not only includes removal of buried teeth but also treatment for fractured facial bones, removal of cancers and the repair of missing tissue and the cosmetic restoration of facial anomalies such as cleft palate or large or small jaws.

DENTITION (see TEETH).

DENTURE: A plate or frame bearing false teeth. It may be complete (replacing all the teeth in one jaw) or partial.

DEODORANTS are substances which remove or lessen objectionable odours. Some, which have a powerful odour, simply cover other smells, but the most effective act by giving off oxygen, so as to convert the objectionable substances into simple and harmless ones.

Varieties: Volatile oils of plants, such as eucalyptus and turpentine, chlorine water and chlorinated lime, peroxide of hydrogen, charcoal, dry earth, sawdust, and potassium permanganate are among the most powerful.

Uses: The main use is to purify sewage, bilgewater, and water- closets. Many powerful deodorants act, at the same time, as disinfectants. They are also used in sick-rooms to cover the smell of discharges, and the like. For the manner of use see under the individual deodorants. (See also PERSPIRATION.)

DEPILATION is the process of destroying hair; substances and processes used for this purpose being known as depilatories. The purpose may be effected in three ways: (1) by removing the hairs at the level of the skin surface; (2) by pulling the hairs out (epilation); (3) by destroying the roots and so preventing the growth of new hairs.

Shaving is the most effective way of removing superfluous hairs. Rubbing morning and night with a smooth pumice-stone is said to be helpful. The alkaline sulphides used as depilatories tend to erode the skin as well as the hairs. Electrolysis and diathermy have a limited use.

DEPOLARIZING NEUROMUSCULAR BLOCKADE (see NEUROMUSCULAR BLOCKADE).

DEPRESSION (see MENTAL ILLNESS).

DEPRESSOR is the name given to a nerve by whose stimulation motion, secretion, or some other function is restrained or prevented: e.g. the depressor nerve of the heart slows the beating of this organ.

DEQUALINIUM CHLORIDE is an antibacterial and antifungal compound which is of value in the treatment of infections of the mouth, gums, and throat, and in certain skin conditions.

DERBYSHIRE NECK is a name for goitre, which was fairly common in Derbyshire. (See GOITRE.)

DERMABRASION, or 'surgical planing', is a method of removing the superficial layers of the skin, which is sometimes useful in the removal of tattoos and superficial blemishes of the skin.

DERMATITIS means inflammation of the skin, though its differentiation from eczema is by no means clear. Indeed, different dermatologists (or skin specialists) use the two terms in quite different ways. For the present purpose only three forms of dermatitis will be considered here: contact dermatitis, light dermatitis, and exfoliative dermatitis. (See also DERMATITIS under OCCUPATIONAL DISEASES.)

ATOPIC DERMATITIS (see NEURODERMATOSES).

CONTACT DERMATITIS is dermatitis caused by contact between the skin and some substance to which the skin is sensitive. The skin eruption may vary from mere redness to severe inflammation of the skin. The onset may be gradual or sudden, depending upon how sensitive the individual is to the incriminating substance. A large range of substances can produce contact dermatitis, including cosmetics such as lipstick, hair dyes, shampoos, perfumes, nail varnish, face powder and rouge; nylon hair nets; rubber sponges; dyes used in clothing; nickel, chromium and rubber, as used in suspenders; contraceptives; paints and varnishes; and plants. So far as plants are concerned, the most important in Britain is the indoor primula, *Primula abconica*; next comes chrysanthemum, anthemis (the stinking mayweed) and the giant hogweed. Medicaments applied to the skin as ointments, lotions and the like are an increasing cause of contact dermatitis. For this reason antibiotics, such as penicillin, are seldom used in the form of such local applications in case they should render the patient sensitive. Not only does this expose patients to the unnecessary discomfort of a contact dermatitis, it may also mean that they can no longer be given the antibiotic in question, when it may be a lifesaving measure. The diagnosis of the condition is usually fairly simple, one of the important factors being the localization of the dermatitis. Thus, if it occurs on the thigh in a woman it may well be due to her suspenders, whereas if it occurs in the armpit it may be due to some dye in clothing or to some deodorant spray. In doubtful cases the diagnosis can usually be settled by what is known as a patch test. This consists of applying a small amount of the suspected sensitizing substance to an area of normal skin. If the individual is sensitive to the substance in question, an area of dermatitis appears beneath the patch in twenty-four to forty-eight hours, and the test is said to be positive.

Prevention consists in the first instance of finding the cause and then making sure the afflicted individual has no further contact with it.

Treatment varies with the severity of the condition. In relatively mild cases the application of calamine lotion is often all that is necessary. In more severe cases this is supplemented by the application of a corticosteroid (q.v.). The area involved should not be washed with soap, but cleaned with olive oil, or an emulsion of water and Emulsifying Ointment, BP. When the condition has become chronic, with thickening and scaliness of the skin, there is often quite intense itching, and the resultant scratching makes the condition worse. In such a case the application of Compound Zinc Paste, BP, to which coal tar has been added, brings relief and aids healing.

DERMATITIS HERPETIFORMIS is a bullous, or bloblike, eruption often mistaken for eczema or scabies. It is associated with a sensitivity to gluten (q.v.). It responds to a gluten-free diet or to the administration of dapsone (q.v.).

LIGHT DERMATITIS, or LIGHT ERUPTION, is a dermatitis, with reddening and blistering of the skin, which occurs on exposure to sunlight. It is recognized by the fact that it occurs on the parts of the body normally exposed to sunlight – the face, neck and hands – and that its incidence is between April and September. It takes two main forms. One is an exaggerated form of sunburn, and this soon passes off. The other occurs in individuals who are photo-allergic. In other words, they have been rendered allergic, or sensitive, to sunlight by some substance. This may be a drug, and the drugs most likely to be responsible are the phenothiazines which include some of the antihistamine drugs and some of the tranquillizers, and the sulphonamides. Eosin in lipstick and perfume in cosmetics may also be the responsible sensitizing agent. In some individuals no sensitizing agent can be implicated, and it is assumed that this form of the condition, sometimes referred to as *polymorphic light eruption*, is due to some innate sensitivity in the individual's skin. It is this form of the condition which is most likely to be seen in children.

Treatment consists of treating the dermatitis as already outlined. To protect the skin a sunscreen, oil or cream should be applied which contains some substance such as titanium dioxide that absorbs the ultra-violet rays in sunlight which cause the trouble. For the unfortunate minority for whom no remedy can be found, the only remedy is the wearing of shady hats, long sleeves and gloves.

EXFOLIATIVE DERMATITIS, or ERYTHRODERMA (q.v.) as it is also known, is a condition which begins with patches of erythema, or reddening of the skin, followed by gradual thickening of the skin which then begins to desquamate, or peel off. It gradually spreads until practically the whole of the body is involved. It is rare before the age of 50, and is three times more common in men than in women. In over half the cases it occurs in people with some other skin condition, usually chronic eczema or psoriasis. In about a third no cause can be found, and in the remainder it develops in patients with Hodgkin's disease (q.v.), mycosis fungoides (q.v.) or chronic leukaemia (see LEUKAEMIA).

Treatment: No matter what the underlying cause, treatment consists of large doses of corticosteroids. (See also SKIN DISEASES.)

DERMATOGLYPHICS is the study of the patterns made by the ridges and crevices of the hands and the soles of the feet. It has become an important study in medicine because of the help it provides in the diagnosis of certain diseases, such as mongolism. It is also proving of value in certain other congenital diseases. Thus, a recent study showed abnormal palmar findings in 64 per cent of patients with congenital heart disease (q.v.) compared with only 17 per cent of patients with acquired heart disease.

DERMATOME: (1) Embryological tissue which has developed from the somites to become the dermis and subcutaneous tissue. The cutaneous area that is derived from each dermatome is supplied by a single dorsal spinal nerve root. (2) A surgical instrument for removing very thin slices of skin for grafting.

DERMATOMYOSITIS is an auto-immune disease, characterized by erythema of the skin and wasting of the muscles.

DERMATOPHYTES: These are fungal infections. They are commonly seen as athlete's foot, scalp ringworm, tinea corporis and nail infection. They are due to fungi that normally inhabit the keratin tissue of the skin, hair and nails.

DERMOGRAPHIA, also known as DERMOGRAPHISM and URTICARIA FACTITIA, is a condition in which tracings made on the skin leave a distinct swollen, reddish mark. It occurs in allergic individuals, in whom the stimulus of scratching the skin produces an excessive amount of histamine. (See ALLERGY.)

DERMOID CYST (see CYSTS).

DESFERRIOXAMINE is a chelating agent which is proving of value in the treatment of iron poisoning and thalassaemia.

DESQUAMATION means the scaling off of the superficial layer of the epidermis.

DETACHED RETINA: Separation of the retina from the choroid in the eye. It may be due to trauma or be secondary to tumour or inflammation of the choroid and causes blindness in the affected part of the retina. It can be treated surgically using photocoagulation.

DETERGENTS are substances which clean the skin surface. This means that, strictly speaking, any soap, or soap-like substance used in washing, is a detergent. At the present day, however, the term is largely used for the synthetic detergents which are now used on such a large scale. These are prepared by the cracking and oxidation of high petroleum waxes with sulphuric acid. The commoner ones in commercial preparations are aryl alkyl sulphate or sulphonate and secondary alkyl sulphate.

In view of their widespread use they appear to cause relatively little trouble with the skin, but more trouble has been reported with the so-called 'biological' detergents that were introduced some years ago. They are so named because they contain an enzyme (q.v.) which destroys protein. As a result they are claimed to remove proteins – stains such as blood, chocolate, milk or gravy, which are relatively difficult for ordinary detergents to remove. Unfortunately these 'biological' detergents may cause dermatitis of the hands. In addition, they have been reported to cause asthma in those using them, and even more so in workers manufacturing them.

DETOXICATION means reduction or removal of the toxic properties of poisons or remedies. (See VACCINE.)

DEVIANCE: Variation from normal. Often used to describe sexual behaviour.

DEVONSHIRE COLIC is caused by drinking cider which has been stored in contact with lead, so that colic comes on as a result of lead poisoning. (See COLIC; LEAD POISONING).

DEXAMETHASONE is a corticosteroid derivative. As an anti- inflammatory agent it is approximately 30 times as effective as cortisone and eight times as effective as prednisolone. On the other hand, it has practically none of the salt-retaining properties of cortisone.

DEXTRAN is the name given to a group of polysaccharides which was first discovered in sugar-beet preparations which had become infected with certain bacteria. A homogeneous preparation of it, with a consistent molecular weight and free from protein, is used as a substitute for plasma for transfusion purposes.

DEXTRIN is a soluble carbohydrate substance into which starch is converted by diastatic ferment or by heat. It is thus contained in toast, the crust of bread, biscuits, and breakfast foods. It is a white or yellowish powder which, dissolved in water, forms mucilage. Animal dextrin, also known as glycogen (q.v.), is a carbohydrate stored in the liver after meals, often in considerable amounts.

DEXTROCARDIA: The heart is situated on the right of the chest in a mirror image of its usual position. This may be associated with similar inversion of the abdominal organs – situs inversus.

DEXTROMORAMIDE is a potent, habit-forming analgesic, or pain-reliever, which is active whether taken by mouth or given by injection.

DEXTROSE is another name for purified grape sugar or glucose.

DIA- is a prefix meaning through or thoroughly.

DIABETES INSIPIDUS is a disease characterized by excessive thirst and the passing of large volumes of urine which have a low specific gravity and contain no abnormal constituents. It is either due to a lack of the antidiuretic hormone normally produced by the hypothalamus and stored in the posterior pituitary gland, or to a defect in the renal tubules which prevents them responding to the antidiuretic hormone vasopressin. When the disorder is due to a vasopressin insufficiency, a primary or secondary tumour in the area of the pituitary stalk is responsible for one third of cases. In another one third of cases there is no apparent cause and such idiopathic cases are sometimes familial. A further one third of cases result from a variety of lesions including trauma, basal meningitis and granulomatous lesions in the pituitary stalk area. When the renal tubules fail to respond to vasopressin this is usually because of a genetic defect transmitted as a sex-linked recessive characteristic and the disease is called nephrogenic diabetes insipidus. Metabolic abnormalities such as hypercalcaemia and potassium depletion render the renal tubule less sensitive to vasopressin and certain drugs such as lithium and tetracycline may have a similar effect.

If the disease is due to a deficiency of vasopressin, treatment should be with the analogue of vasopressin called desmopressin which is more potent than the natural hormone and has less pressor activity. It also has the advantage in that it is absorbed from the nasal mucosa and so does not require to be injected.

Nephrogenic diabetes insipidus cannot be treated with desmopressin. The urine volume can, however, usually be reduced by half by a thiazide diuretic. Diabetes insipidus is a relatively rare condition and must be differentiated from diabetes mellitus (q.v.) which is an entirely different disease.

DIABETES MELLITUS is a condition characterized by a raised concentration of glucose in the blood because of a deficiency in the production and/or action of insulin (q.v.), a pancreatic hormone made in special cells called the islet cells of Langerhans.

Mering and Minkowski in 1889 found that diabetes followed removal of the pancreas from animals. In 1909 it was established that the defect was due to the failure of the pancreas to produce a hormone which was given the name insulin. However it was not until 1921 that two research workers, Banting and Best, first isolated insulin.

Symptoms: Thirst, polyuria, weight loss despite eating, and recurrent infections, e.g. balanitis (q.v.) and vulval infections, are the main symptoms.

However, subjects with non-insulin-dependent diabetes may have the disease for several years without symptoms and diagnosis is often made incidentally or when presenting with a complication of the disease.

Classification INSULIN-DEPENDENT DIABETES

MELLITUS (IDDM) (juvenile-onset diabetes, Type I diabetes) describes subjects with a severe deficiency or absence of insulin production. Insulin therapy is essential to prevent ketosis (q.v.) – a disturbance of the body's acid/base balance and an accumulation of ketones in the tissues. The onset is most commonly during childhood, but can occur at any age. Symptoms are acute and weight loss is common.

NON-INSULIN-DEPENDENT DIABETES MELLITUS (NIDDM) (maturity-onset diabetes, Type II diabetes): this may be further sub-divided into obese and non-obese groups. This type usually occurs after the age of 40 years with an insidious onset. Subjects are often overweight and weight loss is uncommon. Ketosis rarely develops. Insulin production is reduced but not absent.

DIABETES ASSOCIATED WITH OTHER CONDITIONS: (a) Due to pancreatic disease, e.g. chronic pancreatitis; (b) secondary to drugs, e.g. glucocorticoids (q.v.); (c) excess hormone production, e.g. growth hormone (acromegaly, q.v.); (d) insulin receptor abnormalities; (e) genetic syndromes.

GESTATIONAL DIABETES: diabetes occurring in pregnancy and resolving afterwards.

Aetiology: Insulin-dependent diabetes occurs as a result of autoimmune destruction of beta cells within the pancreas. Genetic influences are important and individuals with certain HLA tissue types (HLA DR3 and HLA DR4) are more at risk. However, the risks associated with the HLA genes are small. If one parent has IDDM, the risk of a child's developing IDDM by the age of 25 years is 1·5–2·5 per cent and the risk of a sibling of an IDDM subject's developing diabetes is about 3 per cent.

Non-insulin-dependent diabetes has no HLA association, but the genetic influences are much stronger. The risks of developing diabetes vary with different races. Obesity, decreased exercise and ageing increase the risks of disease development. The risk of a sibling of a NIDDM subject's developing NIDDM up to the age of 80 years is 30–40 per cent.

Treatment of diabetes aims to prevent symptoms, restore carbohydrate metabolism to as near normal as possible and to minimize complications. Concentration of glucose, fructosamine and glycated haemoglobin in the blood are used to give an indication of blood-glucose control.

Insulin-dependent diabetes requires insulin for treatment. Non-insulin-dependent diabetes may be treated with diet, oral hypoglycaemic agents (q.v.) or insulin.

DIET: Many NIDDM diabetics may be treated with diet alone. For those subjects who are overweight, weight loss is important, although often unsuccessful. A diet high in complex carbohydrate, high in fibre, low in fat and aiming towards ideal body weight is prescribed. Subjects taking insulin need to eat at regular intervals in relation to their insulin regime and missing meals may result in hypoglycaemia, a lowering of the amount of glucose in the blood.

ORAL HYPOGLYCAEMICS are used in the treatment of non-insulin- dependent diabetes in addition to diet, when diet alone fails to control blood sugar levels. (a) Sulphonylureas act mainly by increasing the production of insulin. (b) Biguanides, of which only Metformin is available, may be used alone or in addition to sulphonylureas (q.v.). Its main actions are to lower the production of glucose by the liver and improve its uptake in the peripheral tissues.

INSULIN: All insulin is injected – mainly by syringe but sometimes by insulin pump – because it is inactivated by gastrointestinal enzymes. There are three main types of insulin preparation: (a) short action (approximately 6 hours), with rapid onset; (b) intermediate action (approximately 12 hours); (c) long action, with slow onset and lasting for up to 36 hours. Human, porcine and bovine preparations are available. Much of the insulin now used is prepared by genetic engineering techniques from micro-organisms. There are many regimens of insulin treatment involving different combinations of insulin. Regimens vary depending on the requirements of the patients, most of whom administer the insulin themselves. Carbohydrate intake, energy expenditure and the presence of infection are important determinants of insulin requirements on a day-to-day basis.

Complications: The risks of complications increase with duration of disease.

DIABETIC EYE DISEASE: (a) retinopathy, (b) cataract. Regular examination of the fundus enables any abnormalities developing to be detected and treatment given when appropriate to preserve eyesight.

NEPHROPATHY: subjects with diabetes may develop kidney damage which can result in renal failure.

INCREASED RISKS are present of (a) heart disease, (b) peripheral vascular disease and (c) cerebrovascular disease.

NEUROPATHY: (a) Symmetrical sensory polyneuropathy, damage to the sensory nerves that commonly presents with tingling, numbness of pain in the feet or hands. (b) Asymmetrical motor diabetic neuropathy presenting as progressive weakness and wasting of the proximal muscles of legs. (c) Mononeuropathy, individual motor or sensory nerves may be affected. (d) Autonomic neuropathy, which affects the autonomic nervous system, has many presentations, including impotence, diarrhoea or constipation and postural hypotension.

SKIN LESIONS: there are several skin disorders associated with diabetes including (a) Necrobiosis lipoidica diabeticorum usually occurring as an unsightly area on the shin. (b) Ulcers, which most commonly occur on the feet due to peripheral vascular disease, neuropathy and infection. Foot care is very important.

DIABETIC KETOACIDOSIS occurs when there is insufficient insulin present to prevent ketone (q.v.) production. This may occur before the diagnosis of IDDM or when insufficient insulin is being given. The presence of large amounts of ketones in the urine indicates excess ketone production and treatment should be sought immediately. Coma and death may result if the condition is left untreated.

DIABETIC HYPOGLYCAEMIA occurs when amounts of glucose in the blood become low. This may occur in subjects taking sulphonylureas or insulin. Symptoms usually develop when the glucose concentration falls below 2·5 mmol/l. They may, however, occur at higher concentrations in subjects with persistent hyperglycaemia – an excess of glucose – and at lower levels in subjects with persistent hypoglycaemia. Symptoms include confusion, hunger and sweating. Refined sugar followed by complex carbohydrate will return the glucose concentration to normal. If the subject is unable to swallow, glucagon may be given intramuscularly or glucose intravenously, followed by oral carbohydrate, once the subject is able to swallow.

Although there are complications associated with diabetes, many subjects live to an old age. People with diabetes or their relatives can obtain advice from the British Diabetes Association, 10 Queen Anne Street, London W1M 0BD (071-323 1531, fax: 071-637 3644).

DIAGNOSIS is the art of distinguishing one disease from another, and is essential to scientific and successful treatment. The name is also given to the opinion arrived at as to the nature of a disease. It is in diagnosis more than in treatment that the highest medical skill is required, and, for a diagnosis, the past and hereditary history of a case, the symptoms complained of, and the signs of disease found upon examination are all weighed. Many methods of laboratory examination are also used at the present day in aiding diagnosis.

DIALYSIS is the process whereby crystalloid and colloid substances are separated from a solution by interposing a semipermeable membrane, such as cellophane, between the solution and pure water. The crystalloid substances pass through the membrane into the water until a state of equilibrium, so far as the crystalloid substances are concerned, is established between the two sides of the membrane. The colloid substances do not pass through the membrane.

This is the principle upon which the artificial kidney works. (See KIDNEY, ARTIFICIAL.) When, as in the artificial kidney, the patient's blood is used, the process is known as *haemodialysis* (q.v.). An alternative technique is to circulate the dialysing fluid through the abdominal cavity, thus using the peritoneum (q.v.) as the semipermeable membrane. This is the process known as *peritoneal dialysis*.

DIAMORPHINE and DIACETYLMORPHINE are other names for heroin (q.v.).

DIAPHORESIS is another name for sweating. (See PERSPIRATION.)

DIAPHRAGM, or MIDRIFF, is the muscular partition which separates the cavity of the abdomen from that of the chest. It is very thin and is of a dome shape, extending up on the right side to the space beneath the fourth rib, on the left to that beneath the fifth. In contact with its lower surface are, on the right side, the liver, right kidney, and suprarenal body, and to the left the stomach, pancreas, left kidney, suprarenal body, and spleen; while upon its upper surface lies the heart, with a lung on either side. The diaphragm is attached by its edge to the lower margin of the chest all round, and consists of muscular fibres meeting round a trefoil-shaped piece of fibrous tissue in the centre. It completely shuts off the above-named cavities from one another, being pierced only by openings for the gullet, the aorta, and the inferior vena cava, with a few minute openings for nerves and small vessels. The diaphragm is of great importance in respiration, playing the chief part in filling the lungs. During deep respiration its movements are responsible for 60 per cent of the total amount of air breathed and in the horizontal posture, or in sleep, an even greater percentage.

DIAPHYSECTOMY is the operation whereby a part of the shaft of a long bone (e.g. humerus, femur) is excised.

DIAPHYSIS: The shaft of a long bone.

DIAPULSE is a form of pulsed high-frequency electrical energy, consisting of pulsed short-wave bursts of energy of 1000 watts maximum, with an average input of 36 watts. It is used as a form of physiotherapy, particularly in the treatment of severe sprains.

DIARRHOEA or looseness of the bowels is increased frequency, fluidity or volume of bowel movements as compared to the person's customary pattern of bowel movements. Most people have occasional attacks of acute diarrhoea, usually caused by contaminated food or water. Such attacks normally clear up within a day or two, whether or not they are treated. Chronic diarrhoea, on the other hand, may be the result of a serious intestinal disorder or of more general disease.

The commonest cause of acute diarrhoea is food poisoning (q.v.), the organisms involved usually being staphylococcus, clostridium bacteria, salmonella or campylobacter. A person may also acquire infective diarrhoea as a result of droplet infections from adenoviruses or echoviruses. Interference with the bacterial flora of the intestine may cause acute diarrhoea: this often happens to someone who travels to another country and acquires unfamiliar intestinal bacteria. Other infections include bacillary dysentery, typhoid fever and paratyphoid fevers (see ENTERIC FEVERS). Drug toxicity, food allergy, food intolerance and anxiety may also cause acute diarrhoea, and habitual constipation may result in attacks of diarrhoea.

Treatment of diarrhoea in adults depends on the cause. The water and salts (see ELECTROLYTES) lost during a severe attack must be replaced to prevent dehydration. Ready-prepared mixtures of salts can be bought from a chemist. Antidiarrhoeal drugs such as codeine phosphate or loperamide should be used in infectious diarrhoea only if the symptoms are disabling. Antibacterial drugs may be used under medical direction. Persistent diarrhoea – longer than a week – or blood-stained diarrhoea must be investigated under medical supervision.

DIARRHOEA IN INFANTS is such a serious condition that it requires separate consideration. One of its features is that it is usually accompanied by vomiting. Some 10 per cent of the cases in this country are due to the dysentery organisms (q.v.) and will not be considered here. The remainder constitute the group of cases now usually referred to as infantile gastroenteritis. The condition is rare after the age of fifteen months, and the majority of cases occur between the ages of two and four months. The younger the infant, the higher the mortality rate. This is the type of diarrhoea which used to be known as 'summer diarrhoea' because of its high incidence in the late summer, but during recent years this seasonal incidence has tended to disappear. The precise cause is still obscure, but certain strains of the organism known as Escherichia coli (E. coli) are responsible for some cases, whilst in others a virus, often the rotavirus (q.v.), is the cause. One predisposing factor is artificial feeding. The condition is rare in breast-fed babies, and when it does occur in these it is usually less severe. The environment of the infant is also important. The condition is highly infectious and, if a case occurs in a maternity home or a children's hospital, it tends to spread quickly. This is why such an institution is closed to all further admissions if a case of infantile gastroenteritis occurs; and is not opened until the infection has been completely eradicated. A third factor is infection elsewhere in the body, particularly in the ear or the mastoid.

An infant with diarrhoea should not be fed milk but should be given an electrolyte mixture to replace lost water and salts. If the diarrhoea improves within 24 hours, milk can gradually be reintroduced. If diarrhoea continues beyond 36 to 48 hours, a doctor should be consulted. Any signs of dehydration require urgent medical attention; such signs include drowsiness, lack of response, loose skin, persistent crying, glazed eyes and a dry mouth and tongue.

DIASTASE is a mixture of enzymes obtained from malt. These enzymes have the property of converting starch into sugar. It is used in the preparation of predigested starchy foods, and in the treatment of dyspepsia, particularly that due to inability to digest starch adequately. It is also used for the conversion of starch to fermentable sugars in the brewing and fermentation industries.

DIASTASIS is a term applied to separation of the end of a growing bone from the shaft. The condition resembles a fracture, but is more serious because of the damage done to the growing cartilage through which the separation takes place, so that the future growth of the bone is considerably diminished.

DIASTOLE means the relaxation of a hollow organ. The term is applied in particular to the heart, to indicate the resting period between the beats (systole), while blood is flowing into the organ.

DIASTOLIC PRESSURE: The pressure exerted by the blood against the arterial wall during diastole. This is the lowest blood pressure in the cardiac cycle.

DIATHERMY is a process by which electric currents can be passed into the deeper parts of the body so as to produce internal warmth and relieve pain; or, by using powerful currents, to destroy tumours and diseased parts bloodlessly. The form of electricity used consists of high-frequency oscillations, the frequency of oscillation ranging from 10 million to 25,000 million oscillations per second.

The so-called ultra-short-wave diathermy (or short-wave diathermy, as it is usually referred to) has replaced the original long-wave diathermy, as it is produced consistently at a stable wave-length (11 metres) and is easier to apply. In recent years microwave diathermy has been developed, which has a still higher oscillating current (25,000 million cycles per second, compared with 500 million for short-wave diathermy).

When the current passes, a distinct sensation of increasing warmth is experienced and the temperature of the body gradually rises; the heart's action becomes quicker; there is sweating with increased excretion of waste products. The general blood-pressure is also distinctly lowered. The method is used in painful rheumatic conditions, both of muscles and joints, and in severe cases of neuritis, such as sciatica.

By concentrating the current in a small electrode, the heating effects immediately below this are very much increased, and the method may be used to produce the effects of a cautery in surgical conditions. It differs from ordinary forms of cautery because it is cold when brought into contact with the patient, and gradually becomes heated by the current. Its surgical application has been used in treating malignant ulcers, particularly of the mouth, throat, and bladder, where ordinary surgical means are not readily available. (See MICROWAVES.)

DIATHESIS is another name for constitution (q.v.).

DIAZEPAM (see TRANQUILLIZERS, BENZO-DIAZEPINES).

DIBUTYL PHTHALATE is an insect repellent. It is less effective than dimethyl phthalate (q.v.), but has the advantage of being harmless to clothing and resists washing better. When rubbed into clothing it may give protection for up to a fortnight.

DICEPHALUS is the term applied to a fetal 'monster' having two heads.

DICHLOROPHEN is a drug for the treatment of tapeworm infestations. The dose is 70 mg per kg body weight, given as a single dose or in three divided doses eight-hourly.

DICOPHANE is the official name for DDT (q.v.).

DICROTIC pulse is one in which at each heartbeat two impulses are felt by the finger. A dicrotic wave is naturally present in a tracing of any pulse as recorded by an instrument for the purpose, but in health it is imperceptible to the finger. In fevers, a dicrotic pulse indicates considerable prostration, in which the heart continues to beat violently while the small blood-vessels have lost their tone. (See PULSE.)

DIELDRIN is an effective insecticide toxic to a wide range of insects. It is more toxic to man than DDT, and must therefore be handled with care. Its use in the UK is restricted.

DIENOESTROL is a synthetic oestrogen closely related to stilboestrol (q.v.). It is not as potent as stilboestrol, but as it would appear to be less toxic, it may, for this reason, have certain advantages over stilboestrol.

DIET is an environmental factor in the aetiology of several diseases. Variations in morbidity and mortality between population groups are believed to be due, in part, to differences in diet. A balanced diet was traditionally viewed as one which provided at least the minimum requirement of energy, protein, vitamins and minerals needed by the body. However, since nutritional deficiencies are no longer a major problem in developed countries, it seems more appropriate to consider a 'healthy' diet as being one which provides all essential nutrients in sufficient quantities to prevent deficiencies but which also avoids health problems associated with nutrient excesses.

Major diet-related health problems in prosperous communities tend to be the result of dietary excesses, whereas in underdeveloped, poor communities problems associated with dietary deficiencies predominate. Excessive intakes of dietary energy, saturated fats, sugar, salt and alcohol, together with an inadequate intake of dietary fibre, have been linked to the high prevalence of obesity (q.v.), cardiovascular disease, dental caries, hypertension (q.v.), gall-stones (q.v.), non-insulin dependent diabetes mellitus (q.v.) and certain cancers (q.v.) (e.g. breast, endometrium, intestine and stomach) seen in developed nations. Health-promotion strategies in these countries generally advocate a reduction in the intake of fat, particularly saturated fat, and salt, the avoidance of excessive intakes of alcohol and simple sugars, an increased consumption of starch and fibre and the avoidance of obesity. A maximum level of dietary cholesterol is sometimes specified.

Under-nutrition, including protein-energy malnutrition and specific vitamin and mineral deficiencies, is an important cause of poor health in underdeveloped countries. Priorities here centre on ensuring that the diet provides enough nutrients to maintain health.

In healthy people, dietary requirements depend on age, sex and level of physical activity. Pregnancy and lactation further alter requirements. The presence of infections, fever, burns, fractures and surgery all increase dietary energy and protein requirements and can precipitate under-nutrition in previously well-nourished people.

In addition to disease prevention, diet has a role in the treatment of certain clinical disorders, e.g. obesity, diabetes mellitus, hyperlipidaemias, inborn errors of metabolism, food intolerances and hepatic and renal diseases. Therapeutic diets increase or restrict the amount and/or change the type of fat, carbohydrate, protein, fibre, vitamins, minerals and/or water in the diet according to clinical indications. Additionally, the consistency of the food eaten may need to be altered. A commercially available or 'homemade' liquid diet can be used to provide all or some of a patient's nutritional needs if necessary. Although the enteral (by mouth) route is the preferred route for feeding and can be used for most patients, parenteral or intravenous feeding is occasionally required in a minority of patients whose gastrointestinal tract is unavailable or unreliable over a period of time.

DIETETICS: Dietitians apply dietetics, the science of nutrition, to the feeding of groups and individuals in health and disease. They are primarily advisors and teachers. Their training requires a four-year degree course in the nutritional and biological sciences. The role of the dietitian can be divided into four main areas. PREVENTIVE: by liaising with health education departments, schools and various groups in the community. They plan and provide nutrition education programs including in- service training and the production of educational material in nutrition. They are encouraged to plan and participate in food surveys and research projects which involve the assessment of nutritional status.

THERAPEUTIC: they provide advisory services to physicians and surgeons and their patients who require specific dietary therapy as all or part of their treatment. They teach patients in hospitals to manage their own dietary treatment and ensure a supportive follow-up so that they and their families can be seen to be coping with the diet. They advise catering departments on the adaptation of menus for individual diets and on the nutritional value of the food supplied to patients and staff. They advise Social Services departments so that meals on wheels have adequate nutritional value.

INDUSTRY: the advice of dietitians is sought by industry in the production of product information literature, data sheets and professional leaflets for manufacturers of ordinary foods and specialist dietetic food. They give advice to the manufacturers on nutritional and dietetic requirements of their products.

EDUCATION: dietitians are required to teach nutrition and dietetics to student dietitians and students of many other disciplines at universities and colleges.

DIETHYLCARBAMAZINE CITRATE is a derivative of piperazine, which is proving of value in the treatment of filariasis and other parasitic diseases.

DIFFERENTIAL DIAGNOSIS: A list of the possible diagnoses that might explain a patient's symptoms and signs and from which the correct diagnosis will be extracted after further investigations.

DIGESTION, ABSORPTION, AND ASSIMILATION are the three processes by which food is incorporated in the living body. In digestion, the food is softened and converted into a form which is soluble in the watery fluids of the body, or, in the case of fat, into very minute globules. In absorption, the substances formed are taken up from the bowels and carried throughout the body by the blood. In assimilation, these substances, deposited from the blood, are united with the various tissues for their growth and repair. For the maintenance of health each of these must proceed in a regular manner. Transit time through the digestive tract in young and middle-aged people in Britain averages two to four days, all but twelve hours of this being in the colon. Transit time is probably longer in the elderly.

SALIVARY DIGESTION begins as soon as the food enters the mouth. Saliva runs from the minute orifices of the salivary gland ducts, and contains a ferment named ptyalin, which actively changes the starch of bread, potatoes, and the like, into sugar. The object of chewing is not only to bruise the food, and make it more permeable for the gastric juice, but also to mix the starchy parts thoroughly with saliva. This process goes on, after swallowing, for the first

twenty minutes or half-hour that the food remains in the stomach, after which the action of the saliva is checked by the acid of the gastric juice.

GASTRIC DIGESTION begins a little time after the food enters the stomach, the gastric juice exuding rapidly from the openings of the minute glands with which the interior surface of this organ is covered. The gastric juice begins to be secreted even before the food enters the stomach, at the sight and smell of food (psychic secretion). This juice contains ferments or enzymes, named pepsins, which have the power to break down the proteins of food into smaller molecules containing fewer amino-acids and to clot milk. There are also present free hydrochloric acid, which aids the action of the pepsin and prevents putrefaction of the food, and acid salts, such as phosphate of soda, which have a similar action. The slow, churning movements which take place in the walls of the stomach have the effect of thoroughly mixing the food and gastric juice, and, to a slight extent, of breaking up the former. The main function of the stomach is to render the ingested food soluble, and mix it thoroughly with the gastric juice until it assumes a gruel-like consistency. This material, known as *chyme*, is then passed through the pylorus into the intestine. Very soon after soft food has been taken, waves of movement may be seen on X-ray examination, the orifice at the lower end of the stomach (pylorus) opens, and the food is squeezed quickly in small quantities into the bowel; but if any hard food comes in contact with the stomach wall near the exit the orifice at once closes. Gastric digestion of a simple meal of tea, bread, butter and jam should be complete in about an hour, a meal containing milk, eggs or light meat requires three or four hours, while a heavy dinner with soup, meat, fruit, and wine or beer is not entirely treated by the stomach till six or seven hours have elapsed. Hence the English plan of taking the heavy meal of the day (dinner) in the evening is a sound one, giving time during the night for the later stages of digestion.

INTESTINAL DIGESTION: The softened food, or chyme, which leaves the stomach is exposed in the bowels to the action of four factors: (a) bile, (b) pancreatic juice, (c) intestinal juice, (d) bacteria. Bile is collected from the liver and gall-bladder into the common bile-duct, which, together with the duct from the pancreas, opens into the duodenum a short distance from the exit of the stomach. The bile consists mainly of complex salts and pigments, which assist in digesting the fats of the food, and partly of waste products removed from the blood. The pancreatic juice contains four powerful ferments, which have the following effects: lipase breaks down fats into glycerol and fatty acids; amylase completes the digestion of starch; and trypsin and chymotrypsin carry on the breaking down of proteins begun in the stomach. Intestinal juice contains small amounts of enzymes which (1) complete the breakdown of proteins into the constituent amino-acids; (2)

act upon the disaccharides, maltose, sucrose and lactose, converting them into the mono-saccharide glucose; (3) split fats into fatty acids and glycerin. Bacteria are normal inhabitants of both small and large intestine. In the former they have a fermentive, in the latter a putrefactive, action. In the former they act upon carbohydrate to produce acetic, butyric, and lactic acids. In the latter, bacteria decompose protein into such products as histamine, phenol, cresol, indole, skatole. These are no longer believed to be responsible for the ill-effects of constipation. The intestinal bacteria also play an important and valuable role in the manufacture of certain components of the vitamin B complex.

ABSORPTION: The only substance absorbed from the stomach to any extent is alcohol. Water is quickly passed from the stomach into the intestine, and considerable quantities are there absorbed in a few minutes. But it is only after subjection to digestion in the intestine for several hours that the bulk of the food is taken up into the system. The semi-solid chyme which leaves the stomach is converted into a yellowish fluid of creamy consistence called chyle by the action of bile and pancreatic fluid. From this the fats, in the form of a fine emulsion, are taken up by lymph vessels called lacteals, and ultimately reach the blood, while sugars, salts, and amino-acids formed from proteins pass directly into the small blood-vessels of the intestine. The process is facilitated by the extreme unevenness of the intestinal wall, which is folded into many ridges and pockets, while, in microscopic structure, the surface is covered by fine finger-like processes named villi, which are bathed in the fluids passing down the intestine. Further, absorption is probably assisted by the leucocytes, or white cells of the blood, wich are increased in numbers after a meal, and which have the power of wandering out of the blood-stream and taking up particles into their substance. Food materials are absorbed almost exclusively by the small intestine. The large intestine, or colon, absorbs water and salts. The food is passed down the intestine by the contractions of its muscular coat, and, finally, the indigestible residue, together with various waste substances excreted from the liver and intestinal walls, is cast out of the body in the stools.

ASSIMILATION takes place more slowly, the blood circulating through every organ, and each taking from it what is necessary for its own growth and repair. Thus the cells in the bones extract lime salts, muscles extract sugar and protein, and so forth. When the supply of food is much in excess of the immediate bodily requirements it is stored up for future use, fat being deposited in various sites, sugar being converted into glycogen in the liver. The greater bulk of nutriment is assimilated by the muscles for heat production and work, the sugar and amino-acids being built up into a substance which forms the permanent part of the muscle. The substance so formed undergoes chemical changes, and is broken down to form carbonic

1 nerve plexuses
2 serous coat
3 longitudinal muscular coat
4 circular muscular coat
5 submucosa
6 muscularis mucosae
7 crypt of Lieberkühn
8 villus

Section of small intestine (jejunum), showing four of the villi with which the inner surface is covered. Magnified 110 times.

acid, lactic acid and other waste products as the muscle does work. Various hormones, such as insulin, which is an internal secretion of the pancreas, circulate in the blood and are concerned in these processes. For all these processes to function satisfactorily an adequate daily intake of water is necessary; about 1·5 litres (3 pints) are drunk or taken with the food and absorbed daily, a similar amount being discharged from the body in the urine, perspiration, and other excretions.

DIGITALIS is the leaf of the wild fox-glove, *Digitalis purpurea*, gathered when the flowers are at a certain stage, dried, and powdered. The leaf contains several active principles, which can be extracted in various ways. Its action is to strengthen involuntary muscular contraction, particularly that of the muscle fibres in the heart and blood-vessels. It is one of the most valuable remedies we have in cases of disease of the heart, associated with atrial fibrillation. Upon the heart it has the double action of increasing the strength of each beat and of lengthening each intervening pause (diastole), so that the muscle of the damaged organ obtains longer periods for rest and repair. It promotes the excretion of sodium by the kidney and so has a diuretic effect.

Uses: Digitalis may be given as a powder, as tincture, as infusion and also in the form of sugar-coated 'granules' which contain the active principle of the drug. The most common form of administration is the powder given in the form of a tablet. Its action is particularly useful when the heart failure is due to atrial fibrillation, the condition in which the heart rate is wholly irregular. In such cases the digitalis slows the heart rate by abolishing many of the weak heart-beats. (See also DIGOXIN.)

DIGITALIS POISONING may occur from taking medicinal doses over too long a period, or from taking a single overdose. There are nausea and vomiting, and blurring of vision may occur, with objects appearing yellow or green. The heart, which is made slower and more regular by taking small doses, becomes again quicker and more irregular as the result of excessive administration. At the same time breathing gets more difficult, and there may be convulsions or unconsciousness. The amount of urine passed gets less and less, thus causing retention in the system of the drug, which is naturally got rid of by the kidneys.

Treatment: The drug must be stopped. If a single overdose has been swallowed, the stomach should be washed out.

DIGOXIN: One of a number of drugs known as cardiac glycosides. They increase myocardial contractility, depress the conducting tissue while increasing myocardial excitability, and increase activity of the vagus nerve (q.v.). It is usually given orally for the treatment of atrial fibrillation (q.v.) and heart failure. The adverse effects of overdosage (which occur more commonly in people with hypokalaemia, the elderly, and those with renal failure) are vomiting, dysrhythmias, muscle weakness, and visual disturbances. The electrocardiogram has a characteristic appearance.

DI-IODOHYDROXYQUINOLINE is a drug used in the treatment of chronic amoebic dysentery, usually as a supplement to treatment with emetine.

DILATOR: (1) A muscle which has the action of increasing the diameter of an organ or vessel. (2) A drug which usually acts by relaxing smooth muscle to increase the diameter of blood vessels, the bronchial tree, or other organs. (3) An instrument used to increase the diameter of an orifice or organ either to treat a stricture or allow surgical access.

DILTIAZEM (see CALCIUM-CHANNEL BLOCKERS).

DILUENTS are watery fluids of a non-irritating nature, which are given to increase the amount of perspiration or of urine, and carry solids with them from the system. Examples are water, milk, barley-water, and solutions of alkaline salts.

DIMENHYDRINATE, or DRAMAMINE, is a drug which is widely used, with considerable success, in the treatment of travel sickness.

DIMERCAPROL is the official name for BAL (British Anti-Lewisite), the antidote to lewisite poisoning which was discovered during the 1939–45 war. It was subsequently found to be an excellent antidote to poisoning with certain heavy metals, including arsenic, mercury and gold, and it is now widely used for this purpose.

DIMETHYL PHTHALATE is an organic compound which was found, during the 1939–45 war, to be a most effective repellent for mosquitoes. It is also effective against flies, midges, blackflies, mites, fleas and ticks. Available as a cream and as a liquid, it is smeared on the face, arms, hands, legs or other exposed parts of the body. It has to be re-applied every three or four hours. Care must be taken not to allow it to get into the eyes or to come into contact with plastic spectacle-frames. It does not kill, but merely prevents the insect from alighting on the skin.

DINOESTROL (see OESTROGEN).

DIOCTYL SODIUM SULPHOSUCCINATE is a faecal-softening agent that is proving useful in the treatment of constipation in old people.

DIODONE is a complex, organic, iodine-containing preparation. It is used primarily for contrast radiography of the kidney passages, but can also be used for contrast radiography of the biliary tract.

DIOPTRE is a term used in the measurement of the refractive or focusing power of lenses; one dioptre is the power of a lens with a focal distance of one metre and is the unit of refractive power. As a stronger lens has a greater refractive power, this means that the focal distance will be shorter. The strength in dioptres therefore is the reciprocal of the focal length expressed in metres.

DIPHENHYDRAMINE is a widely used antihistamine drug (q.v.).

DIPHENOXYLATE is a drug chemically related to pethidine that is proving of value in the treatment of travellers' diarrhoea by quietening down the gut. It has no anti-infective action.

DIPHTHERIA is an acute infectious disease, which is accompanied by a membranous exudation on the tonsils and back of the throat or pharynx. It is caused by the *Corynebacterium diphtheriae*. Inflammation of the throat is one of the first signs of the disease, and the general symptoms are referable to the absorption of toxins (q.v.) which damage the heart muscle and the nerves. The disease is generally conveyed by direct contagion.

Three strains of *Corynebacterium diphtheriae* are now recognized as causing clinical diphtheria: *gravis*, *intermedius*, and *mitis*. *Gravis* and *intermedius* strains are almost always virulent; about 10 per cent of *mitis* strains are non-virulent.

Although diphtheria can occur at all ages, it is commonest in childhood. The *Schick test* detects the susceptibility of individuals to diphtheria. A minute quantity of toxin is injected into the skin of the arm. Resistant individuals show no reaction, but, in people with little resistance, an area of inflammation is produced on the skin at the site of the injection.

In 1940 a national immunization campaign was launched. The substance injected is diphtheria toxoid, which is diptheria toxin treated so that it is harmless but will stimulate the production of antibodies to the diphtheria bacillus.

Treatment involves the immediate injection of *antitoxin.* In addition, the patient is given penicillin which has a bactericidal action on *C. diphtheriae.* Erythromycin is also effective.

Diphtheria may cause muscle weakness or paralysis which usually recovers without special treatment. If the respiratory muscles are paralysed, it may be necessary to resort to artificial respiration for a time.

DIPHYLLOBOTHRIUM LATUM is a fish tapeworm which infests man and may cause a form of megaloblastic anaemia. (See ANAEMIA.)

DIPLEGIA is extensive paralysis on both sides of the body. (See PARALYSIS.)

DIPLO- is a prefix meaning twofold.

DIPLOCOCCUS is a group of bacterial organisms which have a tendency to occur in pairs: e.g. pneumococci.

DIPLOË is the layer of spongy bone which intervenes between the compact outer and inner tables of the skull.

DIPLOPIA means double vision. It is due to some irregularity in action of the muscles which move the eyeballs, in consequence of which the eyes are placed so that rays of light from one object do not fall upon corresponding parts of the two retinae, and two images are produced. It is a symptom of several nervous diseases, and often a temporary attack follows an injury to the eye, intoxication, or some febrile disease like diphtheria.

DIPROSOPUS is the term applied to a fetus which has two faces instead of one.

DIPSOMANIA is a morbid and insatiable craving for alcohol. (See ALCOHOL.)

DIPYGUS is the term applied to a fetus which has a double pelvis.

DISABLED PERSONS now have a wide range of services available to help them to lead as normal and active a life as possible. Officially, the disabled include those with significant impairment of any kind, including impairment of sight and hearing, learning difficulties, and chronic illness as well as disablement due to accidents and the like.

Financial help is available for the disabled as follows: *Invalidity benefit*, for those who have paid national insurance contributions, is paid for incapacity lasting over 28 weeks. It is not taxable. *Severe disablement allowance* is paid to people aged under 65 who have been incapable of work for 28 weeks, have been in Great Britain for at least 24 of the past 28 weeks and have lived in Britain for at least 10 of the past 20 years. No national insurance contributions are required. Invalidity benefit and severe disablement allowance act as passports to a premium on income support and housing benefit payments. *Attendance allowance* for disabled persons who are dependent on others: for example, needing frequent attention to bodily needs. *Invalid care allowance* for carers of people receiving an attendance allowance. *Mobility allowance* is intended for people aged 5 to 65 (60 for women) who are unable or virtually unable to walk or are both blind and deaf. It can be paid until the person is aged 80. Full details of all these can be had from a local Department of Social Security Office. If asked, someone from the local office will call to see the disabled person in his own home.

Social services are provided by local authority social services departments. They include: practical help in the home (usually through home helps or aids to daily living), assistance in taking advantage of available educational facilities, help with adaptations to the disabled person's house, provision of meals ('Meals on Wheels' or luncheon centres), and help in obtaining a telephone. Many of these facilities will involve the disabled person in some expense, but full details can be obtained from the local social services department which will, if necessary, send a social worker to discuss the matter in the disabled person's home. Owing to lack of funds and staff, many local authority social service departments are unable to provide the full range of services.

Aids to daily living: There is now a wide range of aids for the disabled. Full details and addresses of local offices can be obtained from: Disabled Living Foundation, 380 Harrow Road, London W9 2HU (071-289 6111); British Red Cross, 9 Grosvenor Crescent, London SW1X 7EJ (071-235 5454); National Demonstration Centre, Pinderfields General Hospital, Wakefield, West Yorkshire WF1 4DG (0924-375217, ex. 2510/2263); Disability Scotland, Information Department, Princes House, 5 Shandwick Place, Edinburgh EH2 4RG (031-229 8632, fax: 031-229 5168).

Aids to mobility and transport: The major car manufacturers make specially equipped or adapted cars, and some have official systems for discounts. Details can be obtained from local dealers. Help can also be obtained from Motability, Gate House, West Gate, Harlow, Essex CM20 1HR (0279-635666, fax: 0279 635677) which provides advice to enable the disabled to make the most of the mobility allowance, and financial assistance for buying, adapting or running a car. The disabled travelling in a car, either as a passenger or driver, may be eligible for an orange badge if they have considerable difficulty in walking or if they are blind. It allows the holder some parking concessions, and is obtainable on a doctor's certificate. A wide variety of wheelchairs is available from the Department of Health Appliance Centres which issue them on permanent loan and maintain them.

For help in making full use of these facilities disabled people should consult their general practitioner or local Citizens' Advice Bureau.

DISARTICULATION is the amputation of a bone by cutting through the joint of which the bone forms a part.

DISC: An anatomical term describing a rounded flattened structure. Examples are the cartilagenous disc positioned between two vertebrae (see INVERTEBRAL DISC) and the optic disc. (See EYE.)

DISCHARGE is the term applied to abnormal emissions from any part of the body. It usually applies to purulent material: e.g. the septic material which comes away from an infected ear, or nose.

DISCISSION is the term applied to an operation for destroying a structure by tearing it without removal: e.g. the operation of needling the lens of the eye for cataract.

DISEASE: Any abnormality of bodily structure or function, other than those arising directly from physical injury.

DISINFECTION: Processes by which vegetative organisms, excluding spores, are killed in order to prevent the items disinfected from passing on infection. Equipment, bedlinen and hard surfaces may all be disinfected – the method chosen will depend on the material and size of the object. It should be emphasized that one of the most important procedures in preventing the spread of infection is the careful washing of hands before handling equipment and between treating different patients. Sterilization is different from disinfection in that the methods used kill all living organisms and spores.

Methods of disinfection: (1) Skin, wounds etc. – chlorhexidine (with detergent or spirit); iodine (with detergent or spirit); cetrimide; ethyl alcohol; all must stay in contact with the skin for long enough for bacteria to be killed. (2) Hard surfaces (floors, walls etc.) hypochlorites (i.e. bleaches) with or without detergent; cetrimide; iodine-containing solutions; ethyl alcohol. (3) Equipment – wet or dry heat (e.g. boiling for more than five minutes); submersion in liquid disinfectants for the appropriate time (e.g. glutaraldehyde 2·5 per cent, chlorhexidine in spirit 70 per cent, formaldehyde (irritant), chlorhexidine 0·1 per cent aqueous), hypochlorites.

DISINFESTATION means the destruction of insect pests, especially lice, whether on the person or in dwelling-places.

DISLOCATIONS are injuries to joints of such a nature that the ends of the opposed bones are forced more or less out of connection with one another. Besides displacement of the bones, there is more or less bruising of the tissues around them, and tearing of the ligaments which bind the bones together.

Varieties: Dislocations, like fractures, are divided into simple and compound, the bone in the latter case being forced through the skin. This seldom occurs, since the round head of the bone has not the same power to wound as the sharp end of a broken bone. Dislocations are also divided according as they are (1) congenital, i.e. present at birth in consequence of some malformation, or (2) acquired at a later period in consequence of injury, the great majority falling into the latter class.

Causes: The causes of dislocation are similar to those of fracture, the fact as to whether a bone or a joint gives way depending upon the manner in which force is applied, and still more upon the relative strength of bones and joints. Thus in very young and very old persons dislocations are rare, because the bones are relatively easily broken, and thereby the joints are saved from damage. Congenital dislocations are mainly due to some defect in development of the bones.

Signs and symptoms: The injured limb is useless, but, as a rule, there is little pain, unless the dislocated bone presses upon some nerve trunk. When the limb is compared with that of the opposite side, the joint is found to be unduly prominent in one place, and shows an abnormal hollow in another. Further, there is loss of movement at the joint in question, but no grating (crepitus) as in a case of fracture. Each joint shows further special signs dependent upon its conformation.

Treatment: So far as temporary treatment is concerned, nothing is necessary but a splint, bandage, sling or the like, to keep the injured part moderately quiet, because there is not the same danger of damage to nerves, vessels, and the like, by the rounded head of the bone as by the sharp fragments of a fracture. The greatest care is necessary in reduction, i.e. putting the dislocated bone back in place, for great damage may be done by an unskilled person in the way of breaking the bone, tearing nerves and blood-vessels, or even leaving the bone dislocated in a new direction. After reduction to the natural position, the limb must be fixed for a time so as to prevent a recurrence, which will take place if it be used at once. The length of time depends upon the severity of the injury; as a rule, after about ten days, gentle movements are made to prevent the joint becoming stiff, and the bandages, and the like, left off after about three weeks. But care in using the limb is necessary for much longer.

SHOULDER: This may be reduced in one of two methods. (*a*) By *manipulation*, in which the bone is gently worked back into place by a method too complicated for description here. (*b*) By *extension*. The injured person lies on his back upon a couch or upon the floor. The operator then, sitting down by the injured side opposite the patient's hip and facing towards his shoulder, grasps the limb with one hand by the wrist, with the other above the elbow, while at the same time he places his foot, from which the shoe has been removed, in the armpit, on the edge of the shoulder-blade, to steady it, and give him something against which to pull. He then pulls on the injured arm gently, steadily, and strongly, first in a direction parallel with the injured person's body, and, if this is unsuccessful, at right angles to it, pressing all the while with his foot against the edge of the shoulder-blade. The injured person must at the same time relax all his shoulder muscles. The bone goes into place generally with a snap, and the appearance of the joint is then like that of its fellow.

ELBOW: This joint may be dislocated backwards by a fall on the hand, or forwards by a fall on the point of the elbow. In both cases it is reduced by bending steadily across the knee of the operator, who at the same time pulls on the forearm.

WRIST: This joint is seldom dislocated, and the dislocation is readily replaced by pressure, and is then kept in position by a well-padded splint on the palm and front of forearm. A fracture of the lower end of the radius (Colles's fracture) is sometimes mistaken for a dislocated wrist.

FINGERS AND TOES may be dislocated and are difficult to reduce, because the tight ligaments close round the displaced bone, and because of the difficulty in grasping the finger to pull on it.

This may be overcome by winding strips of sticking-plaster round the finger, or by a device of interlacing tapes known as the 'Indian puzzle'. Dislocation of the thumb at its base is particularly hard to reduce, and may even require an operation to enlarge the opening through which the bone has passed.

HIP: This joint, being extremely strong, is seldom dislocated, and, when dislocated, is very difficult to reduce. The head of the thigh bone usually passes backwards and upwards, so that the limb appears much shortened and the toes turned inward. Reduction is effected by a special form of manipulation, or, failing this, by extension. For the latter, the injured person lying on his back, the limb is pulled straight downwards, one assistant steadying the pelvis by pressing one of his hands upon each iliac spine, and another pulling the whole thigh outwards by means of a towel passed round it as high up as possible. A very steady, powerful pull is necessary if reduction is to be effected.

CONGENITAL DISLOCATION OF THE HIP is commoner in girls than in boys. Its incidence is between 2 and 3 per 1000 births. If detected at, or soon after, birth, the results of treatment are excellent. This is why the routine examination of the newborn baby always includes a careful examination of the hips. Any undue instability of the hip, particularly if accompanied by a clicking sound on movement of the hip, indicates the probable presence of dislocation. When diagnosed within the first few days of life, treatment merely consists of the application for a few months of a simple splint maintaining the hips in abduction and flexion, and the results are excellent. If the condition is not detected at this stage it is often missed until the child starts walking, when she is seen to have a characteristic waddling gait. Treatment at this stage is more complicated and less satisfactory.

KNEE: This joint is very seldom dislocated, and such an injury to it is specially severe, being accompanied by the tearing of strong ligaments.

ANKLE: This joint is hardly ever dislocated, most severe injuries near it being fractures of the leg bones.

SPINE: Dislocation of the spine is only produced by great violence, and is usually combined with fracture. Very often pressure on, or tearing of, the spinal cord takes place, which may produce paralysis of the lower limbs, or even death from shock.

JAW: This joint is sometimes dislocated forwards when the mouth is very widely opened, as in yawning or singing. It can usually be replaced by a person pressing downwards with his thumbs upon the furthest back teeth and at the same time pressing up the chin. He should take care that his thumbs do not get bitten.

DISODIUM CROMOGLYCATE is a drug that is proving of value in the treatment of asthma when given as an inhalation.

DISORIENTATION: Orientation in a clinical sense includes a person's awareness of time and place in relation to himself and others, the recognition of personal friends and familiar places and the ability to remember at least some past experience and to register new data. It is therefore dependent on the ability to recall all learned memories and make effective use of memory. Disorientation can be the presenting feature of both delirium (q.v.) (confusion) and dementia (q.v.); delirium is reversible, developing dramatically, and accompanied by evidence of systemic disease, dementia is a gradually evolving, irreversible condition.

DISPLACEMENT is a term used in psychological medicine to describe the mental process of attaching to one object painful emotions associated with another object.

DISSECTION: (1) The cutting of tissue to separate the structural components for identification or removal during an operation or the study of anatomy. (2) Dissection of an artery involves tearing of the inner part of the wall allowing blood to track through the media occluding the origins of smaller arteries and often leading to vessel rupture.

DISSEMINATED: Spread of disease from its original site throughout an organ or the body. Often used to describe the spread of cancer.

DISSEMINATED SCLEROSIS (see MULTIPLE SCLEROSIS).

DISTICHIASIS is the term applied to the condition in which there are two complete rows of eyelashes in one eyelid (or in both).

DISTOMA is a general term including various forms of trematodes, or fluke-worms, parasitic in the intestine, lung and other organs.

DISTRICT HEALTH AUTHORITY (see NATIONAL HEALTH SERVICE).

DISULFIRAM, the full chemical name of which is tetraethylthiuram disulphide, is used in the treatment of alcoholism. It is relatively nontoxic by itself, but when taken in conjunction with alcohol it produces most unpleasant effects: e.g. flushing of the face, palpitations, a sense of oppression and distress, and ultimately sickness and vomiting. The rationale of treatment therefore is to give the alcoholic subject a course of disulfiram and then demonstrate, by letting him take some alcoholic liquor, how unpleasant are the effects. If the patient is co-operative, the results of treatment are often very satisfactory. It is a form of treatment, however, that is not without risk, and it must therefore be given under skilled medical supervision.

DISUSE ATROPHY: The wasting of muscles after prolonged immobility. This can be seen after lengthy immobilization in a plaster cast and is particularly severe following paralysis of a limb through nerve injury. (See ATROPHY.)

DIURESIS: An increase in the production of urine. This may result from increased fluid intake, decreased levels of antidiuretic hormone, renal disease, or the use of drugs (see DIURETICS).

DIURETICS: Substances which increase urine and solute production by the kidney. They are used in the treatment of heart failure, hypertension, and sometimes for ascites secondary to liver failure. They may work by extra-renal or renal mechanisms.

EXTRA-RENAL: (*a*) Inhibiting release of antidiuretic hormone, e.g. water, alcohol. (*b*) Increased renal blood flow, e.g. dopamine in renal doses. RENAL (*a*) Osmotic diuretics act by 'holding' water in the renal tubules and preventing its reabsorption, e.g. mannitol. (*b*) Loop diuretics prevent sodium, and therefore water, reabsorption, e.g. frusemide. (*c*) Drugs acting on the cortical segment of the Loop of Henle prevent sodium reabsorption, but are 'weaker' than loop diuretics, e.g. thiazides. (*d*) Drugs acting on the distal tubule prevent sodium reabsorption by retaining potassium, e.g. spironalactone.

The potential side-effects of diuretics are hypokalaemia, dehydration, and gout (in susceptible individuals).

DIVERTICULAR DISEASE: The presence of numerous diverticula (sacs or pouches) in the lining of the intestine. These may become inflamed causing pain (diverticulitis).

DIVERTICULITIS is inflammation of diverticula (see DIVERTICULUM) in the large intestine. It is characterized by pain in the left lower side of the abdomen, which has been aptly described as 'left-sided appendicitis' as it resembles the pain of appendicitis but occurs in the opposite side of the abdomen. The onset is often sudden, with fever and constipation. It may, or may not, be preceded by diverticulosis (q.v.). Treatment consists of rest in bed, no solid food but ample fluid, and the administration of tetracycline. Complications are unusual but include abscess formation, perforation of the colon, and severe bleeding.

DIVERTICULOSIS means the presence of diverticula (see DIVERTICULUM) or sacs in the large intestine. Such diverticula are not uncommon over the age of 40, increasing with age until over the age of 70 they may be present in one-third to one-half of the population. They mostly occur in the lower part of the colon, and are predominantly due to muscular hyperactivity of the bowel forcing the lining of the bowel through weak points in the bowel wall, just as the inner tube of a pneumatic tyre bulges through a defective tyre. There is increasing evidence that the low-residue diet of western civilization is a contributory cause. The condition may or may not produce symptoms. If it does, these consist of disturbance of the normal bowel function and pain in the left side in the lower abdomen. If it is causing symptoms, treatment consists of a high-residue diet (see CONSTIPATION) and an agar (q.v.) or methylcellulose (q.v.) preparation.

DIVERTICULUM means a pouch or pocket leading off a main cavity or tube. The term is especially applied to protrusions from the intestine, which may be present either at the time of birth as a developmental peculiarity, or which develop in numbers upon the large intestine during the course of life. The process of formation of these intestinal pockets is known as diverticulosis, and inflammation of them as diverticulitis.

DIZYGOTIC TWINS: Two people born at the same time to the same parents after fertilization of two separate oocytes. They may be of different sexes and are no more likely to resemble each other than any other sibling pairs.

DIZZINESS is a vague symptom and it is important to establish what the individual means by dizziness. It may encompass a feeling of disequilibrium, it may be light-headedness, faintness, a sensation of swimming or floating, an imbalance or unsteadiness or episodes of mental confusion. It may be true vertigo which is an hallucination of movement (see VERTIGO). These symptoms may be due to diseases of the ear, eye, central nervous system, cardiovascular system, endocrine system or they may be a manifestation of psychiatric disease. It is a common symptom in the elderly and by the age of eighty two thirds of women and one third of men have suffered from the condition.

DNA is the abbreviation for deoxy-ribonucleic acid, one of the two types of nucleic acid (q.v.) that occur in nature. It is the fundamental genetic material of all cells, and is present in the nucleus of the cell (q.v.) where it forms part of the chromosome (q.v.) and acts as the carrier of genetic information. The molecule is very large, with a molecular weight of several millions, and consists of two single chains of nucleotides (see NUCLEIC ACID) which are twisted round each other to form a double helix (or spiral). The genetic information carried by DNA is encoded along one of these strands. A gene (q.v.), which represents the genetic information needed to form protein, is a stretch of DNA containing, on average, around 1000 nucleotides paired in these two strands.

To allow it to fulfil its vitally important function as the carrier of genetic information in living cells, DNA has the following properties. It is stable so that successive generations of species maintain their individual characteristics, but not so stable that evolutionary changes cannot take place. It must be able to store a vast amount of information. For example, an animal cell contains genetic information for the synthesis of over a million proteins. It must be duplicated exactly before each cell division to ensure that both daughter cells contain an accurate copy of the genetic information of the parent cells (see CELLS).

DOBUTAMINE is a drug which acts on sympathetic receptors in cardiac muscle and increases the contractility and hence improves the cardiac output but has little effect on the cardiac rate. It is particularly useful in cardiogenic shock. It must be given by intravenous infusion.

DOG BITES (see BITES AND STINGS; RABIES).

DOLICHOCEPHALIC means long-headed and is a term applied to skulls the breadth of which is less than four-fifths of the length.

DONOR INSEMINATION: Use of the semen of an anonymous donor to produce fertilization in cases of infertility where the male partner has oligospermia or impotence. The donor is chosen for ethnic and physiognomic similarity to the male partner and is screened for transmissible diseases (e.g. HIV, syphilis, hepatitis, gonorrhoea, and genetic disorders). Insemination is performed at the time of ovulation by introducing the semen into the upper vagina. Semen may be fresh or have been stored frozen in liquid nitrogen. (See ARTIFICIAL INSEMINATION.)

DONORS: People who donate parts of their bodies for use in other people. Many organs and tissues can be donated. The commonest is blood; but skin, corneas, kidneys, livers, and hearts can all be used. Combined heart and lung transplants are being increasingly used for patients with severe lung diseases, and, if the recipients have a condition such as cystic fibrosis in which the heart is normal, it is sometimes possible for them to receive a heart and lungs from one donor and to donate their own heart to someone else. Recent work has explored the possibility of using pancreatic transplants. Apart from blood, it is unusual for tissue to be taken from living donors. Skin, small pieces of liver, and a kidney can, in theory, be obtained from living donors, but the ethics of this are hotly debated and the situations under which it may be done are tightly controlled.

There are strict regulations about how death should be diagnosed before organs can be removed for transplantation, and potential donors must satisfy the brain-stem death criteria (q.v.), performed twice by two doctors who are independent of the transplant team. There is a great shortage of suitable organs for donation – partly because they must be in excellent condition if the operation is to be a success. Some medical conditions or modes of death make people unsuitable as organ donors. This makes it all the more important that people should be encouraged to donate their organs. People who wish to do so can carry a special card indicating their willingness to become donors in the event of their death. These cards can be obtained from various sources, including hospitals, GPs' surgeries and many public buildings such as libraries.

Information about becoming a blood donor can be obtained from the local branch of the blood transfusion service, or by telephoning the national offices on 071-628 4590.

Those who wish to bequeath their bodies for dissection purposes should get in touch with HM Inspector of Anatomy, Department of Health, Eileen House, 80–94 Newington Causeway, London SE1 6EF (071-972 2964).

Other would-be organ donors may contact the British Organ Donor Society, Balsham, Cambridge CB1 6DL (0223-893636).

DOPA: A precursor of dopamine and noradrenaline. Levodopa is a drug used in the treatment of Parkinson's disease. It can cross the blood-brain barrier and increase the concentration of dopamine in the basal ganglia. It also inhibits prolactin secretion and may be used to treat galactorrhea.

DOPAMINE is a catecholamine (q.v.) and a precursor of noradrenaline (q.v.). Its highest concentration is in that portion of the brain known as the basal nuclei (SEE BRAIN) where its function is to convey inhibitory influences to the extrapyramidal system. There is good evidence that dopamine deficiency is one of the causative factors in Parkinsonism (q.v.).

DORSAL ROOT GANGLIA: These are swellings on the dorsal roots of spinal nerves just proximal to the union of the dorsal and ventral nerve roots. They are situated in the intervertebral formanina and contain the cell bodies of sensory neurones. (See SPINAL COLUMN and SPINAL CORD.)

DORSUM: The back or posterior part of an organ or structure. The dorsum of the hand is the opposite surface to the palm.

DOSAGE: Many factors influence the activity with which drugs operate. Among the factors which affect the necessary quantity are age, weight, sex, idiosyncrasy, genetic disorders, habitual use, disease, fasting, combination with other drugs, the form in which the drug is given, and the route by which it is given.

AGE is but one factor. Normally, a young child requires a smaller dose than an adult. There are, however, other factors to be taken into consideration. Thus, children are more susceptible than adults to some drugs such as morphine, whilst they are less sensitive to others such as atropine. Various methods have been introduced for calculating roughly and quickly the dose generally suitable for a child of any given age. One, for instance, is:

$$\text{adult dose} \times \frac{\text{age next birthday}}{20}$$

Another formula is:

$$\text{adult dose} \times \frac{\text{weight in pounds}}{150}$$

Yet another is:

$$\frac{\text{age} \times \text{adult dose}}{\text{age in years} + 12}$$

Another formula based on the surface area of the child is:

$$\text{adult dose} \times \frac{\text{surface area in square metres}}{1 \cdot 82}$$

There is, however, no simple way of calculating the dose of a drug for an infant child. The body weight is probably the best and simplest, but it must be used with discrimination, bearing in mind the other factors that have to be taken into consideration. An approximate rule of thumb, based on children of average height and weight, and assuming an adult dose of 100 mg is:

Age	Average weight	Dose
years	kg	mg
1	10	25
7	25	50
12	40	75
Adult	70	100

Old people, too, often show an increased susceptibility to drugs. This is probably due to a variety of factors, such as decreased weight in many old people; diminished activity of the tissues and therefore diminished rate at which a drug is utilized; and diminished activity of the kidneys resulting in decreased rate of excretion of the drug.

WEIGHT AND SEX have both to be taken into consideration. Women require slightly smaller doses than men, probably because they tend to be lighter in weight. The effect of weight on dosage is partly dependent on the fact that much of the extra weight of a heavy individual is made up of fatty tissue which is not as active as other tissue of the body. In practice, the question of weight seldom makes much difference unless the individual is grossly overweight or underweight.

IDIOSYNCRASY occasionally causes drugs administered in the ordinary dose to produce unexpected effects. Thus, some people are but little affected by some drugs, whilst in others certain drugs, such as potassium iodide, or atropine, produce excessive symptoms in minute doses. In some cases this may be due to hypersensitiveness, or an allergic reaction, to the drug. This is a possibility that must always be borne in mind, particularly with penicillin. As a rule the individual has had the drug in question previously. Penicillin comes into this category; so much so that an individual who is known to be allergic to penicillin is strongly recommended to carry about with him wherever he goes a card to this effect. The carrying of such a card may well prevent his being given in some emergency a dose of penicillin that could possibly prove fatal.

HABITUAL USE of a drug is perhaps the influence that causes the greatest increase in the dose necessary to produce the requisite effect. The classical example of this is opium and its derivatives. Arsenic is another example that was often encountered in the days when arsenical drugs were one of the great stand-bys in the Pharmacopoeia.

DISEASE may modify the dose of medicines. This can occur in several ways. Thus, in serious illnesses the patient may be more susceptible to drugs, such as narcotics, that depress tissue activity, and therefore smaller doses must be given. Again, absorption of the drug from the gut may be slowed up by disease of the gut, or its effect may be enhanced if there is disease of the kidneys, interfering with the excretion of the drug.

FASTING aids the rapidity of absorption of, and also makes the body more susceptible to the action of, drugs. Partly for this reason, as well as to avoid irritation of the stomach, it is usual to prescribe drugs to be taken after meals, and diluted with water.

COMBINATION OF DRUGS is now frowned upon as it is often difficult to assess what their combined effect may be. In some cases they may have a mutually antagonistic effect, which means that the patient will not obtain full benefit from the prescription. In other cases the combination may have a deleterious effect, whilst in others again the combination may so enhance the effect on the patient as to produce harmful effects.

FORM OF ADMINISTRATION is important in two respects. In the first instance, there is a tendency today to give a drug in the form of the active principle rather than, say, the leaf from which it is obtained as was the case at one time. This means, of course, that a smaller dose of the active principle is required than of the leaf or the tincture. In the second place, it involves the question of whether the drug is given as a tablet, a mixture, a powder or in injectable form. Various factors have to be taken into consideration; but today the common practice is to give a drug in tablet form, mainly because of the convenience of both patient and prescriber.

ROUTE OF ADMINISTRATION naturally affects dosage. In Britain, medicines are given *by mouth* whenever possible, unless there is some degree of urgency, or because the drug is either destroyed in, or is not absorbed from, the gut. In these circumstances, it is given *intravenously*, *intramuscularly* or *subcutaneously*. In some cases, as in cases of asthma or bronchitis, the drug may be given in the form of an *inhalant* (q.v.), in order to get the maximum concentration at the point where it is wanted: that is, in the lungs. If a local effect is wanted, as in cases of diseases of the skin, the drug is applied *topically* to the skin. In some countries there is a tendency to give medicines in the form of a *suppository* which is inserted in the rectum.

Recent years have seen developments whereby the assimilation of drugs into the body can be more carefully controlled. These include, for example, what are known as transdermals, in which drugs are built into a plaster that is stuck on the skin, and the drug is then absorbed into the body at a controlled rate. This method is now being used for the administration of glyceryl trinitrate (q.v.) in the treatment of angina pectoris (q.v.), and of hyoscine hydrobromide in the treatment of travel sickness (q.v.). Another is a new class of implantable devices. These are tiny polymers infused with a drug and implanted just under the skin by injection. They can be tailored so as to deliver drugs at virtually any rate – from minutes to years. A modification of these polymers now being investigated is the incorporation of magnetic particles which allow an extra burst of the incorporated drug to be released in response to an oscillating magnetic field which is induced by a magnetic 'watch' worn by the patient. In this way the patient can switch on an extra dose of drug when this is needed: insulin, for instance, in the case of diabetics. In yet another new development, a core of drug is enclosed in a semi-permeable membrane and is released in the stomach at a given rate. (See also LIPOSOMES.)

GENETIC DISORDERS are now coming to assume an increasing importance. Perhaps the classical example is the individual who suffers from a congenital deficiency of the enzyme known as glucose-6-phosphate dehydrogenase. Such individuals develop an acute haemolytic anaemia (see ANAEMIA) if they are given certain drugs, including phenacetin or a sulphonamide.

DOTHIEPIN is a drug that is being used in the treatment of depression. (See ANTIDEPRESSANTS.)

DOUBLE BLIND TRIAL: A scientific study in which neither the investigators assessing the outcome nor the subjects being treated know which treatment the subject is receiving. The results are analysed after all the data has been collected and the code has been broken.

DOUBLE VISION (see SQUINT).

DOUCHE: An application to the body of a jet of fluid via a pipe or tube. It may be used to clean any part of the body but is used most commonly with reference to the vagina. (Although used as a method of contraception it is ineffective.)

DOWN'S SYNDROME (or MONGOLISM) is a variety of mental subnormality, in which the patient has Mongolian-like eyes, a snub nose, high cheek-bones, a large tongue, a small round skull, and short, thick hands and feet. Another characteristic feature is the palm print, which reveals distinctive markings; the most distinctive of these is the so-called four-finger line. The condition is being increasingly referred to as Down's syndrome (or disease) after Dr. J. L. H. Down, the London doctor who first described it in 1866.

The incidence is approximately 1 per 600 births, but the incidence in the community is lower than this, as many Down's syndrome victims die in infancy. This high death-rate is due partly to the fact that these children have a much higher incidence of other congenital deformities, such as malformations of the heart, than other children, and partly to their lower resistance to infection.

It is much commoner in children born to older women. Thus, the risk of having a Down's child in women over 45 is more than 1 in 60, compared with less than 1 in 1000 in women under 30. Forty per cent of children with Down's syndrome are born to mothers over 40, 30 per cent to those aged 35 to 40. For mothers who give birth to a Down's child when they are younger the chances of a subsequent child being affected is relatively high. Precise figures in this respect can be misleading, and the best advice for a young mother who has had a Down's child, and who wishes to know the risk of her having another, is to go and discuss the matter with her family doctor.

In 95 per cent of cases the cause is the presence of an extra chromosome (q.v.) in the ovum. The cause of this extra chromosome is not known. In the remaining cases the cause is a fault in the division of the germ cells known as translocation.

The degree of mental backwardness varies considerably. Up to a third of all severely mentally handicapped children of school age have Down's syndrome. It has been estimated that 6 per cent of Down's children are probably capable of profiting appreciably from attendance at schools for the educationally handicapped. Practically all who survive to school age gain some benefit. Most eventually acquire some degree of speech, and about 5 per cent learn to read. They practically never learn to write. Most learn to wash, dress and feed themselves, and many are able to run simple errands.

There is no known cure for the condition, but much can be done for them, especially if they can be kept at home rather than sent to an institution. Parents of such children seeking advice and help are recommended to get in touch with the Down's Syndrome Association, 155 Mitcham Road, London SW17 9PG (081-682 4001, fax: 081-682 4012).

DOXORUBICIN is a drug that is proving of value in the treatment of acute leukaemia, lymphoma, and various forms of sarcoma and cancer, including cancer of the bladder. (See CYTOTOXIC.)

DOXYCYCLINE is a wide-spectrum, long-acting antibiotic of the tetracycline group (q.v.), which is active against a wide range of micro-organisms, including the causative organism of scrub typhus.

DRACUNCULIASIS, or DRACONTIASIS, is the disease caused by the guinea-worm, *Dracunculus medinensis*. It has been described as the oldest known human parasite, and is believed to be the Mosaic fiery serpent that harassed the Israelites on the shores of the Red Sea. It is found in India, Arabia, Iran, the Nile valley, East and West Africa, where it afflicts 20–40 million people. The female may attain a length of 120 cm (4 feet). It is transmitted by *Cyclops*, a fresh-water crustacean, and man is infected by drinking contaminated water. The worm causes no trouble for about a year, when it approaches the surface of the body and causes a local painful swelling which is usually accompanied by fever. The essential treatment, i.e. removal of the worm, has changed little since Biblical days. Mebendazole, metronidazole and thiabendazole are proving of value in controlling the disease.

DRAMAMINE is the trade name for dimenhydrinate, a drug widely used in the treatment of travel sickness.

DRAUGHT, or DRAFT, is a small mixture intended to be taken at one dose. It consists generally of two or four tablespoonfuls of fluid.

DREAMS (see SLEEP).

DRENCH is an old term still used in parts of England for a draught of medicine.

DREPANOCYTOSIS is another term for sickle-cell anaemia (q.v.), which is characterized by the presence in the blood of red blood corpuscles sickle-like in shape. The anaemia is a severe one and afflicts black people.

DRESSINGS (see WOUNDS).

DROP ATTACKS are attacks, usually in a middle-aged woman, whose legs suddenly 'give way', so that she falls to the ground without any warning. There is no loss of consciousness. In some cases the loss of tone in the muscles, responsible for the fall, may persist for several hours. In such cases moving the patient or applying pressure to the soles of the feet may restore the tone to the muscles. In most cases, however, recovery is immediate. The cause is probably a temporary interference with the blood supply to the brain. In others there may be some disturbance of the vestibular apparatus which controls the balance of the body. (See EAR.)

DROP-FOOT: This is the inability to dorsiflex the foot at the ankle. The foot hangs down and has to be swung clear of the ground while walking. It is commonly caused by damage to the lateral popliteal nerve or the peroneal muscles.

DROP WRIST: This is the inability to extend the hand at the wrist. It is usually due to damage to the radial nerve which supplies the extensor muscles.

DROWNING: (see APPENDIX: BASIC FIRST AID).

DRUG ABSORPTION: Drugs are usually administered distant to their site of action in the body. They must then pass across cell membranes to reach their site of action. For example – drugs given by mouth must pass across the gut membrane to enter the blood stream and then pass through the endothelium of vessel walls to reach the site of action in the tissues. This process is called absorption and may depend on lipid diffusion, aqueous diffusion, active transport, or pinocytosis – a process in which a cell takes in small droplets of fluid by cytoplasmic engulfment.

DRUG ADDICTION or DEPENDENCE is the compulsion to take a drug repeatedly. Psychological dependence occurs when the drug user craves the drug's desirable effects. Physical dependence occurs when the user has to continue taking the drug to avoid distressing withdrawal or abstinence symptoms. Drug misuse and dependence are surprisingly common, occurring with widely used drugs such as alcohol, caffeine, and nicotine as well as with certain prescribed drugs such as benzodiazepine tranquillizers. Less socially acceptable but frequently misused drugs are described below.

Cannabis, derived from the plant *Cannabis sativa*, is a widely used but illegal recreational drug that does not seem to be addictive. Its two main forms are marijuana – known in the 1960s as 'pot' – which comes from the dried leaves, and hashish which comes from the resin. Cannabis may be used in food and drink but is usually smoked in cigarettes called 'joints' or 'reefers' to induce relaxation and a feeling of well-being. Heavy use can cause apathy and vagueness and may even cause psychosis. Whether or not cannabis leads people to using harder drugs is debatable.

About 1 in 10 of Britain's teenagers misuses volatile substances such as toluene at some time, but only about 1 in 40 does so regularly. These substances are given off by certain glues, solvents, varnishes, and liquid fuels, all of which can be bought cheaply in shops, although their sale to children under 16 is illegal. They are often inhaled from plastic bags held over the nose and mouth. Central-nervous-system excitation, with euphoria and disinhibition, is followed by depression and lethargy. Unpleasant effects include facial rash, nausea and vomiting, tremor, dizziness, and clumsiness. Death from coma and acute cardiac toxicity is a serious risk. Chronic heavy use can cause peripheral neuropathy and irreversible cerebellar damage. (See SOLVENT ABUSE.)

The hallucinogenic or psychedelic drugs include lysergic acid diethylamide (LSD or acid), magic mushrooms, ecstasy (MDMA), and phencyclidine (PCP or 'angel' dust, mainly used in the USA). These drugs have no medicinal uses. Taken by mouth, they produce vivid 'trips', with heightened emotions and perceptions and sometimes with hallucinations. They are not physically addictive but can cause nightmarish bad trips during use and flashbacks (vivid reruns of trips) after use, and can probably trigger psychosis.

Stimulant drugs such as amphetamine and cocaine act like adrenaline and speed up the central nervous system, making the user feel confident, energetic, and powerful for several hours. They can also cause severe insomnia, anxiety, paranoia, psychosis, and even sudden death due to convulsions or tachycardia. Depression may occur on withdrawal of these drugs, and in some users this is sufficiently deterrent to cause psychological dependence. Amphetamine ('speed') is mainly synthesized illegally and may be eaten, sniffed, or injected. Related drugs such as dexamphetamine sulphate (Dexedrine) and diethylpropion hydrochloride (Tenuate, Dospan) are prescribed pills that enter the black market. Cocaine and related drugs are used in medicine as local anaesthetics. Illegal supplies of cocaine ('snow' or 'ice') and its derivative, 'crack', come mainly from South America, where they are made from the plant *Erythroxylon coca*. Cocaine is usually sniffed ('snorted') or rubbed into the gums; crack is burnt and inhaled.

Opiate drugs are derived from the opium poppy, *Papaver somniferum*. They are described as narcotic because they induce sleep. Their main medical use is as potent oral or injectable analgesics such as morphine, diamorphine, pethidine, and codeine. The commonest illegal opiate is heroin, a powdered form of diamorphine that may be smoked, sniffed, or injected to induce euphoria and drowsiness. Regular opiate misuse leads to tolerance (the need to take ever larger doses to achieve the same effect) and marked dependence. The withdrawal syndrome is like a bout of severe gastric flu with painful abdominal cramps. A less addictive oral opiate, methadone, can be prescribed as a substitute that is easier to withdraw.

Some 75,000–150,000 Britons now misuse opiates and other drugs intravenously, and pose a huge public-health problem because

Drugs	Physical Dependence	Tolerance	Over-powering Need	Acquired Desire	Psychic Dependence	Psycho-toxic	Psychotic on Withdrawal	
Morphine-like	+	+	+		+	+	+	
Barbiturates and other hypnotics	+	+	+		+	+	+	+
Cocaine		+		+	+			
Amphetamine	+	+	+	+	+	+		
Cannabis				+	+	+		
LSD and other Hallucinogens		+		+	+	+		
Inhalation Drugs	?		+*	+	+			
Aspirin	?	+*	+	+	+			
Caffeine	+		+	+				
Nicotine		+		+	+			
Alcohol+	+	+	+	+	+			

*Only some of the users display this.

Comparison of the characteristics of drugs of dependence. *The Practitioner.*

injections with shared dirty needles can carry the blood-borne viruses that cause AIDS and hepatitis B. Many clinics now operate schemes to exchange old needles for clean ones, free of charge.

DRUG BINDING: The process of attachment of a drug to a receptor or plasma protein, fat, mucopolysaccharide or other tissue component. This process may be reversible or irreversible.

DRUG CLEARANCE: The volume of blood from which a drug is completely removed in one minute is known as clearance. Renal clearance of a drug is the amount of blood completely cleared of the drug by the kidney in one minute.

DRUG INTERACTIONS: Many patients are on several prescribed drugs, and numerous medicines are available over the counter, so the potential for drug interaction is large. A drug may interact with another by inhibiting its action, potentiating its action, or by simple summation of effects.

The interaction may take place: (*a*) Prior to absorption or administration, e.g. antacids bind tetracycline in the gut and prevent absorption. (*b*) By interfering with protein binding – one drug may displace another from binding sites on plasma proteins. The action of the displaced drug will be increased because more drug is now available, e.g. anticoagulants are displaced by analgesics. (*c*) During metabolism or excretion of the drug – some drugs increase or decrease the activity of liver enzymes which metabolize drugs, thus affecting their rate of destruction, e.g. barbiturates, nicotine, and alcohol all activate hepatic enzymes. Altering the pH of urine will affect the excretion of drugs via the kidney. (*d*) At the drug receptor – one drug may displace another at the receptor affecting its efficacy or duration of action.

DRUG METABOLISM: A process by which the body destroys and excretes drugs, so limiting their duration of action. Phase 1 metabolism consists of transformation by oxidation, reduction, or hydrolysis. In phase 2 this transformed product is conjugated (joined up) with another molecule to produce a water-soluble product which is easier to excrete.

DRUGS: In Britain the supply of drugs is controlled by the Medicines Act. Some drugs are available only on prescription, some both on prescription and over the counter, and some are not available on NHS prescription. When enquiring about drugs that a patient is taking, it is essential to ask about all items bought over the counter and any herbal or traditional remedies that might be used, as these can interact with other prescribed drugs or affect the patient's presenting complaints. Each drug has a single generic name, but many will also have several proprietary (brand) names. It is often much cheaper to prescribe the generic form of a drug, and many doctors, especially in hospitals, do so. Prescriptions for drugs should be written clearly in ink and signed and dated by the prescriber. They should include the patient's name, address and age (obligatory for children under 12), the name of the drug to be supplied, the dose and dose frequency, and the total quantity to be supplied. Any special instructions (e.g. 'after food') should be stated. There are special regulations about the prescription of drugs controlled under the Misuse of Drugs Regulations, 1985 (see CONTROLLED DRUGS). A pharmacist can advise about which drugs are available without prescription, and is able to recommend treatment for many minor complaints. Information about exemption from prescription charges in the NHS can be obtained from health visitors, general practitioners, or social security offices.

DRUGS IN PREGNANCY: Unnecessary drugs during pregnancy should be avoided because of the adverse effect of some drugs on the fetus which have no harmful effect on the mother. Drugs may pass through the placenta and damage the fetus because their pharmacological effects are enhanced as the enzyme systems responsible for their degradation are undeveloped in the fetus. Thus, if the drug can pass through the placenta, the pharmacological effect on the fetus may be great whilst that on the mother is minimal. Warfarin may thus induce fetal and placental haemorrhage and thiazide administration may produce thrombocytopenia in the new born. Many progestogens have androgenic side effects and their administration to a mother for the purpose of preventing recurrent abortion may produce virilization of the female fetus. Tetracycline administered during the last trimester commonly stains the deciduous teeth of the child yellow.

The other dangers of administering drugs in pregnancy are the teratogenic effects. It is understandable that a drug may interfere with a mechanism essential for growth and result in arrested or distorted development of the fetus and yet cause no disturbance in the adult in whom these differentiation and organization processes have ceased to be relevant. Thus the effect of a drug upon a fetus may differ qualitatively as well as quantitatively from its effect on the mother. The susceptibility of the embryo will depend on the stage of development it has reached when the drug is given. The stage of early differentiation, that is from the beginning of the third week to the end of the tenth week of pregnancy, is the time of greatest susceptibility. After this time the risk of congenital malformation from drug treatment is less although the death of the fetus can occur at any time.

DRUNKENNESS (see ALCOHOL).

DUCHENNE MUSCULAR DYSTROPHY: An inherited sex-linked recessive disorder characterized by progressive muscular weakness and wasting. It is the most common muscular dystrophy, occurring in 30 per 100,000 live male births. Spontaneous mutations are common. The calf muscles become bulky (pseudo-hypertrophy). Affected boys develop symptoms in early childhood and die in their teens or early twenties from respiratory infections. Female carriers may be identified by screening for abnormalities of muscle enzymes.

DUCT is the name applied to a passage leading from a gland into some hollow organ, or on to the surface of the body, by which the secretion of the gland is discharged: e.g. the pancreatic duct and the bile duct opening into the duodenum, and the sweat ducts opening on the skin surface.

DUCTLESS GLAND is the term applied to any one of certain glands in the body the secretion of which goes directly into the blood stream and so is carried to different parts of the body. These glands – the pituitary, thyroid, parathyroid, adrenal and reproductive – are also known as the ENDOCRINE GLANDS (q.v.). Some glands may be both duct glands and ductless glands. For example, the pancreas manufactures a digestive juice which passes by a duct into the small intestine. It also manufactures, by means of special cells, a substance called insulin which passes straight into the blood.

DUCTUS ARTERIOSUS is the blood-vessel in the fetus through which blood passes from the pulmonary artery to the aorta, thereby bypassing the lungs, which do not function during intra-uterine life. (See CIRCULATION OF THE BLOOD.) The ductus normally ceases to function soon after birth and within a few weeks is converted into a fibrous cord. Occasionally this obliteration does not occur: a condition known as patent ductus arteriosus. This is one of the more common congenital defects of the heart, and one which responds particularly well to surgical treatment. Closure of the duct can also be achieved in some cases by the administration of indomethacin. (See HEART DISEASES.)

DUCTUS DEFERENS, or VAS DEFERENS, is the tube which carries spermatozoa from the epididimis to the seminal vesicles. (See TESTICLE.)

DUMBNESS (see SPEECH DISORDERS).

DUMPING SYNDROME: A sensation of weakness and sweating after a meal in patients who have undergone gastrectomy (q.v.). Rapid emptying of the stomach and the drawing of fluid from the blood into the intestine has been blamed, but the exact cause is debated.

DUODENAL ILEUS is the term applied to dilatation of the duodenum due to chronic obstruction of the duodenum, caused by an abnormal position of arteries in the region of the duodenum pressing on it.

DUODENAL ULCER has much in common with gastric ulcer. (See STOMACH, DISEASES OF.) The two together are known as peptic ulcers, and in recent years there has been a tendency for the two forms of ulceration to be regarded as modifications of one entity known as peptic ulcer, rather than as separate disease entities.

Part of the reason for this is that, as increasingly detailed statistics have become available, it has become clear that the incidence of the disease (or diseases) has been changing over the last century. Be all that as it may, it is abundantly clear that, as one authority has expressed it, 'peptic ulcer in general is still a large health problem' in Britain, probably as many 'as one in ten of the population suffering at some time or other during his or her lifetime from ulcer-type dyspepsia'.

Duodenal ulcer is ten to fifteen times more common than gastric ulcer. The age incidence of the two forms of ulcer differs. Thus, duodenal ulcer occurs at any age from 20 years onwards, whereas gastric ulcer usually occurs after the age of 40. Duodenal ulcer is three times as common in men as in women; indeed, in some series the ratio between men and women is as high as ten. In gastric ulcer, on the other hand, the sex ratio is less than two men to one woman. Gastric ulcer is rare in women until after the menopause. Here it should be noted that these figures, and the whole of this section, are concerned with chronic peptic ulcer. It is such ulcers that are practically always referred to when mention is made of duodenal or gastric ulcer. Acute peptic ulcers are quite uncommon. Indeed, there is some evidence that they may be an entirely different disease from chronic peptic ulcers. This does not mean, however, that chronic peptic ulcers, whether duodenal or gastric, do not pass through stages when their manifestations can be justifiably described as acute. There is also a different social incidence between the two forms of ulcer. Duodenal ulcer is more common in the upper social classes, although it is to be found in all classes, but gastric ulcer is more common among the lower social classes. There is also a higher incidence of duodenal ulcer in individuals who belong to blood group O. (See BLOOD GROUPS.) Not the least interesting observation in the field of peptic ulcer is that the large increase in incidence since the turn of the century has been due to the increase in duodenal ulcers. There is some statistical evidence that this 'epidemic' is now on the wane, and that the incidence of duodenal ulcer in Britain is beginning to fall.

There is no general consensus of expert opinion as to the precise cause of peptic ulcers. What probably happens is that there is some abrasion, or break, in the lining membrane (or mucosa) of the stomach and/or duodenum, and that it is gradually eroded and deepened by the gastric juice. What is not known, however, is why this only occurs in some people. After all, the probability is that such abrasions occur in everyone of us at some time or other, but it is only in a minority that these develop into peptic ulcers. Equally puzzling is why the acid and pepsin in the gastric juice erode the stomach (or duodenum) lining downwards into the depth of the wall of the stomach (or duodenum), but does not erode, or digest, it all along the surface of the lining. Needless to say, all sorts of theories have been advanced to explain these discrepancies. None is proven, but some are probable, whilst others have practical implications. Thus, mental stress and strain are probably provocative factors, thus explaining the increased incidence of duodenal ulcer in managers and executives. Smoking seems to accentuate, if not cause, duodenal ulcer, and the drinking of alcohol is probably harmful. The apparent association with a given blood group, and the fact that relatives of a patient with a peptic ulcer are unduly likely to develop such an ulcer suggest that there is some constitutional factor.

Symptoms and signs: These are similar in some ways to those of gastric ulcer, but there are certain differences. The presenting symptom is pain in the middle of the upper part of the abdomen, or somewhat to the right. This tends to come on two or three hours after a meal, and to be relieved by taking food (e.g. a glass of milk). It also tends to occur during the night. The pain varies in intensity, and, if not treated, may persist for up to an hour. The appetite is not usually affected, and, though the individual tends to remain thin, there is not usually much loss of weight. Vomiting is not common. When it does occur, it usually means that the ulcer is causing obstruction of the exit of the food from the stomach into the duodenum. The main finding on examination is tenderness over the area of pain, accompanied by stiffening, or guarding, of the overlying muscles. The diagnosis is clinched by the radiological demonstration of what is known as a 'niche' in the duodenum. This niche is the actual ulcer, and it is made visible by giving the individual some radio-opaque substance, such as barium sulphate, to swallow. This fills up the ulcer crater, which is then visible when an X-ray is taken, or when the duodenum is studied by fluoroscopy (q.v.). Direct visualization of the ulcer by fibroscopy has become more popular over recent years. (See FIBREOPTIC ENDOSCOPY.) Another method of examination is gastric analysis. (See TEST MEAL.) In patients with duodenal ulcer this usually reveals a high gastric acidity.

As in the case of a gastric ulcer, the patient with a duodenal ulcer is liable to two complications: perforation of the ulcer, and haemorrhage (see HAEMATEMESIS). If the bleeding from the ulcer is slight, there may be no vomiting of blood (or haematemesis), the blood being passed down the gut. In the course of its passage through the gut it is chemically altered and becomes black in colour. Then, when it is finally passed in the stools, the stools are dark and shiny, or tarry, in appearance. (See MELAENA.)

Treatment consists basically of rest, a diet, and the administration of alkalis. In severe cases a period of rest in bed may be advisable. This in itself has a most beneficial effect. No complicated dietetic regime is called for nowadays. The basis of the diet is the avoidance of all condiments, a minimum of fried food, and something to eat every two hours. The rationale of this is to counteract the increased acidity of the gastric juice. In practice, two-hourly feeding means breakfast, lunch and dinner (or supper), with a glass of milk mid-morning, a snack in mid-afternoon and a snack the last thing at night on going to bed. The basis of the snacks should be milk or something milky. Strong tea and coffee should be avoided, as should smoking. Alcohol is better avoided, but a glass of wine with food will do no harm. There is a large range of alkalis to be chosen from, and the individual choice should be made in conjunction with the family doctor. The management of duodenal ulcers has been revolutionized by the advent of the histamine receptor antagonists which inhibit gastric acid secretion and allow the ulcer to heal. Both cimetidine and rantidine reduce the hyper-acidity of the gastric juice. If the ulcer does not respond to adequate medical treatment along these lines, or if it leads to obstruction of the pylorus (q.v.), then operation is called for. Operation is also indicated should perforation occur. A perforated duodenal (or gastric) ulcer is an emergency, and must be dealt with immediately. The majority of surgeons still favour immediate operation. Should a haemorrhage occur, the treatment depends upon its severity. As a rule, a blood transfusion is called for.

DUODENUM is the first part of the intestine immediately beyond the stomach, so named because its length is about twelve fingerbreadths. (See INTESTINE.)

DUPUYTREN'S CONTRACTURE: A condition of unknown aetiology in which there is progressive thickening and contracture of the palmar fascia with adherence of the overlying skin. A clawing deformity of the fingers, particularly the little and ring fingers, develops. It is associated with liver disease, diabetes, epilepsy, and gout. Treatment is surgical to excise the affected fascia.

DURA MATER is the outermost and strongest of the three membranes or meninges which envelop the brain and spinal cord. In it run vessels which nourish the inner surface of the skull. (See BRAIN.)

DWARF, or DWARFISM, is a term applied to under-development of the body. The causes are either developmental or due to food insufficient in quantity or unsuitable in quality, or to defects in some of the body secretions which can be corrected. The first-named group includes pituitary dwarfism, the subjects being very small people with normally proportioned parts, also achondroplasic dwarfs (see ACHONDROPLASIA) with large globular head and shortened limbs and stumpy fingers. It is now known that in a certain proportion of children of short stature this can be remedied by administration of the growth hormone of pituitary gland (q.v.), provided this is given at an early enough age. All children who by the age of 5 years are at least what is technically known as 'three stand-

ard deviations below the mean' should be referred for examination by specialists to determine whether or not their lack of height is due to lack of growth hormone and therefore likely to respond to treatment with the hormone. In the class of dwarfism which is partly curable, there are included cretins, whose want of growth in mind and body is attributable to a primary defect of the thyroid gland. (See CRETINISM.) In this class are also included various forms of defective growth associated with defects in the secretions of the digestive organs, especially the pancreas; this type of defect, often known as pancreatic infantilism, is mainly confined to a retardation of physical development, while the mental changes are little marked. Another form of dwarfism, associated with a deformity of the bones, is produced by rickets in early life, such persons showing high forehead, great bending of the leg bones, and deformity of the chest. (See RICKETS.)

DYNAMOMETER is an elliptical ring of steel to which is attached a dial and moving index. It is used to test the strength of the muscles of the forearm, being squeezed in the hand, and registering the pressure in pounds or kilograms.

DYS- is a prefix meaning difficult or painful.

DYSARTHRIA is a general term applied when weakness or incoordination of the speech musculature prevents clear pronunciation of words. The individual's speech may sound as if it is slurred or weak. It may be due to damage affecting the centres in the brain which control movements of the speech muscles or damage to the muscles themselves.

Examples of dysarthria may be found in stroke illness, cerebral palsy and the latter stages of Parkinson's disease, multiple sclerosis and motor neurone disease. Whatever the cause a speech therapist can assess the extent of the dysarthria and suggest exercises or an alternative means of communication.

DYSCHEZIA is constipation due to retention of faeces in the rectum. This retention is the outcome of irregular habits, which damp down the normal reflex causing defaecation.

DYSDIADOKOKINESIA means loss of the ability to perform rapid alternate movements, such as winding up a watch. It is a sign of a lesion in the cerebellum.

DYSENTERY, also called bloody flux, is an infectious disease with a local lesion in the form of inflammation and ulceration of the lower portion of the bowels. It occurs in two main forms: bacillary dysentery and amoebic dysentery.
BACILLARY DYSENTERY is found in practically every part of the world.
Cause: The disease may occur sporadically or in

epidemics. The causative organism is the dysentery bacillus, or shigella as it is now known, of which there are several strains, named after their discoverers: Shiga, Flexner and Sonne. In the UK a few thousand cases occur. In Britain in the last two decades the proportion of cases in children has fallen and the seasonal incidence has also changed, with more cases occurring in the summer and autumn. These changes are accounted for by a decrease in the number of cases due to *Shigella sonnei* and an increase in the number of cases due to *Shigella flexneri* because of imported disease. The infection is spread by flies, by direct contact, or by pollution of the water by faeces from infected patients, which contain the bacillus. Epidemics are thus encouraged by overcrowding and insanitary conditions. In the East, uncooked vegetables, especially salads, are a potent source of infection, as are cooks and other foodhandlers who are carriers of the disease. The incubation period is 1 to 7 days. The severity of the disease depends partly upon the strain responsible for the infection. Thus, Shiga infections are usually severe, whilst, except in infants, Flexner and Sonne infections run a more benign course.

The dysentery bacilli affect mainly the large intestine. In mild cases there may be only a catarrh of the intestine with excessive mucoid excretion, whilst in severe cases there may be extensive ulceration involving practically the whole of the large intestine.

Symptoms: These vary from those of a mild attack of diarrhoea to those of an acute fulminating infection. The first symptoms usually consist of colicky pain in the abdomen followed by diarrhoea. There may also be nausea, aching pain in the limbs, and shivery feelings. There is always fever. The number of stools varies, but there may be as many as fifty daily in acute cases. The stools consist mainly of mucus and blood. The duration of the diarrhoea varies from a few days to a fortnight, depending upon the severity of the infection. Diagnosis is established by finding dysentery bacilli in the stools. Complications only occur in severe cases, and consist of perforation of the intestine and severe haemorrhage from the gut. At one time one of the killing diseases of the world, with mortality rates up to 50 per cent during epidemics, the outlook has been entirely altered by the introduction of the sulphonamides, but it is still a serious condition in young infants, old people and the malnourished.

Treatment: PREVENTIVE: This consists of adequate sanitation, the destruction of flies, careful disposal of all garbage, and careful protection of all food from flies. In addition, no carrier of dysentery bacilli should be allowed to handle food.

CURATIVE: Complete rest in bed is essential, and precautions must be taken to ensure that the stools are disposed of without any risk of their spreading the infection. For the first twenty-four hours only water is given. In the case of acutely ill babies or young children it may be necessary to give fluids intravenously, in the form, for example, of 4·3 per cent glucose in 1/5 normal saline, for the first twenty-four hours or so. This is gradually supplemented with milk, milk puddings, and chicken broth, but it is necessary for the diet to be kept light, and to contain as little residue as possible, until the diarrhoea has settled. Purgatives and laxatives are not given. The sheet-anchors of treatment are now the sulphonamides: usually phthalyl-sulphathiazole, succinylsulpha-thizole or sulphadimidine. Alternatively, neomycin may be used. If there is much abdominal pain, morphine may be given during the first day, but usually the application of heat in some form to the abdomen is sufficient.

AMOEBIC DYSENTERY is almost entirely confined to tropical and sub-tropical countries. Around 200 new cases occur annually in England and Wales.

Cause: The causative organism is the *Entamoeba histolytica*. Infection occurs as a result of food, e.g. uncooked vegetables, or drinking water which has been contaminated either by a carrier of the disease or by flies. The amoebae settle in the wall of the large intestine, where they cause first of all inflammatory changes and then ulceration. These ulcers then tend to become infected with other organisms. From the ulcers the amoebae may spread through the portal vein, where they cause abscesses. An amoebic abscess of the liver is not infrequent. More rarely, the amoebae may spread elsewhere, e.g. to the lungs or brain, and cause abscesses. In the latter it may cause meningitis (q.v.) or meningoencephalitis (q.v.). Occasionally a mass may be formed in the colon, known as an amoeboma.

Symptoms: These may appear within a week of infection or be delayed for months or even years. The onset of the disease is usually gradual, with the passage of several stools daily, which ultimately contain blood. Occasionally there may be an acute sudden onset as described for bacillary dysentery. Even in the cases with gradual onset there is loss of weight, with dyspepsia and anaemia. Complications which may occur include perforation of the intestine, haemorrhage from the gut, and abscess formation in the liver, brain, bones or testes. The condition is liable to run a chronic course. Any individual who has been in the tropics and who complains of abdominal pain and dyspepsia should have the stools examined for the presence of *Entamoeba histolytica*, even though there is no history of dysentery.

Treatment: PREVENTIVE: This consists of the protection of food from flies, the avoidance of contamination of water and uncooked vegetables, and steps to ensure that those handling food are not carriers of the amoeba.

CURATIVE: Emetine, for long the great standby in the treatment of amoebic dysentery, has now been largely replaced by the nitroimidazole group of drugs. These include metronidazole, tinidazole, and ornidazole. While these drugs are being taken alcoholic drinks are forbidden as these may produce a psychotic state. A course of one or other of these drugs is followed by a course of diloxamide furoate. In severe cases these drugs may be supplemented with tetracycline. Cure is assessed by the disappearance of symptoms, the return of normal stools and the absence of parasites from the stools on three separate occasions. If an amoebic abscess has formed in the liver this is treated by aspiration following a course of one of the nitroimidazole group of drugs. Aspiration is performed through a wide-bore needle under local anaesthesia.

DYSIDROSIS means disturbance of sweat secretion.

DYSLEXIA is difficulty in reading or learning to read. It is always accompanied by difficulty in writing and particularly by difficulties in spelling correctly. It is a condition which is attracting increasing attention, particularly the form known as specific dyslexia. This is the name given to difficulties in learning to read and write which affect a minority of children exposed to normal educational processes who do not show backwardness in other school subjects. Four per cent of children are said to be affected by it in a severe form, and it is three times more common in boys than in girls.

Parents of such children would be well advised to get in touch with the British Dyslexia Association, 98 London Road, Reading, Berkshire RG1 5AU (0734-668270).

DYSMENORRHOEA means painful menstruation. (See MENSTRUATION.)

DYSPAREUNIA means painful or difficult coitus.

DYSPEPSIA: This is another name for indigestion. It describes a sensation of pain or discomfort in the upper abdomen or lower chest following eating. There may be additional symptoms of heartburn, flatulence, or nausea. There are many causes of dyspepsia including oesophagitis, peptic ulcer, gallstones, hiatus hernia, malignancy of the stomach or oesophagus, and hepatic or pancreatic disease. Occasionally it may be psychological in origin. Treatment depends on the underlying cause but, if there is no specific pathology, avoidance of precipitating foods may be helpful.

DYSPHAGIA is the medical term for difficulty in swallowing.

DYSPHASIA is the term used to describe the difficulties in understanding language and in self-expression, most frequently after stroke (see STROKE), or other brain damage. When there is a total loss in the ability to communicate through speech or writing, it is known as *global aphasia*. Many more individuals have a partial understanding of what is said to them. They are also able to put their own thoughts into words to some extent. The general term for this less severe condition is *dysphasia*. Individuals vary widely, but in general there are two main types of dysphasia. Some people may have a good understanding of spoken language but have difficulty in self- expression; this is called *non-fluent dysphasia*. Others may have a very poor ability to understand speech, but will have a considerable spoken output consisting of jargon words; this is known as *fluent dysphasia*. Similar difficulties may occur with reading, and this is called *dyslexia* (a term more commonly encountered in the different context of children's reading disability). Adults who have suffered a stroke or another form of brain damage may also have difficulty in writing, or *dysgraphia*. The speech therapist can assess the finer diagnostic points. (See SPEECH THERAPY.)

No case is too severe or too mild to be referred to a speech therapist for an assessment. The victim, his relatives and other visitors may be anxious about the effects of the stroke and may find it helpful to have the details of the dysphasic problem explained to them. The speech therapist can help them adjust to the effects of the stroke on communication. Treatment may be conducted on an individual or group basis according to the needs of the individual. It is important for people who come into contact with the dysphasic person to treat him just as they would have done before the stroke: to be patient rather than patronizing.

Dysphasia may come on suddenly and last only for a few hours or days, being due to a temporary block in the circulation of blood to the brain. The effects may be permanent, but although the individual may have difficulty in understanding language and expressing himself, he will be quite aware of his surroundings and may be very frustrated by his inability to communicate with others.

Further information may be obtained from Action for Dysphasic Adults, Canterbury House, Royal Street, London SE1 7LN; and the Stroke Association, CHSA House, Whitecross Street, London EC1Y 8JJ (071-490 7999, fax: 071-490 2686).

DYSPNOEA means difficulty in breathing (see BREATHLESSNESS; ORTHOPNOEA).

DYSTOCIA means slow or painful birth of a child.

DYSTONIA refers to a type of involuntary movement characterized by a sustained muscle contraction, frequently causing twisting and repetitive movements or abnormal postures, and caused by inappropriate instructions from the brain. It is sometimes called torsion spasm, and may be synonymous with athetosis when the extremities are involved. Often the condition is of unknown cause (idiopathic), but an inherited predisposition is increasingly recognized among some cases. Others may be associated with known pathology of the brain such as cerebral palsy or Wilson's disease. The presentation of dystonia may be focal (usually in adults) causing blepharospasm (forceful eye closure), oromandibular dystonia (spasms of the tongue and jaw), cranial dystonia/Meige syndrome/Brueghel's syndrome (eyes and jaw both involved), spastic or spasmodic dysphonia/ laryngeal dystonia (strained or whispering speech), spasmodic dysphagia (difficulty swallowing), spasmodic torti/latero/ante/retrocollis (rotation, sideways, forward or backward tilting of the neck), dystonic writer's cramp or axial dystonia (spasms deviating the torso). Foot dystonia occurs almost exclusively in children and adolescents. In adults, the condition usually remains focal or involves at most an adjacent body part. In children, it may spread to become generalized. The condition has always been considered rare, but commonly is either not diagnosed or mistakenly thought to be of psychological origin. It may, in fact, be half as common as multiple sclerosis. Similar features can occur in some subjects treated with major tranquillizing drugs, in whom a predisposition to develop dystonia may be present.

DYSTROPHY means defective or faulty nutrition, and is a term generally applied to some developmental change in the muscles occurring independently of the nervous system. The best-known forms are those known as *progressive muscular dystrophy*, in which groups of muscles, especially those of the calves and buttocks, undergo a fatty degeneration associated with increase in size but weakness in power; and *adiposogenital dystrophy* associated with defect of the pituitary gland. (See MYOPATHY.)

DYSURIA means difficulty or pain in urination.

E

EAR: The ear is concerned with two functions. The more evident is that of the sense of hearing; the other is the sense of equilibration and of motion. The organ is divided into three parts: (*a*) the external ear, consisting of the auricle on the surface of the head, and the tube which leads inwards to the drum; (*b*) the middle ear, separated from the former by the tympanic membrane or drum, and from the internal ear by two other membranes, but communicating with the throat by the Eustachian tube; and (*c*) the internal ear, comprising the complicated labyrinth from which runs the vestibulocochlear nerve into the brain.
EXTERNAL EAR: The auricle or pinna, shaped in man something like a crumpled-up funnel, is not essential to the sense of hearing, although in animals it appears to play an important part.

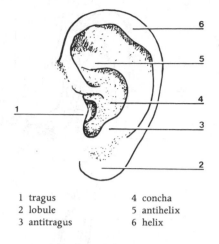

1 tragus	4 concha
2 lobule	5 antihelix
3 antitragus	6 helix

The auricle.

It consists of a framework of elastic cartilage covered by skin, the lobule at the lower end being a small mass of fat. From the bottom of the concha the external auditory (or acoustic) meatus runs inwards for 25 mm (1 inch), to end blindly at the drum. This passage is short in young children, in whom the drum is almost at the surface, and it lengthens as the skull bones develop. The outer half of the passage is surrounded by cartilage, lined by skin, on which are placed fine hairs pointing outwards, and glands secreting a small amount of wax. In the inner half, the skin is smooth and lies directly upon the temporal bone, in the substance of which the whole hearing apparatus is enclosed. The two parts meet at a slight angle, so as to give the whole passage a curve, which can be straightened by pulling the auricle upwards and backwards, when the drum can often be clearly seen by a good light.
MIDDLE EAR: The tympanic membrane, forming the drum, is stretched completely across the end of the passage, being placed rather obliquely, so that it makes an angle of about 60° with the floor. It is about 8 mm (one-third of an inch) across, very thin, and white or pale pink in colour, so that it is partly transparent, and some of the contents of the middle ear shine through it. From this description it can be readily understood how easily it is torn, and how dangerous are blows on the side of the head, and rough manipulations to remove wax. The cavity of the middle ear is about 8 mm (one-third of an inch) wide and 4 mm (one-sixth of an inch) in depth from the tympanic membrane to the inner wall of bone. Although important structures, like the facial nerve which runs down behind it, lie close around, its only important contents are three small bones, the malleus (hammer), incus (anvil), and stapes (stirrup), collectively known as the auditory ossicles, with two minute muscles which regulate their movements, and the chorda tympani nerve which runs across the cavity. The auditory ossicles are of great importance. The

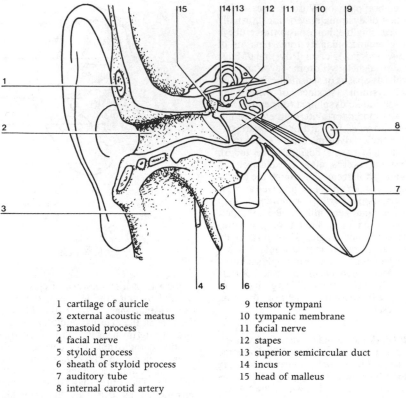

1 cartilage of auricle
2 external acoustic meatus
3 mastoid process
4 facial nerve
5 styloid process
6 sheath of styloid process
7 auditory tube
8 internal carotid artery

9 tensor tympani
10 tympanic membrane
11 facial nerve
12 stapes
13 superior semicircular duct
14 incus
15 head of malleus

The external and middle portions of the right ear from the front.

malleus has a long spicule of bone, the handle, embedded in the substance of the drum, while its head is in contact with the incus. The incus, suspended by one process of bone, has another affixed to the stapes, and the latter fits, by what would in a real stirrup be the footpiece, into one (fenestra vestibuli) of the two openings which lead through the inner wall of the middle ear into the internal ear. Accordingly these three bones form a chain across the middle ear, connecting the drum with the internal ear. Their function is to convert the air-waves, which strike upon the drum, into mechanical movements which can affect the fluid in the inner ear, because air-waves produce little effect upon fluid directly.

The middle ear has two connections which are of great importance as regards disease: in front, it communicates by a passage 37 mm (1½ inches) long, the Eustachian (or auditory) tube, with the upper part of the throat, behind the nose; behind and above, it opens into a cavity known as the mastoid antrum. The Eustachian tube admits air from the throat, and so keeps the pressure on both sides of the drum fairly equal. Serious deafness is produced by its closure, and it also, unfortunately, forms a channel by which acute inflammation, as in measles, can and does spread to the ear. The antrum occupies the interior of the projecting mass of bone, the mastoid process, which is felt on the surface of the head behind the ear; this cavity, along with the middle ear, is separated from the interior of the skull only by a thin plate of bone about the thickness of a playing card. INTERNAL EAR: This consists of a complex system of hollows in the substance of the temporal bone enclosing a membranous duplicate. Between the membrane and the bone is a fluid known as perilymph, while the membrane is distended by another collection of fluid known as endolymph. This membranous labyrinth, as it is called, consists of two parts. The hinder part, comprising a sac, the utricle, and three short semicircular canals opening at each end into it, is the part concerned with the balancing sense; the forward part consists of another small bag, the saccule, and of a still more important part, the cochlear duct, and is the part concerned in hearing. In the cochlear duct is placed the spiral organ of Corti, on which the sound-waves are finally received and by which the sounds are communicated to the cochlear nerve, a branch of the vestibulocochlear nerve, which ends in filaments to this organ of Corti. The essential parts in the organ of Corti are a double row of rods and several rows of cells furnished with fine hairs of varying length. Different musical notes are perhaps appreciated by different rods and hair cells. THE ACT OF HEARING: When sound-waves in the air reach the ear, the drum is alternately pressed in and pulled out, in consequence of which a to-and-fro movement is communicated to the

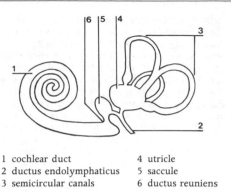

1 cochlear duct   4 utricle
2 ductus endolymphaticus   5 saccule
3 semicircular canals   6 ductus reuniens

The membranous labyrinth.

chain of ossicles. The foot of the stapes communicates these movements to the perilymph. Finally these motions reach the delicate filaments placed in the organ of Corti, and so affect the nerve of hearing, which conveys impressions to the centre in the brain. There are two theories of hearing. The first is that of Helmholtz, who compared the organ of Corti to a piano and presumed that each sound caused a vibration of a corresponding part of Corti's organ. The second and later theory assumes that the entire organ of Corti is thrown into vibration by sounds, and that the nature of the sound is analysed and perceived by the hearing-centre in the brain.

EAR, DISEASES OF: Troubles connected with the ear should be treated early. Mention has been made of the importance of the connection between throat and middle ear by way of the Eustachian tube, both as regards the maintenance of good hearing and as regards the spread of inflammation. There are several simple procedures connected with the management of the ear which demand explanation.
EXAMINATION of the external ear is carried out by placing the person's head in a good light near a window, inclining the head away from the window a little, pulling the auricle upwards and backwards, and if a conical speculum is at hand, introducing this with a gentle screwing movement. The drum and deeper part of the external ear may then be viewed. If available, an electric auriscope is a much more satisfactory means of carrying out the examination.
SYRINGING is done with a large-sized glass or metal syringe provided with a short blunt point (not longer than 25 mm (1 inch), so that no damage to the drum can result). The auricle is pulled gently up and back, while a steady stream from the syringe is directed along the upper wall, and flows out along the lower one. In syringing the ear of a child the point of the syringe should not be inserted within the shallow passage at all.
INFLATION of the middle ear is performed for cases in which the Eustachian tube is partly blocked and the drum indrawn. A catheter is passed along the floor of the nose into the opening of the Eustachian tube in the throat, and forcible inflation made through this by means of a rubber bag (Politzer's bag). Or the bag is used to blow up one nostril, the other being closed, while the Eustachian tube is kept open by one of the following devices. The person swallows a mouthful of water, or pronounces some guttural, such as 'Huck', so as to raise the soft palate and close the opening between the nose and throat; and at this moment the bag is suddenly squeezed. The Eustachian tube may also be inflated by forcibly expelling air from the chest while the mouth and nose are closed. The fact of whether air enters the middle ear becomes plain to the person himself by a click followed by a slight ringing in the ear, and often by improved hearing, as so many people nowadays have learned from experience by clearing their ears while coming in to land in an aircraft.
TUNING-FORK TEST is used to test the internal ear. When a vibrating fork is placed on the centre of the forehead it is heard equally in both ears, the sound being conducted through the bones of the head. If one ear is closed, it is heard better in that ear. Accordingly, if one ear is deaf, and the sound of the fork placed on the forehead is heard better in that ear, the deafness is due to middle ear disease. While if the ear is deaf to the fork when placed on the forehead, as well as when held near the ear, the internal ear or nerve mechanism is at fault.
General symptoms: The following are some of the chief symptoms of ear disease:
DEAFNESS (see DEAFNESS).
EARACHE is most commonly due to acute inflammation in the middle ear, but may also be due to chronic inflammation, or to acute inflammation of the external ear, boils, eczema, wax, or neuralgia affecting the outer ear. Pain in this region may also be caused by carious teeth. The treatment varies with the cause, but the pain may generally be relieved to some extent by applying hot flannel or a hot-water bag to the side of the head. For subsequent treatment see later in this section.
RINGING in the ear, or TINNITUS, is sometimes a very annoying symptom. It may take various forms, but is in general accompanied by catarrh of some part of the ear. Pulsating or throbbing in the ear is sometimes due to bloodlessness, or to large doses of quinine or sodium salicylate, and passes off as the bloodlessness is treated or the drugs producing it are discontinued. Blowing, hissing, and whistling noises, like those made by an escape of steam or by a boiling kettle, are the most common and most annoying forms. Usually they are associated with middle-ear catarrh, but they are often associated with high blood-pressure, and diminish as the general disease is treated. Accompanied by deafness, ringing is not infrequently due to wax. Musical tinnitus sometimes occurs, in which the sound of bells, or of short passages of music, is repeated constantly. It is due to similar causes. A high crescendo musical note, followed by giddiness, is one of the symptoms of Menière's disease (q.v.).

DISCHARGE from the ear may arise in the external ear as the result of eczema, boils, or the irritation caused by a plug of wax or foreign body, but, in the absence of these, comes in the great majority of cases from suppuration in the middle ear through a perforation in the drum. There are two common fallacies regarding this condition. One is that a discharge from the ear is a trifling thing. In reality the presence of suppuration is accompanied usually by increasing deafness, and is attended always by the risk of an abscess in the mastoid antrum, or even within the skull. The other fallacy is that a perforation in the drum necessarily entails great deafness. As a matter of fact, unless the perforation is so large as to interfere with the tension of the drum, it causes little interference with hearing, the real cause of deafness in suppurative middle-ear disease being adhesions which bind down the ossicles and prevent their movements. Treatment depends upon whether the cause of the discharge is in the outer or the middle ear.

OTITIS EXTERNA, or infection of the outer ear, is commonest in tropical countries with a high humidity. Hence the names of 'Singapore ear' and 'Hong Kong ear' that it has been given. It is not uncommon, however, in Britain. Many factors may cause it, including scratching or poking the ears with dirty fingers or with contaminated objects. Badly fitting and infrequently cleaned hearing-aid earpieces are another cause. In some it is the result of spread of infection from the middle ear, whilst quite a number of cases are allergic in origin, the allergic factor often being some ear-drops that have been prescribed in the past. It may be due to a boil, which is discussed elsewhere in this section. It manifests itself by pain in the ear accompanied by a discharge. There is usually also a considerable degree of itching. Deafness develops if the discharge from the infection blocks the meatus.

Treatment consists of careful syringing out of the meatus with normal saline (see ISOTONIC) at a temperature of 38 °C, followed by careful packing of the external ear with some soothing lotion, such as 10 per cent ichthammol in glycerin, or 8 per cent aluminium acetate. Once the acute phase is over, the meatus may be painted with an alcoholic solution of gentian violet or crystal violet. For the pain in the initial stages hot packs or hot applications may be applied to the ear or, simpler and often just as effective, a rubber hot-water bottle. Ear-drops are seldom used nowadays. If the itching is particularly intense at night – which it tends to be – it may be advisable to cover the ear with a gauze bandage, or to wear cotton gloves, to prevent scratching, which may well make the condition worse.

OTITIS MEDIA, or infection of the middle ear, usually occurs as a result of infection spreading up the Eustachian tubes from the nose, throat or one of the sinuses. In other words, it may occur as a complication of a cold, tonsillitis, sinusitis or adenoids. It is above all a disease of children: 1·5 million cases occur every year in Britain. It is not uncommon at the beginning of the swimming season every year, due to the fact that diving and underwater swimming force infected secretions from the nose or throat up through the Eustachian tube into the middle ear. This is most likely to occur after jumping into swimming pools without holding the nose. Pain is always present and, particularly in acute cases of sudden onset, it may be intense and throbbing or sharp in character. It is accompanied by deafness and often tinnitus (q.v.), and the temperature rises. In infants, crying, for which there is no obvious cause, may be the only sign that something is wrong, though this is usually accompanied by some localizing manifestation such as shaking of the head or the infant putting his hand to the ear. Examination of the ear is difficult because it is so tender but when it is carried out it reveals redness, and sometimes bulging, of the ear drum. In the early stages there is no discharge, but in the later stages there may be a discharge from perforation of the ear drum as a result of the pressure created in the middle ear by the accumulated pus.

Treatment consists of the immediate administration of an antibiotic, and the one of choice is usually one of the penicillins: e.g. amoxycillin. While it is taking effect the pain may be eased by the use of heat in the form of a rubber hot-water bottle. If the antibiotic does not quickly bring relief, then it may be necessary to perform the minor operation of myringotomy, or incising the ear drum. This gives immediate relief in those cases in which the middle ear is full of pus; the moment the ear drum is incised, the pus pours out, and the pressure in the middle ear, which has been causing the pain, is relieved. The main complication of otitis media is mastoiditis, which is discussed later in this section. It cannot be too strongly emphasized that, if otitis media is treated immediately with ample doses of the appropriate antibiotic, the chances of any permanent damage to the ear or to hearing is reduced to a negligible degree, as is the risk of any complications such as mastoiditis.

SECRETORY OTITIS MEDIA, or GLUE EAR, is a form of otitis that has come to the fore as the commonest inflammatory condition of the middle ear in children, and one of the commonest causes of the form of deafness known as conduction deafness. (See DEAFNESS.) It is due to a persisting sticky (hence the name of 'glue ear') exudation in the middle ear. It is often associated with enlarged adenoids. If removal of these does not clear the condition, further treatment is needed. If this fails, in bad cases it may be necessary to remove the ossicles and the remains of the ear drum, and so to convert the middle ear into a simple cavity, which can be easily kept clear of infection.

OTOMYCOSIS is infection of the external ear by fungi such as Aspergillus (q.v.) or Candida (q.v.). It is a common condition in tropical and subtropical countries, but is occurring more often in Britain. It is characterized by persisting irritation in the ear and rapid reaccumulation of discharged material in spite of this being repeatedly removed. Treatment consists of cleansing of the external ear by dry mopping, and the application of an anti-fungal agent such as nystatin (q.v.). Drops of 2 per cent salicylic acid in alcohol are sometimes helpful.

WAX in the ear is the commonest cause of deafness, sometimes even of several years' standing. It is removed by syringing with warm water (37 °C) containing two teaspoonfuls of baking soda to a tumblerful of water. If the wax is very hard it should be softened by making the person lie down on his side for half an hour with the affected ear upwards, into which is poured some of this solution, or a few drops of warm olive or castor oil. At the end of half-an-hour the syringing is repeated. In some cases it may be necessary to insert the drops several nights running in order to soften the wax sufficiently. If there is a perforation of the drum, the removal of wax should only be carried out by a specialist.

FOREIGN BODIES, such as peas, gravel, beads or bits of rubber, are often pushed by children into the ear, and are extremely difficult to remove. No attempt to remove such a foreign body should be made until it is known whether it is vegetable in nature (e.g. a pea) or not. The reason for this is that syringing causes a pea to swell up or to become wedged in the ear, difficult to remove and causing exquisite pain. Non-vegetable foreign bodies such as beads, can be removed by syringing or forceps. No attempt should be made by unskilful persons with hairpins, bent wires, or the like, to remove the object, which is apt by such means to be pushed through the ear-drum.

BOILS in the skin lining the outer ear give rise to intense pain. This pain is much relieved by packing the ear lightly with a piece of gauze dipped in a 10 per cent solution of ichthammol glycerin, or in 8 per cent aluminium acetate. Relief is also gained by applying heat to the ear by means of a rubber hot-water bottle. The essential of treatment, however, is a five- day course of penicillin given intramuscularly.

ECZEMA, consisting of a cracked condition of the skin in the ear, with watery discharge and intense irritation, is common, as an acute affection in infants, and as a chronic one in gouty and rheumatic adults and as a sequel to, or accompaniment of, chronic otitis externa.

TUMOURS in the ear are mostly either outgrowths from the surrounding bone or soft polypi. The former may block the passage and interfere with hearing, but have often a narrow neck, so that they can be easily removed. Polypi usually develop as a result of the irritation set up by a chronic discharge, and shrivel up as the discharge is cured, though a large one may have to be removed in order to get to the drum.

MASTOIDITIS is a serious complication of inflammation in the ear, the incidence of which has been dramatically reduced by the introduction of the sulphonamides and penicillin.

The mastoid antrum and its connection with the middle ear have been mentioned under EAR. As a rule, inflammation in this cavity arises by direct spread of a long-standing suppuration from the middle ear, sometimes in consequence of neglect to keep the ear clean and prevent discharge from accumulating. The signs of this condition include swelling and tenderness of the skin behind the ear, redness and swelling inside the ear, pain in the side of the head, feverishness, and a discharge from the ear. Current expert opinion is divided as to the best method of treatment: whether this should be by antibiotics, or by antibiotics plus operation. On the whole, the majority opinion today probably is to reserve operation for those cases which do not respond to a full course of penicillin.

EATING DISORDERS: ANOREXIA NERVOSA, often called the slimmer's disease, is a syndrome characterized by loss of at least a quarter of normal weight, by fear of normal weight and, in women, by amenorrhea. An individual's body image may be distorted so that the sufferer cannot judge real weight and wants to diet even when already very thin.

Anorexia nervosa usually begins in adolescence, affecting about 1–2 per cent of teenagers and college students at any time. It is ten times commoner among women than men and is commonest among daughters of professional couples. Up to 10 per cent of sufferers' sisters also have the syndrome.

The symptoms result from secretive self-starvation, usually with excessive exercise, self-induced vomiting, and misuse of laxatives. An anorexic (or anorectic) person may wear layers of baggy clothes to keep warm and to hide the figure. Fine facial hair called lanugo may grow, perhaps as heat insulation. Starvation can cause serious problems such as anaemia, low blood pressure, slow heart rate, swollen ankles, and osteoporosis. Sudden death from heart arrythmias may occur, particularly if the sufferer misuses diuretic tablets to lose weight and also depletes the body's level of potassium.

There is probably no single cause of anorexia nervosa. Social pressure to be thin seems to be an important factor and has increased over the past 20–30 years, along with the incidence of the syndrome. Psychological theories include fear of adulthood and fear of losing parents' attention.

Treatment should start with the general practitioner who should first rule out other illnesses causing similar signs and symptoms. These include depression and disorders of the bowel, pituitary gland, thyroid gland, and ovaries.

If the diagnosis is clearly anorexia nervosa, the general practitioner may refer the sufferer to a psychiatrist or psychologist. Moderately ill sufferers can be treated by cognitive behaviour therapy. A simple form of this is to agree targets for daily calorie intake and for acceptable body weight. The sufferer and the therapist (the general practitioner or a member of the psychiatric team) then monitor progress towards both targets by keeping a diary of food intake and measuring weight regularly. Counselling or more intensely personal psychotherapy may help too. Severe life-threatening complications will need urgent medical treatment in hospital, including rehydration and feeding using a nasogastric tube or an intravenous drip.

About half of anorectic sufferers recover fully within four years, a quarter improve, and a quarter remain severely underweight with menstrual abnormalities. Recovery after ten years is rare and about 3 per cent die within that period, half of them by suicide.

BULIMIA NERVOSA is a syndrome characterized by binge eating, self-induced vomiting and laxative misuse, and fear of fatness. Unlike anorexia nervosa, it starts at any age from about 16 to 40 and is probably more directly linked with ordinary dieting. Bulimic sufferers say that, although they feel depressed and guilty after binges, the 'buzz' and relief after vomiting and purging are addictive. They often respond well to cognitive behaviour therapy.

Bulimia nervosa does not necessarily cause weight loss because the binges – for example of a loaf of bread, a packet of cereal, and several cans of cold baked beans at one sitting – are cancelled out by purging and by brief episodes of starvation. The full syndrome has been found in about 1 per cent of women but mild forms may be much commoner. In one survey of female college students 13 per cent admitted to having had bulimic symptoms.

Bulimia nervosa rarely leads to serious physical illness or death. But repeated vomiting can cause oesophageal burns, salivary gland infections, small tears in the stomach, and occasionally dehydration and chemical imbalances in the blood. Inducing vomiting using fingers may produce two tell-tale signs – bite marks on the knuckles and rotten, pitted teeth.

Those suffering from this condition may obtain advice from the Eating Disorders Association, Sackville Place, 44 Magdalen Street, Norwich NR3 1JE (0603-621414) and Anorexics Anonymous, 24 Westmoreland Road, London SW13 9RY (081-748 3994).

EBOLA VIRUS DISEASE is another name for VIRAL HAEMORRHAGIC FEVER (q.v.).

EBURNATION is a process of hardening and polishing which takes place at the ends of bones, giving them an ivory-like appearance. It is caused by the wearing away, in consequence of osteoarthrosis, of the smooth plates of cartilage which in health cover the ends of the bones.

ECCHYMOSIS means the discoloured patch resulting from escape of blood into the tissues just under the skin, often from bruising.

ECG (See ELECTROCARDIOGRAM.)

ECHINOCOCCUS is the immature form of a small tapeworm, *Taenia echinococcus*, found in dogs, wolves, and jackals from which human beings become infected, so that they harbour the immature parasite in the form known as hydatid cyst. (See TAENIASIS.)

ECHOCARDIOGRAPHY is the use of ultra-sonics (see ULTRASOUND) for the purpose of examining the heart. By thus recording the echo (hence the name) from the heart of ultra-sound waves it is possible to study, for example, the movements of the heart valves (see HEART), as well as the state of the interior of the heart.

ECHOLALIA is the meaningless repetition, by a person suffering from mental degeneration, of words and phrases addressed to him.

ECHOVIRUSES, of which there are more than 30 known types, occur in all parts of the world. Their full name is Enteric Cytopathogenic Human Orphan (hence the abbreviation, ECHO). They owe their cumbersome full name to the fact that they were originally found in the stools of children without disease. Practically all of them, however, have now been identified with definite diseases. They are more common in children than in adults, and have been responsible for outbreaks of meningitis, common-cold-like illnesses, gastro-intestinal infections, and infections of the respiratory tract. They are particularly dangerous when they infect premature infants, and there have been several outbreaks of such infection in neonatal units, in which premature infants and other seriously ill small babies are nursed. The virus is introduced to such units by mothers, staff and visitors who are unaware that they are carriers of the virus.

ECLAMPSIA is the name applied to convulsions arising in pregnancy. This condition is said to occur in around 50 out of every 100,000 cases of pregnancy. It occurs especially in the later months and at the time of delivery, but a certain proportion of cases occur only after delivery has taken place. The cause is not known although cerebral oedema is thought to occur. In practically all cases the kidneys are profoundly affected.

Symptoms: There are several warning symptoms, such as dizziness, headache, vomiting, and the secretion of albumin in the urine. These pre-eclamptic symptoms may be present for some days or weeks before the seizure takes place, and, if a woman is found to have these during antenatal care, preventive measures must be taken. The seizure consists of rigidity of the body, with unconsciousness, followed by twitching in the face and limbs lasting for one or two minutes and then passing into a state of deep unconsciousness with stertorous breathing. In mild cases there are a few fits at long intervals and the patient recovers consciousness between them, but in severer cases the fits succeed one another so rapidly that there is no appreciable interval. In cases which progress to a fatal termination, the pulse and temperature rise, and cerebral haemorrhage, uraemia or pneumonia may supervene, or the breathing may gradually cease. It accounts for 1 in 12 of all maternal deaths.

Treatment: The treatment of the seizures is that generally applicable to convulsions of any kind, with appropriate sedatives given which may include thiopentone sodium (q.v.) given intravenously. Alternatively a combination of chlorpromazine (q.v.) and pethidine (q.v.) may be used. Magnesium sulphate given intramuscularly sometimes helps to control the fits. The baby's condition should be monitored throughout.

A common presentation of eclampsia is an epileptic fit in the home. The patient should be turned on her side and the airway cleared. The most effective drugs to control eclampsia are intravenous diazepam given slowly or chlormethiazole intravenously, slowly. When the patient is in hospital she should be kept quiet as any stimulus, be it auditory, visual or tactile, may provoke a further epileptiform convulsion. The hypertension should be controlled and urgent Caesarean section undertaken.

ECSTASY is a term applied to a morbid mental condition in which the mind is entirely absorbed in the contemplation of one dominant idea or object, and loses for the time its normal self-control. This condition usually presents itself as a kind of temporary religious insanity, and has frequently appeared as an epidemic.

ECT (See ELECTROCONVULSIVE THERAPY.)

ECTHYMA is the term applied to a pustular eruption accompanied by surrounding inflammation. The pustules burst and discharge, leaving pigmented scars.

ECTO- is a prefix meaning on the outside.

ECTOPIC means out of the usual place. For example, in congenital displacement of the heart outside the thoracic cavity it is said to be ectopic, while an 'ectopic gestation' means a pregnancy outside of the womb.

ECTOPIC BEAT: A heart muscle contraction that is outside the normal sequence of the cardiac cycle. The impulse is generated outside the usual focus of the sinoatrial node (q.v.). Also known as extrasystoles, ectopic beats are called ventricular if they arise from a focus in the ventricles (q.v.) and supraventricular if they arise in the atria (q.v.). They may cause no symptoms and the affected subject may be unaware of them. The beat may, however, be the result of heart disease or may be caused by nicotine or caffeine. If persistent, the individual may suffer from irregular rhythm or ventricular

fibrillation and need treatment with anti-arrhythmic drugs.

ECTROMELIA means the absence of a limb or limbs, from congenital causes.

ECTROPION (see EYE, DISEASE AND INJURIES).

ECZEMA is a term that trips much too lightly off the tongue of doctors and patients alike. So much so that it is sometimes difficult to know what exactly a dermatologist (a skin specialist) means by the term. The confusion is not alleviated when terms such as eczematous dermatitis are used. For ease of description a relatively simplified form of classification will be used here.

Eczema is a reaction of the skin to a wide range of stimulants or irritants, some known, many unknown. In some cases, if not all, there is apparently some constitutional factor that renders the skin vulnerable, so that it responds in this abnormal manner to stimuli which have no effect upon the skin of normal individuals. The two classical criteria of the eruption in eczema are that it itches and that it causes vesication, or blistering, of the skin. Its first manifestation is erythema, or reddening of the skin. This is due to dilatation of the blood-vessels in the skin. The next stage is the formation of vesicles (q.v.) or papules (q.v.); these gradually break down and there is then oozing from the affected area of skin. If the condition persists, the skin tends to become thickened and to start scaling off.

NUMMULAR ECZEMA, or DISCOID ECZEMA as it is sometimes known, consists of coin-shaped areas of eczema, usually on the limbs, which, like all forms of eczema, tend to itch intensely. It is not uncommon in girls when they first start doing manual work, occurring on the back of the hands and fingers, the probability being that the eczema is due to trauma to the skin at work. It also occurs in middle-aged men, usually on the shins, being often aggravated by too frequent hot baths. The outlook for cure is poor, but lotions or pastes containing coal tar are often helpful.

INFECTIVE ECZEMA is a form of eczema that appears on a burn or cut. It comes on suddenly and spreads rapidly. In some cases it is due to sensitivity to the antiseptic that has been applied to the burn or cut. In some instances the eruption may be so severe that admission to hospital may be necessary. Treatment consists of the local application of a corticosteroid (q.v.) combined with an antibiotic. Alternatively, the application of wet dressings of quarter-strength Dilute Hypochlorite Solution, BPC is often effective. Calamine lotion is a soothing local application.

ATOPIC ECZEMA is one of the most widespread and worrying forms of eczema. Atopy means an inherited state of hypersensitivity which may manifest itself as asthma, hay fever or eczema. Hence the name given to this form of eczema.

It is also known as INFANTILE ECZEMA as it starts in infancy at about the age of 3 or 4 months. There is a family history of asthma, hay fever or eczema in about 70 per cent of these infants, and it has been estimated that 3 per cent of all infants suffer from moderate eczema, and that many more probably suffer from a mild degree of it. The condition appears first as red areas or papules on the edge of the scalp, spreading to the face, which soon erupt and start oozing or weeping. In some cases the eruption spreads all over the body and, as it is intensely itchy, the unfortunate infant or child is often worked up into a frenzy and scratches himself until he is bleeding all over. Cold, frosty weather aggravates the condition, as does exposure to heat. Fortunately, parents can console themselves that the outlook is not too gloomy. Many of the children start improving around the age of 2 years, and in one series of 500 cases, only 10 per cent had any appreciable eczema at the age of 10 years. A late appearance of the eczema tends to mean a poor outlook, as does a bad family history of atopy.

Treatment: Local treatment consists of the application of a 1 per cent hydrocortisone ointment (see HYDROCORTISONE). If crusts have formed, these are removed by the application of equal parts of lead diachylon plaster and soft paraffin, applied thickly in strips of lint, and left on for twenty-four hours. Local treatment, however, is only part of the treatment. Equally important is it that parents should not overprotect a baby or child with eczema. He or she must be allowed to lead a perfectly normal life, without any pampering or unnecessary restrictions. The vast majority of children with this form of eczema can eat a normal diet. Only occasionally does such a child prove to be allergic to some particular food. Whether or not soap should be used in washing the baby is an open question. In the more severe cases soap should probably be avoided, and the skin cleaned with Emulsifying Ointment, BP. In cold weather, if there is a tendency for the skin to become dry and crack easily, Oily Cream, BP, may be gently rubbed into the skin at bedtime. If a soap is used for washing, then one of the less alkaline soaps should be used. Adding a processed oatmeal, such as Aveeno Oilated (half a cup per bath of tepid water), to the bath water may help to relieve the itching.

People with eczema and their relatives can obtain advice from the National Eczema Society, 4 Tavistock Place, London WC1H 9RA (071-388 4097).

EDENTULOUS: Lacking teeth: this may be because teeth have not developed or because they have been removed or fallen out.

EDTA: Ethylenediamine tetraacetic acid is used to treat poisoning with metals such as lead and strontium. A chelating agent EDTA is used in the form of sodium or calcium salts. The stable chelate compounds resulting from the treatment are excreted in the urine.

EEG: (See ELECTRO-ENCEPHALOGRAPHY.)

EFFERENT is the term applied to vessels which convey away blood or a secretion from a part, or to nerves which carry nerve impulses outwards from the nerve-centres.

EFFLEURAGE is a form of massage by gentle stroking movements.

EFFORT SYNDROME, also known as Da Costa's syndrome, is a condition in which symptoms occur, such as palpitations and shortness of breath, which are attributed by the patient to disorder of the heart. There is no evidence, however, of heart disease, and psychological factors are thought to be of importance. (See PSYCHOSOMATIC DISEASES.)

EFFUSION means a pouring out of fluid from the vessels in which it is naturally enclosed into the substance of the organs, or into cavities of the body, as a result of inflammation or of injury: for example, pleurisy with effusion, effusions into joints, and effusion of blood.

EGG is a term applied to any animal ovum.

EISENMENGER REACTION: A condition in which the subject suffers from a defect in one of the dividing walls (septum) of the heart and this is accompanied by pulmonary hypertension (q.v.). The defect allows blood low in oxygen to flow from the right to the left side of the heart and be pumped into the aorta, which normally carries oxygenated blood to the body. The patient suffers from cyanosis and has a dusky blue appearance. There is an increase in red blood cells as the body attempts to compensate for the lowered oxygen delivery. The condition requires early surgical repair of the septal defect.

EJACULATION: The expulsion of semen from the penis during orgasm. The stimulation of sexual intercourse or masturbation produces a spinal reflex action that causes ejaculation. The semen comprises several constituents arising from Cowper's gland, the prostate gland, the testicles, and the seminal vesicles and these are discharged in sequence. (See also PREMATURE EJACULATION.)

ELBOW is the joint formed between the humerus above and the radius and ulna below. The humerus has at its lower end a rounded surface, against which the head of the radius moves, and a deep groove to which a saddle-shaped surface at the upper end of the ulna fits. The head of the radius rests upon a projection of the ulna and is bound to it by a stout annular ligament, within which it can rotate. Two important movements take place at this joint: a flail-like backward and forward movement of the radius and ulna moving together upon the humerus, and a rotary movement of the radius on the ulna, by which the lower end of the radius is crossed over the ulna and again brought side by side with it, according as the hand is turned palm downwards and palm upwards. The joint is secured at the sides by strong lateral ligaments, and at the back and front is covered by powerful muscles. The ulnar nerve as it passes down to the forearm has an exposed position behind the inner edge of the humerus at its lower end; this is popularly known as the 'funny- bone'. The elbow is seldom dislocated, but a not uncommon accident consists in the chipping off, through a fall on the elbow, of the olecranon process which forms the point behind the joint.

MINER'S ELBOW, or BEAT ELBOW, is the term applied to an inflammatory condition of the bursa over the point of the elbow, caused by resting the weight of the body on the elbow in hewing coal. The condition corresponds to housemaid's knee in the lower limb, and occurs not only in miners but sometimes in school children and other people who lean upon or bruise the point of the elbow. (See BURSITIS.)

TENNIS ELBOW is a term applied to a pain over the elbow due to mild inflammation in the tendons of the muscles that extend, or straighten, the elbow, caused by strains and jars in playing tennis and similar games. It is not uncommon in the left elbow of right-handed golfers who catch the head of their club in the ground when making a duff shot. Also known as enthesitis, the condition generally clears up spontaneously if games such as tennis, badminton and squash, or clothes wringing, are avoided, though this may be a somewhat slow process, taking up to a year or longer. A quicker result may be obtained by an injection of hydrocortisone (q.v.) into the affected area. The local application of ultrasonics (q.v.) may also be helpful.

PULLED ELBOW is the name applied to a painful condition of the elbow in young children, constituting a slight dislocation of the head of the radius from beneath the ligament which should bind it to the ulna, caused by a jerk of the arm. It is most likely to occur in 1- and 2-year-olds. The condition, which is usually accompanied by loss of power of the arm, may be induced in a variety of ways; by being pulled up when sitting on the floor, when being swung between their parents when walking, when being held firmly by the arm, when in an obstreperous, recalcitrant mood. The pain may occur in the wrist or shoulder. It responds well to manipulation.

ELECTRICAL INJURIES are usually caused by the passage through the body of an electric current of high voltage owing to accidental contact with a live wire or to a discharge of lightning. The general effects produced are included under the term electric shock, but vary greatly in degree. The local effects include spasmodic contraction of muscles, fracture of bones, and in severe cases more or less wide-spread destruction of tissues which may amount simply to burns of the skin or may include necrosis of masses of muscle and internal organs. Fright due to unexpectedness of the shock and pain due to the sudden cramp of muscles are the commonest symptoms and in most cases pass off in a few minutes or less. In more severe cases, especially when the person has remained in contact with a live wire for some time or has been unable to let go of the electrical contact owing to spasmodic contraction of his muscles, the effects are more pronounced and may be those of concussion of the brain or of compression of the brain. (See BRAIN, DISEASES OF.) In still severer cases, death may ensue either from paralysis of the respiration or stoppage of the heart's action. In either instance, the condition may be at first one of suspended animation, and death may not ensue if prompt measures are taken for treatment.

In Britain there are an average of 110 deaths a year from electrocution, half of these occurring in the home.)

Treatment: No electrical apparatus or switch should be touched by anyone who is in metallic contact with the ground, such as through a metal pipe, especially, for example, from a bath. The first necessity in regard to a person through whose body a powerful electric current is passing is to break the current. This can sometimes be done by turning off a switch. If the victim is grasping or in contact with a live wire, the contact may be severed with safety only by someone wearing rubber gloves or rubber boots, but as these are not likely to be immediately available, his hands may be protected by a thick wrapping of dry cloth, or the live wire may be hooked or pushed out of the way with a long wooden stick. If the injured person is unconscious, and especially if breathing has stopped, *artificial respiration should be applied and continued even for hours*, as described in APPENDIX: BASIC FIRST AID, Electrocution. When the patient begins to breathe again, he must be treated for shock: i.e. put to bed and given hot-water bottles and hot drinks. Electrical burns are treated on the same lines as ordinary burns. If the patient shows undue excitement and restlessness, sedatives may be necessary. The local destructive effects of a powerful current, including burns, fractures, and sloughing of large masses of tissue, are treated later by ordinary surgical means, but strong and irritating antiseptics should be avoided. Bleeding from damaged blood-vessels is liable to occur a few days after a severe injury, and is treated by the ordinary means for arrest of haemorrhage.

ELECTROCARDIOGRAM is a record of the variations in electric potential which occur in the heart as it contracts and relaxes. Any muscle in use produces an electric current, but when an individual is at rest the main muscular current in the body is that produced by the heart. This can be recorded by connecting the outside of the body by electrodes with an instrument known as an electrocardiograph. The patient is connected to the electrocardiograph by leads from either the arms and legs or different points on the chest. The normal electrocardiogram of each heart-beat shows one wave corresponding to the activity of the atria and four waves corresponding to the phases of each ventricular beat. Various readily recognizable changes are seen in cases in which the heart is acting in an abnormal manner, or in which one or other side of the heart is hypertrophied. This record therefore forms a useful aid in many cases of heart disease. The main applications of the electrocardiogram are in the diagnosis of myocardial infarction and of cardiac arrhyrthmias.

ELECTROCAUTERY (see CAUSTICS and CAUTERIES).

ELECTROCOCHLEOGRAPHY is a method of recording the activity of the cochlea, the part of the inner ear concerned with hearing. (See EAR.)

ELECTROCONVULSIVE THERAPY: ECT is a controversial treatment for severe depression. Electrical shocks are administered by electrodes placed on the skull to induce seizures of the brain. The patient is given a general anaesthetic and muscle relaxants. Up to 12 treatments may be given over a month and improvement usually shows after the third treatment. Amnesia is often a side-effect of ECT. Widely used at one time, the treatment is now given only to carefully selected patients.

ELECTRO-ENCEPHALOGRAPHY: In the brain there is a regular, rhythmical change of electric potential, due to the rhythmic discharge of energy by nerve cells. These changes can be recorded graphically and the 'brain waves' examined. These records – electro-encephalograms – are useful in diagnosis. For example, the abnormal electro-encephalogram occurring in epilepsy is characteristic of this disease. The normal waves, known as alpha waves, occur with a frequency of 10 per second. Abnormal waves, with a frequency of 7 or less per second, are known as delta waves and occur in the region of cerebral tumours and in the brains of epileptics.

ELECTROLYTES: Substances, for example, potassium chloride, whose molecules split into their constituent electrically charged particles, known as ions, when dissolved in fluid. In medicine the term is customarily used to describe the ion itself. The description 'serum electrolyte concentration' means the amounts of separate ions – for example, sodium and chloride in the case of salt – present in the serum of the circulating blood. Various diseases alter the amounts of electrolytes in the blood, either because more than normal are lost through vomiting or diarrhoea, or electrolytes may be retained because the kidney is not excreting them properly. Measurements of electrolytes are valuable clues to the type of disease and provide a means of monitoring a course of treatment. Electrolyte imbalances can be corrected by administering appropriate substances orally or intravenously or by dialysis (q.v.).

ELECTROMYOGRAPHY: The recording of electrical activity in a muscle using electrodes placed in the fibres. The procedure is used to diagnose muscle and nerve disorders and to assess recovery in certain types of paralysis.

ELECTRON is one of the subatomic particles. (See RADIOTHERAPY.)

ELECTRO-OCULOGRAPHY is a method of recording movements of the eyes, which is proving of value in assessing the function of the retina (see EYE.)

ELECTROPHORESIS means the migration of charged particles between electrodes. A simple method of electrophoresis, known as paper electrophoresis, has been introduced which is proving of value in examining the proteins in body fluids. This method consists in applying the protein-containing solution as a spot or a streak to a strip of filter paper which has been soaked in buffer solution and across the ends of which a potential difference is then applied for some hours.

ELECTRORETINOGRAM: An electroretinogram is the record of an electrical response of visual receptors in the retina (see EYE), which can be measured with corneal electrodes.

ELEPHANTIASIS (synonyms, ELEPHANTIASIS ARABUM, BARBADOS LEG, BOUCNEMIA) is a term applied to a disease which is characterized by gross overgrowth of the skin and subjacent textures. This condition arises from repeated attacks of inflammation of the skin and subcutaneous tissue, and concurrent obstruction of the lymphatic vessels. The common cause in the tropics is infection with certain parasitic worms (filariae) which invade the lymphatic vessels. (See FILARIASIS.) These worms are conveyed to man by mosquitoes. They may attack any portion of the body, but most commonly the leg, which becomes so enlarged and disfigured by the great thickening of its textures as to resemble the leg of an elephant, whence the name of the disease is derived. The thickening is due to excessive increase in the connective tissue, which results from the inflammatory process, and which by pressure on the muscles of the limb causes them to undergo atrophy or degeneration. Hence the limb becomes weak. When affecting the scrotum it often produces a tumour of enormous dimensions. The health ultimately suffers, and serious constitutional disturbance is apt to arise. In elephantiasis of the leg much relief is obtained from the use of elastic bandaging, massage, rest, and elevation of the limb. Prevention must be carried out by destruction of mosquitoes. Promising results are being reported from the use of diethyl-carbamazine in the early stages of the disease.

ELIXIR is a liquid preparation of a potent or nauseous drug made pleasant to the taste by the addition of aromatic substances and sugar. The name was specially applied to several preparations greatly used in the Middle Ages, which had the effect of acting as a tonic to the stomach and relieving constipation, and which were known, for example, as the elixir of Paracelsus, the elixir of long life. The main constituent of all of these was tincture of aloes.

EMACIATION means pronounced wasting, and is a common symptom of many diseases, particularly of those which are associated with a prolonged or repeated rise of temperature, such as tuberculosis. It is also associated with diseases of the alimentary system in which digestion is inefficient, or in which the food is not fully absorbed: for example, in diarrhoea of long-standing, whatever its cause. It is also a marked feature of malignant disease.

EMBALMING (see DEAD, DISPOSAL OF THE).

EMBOLECTOMY: Surgical removal of a clot or embolus to clear an obstruction in an artery. The obstruction may be cleared by inserting a balloon (Fogarty) catheter into the blood vessel or by surgical incision through the arterial wall. Embolectomy may be a life-saving operation when a patient has a pulmonary embolism (q.v.).

EMBOLISM means the plugging of a small blood-vessel by material which has been carried through the larger vessels by the blood stream. It is due usually to fragments of a clot which has formed in some vessel, or to small portions carried off from the edge of a heart-valve when this organ is diseased; but the plug may also be a small mass of bacteria, or a fragment of a tumour, or even a mass of air bubbles sucked into the veins during operations on the neck. The result is usually more or less destruction of the organ or part of an organ supplied by the obstructed vessel. This is particularly the case in the brain, where softening of the brain, with aphasia or apoplexy, may be the result. If the plug is a fragment of malignant tumour, a new growth develops at the spot; and if it is a mass of bacteria, an abscess forms there. Air-embolism occasionally causes sudden death in the case of wounds in the neck, the air bubbles completely stopping the flow of blood. Fat-embolism is a condition which has been known to cause death, masses of fat, in consequence of such an injury as a fractured bone, finding their

way into the circulation and stopping the blood in its passage through the lungs.

EMBROCATIONS are mixtures, usually of an oily nature, intended for external application in cases of rheumatism, sprains, and other painful conditions. Their action is due partly to the massage employed in rubbing in the embrocations, partly to the counter-irritant action of the drugs which they contain. (See LINIMENTS.)

EMBRYO means the fetus in the womb prior to the end of the second month. (See FETUS.)

EMBRYO TRANSFER is the process whereby the initial stages of procreation are produced outside the human body and completed in the uterus or womb. The procedure is also known as EMBRYO TRANSPLANTATION and IN VITRO FER-TILIZATION. It consists of extracting an ovum (or egg) from the prospective mother's body and placing this in a dish where it is mixed with the male partner's semen and special nutrient flu-ids. After the ovum is fertilized by the sperm it is transferred to another dish containing a special nutrient solution. Here it is left for several days while the normal early stages of development (see FETUS) take place. The early embryo (q.v.) as it has then become, is then implanted in the mother's uterus, where it 'takes root' and develops as a normal fetus.

The first 'test-tube baby', to use the popular, and widely used, term for such a child was born by Caesarean section in England on 25 July 1978. Many other children, conceived in this manner, have since been born, and, though only 10 per cent of women conceive at the first attempt, the overall success rate is improving. Embryo transplantation and research are controlled by legislation.

EMESIS means vomiting (q.v.).

EMETICS are drugs or other means which produce vomiting.
Varieties: Emetics are divided into two impor-tant classes: (1) direct emetics, which, being taken by the mouth, irritate the stomach and so cause vomiting, and (2) indirect emetics, which will cause vomiting, even when injected into the blood, by action upon the centre in the brain controlling the act of vomiting. Examples of the first type are sulphate of zinc, mustard in water, alum, sal volatile, copper sulphate, and even copious draughts of warm salt water. In the second class we have apomorphine, ipecacuanha, and tartar emetic; to this class also belong such means as tickling the throat, or presenting evil-smelling substances to the nose.
Uses: Emetics are now rarely used and are contraindicated for several types of poison. They must only be given if the victim is conscious, one drink of salty water, containing sodium chloride (common salt), or a dose of

Ipecacuanha Syrup USP: 15 millilitres followed by 200 millilitres (a tumblerful) of water, should be given. Medical advice should be sought before using emetics for the treatment of poisoning. Emetics in doses too small to produce vomiting are often used in cough mixtures to render the secretions in the bronchial tubes more fluid and therefore more easy to cough up. Wine of ipecacuanha is used for this purpose.

EMETINE is one of the active principles of ipecacuanha. (See IPECACUANHA; DYSENTERY.)

EMICTORY is a drug which provokes the excretion of urine.

EMMETROPIA is a term applied to the normal condition of the eye as regards refraction of light rays. In this state when the muscles in the eyeball are completely relaxed the focusing power is accurately adjusted for parallel rays, so that vision is perfect for distant objects.

EMOLLIENTS are substances which have a softening and soothing effect upon the skin. They include dusting powders such as French chalk, oils such as olive oil and almond oil, and fats such as the various pharmacopoeial preparations of paraffin, suet, and lard. Glycerin is also an excellent emollient.
Uses: They are used in various inflammatory conditions such as eczema, when the skin becomes hard, cracked, and painful. They may be used in the form of a dusting powder, an oil or an ointment.

EMPHYSEMA means an abnormal presence of air in certain parts of the body. In its restricted sense, however, it is generally employed to designate an affection of the lungs, of which there are two forms. In one of these there is over-distension of the air-cells of these organs, and in parts destruction of their walls, giving rise to the formation of large sacs, from the rupture and running together of a number of contiguous air-vesicles. This is much the more common of the two forms and is the one which is usually meant when the term 'emphysema' is used. In the other form the air is infiltrated into the connective tissue beneath the pleura and between the pulmonary air-cells, constituting what is known as *acute interstitial emphysema*.
Causes: Where a portion of the lung has become wasted, or its vesicular structure permanently obliterated by disease, without corresponding falling-in of the chest wall, the neighbouring air-vesicles, or some of them, undergo dilatation to fill the vacuum.
In cases of bronchitis, and especially of bronchial asthma, where numbers of the smaller bronchial tubes become obstructed, the air in the pulmonary vesicles remains imprisoned, the force of expiration being insufficient to expel it; on the other hand, the stronger force of inspi-

ration being adequate to overcome the resistance, the air-cells tend to become more and more distended, and permanent alterations in their structure, including emphysema, are the result.
Emphysema also arises from exertion involving expiratory efforts, during which the glottis is constricted, as in paroxysms of coughing, in straining, and in lifting heavy weights. Whooping-cough is well known as an exciting cause of emphysema.
Smoking is an important cause of emphysema. According to the United States Surgeon General's 1984 report, cigarette smoking is the major cause of chronic obstructive lung disease morbidity and 80 to 90 per cent of cases are attributable to smoking.
Symptoms: In the affected portions of the lungs there are loss of the natural elasticity of the air-cells, destruction of many of the pulmonary capillary blood-vessels, and diminution of aerating surface for the blood. As a consequence there is a strain on the heart and the venous system generally, leading to dilatation of the right side of the heart, and so to oedema. The chief symptom in this complaint is shortness of breath, more or less constant but greatly aggravated by exertion, and by attacks of bronchitis, to which people suffering from emphysema are specially liable. The respiration is of a wheezy character. In severe forms of the disease the patient comes to acquire a peculiar bluish and bloated appearance, and the configuration of the chest is altered, assuming the character known as the *barrel-shaped chest*.
Treatment: The main element in the treatment of emphysema consists in attention to the general condition of the health, and in the avoidance of all causes likely to aggravate the disease or induce its complications. Smoking is of particular importance in this context. The same general plan of treatment as that recommended in asthma and bronchitis is applicable in emphysema. During attacks of urgent breathlessness anti-spasmodic remedies should be given, while inhalation of oxygen will often afford marked and speedy relief.
ACUTE INTERSTITIAL EMPHYSEMA, arising from the rupture of air-cells may occur as a complication of the vesicular form, or separately as the result of some sudden expulsive effort, such as a fit of coughing, or, as has occasionally happened, in parturition. Occasionally the air infiltrates the cellular tissue of the mediastinum, and thence comes to distend the integument of the neck and even the whole surface of the body. This air, however, is rapidly absorbed, and the condition soon subsides.
SURGICAL EMPHYSEMA is the term applied when air is present under the skin. It may get there, for example, if the lungs are wounded through the chest wall, or if the wind-pipe is pierced at any point in its path.

EMPIRICAL treatment is that school of treatment which is founded simply on experience. Because a given remedy has been successful in the treatment of a certain group of symptoms, it is assumed, by those who uphold this principle, that it will be successful in the treatment of other cases presenting similar groups of symptoms, without any inquiry as to the cause of the symptoms or reason underlying the action of the remedy. It is the contrary of 'rational' or 'scientific' treatment. Sometimes a course of treatment must perforce be empirical for want of knowledge.

EMPROSTHOTONOS is the term applied to the spasm of the belly muscles that occurs in tetanus, making the body arch forwards.

EMPYEMA is an accumulation of pus within a cavity, the term being generally reserved for collections of pus within one of the pleural cavities. Since the advent of antibiotics, the condition is relatively uncommon in developed countries. The condition is virtually an abscess, and therefore gives rise to the general symptoms accompanying that condition; but, on account of the thick unyielding wall of the chest, it is unlikely to burst through the surface, and therefore it is of particular importance that the condition should be recognized early, and, as a rule, treated surgically.

The condition most commonly follows an attack of pneumonia. It may also occur in the advanced stage of pulmonary tuberculosis. Empyema also occurs at times through infection from some serious disease in neighbouring organs, such as cancer of the gullet, or follows upon wounds penetrating the chest wall.

EMULSIONS are mixtures containing oily substances in a state of very fine division. The division is effected and the oil kept suspended in the fluid by means of alkalis and sticky ingredients such as albumin, glycerin, or mucilage. Milk is an example of a perfect emulsion of fat globules each surrounded by an envelope of albumin. The various preparations of cod-liver oil are usually emulsified by the aid of glycerin. The oil is not only rendered more devoid of taste, but digestion and absorption are also rendered easier by emulsification.

ENALAPRIL: A drug introduced in 1986 and used to treat hypertension (see ESSENTIAL HYPERTENSION). It reduces the action of angiotensin (q.v.) and this reduces blood vessel constriction.

ENAMEL (see TEETH).

ENCEPHALITIS means inflammation of the brain. It is usually a virus infection, and may occur as a complication of the common infectious diseases, including measles (in which it occurs in around 1 in 1000 cases). ENCEPHALITIS LETHARGICA, also known as SLEEPY SICKNESS and as EPIDEMIC ENCEPHALITIS, and VON ECONOMO'S DISEASE, is a disease that appears from time to time, especially in the spring, in the form of epidemics. There has not been an epidemic in Britain since the late 1920's. It is probably a virus infection, and attacks chiefly the basal ganglia, the cerebrum, and the brain stem. These undergo swelling, haemorrhages, and ultimately destruction of areas of tissue involving both nerve-cells and fibres. The process may involve other parts of the brain, the spinal cord, and even other organs.

Symptoms: The illness begins usually with a rise of temperature and increasing drowsiness or lethargy, which may gradually proceed to a state of complete unconsciousness. In some cases, however, the patient instead of being drowsy passes at first through a stage of restlessness which may amount to maniacal excitement. As a rule the drowsiness deepens gradually over a period of a week or more, and accompanying it there appear various forms of paralysis, shown by drooping of the eyelids, squint, and weakness of one or both sides of the face. The nerves controlling the muscles of the throat are also sometimes paralysed, causing changes in the voice and difficulty in swallowing. In some cases the disease affects the spinal cord, producing severe pain in one or more of the limbs, and it is often followed by partial paralysis. Signs of inflammation are not infrequently found in other organs, and haemorrhages may be visible beneath the skin and may occur in the muscles, or blood may be vomited up or passed in the stools. The effects last usually for many months, the patient remaining easily tired and somnolent or frequently showing rigidity of muscle, mask-like facies, festinant gait (see FESTINATION, and rhythmical coarse tremors, resembling the clinical picture of Parkinsonism (q.v.).

Treatment: There is no specific treatment for the disease unless the virus responsible is the herpes virus when acyclovir is of benefit. During the acute stage the patient must be kept at rest in bed. After the acute stage is over, physiotherapy in the form of massage, passive movements and exercises should be given to control the muscular rigidity.

JAPANESE ENCEPHALITIS is a disease that occurs on the whole of the eastern seaboard of Asia. It is caused by a virus transmitted by a ricefield-breeding mosquito which also causes encephalitis in horses and abortions in pigs. The duration of the disease is variable and convalescence tends to be prolonged. The death-rate, too, is variable and may be as high as 30 per cent in children, in whom it may also cause permanent damage to the nervous system. There is no known drug treatment or any effective vaccine, though in some areas vaccinating pigs against the disease has proved helpful. Treatment therefore consists simply of efficient nursing and maintaining the patient's strength until he or she has overcome the infection.

TICK-BORNE ENCEPHALITIS is a virus infection which occurs in two forms conveyed by different ticks. The Far Eastern form, occurring particularly in Siberia, is transmitted by *Ixodes persulcatus*, causes a severe paralytic form of disease, and carries a mortality rate of over 30 per cent. The virus responsible for the European form is transmitted by *Ixodes ricinus* as a rule, but occasionally through drinking the unboiled milk of infected goats. It has an incubation period of 4 to 14 days, usually runs a relatively mild course, and has a mortality rate of 1 to 2 per cent. It has a seasonal incidence: May–June, and September–October. It occurs over the greater part of Continental Europe, but especially in Austria, Czechoslovakia and Yugoslavia, where it seems to be on the increase. In Yugoslavia around 1500 cases are reported annually though only 10 per cent of these are virologically confirmed. Being a virus infection, there is no known drug therapy, but promising results are being obtained from a vaccine now under trial.

ENCEPHALOID is the name applied to a form of cancer which, to the naked eye, resembles the tissue of the brain.

ENCEPHALOMYELITIS means inflammation of the substance of both brain and spinal cord.

ENCEPHALOPATHY is the term used to describe certain conditions in which there are signs of cerebral irritation without any localized lesion to account for them. The two best examples are *hypertensive encephalopathy* and *lead encephalopathy*. In the former, which occurs in the later stages of chronic glomerulonephritis, or uraemia (q.v.), the headache, convulsions, and delirium which constitute the main symptoms are supposed to be due to a deficient blood-supply to the brain. In the latter the symptoms are probably due to spasm of the arteries in the brain.

ENCHONDROMA means a tumour formed of cartilage. (See TUMOUR.)

ENCYSTED means enclosed within a bladder-like wall. The term is applied to parasites, collections of pus, etc., which are shut off from surrounding tissues by a membrane or by adhesions.

ENDARTERITIS means inflammation of the inner coat of an artery. (See ARTERIES, DISEASES OF.)

ENDEMIC is a term applied to diseases which exist in particular localities or among certain races. Some diseases, which are at times epidemic over wide districts, have a restricted area where they are always endemic, and from which they spread. For example, both cholera and plague are endemic in certain parts of Asia.

ENDO- is a prefix meaning situated inside.

ENDOCARDITIS Inflammation of the lining, valves and muscle of the heart. The main causes are bacterial and virus infections and rheumatic fever and the condition occurs most often in patients whose endocardium is already damaged by congenital deformities or whose immune system has been suppressed by drugs. Infection may be introduced into the bloodstream during dental treatment or surgical procedures, especially on the heart or on the gastrointestinal system. Treatment is with large doses of antibiotic drugs.

ENDOCRINE GLANDS are organs whose function is to secrete into the blood or lymph substances known as hormones which play an important part in general chemical changes or the activities of other organs at a distance. Some organs have a double function, such as the pancreas, which pours digestive secretions by a duct into the intestine, and, at the same time, has an endocrine or internal secretion (insulin) which is secreted direct into the blood. Various diseases arise as the result of defects or excess in the internal secretions of the different glands. The chief endocrine glands are the thyroid, adrenal, pituitary, parathyroid, pancreas, ovaries, and testicles.

THYROID GLAND: This gland, situated in front of the neck, produces a secretion which has an important effect in regulating the general metabolism of the body. When it is defective, the conditions known as myxoedema and cretinism result; whilst excess of the secretion is associated with thyrotoxicosis. The active principle of this secretion is thyroxine and this is used in patients in whom the secretion is defective.

ADRENAL GLANDS: These two glands, also known as SUPRARENAL GLANDS, lie immediately above the kidneys. The central or medullary portion of the glands forms the secretions known as adrenaline or epinephrine, and noradrenaline. Adrenaline acts upon structures innervated by sympathetic nerves; its action is therefore said to be sympathomimetic. Briefly, the blood-vessels of the skin and of the abdominal viscera (except the intestines) are constricted, and at the same time the arteries of the muscles and the coronary arteries are dilated; systolic blood-pressure rises; blood-sugar increases; the metabolic rate rises; muscle fatigue is diminished. Adrenaline can be synthetically prepared in the laboratory. This substance is widely used in medicine in 1 in 1000 solutions, for the purpose of checking bleeding, relieving congestion of mucous membranes, for the relief of asthma, and in the treatment of anaphylactic shock. The superficial or cortical part of the glands produce a series of chemical substances which have as their basis a complicated steroid nucleus. The best known of these are aldosterone, cortisone, hydrocortisone, and deoxycortone acetate. These substances are essential for the maintenance of life. It is the absence of these substances, due to atrophy or destruction of the suprarenal cortex, that is responsible for the condition known as Addison's disease (q.v.).

PITUITARY GLAND: This gland is attached to the base of the brain and rests in a hollow on the base of the skull immediately above the hinder part of the throat. The pituitary gland is the most important of all endocrine glands and has been called the conductor of the endocrine orchestra. It consists of two embryologically and functionally distinct lobes. The function of the anterior lobe depends on the secretion by the hypothalamus (q.v.) of certain 'neuro-hormones' which are carried down the infundibular stalk in the hypophyseal portal system. These neuro-hormones are secreted into the portal venous system flowing from the median eminence of the hypothalamus to the anterior lobe of the pituitary gland and control the secretion of the pituitary trophic hormones. The hypothalamic centres involved in the control of specific pituitary hormones appear to be anatomically separate. Through the pituitary trophic hormones the activity of the thyroid, adrenal cortex and the sex glands is controlled. A reciprocal relationship between the anterior pituitary and the target glands exists. The liberation of trophic hormones is inhibited by a rising concentration of the circulating hormone of the target gland and stimulated by a fall in its concentration. Six trophic hormones are formed by the anterior pituitary. Growth hormone and prolactin are simple proteins formed in the acidophil cells. Follicle-stimulating hormone, luteinizing hormone and thyroid-stimulating hormone are glycoproteins formed in the basophil cells. Adrenocorticotrophic hormone (ACTH), although a polypeptide, is derived from basophil cells. The chromophobe cell, once thought to be inactive, is in fact the stem cell and 50 per cent of chromophobe adenomas secrete prolactin.

All these pituitary hormones are polypeptides. When used therapeutically they cannot be given by mouth, as they would be digested in the gastro-intestinal tract. They are therefore prepared in powder form for intramuscular injection. The powder should be dissolved carefully, and after injection the site should be massaged to ensure efficient absorption.

The posterior pituitary lobe, or neuro-hypophysis, is closely connected with the hypothalamus by the hypothalmic-hypophyseal tracts. It is concerned with the production or storage of oxytocin and vasopressin (the anti-diuretic hormone).

PITUITARY HORMONES: Rapid advances have taken place in the past decade in the methods of assay of pituitary hormones and in the production and preparation of these hormones for clinical use. Growth hormone, gonadotrophic hormone, adrenocorticotrophic hormone and thyrotrophic hormones can be assayed in blood or urine by radio-immuno-assay techniques. Growth hormone extracted from human pituitary glands obtained at autopsy was available for clinical use until 1985 when it was withdrawn as it is believed to carry the virus responsible for Creutzfeldt-Jakob disease. However growth hormone produced by DNA recombinant techniques is now available as Somatonorm.

Human pituitary gonadotrophins are readily obtained from post-menopausal urine. Commercial extracts from this source are available and are effective for treatment of infertility due to gonadotrophin insufficiency.

The adrenocorticotrophic hormone is extracted from animal pituitary glands and has been available therapeutically for many years. It is used as a test of adrenal function, and, under certain circumstances, in conditions for which cortico-steroid therapy is indicated. The pharmacologically active polypeptide of ACTH has now been synthesized. It is called tetracosactrin, and as it is a pure substance it is prescribed by weight. Thyrotrophic hormone is also available but it has no therapeutic application. Melanocyte-stimulating hormone (MSH) does not occur in the human pituitary.

HYPOTHALAMIC RELEASING HORMONES which affect the release of each of the six anterior pituitary hormones have been identified. Their blood levels are only one- thousandth of those of the pituitary trophic hormones. The release of thyrotrophin, adrenocorticotrophin, growth hormone, follicle-stimulating hormone and luteinizing hormone is stimulated whilst release of prolactin is inhibited. The structure of the releasing hormones for TSH, FSH-LH, GH and, most recently, ACTH is known and they have all been synthesized. Thyrotrophin-releasing hormone (TRH) is already in clinical use as a diagnostic test of thyroid function but it has no therapeutic application. FSH-LH-releasing hormone provides a useful diagnostic test of gonadotrophine reserve in patients with pituitary disease and is now used in the treatment of infertility and amenorrhoea in patients with functional hypothalamic disturbance. As this is the commonest variety of secondary amenorrhoea the potential use is great. The therapeutic use of GH-releasing hormone and corticotrophin releasing hormone has yet to be established. Most cases of congenital deficiency of GH, FSH, LH and ACTH are due to defects in the hypothalamic production of releasing hormone and are not a primary pituitary defect, so that the therapeutic implication of this recently synthesized group of releasing hormones is considerable.

Galactorrhoea (q.v.) is frequently due to a microadenoma of the pituitary and less frequently results from impairment of the tonic inhibition exerted on the pituitary by the hypothalamus. Dopamine is the prolactin-release inhibiting hormone. Its duration of action is short so its therapeutic value is limited. However, bromocriptine is a dopamine agonist with a more prolonged action and is effective treatment for galactorrhoea whether this is due to a prolactin-secreting adenoma or to impairment of the tonic inhibition exerted by the prolactin-release inhibiting hormone.

PARATHYROID GLANDS: These are four minute glands lying at the side of, or behind, the thyroid. They have a certain effect in controlling the absorption of lime salts by the bones and other tissues. When their secretion is defective, tetany occurs.

PANCREAS: This gland is situated in the upper part of the abdomen and, in addition to the digestive ferments which it produces, a substance known as insulin is absorbed from it into the circulating blood. This has the effect of adapting sugary foods for incorporation in the muscles and other tissues that particularly require such foodstuffs. Lack of it is followed by the production of the disease known as diabetes mellitus.

OVARIES AND TESTICLES: In addition to their main function of producing reproductive cells, these organs secrete substances which have a general effect upon the other bodily tissues.

The ovary secretes at least two hormones, known, respectively, as oestradiol (follicular hormone) and progesterone (corpus luteum hormone). Oestradiol develops (under the stimulus of the anterior pituitary lobe) each time an ovum in the ovary becomes mature, causes extensive proliferation of the endometrium lining the uterus, a stage ending with shedding of the ovum about 14 days before the onset of menstruation. The corpus luteum, which then forms, secretes both progesterone and oestradiol. Progesterone brings about great activity of the glands in the endometrium. The uterus is now ready for the nesting of the ovum if it is fertilized. If fertilization does not occur, the corpus luteum degenerates, the hormones cease acting, and menstruation takes place.

The hormone secreted by the testicles is known as testosterone. It is responsible for the growth of the male secondary sex characteristics.

ENDOCRINOLOGY: The study of the endocrine system, the substances (hormones) it secretes and its disorders (see ENDOCRINE GLANDS.)

ENDOGENOUS: Coming from within the body. Endogenous depression, for instance, occurs as a result of causes inside a person.

ENDOMETRIOSIS is the condition in which the endometrium (i.e. the cells lining the interior of the uterus) is found in other parts of the body. The most common site of such misplaced endometrium is the muscle of the uterus. The next most common site is the ovary, followed by the peritoneum (q.v.) lining the pelvis (q.v.), but it also occurs anywhere in the bowel. The cause is not known. It never occurs before puberty and seldom after the menopause. The main symptoms it produces are menorrhagia (q.v.), dyspareunia (q.v.), painful menstruation and pelvic pain. Treatment is usually by removal of the affected area, but in some cases satisfactory results are obtained from the administration of progestogens (q.v.) such as norethisterone (q.v.), norethynodrel (q.v.) and danazol (q.v.).

ENDOMETRITIS means inflammation of the mucous membrane lining the womb. (See UTERUS, DISEASES OF.)

ENDOMETRIUM is the mucous membrane which lines the interior of the uterus.

END ORGAN: A structure at the end of a peripheral nerve that acts as receptor for a sensation. For example, the olfactory nerves have end organs that pick up smells.

ENDORPHINS are peptides (q.v.) produced in the brain which have a pain-relieving action. Hence their alternative name of opiate peptides. Their name is derived from *endo*genous mor*phine*. They have been defined as endogenous opiates or any naturally occurring substances in the brain with pharmacological actions resembling opiate alkaloids such as morphine. There is some evidence that the pain-relieving action of acupuncture (q.v.) may be due to the release of these opiate peptides. It has also been suggested that they may have an anti-psychotic action and therefore of value in the treatment of major psychotic illnesses such as schizophrenia.

ENDOSCOPE: A tube-shaped instrument inserted into a cavity in the body to investigate and treat disorders. It is flexible and equipped with lenses and a light source. Examples of endoscopes are the cystoscope for use in the bladder, the gastroscope for examining the stomach and the arthroscope for looking into joints. (See FIBREOPTIC ENDOSCOPY.)

ENDOTHELIUM is the membrane lining various vessels and cavities of the body, such as the pleura, pericardium, peritoneum, lymphatic vessels, blood-vessels, and joints. It consists of a fibrous layer covered with thin flat cells, which render the surface perfectly smooth and secrete the fluid for its lubrication.

ENDOTOXIN: A poison produced by certain bacteria that is released after the micro-organisms die. Endotoxins can cause fever and shock, the latter by rendering the walls of blood vessels permeable so that fluid leaks into the tissues, with a consequent sharp fall in blood pressure.

ENDOTRACHEAL INTUBATION: Insertion of a rubber or plastic tube through the nose or mouth into the trachea. The tube often has a cuff at its lower end which, when inflated, provides an airtight seal. This allows an anaesthetist to supply oxygen or anaesthetic gases to the lungs and know exactly how much the patient is receiving. Endotracheal intubation is necessary to undertake artificial ventilation of a patient.

ENEMA means an injection of fluid into the bowel.

Uses: PURGATIVE ENEMAS are given generally in large bulk, so as to distend the rectum; they also contain various stimulating substances. For an adult, 450 to 900 ml (1 to 2 pints) are injected, for a young child about 170 ml (6 ounces). The process of injection should be slow, and the person should retain the enema as long as he can, in order to obtain the maximum effect. The water should be tepid: about 38 °C (100 °F). The usual constituent is soft green soap BP, 14 g (½ ounce) in 450 ml (1 pint) of water. Yellow soap is also satisfactory. In some cases an olive-oil enema is preferred, or a glycerin enema of equal parts of glycerin and water). To expel flatulence, two tablespoonfuls of turpentine may be added to each pint of warm water. The frequent use of enemas is unhealthy, as they ultimately increase the constipation.

DISPOSABLE ENEMAS are largely supplanting the traditional soap-and-water enemas – largely on account of their convenience. The ingredients, usually sodium diphosphate and sodium phosphate in the case of a purgative enema, are contained in around 100 ml of solution in a small plastic bag with tube and plug.

MINIATURE ENEMAS are in increasing use. Their great advantage is that they are of a much smaller volume – only 2 millilitres, and therefore much more comfortable for the patient. They are also prepared much more easily and are supplied ready made up in a plastic container with a soft nozzle. They may be self-administered. As a rule, a movement of the bowels occurs within fifteen minutes. A widely used formula for such a miniature enema is: 5 mg of bisacodyl; 0·5 millilitre of glycerin; made up to 2 millilitres with Sulphated Castor Oil BPC.

Mode of administration: Nutrient enemas are administered by means of a rubber tube 90 to 120 cm (3 or 4 feet) in length, with a funnel at one end, and soft rubber nozzle, with rounded end, at the other. For purgative enemas, the rubber syringe with a ball in the centre may be used, and for small enemas a rubber bag which contains the exact amount required. In all cases the old bone or metal nozzle should be replaced by a soft rubber one, because much pain and injury may be inflicted by a rigid one carelessly or forcibly introduced.

The patient lies upon his left side with the hips raised on a thick pillow, and should remain so after the enema has been given. The nozzle is oiled, introduced forwards and upwards with a screwing motion, and should be passed gently up for 75 or 100 mm (3 or 4 inches). The fluid is now pumped, or, if a tube and funnel is used, allowed to flow gently in by raising the funnel.

ENGAGEMENT: The event during pregnancy when the presenting part of the baby, usually the head, moves down into the mother's pelvis.

ENKEPHALINS are peptides that have a pain-killing effect similar to that of endorphins (q.v.). Produced by certain nerve endings and in the brain, enkephalins (also spelt encephalins) are also believed to act as a sedative and mood changer.

ENOPHTHALMOS is a term applied to abnormal retraction of the eye into its socket: for example, when the sympathetic nerve in the neck is paralysed.

ENSURE (see ENTERAL FEEDING).

ENTAMOEBA (see AMOEBA).

ENTERAL FEEDING: In severely ill patients the metabolic responses to tissue damage may be sufficient to cause a reduction of muscle mass and of plasma proteins. This state of catabolism may also impair the immune response to infection and delay the healing of wounds. It is probable that as many as one half of patients who have had a major operation a week previously show evidence of protein malnutrition. This can be detected clinically by a loss of weight and a reduction in the skinfold thickness and arm circumference. Biochemically the serum albumin falls as does the lymphocyte count. The protein reserves of the body fall even more dramatically when there are sepsis, burns, acute pancreatitis or renal failure.

The purpose of enteral feeding is to give a liquid, low residue food through a naso-gastric feeding tube. It has the advantage over parenteral nutrition that the septic complications of insertion of catheters into veins are avoided. It is also much cheaper. Enteral feeding may either take the form of intermittent feeding through a large-bore naso-gastric tube or continuous gravity feeding through a fine-bore tube.

A number of proprietary enteral foods are available and these avoid the necessity of nursing or dietetic staff making up the preparations. Some of these proprietary feeds contain whole protein as the nitrogen source. Others, and these are called elemental diets, contain free amino acids. Clinifeed, Ensure, Isocal and Triosorbon all contain whole protein whilst Flexical contains 70 per cent amino acids and 30 per cent oligopeptides; Vivonex contains amino acids only. Diarrhoea is the most common problem with enteral feeding and it tends to occur when enteral feeding is introduced too rapidly or with too strong a preparation.

ENTERALGIA is another name for colic.

ENTERIC-COATED: A description of tablets covered in material that allows them to pass through the stomach and enter the intestine unaltered. Drugs coated in this way are those whose action is reduced or stopped by acid in the stomach.

ENTERIC FEVERS are typhoid fever and paratyphoid fever.

Until the middle of the last century typhoid was not distinguished from typhus fever. Subsequently all doubt upon the subject was removed by the careful clinical and pathological observations made by Sir William Jenner at the London Fever Hospital (1849–51). At the end of the nineteenth century it was noticed that cases of fever resembling typhoid but of shorter duration occurred, and these were found to be due to bacilli resembling the typhoid bacillus and are known as paratyphoid fevers. This group of fevers, again, has a resemblance, both as regards symptoms and as regards the causal bacteria, to cases of food-poisoning and dysentery.

Causes: A bacillus, discovered first by Eberth in 1880, and known as *Salmonella typhi*, is the cause of typhoid fever. (See BACTERIOLOGY.) The bacilli responsible for cases of paratyphoid fever are known as *Salmonella paratyphi A* and *Salmonella paratyphi B*, the latter being the commoner. Other bacilli which do not altogether correspond to either of these are also responsible for mild attacks of fever, sometimes grouped as paratyphoid C.

TYPHOID FEVER: Where the discharges, sheets, etc., from typhoid patients are carefully disinfected, there is little risk of direct spread from person to person. In many hospitals patients with typhoid are therefore treated in the general wards, with little or no risk to the other patients, provided certain precautions are taken.

All insanitary conditions in respect of drainage of houses and localities furnish the most ready means for the spread of the contagion of typhoid fever. The most certain means of preventing its appearance or checking its spread are: the water- carriage system of sewage disposal; prevention of pollution of water-supplies, food, milk, and shell-fish with human excreta; chlorination of drinking water; pasteurization of milk; control of the house-fly; personal cleanliness; detection of carriers of enteric bacilli. The bacillus resides in the stools and urine of typhoid patients. Thus, in badly laid drains, where the contents stagnate, the bacillus may increase indefinitely, and, by the contamination of drinking-water in places where wells or cisterns are exposed to sewage pollution, convey infection to a whole community. Dust may also act as the medium which conveys the bacilli in cases in which the discharges of a typhoid patient or the sewage are allowed to dry, and so get blown into drinking-water or on to food. Milk may readily be contaminated by the bacillus and form the cause of an epidemic, when a case of the fever has occurred in a dairy. The source of an epidemic has also been traced to the eating of oysters taken from oyster- beds near which contaminated sewage is discharged. During an epidemic flies may also form a means of contamination between uncovered stools and uncovered food. It may therefore be said that the spread of typhoid fever depends upon food or drink contaminated by a bacillus which is derived more or less directly from the discharges of previous typhoid cases.

The incubation period is usually ten to fourteen days, but may be as short as five days or as long as twenty-one days.

The chief symptoms will be better understood by a brief reference to the principal changes that take place in the body during the disease. The bowels are chiefly affected, particularly the lower end of the small intestine, where the Peyer's patches on the inner surface of the bowel (see INTESTINE) pass through changes that bear a distinct relation to the symptoms exhibited by the patient during the course of the disease. (1) During the first eight or ten days of the illness these patches, which in health are comparatively indistinct, become enlarged and prominent as the result of inflammation. (2) During the second week of the fever these enlarged patches undergo a process of sloughing, being cast off either in fragments or *en masse*. (3) From the second week onwards during the remainder of the fever, and even into the stage of convalescence, the ulcers formed by this process remain open, though slowly healing. The ulcers vary in size according to the Peyer's patches that have sloughed away, and they may be few or many in number. They are frequently, but not always, oblong in shape, with their long axis in that of the bowel, and they have somewhat thin and ragged edges. They may extend through the thickness of the bowel to the peritoneal coat, and they may perforate this, or may erode blood-vessels in their progress. (4) During convalescence the ulcers usually heal, leaving no contraction in the wall of the bowel.

The mesenteric glands associated with the intestine become enlarged, but usually subside without abscess formation as recovery takes place. The spleen becomes soft and enlarged, this enlargement being a useful guide to the physician in cases which are difficult to diagnose. As in other fevers, the muscular tissues soften and waste, and various complications affecting other organs may arise.

Symptoms: The symptoms at the *onset* of typhoid fever are much less marked than those of most other fevers, and the disease in the majority of instances sets in somewhat insidiously. Indeed, it is no uncommon thing for patients with this fever to go about for a considerable time after it has begun. The most marked of the early symptoms are headache, lassitude, and discomfort, together with sleeplessness and feverishness, particularly at night; this last symptom is that by which the disease is most readily detected in its early stages. Bleeding from the nose is also an early symptom in many cases. The course of *the temperature* is one of the important diagnostic features. During the first week it rises about 1·2 °C in the evening and falls 0·7 °C in the morning so that by the end of the first week it has reached a plateau of 38·8 to 40 °C (102 to 104 °F). Because of this feature of rising by steps, so to speak, it is known as a step-ladder temperature. During the second week the daily range of temperature is comparatively small, a slight morning remission being all that is observed. In the third week the same condition continues more or less; but frequently a slight tendency to lowering may be discerned, particularly in the morning temperature, and the fever gradually dies down as a rule between the twenty-first and twenty-eighth day, although it is liable to recur in the form of a relapse. Although during the earlier days of the fever the patient may be able to move about, he feels languid and uneasy; and usually before the first week is over he has to take to bed, and soon the effects of the attack become more apparent. He is restless, hot, and uncomfortable, particularly as the day advances, and his cheeks show a red flush, especially in the evening or after taking food. The *pulse* in an ordinary case, although more rapid than normal, is not accelerated to an extent corresponding to the height of the temperature, and, at least in the earlier stages of the fever, is rarely above 100 a minute. In severe and protracted cases, where there is evidence of extensive intestinal ulceration, the pulse becomes rapid and weak. The *tongue* has at first a thin whitish fur and is red at the tip and edges. It tends, however, to become dry, brown or glazed-looking, and fissured transversely, while sordes may be present about the lips and teeth. There is much thirst, and, in some cases, vomiting.

From an early period in the disease *abdominal symptoms* show themselves and are often of great help in diagnosis. The abdomen is somewhat distended, and pain accompanying some gurgling sounds may be elicited on light pressure about the lower part of the right side close to the groin – the region corresponding to that portion of the intestine in which the morbid changes already referred to are progressing. *Diarrhoea* is a common but by no means constant symptom. When present, it may be slight in amount, or, on the other hand, extremely profuse, and it corresponds, as a rule, to the severity of the intestinal ulceration, and to the nature of the diet which the patient has been taking. The discharges are highly characteristic, being of light-yellow colour, resembling 'pea soup' in appearance. Sometimes, especially in milder cases, constipation is found instead of diarrhoea. Should intestinal haemorrhage occur, the stools may be dark brown, or composed entirely of blood. Enlargement of the spleen and liver can usually be made out by the physician. The urine is scanty and high-coloured. When the fever is well developed from the second week onwards, the *blood* shows a well-marked feature known as the Widal reaction. (See AGGLUTINATION.)

About the beginning, or during the course, of the second week of the fever, an *eruption* often makes its appearance on the skin. It consists of small isolated spots, oval or round in shape, of a pale pink or rose colour, which are seen chiefly upon the abdomen, chest, and back, and they come out in crops, which continue for four or five days and then fade away. At first they are slightly elevated, and disappear on pressure. In some cases they are very few in number,

and their presence is made out with difficulty; but in others they are numerous and sometimes show themselves upon the limbs as well as upon the body. They do not appear to have any relation to the severity of the attack, and in a large proportion of cases (particularly in children) they are entirely absent. Besides this eruption there are often numerous very faint bluish patches or blotches about half an inch in diameter, chiefly upon the body and thighs. When present, the rose-spots, as they are known, continue to come out in crops till nearly the end of the fever, and they may reappear should a relapse subsequently occur.

These various symptoms persist throughout the third week, usually, however, increasing in intensity. The patient becomes prostrated and emaciated; the tongue is dry and brown, the pulse quickened and feeble, and the abdominal symptoms more marked; while nervous disturbance is exhibited in delirium, in tremors and jerkings of the muscles (*subsultus tendinum*), in drowsiness, and occasionally in 'coma vigil'. (See TYPHUS FEVER.) In severe cases the exhaustion reaches an extreme degree, but even in such instances the condition should not be regarded as hopeless. In favourable cases a change for the better may be expected between the twenty-first and twenty-eighth days, although it takes place by a lysis or gradual subsidence of the symptoms (the morning and evening temperatures descending, the pulse becoming stronger, the diarrhoea passing off, the tongue becoming clean, etc.), not by a crisis as in typhus fever or pneumonia. Convalescence proceeds slowly, and relapses are apt to occur (due often to errors in diet). Such relapses may prolong the fever for two or three months, though this is not common.

Abscesses sometimes arise, especially in connection with inflammation in the periosteum of the bones, found after the patient has been convalescent for some time, and these form a troublesome and prolonged complication. Stiff back, known as 'typhoid spine', is an occasional sequel to this disease, due either to inflammation in the spine or more commonly to changes in the muscles with development of fibrous tissue, causing the patient for long, it may be for years, to suffer from severe 'rheumatic' pains. Inflammation of the bile passages, with retention of the bacilli in these and their constant discharge in the stools, is also an occasional sequel; and, although this may cause no trouble to the patient, it renders him a source of danger to others as a 'carrier' of the disease. (See INFECTION.)

When death takes place, it is generally due to one of the following causes: (1) exhaustion in the second or third week or later; (2) haemorrhage from the bowels; (3) perforation of an ulcer and the onset of peritonitis; (4) excessive rise of temperature; (5) complications, such as inflammation of the lungs.

Treatment: The preventive treatment includes all the municipal and domestic measures that aim at securing pure supplies of water and milk and well-laid drains. Inoculation with anti-typhoid vaccine is a precaution which ought to be adopted by people travelling to Africa, Asia, South America, or any country around, or any island in, the Mediterranean, or in the Balkans. It should be repeated every three years. (See VACCINE.)

When an outbreak of typhoid fever occurs in a family, the source of the milk supply especially should be scrutinized. The discharges of a typhoid patient should be mixed so soon as passed with a strong disinfectant. (See DISINFECTION.) Similar care should be taken to sterilize all sheets, towels, etc., soiled by the patient. Special care is necessary on the part of those in attendance on a typhoid-fever patient to cleanse the hands at once after touching the patient, and especially after they have become in any way soiled by contact with his discharges.

The use of chloramphenicol has transformed a fever that lasted three to four weeks into a sharp febrile illness of three to four days. This means that diet is not so important as it was, but milk, or milk dishes, are still the great standby.

Penicillin (q.v.) is also proving of value, but the relative value of these two antibiotics has not been determined. Whichever is used, however, it is still necessary to keep the patient in bed for three weeks, and to keep him on a bland nutritious diet during this period. Otherwise complications may arise. The patient should be considered infective until six consecutive specimens of stools and urine are found to be negative on bacteriological examination.

In the convalescent stage, and even after apparently complete recovery, the utmost care should be observed by the patient as to diet, all hard and indigestible substances being dangerous from their tendency to irritate or reopen unhealed ulcers and bring on a relapse of the fever or cause a sudden perforation. Lastly, the general health demands careful attention for a length of time.

PARATYPHOID FEVER is a continued fever which closely resembles mild attacks of typhoid and which, like typhoid fever, is due to one or more members of the genus *Salmonella*.

Causes: Paratyphoid fever is due to infection with one of three micro-organisms: *Salmonella paratyphi A, B,* or *C*. These organisms closely resemble that of typhoid fever in appearance and some of its reactions. The infection is usually conveyed by a 'carrier' case who has already had the disease, or it is due to contaminated food or water.

Symptoms resemble those found in a mild case of typhoid fever. The incubation period is shorter (one to ten days), and rose spots are seen less commonly. The onset of the disease is often more sudden than in typhoid fever, but the fever tends to be less prolonged and less severe.

Treatment is the same as for typhoid fever.

ENTERITIS means inflammation of the intestines. (See DIARRHOEA; INTESTINE, DISEASES OF.)

ENTEROBIASIS is infection with *Enterobius vermicularis*, the threadworm, or pinworm as it is known in the USA. It is the most common of all the intestinal parasites in Britain and the least harmful. The male is about 6 mm (¼ inch) in length and the female about 12 mm (½ inch) in length. Each resembles a little piece of thread. These worms live in considerable numbers in the lower bowel, affecting children particularly. They cause great irritation round the anus, especially in the evening when the female worm emerges from the anus to lay its eggs and then dies. Apart from this irritation around the anus, they seldom cause any symptoms. The most effective form of treatment is either viprynium embonate or piperazine citrate.

ENTEROCELE means a hernia of the bowel. (See HERNIA.)

ENTEROGASTRONE is a hormone derived from the mucosal lining of the small intestine which inhibits the movements and secretion of the stomach.

ENTEROKINASE is the enzyme (q.v.) secreted in the duodenum (q.v.) and jejunum (see INTESTINE) which converts the enzyme, trypsinogen, secreted by the pancreas (q.v.) into trypsin (q.v.). (See also DIGESTION.)

ENTEROPTOSIS means a condition in which, owing to a lax condition of the mesenteries and ligaments which support the bowels, the latter descend into the lower part of the abdominal cavity.

ENTEROSTOMY means an operation by which an artificial opening is formed into the intestine.

ENTEROVIRUSES are a family of viruses which include the poliomyelitis, coxsackie and echo groups of viruses. Their importance lies in their tendency to invade the central nervous system. They receive their name from the fact that their mode of entry into the body is through the gut.

ENTOMOPHOBIA is excessive fear of insects, particularly spiders, mites and other anthropods.

ENTONOX: A proprietary analgesic drug taken by inhalation and comprising half nitrous oxide and half oxygen. It is valuable in providing relief to casualties who are in pain as it provides analgesia without making them unconscious. Entonox is also used in obstetric practice.

ENTROPION (see EYE, DISEASE AND INJURIES).

ENURESIS means the unconscious or involuntary passage of urine. (See NOCTURNAL ENURESIS.)

ENZYME is the name applied to a chemical ferment produced by living cells. The first enzyme was obtained in a reasonably pure state in 1926 and shown to be a protein. Since then several hundred enzymes have been obtained in pure crystalline form. Many more have been purified to less exacting standards and all have been proved to be proteins. They are present in the digestive fluids and in many of the tissues, and are capable of producing in small amount the transformation on a large scale of various compounds. Indeed, they are an integral, essential component of what might be described as the *modus operandi* of the body. Examples of enzymes are found in the ptyalin of saliva and diastase of pancreatic juice which split up starch into sugar, the pepsin of the gastric juice and the trypsin of pancreatic juice which break proteins into simpler molecules and eventually into the constituent amino-acids, the thrombin of the blood which causes coagulation.

EOSINOPHIL is any cell in the body with granules in its substance that stain easily with the dye eosin. About 2 per cent of the white cells of the blood are eosinophils.

EOSINOPHILIA means an abnormal increase in the number of eosinophils in the blood. It occurs in Hodgkin's disease, in asthma and hay fever, in some skin diseases, and in parasitic infestation.

EPHEDRINE is an alkaloid derived from a species of *Ephedra* or prepared synthetically, much used for asthma and other allergic disorders, in doses of 15 to 60 mg. It is similar to adrenaline in pharmacological action.

EPHELIS is a freckle (q.v.). *Ephelis ab igne* is the dark-brown pigmentation produced on the legs by constant exposure of them to a fire. A similar discoloration of the skin of the abdomen may be produced by constant use of a hot-water bottle.

EPI- is a prefix meaning situated on or outside of.

EPICANTHIC FOLD: A vertical skinfold that runs from the upper eyelid to the side of the nose. These folds are normal in oriental races but uncommon in others, although babies may have a temporary fold that disappears. Folds are present in people with Down's Syndrome.

EPIDEMIC is a term applied to a disease which affects a large number of people in a particular locality at one time. The term is, in a sense, opposed to endemic, which means a disease always found in the locality in question. A disease may, however, be endemic as a rule – for example, malaria in swampy districts, and may become at times epidemic, when an unusually large number of people are affected.

As a rule an epidemic disease is infectious from person to person, but this is not necessarily the case, since many persons in a locality may simply be exposed to the same cause at one time; for example, outbreaks of lead-poisoning are epidemic in this sense.

The laws which govern the outbreak of epidemics are by no means fully understood. Infected food supplies, such as drinking water contaminated by the evacuations of persons sick of cholera or typhoid fever, or milk tainted by the organism of scarlet fever have been traced as the cause of outbreaks of these diseases. The migrations of certain animals, such as rats, are in some cases responsible for the spread of plague, from which these animals die in great numbers. Certain epidemics come with regularity at certain seasons. Thus scarlet fever and diphtheria are autumnal complaints, and produce their epidemics in September, October and November. Whooping-cough, on the other hand, is a spring complaint, and very few cases occur in autumn. Measles produces two epidemics, as a rule, one in winter and one in March. Influenza, the common cold, and other infections of the upper respiratory tract, such as sore throat, occur predominantly in the winter.

There is another variation, both as regards the number of persons affected and the number who die in successive epidemics: the severity of successive epidemics rising and falling over periods of five or ten years.

EPIDEMIC ENCEPHALITIS is another term for ENCEPHALITIS LETHARGICA (see ENCEPHALITIS).

EPIDEMIOLOGY: The study of disease as it affects groups of people. Originating in the study of epidemics of diseases like cholera, plague and smallpox, epidemiology is an important discipline which contributes to the control not only of infectious diseases but also of conditions such as heart disease and cancer. Their distributions in populations can provide important pointers to possible causes. The relation between the environment and disease is an essential part of epidemiology.

EPIDERMIS: The outer layer of the skin, which forms the protective covering of the body. Comprising four layers, the epidermis constantly renews itself, with the bottom or germinative layer producing new cells and the top layer, stratum corneum, made up of dead cells which are regularly worn off. The cells of the two intermediate layers are gradually impregnated with keratin, a horny substance which gives the epidermis its toughness.

EPIDURAL ANAESTHESIA (see ANAESTHESIA).

EPIDYDIMIS is an oblong body attached to the upper part of each testicle, composed of convoluted vessels and ducts. It is liable to be the seat of tuberculous and other inflammation. (See TESTICLE.)

EPIGASTRIUM is the region lying in the middle of the abdomen over the stomach.

EPIGLOTTIS is a leaf-like piece of elastic cartilage covered with mucous membrane, which stands upright between the back of the tongue and the glottis, or entrance to the larynx. In the act of swallowing, it prevents fluids and solids from passing off the back of the tongue into the larynx.

EPIGLOTTITIS: Acute epiglottitis is an acute inflammatory oedema of the epiglottis, due to *Haemophilus influenzae*, which causes laryngeal obstruction due to swelling and immobilization of the epiglottis. It is a disease predominantly of children, occurs usually in the winter, and may prove rapidly fatal.

EPIGNATHUS is a mal-development of the fetus in which the deformed remains of one twin are united to the upper jaw of the other.

EPILATION means the removal of hair by the roots. (See DEPILATION.)

EPILEPSY, or FALLING SICKNESS, is a nervous disorder characterized by a fit of sudden loss of consciousness, attended with convulsions. There may, however, exist manifestations of epilepsy much less marked than this, yet equally characteristic of the disease. On the other hand, it is to be borne in mind that many other attacks of a convulsive nature have the term 'epileptiform' applied to them because they resemble epilepsy.

There are two well-marked varieties of the epileptic seizure. To these the terms, *le grand mal* and *le petit mal*, are generally applied. The former of these is that which attracts most attention, being what is generally known as an epileptic fit. In addition to these two forms there is a type known as *Jacksonian epilepsy*, in which the seizure consists of convulsive movements starting in a single muscle or group of muscles, consciousness being in general retained. Cases of this type shade off, however, into *grand mal*, and indeed the subjects of Jacksonian epilepsy may, at a later stage, be affected by typical seizures of severe type.

Incidence: It is estimated that in England and Wales there are around 290,000 epileptics: 190,000 adults and 100,000 children under the age of 16 years. It is also estimated that approximately 33,000 new cases occur every year. Probably one person in 20 has a fit of

some sort in the course of a lifetime, but only one in 8 of those who have a fit will suffer from chronic epilepsy: that is, have a continuing liability to fits. The onset of epilepsy occurs before the age of 5 in nearly a quarter of the cases, and before school-leaving age in more than half.

Causes: Epilepsy has many causes. It may be a manifestation of a space-occupying lesion within the cranium such as a cerebral tumour, a cerebral haemorrhage, a scar from a previous cerebral thrombosis or an inflammation such as encephalitis. It may also be a manifestation of a metabolic disturbance, such as hypoglycaemia, hypokalaemia, hypocalcaemia or hypoxia. When it is idiopathic the onset usually occurs during infancy or at puberty. The diagnosis is usually made clinically and is confirmed by an electro-encephalogram (q.v.) in which characteristic changes are seen in epilepsy.

Symptoms: Although in most instances an epileptic attack comes on suddenly, it is in some cases preceded by certain premonitory indications or warnings. These are of very varied character, and may be in the form of some temporary change in the disposition, such as unusual elevation or depression of spirits, or of some alteration in the look. Besides these general symptoms, there are often peculiar sensations which immediately precede the onset of the fit, and to such the name of *aura epileptica* is applied. The so-called aura, which occurs in over 50 per cent of cases, may be of mental character, in the form of an agonizing feeling of momentary duration; of sensory character, in the form of pain in a limb or in some internal organ, such as the stomach; or an unusual feeling connected with the special senses, such as a strange smell or extraordinary vision; or of a motor character, in the form of contractions or trembling in some of the muscles. The aura may be so distinct and of such duration as to enable the patient to lie down or seek a place of safety before the attack comes on.

The seizure is usually preceded by a loud scream or cry, which is not to be ascribed, as was at one time supposed, to terror or pain, but is due to the convulsive action of the muscles of the larynx, and the expulsion of air through the narrowed glottis. If the patient is standing he immediately falls, and often sustains serious injury. Unconsciousness is complete, and the muscles generally are in a state of stiffness or tonic contraction, which may be found to affect those on one side of the body in particular. The head is turned towards one or other shoulder, the breathing is for the moment arrested, the countenance first pale then livid, the pupils dilated, and the pulse rapid. This, the first stage of the fit, generally lasts for about half-a-minute, and is followed by the state of clonic (i.e. tumultuous) spasm of the muscles, in which the whole body is thrown into violent agitation. The eyes roll wildly, the teeth are gnashed together, and the tongue is often severely bitten. The breathing is noisy, and foam (often tinged with blood) issues from the mouth, while even the contents of the bowels and bladder may be ejected. This stage lasts for a period varying from a few seconds to several minutes, when the convulsive movements gradually subside and relaxation of the muscles takes place, together with partial return of consciousness, the patient looking confusedly about him and attempting to speak. This, however, is soon followed by drowsiness and stupor, which may continue for several hours. When he awakes either apparently quite recovered, or fatigued and depressed, he is occasionally in a state of excitement which sometimes assumes the form of mania.

Epileptic fits of this sort succeed each other with varying degrees of frequency, and occasionally though not frequently with regular periodicity. In some people they only occur once in a lifetime, or once in the course of many years, while in others they return every week or two, or even are of daily occurrence, and sometimes there are numerous attacks each day. Occasionally there occurs a constant succession of attacks extending over many hours, and with such rapidity that the patient appears as if he had never come out of the one fit. The term *status epilepticus* is applied to this condition, which sometimes has fatal results. In many epileptics the fits occur during the night as well as during the day, but in some instances they are entirely nocturnal, and in such cases the disease may long exist and yet remain unrecognized either by the patient or by the physician, until observed and described by some other person.

The other variety of epilepsy, to which the name *le petit mal* is given, differs from that just described in the absence of the convulsive spasms. It consists essentially in the sudden arrest of consciousness, which is of short duration, and may be accompanied by staggering or some alteration in position or motion, or may simply exhibit itself in a look of absence or confusion, and, should the patient happen to be engaged in conversation, by an abrupt termination of the act. In general, it lasts a few seconds, and the individual resumes his occupation without perhaps being aware of anything having been the matter. In some instances there is a degree of spasmodic action in certain muscles which may cause the patient to make some unexpected movement, such as turning half round, or walking abruptly aside, or may show itself by some unusual expression of countenance, such as squinting or grinning. There may be some amount of aura preceding such attacks, and also of faintness following them.

There is another sequel of an epileptic fit, particularly *petit mal*, which may have medicolegal implications. This is what is known as *post-epileptic automatism*. In this state, following an attack, an epileptic may carry out or perform some action of which he is entirely unaware when he recovers. Thus, he may proceed to undress himself no matter where he may be, or he may pick up the first thing he lays his hands on, or he may attack someone. An interesting feature of this phenomenon is that the action performed by any one epileptic is stereotype: that is, it is always the same odd action he performs. The possible medico-legal implications of this automatism are obvious.

Treatment: During the fit, little can be done beyond preventing the patient as far as possible from injuring himself while unconsciousness continues. Tight clothing should be loosened, and a cork or pad inserted between the teeth if possible, to prevent biting of the tongue. This, however, should never be done forcibly; otherwise teeth may be broken, and, as has been said, 'broken teeth are worse than a bitten tongue'. Unprotected fingers should never be put in the patient's mouth. When the fit is over, the patient should be allowed to sleep, and have the head and shoulders well raised.

Of medicinal remedies, the most commonly used is phenytoin, which is tending to replace phenobarbitone, either alone or in combination with one of the increasing number of other drugs being introduced for the treatment of epilepsy. The bromides, originally the great stand-by in the treatment of epilepsy, are seldom used for this purpose at the present day. Other drugs that have proved of value include methoin and primidone. In severe cases which do not respond satisfactorily to one or more of these drugs, there is a further choice of drugs including carbamazepine, clonazepam, and sodium valproate. One of the most effective drugs for controlling *petit mal* is troxidone. The secret of success in controlling epilepsy is to remember that every case must be considered individually, and that once a successful means of control has been established, it should not be altered unless there is some special reason for so doing. Alcohol is strictly forbidden. A worrying feature, however, now attracting attention, is the increased rate of congenital malformations in children born to treated epileptic mothers. This is estimated to be about three times the normal rate.

As few restrictions as possible should be placed on the activities of an epileptic. This particularly applies to children. Unless the fits are severe and frequent, the child should be allowed to lead as normal a life as possible. Car driving licences can now be issued in suitable cases to people with epilepsy who, on the basis of medical evidence, have been free from attacks for at least two years, with or without treatment, or who for more than three years have had a history of attacks only during sleep. Heavy goods vehicle driving licences can now be issued to people who have been free from any epileptic attack since reaching the age of five.

Epileptic colonies have been established, where people seriously afflicted in this way can carry out productive work under safe conditions. These colonies are particularly useful for the 20 per cent or so of epileptics who are mentally retarded.

Patients with epilepsy and their relatives can obtain further advice and information from the British Epilepsy Association, Anstey House, 40

Hanover Square, Leeds LS3 1BE (0532–439393); or The Epilepsy Association of Scotland, 48 Govan Road, Glasgow G51 1JL (041-427 4911, fax: 041-427 7414).

EPILOIA (see TUBEROSE SCLEROSIS).

EPIPHORA (see EYE, DISEASE AND INJURIES OF).

EPIPHYSIS means the spongy extremity of a bone, attached to it for the purpose of forming a joint with the similar process of another bone. An epiphysis is covered on its surface by cartilage, is developed from a distinct centre of ossification, and in a young person is connected with the shaft of the bone by a plate of cartilage that disappears in the adult. Separation of an epiphysis is a form of fracture which sometimes occurs in children, and is apt to be more serious than a break through bony tissue because it involves damage to the plate of growing cartilage, so that, although union takes place readily, the subsequent growth of the bone may be interfered with and the full growth of the limb may afterwards fail to be attained.

EPIPHYSITIS means inflammation of an epiphysis.

EPISIOTOMY is the operation of cutting the outlet of the vagina in childbirth so as to facilitate the birth of the child.

EPISTAXIS means bleeding from the nose. (See HAEMORRHAGE.)

EPITHELIOMA is a tumour of malignant nature arising in the epithelium covering the surface of the body. (See CANCER.)

EPITHELIUM is the cellular layer which forms the epidermis on the skin, covers the inner surface of the bowels, and forms the lining of ducts and hollow organs, like the bladder. It consists of one or more layers of cells which adhere to one another, and is one of the simplest tissues of the body. It is of several forms: for example, the epidermis is formed of scaly epithelium, the cells being in several layers and more or less flattened. (See SKIN.) The bowels are lined by a single layer of columnar epithelium, the cells being long and narrow in shape. The air passages are lined by ciliated epithelium: that is to say, each cell is provided with lashes which drive the fluid upon the surface of the passages gradually upwards.

EPIZOÖTIC is a term applied to any disease in animals which diffuses itself widely. The term corresponds to the word epidemic as applied to human beings. In plague, for example, an epizöotic in rats usually precedes the epidemic in human beings.

Diagram of ciliated epithelium (1) and pseudostratified columnar ciliated epithelium (2).

1 squamous epithelium seen in section
2 squamous epithelium seen in face view
3 cuboidal and columnar epithelium in face view
4 stratified, squamous, non-keratinized epithelium
5 stratified, squamous, keratinized epithelium
6 transitional epithelium
7 columnar epithelium
8 cuboid epithelium

Diagram of various types of epithelium.

EPSOM SALTS is the popular name for magnesium sulphate, which is perhaps the most commonly used saline purgative.

EPSTEIN BARR VIRUS: The virus that causes GLANDULAR FEVER or infectious mononucleosis. It is similar to the viruses that cuase herpes and is associated with Burkitt's Lymphoma (q.v.).

EPULIS is a term applied to any tumour connected with the jaws. (See MOUTH, DISEASES OF.)

EQUINE OESTROGENS (see OESTROGEN).

ERB'S PARALYSIS is a form of paralysis of the arm due to stretching or tearing of the fibres of the brachial nerve plexus. Such damage to the brachial plexus may occur during birth, and it is found that the arm lies by the side of the body with elbow extended, forearm pronated, and the fingers flexed. The infant is unable to raise the arm.

ERECTION: The rigid state of the penis when it responds to sexual stimulus. An erection is necessary for satisfactory intercourse to occur. As a result of sexual arousal the three cylinders of erectile tissue in the penis become engorged with blood, lengthening, raising and hardening the penis. Muscles surrounding the blood vessels contract and retain the blood in the penis. Erections also occur during sleep and in young boys. Inability to have or maintain an erection is one cause of impotence.

ERETHISM is the psychic disturbance that is one of the manifestations of chronic mercury poisoning (see MERCURY). It is characterized by irritability, self-consciousness, shyness, timidity, embarrassment, lack of concentration, depression and resentment of criticism. It was this condition that gave rise to the phrase, 'mad as a hatter', as chronic mercurial poisoning used to be one of the occupational hazards of the hat-making industry.

ERGOMETRINE is one of the active constituents of ergot (q.v.). It has a powerful action in controlling the excessive bleeding from the womb which may occur after childbirth. The official *British Pharmacopoeia* preparation is Ergometrine Maleate.

ERGOSTEROL is a sterol found in yeasts and fungi and in plant and animal fat. Under the action of sunlight or ultra-violet rays it produces vitamin D_2. The substance produced in this way is known as calciferol, and is used for the prevention and cure of rickets and osteomalacia. A similar change in the ergosterol of the skin is produced when the body is freely exposed to sunlight. Calciferol is probably not so active as, and differs chemically from, the vitamin D occurring in fish-liver oils.

ERGOT is the spawn of *Claviceps purpurea*, a fungus which grows in the grain of rye. It contains several active principles, including the alkaloids, ergometrine, ergotoxine and ergotamine. Ergot causes prolonged contraction of unstriped muscle fibres all over the body, particularly the muscle fibres of the blood-vessels and of the womb. This action on the womb makes the drug of great value in midwifery, and it has been in use in midwifery since the 16th century.
Uses: Ergot is used mainly to check haemorrhage, particularly that which is apt to follow upon childbirth. It is also given in small doses for some time after childbirth to reduce the

womb to its proper size in cases in which this is not taking place naturally.

ERGOTAMINE is one of the alkaloids in ergot. In the form of ergotamine tartrate it is most effective in the treatment of migraine (q.v.). It is usually given by mouth. Its continued use is not without risk, occasionally leading to gangrene of the tips of the fingers, so it should only be used under medical supervision. It has also been used for the relief of the itching of the skin which is sometimes such a troublesome feature of uraemia (q.v.).

ERGOT POISONING or ERGOTISM occasionally results from eating bread made from diseased rye. Several terrible epidemics (*St Anthony's Fire*), characterized by intense pain and hallucinations, occurred in France and Germany during the Middle Ages (cf ERYSIPELAS). Its symptoms are the occurrence of spasmodic muscular contractions, and the gradual production of gangrene in parts like the fingers, toes and tips of the ears.

EROSION means a process of gradual wearing down of structures in the body. The term is applied to the effect of tumours, when they cause destruction of tissue in their neighbourhood without actually growing into the latter: for example, an aneurysm may erode bones in its neighbourhood. The term is also applied to minute ulcers, for example, erosions of the stomach, caused by extreme acidity of the gastric juice.
DENTAL EROSION is the loss of tooth substance due to a cause other than decay or trauma. This is usually due to the presence of acid, e.g. frequent vomiting or the excessive intake of citrus fruits. The teeth appear very smooth and later develop saucer-shaped depressions.

ERUCTATION, or belching, is the sudden escape of gas or of portions of half-digested food from the stomach up into the mouth.

ERUPTION or RASH, means an outbreak, in a scattered form, upon the surface of the skin, usually raised and red, or it may be covered with scales, or crusts, or vesicles containing fluid. The appearance of an eruption depends, to a certain extent, upon the nature of the disease, or other source of irritation, which causes it: for example, the eruption of measles is always distinguishable from that of chickenpox. But the same disease may also produce different eruptions in different people or in the same person in different states of health, or even on different parts of the body at one time.

Eruptions may be acute or chronic. Most of the acute eruptions belong to the exanthemata (q.v.): i.e. they are bright in colour and burst out suddenly like a flower. These are the eruptions of scarlet fever, measles, German measles, smallpox and chickenpox. In general the severity of these diseases can be measured by the amount of eruption, but in cases in which the eruption is suppressed, or, as it is popularly termed, 'goes in', the disease is apt to be serious.

Some eruptions are very transitory, like nettle-rash, appearing and vanishing again in the course of a few hours.

(For chronic eruptions see SKIN DISEASES.)

ERYSIPELAS: (synonyms, *the Rose, St Anthony's Fire*) is a disease characterized by diffuse inflammation of the skin, attended with fever. In the Middle Ages this disease was confused with ergot poisoning.

Causes: It has long been known that the disease is of a highly infectious nature. The infecting organism is the *Streptococcus pyogenes*. Erysipelas is slightly commoner in women than in men, and is commonest between the ages of 50 and 60.

Symptoms: When erysipelas is of moderate character, there is simply a redness of the skin, which feels somewhat hard and thickened, and upon which there often appear small vesicles. This redness, though at first circumscribed, tends to spread and affect the neighbouring sound skin, until an entire limb or a large area of the body may become involved in the inflammatory process. There is usually considerable pain, with heat and tingling in the affected part.

Treatment: The patient must be isolated, and great care must be taken to ensure that the infection is not transmitted to others by those in attendance on the patient. The outlook has changed considerably for the better since the introduction of penicillin, which should be given in full doses as soon as the condition is recognized. For local application the best preparations are either cold compresses of a saturated solution of magnesium sulphate or a 10 per cent solution of ichthyol in water.

ERYTHEMA is a general term signifying several conditions in which areas of the skin become congested with blood, and consequently a red eruption appears. The eruption is accompanied by tingling, and often by itching and pain.

Causes: It may be due to heat, such as exposure to the sun, or the constant exposure, by cooks or iron-workers, of the face, hands or legs to a blazing fire. *Erythema ab igne* is the reddening of the skin of the leg producing a net-like pattern that is found in people who sit huddled over the fire. Another form, known as *erythema pernio*, is due to exposure to cold and wet. (See CHILBLAINS.) A variety, which appears, usually on the front of the legs, in the form of red or livid, tender swellings, often over 2·5 cm in breadth, is known as *erythema nodosum*, and is a hypersensitivity reaction to infection with the streptococcus or mycobacterium tuberculosis. It is also a manifestation of sarcoidosis and may be an allergic reaction to the sulphonamide drugs. Children and young adults, especially women, may also suffer from a severer form, which begins as red blotches on the hands, and, spreading up the arms to the body, produces lumps and vesicles, or even large blebs full of fluid. This form, on account of the diversity of the appearances in different parts, is known as *erythema multiforme*. The cause in some cases is a virus. It also occurs as a drug-rash from the use of such drugs as sulphonamides and barbiturates. *Erythema infectiosum*, or slapped cheek disease, is characterized by a fiery red rash on the cheeks: hence its alternative name. It occurs in children, in the spring. The rash, which spreads to the rest of the body, lasts for up to three weeks. Although highly infectious, the causative organism, probably a virus, has not been discovered.

ERYTHRASMA is a reddish-brown macular eruption of the skin, caused by a micro-organism known as *Nocardia minutissima*.

ERYTHROBLASTOSIS FOETALIS (see HAEMOLYTIC DISEASE OF THE NEW-BORN).

ERYTHROBLASTS: A series of nucleated cells in the bone marrow that go through various stages of development until they form erythrocytes (q.v.). They may appear in the blood in certain diseases.

ERYTHROCYTE: The red, saucerlike cell in the blood that carries oxygen to the tissues and carbon dioxide waste away from them. Erythrocytes, which have no nuclei, are formed during erythropoesis (q.v.) from erythroblast (q.v.) cells in the bone marrow (q.v.) and each mm^3 of blood contains 5 million of them. They are by far the largest constituent among the blood cells and they contain large amounts of the oxygen carrier haemoglobin. They have a life of about 120 days after which they are absorbed by macrophages (q.v.), the blood's scavenging cells. Most components of the erythrocytes including the red pigment haemoglobin (q.v.) are reused, though some of the pigment is broken down to the waste product bilirubin (q.v.).

ERYTHROCYTE SEDIMENTATION RATE (see ESR).

ERYTHRODERMA: An abnormal inflammation, thickening and flaking of the skin of the body. Also called exfoliative dermatitis, this condition occurs most commonly after the age of 50 and affects men more often than women, sometimes developing from a previously existing skin disease such as eczema or psoriasis. About two-thirds of patients recover after two or three months, a few develop chronic erythroderma and some patients die from complications.

ERYTHROEDEMA: Other terms for this condition are ACRODYNIA and PINK DISEASE. This is a disease of infants with the following features: restlessness, weakness, neuritis and swelling and redness of the face, fingers and toes. In the vast majority of cases it is a manifestation of mercurial poisoning, often due to the infant's having been given teething powders containing a mercurial laxative.

ERYTHROMELALGIA, or RED NEURALGIA, is a condition in which the fingers or toes, or even larger portions of the limbs, become purple, bloated in appearance, and very painful. In people suffering from the condition, which is not a common one, the attacks come and go, being worse in summer (unlike chilblains), and worse on exertion or when the affected parts are warmed or allowed to hang down. The condition may appear without apparent cause, but is often associated with vascular diseases, such as hypertension and polycythaemia vera. It also occurs in association with certain diseases of the central nervous system, and in cases of metallic poisoning: e.g. arsenic, mercury and thallium. Treatment is unsatisfactory. Residence in a moderate climate, the wearing of light-weight stockings or socks, and sandals, and the avoidance of excessive heat help to relieve the discomfort. Aspirin also gives marked relief.

ERYTHROMYCIN is an antibiotic derived from *Streptomyces erythreus*. Its antibacterial range of activity is comparable to that of penicillin, and it is effective when taken by mouth.

ERYTHROPOEISIS: The process by which erythrocytes or red blood cells are produced. The initiating cell is the haemopoietic stem cell from which an identifiable proerythroblast develops. This goes through several stages as a normoblast before losing its nucleus to become an erythrocyte. This process takes place in the blood-forming bone-marrow tissue.

ERYTHROPOIETIN is the protein, produced mainly in the kidney, that is the major stimulus for the production of erythrocytes, or red blood corpuscles. (See BLOOD.)

ESCHAR is a piece of the body killed by heat or caustics.

ESCHERICHIA is the generic name given to the group of gram-negative, rod-shaped bacteria found as normal inhabitants of the lower bowel: e.g. *Escherichia coli*.

ESERINE is another name for physostigmine (q.v.).

ESMARCH'S BANDAGE is a rubber bandage which is applied to a limb from below upwards in order to drive blood from it. The bandage is used when operating on a limb as it reduces bleeding.

ESR: The ESR or erythrocyte sedimentation rate is a test that measures the rate at which red blood cells settle out of suspension in blood plasma. In certain diseases, such as infection and malignancy, the amount of proteins in the plasma increases; the result is that red cells settle out more quickly and this test is used to show whether disease is present.

ESSENCES are strong solutions of an active substance. Some of these are made by solution in water, but the aromatic essences are usually solutions of volatile oils (e.g. essence of peppermint), in rectified spirit of the strength 1 in 5.

ESSENTIAL AMINO ACIDS are amino acids that are essential for the body to grow and develop normally but which the body is unable to produce. Nine essential amino acids exist – histidine, isoleucine, leucine, lysine, methionine, phenylalanine, threonine, tryptophan, and valine – and they are present in foods rich in protein: dairy products, eggs, meat, and liver.

ESSENTIAL FATTY ACIDS: Three acids – arachidonic, linolenic and tinoleic – essential for life which the body cannot produce. They are found in natural vegetable and fish oils and their functions are varied. EFAs have a vital function in fat metabolism and transfer and they are also precursors of prostaglandins (q.v.).

ESSENTIAL HYPERTENSION is the most common form of high blood- pressure. Other causes of a high blood-pressure include kidney disease, especially glomerulonephritis; certain diseases of the endocrine glands; and a congenital abnormality of the aorta known as coarctation of the aorta.
Cause: In spite of its being such a common condition, the cause of essential hypertension is still obscure. It has been recognized for a long time that arteriosclerosis and hypertension often occur together, and at one time it was considered that the arteriosclerosis was the primary lesion and that the raised blood-pressure was a compensatory effort on the part of the heart to maintain an adequate circulation of blood through the thickened and narrowed arteries. This view is now considered to be wrong, and the general consensus of opinion is that the raised blood-pressure is the cause of the arteriosclerosis in these cases, although it must be remembered that arteriosclerosis can occur without hypertension. At the present moment it is generally believed that the primary lesion in essential hypertension is spasm of the smaller arteries (or arterioles). What is still undecided

is what is responsible for this spasm. We know that such spasm can be produced by adrenaline and that adrenaline is produced by emotional, mental and physical strain. On the other hand, it has never been possible to demonstrate an excess of adrenaline in the blood of people with hypertension, nor does this theory explain why only some people exposed to strain develop hypertension. Although we still do not know why this spasm of the arterioles is produced in the first instance, there is now evidence that spasm of the arteries to the kidneys results in the production of a substance called *renin* (q.v.) which produces a rise in the blood-pressure. It is therefore possible that the course of events in essential hypertension is as follows: spasm of arterioles → renin → hypertension → arteriosclerosis of kidneys. It must be realized, however, that this is a marked simplification of a most complicated problem, but it is useful as a working basis.

The following are among some of the other factors known about essential hypertension. It is much more common among western races than among eastern races. There is a strong hereditary factor. It is more common in males than in females, and it is rare under the age of 40 years. The highest incidence is between the ages of 50 and 60 years. It is also more common among obese individuals than among those who are normal in weight or under- weight. There is no evidence that the consumption of meat has anything to do with essential hypertension.

Symptoms: Essential hypertension may be present without any symptoms whatsoever, and the condition may be discovered accidentally during a routine medical examination. The basis for a diagnosis of hypertension is usually taken to be a systolic pressure which is persistently greater than 150 mm of mercury and a diastolic pressure which is persistently greater than 95 mm of mercury. The emphasis is upon the persistence of the raised pressure, because it is not unusual for the blood- pressure in a normal individual to be raised temporarily by excitement. Even the mere recording of it may be sufficient to raise it quite considerably. From the point of view of prognosis, the height of the diastolic pressure is much more important than that of the systolic pressure.

When essential hypertension is accompanied by symptoms, these usually consist of headache, ringing in the ears (tinnitus) and giddiness. When headache is present, it is often in the back of the head and often worst on wakening in the morning, wearing off during the course of the day, and then becoming worse again towards evening.

When essential hypertension runs its natural course, it usually causes death in the end as a result of heart failure, but a proportion of its victims die of a stroke, or myocardial infarction, whilst some die of failure of the kidneys. To a certain extent it is true to say that the earlier the onset of essential hypertension, the poorer the expectation of life, but many people with this condition live to a ripe old age.

Treatment: As the cause of hypertension is not known there is no specific treatment. However over recent years a large number of drugs which are effective in lowering peripheral resistance and hence lowering blood pressure have been introduced. Most of the newer hypotensive drugs are without serious side effects and so have replaced the old ganglion-blocking drugs such as bretylium tosylate, mecamylamine and the methonium compounds. The first line drugs are probably still the benzothiadiazine diuretics and the beta adreno-receptor blocking drugs. The thiazide diuretics both reduce the circulating blood volume and hence the blood pressure and also, as a result of sodium depletion, render the arterioles less sensitive to the vaso-constrictor effects of noradrenaline. They may however cause hypokalaemia and hyperuricaemia, reduce carbohydrate tolerance and pre-dispose to hyperlipidaemia. The beta adreno-receptor-blocking drugs are also effective in lowering the blood pressure by reducing peripheral resistance. They are, however, contra-indicated in patients with asthma or obstructive airways disease. The more recently introduced calcium-channel blockers such as nifedipine are effective vaso-dilators and hence hypotensive drugs. Alpha-receptor-blocking drugs such as prazosin also have a place in the management of hypertension and hydralazine is another effective vaso-dilator independent of any alpha-receptor blockade. The angiotensin-converting enzyme inhibitors are potent hypotensive drugs that have been recently introduced. Captopril was the first of these angiotensin inhibitors and enalopril was introduced in 1985.

Since the introduction of these potent hypotensive agents the incidence of cardiac failure, renal disease and strokes complicating hypertension have been drastically reduced. Nevertheless other commonsense measures should still be pursued. The patient who is overweight must reduce weight and life style should be adjusted so that relaxation is possible at weekends. Excess salt intake should be avoided.

ESTER is an organic compound formed from an alcohol and an acid by the removal of water.

ETHACRYNIC ACID is a potent diuretic (q.v.), with a rapid onset, and a short duration (4 to 6 hours), of action. (See BENZOTHIADIAZINES, DIURETICS.)

ETHAMBUTOL is a synthetic drug which is proving of value in the treatment of tuberculosis.

ETHAMIVAN is chemically similar to nikethamide (q.v.) and has a similar action in stimulating the respiratory centre.

ETHANOL is another name for ethyl alcohol. (See ALCOHOL.)

ETHER is a colourless, volatile, highly inflammable liquid formed by the action of sulphuric acid upon alcohol, with the aid of heat. Ether boils below the body temperature, and so, when sprayed over the skin, rapidly evaporates. It dissolves many substances, such as fats, oils and resins, better than alcohol or water, and is accordingly used in the preparation of many drugs.
Uses: Externally it is used as a cleansing agent before operations. By inhalation it is used as a general anaesthetic. (See ANAESTHESIA.) Internally it is used occasionally for relieving pain such as colic.

ETHICS COMMITTEES: It is now generally agreed that research investigations on human beings should be governed by codes, such as those of the World Medical Association (Declaration of Helsinki) and of the Medical Research Council of Britain. Ethics committees developed in this country when the Royal College of Physicians, in 1967, recommended that clinical research investigations should be the subject of ethical review. The Medical Research Council requires ethical review of projects prior to making a grant and some scientific journals require it as a condition of publication. The objectives of ethics committees are to facilitate medical research in the interest of society, to protect subjects of research from possible harm, to preserve their rights and to provide reassurance to the public that this is being done. Ethics committees comprise medical, nursing and lay members. Ethics committees have now been established in most district health authorities in this country.

ETHINYLOESTRADIOL is a highly active oestrogen (q.v.), which is about twenty times as active as stilboestrol (q.v.). It is active when given by mouth. (See OESTROGEN.)

ETHISTERONE is the name approved by the *British Pharmacopoeia* for the orally active analogue of progesterone. It is given in certain cases of menorrhagia and habitual abortion, where a deficient secretion of the corpus luteum is suspected. (See PROGESTERONE.)

ETHMOID is a bone in the base of the skull which separates the cavity of the nose from the membranes of the brain. It is a spongy bone with numerous cavities or sinuses.
   Suppuration in the ethmoidal sinuses is sometimes responsible for inflammation in neighbouring parts such as the eye.

ETHOGLUCID is an alkylating agent (q.v.), which is proving of value in the treatment of cancer.

ETHOSUXIMIDE is a drug that is proving of value in the treatment of the form of epilepsy known as petit mal.

ETHYL CHLORIDE is a gas at ordinary temperatures and pressures, but is liquefied by slight compression. It is extremely volatile, and rapidly produces freezing of the surface, when sprayed upon it. Accordingly it is used to produce insensibility to pain for small and short operations. It is put up in graduated glass or metal tubes, with a fine nozzle. The tube is warmed by the hand and the liquid jets out in a fine spray which evaporates at once and so freezes the skin upon which it is sprayed. At one time it was used by inhalation to produce general anaesthesia for very brief operations, and to induce anaesthesia in patients in whom the anaesthesia is subsequently to be maintained by some other anaesthetic such as nitrous oxide or ether, but is seldom used now for this purpose.

ETHYLENE is a colourless inflammable gas used as an anaesthetic.

ETHYLOESTRENOL (see ANABOLIC STEROIDS).

ETIDRONATE is one of a group of substances known as diphosphonates which are proving of value in the treatment of Paget's disease of bone (q.v.). One of its practical advantages is that it is taken by mouth, and not by injection as is the case with calcitonin.

ETIOLOGY, or AETIOLOGY, means the group of conditions which form the cause of any disease.

EU- is a prefix meaning satisfactory or beneficial.

EUCALYPTUS, or BLUE-GUM (*Eucalyptus globulus*), is a tree, originally a native of Australia, and now grown all over the world. Its important constituent, oil of eucalyptus, is an oil of pleasant smell and spicy taste, which is obtained by distillation from the leaves of the tree. Similar oils are obtained in varying amount from most species of gum-trees, some of which have peculiar and fragrant odours. Groves of eucalyptus trees exert a marked influence upon the soil and air in their neighbourhood. The trees, which reach a great size, and have wide-spreading roots, remove much moisture from the soil, and have accordingly a powerful action in drying up swampy ground. The oil constantly exhaled from the leaves has the power of oxidizing and destroying large quantities of the foul gases which emanate from swamps, and of checking to some extent the growth of microbes. Accordingly these trees have a beneficial influence upon unhealthy districts in which they are planted.
Uses: The oil is used as a disinfectant and deodorant. It is also used as an inhalation or internally in bronchitis and in coryza.

EUGENICS is the study and cultivation of conditions that may improve the human race, in particular the detection and elimination of genetic disease.

EUSOL, which stands for Edinburgh University Solution, is a solution of 12·5 g of boric acid and 12·5 g of chlorinated lime in 1 litre of water. It was introduced during the 1914–18 War as an antiseptic for the treatment of wounds, and proved to be one of the most valuable antiseptics then available. Although largely replaced by modern antiseptics, and the introduction of the sulphonamides (q.v.) and antibiotics, it is still a useful dressing for infected wounds.

EUPHORIA: A feeling of well-being. This may occur normally, for instance, when someone has passed an examination. In some neurological or psychiatric conditions, however, patients may have an exaggerated and quite unjustified feeling of euphoria. This is then a symptom of the underlying condition. Euphoria may also be drug induced – by drugs of addiction or by therapeutic drugs such as corticosteroids.

EUPHORIANTS are drugs which induce a state of euphoria or well-being.

EUSTACHIAN TUBES are the passages, one on each side, leading from the throat to the middle ear. Each is about 38 mm (1½ inches) long and is large at either end, though at its narrowest part it only admits a fine probe. The tubes open widely in the act of swallowing or yawning. The opening into the throat is situated just behind the lower part of the nose, so that a catheter can be passed through the corresponding nostril into the tube for inflation of the middle ear. (See also EAR; NOSE.)

EUTHANASIA means the procuring of an easy and painless death. It has been advocated in some quarters that a medical practicioner should have the power to put to death painlessly, by means of such drugs as morphine, any person suffering from a painful, distressing and incurable disease the outcome of which is inevitably fatal, the patient or his relatives consenting. Various legal safeguards have been proposed, but there are obvious moral and religious – not to mention medical – objections to the recognition of such a procedure.

EVACUANT is a name for a purgative medicine.

EWING'S SARCOMA: An uncommon but very malignant cancer of the bone in children and young adults, the condition was first identified as different from osteosarcoma (q.v.) by Dr J. Ewing in 1921. It usually occurs in the limbs or pelvis and soon spreads to other parts of the body. Treatment is radiotherapy and anticancer drugs. Since the use of the latter the number of patients who survive for five years or more has much improved.

EXANTHEMATA is an old name used to classify the acute infectious diseases distinguished by a characteristic eruption. (See ERUPTION.)

EXCHANGE TRANSFUSION: A method of treating new-born infants with haemolytic disease (q.v.). blood is taken out of the baby through the *umbilical* vein and is replaced with the same quantity of blood from a donor that is compatible with the mother's blood. The procedure is repeated several times to get rid of damaged cells while maintaining the infant's blood volume and keeping its red cell (erythrocyte) count constant.

EXCIPIENT means any more or less inert substance added to a prescription in order to make the remedy as prescribed more suitable in bulk, consistence, or form for administration.

EXCISION means literally a cutting out, and is a term applied to the removal of any structure from the body, when such removal necessitates a certain amount of separation from surrounding parts. For example, one speaks of the excision of a tumour, of a gland, of a joint. When an opening is simply made into the body the term incision is used. When a limb, or part of one, is removed, the term amputation is employed.

EXCITEMENT (see DELIRIUM; HYSTERIA; MENTAL ILLNESS).

EXCORIATION means the destruction of small pieces of the surface of skin or mucous membrane. (See CHAFING OF THE SKIN.)

EXCRETA: Waste substances discharged from the body, in particular faeces.

EXERCISE is a matter of great importance in the maintenance of health at all ages, but particularly for those who are normally engaged in sedentary occupations.
EFFECTS OF EXERCISE: The right amount of the right type of exercise results in all parts of the body working at their best. The muscles are firm in tone, strong and working at maximum efficiency, so that the onset of fatigue, with its accompanying aching and soreness, is postponed. The heart, too, works more efficiently, pumping more blood round the body. For instance, when an individual is resting, the output of the heart per minute is 5 litres. When running at 12 km (7½ miles) per hour, this shoots up to around 25 litres: a five-fold increase. This increased volume of blood dealt with by the heart per minute is achieved with

increasing efficiency, as is shown by the fact that at each contraction the heart expels 150 millilitres, compared with 70 millilitres at rest. The lungs also function more efficiently. Again taking the example of the individual running at 12 km (7½ miles an hour), the amount of oxygen used up increases twelvefold, although the output of the heart has only increased five-fold. The digestive tract, including the liver, also functions better, partly because it is not being overloaded by unnecessary food. The increased expenditure of energy involved in exercise ensures that the food eaten is metabo-lized, or used up, immediately to cope with the increased energy demands. The nervous system also works more efficiently, reflexes becoming brisker and the muscles thereby being able to respond more promptly and more effectively to any special stress or strain. Finally, possibly more imponderable but nevertheless of great practical importance, there is considerable emotional benefit. The individual feels more satisfied with life, is less affected by the normal worries of life in so far as he can forget them in exercising himself – whether this is in some form of athletics or games, or merely tramping the countryside – and when he falls into bed at night his physical tiredness, combined with his emotional peace of mind, allows him to fall asleep – and sleep soundly.

LACK OF EXERCISE: Failure to take adequate exercise affects the body adversely at all ages. In children it leads to slouching, faulty posture and flabbiness of the muscles. In adult life, and particularly in middle age, lack of exercise leads to the putting on of weight, with all the hazards to life that this involves (see OBESITY), constipa-tion, not to mention dyspepsia as often as not due to overeating. What is of even more serious import is that there is an increased tendency to atherosclerosis (q.v.) and coronary thrombosis (q.v.).

OVER-EXERCISE seldom does any permanent harm except in the rapidly growing adolescent and in the old, provided the individual is healthy. For instance, there is no evidence that a healthy heart can be damaged by exercise. The circulatory system is so adaptable that, if there is any possibility of undue strain being placed upon the heart, certain mechanisms come into play which cause giddiness or faint-ing, so that the exercise in question is automati-cally stopped before any real harm is done. On the other hand, should there be any undetected disease of the heart, then undue exercise may produce permanent harm. This is why a careful medical examination is an essential preliminary to any severe form of exercise. This is particu-larly important, indeed essential, in the case of school children.

The secret of success is moderation. The man in his fifties or sixties must realize that he can no longer do many of the things that he did when he was thirty years younger. If he bears this in mind, there is little chance of his damaging himself by exercise. For instance, if he finds that an afternoon's tennis begins to make him uncomfortably breathless, then he should give up the game for a less exacting one, or alternatively be satisfied with one or two sets instead of several.

In the case of adolescents and young adults, the wise rule is to ensure that the individual, and particularly his heart, is sound, and then to insist upon his undergoing a careful course of training before embarking upon any severe form of exercise such as running or football.

EXFOLIATION means the separation, in lay-ers, of pieces of dead bone or skin.

EXOCRINE GLAND: A gland that secretes its products through a duct to the surface of the body or of an organ. The sweat glands in the skin and the salivary glands in the mouth are examples. The secretion is set off by a hormone (q.v.) or a neurotransmitter (q.v.).

EXOGENOUS: Arising outside the body. For example, exogenous depression is an illness caused by an outside factor such as the death of a close relative. Or an illness may occur because of something eaten in the diet.

EXOMPHALOS is the term applied to a hernia formed by the projection of abdominal organs through the umbilicus.

EXOPHTHALMIC GOITRE is a disease in which there is overactivity of the thyroid gland, protrusion of the eyes, and other symptoms. (See GOITRE.)

EXOPHTHALMOS, or PROPTOSIS, refers to forward displacement of the eyeball and must be distinguished from retraction of the eyelids, which causes an illusion of exophthalmos. Lid retraction usually results from activation of the autonomic nervous sytem. Exophthalmos is a more serious disorder caused by inflammatory and infiltrative changes in the retro-orbital tissues and is essentially a feature of Graves' disease (q.v.), though it has been described in chronic thyroiditis. Exophthalmos commonly starts shortly after the development of thyrotoxicosis but may occur months or even years after hyperthyroidism has been success-fully treated. Only 3 per cent of patients with Graves' disease develop severe exophthalmos. The degree of exophthalmos is not correlated with the severity of hyperthyroidism even when their onset is simultaneous. Some of the worst examples of endocrine exophthalmos occur in the euthyroid state and may appear in patients who have never had thyrotoxicosis; this disor-der is named ophthalmic Graves' disease. The exophthalmos of Graves' disease is due to auto-immunity. Antibodies to surface antigens on the eye muscles are produced and this causes an inflammatory reaction in the muscle and retro-orbital tissues.

Exophthalmos may also occur as a result of a tumour at the back of the eye, pushing the eyeball forwards. In this situation it is always unilateral.

EXOSTOSIS means an outgrowth from a bone; it may be due to chronic inflammation, constant pressure or tension on the bone, or tumour-formation. (See BONE, DISEASES OF.)

EXPECTANT is a form of treatment in which the cure of the patient is left mainly to nature, while the physician simply watches for any unsatisfactory developments or symptoms, and relieves them if they occur.

EXPECTORANTS are drugs which assist the removal of secretions from the air passages. Most drugs used as expectorants have a complicated mode of action. (1) Some act chiefly by making the secretion in the bronchial tubes more watery, and therefore less sticky; (2) others have exactly the opposite action, drying up the secretion where it is very copious; (3) a third group assists the act of coughing in feeble people, and so helps the removal of secretion; (4) those in a fourth group soothe the lining membrane of the air passages and quiet ineffectual coughing. These drugs are combined in various ways in bronchitis and other chest conditions. For example, those in the first group are used in the early stages of acute and in chronic bronchitis, those in the next group are better for later stages of acute bronchitis, those of the third group are used for aged persons with pneumonia and bronchitis, and the members of the fourth group are applicable to a constant hacking cough.

EXPECTORATION means either material brought up from the chest by the air passages, or the act by which it is brought up.

EXPIRATION: (1) Breathing out air from the lungs. (2) The act of dying.

EXSANGUINATE: The removal of blood from the body. This may occur as the result of a serious accident in which the victim bleeds extensively. Rarely it may happen that bleeding becomes uncontrollable during an operation.

EXTENSION is the process of straightening or stretching a limb. In cases of fractured limbs, extension is employed during the application of splints, in order to reduce the displacement caused by the fracture, and prevent movement of the broken ends of bone. It is effected by gently and steadily pulling upon the part of the limb beyond the fracture. Extension of a more permanent type is used in the after-treatment of some fractures, as well as in diseases of the spine, by placing the patient upon an inclined bed and affixing weights to his lower limbs or to his head by means of adhesive plaster or of straps. A similar procedure is often adopted in

tuberculous disease of the knee or hip, to prevent the starting pains, which are apt to occur as the affected person is dropping off to sleep.

EXTRA- is the Latin prefix meaning outside of, or in addition, such as extra-capsular, meaning outside the capsule of a joint, and extrasystole, meaning an additional contraction of the heart.

EXTRACTS are preparations, usually of a semi-solid consistence, containing the active parts of various plants extracted in one of several ways. In the case of some extracts the juice of the fresh plant is simply pressed out and purified; in the case of others the active principles are dissolved out in water, which is then to a great extent driven off by evaporation; other extracts are similarly made by the help of alcohol, and in some cases ether is the solvent.

EXTRADURAL: Outside the dura mater (q.v.), the outermost of the three membranes that cover the brain and spinal cord (qq.v.). The extradural or epidural space is the space between the vertebral canal and the dura mater of the spinal cord (see ANAESTHESIA: epidural).

EXTRASYSTOLE is a term applied to premature contraction of one or more of the chambers of the heart. A beat of the heart occurs sooner than it should do in the ordinary rhythm and is followed by a longer rest than usual before the next beat. In an extrasystole the stimulus to contraction arises in a part of the heart other than the usual. Extrasystoles often give rise to an unpleasant sensation as of the heart stumbling over a beat, but their occurrence is not usually serious.

EXTRAVASATION means an escape of fluid from the vessels or passages which ought to contain it. Extravasation of blood due to tearing of vessel walls is found in apoplexy, and in the commoner condition known as a bruise. Extravasation of urine takes place when the bladder or the urethra is ruptured by a blow on the abdomen or on the crutch (or perineum), or torn in a fracture of the pelvis.

EXTRINSIC: (1) Originating outside the body. (2) Extrinisc muscle is one whose origin is some way from the part of the body it acts on – for example, the muscles controlling the movement of the eyeball which are attached to the bony orbit in which the eye sits.

EXUDATION means the process in which some of the constituents of the blood pass slowly through the walls of the small vessels in the course of inflammation, and also means the accumulation resulting from this process. For example, in pleurisy the solid, rough material deposited on the surface of the lung is an exudation.

EYE: The eye is the sensory organ of sight. It is an elaborate photoreceptor detecting information, in the form of light, from the environment and transmitting this information by a series of electro-chemical changes to the brain. The visual cortex is the part of the brain that processes this information (i.e. the visual cortex is what 'sees' the environment). There are two eyes, each a roughly spherical hollow organ held within a bony cavity (the orbit). Each orbit is situated on the front of the skull, one on each side of the nose. The eye consists of an outer wall of three main layers and a central cavity divided into three.

The outer coat consists of the opaque *sclera* posteriorly and the clear *cornea* anteriorly; their junction is called the *limbus*.

(a) SCLERA: This is white, opaque, and constitutes the posterior five-sixths of the outer layer. It is made of dense fibrous tissue. The sclera is visible anteriorly, between the eyelids, as the 'white of the eye'. Posteriorly and anteriorly it is covered by Tenons capsule, which in turn is covered by transparent conjunctiva. There is a hole in the sclera medial to the posterior pole of the eye through which nerve fibres from the retina leave the eye in the optic nerve. Other smaller nerve fibres and blood vessels also pass through the sclera at different points.

(b) CORNEA: This constitutes the transparent colourless anterior one-sixth of the eye. It is transparent in order to allow light into the eye and is more steeply curved than the sclera. Viewed from in front, the cornea is roughly circular. Most of the focusing power of the eye is provided by the cornea (the lens acts as the 'fine adjustment'). It has an outer *epithelium*, a central *stroma* and an inner *endothelium*. The cornea is supplied with very fine nerve fibres which make it exquisitely sensitive to pain. The central cornea has no blood supply – it relies mainly on aqueous humour for nutrition. Blood vessels and large nerve fibres in the cornea would prevent light entering the eye.

(c) LIMBUS is the junction between cornea and sclera. It contains the *trabecular meshwork*, a sieve-like structure through which aqueous humour leaves the eye.

The middle coat (uveal tract) consists of the *choroid, ciliary body* and *iris*.

(a) CHOROID: A highly vascular sheet of tissue lining the posterior two-thirds of the sclera. The network of vessels provides the blood supply for the outer half of the retina. The blood supply of the choroid is derived from numerous *ciliary vessels* which pierce the sclera in front and behind.

(b) CILIARY BODY: A ring of tissue extending 6 mm back from the anterior limitation of the sclera. The various muscles of the ciliary body by their contractions and relaxations are responsible for changing the shape of the lens during accommodation. The ciliary body is lined by cells that secrete aqueous humour. Posteriorly the ciliary body is continuous with the choroid, anteriorly it is continuous with the iris.

(c) IRIS: A flattened muscular diaphragm that is attached at its periphery to the ciliary body and has a round central opening, the *pupil*. By contraction and relaxation of the muscles of the iris the pupil can be dilated or constricted (dilated in the dark or when aroused, constricted in bright light and for close work). The iris forms a partial division between the *anterior chamber* and the *posterior chamber* of the eye. It lies in front of the lens and forms the back wall of the anterior chamber. The iris is visible from in front, through the transparent cornea, as the 'coloured part of the eye'. The amount and distribution of iris pigment determine the colour of the iris. The pupil is merely a hole in the centre of the iris and appears black.

The inner layer: The RETINA is a multi-layered tissue (ten layers in all) which extends from the edges of the optic nerve to line the inner surface of the choroid up to the junction of ciliary body and choroid. Here the true retina ends at the *ora serrata*. The retina contains light sensitive cells of two types: (i) *cones*: Cells that operate at high and medium levels of illumination. They subserve fine discrimination of vision and colour vision. (ii) RODS: Cells that function best at low light intensity and subserve black and white vision.

The retina contains about 6 million cones and about 100 million rods. Information from them is conveyed by the nerve fibres which are in the inner part of the retina to leave the eye in the optic nerve. There are no photoreceptors at the optic disc (the point where the optic nerve leaves the eye) and therefore there is no light perception from this small area. The optic disc thus produces a physiological blind spot in the visual field.

The retina can be subdivided into several

1 fovea	8 conjunctiva
2 optic nerve	9 iris
3 sclera	10 cornea
4 choroid	11 lens
5 retina	12 anterior chamber
6 ora serrata	13 posterior chamber
7 ciliary muscle	(vitreous body)

Diagram of the left eye from above.

areas: (a) PERIPHERAL RETINA contains mainly rods and a few scattered cones. Visual acuity from this area is fairly coarse. (b) MACULA LUTEA, so called because histologically it looks like a yellow spot. It occupies an area 4 5 mm in diameter lateral to the optic disc. This area of specialized retina can produce a high level of visual acuity. Cones are abundant here but there are few rods. (c) FOVEA CENTRALIS: A small central depression at the centre of the macula. Here the cones are tightly packed, rods are absent. It is responsible for the highest levels of visual acuity.

1 pigment cells	5 axon
2 cone	6 ganglion cells
3 rod	7 axon to optic
4 felt-work of dendrons	nerve

Diagrammatic section of the retina.

The chambers of the eye: There are three, *anterior* and *posterior chambers* and the *vitreous cavity*. The ANTERIOR CHAMBER is limited in front by the inner surface of the cornea, behind by the iris and pupil. It contains a transparent clear watery fluid, the *aqueous humour*. This is constantly being produced by cells of the ciliary body and constantly drained away through the trabecular meshwork. The trabecular meshwork lies in the angle between the iris and inner surface of the cornea. The POSTERIOR CHAMBER: A narrow space between the iris and pupil in front and the lens behind. It too contains aqueous humour in transit from the ciliary epithelium to the anterior chamber, via the pupil. The VITREOUS CAVITY: The largest cavity of the eye. In front it is bounded by the lens and behind by the retina. It contains *vitreous humour*. The *lens* is transparent, elastic and biconvex in cross section. It lies behind the iris and in front of the vitreous cavity. Viewed from the front it is roughly circular and about 10 mm

in diameter. The diameter and thickness of the lens vary with its accommodative state. The lens consists of (a) *capsule*: a thin transparent membrane surrounding the cortex and nucleus; (b) *cortex*: This is made up of newly made lens fibres that are relatively soft. It separates the capsule on the outside from the nucleus at the centre of the lens; (c) *nucleus*: The dense central area of old lens fibres that have become compacted by new lens fibres laid down over them. The *zonule* consists of numerous radially arranged fibres attached between the ciliary body and the lens around its circumference. Tension in these zonular fibres can be adjusted by the muscles of the ciliary body, thus changing the shape of the lens and altering its power of accommodation. The *vitreous humour* is a transparent clear jellylike structure made up of a network of collagen fibres suspended in a viscid fluid. Its shape conforms to that of the vitreous cavity within which it is contained, i.e. it is spherical except for a shallow concave depression on its anterior surface. The lens lies in this depression.

Eyelids: These are multilayered curtains of tissue whose functions include spreading of the tear film over the front of the eye to prevent desiccation, protection from injury or external irritation and to some extent to control light entering the eye. Each eye has an upper and lower lid which form an elliptical opening (the *palpebral fissure*) when the eyes are open. The lids meet at the *medial canthus* and *lateral canthus* respectively. The inner medial canthus is fixed, the lateral canthus is more mobile. An *epicanthus* is a fold of skin which covers the medial canthus in oriental races. Each lid consists of several layers. From front to back they are: very thin skin, a sheet of muscle (*orbicularis oculi* whose fibres are concentric around the palpebral fissure and which produce closure of the eyelids), the orbital septum (modified near the lid margin to form the *tarsal plates*) and, finally, lining the back surface of the lid, the conjunctiva (known here as *tarsal conjunctiva*). At the free margin of each lid are the eyelashes, the openings of tear glands which lie within the lid and the *lacrimal punctum*. Toward the medial edge of each lid in an elevation known as the *papilla*. The lacrimal punctum opens into this papilla. The punctum forms the open end of the *cannaliculus*, part of the tear-drainage mechanism.

Orbit: The bony cavity within which the eye is held. The orbits lie one on either side of the nose, on the front of the skull. They afford considerable protection for the eye. Each is roughly pyramidal in shape, with the apex pointing backwards and the base forming the open anterior part of the orbit. The bone of the anterior orbital margin is thickened to protect the eye from injury. There are various openings into the posterior part of the orbit, namely the *optic canal* which allows the optic nerve to leave the orbit en route for the brain, the *superior orbital fissure* and *inferior orbital fissure* which allow passage of nerves and blood vessels to and from the orbit. The most important structures holding the eye within the orbit are the *extra-ocular muscles*, a *suspensory ligament* of connective tissue that forms a hammock on which the eye rests and which is slung between the medial and lateral walls of the orbit. Finally, the *orbital septum*, a sheet of connective tissue extending from the anterior margin of the orbit into the lids, helps keep the eye in place. A pad of fat fills in the orbit behind the eye and acts as a cushion for the eye.

Conjunctiva: A transparent mucous membrane that extends from the limbus over the anterior sclera or 'white of the eye'. This is the *bulbar* conjunctiva. The conjunctiva does not cover the cornea. Conjunctiva passes from the eye on to the inner surface of the eyelid at the *fornices* and is continuous with the *tarsal* conjunctiva. The *semilunar fold* is the vertical crescent of conjunctiva at the medial aspect of the palpebral fissure. The *caruncle* is a piece of modified skin just within the inner canthus.

Eye muscles (extra ocular muscles): There are six in all, the four rectus muscles (superior, inferior, medial and lateral rectus muscles) and two oblique muscles (superior and inferior oblique muscles). The muscles are attached at various points between the bony orbit and the eyeball. By their combined action they move the eye in horizontal and vertical gaze. They also produce torsional movement of the eye (i.e. clockwise or anticlockwise movements when viewed from the front).

Lacrimal apparatus: There are two components, a tear production system, namely the lacrimal gland and accessory lacrimal glands, and a drainage system.

LACRIMAL GLAND is located below a small depression in the bony roof of the orbit. Numerous tear ducts open from it into predominantly the upper lid. *Accessory lacrimal glands* are found in the conjunctiva and within the eyelids. The former open directly on to the surface of the conjunctiva, the latter on to the eyelid margin.

LACRIMAL DRAINAGE SYSTEM consists of (a) *Punctum*: an elevated opening toward the medial aspect of each lid. Each punctum opens into a cannaliculus. (b) *Cannaliculus*: a fine tube- like structure running within the lid, parallel to the lid margin. The cannaliculus from upper and lower lid join to form a common cannaliculus which opens into the lacrimal sac. (c) *Lacrimal sac*: a small sac on the side of the nose which opens into the nasolacrimal duct. During blinking the sac sucks tears into itself from the cannaliculus. Tears then drain by gravity down the nasolacrimal duct. (d) *Nasolacrimal duct*: A tubular structure which runs down through the wall of the nose and opens into the nasal cavity.

Tears keep the front of the eye moist; they also contain nutrients and various components to protect the eye from infection. Crying results from excess tear production. The drainage system cannot cope with the excess and therefore tears overflow on to the face. Newborn babies do not produce tears for the first three months of life.

Visual pathway: Light stimulates the rods and cones of the retina. Electrochemical messages are then passed to nerve fibres in the retina and then via the *optic nerve* to the *optic chiasm*. Here information from the temporal (outer) half of each retina continues to the same side of the brain. Information from the nasal (inner) half of each retina crosses to the other side within the optic chiasm. The rearranged nerve fibres then pass through the *optic tract* to the *lateral geniculate body*, then the *optic radiation* to reach the *visual cortex* in the occipital lobe of the brain.

EYE, DISEASE AND INJURIES: Diseases affecting the eye are numerous and varied. The eye has its own group of disorders that affect one or more of the ocular structures but have no effect on the rest of the body. In addition a wide variety of systemic diseases produce changes in the eye. By careful examination of the eye it is therefore possible to assist diagnosis of many diseases affecting the body as a whole. Some of these disorders are dealt with below. The subjects of *artificial eyes* (see under PROSTHESES); CATARACT; GLAUCOMA; RETINA, DISORDERS OF; SQUINT; and UVEITIS; are dealt with under these headings.

Conjunctiva (disorders of)

CONJUNCTIVITIS: An inflammation of the conjunctiva. There are many causes including *bacteria, viruses, allergy* and *chlamydia*. Symptoms and signs vary depending on the cause. (The conjunctiva may become infected in disorders of the cornea or iris. This is not true conjunctivitis.)

Bacterial conjunctivitis: Almost any bacteria can be involved, the commonest being *streptococci* and *staphylococci*. The patient complains of a mild grittiness or itching, redness of the eye and a yellow discharge (pain and photophobia are *not* features of bacterial conjunctivitis). One eye is involved first but both eyes are invariably affected within a few hours. The conjunctiva is most inflamed in the conjunctival fornices (that area of the 'white of the eye' furthest from the cornea). The disorder is self limiting but recovery can be accelerated with treatment. Topical antibiotic drops (e.g. chloramphenicol eye drops) are usually effective within a day or two.

Viral conjunctivitis: There are numerous types of viruses causing conjunctivitis. One of the commonest is the group of *adenoviruses* (there are currently 31 recognized types). Symptoms include redness, watering, discomfort (which may be marked) and photophobia. Usually one eye is affected (although both may be). There is conjunctival swelling (chemosis), subconjunctival haemorrhages (see later), keratitis and pre-auricular lymph node enlargement. There may be an associated upper respiratory tract infection with fever, sore throat, coughing and feeling generally unwell. Adenoviral conjunctivitis is common, highly infectious and occurs in epidemic form (*epidemic keratoconjunctivitis*). Treatment involves the relief of symptoms as there is no active cure. It recovers spontaneously over a variable period of time. It is important that patients keep soap, towels and hairbrushes to themselves and avoid close contact with others in order to limit the chances of spreading the disorder. *Molluscum contagiosum* (see MOLLUSCUM CONTAGIOSUM) is a viral skin infection which usually affects children. Conjunctivitis can occur if the virus affects the eyelids. *Acute haemorrhage conjunctivitis* is caused by a *picornavirus*. It is highly contagious, self limiting and produces subconjunctival haemorrhages, keratitis and enlarged lymph nodes in front of the ear.

Allergic conjunctivitis: This includes *Vernal keratoconjunctivitis*. This common disorder affects children and young adults. It is recurrent with most frequent episodes in spring. Symptoms include itching and watering of the eyes with or without pain, photophobia and discharge. The most marked feature is large flat elevations of the conjunctiva of the upper eyelid, visible on turning the lid inside out. Treatment is with sodium cromoglycate drops or steroid drops. *Hay-fever conjunctivitis* causes a pale swelling of the conjunctiva giving it a jellylike appearance. The condition may be otherwise symptom free or give rise to mild itching. Treatment is with sodium cromoglycate drops.

Chlamydia conjunctivitis: There are various disorders of the conjunctiva produced by chlamydia including (i) *Adult inclusion conjunctivitis*: this occurs two weeks or so following sexual intercourse with an infected partner. There is a mucopurulent discharge from both eyes, and conjunctival follicles (visible with a slit lamp microscope), conjunctival oedema, keratitis and pre-auricular lymph-node enlargement are common. Treatment is with tetracycline tablets for both patient and sexual partners. The patient should also be treated with tetracycline eye drops. (ii) *Trachoma* is caused by *Chlamydia trachomatis*. It is common in the Third World and is the leading cause of preventable blindness worldwide. It is seen in Great Britain in predominantly immigrant populations in its inactive form. The organism is transmitted by flies and causes inflammation of the conjunctiva and cornea with resultant scarring. Treatment of the active disease is with tetracycline tablets and tetracycline eye drops. *Ophthalmia neonatorum*: Inflammation of the conjunctiva occurring within the first month of life. It can be caused by *chlamydia* (the commonest cause) or *gonococcal infection* which can result in perforation of the cornea). These two types of infection occur by passage through the mother's infected birth canal. Other causes include *bacteria*, *herpes simplex* or inflammation induced by *eye drops*. Treatment is of the underlying cause, e.g. tetracycline for chlamydia, penicillin for gonorrhoea, and acycloguanosine ointment for herpes simplex.

SUBCONJUNCTIVAL HAEMORRHAGE: Bleeding under the conjunctiva. Because the conjunctiva is transparent, the white of the eye becomes bright red either in part, or totally. Usually it occurs spontaneously in elderly people due to increased fragility of the blood vessels. Subconjunctival haemorrhages can also occur in conjunctival inflammation or as a result of injury. Treatment of the haemorrhage itself is unnecessary as it will disappear over a few days.

Cornea (disorders of):

ARCUS SENILIS: A very common finding in elderly people. Deposits of fat in the peripheral circumference of the cornea appear as a white crescent or a complete ring. It is a normal ageing change (see AGE, NATURAL CHANGES IN). Occasionally an arcus can occur in the young. In this group there may be an association with raised blood lipid levels.

CORNEAL DYSTROPHIES: A group of inherited disorders of the cornea. They are bilateral, usually developing during adolescence and progressing slowly throughout life. They cause opacification of the cornea to a greater or lesser degree. Many do not interfere with vision, those that do may require a *corneal graft* (see CORNEAL GRAFT).

KERATITIS: An inflammation of the cornea. There are numerous causes, only a few of which are dealt with below.

Bacterial keratitis: Bacteria may reach the cornea from an infection of the conjunctiva, the eyelids, lacrimal system, or may be introduced by, for example, a foreign body. For bacterial infection of the cornea to occur there must first be some damage to the corneal epithelium (the exception is *gonorrhoea*). The commonest bacterial causes of keratitis include *staphylococci*, *streptococci*, *pseudomonas* and *enterobacteria*. The eye becomes intensely red and painful with a yellow discharge. There is damage to the corneal epithelium with suppuration of the corneal stroma. The latter results in opacification of the cornea. Blood vessels may grow into the cornea from the limbus. Pus develops within the anterior chamber (*hypopyon* – pus in the anterior chamber). Bacterial keratitis is an extremely serious condition which can rapidly lead to blindness. Treatment is urgent and requires admission to hospital, the administration of intensive antibiotic drops and antibiotic tablets.

Viral keratitis: *Herpes simplex* is a virus that causes infection of the eyes, skin, lips and genitalia. Primary infection occurs during early childhood and thereafter recurrent infection can occur throughout life at variable intervals. Recurrences may be brought on by poor general health, injury, the effect of ultraviolet light on the eye. If the dendritic ulcer involves the central cornea, patients may experience blurred vision. The corneal stroma may also become involved, invariably resulting in blurred vision due to the development of a *disciform keratitis*. Treatment is with acycloguanosine ointment to kill the active virus. Very weak steroids can be used under *strict supervision* by an eye specialist to reduce inflammation in cases of disciform keratitis. Recurrent attacks can lead to dense scarring of the cornea; fortunately this is not common since the introduction of anti-viral drugs. A severely scarred cornea can be replaced with a corneal graft (see CORNEAL GRAFT).

Systemic viral illness such as *measles*, *mumps* and *chickenpox* can also affect the cornea.

Exposure keratitis If the front of the eye becomes dry, desiccation and ulceration of the cornea can occur with the possibility of secondary bacterial infection – a potentially blinding condition. During the action of blinking tears are spread over the front of the eye keeping it moist. If the eyelids are prevented from spreading the tear film, exposure of the eye results. Some causes include: (a) *Facial nerve palsy*: the muscles of the face, including orbicularis oculi, are paralysed and unable to close the eyelids. (b) *Scarring*: this can cause distortion and restriction of movement of the eyelids. (c) *Proptosis*, a condition in which the eye is pushed forward for a variety of reasons. The lids cannot then close over the eye.

Peripheral corneal ulceration can occur in a number of conditions including *focal desiccation* (called a *dellen*), *hypersensitivity* to bacteria, or as a complication of one of the *connective tissue disorders*.

KERATOCONUS: The normal symmetrical curve of the cornea is distorted due to abnormal thinning and subsequent forward bulging of the central cornea. This bulging results in deterioration of the vision. Mild forms can be corrected with spectacles, the more severe forms with contact lenses. The most severe forms require corneal grafting because they cannot be corrected either with glasses or with contact lenses – the cornea becomes so distorted that contact lenses fall off.

Eyelids (disorders of):

BLEPHARITIS: A chronic inflammation of the margin of the eyelids. It frequently begins in childhood, although it does not cause much trouble until later life. The cause is a combination of staphylococcal infection, seborrhoeic dermatitis and concurrent dry eyes due to a reduction in the aqueous component of the tear film. The lid margins may become reddened, scales may appear around the lashes, the lashes may point in different directions or may fall out. Less commonly focal ulceration of the skin of the lids can occur. The conjunctiva and cornea may become involved. Treatment is aimed at relieving the symptoms of burning and redness of the eyelids. Cleaning the eyelids with a solution of sodium bicarbonate may help, as does the use of antibiotic eye drops and artificial tear drops. It is difficult to cure but not dangerous.

BLEPHAROSPASM: An involuntary repeated twitching or even full closure of the eyelids due to spasm of the orbicularis oculi muscle (see EYE: eyelids). It usually affects the elderly although it may occur as a transient episode in younger people. When marked it is cosmetically unsightly and may even interfere with vision. Some patients improve with drugs, some recover following injections of local anaesthetic into the eyelids, others may require surgery.

CHALAZION (CYST OF MEIBOMIAN GLAND): Meibomian glands are present in the eyelids. A chalazion is a chronic inflammation of these glands. The cysts may be single or multiple.

They are slowly enlarging painless non-red swellings in the eyelids. They may become secondarily infected, in which case they become red and painful. A chalazion usually resolves spontaneously over several months or may be removed surgically if infected or cosmetically unsightly. A small incision is made on the under surface of the lid and the contents of the cyst removed. The procedure takes a few minutes and can be done under local anaesthetic.

ECTROPION: The lid turns outwards. It is far more common in the lower than upper lid. Symptoms include watering of the eye and an unsightly appearance. Treatment is surgical.

ENTROPION: The lid turns inwards. Again the lower lid is usually involved. The eyelashes rub against the eye and cause irritation. Treatment is surgical.

PTOSIS: Drooping of the upper lid. This may be minor, or be complete so that the eye is shut. Ptosis may result from damage or weakness of the muscles lifting the lid, or the nerve supply of those muscles, or may be due to mechanical restriction of lid opening, such as by scarring or the presence of a large (and therefore heavy) cyst or lid tumour, pulling the lid down. Treatment depends on the cause of the ptosis. Some patients may benefit from surgery.

STYE: An acute purulent inflammation of an eyelash follicle. A small abscess results. Styes are common and present as a localized red swelling at the lid margin which appears to surround an eyelash. They are often multiple and are usually due to staphylococcal infection. Treatment includes hot compresses, removal of the eyelash to allow the pus to drain and antibiotic drops or ointment (chloramphenicol).

Eye injuries These may be trivial, or so severe as to cause blindness or loss of the eye. Anyone involved in tasks where an eye injury could be expected (e.g. welding, grinding, drilling) should wear appropriate protective goggles or visor.

Sub-conjunctival haemorrhage (see above).

Black eye (or periorbital haematoma) is bruising of the skin of the lids due to an injury around the eye, or to the forehead. Most cases occur without any damage to the eye itself and settle within a week or so. No treatment is required for the bruising.

Corneal foreign bodies constitute 25 per cent of eye injuries. They may arise from dust blowing into the eye or from material thrown from mechanical tools such as drills or even a hammer and chisel. Corneal foreign bodies can cause intense irritation, photophobia and watering of the eye. Treatment involves removal of the foreign body, the application of antibiotic drops or ointment and a patch over the eye until the cornea heals (24 hours in most cases).

Sub-tarsal foreign body (i.e. a foreign body under the lid): As the lid blinks, the foreign body is dragged across the cornea, scratching it. Causes, symptoms and treatment are the same as for corneal foreign bodies.

Corneal abrasions: These are losses of corneal epithelium due to an injury. They are painful and cause watering and redness of the eye. Most are small and heal quickly, usually with

no long-term effects. Treatment consists of the application of antibiotic drops or ointment and wearing a patch until the abrasion heals.
Corneal ulcer In ophthalmic terms this is an infection of the cornea.
Blunt injury may result in damage to the interior of the eye. Bleeding from the iris or ciliary body results in blood in the anterior chamber (a *hyphema*). The iris may be torn in a blunt injury. More serious is the possibility of development of a cataract or dislocation of the lens. The retina may become swollen (*commotio retinae*) or detached (see RETINA, DISORDERS OF). Bleeding into the vitreous from the retinal or choroidal vessels can occur. A certain amount of spontaneous recovery will occur but complications such as *cataract, retinal detachment* or *glaucoma* may require surgery. These three complications are the commonest long-term problem resulting from eye injury.
Lacerating injury: This is a serious condition, there is initial damage at the time of injury with possible prolapse of the contents of the eye through the laceration (e.g. iris, lens, vitreous); in addition infection may gain access to the eye through the penetrating injury. Surgical repair of the injury aims to try and restore the eye to as near anatomically normal as possible and to minimize the risk of infection. This is a matter of some urgency. Foreign bodies within the eye should be removed if they are likely to cause further damage (e.g. bits of wood, copper, iron). Other materials (glass and perspex) can be left alone if they are not easily accessible or if their removal would cause further damage.
Chemical injury: Acids coagulate the proteins of the cornea and sclera producing a barrier that can limit the spread of the acid. Alkali are more dangerous in that they destroy normal barriers and can enter the eye resulting in damage that may be progressive for several days after injury. Treatment is immediate and requires copious irrigation of the eye with water with subsequent treatment to try and minimize the complications that can occur.
Radiant energy injuries: *Ultraviolet light* is almost entirely absorbed by the cornea. Excessive exposure to UV light results in a painful watery red eye. On examination there are hundreds of tiny punctate abrasions on the exposed cornea. *Arc eye* and *snow blindness* result from excessive exposure to UV light. *Infra-red* light can result in cataract formation.
Nystagmus: An involuntary rhythmic, oscillatory movement of the eyes. The movements may be horizontal, vertical or torsional. Nystagmus may occur as an isolated finding in a benign form (congenital nystagmus) or may accompany severe disease of the nervous system, or intoxication with certain drugs including alcohol. Some individuals can induce short bursts of voluntary nystagmus. Nystagmus can also be induced by irritation of the middle ear either by disease, or by water in the ear. Nystagmus was previously thought to be associated with poor lighting (hence 'miner's nystagmus'). This is no longer thought to be true.

Sclera and Episclera (disorders of):
EPISCLERITIS: An inflammation of the episclera (the most superficial layer of the sclera). It typically affects young adults, is common, benign and resolves spontaneously. It may be recurrent but is not associated with systemic disease. Treatment is not usually necessary as it recovers spontaneously in a day or two. Steroid eye drops can speed recovery (see EYE DROPS).
SCLERITIS: An inflammation of the sclera. It is uncommon, occurs in middle age and affects women more than men. It can be bilateral and recurrent, may be painful and can result in blindness due to complications of scleritis. Systemic diseases associated with scleritis include *rheumatoid arthritis, connective tissue disorders* generally, *sarcoidosis, ulcerative colitis, ankylosing spondylitis* and *Bechet's disease*. Treatment is with anti-inflammatory drugs (indomethacin, oxyphenbutazone or steroids).
'Watery eye': This may be due to excessive production of tears (lacrimation) as in crying or irritation of the eye. Treatment is aimed at removal of the cause of irritation. It may also be due to inadequate tear drainage so that tears overflow on to the cheek (*epiphora*). Epiphora may result from the punctum of the lower lid turning out from the eye (as in ectropion). Treatment is to turn the lid back inwards so that the punctum is once more in contact with the eye. More commonly epiphora results from an obstruction in the lacrimal drainage system; commonly this occurs because the cannaliculi become narrowed. Occasionally obstruction of the nasolacrimal duct can result in infection of the lacrimal sac (dacryocystitis). A red painful swelling occurs at the side of the nose which may or may not be made smaller (temporarily) by pressing on it. Pressure on the swelling may result in regurgitation of pus through the puncta on to the eyelids. Treatment is to relieve the obstruction. This may be relatively simple if the obstruction can be cleared by dilating the punctum. If infection has occurred, it must first be overcome by antibiotic tablets and drops, followed by surgery to create a channel between the lacrimal sac and the inside of the nose which bypasses the blocked nasolacrimal duct.
Xerophthalmia: A condition in which the conjunctiva and cornea become dry due to a deficiency of vitamin A. It is seen in Third World countries, but is rare in Great Britain. It may present with night blindness and progress to complete blindness.

EYE DROPS (AND OINTMENT) are used extensively in the treatment of eye disease. They should be used as instructed by the prescribing physician. Most can be used for one month after the bottle has been opened but should then be discarded and a repeat prescription obtained if necessary. Any eye drops or ointment can have side effects and any difficulty with them should be referred to the prescribing physician.

EYE STRAIN (see REFRACTION).

F

FACE is that part of the head extending from the forehead to the chin. It is supported by 14 bones: 2 nasal bones. 2 superior maxillae which carry the upper teeth. 2 lacrimal bones, 2 zygomatic bones, 2 palatine bones, 2 nasal bones at the sides of the nose, the vomer, forming a partition between the nostrils, and the mandible carrying the lower teeth. The lower jaw forms a joint of hinge-shape with the temporal bones of the skull, whilst the other bones of the face are firmly fixed together by sutures. The face in man is relatively small, as compared with that in lower animals, on account of the development of the cranium containing the brain. For the same reason, the face has an almost vertical direction instead of being sloped backwards as in animals.

The general character of the features depends chiefly upon the presence of air spaces in the frontal bone, situated immediately behind the eyebrows and in the upper jaw-bones. The varying expressions which are connected with the emotions and the general expression denoting character are chiefly due to the action of numerous thin muscles situated around the openings of the eyes, nose, and mouth. (See MUSCLE.) These are controlled by the 7th cranial nerve, which springs from the hinder part of the brain, passes through the skull to the ear, and, emerging immediately below the latter, passes forward on to the face round the edge of the lower jaw. In this position it is liable to be wounded or injured by such conditions as cold, then giving rise to a flat and expressionless appearance of one side of the face known as *Bell's palsy* (or *paralysis*) or *facial paralysis*. (See BELL'S PALSY.) The sensory nerve of the face is the 5th cranial nerve, which originates from the neighbouring part of the brain and within the skull divides into three portions called, respectively, ophthalmic, maxillary, and mandibular divisions. Each of these sends branches on to the face through a notch that can be felt near the inner end of the eyebrow, through an opening immediately beneath the eye, and through another opening near the middle of the chin. On their way to the face these nerves

1 greater wing of sphenoid bone	8 maxilla
2 lesser wing of sphenoid bone	9 zygomatic bone
3 lacrimal bone	10 superior orbital fissure
4 nasal bone	11 squamous part of temporal bone
5 vomer	12 supra-orbital foramen
6 anterior nasal spine of maxilla	13 parietal bone
7 mandible	14 frontal bone

The skull from the front.

supply the parts about the eye, the teeth, and the muscles which move the lower jaw in chewing. The various parts of this nerve are subject to a particularly painful form of neuralgia, known sometimes as tic douloureux. (See NEURALGIA.)

The face is liable to certain deformities, of which hare-lip and cleft palate are the principal. (See PALATE, MALFORMATIONS OF.) The skin of the face, which has an unusually free blood supply, bleeds with great freedom when wounded, but, for the same reason, wounds heal with special rapidity and freedom from suppuration. The contraction of scars after severe injuries, such as burns, sometimes leads to marked deformity of the eyelids, mouth, and nose. The skin condition known as acne (see ACNE) is common in young people about the chin and brow, disappearing as age advances. Boils, carbuncles, and other infectious conditions often occur on the face, and, when situated about the upper lip, present a considerable degree of danger from the liability of the infection to spread to the interior of the head. The tuberculous disease known as lupus is more frequent on the face than in any other situation and may lead to unsightly ulceration and scarring. Certain simple tumours, particularly sebaceous cysts and naevi or birth marks, commonly affect the skin in this region, and cancer, in the form of epithelioma, is not uncommon in the later stages of life about the margins of the lip, nostril, or eyelid. This is also one of the commonest sites of the slow-growing form of cancer known as rodent ulcer.

FACIAL NERVE is the seventh cranial nerve, and supplies the muscles of expression in the face, being purely a motor nerve. It enters the face immediately below the ear after splitting up into several branches. (See BELL'S PALSY.)

FACIES is a term applied to the expression or appearance of the face, which often gives indications of the presence of disease in other parts of the body. Thus the *abdominal facies* is a pinched, anxious expression associated with severe disease in the abdomen. The *cardiac facies* is a condition present in some valvular defects of the heart, showing bright purplish cheeks and lips, with a sallow hue of the rest of the face. The *typhoid facies* is a vacant, bewildered, and apathetic expression seen in typhoid fever and other debilitating diseases. The *Hippocratic facies* is a cast of countenance originally described by Hippocrates, in which the face is drawn, pinched, and livid, indicating approaching death. Anxiety and depression are often reflected in the facial expression.

FAECES is another name for the stools. (See CONSTIPATION; DIARRHOEA; STOOLS.)

FAINTING, or SYNCOPE, is a temporary loss of consciousness caused by inadequate brain perfusion. It may be preceded by nausea, sweating, loss of vision, and ringing in the ears. It is most often caused by pooling of blood in the extremities, which reduces venous return and thus cardiac output. This may be caused by hot weather or prolonged standing. Occasionally fainting on standing occurs in people with low blood pressure, autonomic neuropathy (in which normal vasomotor reflexes are absent), or those taking antihypertensive drugs. A prolonged rise in intrathoracic pressure caused by coughing, micturition, or the valsalva manoeuvre also impedes venous return and may cause fainting. Hypovolaemia produced by bleeding, prolonged diarrhoea, or vomiting may also cause fainting. Fainting is also produced by severe pain or emotional upset. Cardiac causes, such as severe stenotic valve disease or rhythm disturbances (particularly complete heart block or very rapid tachycardias), may result in fainting. Treatment must be directed towards the underlying cause, but immediate first aid consists of laying the patient down and elevating the legs.

FALLING SICKNESS is an old name for epilepsy. (See EPILEPSY.)

FALLOT'S TETRALOGY: A hereditary defect of the heart in which intraventricular septal defect, pulmonary stenosis, right ventricular hypertrophy and a wrongly positioned aorta occur. It is usually treatable by surgery.

FALLOPIAN TUBES, or UTERINE TUBES, are tubes, one on each side, which are attached at one end to the womb, and have the other unattached but lying close to the ovary. Each is between 10 to 12·5 cm (4 to 5 inches) long, large at the end next the ovary, but communicating with the womb by an opening which admits only a bristle. These tubes conduct the ova from the ovaries to the interior of the womb. Blockage of them by a chronic inflammatory process resulting from infection is a not uncommon cause of infertility in women.

FALSE MEMBRANE is the name given to the deposit which forms upon the walls of the air passages in cases of diphtheria. It consists partly of fibrin derived from the blood, partly of the destroyed surface of the mucous membrane upon which it rests, and it contains bacteria in enormous numbers. If it is removed, it leaves a raw and bleeding surface upon which new membrane quickly forms.

FAMILY HEALTH SERVICES AUTHORITY: An appointed committee that is responsible for the provision of local medical, dental, pharmaceutical and ophthalmic services in the NATIONAL HEALTH SERVICE. There are over two hundred of these committees in the United Kingdom and they are responsible to regional health authorities.

FANGO is the name of a kind of mud, derived from thermal springs at Battaglio in Italy, which is applied warm to gouty and rheumatic joints.

FANSIDAR is a combination of pyrimethamine (q.v.) and sulfadoxine (q.v.) which is being used for the prevention of malaria (q.v.). It has the advantage of needing to be taken only once a week, or even only once a fortnight. It should not be taken by pregnant women, nor by those hypersensitive to sulphonamides.

FARCY is another name for glanders. (See GLANDERS.)

FARMER'S LUNG is a form of external allergic alveolitis (see ALVEOLITIS) caused by the inhalation of dust from mouldy hay or straw.

FASCIA is the name applied to sheets or bands of fibrous tissue which enclose and connect the muscles.

FASCIITIS is inflammation of fascia (q.v.). The commonest site for it is the sole of the foot where it is known as plantar fasciitis. It is characterized by gnawing pain. There is no specific treatment, but it usually clears up spontaneously though over a considerable time. Gentle massage may be helpful in easing the pain.

FASCIOLIASIS is the disease caused by the liver fluke, *Fasciola hepatica*. This is found in sheep, cattle and other herbivorous animals, in which it is the cause of the condition known as liver rot. It measures about 35 × 13 mm, and is transmitted to man from the infected animals by snails. In Britain it is the commonest disease found in animal slaughterhouses. The danger to man is in eating vegetables, particularly wild watercress, that have been infected by snails. There have been several outbreaks of fascioliasis in Britain due to eating contaminated wild watercress. Much larger outbreaks of fascioliasis due to eating wild watercress have also been reported in France. The disease is characterized by fever, dyspepsia, heavy sweating, loss of appetite, abdominal pain, urticaria, and a troublesome cough. In the more serious cases there may be severe damage to the liver with or without jaundice. The diagnosis is clinched by the finding of the eggs of the fluke in the stools. The two drugs used in treatment are bithionol and chloroquine. Even though many cases are quite mild and recover spontaneously, prevention is particularly important. This consists primarily of never eating wild watercress, as this is the main cause of infestation. Lettuces have also been found to be infested.

FASTIGIUM means the highest temperature reached in a feverish state.

FASTING means the abstention from, or deprivation of, food and drink.

If food and drink is entirely suspended two results quickly follow: the body becomes thinner and lighter as it draws upon its stored-up nourishment, and also the temperature gradually falls. If water is taken, the process of using up the fat and muscles in order to maintain the activity of the heart, lungs, and other vital organs, proceeds to an extreme extent, and the body becomes very emaciated before death.

After prolonged fasting the return to food should be gradual, and no heavy meal should be taken for a day or two.

FAT as a food has more energy-producing power weight for weight than any other food. Animal fat is a mixture in varying proportions of stearic, palmitic, and oleic acids combined with glycerin. Butter contains about 80 per cent of fat, ordinary cream contains 20 per cent fat, and rich cream 40 per cent, whilst olive oil is practically a pure form of fat. Fat requires, when taken to a large extent in the diet, to be combined with a certain proportion of either carbohydrate or protein in order that it may be completely consumed, otherwise harmful products, known as ketones, are apt to be formed in the blood. Each gram of fat has an energy-producing equivalent of 9·3 Calories.

From the medical point of view, fats are divided into saturated fats, that is, animal fats and dairy produce, and unsaturated fats which include vegetable oils from soya bean, maize and sunflower, and marine oils from fish (eg. cod-liver oil). (See ADIPOSE TISSUE; LIPID; OBESITY.)

FATIGUE is brought about in two ways. In the first place muscles become fatigued by the lactic acid accumulating in them as the result of their activity. For the removal of lactic acid in the recovery phase of muscular contraction oxygen is needed. If the supply of oxygen is not plentiful enough, or cannot keep pace with the work the muscle is doing, then lactic acid accumulates and fatigue results. There is also a nervous element in muscular fatigue: it is diminished by stimulation of the sympathetic nervous system. (See MUSCLE.)

INDUSTRIAL WORKERS: Many factors enter into the maintenance of efficiency and the avoidance of fatigue, mental and physical. Intensity and direction of illumination, ventilation, temperature and humidity of the air, adequate diet, posture at work, rest pauses, monotony, and, above all, hours of work are among some of these factors. There is a level beyond which the human machine can no longer produce work satisfactorily. If this is exceeded it is shown by a reduction in the quantity and quality of the work done. If work is done under conditions of fatigue, damage to health results and accidents may occur. The shortening of unduly long hours of labour under improved hygienic conditions is followed by increased productive efficiency.

FAT NECROSIS: In injury to, or inflammation of, the pancreas the fat-splitting enzyme in it may escape into the abdominal cavity, causing death of fat-containing cells.

FATTY DEGENERATION: As a result of anaemia, interference with blood or nerve supply, or because of the action of various poisons, body cells may undergo abnormal changes accompanied by the appearance in their substance of fat droplets.

FAUCES is the somewhat narrowed opening between the mouth and throat. It is bounded above by the soft palate, below by the tongue, and on either side by the tonsil. In front of, and behind, the tonsil are two ridges of mucous membrane, the anterior and posterior pillars of the fauces.

FAVISM is a haemolytic anaemia, attacks of which occur within an hour or two of eating broad beans (*Vicia fava*). It is a hereditary disease due to lack of an essential enzyme called glucose-6-phosphate dehydrogenase which plays an important part in the metabolism of glucose and is necessary for the continued integrity of the red cell. This defect is inherited as a sex-linked dominant trait, and the red cells of patients with this abnormality have a normal life span until challenged by certain drugs or fava beans when the older cells are rapidly destroyed, resulting in haemolytic anaemia. Fourteen per cent of American Negroes are affected and 60 per cent of Yemenite Jews in Israel. The perpetuation of the gene is due to the greater resistance against malaria that it carries. Severe and even fatal haemolysis has followed the administration of the antimalarial compounds pamaquine and primaquine in sensitive individuals. These red cells are sensitive not only to fava beans and primaquine but also to sulphonamides, acetanilide, phenacetin, para-aminosalicyclic acid, nitrofurantoin, probenecid and vitamin K analogues.

FAVUS is another name for honeycomb ringworm. (See RINGWORM.)

FEBRILE: Having a fever. Describes a patient whose body temperature is greater than normal (36·9–37·8 °C).

FEMINIZATION: The development of a feminine appearance in a man, often the result of an imbalance in the sex hormones.

FEMORAL: Appertaining to the femur or the region of the thigh. Thus named are the femoral nerve, artery, vein, and canal.

FEMUR is the bone of the thigh, and is the longest and strongest bone in the body. As the upper end is set at an angle of about 120 degrees to the rest of the bone, and since the weight of the body is entirely borne by the two femora, fracture of one of these bones close to its upper end is a common accident in old people, whose bones are becoming brittle. The femur fits, at its upper end, into the acetabulum of the pelvis, forming the hip-joint, and, at its lower end, meets the tibia and patella in the knee-joint.

FENBUFEN (see NON-STEROIDAL ANTI-INFLAMMATORY DRUGS).

FENESTRATION is the operation whereby a new opening is made into the labyrinth of the ear. It has proved most valuable in restoring hearing to patients with otosclerosis (q.v.), particularly in young people with this disease.

FENFLURAMINE is an anorexiant drug, introduced to aid the slimming process by suppressing or reducing appetite. Although less likely to become a drug of addiction than some of the other anorexiant drugs, it is not without its risks and must only be used under skilled medical supervision. One of its disadvantages is that in some people it induces an increased frequency of dreaming or even nightmares.

FENNEL is the seed-like fruit of *Foeniculum vulgare* used as a carminative: i.e. to relieve griping, flatulence, and distension of the stomach. Fennel water used to be a popular remedy for griping.

FENOTEROL is a drug that is proving useful by inhalation in the treatment of asthma.

FERRUM is the Latin name for iron.

FERTILIZATION: The process by which male and female gametes (spermatozoa and oöcytes respectively) fuse to form a zygote which develops by a complex process of cell division and differentiation into a new individual of the species. In humans fertilization occurs in the fallopian tubes. Sperm deposited in the upper vagina traverse the cervix and uterus to enter the fallopian tube. Many sperm attempt to penetrate the zona pellucida surrounding the oöcyte, but only one is able to penetrate the oöcyte proper and this prevents any other sperm entering. Once the sperm has entered the oöcyte, their nuclei fuse before the zygote begins to divide.

FESTER is a popular term used to mean any collection or formation of pus. It is applied to both abscesses and ulcers. (See ABSCESS; ULCER; WHITLOW.)

FESTINATION is the term applied to the involuntary quickening of gait seen in some nervous diseases, especially in PARKINSONISM (q.v.).

FETISHISM: This is a form of sexual deviation in which the person becomes sexually stimulated by parts of the body, such as the feet, which are not usually regarded as erotogenic.

FETUS is the name given to the unborn child after the eight week of development. The human being, like the young of all animals, begins as a single cell, the *ovum*, in the ovary. After fertilization with a spermatozoon the ovum becomes embedded in the mucous membrane of the uterus, its covering being known as the decidua. Increase in size is rapid, and development of complexity is still more marked. The original cell divides again and again to form new cells, and these become arranged in three layers, known as the ectoderm, mesoderm, and endoderm. From the first are produced the skin, the brain and spinal cord, and the nerves; from the second the bones, muscles, blood-vessels, and connective tissues; while the third develops into the lining of the digestive system and the various glands attached to it.

The ovum produces not only the fetus but several membranes and appendages which serve it till birth, and are then cast away. The embryo develops upon one side of the ovum, its first appearance consisting of a groove, the edges of which grow up and join to form a tube, which in turn develops into the brain and spinal cord. At the same time, a part of the ovum beneath this is becoming pinched off to form the body, and within this the endoderm forms a second tube, which in time is changed in shape and lengthened to form the digestive canal. From the gut there grows out very early a process called the allantois, which attaches itself to the wall of the womb, forming later on the navel-string and afterbirth, by which nourishment is gained for growth. (See AFTERBIRTH.)

The remainder of the ovum, which within two weeks of conception has increased to about 2 mm (1/12 inch) in size, splits into an outer and inner shell, from the outer of which are developed two covering membranes, the chorion and amnion, while the inner constitutes the yolk sac, attached by a pedicle to the developing gut of the embryo. From two weeks after conception onward, the various organs and limbs appear and grow, the name of *embryo* being applied to the developing being while almost indistinguishable in appearance from the embryo of other animals, till the middle of the second month, when it begins to show a distinctly human form. After this stage it is called the *fetus*. The property of 'life' is present from the very beginning, although the movements of the fetus are not felt by the mother till the fifth month.

During the first few days after conception the eye begins to be formed, beginning as a cup-shaped outgrowth from the mid-brain, its lens being formed as a thickening in the skin. It is very soon followed by the beginnings of the nose and ear, both of which arise as pits on the surface, which increase in complexity, and are joined by nerves that grow outward from the brain. These three organs of sense have practically their final appearance as early as the beginning of the second month.

As already stated, the body closes in from behind forward, the sides growing forward from the spinal region. In the neck, the growth takes the form of five arches, similar to those which bear gills in fishes. From the first of these the lower jaw is formed, from the second the hyoid bone, all the arches uniting, and the gaps between them closing up by the end of the second month. At this time the head and neck have assumed quite a human appearance.

The digestive canal begins as a simple tube running from end to end of the embryo, but it grows in length and becomes twisted in various directions to form the stomach and bowels. From this tube also the lungs and the liver arise as two little buds, which quickly increase in size and complexity. The kidneys also appear very early, but go through several changes before their final form is reached.

The genital organs appear late. The swellings, which form the ovary in the female and the testicle (or testis) in the male, are produced in the region of the loins, and gradually descend to their final positions. The outward organs are exactly similar in the two sexes till the end of the third month, and the sex is not clearly distinguishable till late in the fourth month.

The blood-vessels appear in the ovum even before the embryo. The heart, originally double, forms as a dilatation upon the arteries which later produce the aorta. These two hearts later fuse into one. (For the circulation in the fetus, see CIRCULATION OF BLOOD.)

The limbs appear about the end of the third week as buds which increase quickly in length and split at their ends into five parts, for fingers or toes. The bones at first are formed of cartilage, in which true bone begins to appear during the third month.

The following table gives the average size and weight of the fetus at different periods:

Age	Length	Weight
4 weeks	5 mm	1·3 grams
3 months	8 to 9 cm	30 to 60 grams
5 months	15 to 25 cm	170 to 340 grams
7 months	32 to 35 cm	1360 to 1820 grams
Birth	45 to 60 cm	3200 grams

Approximate length and weight of the fetus at different periods.

FEVER is the condition of the body characterized by a rise in temperature. It is one of the most common accompaniments of diseases in general, and serves to make the distinction between *febrile* and *non-febrile* ailments.

Causes: The cause of fever is the release of an endogenous pyrogen by phagocytic cells called monocytes and macrophages. The cause of the fever is a small protein which is produced in response to a variety of infectious, immunological and neoplastic stimuli. The lymphocytes play a part in fever production because they recognize the antigen and release substances called lymphokines and these lymphokines promote the production of endogenous pyrogen. The pyrogen then acts on the thermo-regulatory centre in the hypothalamus and this results in an increase in heat generation and a reduction in heat loss, resulting in a rise in body temperature.

In many cases the fever must be regarded as only secondary to, and symptomatic of, the disordered state with which it is found associated. For example, a certain amount of fever may arise in consequence of some nervous shock. But there is a large class of diseases in which fever is the predominant factor, and which arise from the formation in the system of something of the nature of a poison (toxin), upon which all the symptoms depend. To such diseases, the term primary or specific fevers is applied; they include typhoid fever, scarlet fever, diphtheria. These diseases depend on the growth of bacteria in the blood or tissues of the body, the toxins being formed by the activity of these organisms.

In considering the general subject of fever, regard must be had in particular to the two main features of the febrile process: the abnormal elevation of temperature, and the changes affecting the tissues of the body in reference thereto.

The average temperature of the body in health ranges between 36·9 and 37·5 °C (98·4 and 99·5 °F). It is liable to slight variations from such causes as the ingestion of food, the amount of exercise, the menstrual cycle, and the temperature of the surrounding atmosphere. There are, moreover, certain appreciable daily variations, the lowest temperature being between the hours of 01.00 and 07.00 hours, and the highest between 16.00 and 21.00 hours, with trifling fluctuations during these periods. (See TEMPERATURE.)

The development and maintenance of heat within the body are generally regarded as depending on the destructive oxidation of all its tissues, consequent on the changes continually taking place in the processes of nutrition. In health this constant tissue disintegration is exactly counterbalanced by the introduction of food, whilst the uniform normal temperature is maintained by the due adjustment of the heat thus developed, and of the processes of exhalation and cooling which take place, especially from the lungs and skin. In the febrile state this relationship is no longer preserved, the tissue waste being greatly in excess of the food supply, while the so-called 'law of temperature' is in abeyance. In this condition the body wastes rapidly, the loss to the system being chiefly in the form of nitrogen compounds (eg. urea). In the early stage of fever a patient excretes about three times the amount of urea that he would excrete on the same diet if he were in health – the difference being that in the latter condition he discharges a quantity of nitrogen equal to that taken in with the food, whilst in the fevered state he wastes the store of nitrogen contained in the tissues and the blood. The amount of fever is estimated by the degree of elevation of the temperature above the normal standard. When it reaches as high a point as 41·1 °C (106 °F) the term hyperpyrexia (excessive fever), is applied, and is regarded as indicating a condition of danger; while, if it exceeds 41·7 or 42·2 °C (107 or 108 °F) for any length of time, death almost always results.

Symptoms: The onset of a fever is usually marked by a rigor or shivering, which may exist only as a slight but persistent feeling of chilliness, or, on the other hand, be of a violent character, and, as occasionally happens with children, find expression in the form of well-marked convulsions. Although termed the *cold stage* of fever, in this condition the temperature of the body is really increased. There are, besides, various accompanying feelings of illness, such as pain in the back, headache, sickness, thirst, and great lassitude. In all cases of febrile complaints it is of importance for the physician to note the first occurrence of shivering, which in general fixes the beginning of the attack. This stage is soon followed by the full development of the febrile condition, the *hot stage*. The skin now feels hot and dry, and the temperature, always elevated above the normal standard, will often be found to show daily variations corresponding to those observed in health – namely, a rise toward evening, and a fall in the morning. There is a relative increase in the rate of the pulse and quickness of breathing. The tongue is dry and furred; the thirst is intense, while the appetite is gone; the urine is scanty, of high specific gravity, containing a large quantity of solid matter, particularly urea, the excretion of which, as already stated, is increased in fever; while, on the other hand, certain of the saline ingredients, such as chlorides, are often diminished. The bowels are in general constipated, but they may be relaxed, especially if the gut is the primary site of infection, as in typhoid fever. The nervous system participates in the general disturbance, and sleeplessness and disquietude are common accompaniments, and there may be delirium. The wasting of the muscles, and corresponding loss of strength, may be marked, and continue even although considerable quantities of nutriment may be taken.

The decline of the fever takes place either by the occurrence of a *crisis*, i.e. a sudden termination of the symptoms, or by a more gradual subsidence of the temperature, technically termed a *lysis*. If death ensues, this is due to failure of the vital centres in the brain or of the heart, as a result of either the infection or hyperpyrexia. Such terminal failure may be gradual, the patient passing into what is sometimes known as the *typhoid state* (a condition of extreme prostration, associated with low delirium or coma). In other cases death occurs suddenly after slight exertion, as a result of the additional strain on the heart.

Certain well-marked types of fever are recognized. The term *continued fever* is applied to those forms in which the febrile temperature persists for a more or less definite period, uninterrupted by any distinct intermission till the crisis is reached. To this type belong typhus and typhoid fevers, and the eruptive fevers or exanthemata: e.g smallpox, measles, and scarlet fever. *Relapsing fever* is a form of continued fever, the chief characteristic of which is the occurrence in about a week after the crisis of a distinct relapse and repetition of all the symptoms. Occasionally second and third relapses take place.

The term *remittent* is applied to those forms of fever the course of which is interrupted by a short, usually daily, diminution of the fever, followed by a recurrence of all the symptoms. Such fevers are chiefly met in tropical climates, but occasionally continued fevers assume this form, particularly in children.

In *intermittent fever* there is a distinct periodic subsidence of the symptoms, which, according to its duration, characterizes the variety as *quotidian* (where the paroxysm recurs in twenty-four hours), *tertian* (in forty-eight hours), *quartan* (in seventy-two hours).

Treatment: Fever is a symptom, and the correct treatment is therefore that of the underlying condition. Occasionally, however, it is also necessary to try and reduce the temperature by more direct methods. For this latter purpose it will be sufficient to refer to two methods: namely, the external application of cold and the administration of antipyretic remedies. The former of these methods is accomplished by means of baths, in which the patient is placed, the water being somewhat below the febrile temperature and gradually cooled down by the addition of cold water till a temperature of from 15·5 to 21 °C (60 to 70 °F) is reached. The cooler the bath the longer the effect lasts. Sponging with cold water and the wet pack are other methods used to reduce temperature and exert a soothing influence. (See COLD, USES OF.)

Certain drugs possess the power of reducing the temperature by their action on the heat-regulating centres in the brain, thereby causing an increased loss of heat through dilatation of the blood-vessels in the skin. These drugs include sodium salicylate, aspirin and quinine.

FEVERFEW: The leaf of *Chrysanthemum parthenium* which is an old herbal treatment for the relief of fever. It has also been used for the prevention of migraine (q.v.). Its side-effects are not common, but include itching, mouth ulcers and indigestion. It should not be taken by pregnant women.

FIBRE, DIETARY (see ROUGHAGE).

FIBREOPTIC ENDOSCOPY has transformed the management of gastro-intestinal disease. In chest disease fibreoptic bronchoscopy has now replaced the rigid wide-bore metal tube which was previously used for examination of the tracheo-bronchial tree. The principle of fibreoptics is that a light from a cold light source passes down a bundle of quartz fibres to illuminate the lumen of the gastro-intestinal tract or the bronchi. The reflected light is returned to the observer's eye via the image bundle which may contain up to 20,000 fibres. The tip of the instrument can be angulated in both directions and finger-tip controls are provided for suction, air insufflation and for water injection to clear the lens or the mucosa. The oesophagus, stomach and duodenum can be visualized. Furthermore, visualization of the pancreatic duct and direct endoscopic cannulation is now possible, as is visualization of the bile duct. Fibreoptic colonoscopy can visualize the entire length of the colon and it is now possible to biopsy polyps or suspected carcinomas and to perform polypectomy. The flexible smaller fibreoptic bronchoscope has many advantages over the rigid tube and extends the range of view to all segmental bronchi and enables biopsy of pulmonary parenchyma itself. A biopsy forceps can be directed well beyond the tip of the bronchoscope itself and the more flexible fibreoptic instrument causes less discomfort to the patient.

FIBRILLATION is a term applied to rapid contraction or tremor of muscles, especially to a form of abnormal action of the heart muscle in which individual bundles of fibres take up independent action. It is believed to be due to a state of excessive excitability in the muscle associated with the stretching which occurs in dilatation of the heart. Fibrillation is distinguished as atrial or ventricular, according as the muscle of the atria or of the ventricles is affected. In atrial fibrillation the heart beats and the pulse become extremely irregular, both as regards time and force. When the atrium is fibrillating there is no significant contraction of the atrial muscle but the cardiac output is maintained by ventricular contraction. In ventricular fibrillation there is no significant contractile force so that there is no cardiac output and the patient is essentially dead. If the ventricular fibrillation takes place in hospital resuscitation and de-fibrillation can be applied and the normal cardiac function restored.

FIBRIN is a substance formed in the blood as it clots. Its formation indeed causes clotting. The substance is produced in threads. After the threads have formed a close meshwork through the blood, they contract, and produce a dense felted mass. The substance is formed not only from shed blood but also from lymph which exudes from the lymph-vessels. Thus fibrin is found in all inflammatory conditions within serous cavities like the pleura, peritoneum, and pericardium, and forms a thick coat upon the surface of the inflamed membranes. It is also found in inflamed joints, and in the lung as a result of pneumonia. (See COAGULATION.)

FIBRIN FOAM is one of a series of absorbable haemostatics introduced into surgical use. A haemostatic is a preparation which arrests bleeding, and the great advantage of an absorbable haemostatic is that it produces no irritation in the tissues into which it is introduced and that it does not need to be removed after the bleeding is arrested, but is gradually absorbed by the tissues. Fibrin foam is a spongy material which is soaked in a solution of thrombin immediately before use. Other absorbable haemostatics now in use include oxidized cellulose which is prepared as a gauze, and calcium alginate (derived from seaweed) which is prepared as a gauze and as wool. These absorbable haemostatics, which constitute a great advance in surgery, are of particular value in operations on the brain and in operations on blood-vessels and nerves.

FIBRINOGEN is the soluble protein in the blood which is the precursor of fibrin (q.v.), the substance in blood-clot.

FIBROADENOMA: A benign tumour of glandular epithelium containing fibrous elements. The commonest benign tumour of the breast, often occurring in young women.

FIBROCYSTIC DISEASE OF THE PANCREAS, (see CYSTIC FIBROSIS).

FIBROID is a term sometimes applied to tumours of the womb consisting partly of muscular and partly of fibrous tissue. (See UTERUS, DISEASES OF.)

FIBROMA is a tumour consisting of fibrous tissue. (See TUMOUR.)

FIBROSING ALVEOLITIS: In this disease there is diffuse fibrosis of the alveolar wall. This causes loss of lung volume with both forced expiratory volume and vital capacity affected but the ratio between them remaining normal. The patient complains of cough and progressive dyspnoea. Typically the patient will be cyanosed, clubbed, and have crackles in the mid and lower lung fields. Blood gases will reveal hypoxia and, in early disease, hypocapnia (due to hyperventilation). There is an association with rheumatoid arthritis (q.v.) (about ⅛ cases). Systemic lupus erythamatosis, and systemic sclerosis. Certain drugs, e.g., bleomycin, busulphan, hexamethonium, high concentrations of oxygen, and inhalation of cadmium fumes may also cause this condition.

FIBROSIS means the formation of fibrous or scar tissue, which is usually due to either infection or deficient blood supply.

FIBROSITIS, also known as MUSCULAR RHEUMATISM describes pain and muscular stiffness

and inflammation affecting the soft tissues of the arm, legs and trunk. The cause is unknown but may include immunological factors, muscular strain and psychological stress. Treatment is usually palliative.

FIBROUS DYSPLASIA is a rare disease in which areas of bone are replaced by fibrous tissue (q.v.). This renders the bone fragile and liable to fracture. It may involve only one bone, usually the thigh bone, or femur (q.v.), or several bones. This latter form of the disease may be accompanied by pigmentation of the skin and the early onset of puberty. There is another form of the disease known as cherubism because of the appearance it gives to the face, in which the abnormality of bone is confined to the upper and lower jaw-bones (the maxilla and mandible). The cause of the disease is not known.

FIBROUS TISSUE is one of the most abundant tissues throughout the body. White fibrous tissue consists of fibres of a substance known as collagen, which yields gelatine on being boiled. Between these fibres lie flattened or star-shaped cells, by which the fibres are produced. The fibres, like the cells, are of microscopic size, and are grouped into bundles which are held together by other fibres running round them. Yellow fibrous tissue is a rarer form, and consists of bundles of long yellow fibres, formed from a substance known as elastin. White fibrous tissue is very unyielding and forms sinews, ligaments, the material which binds muscle fibres together, the substance of the true skin. It is also the tissue which is laid down in the repair of wounds, or as a result of inflammation, and so forms the tissue composing a scar. It has the property of contracting and becoming denser as time goes on, and hence the puckering seen in scars, and the contraction resulting from burns and inflammation. Yellow fibrous tissue is highly elastic, and so is found in the walls of arteries, and in ligaments, like that on the back of the neck, which are often stretched. (See also ADHESION; SCAR; WOUNDS.)

FIBULA is the slender bone upon the outer side of the leg.

FILARIASIS is the name given to a group of tropical diseases in which minute Nematode worms, called filariae, are found in the blood. The estimated prevalence is 250 million cases. The most widespread of these is Bancroftian filariasis, so called after Dr Joseph Bancroft. The causative worm is *Wuchereria bancrofti*, also known as *Filaria bancrofti*. This is a threadlike worm which is transmitted by certain mosquitoes. It is named after Wucherer, who discovered microfilariae in the urine of a filarial patient in Brazil in 1866 and Bancroft, who first described the adult worms in Australia in 1876. The adult female worm measures up to 100 millimetres in length. One of the striking features of these worms is that they are found in the circulating blood in large numbers in the evening, whilst during the day they disappear from the blood-stream. Its geographical distribution is widespread in warm countries, but it is most prevalent in India. It is also found in Sri Lanka, South East Asia, China, New Guinea, tropical Africa, Egypt, many Pacific islands, and parts of the West Indies and Central and South America.

The form of filariasis produced by *W. bancrofti* is characterized by inflammation and blockage of the lymphatics. In the early stages this leads to enlargement of the lymphatic glands. There is also involvement of the testicles, which become painful and enlarged, and this is accompanied by the formation of a hydrocele. Repeated inflammation of the lymphatic vessels ultimately leads to their blockage and this is responsible for the most characteristic of the later stages of the disease – elephantiasis, i.e. gross enlargement of the lower limbs and the scrotum. This may be so marked that the leg may attain a circumference of several feet, whilst the scrotum may weigh 23 kg. Elephantiasis may occur elsewhere in the body, e.g the arms, but not very commonly. (See ELEPHANTIASIS.)

Treatment: Encouraging results are being obtained, particularly in early cases, from the use of diethylcarbamazine. Surgery is required for the treatment of elephantiasis. Prevention consists primarily of (*a*) destroying the mosquitoes which transmit the worm, and (*b*) protection of the individual against mosquito bites by the use of mosquito nets and repellents.

FINGERS consist of three bones called phalanges united by hinge-joints and strong ligaments. The thumb, like the great toe, differs from the others in having only two bones. These are bent or flexed, and straightened or extended by powerful sinews, two in front and two behind, which are brought into action by the contraction of muscles in the forearm. The sinews are enveloped in complicated synovial sheaths, through which they slide without friction, and are attached to the bases of the middle and end phalanges, back and front.

Running up each side of each finger are two small arteries and two small nerves, which supply the various structures and especially the overlying skin. The skin of the fingers is specially strong and particularly sensitive, and the end of the finger has a highly specialized part, the nail (see SKIN). Each finger is set upon a bone, the metacarpal, which lies in the substance of the hand between the finger and the carpus or wrist.

FINSEN LIGHT (see LIGHT TREATMENT).

FIRST AID: Courses of instruction in first aid comprise six to twelve sessions, each of about two hours' duration. Syllabuses of instruction are published by various organizations, the principal ones being the British Red Cross, the St John Ambulance Association, and the St Andrew's Ambulance Association. For full details reference should be made to the secretary of one of these associations: British Red Cross, 9 Grosvenor Crescent, London, SW1X 7EJ (071-235 5454); St John Ambulance, 1 Grosvenor Crescent, London, SW1X 7EF (071-235 5231, fax: 071-235 0796); St Andrew's Ambulance Association, Strachan House, 16 Torphichen Street, Edinburgh EH3 8JB (031-229 5419).

(For subjects connected with first-aid, see under BANDAGES; BURNS AND SCALDS; CONVULSIONS; FAINTING; FRACTURES; HAEMORRHAGE; POISONS; WOUNDS; APPENDIX: BASIC FIRST AID.)

FISSURE is a term applied both to clefts of normal anatomical structure and also to small narrow ulcers occurring in skin and mucous membrane. The latter type of fissure occurs especially at the corners of the mouth and at the anus. (See LIPS; RECTUM, DISEASES OF.)

FISTULA is an unnatural, narrow channel, leading from some natural cavity, such as the duct of a gland, or the interior of the bowels, to the surface. Or it may be a communication between two such cavities, where none should exist, as, for example, a direct communication between the bladder and bowel.

Cause: Sometimes a child is born with a fistula, as a result of some defect in development, for example, a fistula from the thyroid gland to the surface; but, as a rule, the cause of the formation is either disease or injury. Often, the blockage of the duct of a gland leads to a fistula and the escape of the secretion from the gland on to the surface. Thus a salivary fistula may form on the face as a result of blockage by a concretion of the salivary duct in the cheek, and saliva then runs out on the cheek instead of into the mouth. Injury may also be the cause. For example, if the pelvis is fractured, the urethra may be torn across, so that urine, instead of being properly voided, passes among the tissues, and, by a process of suppuration, gradually bursts its way out through the skin, forming a permanent urinary fistula. A fistula from the bowel or bladder occasionally arises in women as a result of injury during protracted childbirth. Disease is another cause; thus an abscess may form at the side of the lower end of the bowel, and, bursting into the bowel on one side, and through the skin on the other, forms a fistula. This fistula in ano, as it is known, forms the most important variety of fistula. The abscess which produces the fistula may be tuberculous or an acute abscess due to other micro-organisms. (See ABSCESS, ACUTE.) Sometimes a fish-bone or pin, which has been swallowed, travels through the whole digestive canal without doing damage, till it reaches this point, where it lodges and produces a fistula.

Treatment: As a rule, a fistula is extremely difficult to close, especially after it has persisted for some time. The treatment consists in an operation to restore the natural channel, be it salivary duct, or urethra, or bowel. This is effected by appropriate means in each locality, and when it is attained the fistula heals quickly under simple dressings.

Fistula in ano is a very troublesome condition, and is kept from healing by the constant entrance into it of material from the bowel. It is only to be cured by dividing the tissues which separate it from the bowel, and, each day, after the bowels move, packing the wound in such a way as to compel it to heal gradually from its deepest part. The process of healing is therefore a tedious one.

FIT is a popular name for a sudden convulsive seizure, although the term is also extended to include sudden seizures of every sort. During the occurrence of a fit of any sort the chief object should be to prevent the patient from doing any harm to himself by the convulsive movements. The person should therefore be laid flat, and the head supported on a pillow or other soft material. To prevent the tongue from being bitten, some object of moderate hardness may be placed between the teeth. (See CONVULSIONS; ECLAMPSIA; EPILEPSY; FAINTING; HYSTERIA; STROKE; URAEMIA.)

FLACCID: Relaxed or lacking in stiffness. Used to describe muscles that are not contracting (or following denervation) and organs, e.g. the penis, that are lying loose, empty, or with wrinkles. The opposite of firm or erect.

FLAIL CHEST (see FRACTURES).

FLAP: A section of tissue (usually skin) separated from underlying structures but still attached to its distal end by a pedicle through which it receives its blood supply. The free end may then be sutured into a new position to cover a defect caused by trauma or excision of diseased tissue. A free flap involves detachment of a section of tissue, often including bone and muscle, to a distant site where the artery and vein supplying it are anastomosed to adjacent vessels and the tissue is sutured into place.

FLAT-FOOT, or PES PLANUS, is a deformity of the foot in which its arch sinks down so that the inner edge of the foot comes to rest upon the ground.
Causes: Most cases occur in young people in whom the ligaments which support the arch are still soft. It also tends to develop in obese middle-aged individuals who have to stand about a great deal without actually exercising the muscles.
Symptoms: There is pain along the instep and beneath the outer ankle, the foot is stiff and broad, walking is tiresome, and the toes turn far out.
Treatment: Change of occupation to one which allows sitting is sometimes necessary. In early cases the leg muscles may be strengthened by tiptoe exercises performed for ten minutes night and morning. A pad to support the arch may have to be worn inside the shoe. In severe cases surgical correction may be necessary.

FLATULENCE means a collection of gas in the stomach or bowels. In the former case the gas is expelled from time to time in noisy eructations by the mouth; in the latter case it may produce unpleasant rumblings in the bowels, or be expelled from the anus.
Causes: When gas is found in large amount in the bowels its production is usually due to fermentation set up by bacteria. Marsh gas and hydrogen are formed from the cellulose of vegetables, sulphuretted hydrogen and carbon disulphide from eggs, peas, and other articles of diet containing much sulphur. Many cases of flatulence are much aggravated by a habit of gulping mouthfuls of air.
Treatment: Flatulence in the stomach is treated by relieving the dyspepsia which causes it. It may also be relieved, or eased, by the administration of carminatives (q.v.). In many cases the flatulence is aggravated by a nervous condition which must receive appropriate treatment. If the flatulence is due to, or aggravated by, the habit of swallowing air, the patient must, by taking a careful note of the occcasions when he does this almost unconsciously, break himself of this habit. When this is done the flatulence often passes off. In cases of intestinal flatulence, articles of diet which tend to decompose, e.g. green vegetables and starchy foods, should be avoided, and the food should be light and quickly digestible.

FLAVINE (see ANTISEPTICS).

FLEAS (see INSECTS IN RELATION TO DISEASE).

FLEXIBILITAS CEREA is an abnormal state in which the limbs remain in any position into which they are moved.

FLEXION means bending, and is a term applied either to the bending of joints or to an abnormal shape of organs.

FLEXOR: A muscle that causes bending of a limb or other body part.

FLEXURE: A bend in an organ or body part. The term is used, for example, to describe the skin on the inner aspect of the elbow or knee as in the 'hepatic flexure' of the colon.

FLIES (see INSECTS IN RELATION TO DISEASE).

FLOODING is a popular name for an excessive blood-stained discharge from the womb. (See

MENSTRUATION.) In the majority of cases flooding is the sign of a miscarriage. (See ABORTION.)

FLUCLOXACILLIN (see PENICILLIN, ANTIBIOTIC).

FLUCTUATION is a sign obtained from collections of fluid by laying the fingers of one hand upon one side of the swelling, and, with those of the other, tapping or pressing suddenly on a distant point of the swelling. The thrill communicated from one hand to the other through the fluid is one of the most important signs of the presence of an abscess, or of effusion of fluid into joints or into the peritoneal cavity.

FLUCYTOSINE is a drug that is proving of value in the treatment of certain fungal infections such as candidiasis (see CANDIDA) and cryptococcosis (q.v.).

FLUFENAMIC ACID is a drug with analgesic, anti-inflammatory and anti-pyretic actions which is proving of value in the treatment of osteoarthrosis and rheumatoid arthritis.

FLUKES are a variety of parasitic worms. (See FASCIOLIASIS.)

FLUOCINOLONE is a corticosteroid for application to the skin as a cream, lotion or ointment. It is more potent than hydrocortisone. It must not be given by mouth.

FLUORESCEIN is a dye which has the special property of absorbing blue-light energy and emitting this energy as green light. This property is made use of in examining the cornea for scratches or ulceration and it is also used to detect abnormally permeable (or leaking) blood vessels in the retina and iris – especially in diabetic retinopathy and diseases of the macula.

FLUORINE, one of the halogen series of elements. In the form of fluoride it is one of the constituents of bone and teeth. Supplementing the daily intake of fluorine diminishes the incidence of dental caries. American and British evidence indicates that people who, throughout their lives, have drunk water with a natural fluorine content of 1 part per million, have less dental caries than those whose drinking water is fluorine free. All the available evidence indicates that this is the most satisfactory way of giving fluorine, and that if the concentration of fluorine in drinking water does not exceed 1 part per million, there are no toxic effects.

FLUOROSCOPE is an apparatus for rendering X-rays visible after they have passed through the body by projecting them on a screen of calcium tungstate. The technique of using it is known as FLUOROSCOPY. It provides a method of being able to watch, for instance, the beating of the heart, or the movements of the intestine after the administration of a barium meal. (See X-RAYS.)

FLUOROURACIL is a drug that is proving of value when given intravenously, in the treatment of recurrent and inoperable carcinoma of the colon and rectum, as well as secondaries from cancer of the breast. (See CYTOTOXIC.)

FLUPENTHIXOL is a tranquilizer that is proving of value in the treatment of schizophrenia (see MENTAL ILLNESS).

FLUPHENAZINE is one of the phenothiazine derivatives of value as an anti-psychotic drug. (See NEUROLEPTICS.)

FLURAZEPAM (see BENZODIAZEPINES).

FLURBIPROFEN is a drug that is proving of value in the treatment of rheumatoid arthritis and ankylosing spondylitis. (See NON-STEROIDAL ANTI-INFLAMMATORY DRUGS.)

FLUSPIRILENE is a tranquilizer that is used in the treatment of schizophrenia (see MENTAL ILLNESS). It is given by intramuscular injection, and the effect of one injection lasts for six to fifteen days.

FLUTTER, or ATRIAL FLUTTER, is the term applied to a form of abnormal cardiac rhythm, in which the atria contract at a rate of between 200 and 400 beats a minute, and the ventricles more slowly. The abnormal rhythm is the result of a diseased heart.

FLUX means an excessive discharge from any of the natural openings of the body. 'Bloody flux' is a popular name for dysentery, 'white flux' or 'whites' for leucorrhoea.

FOETOR OF THE BREATH (see BREATH, DISORDERS OF).

FOETUS (see FETUS)

FOLIC ACID, one of the constituents of the vitamin B complex, derives its name from the fact that it is found in many green leaves, including spinach and grass. It has also been obtained from liver, kidney, and yeasts. In 1945 it was synthesized by American workers, who proposed that the chemical name should be pteroylglutamic acid. It has proved of value in the treatment of macrocytic anaemias, particularly those associated with sprue and nutritional deficiencies.

FOLIUM is the latin term for leaf: e.g. digitalis folium is digitalis leaf. (Plural: folia.)

FOLLICLE is the term applied to a very small sac or gland: e.g. small collections of adenoid tissue in the throat and the small digestive glands on the mucous membrane of the intestine.

FOLLICLE-STIMULATING HORMONE: A hormone produced by the anterior pituitary gland (see PITUITARY GLAND) which stimulates the formation of follicles in the ovary each menstrual cycle and of spermatocytes in the testis. It is under hypothalamic control and in the female there is feedback inhibition by oestrogens from the developing follicle.

FOLLICULAR HORMONE (see OESTRADIOL).

FOMENTATION (see also POULTICES) is any warm application to the surface of the body in the form of a cloth. Usually the fomentation cloth is heated by being wrung out of hot water, but the term is also applied to dry applications and to hot cloths upon which various drugs are sprinkled.

FOMITES is a term used to include all articles which have been brought into sufficiently close contact with a person sick of some infectious disease to retain the infective material and spread the disease. For example, clothes, bedding, carpets, toys, books, may all be fomites till disinfected.

FONTANELLE is the term applied to areas on the head on which bone has not yet formed. The chief of these is the anterior fontanelle, situated on the top of the head between the frontal and two parietal bones. In shape it is four-sided, about 25 mm (1 inch) square at the time of birth, gradually diminishing until it is completely covered by bone, which should happen by the age of 18 months. The pulsations of the brain can be readily felt through it. Delay in its closure is particularly found in cases of rickets, as well as in other states of defective development. The fontanelle becomes more tense than usual in acute fevers, whooping-cough, and bronchitis, and tends to bulge in cases of hydrocephalus. It becomes unusually depressed in all cases of diminished vitality, such as that due to diarrhoea or wasting from any cause.

FOOD (see BREAD; CANNED FOODS; CEREAL; DIET; DIGESTION; FAT; INFANT FEEDING; MILK; NUTRITION; PROTEIN; VITAMIN).

FOOD INTOLERANCE: Most cases of food intolerance are not due to allergy. The most common cause of an aversion to food is psychological. Patients with a history of neurotic ill health may develop an obsessional aversion first to one food and then to another. Other cases of food intolerance are due to idiosyncrasy, that is a genetic defect in the patient, such as alactasia, where the intestine lacks the enzyme that digests milk sugar with the result that individuals so affected develop diarrhoea when they drink milk. Intolerance to specific foods, as distinct from allergy, is probably quite common and may be an important factor in the aetiology of the irritable bowel syndrome.

For the diagnosis of true food allergy it is necessary to demonstrate that there is a reproducible intolerance to a specific food and then that there is evidence of an abnormal immunological reaction to it. Occasionally the allergic response may not be to the food itself but to food contaminants such as penicillin, or to food additives such as tartrazine. There may also be reactions to foods which have pharmacological effects, such as caffeine in strong coffee or histamine in fermented cheese, or such reactions may be due to the irritant effect on the intestinal mucosa, especially if it is already diseased, by highly spiced curries. Of those patients who believe that their symptoms are provoked by food, probably only two out of every ten can be shown to have a true food intolerance and one in ten to have an immunological basis which would justify the diagnosis of food allergy.

FOOD POISONING is characterized by vomiting, diarrhoea, and abdominal pain and results from eating food contaminated with metallic or chemical poisons, or certain micro-organisms, or microbial products. Alternatively, the foods may contain natural poisons (for examples, undercooked red kidney beans or fish of the scrombroid family (mackerel and tuna)). Food poisoning caused by chemical or metallic substances usually occurs rapidly, within minutes or a few hours of eating. Among micro-organisms, bacteria are the leading cause of food poisoning, particularly *Staphylococcus aureus*, *Clostridium perfringens* (formerly *Cl. welchii*), *Salmonella* spp. and *Campylobacter jejuni*.

Staphylococcal food poisoning occurs after food such as meat products, cold meats, milk, custard, and egg products become contaminated before or after cooking, usually through incorrect handling by humans who carry *S. aureus*. In the food the bacteria produce an enterotoxin, which causes the symptoms of food poisoning one to eight hours after ingestion. The toxin can withstand heat; thus subsequent cooking of contaminated food will not prevent illness.

Heat-resistant strains of *Cl. perfringens* cause food poisoning associated with meat dishes, soups, or gravy that results when dishes cooked in bulk are left unrefrigerated for prolonged periods before consumption. The bacteria are anaerobes and form spores; the anaerobic conditions in these cooked foods allow the germinated spores to multiply rapidly during cooling, resulting in heavy contamination. Once ingested, the bacteria produce enterotoxin in the intestine, causing symptoms within eight to twenty-four hours.

Many different types of Salmonella (about 2000) cause food poisoning or enteritis, from eight hours to three days after ingestion of food in which they have multiplied. *S. brendeny, S. enteritidis, S. heidelberg, S. newport* and *S. thompson* are among those commonly causing enteritis. Salmonella infections are common in domesticated animals such as cows, pigs and poultry, whose meat and milk may be infected, although the animals may show no symptoms. Duck eggs may harbour Salmonella (usually *S. typhimurium*), arising from surface contamination with the bird's faeces, and foods containing uncooked or lightly cooked hen's eggs, such as mayonnaise, have been associated with outbreaks of enteritis. The incidence of human *S. enteritidis* infection has been increasing (fifteenfold in England and Wales, from 1,101 to 15,000 cases annually between 1982 and 1987), with a sharp rise in phage type-4 isolates. A serious source of infection seems to be poultry meat and hen's eggs.

Although Salmonella are mostly killed by heating at 60 °C for 15 minutes, contaminated food requires considerably longer cooking and, if frozen, must be completely thawed beforehand, to allow even heating at a sufficient temperature.

Enteritis due to *Campylobacter jejuni* is usually self limiting, lasting one to three days. Since reporting of the disease began in 1977, in England and Wales its incidence has increased from 1,349 reports initially to 12,822 in 1982 to more than 34,500 in 1990. Outbreaks have been associated with unpasteurized milk: the main source seems to be infected poultry.

Food poisoning associated with fried or boiled rice is due to *Bacillus cereus*, whose heat-resistant spores survive cooking. An enterotoxin is responsible for the symptoms, which occur two to eight hours after ingestion and resolve after eight to twenty- four hours.

Viruses are emerging as an increasing cause of some outbreaks of food poisoning from shellfish (cockles, mussels, and oysters).

Public-health measures to control the incidence of food poisoning include agricultural aspects of food production, implementing standards of hygiene in abattoirs, and regulating the environment and process of industrial food production, handling, transportation, and storage.

FOOT is that portion of the lower limb situated below the ankle-joint. Its structure is similar to that of the hand. There are seven tarsal bones, of which the talus, supporting the leg bones, and the calcaneus, forming the heel, are the largest. The others are the navicular, three cuneiform, and the cuboid bones. Then comes a row of five metatarsal bones (known together as the metatarsus), and finally fourteen phalanges contained in the toes, the great toe having two only, while each of the others has three. The

1 perforating branches	4 medial plantar
of plantar arch	5 plantar arch
2 lateral planta	6 plantar metatarsal
3 posterior tibial	7 adductor hallucism

Arteries of the foot.

arrangement of the arteries and nerves is similar to the found in the hand and fingers.

The arch of the foot is a most important structure. The bones are so arranged that the sole is hollow both from before back and from side to side. In walking, the outer edge only, at the middle of the sole, should touch the ground. The arch is further supported by a short plantar ligament situated in the hollow of the arch, running from the calcaneus to the cuboid bone, and by a long plantar ligament situated nearer the surface. It is also slung up by two sinews on either side, coming from muscles in the leg, the two tibial muscles on the inner side, and the two peroneal muscles on the outer side. When this arch gives way, flat-foot (q.v.) is the result.

1 calcanean tuberosity	7 intermedial
2 calcanus	8 medial
3 cuboid	9 lateral
4 metatarsals	10 navicular
5 5 phalanges	11 talus
6 cuneiforms	

Bones of the foot as seen from above (i.e. superior aspect).

For diseases of the foot see BONE, DISEASES OF; CHAFING OF THE SKIN; CHILBLAIN; CLAW-FOOT; CLEFT-FOOT; CLUB-FOOT; CORNS AND BUNIONS; DROP-FOOT; FLAT-FOOT; GOUT; HALLUX RIGIDUS; HALLUX VALGUS; MALLET TOE; METATARSUS for metatarsus varus; METATARSALGIA; NAILS, DISEASES OF.

FORAMEN is the Latin term for a hole. It is especially applied to natural openings in bones, such as the foramen magnum, the large opening in the base of the skull through which the brain and spinal cord are continuous.

FORCED DIURESIS: A means of encouraging the renal excretion of a compound by altering the pH and increasing the volume of the urine. Occasionally used after drug overdoses, but potentially dangerous, and so only suitable where proper intensive monitoring of the patient is possible. Excretion of acid compounds, such as salicylates, can be encouraged by raising the pH of the urine to 7·5–8·5 by the administration of an alkali such as bicarbonate (forced alkali diuresis) and that of bases, such as amphetamines (q.v.), by lowering the pH of the urine to 5·5–6·5 by giving an acid such as ammonium chloride (forced acid diuresis).

FORCED FEEDING (see GAVAGE).

FORCEPS: Surgical instruments with a pincerlike action which are used for grasping objects firmly. There are many different designs for different uses. Obstetric forceps are designed to fit around the infant's head and allow traction to be applied to aid its delivery.

FORENSIC MEDICINE: That branch of medicine concerned with matters of law and the solving of crimes, for example, by determining the cause of a death in suspicious circumstances or identifying a criminal by examining tissue found at the scene of a crime.

FORESKIN (see PREPUCE).

FORGETFULNESS in many people is inborn; in others it arises as the result of some disease. Memory involves the mental retention of an event and its reproduction (see MEMORY).

Forgetting may sometimes be an active process. Painful memories may be repressed out of consciousness, and, buried in the 'unconscious mind', may be the source of anxiety and neurotic behaviour.

There are certain changes in which memory becomes impaired. Chief among these is old age. (See AGE, NATURAL CHANGES IN.) Dementia and concussion may also produce loss of memory. (See BRAIN, DISEASES AND INJURIES OF; MEMORY.)

FORMALDEHYDE: The *British Pharmacopoeia* preparation, Formaldehyde Solution, also known as FORMALIN, contains 34 to 38 per cent formaldehyde in water. It is a powerful antiseptic, and has also the power of hardening the tissues. The vapour is very irritating to the eyes and nose.

Uses: For disinfection it is largely used in the form of a spray. It can also be vaporized by heat. One of its advantages is that it does not damage metals or fabrics. In 3 per cent solution in water it is used for the treatment of warts on the palms of the hands and the soles of the feet.

FORMULARY: A list of formulae used as drugs and other medical preparations.

FOSSA is a term applied to various depressions or holes, both on the surface of the body and in internal parts, such as the iliac fossa in each lower corner of the abdomen, and the fossae within the skull which lodge the different parts of the brain.

FOVEA: A small depression. In the eye this is an area near the fundus which contains predominantly cones and is the area with greatest visual acuity (see EYE; VISION).

FOXGLOVE (see DIGITALIS).

FRACTURES occur when there is a break in the continuity of the bone. This happens either as a result of violence or because the bone is unhealthy and unable to withstand normal stresses.

Simple fracture refer to fractures where the skin remains intact or merely grazed. *Compound fractures* have at least one wound which is in communication with the fracture which means that bacteria can enter the fracture site and cause infection. A compound fracture is also more serious because there is greater potential for blood loss. Compound fractures usually need hospital admission, antibiotics and careful reduction of the fracture. Debridement (cleaning and excising dead tissue) in a sterile theatre may also be necessary.

The type of fracture depends on the force which has caused it. Direct violence occurs when an object hits the bone often causing a transverse break – which means the break runs horizontally across the bone.

Indirect violence occurs when a twisting injury to the ankle, for example, breaks the calf bone (the tibia) higher up. The break may be more oblique. A fall on the outstretched hand may cause a break at the wrist, in the humerus or at the collar-bone depending on the force of impact and age of the person.

Fatigue fractures occur after the bone has been under recurrent stress. A typical example is the March fracture of the second toe which army recruits suffer from after long marches.

Pathological fractures occur in bone which is

already diseased, for example, by osteoporosis in post-menopausal women. A woman has a one-in-two chance of suffering from an osteoporotic fracture in her lifetime. These fractures are typically crush fractures of the vertebrae, fractures of the neck of the femur, and Colles fractures (wrist). Pathological fractures also occur in bone which has secondary-tumour deposits.

Greenstick fractures occur in young children whose bones are soft and bend in response to stress rather than break. The bone tends to buckle on the side opposite to the force. These fractures heal quickly but still need any deformity corrected and plaster of Paris to maintain the correction.

Complicated fractures involve damage to important soft tissue such as nerves, blood vessels or internal organs. In these cases the soft-tissue damage needs as much attention as the fracture site.

Comminuted fractures occur when a fracture has more than two fragments. It usually means the injury was more violent and that there is more risk of vessels and nerves' being damaged. These fractures are unstable and take longer to unite. Rehabilitation tends to be protracted.

Depressed fractures are most commonly found in skull fractures. A fragment of bone is forced inwards so that it lies lower than the level of the bone surrounding it. It may damage the brain beneath it.

Hair-line fractures occur when the bone is broken but the force has not been severe enough to cause visible displacement. These fractures may be easily missed.

Symptons and signs: The fracture site is usually painful, swollen and deformed. There is asymmetry of contour between limbs. The limb is held uselessly. If the fracture is in the upper limb, the arm is usually supported by the patient, if it is in the lower limb the patient is not able to bear weight on it. The limb may appear short because of muscle spasm.

Examination may reveal crepitus – a bony grating – at the fracture site. The diagnosis is confirmed by radiography.

Healing of fractures (union) begins with the bruise around the fracture's being resorbed and new bone-producing cells and blood vessels migrating into the area. Within a couple of days they form a bridge of primitive bone across the fracture. This is called *callus*.

The callus is replaced by woven bone which gradually matures as the new bone remodels itself. Treatment of fractures is designed to ensure this process occurs with minimal residual deformity to the bone involved.

Treatment is initially to relieve pain and may involve temporary splinting of the fracture site. Reducing the fracture means restoring the bones to their normal position and this is particularly important at the site of joints where any small displacement may limit movement considerably. A Potts fracture at the ankle joint, for example, may also lead to early osteoarthritis if the congruity of the joint is not fully restored.

In children it is possible to accept a higher degree of deformity at the fracture site because childrens' bones re-model so well.

Reduction may be done under a general anaesthetic which relaxes muscles and makes manipulation easier. Traction, which means sustained but controlled pulling on the bone, then restores the fragments of the fracture into their normal position. They are then kept in position with plaster of Paris. If closed traction does not work, then open reduction of the fracture may be needed. This may involve fixing the fracture with internal-fixation methods, using metal plates, wires or screws.

This holds the fracture site in a rigid position with the two ends closely opposed. The system developed by the Association for the Study of Internal Fixation (ASIF) has changed the philosophy of fracture healing by encouraging early mobilization after fractures.

External fixators are usually metal devices applied to the outside of the limb to support the fracture site. They are useful in compound fractures where internal fixators are at risk of becoming infected.

Consolidation of a fracture means that repair is complete. The time taken for this depends on the age of the patient, the bone and the type of fracture. A wrist fracture may take six weeks, a femoral fracture three to six months in an adult.

Complications of fractures are fairly common. In *non-union* the fracture does not unite usually because there has been too much mobility around the fracture site. Treatment may involve internal fixation. *Mal-union* means that the bone has healed with a persistent deformity and the adjacent joint may then develop early osteoarthritis. Sudeck's atrophy typically occurs after the plaster of Paris cast has been removed from Colles fractures of the wrist. The fingers remain swollen and the wrist is tender. It tends to resolve after six months.

Myositis ossificans commonly occurs at the elbow after a fracture. A big mass of calcified material develops round the fracture site which restricts elbow movements. Late surgical removal (after six to twelve months) is recommended.

Fractured neck of femur (q.v.) typically affects elderly women after a trivial injury. The bone is usually osteoporotic. The leg appears short and is rotated outwards. Usually the patient is unable to put any weight on the affected leg and is in extreme pain. The fractures are classified under Garden's classification which identifies the fractures most likely to result in cutting off the blood supply to the femoral head. Most of these fractures of the neck of femur need fixing by metal plates or hip replacements as immobility in this age group has a mortality of nearly 100 per cent.

In fractures of the *spinal column* (q.v.) mere damage to the bone, as in the case of the so-called compression fracture, in which there is no damage to the spinal cord, is not necessarily serious. If, however, the spinal cord is damaged, as in the so-called fracture dislocation, the accident may be a very serious one, the usual result being paralysis of the parts of the body below the level of the injury. Therefore the higher up the spine is fractured, the more serious the consequences. The injured person should not be moved till skilled assistance is at hand, or, if he must be removed, this should be done on a rigid shutter or door, not on a canvas stretcher or rug, and there should be no lifting which necessitates bending of the back. In such an injury an operation designed to remove a displaced piece of bone and free the spinal cord from pressure is often necessary and successful in relieving the paralysis. Dislocation or subluxation (q.v.) of the spine is not uncommon in certain sports, particularly rugby. Anyone who has had such an injury in the cervical spine (i.e. in the neck) should be strongly advised not to return to any form of body-contact sport or vehicular sport.

Simple fissured fractures and depressed fractures of the skull often follow blows or falls on the head, and may not be serious, though there is always a risk of damage which is potentially serious to the brain at the same time.

Injury to the spine: compression fracture with no involvement of spinal cord. Dotted lines indicate outline of undamaged spinal cord.

Injury to the spine: fracture dislocation with cord involvement. Dotted lines indicate outline of damaged spinal cord.

Compound fractures may result in infection within the skull, and if the skull is extensively broken and depressed, surgery is usually required to check any intercranial bleeding or to relieve pressure on the brain. Another risk of fracture is that some of the small arteries on the inner surface of the skull may be torn and may bleed, thus causing compression of the brain. For this reason also the skull is often trephined (q.v.).

JAW: The lower jaw is often fractured by a blow on the face. There is generally bleeding from the mouth, the gum being torn. Also there are pain and grating sensations on chewing, and unevenness in the line of the teeth. The treatment is simple, the line of teeth in the upper jaw forming a splint, against which the lower jaw is bound, with the mouth closed.

FRAMYCETIN is an antibiotic derived from *Streptomyces decaris*. It is active against a wide range of organisms, when taken by mouth or applied locally in infections of the skin.

FRECKLES, or SUMMER-SPOTS, are small yellow or brown spots which appear on the exposed parts of the body during hot or windy weather. They appear especially in people with fair skin and red hair. They consist of small pigmented areas in the deeper part of the epidermis, which are stimulated to increased development by exposure.

FREMITUS is a sensation which is communicated to the hand of an observer when it is laid upon the chest in certain diseases of the lungs and heart. Friction fremitus is a grating feeling communicated to the hand by the movements of lungs or heart when the membrane covering them is roughened, as in pleurisy or pericarditis. Vocal fremitus means the sensation felt by the hand when a person speaks; it is increased when the lung is more solid than usual. The 'thrills' felt over a heart affected by valvular disease are also varieties of fremitus.

FREUD'S THEORY is the term applied to a theory that emotional and allied diseases are due to a psychic injury or trauma, generally of a sexual nature, which did not produce an adequate reaction when it was received and therefore remains as a subconscious or 'affect' memory to trouble the patient's mind. As an extension of this theory Freudian treatment consists in encouraging the patient to tell everything that happens to be associated with trains of thought which lead up to this memory, thus securing a 'purging' of the mind from the original 'affect memory' which is the cause of the symptoms. This form of treatment is also called psychocatharsis or abreaction. The general term, psychoanalysis, is applied, in the first place, to the *method* of helping the patient to recover buried memories by free association of thoughts. In the second place, the term is applied to the body of psychological knowledge and theory accumulated and devised by Sigmund Freud (1856–1939) and his followers. The term 'psychoanalyst' should be applied only to those who have had a strict Freudian training, not to anyone who happens to practise psychotherapy.

FRIARS' BALSAM (see BALSAMS).

FRICTION is the name given either to the fremitus felt, or to the grating noise heard, when two rough surfaces of the body move over one another. It is characteristically obtained over the chest in cases of dry pleurisy.

FRIEDREICH'S ATAXIA is a hereditary disease resembling locomotor ataxia, and due to degenerative changes in nerve tracts and nerve cells of the spinal cord and the brain. It occurs usually in children, or at any rate before the twentieth year of life, and affects often several brothers and sisters. Its chief symptoms are unsteadiness of gait, with loss of the knee jerks, followed later by difficulties of speech, tremors of the hands, head, and eyes, deformity of the feet, and curvature of the spine. There is often associated heart disease. The sufferer gets gradually worse, but may live, more or less helpless, for twenty or thirty years.

FRÖHLICH'S SYNDROME is a condition in children characterized by obesity, physical sluggishness, and retarded sexual development. It is the result of disturbed pituitary function.

FRONTAL BONE is the bone which forms the forehead and protects the frontal lobes of the brain. Before birth, the frontal bone consists of two halves, and this division may persist throughout life, a deep groove remaining down the centre of the forehead. Above each eye is a heavy ridge in the bone, most marked in men, and, behind this, in the substance of the bone, is a cavity on each side, the frontal sinus, which communicates with the nose. Catarrh in these cavities produces the frontal headache characteristic of a 'cold in the head', and suppuration may occur in them, producing discharge from the nose. (See NOSE, DISEASES OF.)

FRONTAL LOBE: The anterior part of the cerebral hemisphere as far back as the central sulcus. It contains the motor cortex and the parts of the brain concerned with personality, behaviour and learning. (See BRAIN.)

FROSTBITE results from the action of extreme cold. In mild cases, the condition sometimes known as frostnip, the skin on exposed parts of the body, such as the cheeks or nose, becomes white and numb with a sudden and complete cessation of cold and discomfort. In more severe cases blisters develop on the frozen part, and the skin then gradually hardens and turns black until the frozen part, such as a finger, is covered with a black shell of dead tissue. Swelling of the underlying tissue occurs and this is accompanied by throbbing and aching. If, as is often the case, only the skin and the tissues immediately under it are frozen, then in a matter of months the dead tissue peels off, leaving behind it shiny red babyskin, as it is known, which at first is exquisitely tender. In the most severe cases of all, muscles, bone and tendon are also frozen, and the affected part becomes cold, swollen, mottled and blue or grey. There may be no blistering in these severe cases. At first there is no pain, but in time shooting and throbbing pains usually develop.

Prevention: This consists of wearing the right clothing and never venturing on even quite short expeditions in cold weather, particularly on mountains, without taking expert advice as to what should be worn.

Treatment: Frostnip is the only form of frostbite that should be treated on the spot. As it usually occurs on exposed parts, such as the face, each member of the party should be on the look out for it in the other. The moment whitening of the skin is seen, the individual should seek a place sheltered from the wind, or turn his back on the wind, and warm the affected part by covering it with his warm hand or a glove until the normal colour and consistency of the affected part are restored. In more severe cases treatment should only be given in hospital or a well-equipped camp. In essentials this consists of warming the affected part, preferably in a container filled with water at 44 °C. This temperature must not be exceeded. If there is no thermometer available, the alternative is a normal unfrostbitten finger. If the water is too hot for comfort, then cold water should be added. If no container is available, the alternative is hot water poured over towels or a cloth wrapped round the affected part. Rewarming should be done for spells of twenty minutes at a time. If facilities are not available for warming in this way, the alternative is to place the affected part in contact with a warm abdomen or armpit, or held in warm air. It should never be placed near an open fire. Generalized warming of the whole body may also be necessary, and this is achieved by giving hot drinks, and putting the victim in a sleeping bag. Extra heat may be supplied by his companions lying alongside him – either in their own sleeping bags, or by one getting into the same sleeping bag. After rewarming, the part should be very gently cleaned. Blisters should not be pricked. Antibiotics may be given to reduce the risk of infection. An important point to bear in mind is that no one should be allowed to walk on a thawed, or partly thawed, foot, as this will almost certainly do irreparable damage. On the other hand, walking on frostbitten feet for a period does not appear to increase the liability to further damage.

The treatment of frostbite which has resulted in gangrene is given under GANGRENE.

FROZEN SHOULDER is a painful condition of the shoulder accompanied by stiffness and considerable limitation of movement. The usual age-incidence is between 50 and 70. The cause is not known. There is no specific treatment, but there is practically always complete recovery, even though this may take twelve to eighteen months.

FRUCTOSE is another name for laevulose, or fruit sugar, which is found along with glucose in most sweet fruits. It is sweeter than sucrose (cane or beet sugar) and this has led to its use as a sweetener.

FRUSEMIDE is a potent diuretic (q.v.) with a rapid onset (30 minutes), and short duration, of action. (See BENZOTHIADIAZINES, DIURETICS.)

FUGUE literally means flight and it is used to describe the mental condition in which an individual is suddenly seized with an unconscious motivation to flee from some intolerable reality of everyday existence. This usually involves some agonizing interpersonal relationship. As a rule, it lasts for a matter of hours or days, but may go on for weeks or even months. During the fugue the individual seldom behaves in a particularly odd manner though he may be considered somewhat eccentric. When it is over there is no remembrance of events during the fugue.

FUMIGATION is a means of disinfection by the vapour of powerful antiseptics. (See DISINFECTION).

FUNCTIONAL DISEASES (see PSYCHOSOMATIC DISEASES).

FUNDUS: (1) The base of an organ or that part remote from its opening. (2) Point on the retina opposite the pupil through which nerve fibres and blood vessels traverse the retina (see EYE).

FUNGAL DISEASES: Infections caused by fungal organisms (see FUNGUS; MICROBIOLOGY).

FUNGUS: A simple plant that is parasitic on other plants and animals. Included in this group are mildews, moulds, mushrooms, toadstools and yeasts. Unlike other plants they do not contain the green pigment chlorophyll. Most of the world's 100,000 different species are harmless or even beneficial to humans. Yeasts are used in the preparation of food and drinks and antibiotics are obtained from some fungi. A few, however, can cause fatal disease and illness in humans.

FUNGUS-POISONING: Several diseases are due to the growth of minute fungi in the tissues of the body; for example, actinomycosis (caused by the ray-fungus), ringworm, and Madura foot of India. As to the large fungi, or mushrooms as they are often called, although they grow in dead and decaying material, they do not infest the living body, but many of them contain a poisonous alkaloid known as muscarine, others a body called phallin, both of which are poisons when swallowed. About 2000 of these larger fungi grow in England, of which 200 are edible. There are about a dozen which are classified as poisonous, but several of these cause no more than indigestion. The most poisonous of all is the 'death cap' or *Amanita phalloides*. In the USA it is responsible for over 90 per cent of deaths from mushroom poisoning. The fatal dose is three mushrooms (50 grams), and one in three cases proves fatal. The distinguishing features of this fungus are that it has a yellowish green cup, the gills are white and at the base of the stem, or stalk, there is a cup, or volva. These features distinguish it from the common edible mushroom (*Psalliota campestris*), which has brownish purple gills and no cup at the base of the stem. Other poisonous mushrooms include *Amanita virosa, Amanita vernu,* and *Amanita muscaria*. Deaths from mushroom poisoning are rare in England but more common in Continental Europe. Many fungi cause gastrointestinal irritation without being dangerously toxic.

Symptoms: There is usually a latent period of 8 to 12 hours before the onset of symptoms. Initially these consist of severe abdominal pain, vomiting and violent diarrhoea. These usually respond to treatment but in serious cases are followed in 2 or 3 days by the onset of jaundice, circulatory failure, failure of the kidneys, and widespread haemorrhage, leading on in fatal cases to liver failure and death.

Treatment: The first thing to do is to wash out the stomach. A duodenal tube is then passed into the duodenum, the contents of which are aspirated every hour. This is done as it has been shown that the poisonous toxins accumulate here for up to 36 hours. Addition of charcoal to the washing-out fluid is useful as it binds the toxins. Ample fluids must be given to compensate for the fluid lost in the vomiting and stools. Drugs that are given to counteract the effect of the toxins include penicillin, and silymarin, which is prepared from milk thistle (*Silybum marianum*). In all serious cases atropine should be administered, since it forms a direct antidote to muscarine.

FURUNCLE is another name for a boil. (See BOILS.)

FUSIDIC ACID is an antibiotic derived from the fermentation products of the fungus, *Fusidium coccineum*. It is particularly active against staphylococci, including those which are resistant to penicillin.

G

GABA: Gamma aminobutyric acid is an amino acid that occurs in the central nervous system, mainly in the brain tissue. It is a chemical substance that transmits inhibitory impulses from nerve endings across synapses to other nerves or tissues.

GAG: A device that when placed between a person's teeth keeps the mouth open.

GAIT, the way in which an individual walks, is an important sign of health and disease. Children, as a rule, begin to walk between the ages of twelve and eighteen months, having learned to stand before the end of the first year. If a normal-sized child shows no ability to make movements by this time the possibility of his being mentally retarded must be borne in mind, and if the power of walking is not gained by the time the child is a year and a half old, rickets, cerebral palsy, or a malformation of the hip-joint must be excluded. (See RICKETS; PARALYSIS.)

In *hemiplegia*, or paralysis down one side of the body following a stroke (q.v.), the person drags the paralysed leg.

Steppage gait occurs in certain cases of alcoholic neuritis, tertiary syphilis (tabes) and other conditions where the muscles that raise the foot are weak and the toes in consequence droop. The person bends the knee and lifts the foot high, so that the toes may clear obstacles on the ground. (See DROP-FOOT.)

In *locomotor ataxia* (q.v.) or tabes dorsalis the sensations derived from the lower limbs are blunted, and consequently the movements of the legs are uncertain and the heels planted on the ground with unnecessary force. When the person tries to turn or stands with the eyes shut he may fall over. When he walks he feels for the ground with a stick or keeps his eyes constantly fixed upon it.

In *spastic paralysis* the limbs are moved with jerks. The foot first of all clings to the ground and then leaves it with a spasmodic movement, being raised much higher than necessary.

In Parkinsonism (q.v.) the movements are tremulous, and as the person takes very short steps, he has the peculiarity of appearing constantly to fall forward, or to be chasing himself.

In *St Vitus's dance* (*chorea*) (q.v.) the walk is bizarre and jerky, the affected child often seeming to leave one leg a step behind him, and then, with a screwing movement on the other heel, go on again.

GALACTOCELE is a cyst-like swelling in the breast which forms as a result of obstruction in the milk-duct draining the swollen area.

GALACTORRHOEA is a recurrent or persisting discharge of milk from the breast.

GALACTOSAEMIA is a hereditary disease due to the lack of the enzyme which normally converts galactose, the sugar derived from lactose, or sugar-milk, into glucose. The incidence is around 1 in 75,000 births. Soon after birth the affected baby becomes jaundiced and lethargic. If he survives and is not treated, he becomes mentally retarded. Treatment consists basically of a diet free of lactose. Special lactose-free milks are now available.

GALACTOSE: A constituent of lactose, galactose is a simple sugar that is changed in the liver to glucose. A rare genetic metabolic disease, galactosaemia (q.v.), results in infants' being unable to do this conversion because the enzyme necessary for the reaction is absent.

GALL is another name for bile. (See BILE.)

GALL-BLADDER (see LIVER).

GALL-BLADDER, DISEASES OF: The gall-bladder rests on the underside of the liver and joins the common hepatic duct via the cystic duct to form the common bile duct. The gall-bladder acts as a reservoir and concentrator of bile, alterations in the composition of which may result in the formation of gall-stones, the commonest disease of the gall-bladder.

Gall-stones affect 22 per cent of women and 11 per cent of men. The incidence increases with age, but only about 30 per cent of those with gall-stones undergo treatment as the majority of cases are asymptomatic. There are three types of stone: cholesterol, pigment and mixed, depending upon their composition; stones are usually mixed and may contain calcium deposits. The cause of most cases is not clear but sometimes gall-stones will form around a 'foreign body' within the bile ducts or gall-bladder, such as suture material or the corpse of a parasite.

In *biliary colic* muscle fibres in the biliary system contract around a stone in the cystic duct or common bile duct producing pain in the right upper quarter of the abdomen, with nausea and occasionally vomiting. Gall-stones small enough to enter the common bile duct may block the flow of bile and cause *jaundice*. Blockage of the cystic duct may lead to *acute cholecystitis*; the gall-bladder wall becomes inflamed resulting in pain in the right upper quarter of the abdomen, fever and an increase in the white blood cell count. There is characteristically tenderness over the tip of the right ninth rib on deep inhalation (Murphy's sign). Infection of the gall-bladder may accompany the acute inflammation and occasionally an empyema of the gall-bladder may result. The elderly are particularly prone to complications of acute cholecystitis, including perforation of the gall-bladder and the formation of an abnormal connection with the small intestine (fistula). *Chronic cholecystitis* is a more insidious form of gall-bladder inflammation, producing non-specific symptoms of abdominal pain, nausea and flatulence which may be worse after a fatty meal.

Diagnosis of gall-stones is usually on the basis of the patients' reported symptoms, although asymptomatic gall-stones are often an incidental finding when investigating another complaint. Confirmatory investigations include abdominal radiography – although many gall-stones are not calcified and thus do not show up on these images; ultrasound scanning (see ULTRASOUND), oral cholecystography, which entails a patient's swallowing a substance opaque to X-rays which is concentrated in the gall-bladder, and endoscopic retrograde cholangiopancreatography (ERCP) – a technique in which an endoscope (q.v.) is passed into the duodenum and a contrast medium injected into the biliary duct.

Treatment of gall-stone disease is now available in several forms. Biliary colic is treated conservatively with bed rest and injection of morphine-like analgesics. Once the pain has subsided, the patient may then be referred for further treatment as outlined below. Acute cholecystitis is treated by surgical removal of the gall-bladder within 2–3 days of admission to hospital. There are two techniques available for this procedure; firstly, conventional cholecystectomy in which the abdomen is opened and the gall-bladder cut out and, secondly, laparoscopic cholecystectomy in which fibreoptic instruments called endoscopes (see FIBREOPTIC ENDOSCOPY) are introduced into the abdominal cavity via several small incisions. Laparoscopic surgery has the advantage of reducing the patient's recovery time. Gall-stones may be removed during ERCP, they can be dissolved using ultrasound waves (lithotripsy) or tablet therapy (dissolution chemotherapy), Pigment stones, calcified stones or stones larger than 15 mm in diameter are not suitable for this treatment, which is also less likely to succeed in the overweight patient. Drug treatment is prolonged but stones may disappear completely after two years. Stones may reform on stopping therapy. The drugs used are derivatives of bile salts, particularly chenodeoxycholic acid; side-effects include diarrhoea and liver damage.

Other disorders of the gall-bladder are rare. *Polyps* may form and, if symptomatic, should be removed. Malignant change is rare. *Carcinoma* of the gall-bladder is a disease of the elderly and is almost exclusively associated with gall-stones. By the time such a cancer has produced symptoms, the prognosis is bleak: 80 per cent of these patients die within one year of diagnosis. If the tumour is discovered early, 60 per cent of patients will survive five years.

GALLS, or NUTGALL, is the name of an excrescence growing upon oaks and containing a large quantity of tannic acid which gives the galls a strongly astringent action. Galls are chiefly used in the form of ointment of galls, and ointment of galls with opium, for application to bleeding piles.

1 stone in cystic duct
2 stone in Hartmann's pouch
3 gall-bladder
4 silent stones
5 ampulla of Vater
6 stone in common bile duct
7 bile duct
8 hepatic ducts

Diagram showing various positions of gall-stones.

GALL-STONES (see GALL-BLADDER, DISEASES OF.)

GAMETE is a sexual or germ cell: for example, an ovum (q.v.) or spermatozoon (q.v.).

GAMETE INTRAFALLOPIAN TRANSFER (GIFT) (see ARTIFICIAL INSEMINATION).

GAMGEE TISSUE is a surgical dressing composed of a thick layer of cotton-wool between two layers of absorbent gauze, introduced by the Birmingham surgeon, Sampson Gamgee (1828–1886).

GAMMA BENZENE HEXACHLORIDE is a drug that is used in the treatment of pediculosis (q.v.) and scabies (q.v.).

GAMMA-GLOBULIN: It has been known for a long time that the protective antibodies of the body are closely associated with the proteins of the blood. Gamma-globulin is a concentrated solution of the antibody fraction of human blood which has proved of great value in providing immunity against certain infectious diseases, particularly measles. It is of little value once the disease is begun but, if given before the disease manifests itself, it either prevents its onset or modifies its severity very considerably.

GAMMA RAYS: Short-wavelength penetrating electromagnetic rays produced by some radioactive compounds. More powerful than X-rays, they are used in certain radiotherapy (q.v.) treatments and to sterilize some materials.

GAMMEXANE is the proprietary name for a synthetic insecticide which is a formulation of benzene hexachloride. It is active against a large range of insects and pests, including mosquitoes, fleas, lice, cockroaches, house-flies, clothes moths, bed-bugs, ants, and grain pests.

GANGLION is a term used in two senses. In anatomy, it means an aggregation of nerve-cells found in the course of certain nerves (see NERVES). In surgery, it means an enlargement of the sheath of a tendon, containing fluid. The latter occurs particularly in connection with the sinews in front of, and behind, the wrist.

Causes: The cause of these dilatations on the tendon-sheaths is either some irregular growth of the synovial membrane which lines them and secretes the fluid that lubricates their move-ments, or the forcing out of a small pouch of this membrane through the sheath in conse-quence of a strain. In either case a bag-like swelling forms, whose connection with the synovial sheath becomes cut off, so that synovial fluid collects in it and distends it more and more.

Symptoms: A soft, elastic, movable swelling forms, most often on the back of the wrist. When noticed first it is perhaps the size of a pea, and its connection with a tendon can easily be made out. It may remain this size for many years and occasion no trouble at all, but generally a ganglion gives a peculiar feeling of weakness to the wrist, and on account of its size or position it may be very inconvenient. A ganglion which forms in connection with the flexor tendons in front of the wrist sometimes attains a large size, and extends down the sinews to form another swelling in the palm of the hand.

Treatment: Sudden pressure with the thumbs may often burst a ganglion and disperse its contents beneath the skin, after which it should be prevented from refilling by bandaging the part tightly, a very efficient pad being made by wrapping up a large coin in a piece of lint. If it cannot be burst, there only remains the opening of the ganglion, with scraping of its interior. As the ganglion may disappear spontaneously there should be no rush to remove it unless it is causing inconvenience or pain.

GANGRENE, or MORTIFICATION, means the death of a part of the body sufficiently large to be seen. When the process is slow and superfi-cial, only microscopic parts dying in succession, the process is called ulceration, whilst the term necrosis is usually restricted to the death of internal parts, particularly of bones. There are two varieties of gangrene, dry and moist, dry gangrene being a process of mummification, in which, as a rule, the circulation simply stops, and the part, so to speak, withers up; whilst in moist gangrene there is inflammation accom-panied by putrefactive changes. The dead part, when formed of soft tissues, is known as a slough, and, when part of a bone, is called a sequestrum.

Causes: Certain diseases which lessen the strength and vitality of the tissues throughout the body render them more liable to die when subjected to injury. Chief among these is diabetes mellitus. The nervous system, too, exerts an important influence over the nutrition and repair of the body, so that where it is diseased a quite trifling injury may produce gangrene of the injured part: for example, in paralysis bed sores are apt to form, owing to the mere pressure of the body on the bed.

Direct injury is perhaps the commonest cause. If a limb is badly crushed, or frozen, or burned by heat or powerful chemicals, it may not recover.

Interference with the nutrition of a part by the gradual closure of the arteries, which may occur in old age; by their sudden closure in Raynaud's disease, or after the eating of dis-eased rye (see ERGOT POISONING); or by pro-longed mechanical compression, may also cause it.

Infection by bacteria is another, and the most serious, cause, although fortunately it is rare and seldom occurs save in people of very low vitality. The hospital gangrene, so much dreaded by surgeons last century, belonged to this type, but is now practically unknown, thanks to aseptic surgery.

Symptoms: *Dry gangrene* usually comes on in old people with diseased arteries, and is pre-ceded by pain in the affected limb, which gradually becomes a dusky red colour and later brown and black. The line between the dead and living tissues is quite sharp (line of demar-cation), and marked by a red ring, where a slight degree of inflammation is going on. There is some smell, especially if care is not taken to keep the foot or other affected part absolutely dry. There is little or no pain after gangrene has occurred, nor any fever, and the red ring gradually deepens till the gangrenous part drops off in the course of some months.

Moist gangrene is the more common form, and is accompanied by putrefaction. The part becomes swollen, livid, and covered with blebs; later it turns bluish-green and black in places. The smell is very offensive, and much fluid is effused from the decaying tissues, speedily soaking the dressings applied. There is not much pain, but the general symptoms are apt to be very serious, and there is then high fever. In the latter case the person may die of blood-poisoning, and in any case the line of demarca-tion is not definite, and the gangrene is apt to extend up the limb.

Gas gangrene is a form which may occur when wounds are infected with soil from highly cultivated fields. Gas-producing bacilli (eg. *Clostridium welchii*) from the soil then grow with great rapidity in the wound, and the gas spreads along the spaces in the muscles and connective tissues. Some of these bacilli grow only in the absence of oxygen, so that incisions to admit the air, together with application of oxidizing agents, and the use of gas-gangrene antitoxin, check their spread. In this form speedy amputation may be necessary. Experience gained in the 1939–45 War clearly demonstrated the value of penicillin, in conjunction with surgery, in the treatment of this condition. **Treatment**: The dry form must be kept dry by wrapping in cotton-wool, and, when the line of demarcation has distinctly formed, amputation may be performed close above it. In the moist form, which is not spreading quickly, the surgeon also waits till he can see clearly how much is to become gangrenous, and an attempt is made to control any infection by means of antibiotics. The gangrenous area is left dry. When small parts, like the fingers, become gangrenous after frostbite, they may be treated by applying on lint some simple antiseptic ointment, such as boric acid ointment, containing a small amount of eucalyptus or other volatile oil, to subdue the smell. (See also FROSTBITE.)

GARGLES: Gargling is a process by which various substances in solution are brought in contact with the throat without being swallowed. The watery solutions used for the purpose are called gargles. Gargles are used in the treatment of infections of the throat: i.e. 'sore throat', pharyngitis, and tonsillitis.

GARGOYLISM, or HURLER'S SYNDROME, is a rare condition due to lack of a specific enzyme (q.v.). It is a progressive disorder usually leading to death before the age of 10 years. The affected child is usually normal during the first few months of life. Mental and physical deterioration then set in. The characteristic features include coarse facial features (hence the name of the condition), dwarfism, chest deformity, stiff joints, clouding of the cornea, enlargement of the liver and spleen, deafness, and heart murmurs, with mental deterioration. It occurs in about 1 in 100,000 births.

GAS (see ANAESTHESIA; CARBON MONOXIDE; NITROUS OXIDE GAS).

GAS GANGRENE (see GANGRENE).

GASTRECTOMY is an operation for removal of the whole or part of the stomach.

GASTRIC means anything connected with the stomach, such as gastric ulcer.

GASTRIC LAVAGE: A technique of washing out the stomach with warm water or saline to remove the contents. It is usually done when a person, often a child, has eaten something such as poisonous berries that are potentially harmful. It is also used for treating people who have taken an overdose of drugs. The procedure should be done only by an experienced nurse or doctor.

GASTRIC ULCER (see STOMACH, DISEASES OF).

GASTRIN: A hormone produced by the mucous membrane (q.v.) in the pyloric part of the stomach (q.v.). The arrival of food stimulates production of the hormone which in turn stimulates the production of gastric juice.

GASTRITIS is inflammation of the stomach. (See DYSPEPSIA.)

GASTROCNEMIUS is the large double muscle which forms the chief bulk of the calf, and ends below in the tendo calcaneus.

GASTROENTERITIS is inflammation of the stomach and intestines. Its main symptoms are vomiting and diarrhoea. (See DIARRHOEA.)

GASTROENTEROSTOMY is an operation performed usually in order to relieve some obstruction to the outlet from the stomach, and consists in making one opening in the lower part of the stomach, another in a neighbouring loop of the small intestine, and stitching the two together.

GASTROSCOPE is an instrument for viewing the interior of the stomach, by means of a special arrangement of light and mirrors attached to a hollow tube, which is introduced into the stomach via the mouth and gullet. A special camera attachment makes it possible to photograph the interior of the stomach. The modern instruments are fully flexible, transmitting an image through a fibreoptic bundle or by a small videocamera. The operator can see and photograph all areas of the stomach and also take biopsy specimens when required. (See FIBREOPTIC ENDOSCOPY.)

GASTROSTOMY is an operation on the stomach by which, when the gullet is blocked by a tumour or other cause, an opening is made from the front of the abdomen into the stomach, so that fluid food can be passed into the organ.

GAUCHER'S DISEASE is a disease characterized by abnormal storage of lipoids, particularly in the spleen, bone marrow, and liver. This results in enlargement of the spleen and the liver, particularly the former, and anaemia. It runs a chronic course. There is no curative treatment, but splenectomy (removal of the spleen) is often helpful.

GAVAGE means forced feeding by a soft rubber tube in cases when a person cannot swallow owing to weakness or other cause, or when an insane person refuses food. The tube, in the former case, is passed through the mouth into the stomach, and in the latter case a small tube is often simply passed through one nostril into the back of the throat, from which the person must automatically swallow food. By this means only liquid food, like strong soup, whipped eggs, or milk, can be administered. (See ENTERAL and PARENTERAL NUTRITION.)

GEL is the term applied to a colloid substance which is firm in consistence although it contains much water: e.g ordinary gelatin.

GELATIN is derived from collagen (q.v.), the chief constituent of connective tissue. It is a colourless transparent substance which dissolves in boiling water, and on cooling sets into a jelly. Such a jelly is a pleasant addition to the invalid diet, especially when suitably flavoured, but it is of relatively little nutritive value as not more than 1 ounce can be taken in the day: i.e. the amount required to make one pint of jelly. Although it is a protein, it is lacking in several of the vital amino-acids. The ordinary household 'stock' made from boiling bones contains gelatin. Mixed with about two and a half times its weight of glycerin, gelatin forms a soft substance used as the basis for many pastilles and suppositories.

GENERAL PARALYSIS OF THE INSANE, also known as GPI, GENERAL PARALYSIS, DEMENTIA PARALYTICA, is a late manifestation of syphilis in which both bodily and mental powers degenerate; though in some cases the bodily symptoms are for a time most marked, whilst in others the mental change appears first. The disease usually begins eight to twenty years after infection – namely, between the ages of 30 and 50 years. It is much commoner among males than among females. Occasionally it is found in adolescents, when it is due to congenital syphilis.

When a person dies in an advanced stage of the disease, certain very marked changes are found in the brain and its membranes.

Symptoms come on insidiously, as a rule, and the disease is often far advanced before it is recognized.

The first stage is characterized by slight physical symptoms, which generally escape the notice of the affected person's friends, such as tremors of the tongue and facial muscles in speaking, transient paralysis of eye muscles producing slight squint and double vision for a time, stammering over difficult words. The physical signs are apt to be masked by the peculiar state of mental exaltation which sometimes ushers in the disease. These delusions often go further and the patient believes himself to be very rich or identifies himself with some well-known personality.

Great emotionalism is another feature, and the affected person is easily excited to tears or to laughter while the memory at the same time fails and the patient becomes notably absent-minded. Important early signs, in addition to the mental excitement or mental enfeeblement,

are diminished reaction of the pupil of the eye to light, and alteration of the knee-jerks and other reflexes. In the second stage the physical weakness becomes more and more marked. The mind, too, becomes quite clouded, and unfit to sustain the simplest exercise. In the third stage the mental failure is profound, and the sufferer cannot recognize even his nearest relatives.

The whole course of the disease lasts usually only two to three years, and, though occasional remissions take place, which may prolong life to ten years or more, there is little ground for hope unless effective treatment is instituted at as early a stage as possible.

Treatment: Recognition of general paralysis at a very early stage is important. In the first place, treatment at this stage affords considerable prospect of stopping the progress of the disease. In the second place, the person suffering from an early stage of this disease is liable through mental weakness to transact his affairs badly. The most effective form of treatment is penicillin, particularly if given early enough.

In the late stages of GPI the patient's mental condition is such that residential care is either desirable or necessary.

GENERAL PRACTITIONER: The doctor who provides primary medical care and is usually the initial contact for a person who is seeking treatment. In the National Health Service the general practitioner (GP) or family doctor provides 90 per cent of the medical care for the population. Most illnesses are treated by the GP and, except when emergency patients go direct to hospital, he or she advises whether a patient should see a specialist. This gatekeeper function in the NHS helps to ensure that expensive hospital facilities are used only by those patients who really need them. GPs usually see patients in their surgeries but will also visit them at home when necessary. Around 70 per cent of GPs, of whom there are over 33,000 in the United Kingdom, work in partnerships of two or more, covering each other's work, and on average they each look after 1,900 patients. They are responsible to local family health service authorities (q.v.) and are paid in part by capitation fees according to the number of patients registered with them and in part by item of service fees. Almost every person in the country is registered with a GP, who is also allowed to do private practice.

GENERIC DRUG: A medicinal drug that is sold under its official (generic) name instead of its proprietary (patented brand) name. NHS doctors are advised to prescribe generic drugs where possible as this enables any suitable drug to be dispensed, saving delay to the patient and the sometimes expense to the NHS.

GENES, of which there are more than 100,000 in a human being, are the biological units of heredity. They are arranged along the length of the chromosomes (q.v.). (See HEREDITY.)

DOMINANT GENES: A dominant characteristic is an effect which is produced whenever the gene is present. If a disease is due to a dominant gene those affected are heterozygous, that is they only carry the gene in one of the pair of chromosomes concerned. Affected people married to normal individuals transmit the gene directly to one half of the children. In the ABO blood group system A and B are dominant over O. Huntington's chorea is due to the inheritance of a dominant gene, as is neurofibromatosis. Another dominantly inherited condition is multiple polyposis of the colon. Haemolytic disease of the newborn, due to Rhesus (Rh) incompatibility, is the commonest genetically determined disease in this country. The Rh antigen is a dominant characteristic which in haemolytic disease of the newborn is inherited from the father. The mother, being Rh negative, may develop antibodies against antigen present in the fetal red cells if they enter the maternal circulation and these antibodies may give rise to the disease in the fetus.

Achondroplasia is an example of a dominant mutation, for the majority of affected people have normal parents and siblings. However the chances of the children of a parent with achondroplasia being affected are one in two, as with any other dominant characteristic. Other diseases inherited as dominant characteristics include spherocytosis, haemorrhagic telangiectasia and polycystic kidney. Further examples are listed below:

RECESSIVE GENES: If a disease is due to a recessive gene, those affected must have the gene on both members of the chromosome pair (ie. be homozygous). The possession of a single recessive gene does not result in overt disease and the bearer usually carries this potentially unfavourable gene without knowing it. If he marries another carrier of this recessive gene there is a one in four chance that their children will receive the gene in double dose and so have the disease. If an individual sufferer from a recessive disease marries an apparently normal person who is a heterozygous carrier of the same gene, one half of the children will be affected and the other half will be carriers of the disease. The commonest of such recessive conditions in Britain is fibrocystic disease of the pancreas, which affects about one child in two thousand. It can be calculated that 5 per cent of the population must carry the gene.

Most of the inborn errors of metabolism, such as phenylketonuria, galactosaemia and congenital adrenal hyperplasia, are due to recessive genes. Further examples are listed above. There are characteristics which may be incompletely recessive, that is, neither completely dominant nor completely recessive and the heterozygote, who bears the gene in a single dose, may have a slight defect whilst the homozygote, with a double dose of the gene has a severe illness. There are certain mild bony defects in the heterozygote such as the shortening of the middle phalanx of the second finger and toes in brachy- phalangia which results in gross deformity of the skeleton in the homzygote.

The sickle cell trait is a result of the sickle cell gene in single dose and sickle cell anaemia is the consequence of a double dose. Thalassaemia minor and major demonstrate a similar incompletely recessive characteristic.

SEX-LINKED GENES: If a condition is sex-linked, affected males are homozygous for the mutated gene as they carry it on their single X chromosome. The X chromosome carries many genes while the Y chromosome bears few genes, if any, other than those determining masculinity. The genes on the X chromosome of the male are thus not matched by corresponding genes on the Y chromosome. There is thus no chance of the Y chromosome neutralizing any recessive trait on the X chromosome. A recessive gene can therefore produce disease since it will not be suppressed by the normal gene of the homologous chromosome. The same recessive gene on the X chromosome of the female will be suppressed by the normal gene on the other X chromosome. Such sex-linked conditions include haemophilia, Christmas disease, the severe form of Duchenne type of muscular dystrophy and nephrogenic diabetes insipidus. If the mother of an affected child has another male relative affected she is a heterozygote carrier; half her sons will have the disease and half her daughters will be carriers. The sister of a haemophiliac thus has a 50-per-cent chance of being a carrier. An affected male cannot transmit the gene to his son because the X chromosome of the son must come from the mother; all his daughters however will be carriers as the X chromosome of the father must be transmitted to all his daughters. Hence sex-linked recessive characteristics cannot be passed from father to son. Sporadic cases may be the result of a fresh mutation in which case the mother is not a carrier and is not likely to have further affected children. It is probable that one-third of haemophiliacs arise as a result of mutation and these patients will be the first in their families to be affected. Sometimes the carrier of a sex-linked recessive gene can be identified. A proportion of haemophilia carriers reveal haematological abnormalities and carriers of the sex-linked variety of retinitis pigmentosa can be detected by ophthalmoscopic examination.

A few rare disorders are due to dominant genes carried on the X chromosome. An example of such a condition is familial hypophosphataemia with vitamin D resistant rickets. Glucose phosphate dehydrogenase deficiency is due to a sex-linked incompletely dominant gene.

Many hundreds of conditions are due to mutations of genes on the autosomes and more than sixty conditions are due to gene mutations on the X chromosomes. Gene mutations duplicate themselves at cell division in the same way as normal genes. As a result of these mutations a number of alternative forms for a given gene exist and these are called alleles. In many inherited conditions the disease is due to the combined action of several genes and the genetic element is then called multi-factorial. In this situation there will be an increased incidence of the disease in the families concerned but it will not follow the Mendelian ratio. The greater the number of independent genes involved in determining a certain disease, the more complicated will be the pattern of inheritance. Furthermore, many inherited disorders are the result of a combination of genetic and environmental influences. Diabetes mellitus is the most familiar example of such multifactorial inheritance. The predisposition to develop diabetes is an inherited recessive character although the gene is not always able to express itself: this is called incomplete penetrance. Whether or not the individual with the genetic predisposition towards the disease actually develops diabetes will also depend on environmental factors. Diabetes is more common in the relatives of diabetic patients and even more so amongst identical twins. However as the incidence of diabetes amongst the children of marriages between diabetic patients is well below 100 per cent, the gene does not receive complete functional expression. Non-genetic factors which are of importance in precipitating overt disease are obesity, excessive intake of carbohydrate foods and pregnancy. The influence of diet was made apparent during the two world wars when the mortality rate for diabetes mellitus showed a fall throughout Europe.

Schizophrenia is another example of the combined effects of genetic and environmental influences in precipitating disease. The risk of schizophrenia in a child, one of whose parents has the disease, is one in ten, but this figure is modified by the early environment of the child.

The capacity of genes for replication has recently been explained in terms of the structure of the deoxyribonucleic acid (DNA) molecule, which consists of a long double spiral with thousands of mononucleotides, each containing sugar, phosphoric acid and bases. A single change in the base sequence causes a permanent change in genetic information and provides a chemical explanation of mutations. Genes control the production of specific proteins. The proteins are either structural proteins in the cell and thus a definitive product of the gene or they act as enzymes and are thus a link in the biochemical reaction in the body.

GENETIC CODE: A human being originates in the union of two gametes, the ovum and the sperm. These two cells contain all that the new individual can inherit from his parents. The hereditary elements or genes are carried on the chromosomes, which are present in the cell nucleus. Man has 46 chromosomes, comprising two sex chromosomes and 44 autosomes. The autosomes, which are somatic or non-sex chromosomes, can be matched according to their size and shape and arranged in 22 homologous pairs. In the female the pair of sex chromosomes are equal in size and are called XX. In the male the pair are unequal and are called XY. Every somatic cell of the male contains 44 autosomes and one X and one Y chromosome;

every somatic cell of the female contains 44 autosomes and two X chromosomes. The hereditary elements themselves are the genes and are arranged in a linear manner along the length of the chromosomes. The chromosomes are long filaments, which during division become coiled and interwoven like spiral springs. Genes are responsible for the protein synthesis of the cell. They instruct the cell how to make a particular polypeptide chain for a particular protein.

Genes carry in coded form the detailed specifications for the thousands of kinds of protein molecules the cell requires for its existence, for its enzymes, for its repair work and for its reproduction. These proteins are synthesized from the 20 natural amino acids, which are uniform throughout nature and which exist in the cell cytoplasm as part of the metabolic pool. The protein molecule consists of amino acids joined end to end to form long polypeptide chains. An average chain contains 100 to 300 amino acids. The sequence of bases in the nucleic acid chain of the gene corresponds in some fundamental way to the sequence of amino acids in the protein molecule, and hence it determines the structure of the particular protein. This is the genetic code. Deoxyribonucleic acid (DNA) is the bearer of this genetic information.

DNA has a long backbone made up of repeating groups of phosphate and the sugar deoxyribose. To this backbone four bases are attached as side groups at regular intervals. These four bases are the four letters used to spell out the genetic message. They are adenine, thymine, guanine and cystosine (A, T, G and C in the figure below). The molecule of DNA is made up of two chains coiled round a common axis to form what is called a double helix. The two chains are held together by hydrogen bonds between pairs of bases. Since adenine only pairs with thymine and guanine only with cystosine, the sequences of bases in one chain fixes the sequence in the other. Several hundred bases would be contained in the length of DNA of a typical gene. If the message of the DNA base sequence is a continuous succession of thymine, the ribosome will link together a series of the amino acid phenylalanine. If the base sequence is a succession of cytosine the ribosome will link up a series of prolines. Thus each amino acid has its own particular code of bases. In fact each amino acid is coded by a word consisting of three adjacent bases. In addition to carrying genetic information, DNA is able to synthesize or replicate itself and so pass this information on to daughter cells.

All DNA is part of the chromosome and so it remains confined to the nucleus of the cell. Proteins are synthesized by the ribosomes which are in the cytoplasm. DNA achieves control over protein production in the cytoplasm by directing the synthesis of ribonucleic acid (RNA). Most of the DNA in a cell is inactive, otherwise the cell would synthesize simultaneously every protein that the individual was capable of forming. When part of the DNA structure becomes 'active' it acts as a template for the riboneucleic acid (RNA) which itself acts as a template for protein synthesis when it becomes attached to the ribosome. Ribonucleic acid exists in three forms. Firstly 'messenger RNA' carries the necessary 'message' for the synthesis of a specific protein, from the nucleus to the ribosome. Secondly, 'transfer RNA' collects the individual amino acids, which exist in the cytoplasm as part of the metabolic pool, and carries them to the ribosome. Thirdly, there is RNA in the ribosome itself.

RNA has a similar structure to DNA, but the sugar is ribose instead of deoxyribose, and uracil replaces the base thymine. Before the ribosome can produce the proteins, the amino acids must be lined up in their correct sequence on the messenger RNA template. This alignment is carried out by transfer RNA, of which there is a specific form for each individual amino acid. Transfer RNA can not only recognize its specific amino acid but also identify the position it is required to occupy on the messenger RNA template. This is because each transfer RNA has its own sequence of bases and recognizes its site on the messenger RNA by pairing bases with it. The ribosome then travels along the chain of messenger RNA and links the amino acids, which have thus been arranged in the requisite order, by peptide bonds and the protein is released.

Proteins are important for two main reasons. Firstly, all the enzymes of living cells are made of protein. One gene is responsible for one enzyme. Genes thus control all the biochemical processes of the body and are responsible for the inborn difference between human beings. Secondly, proteins also fulfil a structural role in the cell so that genes controlling the synthesis of structural proteins are responsible for morphological differences between human beings.

During ordinary somatic or mitotic division each chromosome divides longitudinally, duplicating itself with an exact copy of all the genes it bears. When the cell divides, each double chromosome separates, one half passing to each of the two daughter cells, so that the two daughter cells contain exact replicas of the 23 pairs of chromosomes of the mother cell. In the formation of the gametes (ovum and sperm) a special kind of cell division takes place, called meiosis (q.v.) or reduction division, in which two divisions of the nucleus occur and only one division of the chromosomes so that the number of chromosomes in the gametes is half that of the somatic cells. The gamete thus receives only one member of each pair of chromosomes from the parent cell.

It was not until 1956 that the number of chromosomes in the human cell was established as 46. The morphology of the human chromosomes has only been appreciated since the discovery that colchicine has the property of stopping mitosis at the stage of the metaphase when the chromosomes assume their most visible form. Tissue culture provides a source of dividing cells, whose mitosis may be arrested by colchicine. The cells used are white blood cells which are incubated in their plasma with an added synthetic culture medium. There is as yet no known way of producing meiosis artificially. Chromosomes can be seen quite clearly under a microscope and arranged in order of decreasing size. Variations in size, the position of the centromere and specific characteristics of shape enable the 22 pairs of autosomes to be identified and numbered from 1–22. The paired sex chromosomes are of equal length in the female (XX) but of unequal length in the male (XY). The longest chromosome is 7–8 microns in length and the shortest about 1–5 microns.

In 1949 it was discovered that cells of females had a nucleolar satellite, which stains readily with certain dyes, whereas no such body could be detected in the cells from males. This is because the two X chromosomes in the female contain more chromatin than the XY pair in the male and are therefore more visible when stained. It is believed that one X chromosome remains condensed and physiologically inactive when a cell is not dividing and this forms the sex chromatin characteristic of female cell nuclei. The sex chromatin is not a complete index of sexual genetic makeup. All that can be inferred is whether an individual does or does not carry two X chromosomes. It does not indicate whether the normal Y chromosome is present. This sex chromatin body can be identified in 30 to 60 per cent of cells in the female. Buccal smears and biopsies of skin are the most favoured sources of cells as these cells have an open nucleus, though polymorphonuclear granulocytes can also be used. As the chromatin body (or drumstick of the polymorph) is formed from part of the X chromosome of the female cell, it is not present in cells, which carry only one X chromosome, such as those of normal males or patients with Turner's syndrome (XO). If a cell carries three X chromosomes two chromatin bodies will be visible in the cells.

Recently it has become possible to identify the Y chromosome. The anti-malarial drug quinacrine has been shown to be extremely useful for staining chromosomes with a fluorescence that is clearly visible through an ultraviolet microscope. The Y chromosome fluoresces intensely and this fluorescence is even visible in non-dividing (interphase) cells. Quinacrine is thus a reliable way of sexing human cells whether they are resting or dividing.

GENETIC COUNSELLING is the procedure whereby advice is given to couples wishing to have children, as to the likelihood of their having congenitally abnormal children. It is a procedure which is assuming enhanced value now that by means of antenatal diagnosis it is possible in certain cases to tell in the early stages of pregnancy whether or not the unborn child is abnormal: for example, whether or not he or she has Down's syndrome. There are now over twenty genetic advisory centres in the United Kingdom, to which patients can be referred by their family doctors.

GENETIC ENGINEERING, or recombinant DNA technology, has only developed in the past decade or so; it is the process of changing the genetic material of a cell. Genes from one cell, for example a human cell, can be inserted into another cell, usually a bacterium, and made to function. It is now possible to insert the gene responsible for the production of human insulin, human growth hormone and interferon from a human cell into a bacterium. Segments of DNA for insertion can be prepared by breaking long chains into smaller pieces by the use of restriction enzymes. The segments are then inserted into the affecting organism, usually the bacteria *Escherichia coli* by using plasmids and bacteriophages. Plasmids are small packets of DNA that are found within bacteria and can be passed from one bacterium to another. Already genetic engineering is contributing to easing the problems of diagnosis. At the present time beta-thalassaemia can be diagnosed ante-natally by obtaining a sample of fetal blood at 15 weeks gestation. DNA analysis and the production of monoclonal antibodies (q.v.) are other applications of genetic engineering.

GENETIC FINGERPRINTING: This technique shows the relationships between individuals. For example, it can be used to prove maternity or paternity of a child. The procedure is also used in forensic medicine whereby any tissue left behind by a criminal at the scene of a crime can be compared genetically with the tissue of a suspect. DNA (q.v.), the genetic material in living cells, can be extracted from blood, semen, and other body tissues. The technique, pioneered in Britain in 1984, is now widely used.

GENETICS is the science which deals with the origin of the characteristics of an individual or the study of heredity.

GENETIC SCREENING: A screening procedure that tests whether a person has a genetic make-up that is linked with a particular disease. If so, the person may either develop the disease or pass it on to his or her offspring. When an individual has been found to carry a genetically linked disease, he or she should receive genetic counselling (q.v.) from an expert in inherited diseases. (See GENES.)

GENITALIA are the organs of reproduction.

GENITO-URINARY MEDICINE: the branch of medicine that deals with sexually transmitted diseases (see VENEREAL DISEASES).

GENITO-URINARY TRACT consists of the kidneys, ureters, bladder, and urethra and, in the male, the genital organs.

GENOME is a complete set of chromosomes derived from one parent, or the total gene complement of a set of chromosomes.

GENOTYPE: All of an individual's genetic information that is encoded in his or her chromosomes (q.v.). It also means the genetic information carried by a pair of alleles which controls a particular characteristic. (See GENES.)

GENTAMICIN is an antibiotic derived from a species of micro-organisms, *Micromonospora purpurea*. Its main value is that it is active against certain micro-organisms such as *Pseudomonas pyocyanea*, *E. coli* and *Aerobacter aerogenes* which are not affected by other antibiotics, as well as staphylococci which have become resistant to penicillin.

GENTIAN VIOLET, or CRYSTAL VIOLET, is a dye belonging to the rosaniline group. Gentian violet is a good superficial antiseptic. It is used in the treatment of burns, either alone or in conjunction with brilliant green and proflavine. Applied to a burn, gentian violet forms a tough pliable film.

GENU VALGUM is the medical term for knock-knee (q.v.).

GENU VARUM is the medical term for bow leg (q.v.).

GERIATRICS is that branch of medicine which treats of the disorders and diseases associated with old age.

GERMAN MEASLES, or RUBELLA, is an acute infectious disease of a mild type, which may sometimes be difficult to differentiate from mild forms of measles and scarlet fever. It is also known by the name of rötheln. The term, 'german', has no geographical significance. It comes from 'germane' meaning akin to. Rubella comes from the Latin, *rubellus* meaning red.
Cause: The cause of infection is a virus. It is spread by close contact with infected individuals, and is infectious for a week before the rash appears and at least four days afterwards. It occurs in epidemics every three years or so, predominantly in the winter and spring. Children are more likely to be affected than infants. One attack gives permanent immunity. The incubation period is usually 14 to 21 days.
Symptoms are very mild, and the disease is not at all serious. On the day of onset there may be shivering, headache, slight catarrh with sneezing, coughing and sore throat, very slight fever, not above 37·8 °C (100 °F), and at the same time the glands of the neck become enlarged. These symptoms are usually slight. Within 24 hours of the onset a pink, slightly raised eruption appears, first on the face or neck, then

on the chest, and the second day spreads all over the body. The appearance of the rash is intermediate between that of measles and scarlet fever, being less blotchy, and remaining more as minute pink spots than the rash of measles, and the spots being more definite than the fairly uniform redness of scarlet fever. The rash is very bright on some parts of the body, while other parts are almost entirely free. The duration of the rash is variable. It may last for the greater part of a week, and, as it disappears, fine bran-like scales separate from the surface. The most distinguishing feature of this disorder is a well-marked but transient enlargement of the glands in the neck.

An attack of German measles during the early months of pregnancy may be responsible for congenital defects in the fetus, and it is for this reason that the disease has assumed such great importance in recent years. The incidence of such defects is not precisely known, but probably around 20 per cent of children, whose mothers have had German measles in the first three months of the pregnancy, are born with congenital defects. These defects take a variety of forms, but the most important ones are: low birth weight with retarded physical development; malformations of the heart; cataract, and deafness.

Treatment: The only treatment necessary is confinement to bed so long as there are any symptoms. Infectivity ceases within four days provided there are no symptoms. Children who develop the disease should not return to school until they have recovered, and in any case not before four days have passed from the onset of the rash. In view of the mildness of the disease, contacts are seldom kept in quarantine, but they should be carefully watched from the tenth to the twenty-first day from exposure to infection.

In view of the possible effect of the disease upon the fetus, particular care should be taken to isolate pregnant mothers from contact with infected subjects. As the risk to the fetus is particularly high during the first sixteen weeks of pregnancy, any pregnant mother exposed to infection during this period should be given an intramuscular injection of gamma-globulin (q.v.). Female members of school staff who have not had the disease or been vaccinated against it, who might probably become pregnant should be recommended not to attend the school until the risk of infection is over. A vaccine is now available which should make it possible to give a girl an immunity to the disease before she attains adult life, and it is now officially recommended that such vaccination should be offered to all girls between 11 and 14 years of age. It is also recommended that all women of childbearing age, who have been shown by a simple laboratory test not to have had the disease, should be vaccinated, always provided the woman is not pregnant at the time and has not been exposed to the risk of pregnancy during the previous eight weeks.

GERMS (see MICROBIOLOGY).

GESTATION is another name for pregnancy.

GIARDIASIS is a condition caused by a parasitic organism known as *Giardia lamblia*, which is found in the duodenum (see INTESTINE) and the upper part of the small intestine. This organism is usually harmless, but is sometimes responsible for causing diarrhoea. Over 3000 cases a year are reported in Britain. In most of these the infection has been acquired from drinking untreated water in the Middle East or Russia. The illness develops one or two weeks after exposure to infection, and usually starts as an explosive diarrhoea, with the passage of pale fatty stools, abdominal pain and nausea. It responds well to metronidazole or mepacrine.

GIDDINESS (see VERTIGO).

GIGANTISM (see ACROMEGALY).

GINGIVITIS means inflammation of the gums. (See TEETH, DISEASES OF.)

GIPPY TUMMY (see TRAVEL SICKNESS).

GLANDERS, or EQUINIA, is a specific infectious disease to which certain animals, chiefly those possessing an undivided hoof – such as horses, asses, and mules – are liable, and communicable by them to man. The term farcy is also used to designate a variety of the disease in which the lymphatic glands are first and chiefly affected. Glanders is a rare form of disease in man. It occurs chiefly among those who from their occupation are in contact with horses and seems to be produced either by direct inoculation of the organism from a diseased animal into the broken skin or by inhalation. The cause of glanders is a short rod-shaped organism, known as the *Loefflerella mallei*. It has been eradicated from Britain, but still occurs in Eastern Europe and Asia.

In the untreated acute form of the disease, the case generally terminates fatally in a period varying from two or three days to as many weeks. A chronic form of glanders and farcy is more common, in which the symptoms advance much more slowly, and are attended with relatively less constitutional disturbance. Around 30 to 50 per cent of patients with chronic glanders survive without treatment. Promising results have been reported from the use of sulphonamides, penicillin and streptomycin.

GLANDS are divisible into several classes. In the first place, the term is applied to organs like the liver, pancreas, and kidneys, which produce a secretion; but in general the term is limited to smaller structures concerned in the production of some excretion from the body, or of some substance needful to its working. These latter

Various types of glands; 1 simple tubular (e.g. intestinal glands); 2 simple coiled tubular (e.g. sweat glands); 3, 4 simple branched tubular (e.g. gastric glands); 5 simple alveolar; 6 simple branched alveolar (e.g. sebaceous glands); 7 compound (e.g. salivary and mammary glands). The secretory part of the gland is black.

are divided into two quite distinct groups: (1) glands which produce some form of secretion or excretion; (2) lymphatic glands.

(1) SECRETING AND EXCRETING GLANDS comprise glands in almost all parts of the body, which vary much in appearance, in size, and in the character of the substances they produce. The skin, for example, is richly supplied with sebaceous glands, which secrete an oily material, and with sweat glands, which are placed in rows whose openings can be seen with a weak magnifying lens upon the ridges of the palms and soles. The lining membrane of the stomach is made up of long tubular glands set closely side by side, and in these the gastric juice is formed. The structure of the mucous membrane in the intestine is much the same. In all these mucous membranes there are situated other glands, generally formed each of a small mass of twisted tubes, which secrete a clear shining fluid known as mucus, that gives to these membranes their soft, smooth appearance and their name. The glands so far mentioned are all of microscopic size, but there are many of large dimensions. The parotid gland, situated just in front of the ear, the submaxillary gland, which can be easily felt, of the size of a chestnut beneath the jaw, and the sublingual gland, which can be seen beneath the tongue, are occupied in producing saliva, and known as salivary glands. The breasts or mammary glands are a pair of large glands situated in the skin over the front of the chest, and secrete milk. The thyroid gland, situated in front of the neck,

has no outlet to the exterior, but produces an important secretion which is absorbed by the blood and carried throughout the body. The suprarenal glands situated immediately above the kidneys act under similar conditions. Many of the glands which have an outlet through which one secretion comes, such as the pancreas and testes, also produce what is called an internal secretion that is absorbed by the blood, and exerts a profound effect upon general nutrition and metabolism.

Glands which produce an internal secretion are known as endocrine glands. (See ENDOCRINE GLANDS.)

(2) LYMPHATIC GLANDS are scattered all through the body in connection with the system of lymphatic vessels. They vary much in size, from that of microscopic masses to that of large beans, but they have essentially the same structure everywhere. Round each gland is a fibrous tissue capsule, from which partitions and bands run into the gland to join one another and give it cohesion. In the meshes of these lie enormous numbers of lymph corpuscles in the circulating blood. These corpuscles are arranged in masses round which the lymph circulates freely. Numbers of lymph-vessels (afferent vessels) pierce the capsule of the gland, and the lymph, after passing from them, percolates through the gland and leaves its central part, carrying with it many corpuscles, by a few larger lymph-vessels (efferent vessels). The vessels leaving one gland pass on to enter another, the glands being, as a rule, arranged in chains.

Structure of a lymph gland: 1 afferent lymphatic; 2 capsule; 3 cortical lymph
follicle; 4 lymph sinus; 5 trabecula; 6 efferent lymphatic.

In the limbs the lymph-vessels pass from the foot and hand up to the knee and elbow, respectively, before they encounter glands. A few glands are situated in the bend of each of these joints, and the vessels passing from these reach large chains of glands in the groin and armpit, respectively. The chains of glands beneath the jaw and down each side of the neck are known to everyone from the frequency with which they become inflamed and swollen. Inside the abdomen small lymph vessels known as lacteals collect certain parts of the food from the intestine, and pass their contents through mesenteric glands, situated deep in the abdominal cavity. Deep in the chest, too, lie many large bronchial glands, receiving lymphatics from the lungs. The lymph-vessels from the lower limbs and abdomen, after passing through numerous glands, unite into a single trunk, about the size of a quill, called the thoracic duct, which passes upwards through the chest, collecting the lymphatics of the chest, left arm, and left side of the neck, to open into the veins on the left side of the neck. A shorter lymphatic vessel collects the lymphatics from the right side of the chest, right arm, and right side of the neck, opening into the veins of the right side. The point where the lymphatic system on each side opens into the venous system is at or close to the point of union of the subclavian vein with the internal jugular vein. By means of these connections the lymph corpuscles formed in the glands may reach the blood. Beyond forming these corpuscles, the glands have another function, acting as a species of filters upon the lymph circulation, and keeping back micro-organisms and other dangerous impurities from entering the blood circulation.

GLANDS, DISEASES OF: The diseases of the chief secreting glands are described under various headings, and reference is made here only to diseases of the lymphatic glands. Most of the diseases which affect these glands are of an inflammatory nature, various poisonous substances lodging in them in the attempt to pass through the system by way of the lymphatic vessels. (See also ENDOCRINE GLANDS.)

SIMPLE ENLARGEMENT AND SUPPURATION OF A GLAND is the commonest condition. This is generally the result of a wound or other source of infection in the area drained by the lymphatic vessels going to the gland. For example, any source of irritation about the head, such as lice or eczema, is apt to produce swelling of the glands behind the ear and down the neck; or a wound of the foot or hand to cause inflammation of the glands in the groin or armpit, respectively.

Treatment: The object at first is to prevent suppuration of the enlarged and inflamed gland. For this purpose the source of irritation must be removed by opening the gumboil, cleaning the head, dressing the wound of the foot, etc. If the infection is due to a penicillin-sensitive organism, penicillin should also be given unless the infection is very mild. The gland itself is best left entirely alone, or at most kept supported and at rest by a pad and flannel bandage. If the swelling becomes soft and the skin over it reddened, suppuration is taking place, and the condition must be treated as an acute abscess. (See ABSCESS, ACUTE.)

TUBERCULOUS GLANDS, or SCROFULA, is a disease of childhood, especially in the neck. In many cases the glands become infected by the tubercle bacillus, *Mycobacterium tuberculosis*, through the tonsils. The chain of glands under the jaw and that running up and down the neck become affected in most cases, whilst in others the glands inside the abdomen are diseased, producing the condition of wasting known as tabes mesenterica. The condition progresses very slowly, as a rule, the glands enlarging for some months, then becoming matted together, to form an irregular mass, which softens, reddens here and there, and finally bursts through the skin to produce sinuses, which may go on discharging for years, healing finally with red, puckered, unsightly scars.

Treatment: Tuberculous glands are often the result of infection with the bovine tubercle bacillus. Therefore, one of the most important preventive measures is to see that children drink only milk that has been pasteurized. In the first stage, while the glands are simply enlarging, general treatment to improve the constitution is required, as well as the administration of anti-tuberculous drugs.

The use of anti-tuberculous drugs means that in many cases the infection can be brought satisfactorily under control.

CANCER, when it is present in any organ, may sooner or later affect the neighbouring lymphatic glands. It is by way of the lymphatic system that cancer usually spreads to parts at a distance, and glands in a part of the body far removed from the original cancer may become affected, while the intervening tissues remain healthy. This is the chief reason for the recurrence of cancer after apparently complete removal. As an example of this, it may be noted that the glands on the left side of the neck are prone to be diseased as a result of cancer in the stomach; those in the armpit may become affected early in cancer of the breast.

OTHER CONDITIONS which produce enlargement of glands are the venereal diseases, leukaemia, and the disease known as lymphadenoma, or Hodgkin's disease. (See also BUBO.)

GLANDULAR FEVER (see MONONUCLEOSIS).

GLANS: The term applied to the ends of the penis (q.v.) and the clitoris (q.v.). In the penis the glans is the distal helmet-shaped part that is formed by the bulbous corpus spongiosum (erectile tissue). In an uncircumcised man the glans is covered by the foreskin or prepuce when the penis is flaccid.

GLASGOW COMA SCALE: A method developed by two doctors in Glasgow that is used to assess the depth of coma or unconsciousness suffered by an individual. The scale is split into three groups: eye opening, motor response, and verbal response, with the level of activity within each group given a score. A person's total score is the sum of the numbers scored in each group and this provides a reasonably objective assessment of the patient's coma state.

GLAUCOMA is a term used to describe a group of disorders characterized by the intra-ocular pressure being so high as to damage the nerve fibres in the retina and optic nerve as it leaves the eye. Glaucoma is usually classified as being either open-angle glaucoma or narrow-angle glaucoma. *Open-angle glaucoma* is a chronic, slowly progressive, usually bilateral disorder. It occurs in 1 in 200 of people over 40 and amounts for 20 per cent of those registered blind in Great Britain. Symptoms are virtually non-existent until well into the disease, when the patient may experience visual problems. It is not painful. The characteristic findings are that the intra-ocular pressure is raised (normal pressure is up to 21 mm Hg) causing cupping of the optic disc and a glaucomatous visual-field loss. The angle between the iris and the cornea remains open. Treatment is aimed at decreasing the intra-ocular pressure initially by drops and tablets. Surgery may be required later. A *trabeculectomy* is an operation to create a channel through which fluid can drain from the eye in a controlled fashion in order to bring the pressure down. *Narrow-angle glaucoma* affects 1 in 1000 people over 40 years of age and is more common in women. Symptoms may start with coloured haloes around street lights at night. These may then be followed by rapid onset of severe pain in and around the eye accompanied by a rapid fall in vision. One eye is usually affected first; this alerts the surgeon so that action can be taken to prevent a similar attack in the other eye. Treatment must be started as an emergency with intensive drops and tablets to bring the pressure down. This is followed by surgery to prevent recurrence. Acute narrow-angle glaucoma occurs because the peripheral iris is pushed against the back of the cornea. This closes off the angle between iris and cornea through which aqueous humour drains out of the eye. Since the aqueous humour cannot drain away, it builds up inside the eye causing a rapid increase in pressure.

GLEET means a chronic form of gonorrhoea.

GLENOID is the term applied to the shallow socket on the shoulder-blade into which the humerus fits, forming the shoulder-joint.

GLIBENCLAMIDE is a drug which stimulates the beta cells of the pancreas to liberate insulin, and is thereby proving of value in some cases of diabetes mellitus (q.v.). (See SULPHONYLUREAS.)

GLICLAZIDE (see SULPHONYLUREAS).

GLIOMA is a tumour which forms in the brain or spinal cord, composed of neuroglia, which is the special connective tissue that in these organs supports the nerve-cells and nerve-fibres.

GLIPIZIDE (see SULPHONYLUREAS).

GLIQUIDONE (see SULPHONYLUREAS).

GLOBIN: A protein which when it combines with haem forms haemoglobin (q.v.), the molecule found in the red blood cell that carries oxygen and carbon dioxide.

GLOBULIN is a class of proteins which are insoluble in water and alcohol and soluble in weak salt solution. (See also GAMMA-GLOBULIN.)

GLOBUS is a term applied generally to any structures of ball shape, but especially to the sensation of a ball in the throat causing choking, which forms a common symptom of hysteria.

GLOMERULAR FILTRATION RATE: The kidney filters a large volume of blood – 25 per cent of cardiac output or around 1300 ml – through its two million glomeruli (q.v.) every minute. The glomeruli filter out cell, protein, and fat-free fluid which, after reabsorption of certain chemicals, is excreted as urine. The rate of this ultrafiltration process, which in health is remarkably constant, is called the glomerular filtration rate (GFR). Each day nearly 180 litres of water plus some small molecular-weight constituents of blood are filtrated. The GFR is thus an indicator of kidney function. The most widely used measurement is creatinine (q.v.) clearance and this is assessed by measuring the amount of creatinine in a 24-hour sample of urine and the amount of creatinine in the plasma; a formula is applied that gives the GFR.

GLOMERULONEPHRITIS describes a bilateral non-suppurative disease of the kidneys, affecting primarily the glomerulus. Usually all the glomeruli are involved. On the rare occasions when only a limited number of glomeruli are affected the disorder is known as focal or segmental glomerulonephritis. When the disease presents abruptly the term acute glomerulonephritis is used.
Cause: The disease is the result of the depositing of immune complexes in the capillary wall of the glomerulus. The activation of complement as a result leads to a combination of inflammation and coagulation which damages the glomeruli. This may resolve completely or it may lead to progressive scarring and obliteration of the glomeruli as occurs in chronic glomerulonephritis.

By studying the histology of the kidney from renal biopsy specimens three histological varieties have been recognized. These are: (*a*) minimal change glomerulonephritis; (*b*) proliferative glomerulonephritis, and (*c*) membranous glomerulonephritis. These three varieties are dependent on the differing ways in which the glomerulus reacts to injury. The most common antigen responsible for the development of soluble immune complexes is the streptococcus. This is the bacteria which causes acute tonsillitis and scarlet fever. Rarer forms of glomerular disease caused by immune complexes occur in systemic lupus erythematosis and polyarteritis and in the course of some tumours which provoke circulating antibodies.
Symptoms and Treatment: Glomerulonephritis can present in a number of different ways. The syndrome of acute nephritis following a streptococcal throat infection is the most common. It usually presents with swelling of the face and the eyelids and to a less extent the rest of the body. The urinary output is reduced and the urine contains blood and albumin. There is nearly always a rise in the blood pressure. The disease most commonly occurs in children and adolescents and the onset is abrupt with malaise, fever and sometimes pain in the loins. Ninety per cent of children with this form of acute nephritis make a complete and permanent recovery. A few patients will develop a rapidly progressive nephritis leading to renal failure. Some patients appear to make a good initial recovery but continue to pass protein in the urine although they may feel well within themselves. If the protein loss in the urine exceeds the liver's ability to produce the protein the plasma level will fall and a nephrotic syndrome will result. The rationale of medical treatment of this disorder is to maintain the water and electrolyte balance of the body and to provide adequate calories until the spontaneous recovery of renal function occurs. In view of the hypertension it is important to restrict the intake of salt. Initially when the patient is oliguric the amount of fluids taken by mouth must be restricted. As the urinary output increases the fluid intake can also be increased. The amount of fluid allowed is estimated as 500ml plus a volume equal to the amount of urine passed in the previous 24 hours. Penicillin is probably advisable to clear streptococci from the throat. No other drug influences the course of acute glomerulonephritis. As has been mentioned acute nephritis may be a manifestation of systemic lupus erythematosis, polyarteritis nodosa, anaphylactic purpura or Goodpasture's syndrome and then the treatment is that of the primary disorder.

When nephritis is due to the minimal change lesion or membraneous glomerulonephritis the onset is more insidious. Because these conditions are associated with an increase in the permeability of the glomerulus and hence proteinuria the clinical presentation is usually as a nephrotic syndrome. This is a syndrome characterized by a heavy proteinuria, hypoalbuminaemia and peripheral oedema. The nephrotic syndrome may be the result of a primary nephritis or it may occur secondary to diabetic renal damage, amyloid disease, malaria or systemic lupus erythematosis. The management of the oedema is by diuretics.

When the nephrotic syndrome is secondary to other diseases the management is the control of those diseases. When it is the result of primary renal disease corticosteroids are often of benefit, especially in the minimal change lesion. Immunosuppressive drugs such as azathioprine may also be indicated. If hypertension is present it will require treatment in its own right.

Chronic glomerulonephritis results when proliferative glomerulonephritis becomes progressive and in most cases of membranous glomerulonephritis. The clinical symptoms are those of chronic renal failure, usually associated with hypertension, polyuria, loss of energy, nausea and vomiting: anaemia is usually present. Muscle and bone pain frequently result due to osteomalacia. The disease progresses relentlessly as a rule and the only effective treatment is dialysis or renal transplantation.

GLOMERULUS is a small knot of blood-vessels about the size of a sand grain, of which around 1,000,000 are found in each kidney, and from which the excretion of fluid out of the blood into the tubules of the kidney takes place.

GLOSSITIS means inflammation of the tongue.

GLOSSOPHARYNGEAL nerve is the ninth cranial nerve, which in the main is a sensory nerve, being the nerve of taste in the posterior third of the tongue and the nerve of general sensation for the whole upper part of the throat and middle ear. It also supplies the parotid gland and one of the muscles on the side of the throat.

GLOTTIS is the narrow opening at the upper end of the larynx. The glottis is made up of the true vocal cords. (See AIR PASSAGES; CHOKING; LARYNX.)

GLUCAGON is a hormone secreted by the alpha cells of the islets of Langerhans in the pancreas, which increases the amount of glucose in the blood. This it does by promoting the breakdown of liver glycogen (glycogenolysis). It is secreted in response to a lowered blood sugar and is used therapeutically to treat hypoglycaemia (q.v.).

GLUCOCORTICOIDS is the group of steroid hormones produced by the adrenal cortex, which includes cortisol and cortisone (q.v.), and which particularly affect protein, fat and carbohydrate metabolism.

GLUCONEOGENESIS means the formation of sugar from amino-acids in the liver.

GLUCOSE (DEXTROSE; GRAPE SUGAR) is the form of sugar found in honey and in grapes and some other fruits. It is also the form of sugar circulating in the blood stream and the form into which all sugars and starches are converted in the small intestine before being absorbed. Glucose is a yellowish-white crystalline substance soluble in water and having the property of turning the ray of polarized light to the right. It is often given to patients as an easily assimilated form of carbohydrate. It has the further practical advantage in this context of not being nearly as sweet-tasting as cane sugar and therefore relatively large amounts can be consumed without sickening the patient. For patients unable to take food by the mouth, glucose is sometimes administered in the form of an enema consisting of 5 per cent of glucose in normal saline fluid, or 28·5 grams (1 ounce) of glucose to 570 ml (1 pint) of water. The same fluid, when carefully sterilized, may be injected beneath the skin or directly into the veins, and is quickly absorbed. (See SUGAR; URINE.)

GLUCOSE-TOLERANCE TEST: A way of assessing the body's efficiency at metabolizing glucose (q.v.). The test is used in diagnosing diabetes mellitus (q.v.). The patient is starved for up to 16 hours after which he is fed glucose by mouth. The concentrations of glucose in the blood and urine are then measured at half-hour intervals over two hours.

GLUCOSIDE is a glycoside (q.v.) formed from glucose.

GLUE EAR is another name for secretory otitis media. (See EAR, DISEASES OF.)

GLUE SNIFFING (see SOLVENT ABUSE).

GLUTEAL is the name applied to the region of the buttock and the structures situated in it, such as the gluteal muscles, arteries, and nerves.

GLUTEN is the constituent of wheat-flour which forms an adhesive substance on addition of water, and allows the 'raising' of bread. It can be separated from the starch of flour, and being of a protein nature is used to make bread for those diabetics who are debarred from starchy and sugary foods.

It is also responsible for certain forms of what is now known as the malabsorption syndrome (q.v.). In these cases an essential part of treatment is a gluten-free diet.

GLUTETHIMIDE is a non-barbiturate hypnotic, which induces sleep fairly rapidly, and whose effects last about six hours.

GLUTEUS: Three gluteal muscles form each buttock. The gluteus maximus is the large powerful muscle that gives the buttocks their rounded shape. The remaining two muscles are the gluteus medius and gluteus minimus and together the three muscles are responsible for moving the thigh.

GLYCERIN, or GLYCEROL, is an alcohol, $C_3H_8O_3$, which occurs naturally in combination with organic acids in the form of fats or triglycerides. It is a clear, colourless, thick liquid of sweet taste. It dissolves many substances, and it has a great power of absorbing water, in consequence of which, in the pure state, it diminishes congestion in surfaces with which it is brought in contact.
Uses: Glycerin has many varied uses. Numerous substances, such as carbolic acid, tannic acid, alum, borax, boric acid, starch, are dissolved in it for application to the body. It is frequently applied along with other remedies to inflamed areas for its action in extracting fluid and thus diminishing inflammation.

Mixed with an equal quantity of water it forms a useful mouth-wash when the tongue and gums are furred or dry, and, as a spray, is one of the best ways of relieving the discomfort of laryngitis. It is also useful for application to the skin in order to prevent chapping in cold weather, and to protect and heal all sorts of small abrasions.

Internally, pure glycerin, in doses of 1 or 2 teaspoonfuls, acts as a laxative, administered either by the mouth or as an enema. For its pleasant taste it is added to various medicines. It is mixed with gelatin to form a basis for pastilles. (See GELATIN.)

GLYCEROL is another name for glycerin (q.v.).

GLYCERYL TRINITRATE is a drug which is used in the treatment of angina pectoris (q.v.). Also known as TRINITRIN and NITROGLYCERIN, it is a thick oily liquid of sweet taste and explosive properties. When a small quantity is taken internally it produces marked effects in about two minutes, relaxing the smaller arteries, capillaries (q.v.) and veins so as to cause the skin to flush visibly, quickening the pulse, and causing a sense of fullness all over the body and throbbing in the head. It greatly lessens the blood pressure and temporarily relaxes all muscle, whether striped or unstriped.
Uses: This sudden action in relaxing muscle fibres and lessening blood-pressure proves very valuable in conditions where serious effects are produced by spasm, particularly in angina pectoris, but also in bronchial asthma (due in part to spasm of the small bronchial tubes), in gall-stone and renal colic, and in the vomiting of seasickness. In these it diminishes the spasmodic condition and gives relief.

It is used in the form of glyceryl trinitrate tablets B.P., each containing 500 micrograms made up with chocolate. These should not be swallowed intact, but allowed to melt in the mouth before being swallowed. As these tablets quickly lose their strength, they are prescribed in a special glass bottle tightly sealed with a foil-lined cap, and it is essential that the cap is screwed tightly back on to the bottle each time after a tablet is removed. (See ANGINA PECTORIS.)

Other substances have a similar action. Sodium nitrite and potassium nitrite are used in doses of 200 to 500 mg, and have the advantage of producing their effect more slowly and more permanently. Erythrol tetranitrate has a similarly prolonged effect. Glyceryl trinitrate spray – administered under the tongue – may also be used for its quick effect.

GLYCO- is a prefix meaning of the nature of, or containing, sugar.

GLYCOGEN, or ANIMAL STARCH, is a carbohydrate substance found specially in the liver, as well as in other tissues. It is the form in which carbohydrates taken in the food are stored in the liver and muscles before they are converted into glucose as the needs of the body require.

GLYCOSIDE is a compound of a sugar and a non-sugar unit. Glycosides are widespread throughout nature and include many important drugs such as digoxin.

GLYCOSOLATED HAEMOGLOBIN (HBA1): Normal haemoglobin on chromatography separates into the major component HBA, which accounts for 94 per cent of the total, and HBA1. HBA1 has the same structure as HBA except that a glucose group is attached to the terminal amino-acid of the beta chain. The rate of synthesis of HBA1 is a function of the blood glucose concentration. The red blood cell lives for 120 days and as HBA1 accumulates throughout the life of the erythrocyte its concentration is related to the mean blood glucose concentration over the previous three months. It is thus a very useful test for the overall control of the blood glucose in diabetes mellitus (q.v.).

GLYCOSURIA means the presence of sugar in the urine. By far the most common cause of glycosuria is diabetes mellitus, but it may also occur as a result of a lowered renal threshold for sugar when it is called renal glycosuria, and is not indicative of disease.

GOBLET CELL: A columnar secretory cell occurring in the epithelium of the respiratory and intestinal tracts. The cells produce the main constituents of mucus (q.v.).

GOITRE is a term applied to a swelling in the front of the neck caused by an enlargement of the thyroid gland. The thyroid lies between the skin and the front of the windpipe and in health is not large enough to be seen. The four main varieties of goitre are the simple goitre, the nodular, the lymphadenoid goitre and the toxic goitre.
SIMPLE GOITRE is a benign enlargement of the thyroid gland with normal production of hormone. It is a physiological response to maintain the synthesis of thyroid hormone. It may occur sporadically, but in certain geographical areas of the world it is found more frequently and it is then referred to as 'endemic'. It may be the result of a deficiency of iodine, which is essential for thyroid hormone production. If iodine intake is deficient and the production of thyroid hormone is threatened, the anterior pituitary secretes increased amounts of thyrotrophic hormone with consequent hyperplasia of the thyroid gland. The prevalence of endemic goitre can be, and has been, reduced by the iodinization of domestic salt in many countries. Simple goitres commonly occur at puberty, during pregnancy and at the menopause, which are times of increased demand for thyroid hormone. They may also result from defective utilization of iodine in the synthesis of thyroxine. The immediate cause of simple goitre is increased production of thyrotrophic hormone by the pituitary. The only effective treament is

thyroid replacement therapy to suppress the enhanced production of thyrotrophic hormone. NODULAR GOITRES do not respond as well as the diffuse goitres to thyroxine treatment. They are usually the result of alternating episodes of hyperplasia and involution which lead to permanent thyroid enlargment. The only effective way of curing a nodular goitre is to excise it and thyroidectomy should be recommended if the goitre is causing pressure symptoms or if there is a suspicion of malignancy.

LYMPHADENOID GOITRES are due to the production of antibodies against antigens in the thyroid gland. They are an example of an auto-immune disease. They tend to occur in the 3rd and 4th decade and the gland is much firmer than the softer gland of a simple goitre. Lymphadenoid goitres respond to treatment with thyroxine.

TOXIC GOITRES are usually the result of Graves' disease (q.v.), though much less frequently autonomous nodules of a nodular goitre may be responsible for the increased production of thyroxine and render the patient hyperthyroid (toxic). Graves' disease is also an auto-immune disease in which an antibody is produced that stimulates the thyroid to produce excessive amounts of hormone, making the patient thyrotoxic.

GOLD SALTS are used in the treatment of rheumatoid arthritis. Gold may be administered in various forms, such as sodium aurothiomalate. It is injected in very small doses intramuscularly and produces a reaction in the affected tissues which leads to their scarring and healing. If gold is administered in too large quantities skin eruptions, albuminuria, metallic taste in the mouth, jaundice, and feverishness may be produced, so that it is necessary to prolong a course of this remedy over many months in minute doses. Routine blood and urine tests are also necessary in order to detect any adverse or toxic effect at an early stage.

GOLFER'S ELBOW is a term applied to a condition comparable to tennis elbow. It is not uncommon in the left elbow of right-handed golfers who catch the head of their club in the ground when making a duff shot. (See ELBOW.)

GONAD is a gland which produces a gamete; an ovary or a testis. There are four stages of sexual development: (1) gonadal differentiation, (2) development of internal genitalia, (3) external genital differentiation, (4) puberty.

The testis and ovary both develop from the undifferentiated gonad which appears in the fourth week of gestation. This indifferent gonad has a cortex and a medulla. In the presence of a Y chromosome the medulla of this structure evolves into a testis and the cortex regresses. In the presence of two X chromosomes the cortex differentiates into an ovary and the medulla regresses. (See GENETIC CODE.)

The internal genitalia also develop from separate primitive structures that transiently co-exist in embryos of both sexes. In the male the Wolffian ducts give rise to the vas deferens, the seminal vesicles and the epididymus, and the Mullerian ducts regress (the prostatic utricle is a remnant). In the female the Mullerian ducts fuse to produce the Fallopian tubes, the uterus and the upper vagina, and the Wolffian ducts regress. The development of the Wolffian ducts and the suppression of the Mullerian ducts requires the presence of a functioning fetal testis from which an 'inducer' diffuses locally to both suppress the Mullerian ducts and stimulate the development of the Wolffian ducts. This inducer is not androgen which is unable to suppress the Wolffian ducts. In the absence of this substance the duct system differentiates along feminine lines irrespective of the genetic sex. Thus if there is no gonad, as in gonadal agenesis, the ducts will develop along female lines. Jost showed in 1947 that surgical castration of the animal fetus before the time of sexual differentiation prevented masculinization and all the litters grew up as apparent females. The developing testis was thus essential for masculinity but the ovary was not essential for feminity. The female form, both internal and external, was that of the neuter sex.

The third stage of sexual development, namely the differentiation of the external genitalia, also involves development from primitive structures common to both sexes. In the female the genital folds become the labia minora, the genital swellings the labia majora and the genital tubercule the clitoris, whilst in the male under the influence of androgens the shaft of the penis, the glans penis and the scrotum are respectively developed. Failure of the genital folds to fuse correctly in the male results in hypospadias. Thus both in the development of the internal genitalia and the external genitalia differentiation to the male form requires a positive influence, otherwise development follows the female pattern.

The final stage of sexual development is puberty when pituitary gonadotrophin production increases to adult levels, and secondary sex characteristics appear.

GONADOTROPHINS, or GONADOTROPHIC HORMONES, are hormones that control the activity of the gonads (i.e. the testes and ovaries). In the male they stimulate the secretion of testosterone and the production of spermatozoa. In the female they stimulate the production of ova and the secretion of oestrogen (q.v.) and progesterone (q.v.). There are two gonadotrophins produced by the pituitary gland. *Chorionic gonadotrophin* is produced in the placenta and excreted in the urine.

GONORRHOEA is an inflammatory disease affecting especially the mucous membrane of the urethra in the male and that of the vagina in the female, but spreading also to other parts. It is the most common of the venereal diseases (q.v.). According to the World Health Organization, 200 million new cases are notified annually in the world. In England in 1988, there were nearly 19,000 cases.

Causes: The disease is directly contagious from another person already suffering in this manner, usually by sexual intercourse, but occasionally it is conveyed by the discharge on sponges, towels or clothing as well as by actual contact. The infecting agent is the gonococcus or *Neisseria gonorrhoeae*. This is found in the discharge expressed from the urethra, which may be spread as a film on a glass slide, suitably stained, and examined under the microscope; or a culture from the discharge may be made on certain bacteriological media and films from this, similarly examined under the microscope. Since discharges resembling that of gonorrhoea accompany other forms of inflammation, the identification of the organism is of great importance.

Symptoms: These differ considerably, according to whether the disease is in an acute or a chronic stage. In *men*, after an incubation period of between two and ten days, irritation in the urethra, scalding pain on passing water, and a viscid yellowish-white discharge appear; the glands in the groin often enlarge and may suppurate. The urine when passed is hazy and is often found to contain yellowish threads of pus visible to the eye. After some weeks, if the condition has become chronic, the discharge is clear and viscid, there may be irritation in passing urine, and various forms of inflammation in neighbouring organs may appear, the testicle, prostate gland and bladder becoming affected. At a still later stage the inflammation of the urethra is apt to lead to gradual formation of fibrous tissue around this channel. This contracts and produces narrowing, so that the passage of water becomes difficult or may be stopped for a time altogether (the condition known as stricture). Inflammation of some of the joints is a common complication in the early stage, the knee, ankle, wrist, and elbow being the joints most frequently affected, and this form of 'rheumatism' is very intractable and liable to lead to permanent stiffness. The fibrous tissues elsewhere may also develop inflammatory changes, causing lumbago, pain in the foot, etc. In occasional cases, during the acute stage, a general blood-poisoning results, with inflammation of the heart-valves (endocarditis) and abscesses in various parts of the body. The infective matter occasionally is inoculated accidentally into the eye producing a very severe form of conjunctivitis. In the newly born child this is known as *ophthalmia neonatorum* and until recently was one of the chief causes of blindness. (See EYE, DISEASE AND INJURIES.)

In women the course and complications of the disease are somewhat different. It begins with a yellow vaginal discharge, pain on passing water, and very often inflammation or abscess of the Bartholin's glands, situated close to the vulva or opening of the vagina. The chief seriousness, however, of the disease is due to the spread of inflammation to neighbouring organs, the uterus, Fallopian tubes, and ovaries, causing permanent destructive changes in these, and leading occasionally to peritonitis through the Fallopian tube, with a fatal result. Many cases of prolonged ill-health and sterility or recurring miscarriages are due to these changes.

Treatment: The chances of cure are better the earlier treatment is instituted. The treatment of gonorrhoea was revolutionized by the introduction of the sulphonamides. These, in turn, have now been replaced by the antibiotics. Penicillin is now the antibiotic of choice: a single injection of 2·4 or 4·8 mega units of procaine penicillin. Unfortunately, the gonococcus is liable to become resistant to penicillin. In patients who are infected with penicillin-resistant organisms, one of the other antibiotics is used. In all cases it is essential that bacteriological investigation should be carried out at weekly intervals for three or four weeks, to make sure that the patient is cured.

GOUT is a constitutional disorder connected with excess of uric acid in the blood, and manifesting itself by inflammation of joints with deposition therein of urate of soda, and also by morbid changes in various important organs.

Causes: The cardinal feature of gout is the presence of an excessive amount of uric acid, and its deposition in the joints in the form of sodium monourate. The cause of this excess of uric acid is not known. Uric acid is formed in the system in the processes of nutrition, and is excreted by the kidneys, the amount passing off in the urine being 0·1 to 2 grams daily. In the healthy human subject the blood contains 3 to 6 mg per 100 millilitres, but in gout it is increased, both before and during the acute attack, while in chronic gout the amount in the blood and elsewhere in the body is always above the normal level.

Gout is in a marked degree hereditary. A family history of the disease is obtained in from 50 to 80 per cent of cases. Gout is said to affect the sedentary more readily than the active, but this cannot be taken as a constant rule. On the other hand, inadequate exercise, habitual overindulgence in animal food and rich dishes, and especially in alcoholic drinks, are undoubtedly important precipitating factors in the production of the disease. These, however, are no more than precipitating factors, and the disease can occur in vegetarians and teetotallers.

Gout is more common in mature age than in the earlier years of life, being infrequent before the age of 40, but it may occasionally affect very young people in whom there is a strong family history. About 95 per cent of patients are males. In women it most often appears after the cessation of the menses.

Symptoms: An attack of gout may appear without warning, or there may be premonitory symptoms. On the night of the attack, the patient retires to rest apparently quite well, but about two or three o'clock in the morning is awakened by a painful feeling in the foot, most commonly in the ball of the great toe, but it may be in the instep or heel, or in the thumb. With the pain there often occurs a distinct shivering, followed by feverishness. The pain soon becomes of an agonizing character.

When the affected part is examined it is found to be swollen and of a deep red hue. The skin is tense and glistening, and the surrounding veins are more or less distended. After a few hours there is a remission of the pain, slight perspiration takes place, and the patient may fall asleep. The pain, however, returns next night, and these nocturnal exacerbations occur with greater or less severity during the continuance of the attack, which generally lasts for a week or ten days. As the symptoms decline, the swelling and tenderness of the affected joint abate, but the skin over it pits on pressure for a time, and with this there is often associated slight desquamation of the skin. It is rare that the first is the only attack of gout, although by care and treatment recurrences may be warded off. In the earlier recurrences the same joints as were the original seat of the gouty inflammation suffer again, but in the course of time others become implicated, until in advanced cases scarcely any joint escapes, and the disease becomes chronic. When gout assumes this form, the frequently recurring attacks are usually attended with less pain, but chalk-stones, or tophi, are gradually formed round the affected joints. These deposits, which are highly characteristic of gout, at first occur in the form of a semi-fluid material, consisting for the most part of bi-urate of soda, which gradually becomes more dense, and ultimately quite hard. In some cases of chronic gout the deposit is so slight as to be barely appreciable externally, but on the other hand it occasionally causes great enlargement of the joints, and fixes them in a flexed or extended position which renders them entirely useless. Any of the joints may be thus affected, but most commonly those of the hands and feet. The deposits occur in other structures besides those of joints, such as along the course of tendons, underneath the skin and periosteum, in the sclerotic coat of the eye, and especially on the cartilages of the external ear. When bi-urate of soda is largely deposited in joints the skin sometimes gives way, and the concretion is exposed.

A variety of urinary calculus – the uric acid stone – formed by concretions of this substance in the kidneys is a not infrequent occurrence in connection with gout; hence the well-known association of this disease and gravel (q.v.).
Treatment: During the acute attack the affected part should be kept at perfect rest, and be enveloped in cotton-wool covered with oil-silk. The medicinal agent upon which most reliance was placed was colchicum. The first known record of the use of this drug, which is said to derive its name from Colchis in Asia Minor, is in the Eber papyrus of around 1500 BC. The mode of action of colchicum is uncertain, but it is probable that it has simply a special sedative action upon the gouty inflammation

without affecting the excretion of uric acid. It is usually administered as colchicine, which is the active principle of the drug and was first isolated in 1820. In cases which do not respond satisfactorily to colchicine, one of the non-steroidal anti-inflammatory drugs such as indomethacin should be used. For the long-term management and prevention a uricosuric agent such as probenecid should be used or an xanthine oxidase inhibitor such as allopurinol which prevents the formation of uric acid.

GRAFT is the term applied to a piece of tissue removed from one person or animal and implanted in another, or the same, individual in order by its growth to remedy some defect. Skin grafts are commonly used. Bone grafts are also used to replace bone which has been lost by disease: for example, a portion of rib is sometimes removed in order to furnish support for a spine weakened by disease, after the disease has been removed. Also, the bone of young animals is used to afford additional growth and strength to a limb bone which it has been necessary to remove in part on account of disease or injury. Vein grafts are used to replace stretches of arteries which have become blocked, particularly in the heart and lower limbs. The veins most commonly used for this purpose are the saphenous veins of the individual in question provided they are healthy. An alternative is specially treated umbilical vein. (See SKIN-GRAFTING.)

GRAFT VERSUS HOST DISEASE (GVHD): A condition that is a common complication of bone marrow transplant. It results from certain lymphocytes (q.v.) in the transplanted marrow attacking the transplant recipient's tissues, which they identify as 'foreign'. GVHD may appear soon after a transplant or develop several months later. The condition, which is fatal in about a third of victims, may be prevented by immuno-suppressant drugs such as cyclosporin (see IMMUNO-SUPPRESSION).

GRAM, or GRAMME, is the unit of weight in the metric system and is equal to a little over 15·4 grains. For purposes of weighing food, 30 grams are usually taken as approximately equal to 1 ounce.

GRAM'S STAIN, named after the bacteriologist, H. C. J. Gram, who first described it in 1884, is one of the most valuable methods of differentiating certain micro-organisms. The principle involved depends upon the fact that certain bacteria, when treated with a dye such as gentian violet and then with iodine, fix the dye, whereas other bacteria do not. Those bacteria, such as the pneumococcus, that fix the dye are known as Gram-positive, whilst those that do not fix it, e.g. the gonococcus, are said to be Gram-negative.

GRAND MAL is the name applied to a convulsive epileptic attack, in contrast to petit mal, which includes the milder forms of epilepsy (q.v.).

GRANULATIONS are small masses of formative cells containing loops of newly formed blood-vessels which spring up over any raw surface, as the first step in the process of healing of wounds. (See ULCER; WOUNDS.)

GRANULOCYTE: White blood cells which, when stained with Romanowsky stains containing thiazine dyes and eosin, are found to contain granules in their cytoplasm. The colour of the granules enables the cells to be further classified as basophils, eosinophils, and neutrophils (qq.v.).

GRANULOMA is a tumour or new growth made up of granulation tissue. This is caused by various forms of chronic inflammation, such as syphilis and tuberculosis.

GRAVEL is the name applied to any sediment which falls down in the urine, but particularly to small masses of uric acid. It produces various unpleasant symptoms. (See BLADDER, DISEASES OF; GOUT; URINE.)

GRAVES' DISEASE is a syndrome consisting of diffuse goitre, hyperthyroidism and eye signs and is due to the production of various auto-antibodies. The hyperthyroidism is due to the production of antibodies to the TSH receptor which stimulate the receptor with resultant production of excess thyroid hormones. The goitre is due to antibodies that stimulate the growth of the thyroid gland. The exophthalmos is due to another immunoglobulin called the ophthalmopathic immunoglobulin which is an antibody to a retro-orbital antigen on the surface of the retro-orbital eye muscles. This provokes inflammation in the retro-orbital tissues which is associated with the accumulation of water and mucopolysaccharide which fills the orbit and causes the eye to protrude forwards.

Although Graves' disease may affect any age group the peak incidence is in the 3rd decade. Females are affected ten times as often as males. The prevalence in females is one in 500. As with many other auto-immune diseases, there is an increased prevalence of auto-immune thyroid disease in the relatives of patients with Graves' disease. Some of these patients may have hypothyroidism and others thyrotoxicosis. Patients with Graves' disease may present with a goitre or with the eye signs or, most commonly, with the symptoms of excess thyroid hormone production. Thyroid hormone controls the metabolic rate of the body so that the symptoms of hyperthyroidism are those of excess metabolism. Patients thus lose weight despite a good appetite. They become

intolerant of heat and sweat more than previously. The heart rate is rapid so that patients may be aware of palpitations or shortness of breath. There is excess stimulation of the central nervous system so that patients become irritable, hyperactive and develop tremor. They commonly also develop muscle weakness due to a myopathy. This tends to affect the girdle muscles so that patients may have difficulty getting out of chairs or climbing stairs or combing their hair. In addition to the prominence of the eyes due to exophthalmos there may also be swelling of the eyelids and congestion of the conjunctiva, and paralysis of the eye muscles leading to double vision. Some patients with exophthalmos also develop pre-tibial myxoedema. This is a localized involvement of the skin with infiltration of muco polysaccharide which occurs in the front of the shins but may extend to the dorsum of the foot and even to the toes.

The diagnosis of Graves' disease is confirmed by the measurement of the circulating levels of the two thyroid hormones, thyroxine and tri-iodothyronine.

Treatment: There are three effective treatments for Graves' disease. (1) Antithyroid drugs: these drugs inhibit the iodination of tyrosine and hence the formation of the thyroid hormones. The most commonly used drugs are carbimazole, propylthiouricil and methimazole. They will control the excess production of thyroid hormones in virtually all cases. Once the patient has been rendered euthyroid the dose can be reduced to a maintenance dose and is usually continued for two years. The disadvantage of antithyroid drugs is that even after two years' treatment nearly half the patients will relapse and will then require more definitive therapy.

(2) Partial thyroidectomy: removal of three-quarters of the thyroid gland is effective treatment of the hyperthyroidism of Graves' disease. It is the treatment of choice in those patients with large goitres. The patient must however be rendered euthyroid before surgery is undertaken, or thyroid crisis and arrhythmias may complicate the operation.

(3) Radioactive iodine therapy: this has been in use for more than 30 years. It is an effective means of controlling hyperthyroidism and does not require admission to hospital but merely the taking of a tasteless, colourless drink. One of the disadvantages of radioactive iodine is that the incidence of hypothyroidism is much greater than with other forms of treatment. The incidence of hypothyroidism increases as the years pass and after 20 years the incidence approaches 80 per cent of patients. However the management of hypothyroidism is simple and requires only the taking of thyroxine tablets, so that, provided the patients are followed up and the hypothyroidism is diagnosed, this presents little problem. There is no evidence of any increased incidence of cancer of the thyroid or leukaemia following radio-iodine therapy over the 30 years that it has been used. It has been the pattern in Britain to reserve radio-iodine treatment to those over the

age of 35 or those whose prognosis is unlikely to be more than 30 years as a result of cardiac or respiratory disease.

GRAVID means pregnant.

GREENSTICK FRACTURE is an incomplete fracture, in which the bone is not completely broken across. It occurs in the long bones of children and is usually due to indirect violence. (See FRACTURES.)

GREY MATTER: Those parts of the brain and spinal cord that comprise mainly the interconnected and tightly packed nuclei of nerve cells. The tissue is darker than that of the white matter, which is made of *axons* from the nerve cells. In the brain grey matter is mainly found in the outer layers of the cerebrum, which is the zone responsible for advanced mental functions. The inner core of the spinal cord is made up of grey matter.

GRIPES is a popular name for the colic of infants, generally due to irregular feeding. (See COLIC.)

GRISEOFULVIN is an antibiotic obtained from *Penicillium griseofulvum Dierckse*, which is proving of value in the treatment of various forms of ringworm.

GROIN is the region which includes the upper part of the front of the thigh and lower part of the abdomen. A deep groove runs obliquely across it, which corresponds to the inguinal ligament, and divides the thigh from the abdomen. The principal diseased conditions in this region are enlarged glands (see GLANDS), and hernia (q.v.).

GROMMET is a small bobbin-shaped tube used to keep open the incision made in the ear drum in the treatment of secretory otitis media. It acts as a ventilation tube by allowing the Eustachian tube to recover its normal function. (See EAR, DISEASES OF; EUSTACHIAN TUBES.)

GROUP THERAPY: Psychotherapy in which at least two, but more commonly up to ten patients as well as the therapist, take part. The therapist encourages the patients to analyse their own and the others' emotional and psychological difficulties. Group therapy is also used to help patients with the same condition, for instance, alcoholism or compulsive gambling. They discuss their problems for perhaps an hour twice a week and explore ways of resolving them.

GROWING PAINS occur in children during the course of development most commonly in the legs and back. As often as not they are of no significance, but they must not be entirely ignored because they may on occasion be the first manifestation of rheumatic fever. Severe pains in young children are occasionally due to actual disease in a bone, either of tuberculous nature or caused by acute inflammation (osteomyelitis), and special attention is required in such cases.

GROWTH is a popular term applied to any new formation in any part of the body. (See CANCER; CYSTS; GANGLION; TUMOUR.) For growth of children, see WEIGHT AND HEIGHT.

GROWTH HORMONE: A product of the anterior part of the pituitary gland that promotes normal growth and development in the body by changing the chemical activity in the cells. The hormone activates protein production in the muscle cells as well as the release of energy from the metabolism of fats. Its release is controlled by the contrasting actions of growth-hormone releasing factor and somatostatin. If the body produces too much growth hormone before puberty gigantism (q.v.) results; in adulthood the result is acromegaly (q.v.). Lack of growth hormone in children causes dwarfism (q.v.).

GUANETHIDINE is one of the hypotensive drugs which act by inhibiting the action of the sympathetic nervous system (q.v.).

GUINEA-WORM (see DRACUNCULIASIS).

GULLET, or OESOPHAGUS, is the tube down which food passes from the throat to the stomach. (See OESOPHAGUS.)

GUM is a complex viscid substance which exudes from the stems and branches of various trees, and consists principally of arabin or bassorin. The two best-known gums are gum acacia and gum tragacanth. Gum-resins such as asafoetida, galbanum, and myrrh also contain resin.

A grommet

GUMBOIL is a painful condition of inflammation, ending sometimes as an abscess, situated about the root of a carious tooth.

GUMMA means a hard swelling situated usually in connective tissue, although it may be in internal organs, muscle, or brain, and resulting from syphilis. The swelling is usually painless but it may produce very marked symptoms by interference with the organ in which it is situated. A gumma generally disappears speedily when the treatment appropriate to syphilis is administered.

GUMS, DISEASES OF (see MOUTH, DISEASES OF; TEETH, DISEASES OF).

GYNAECOLOGY is the branch of medical science which deals with diseases peculiar to women.

GYNAECOMASTIA is the term used for describing an abnormal increase in size of the male breast.

GYRUS is the term applied to a convolution of the brain.

H

H₂ RECEPTOR ANTAGONISTS: Drugs that block the action of HISTAMINE (q.v.) at the H_2 receptor (which mediates the gastric and some of the cardiovascular effects of histamine). Histamine increases the secretion of acid by the stomach, and these drugs therefore decrease the basal and stimulated acid production of the stomach. They are used in the treatment of peptic ulcers, reflux inflammation of the oesophagus (q.v.), and Zollinger Ellison syndrome.

HABIT SPASM (see CRAMP).

HAEMANGIOMA is a benign tumour composed of tortuous dilated blood-vessels.

HAEMARTHROSIS denotes bleeding into, or the presence of blood in, a joint.

HAEMATEMESIS means vomiting of blood. Blood brought up from the stomach is generally dark in colour, and is often so far digested as to form small brown granules resembling coffee grounds. Vomiting of blood is one of the chief symptoms of peptic ulcer, but it may also occur in gastritis, especially when this is due to the action of irritant poisons or alcohol, and cancer of the stomach. It should always be remembered that the blood may come from the nose or throat, and, after being swallowed, provoke vomiting. (See HAEMORRHAGE.)

HAEMATOCOELE means a cavity containing blood. Generally as the result of an injury which ruptures blood-vessels, blood is effused into one of the natural cavities of the body, or among loose cellular tissue, producing a haematocoele.

HAEMATOCOLPOS is the condition in which menstrual blood is held up in the vagina as a result of an imperforate hymen.

HAEMATOCRIT: An expression of the fraction of blood volume occupied by the red cells. It is determined by centrifuging a sample of blood in a capillary tube and measuring the height of the resulting packed cells as a percentage of the total sample height.

Normal values: males 42–52%
                 females 32–47%

HAEMATOLOGY is the study of diseases of the blood.

HAEMATOMA means a collection of blood forming a definite swelling. It is found often upon the head of new-born children after a protracted and difficult labour. It may occur as the result of any injury or operation.

HAEMATOXYLON, or LOGWOOD, is the wood of *Haematoxylon campechianum*, which is used as a dye in staining tissues in histology. As it has a mildly astringent action, it is used for checking diarrhoea.

HAEMATURIA means the condition of blood in the urine. (See URINE.) The blood may come from any part of the urinary tract. When the blood comes from the kidney or upper part of the urinary tract, it is usually mixed throughout the urine, giving the latter a brownish or smoky tinge. This condition is usually the result of acute or subacute glomerulonephritis, or it may be present in persons suffering from high blood-pressure or pyelitis (q.v.). Blood may also appear in the urine from time to time in considerable quantites when a stone or gravel is present in the pelvis of the kidney setting up irritation, especially when the person undergoes unwonted exercise. The blood may also originate from the bladder in cases in which this is inflamed, and is then present in smaller quantities as a rule. The presence of a stone in the bladder is also productive of blood, and in either of the latter cases the urine is generally turbid from admixture with pus. A condition which leads to the passage of bright red blood at occasional intervals is the presence of a species of warty growth (papilloma) on the wall of the bladder. Blood may also be derived from the urethra following some inflammatory condition in this passage, or injury to it as by a fracture of the pelvic bones. Occasionally the bleeding may be due to purpura.

The recognition of the site of the haemorrhage is important in relation to the measures to be adopted for its treatment. This can often be made out by the character of the blood, whether intimately mixed with the urine or in the form of clots, also by the shape of the clots, and by the presence of other abnormal constituents in the urine. For the final diagnosis, examination of the interior of the bladder by the cystoscope and the passage of fine catheters up the ureters to the kidneys is often of importance.

HAEMIC MURMUR is a term applied to unusual sounds heard over the heart and large blood-vessels in severe cases of anaemia. They disappear as the condition is recovered from. Murmurs of this type are to be distinguished from 'organic murmurs', which are due to some disease of the heart-valves or vessel walls.

HAEMOCHROMATOSIS, or BRONZED DIABETES, is a disease in which cirrhosis of the liver, enlargement of the spleen, pigmentation of the skin, and diabetes mellitus are associated with the abnormal and excessive deposit in the organs of the body of the iron-containing pigment, haemosiderin.

HAEMOCYTOMETER is an instrument for counting corpuscles in the blood.

HAEMODIALYSIS is the principle used in the artificial kidney (see KIDNEY, ARTIFICIAL), whereby the patient's blood is circulated through a cellophane tube, on the other side of which is a dialysing solution containing electrolytes in the concentration they should be in normal blood, but no urea. In this way the patient's blood is restored to its normal state as it would were it passing through normally functioning kidneys. (See also DIALYSIS.)

HAEMOFILTRATION: A means of removing excess fluid, electrolytes and some waste products from the blood in patients with acute renal failure. The filter usually consists of a cylinder containing a large number of microtubules which are made from a membrane which is permeable to water and small molecules (molecular weight<12,000). Blood from the patient is passed through the cylinder where water and solutes pass out of the blood and through the membrane by convection before the blood is returned to the patient. The process is continuous via an extracorporeal (outside the body) circulation. As the system removes large volumes of water and electrolytes from blood, these are replaced by intravenous infusion of a balanced salt solution (the volume is calculated to produce an overall negative, positive or static fluid balance each day).

HAEMOGLOBIN is the colouring material which produces the red colour of blood. It is a chromoprotein, made up of a protein called globin and the iron-containing pigment, haemin. When separated from the red blood corpuscles, each of which contains about 600 million haemoglobin molecules, it is crystalline in form. It exists in two forms: simple haemoglobin, found in venous blood, and oxyhaemoglobin, which is a loose compound with oxygen, found in arterial blood after the blood has come in contact with the air in the lungs. This oxyhaemoglobin is again broken down as the blood passes through the tissues, which take up the oxygen for their own use. This is the main function of haemoglobin: to act as a carrier of oxygen from the lungs to all the tissues of the body. When the haemoglobin leaves the lungs it is 97 per cent saturated with oxygen. When it comes back to the lungs in the venous blood it is 70 per cent saturated. The oxygen content of 100 millilitres of blood leaving the lungs is 19·5 millilitres, and that of venous blood returning to the lungs is 14·5 millilitres. Thus each 100 millilitres of blood delivers 5 millilitres of oxygen to the tissues of the body. Human male blood contains 13 to 18 grams of haemoglobin per 100 millilitres. In women, there are 12 to 16 grams per 100 millilitres. A man weighing 70 kilograms (154 pounds) has around 770 grams of haemoglobin circulating in his red blood corpuscles.

HAEMOGLOBINOPATHIES: Haemoglobin (q.v.) is a pigment composed of an iron protoporphyrin complex combined with a protein globin. It is the globin portion which varies in different types of haemoglobin. Impairment of adult haemoglobin formation is the characteristic abnormality of the haemoglobinopathies, which are hereditary haemolytic anaemias, genetically determined and related to race. The haemoglobin may be abnormal because: (1) there is a defect in the synthesis of normal adult haemoglobin and this occurs in thalassaemia when there may be an absence of one or both of the polypeptide chains characteristic of normal adult haemoglobin, or (2) an abnormal form of haemoglobin such as haemoglobin S, that of sickle-cell disease, is formed instead of adult haemoglobin. This abnormality may involve as little as one amino acid of the 300 in the haemoglobin molecule. In sickle-cell haemoglobin one single amino acid molecule, that of glutamic acid, is replaced by another, that of valine, and this results in such a deficient end product that the ensuing disease is frequently rapidly fatal.

HAEMOGLOBINURIA means the presence of blood pigment in the urine caused by the destruction of blood corpuscles in the bloodvessels or in the urinary passages. It produces in the urine a dark red or brown colour. In some people this condition, known as intermittent haemoglobinuria, occurs from time to time, especially on exposure to cold. It is also produced by various poisonous substances taken in the food. It occurs in malarious districts in the form of one of the most fatal forms of malaria: blackwater fever (q.v.). (See also MARCH HAEMOGLOBINURIA.)

HAEMOLYSIS means the breaking up of blood corpuscles by the action of poisonous substances, usually of a protein nature, circulating in the blood, or by certain chemicals. It occurs, for example, gradually in some forms of anaemia and rapidly in poisoning by snake venom.

HAEMOLYTIC DISEASE OF THE NEW-BORN: A serious disease of the new-born characterized by haemolytic anaemia and jaundice (qq.v.). It may be associated with oedema, and if there is a great deal of fluid in the PERICARDIAL, PLEURAL, and PERITONEAL cavities the condition is known as Hydrops foetalis. If jaundice appears within 24 hours of birth it is likely to be due to blood-group incompatibility between the mother and baby. The commonest cause of haemolytic disease of the new-born is rhesus incompatibility (see BLOOD GROUPS) – a previously sensitized rhesus-negative mother produces antibodies which cause haemolysis (destruction of the blood cells) in her rhesus-positive baby.

The infant's serum bilirubin (q.v.) concentration should be plotted regularly so that treatment can be given before levels likely to cause brain damage occur. Safe bilirubin concentrations depend on the age of the child, and reference charts should always be used.

High bilirubin concentrations may be treated with phototherapy. The infant, with its eyes suitably protected, is nursed under ultraviolet light. Extra fluid is given to prevent dehydration and to improve bilirubin excretion by shortening the gut transit time. Severe jaundice and anaemia may require exchange transfusion (see TRANSFUSION OF BLOOD). Haemolytic disease of the new-born secondary to rhesus incompatibility has become less common since the introduction of anti-D. This antibody should be given to all rhesus-negative women at any risk of a fetomaternal transfusion, to prevent them from mounting an antibody response. Anti-D is given routinely to rhesus-negative mothers after the birth of a rhesus-positive baby, but doctors should also remember to give it after threatened abortions, antepartum haemorrhages, miscarriages, and terminations of pregnancy.

HAEMOLYTIC URAEMIA SYNDROME: A disease of children resulting in acute oliguric (q.v.) renal failure. A febrile illness of the gastrointestinal or respiratory tracts is followed by intravascular coagulation of blood which results in haemolysis (q.v.), anaemia (q.v.), thrombocytopaenia (q.v.) and renal failure (resulting from fibrin deposition in renal arterioles and glomerular capillaries).

The death rate is 2–10 per cent and the majority of patients survive without renal failure. The longer the period of oliguria the greater the risk of chronic renal failure.

Treatment is supportive with replacement of blood and clotting factors, control of hypertension (q.v.) and careful observance of fluid balance.

HAEMOPHILIA: An inherited disorder of blood coagulation which results in prolonged bleeding even after minor injury. There is a deficiency of Factor VIII, an essential clotting factor in the coagulation cascade – the complex series of biochemical events that lead from injury of the wall of a blood vessel to the formation of a blood clot that checks bleeding. It is a sex-linked recessive disorder (though a small number of cases arise by spontaneous mutation) so that females carry the disease, half their sons will be affected and half their daughters will be carriers. The sons of haemophiliacs are unaffected but half their daughters will be carriers. Haemophilia affects approximately 1:4,000 of the UK population but only 1:20,000 is severely affected. Severity of the disease depends upon the percentage, compared with normal, of Factor VIII activity present. Less than 1 per cent and there will be spontaneous bleeding into joints and muscles; 1–5 per cent and there will be occasional spontaneous bleeding and severe bleeding after minor injury; 5–25 per cent and there will only be severe bleeding after major injury. Before treatment was available, severe haemophiliacs suffered from severe pain and deformity from bleeds into joints and muscles. Bleeding also occurred into the gut, kidney and brain and few survived past adolescence.

Freeze-dried Factor VIII may be kept in domestic refrigerators. Haemophiliacs can use it to abort minor bleeds by reconstituting it and injecting it intravenously. More major bleeding or preparation for surgery involves raising Factor VIII levels to 30–100 per cent by giving cryoprecipitate.

With treatment most haemophiliacs lead normal lives, though obviously dangerous or contact sports should be avoided.

There is a National Haemophilia Register and each registered sufferer carries a card with details about his condition. Information may also be obtained from NHS haemophilia centres and the Haemophilia Society, 123 Westminster Bridge Road, London SE1 7HR (071-928 2020).

HAEMOPHILUS: A genus of Gram negative, rod-like, aerobic, parasitic bacteria. They are found in the respiratory tract, and most are pathogenic.

HAEMOPOIESIS: The formation of blood.

HAEMOPTYSIS means the spitting up of blood from the lower air passages. The blood is usually coughed or gently hawked up, it may be in mouthfuls at a time, and is bright red and frothy, thus differing from the blood brought up from the stomach. Generally the condition results from some disease of the heart or lungs. It should be remembered, however, that in elderly people haemoptysis may be due to a varicose condition of the small veins in the throat, not to haemorrhage in the lungs; while in young people this condition is often due to bleeding from the nose, in which, owing to the position of the head, the blood happens to run backwards instead of forwards through the nostrils. (See HAEMORRHAGE; TUBERCULOSIS.)

HAEMORRHAGE means any escape of blood from the vessels which naturally contain it. It may occur from a wound of the skin, in which case it escapes externally, or into some internal cavity such as the stomach or bowels, or may simply be poured out into the tissues in consequence of a blow or similar injury; but, in all cases alike, the blood escaping from the vessels is lost to the circulation. Haemorrhage is classified according to the vessels from which it occurs, as *arterial*, in which case the blood is bright and appears in jets or spurts, corresponding to the heart-beats; *venous*, when it comes from veins, is dark, and wells up gradually into the wound; *capillary*, when it flows merely from torn capillaries, and comes in a gentle ooze out of the general surface of the wound. The immediate result of a severe haemorrhage is great anaemia, so that in extreme cases the bodily organs may be unable to continue their functions, and the person dies in consequence, with symptoms of shock.

In general, arterial haemorrhage is the most serious, and if a large artery, such as the femoral, is wounded, the person concerned may bleed to death in a few minutes. Venous haemorrhage is so easily checked by slight pressure, and the valves in the veins so effectively prevent blood from running backwards in these vessels, that this form is not dangerous to life except in the case of ruptured varicose veins of the leg, or when a serious internal injury is received. Capillary haemorrhage stops so quickly, that only in the case of the disease known as haemophilia (q.v.) is it of serious import. The following terms are applied to haemorrhage from special sites: *haematemesis*, bleeding from the stomach; *haemoptysis*, bleeding from the lungs; *epistaxis*, bleeding from the nose; and *haematuria*, bleeding from the kidney or urinary passages. (See these headings.) Haemorrhage is also classed as primary, reactionary, and secondary. (See WOUNDS.)

Natural arrest: When a small artery is cut across, the bleeding stops in consequence of changes in the wall of the artery on the one hand, and in the constitution of the blood on the other. Every artery is surrounded by a fibrous sheath, and when cut, the vessel retracts some little distance within this sheath, in consequence of the shortening of its muscle fibres; and further, by the same process the end contracts so as to form an opening of smaller size than the rest of the vessel. In the space between the end of the vessel and its sheath, and afterwards for some distance up the interior of the narrowed artery, blood-clot quickly forms by the following process, and rapidly blocks the open end of the vessel. When blood is shed so as to come in contact with any surface other than the smooth lining of blood-vessels, the fibrinogen which is dissolved in its fluid becomes converted into threads of fibrin through combination with the lime salts of the blood, and the action of a chemical given off probably by the blood platelets. These threads of fibrin slowly contract and develop into a dense felt-work, in the meshes of which the corpuscles are held, and in this way a blood-clot of increasing hardness is produced, within and round the ends of the injured vessels. This chain of events is called the coagulation cascade. When an artery is only partially severed it is evident that contraction and retraction within the sheath cannot take place, and accordingly bleeding is apt to be more serious than when the vessel is completely cut across. Again, if an artery is torn across or twisted instead of cut, the opening at its end is still more narrowed, and the blood clots more rapidly on the ragged surface than it would do upon a clean cut, so that haemorrhage from a torn or bruised wound is in general much smaller in amount than from a stab or cut. The natural arrest of bleeding is usually described therefore as depending upon four factors: (*a*) the retraction, and (*b*) the contraction of the cut artery: (*c*) the external, and (*d*) the internal clot formed by the blood. For the means by which circulation is subsequently carried on after an artery is cut, see ANASTOMOSIS.

Control of external haemorrhage: Four main principles are applicable in the control of a severe external haemorrhage: (*a*) direct pressure on the bleeding point or points; (*b*) elevation of the wounded part; (*c*) pressure on the main artery of supply to the part; and (*d*) application of substances known as styptics, which contract the vessels or aid the coagulation of the blood.

(*a*) DIRECT PRESSURE may be made with the finger, which is the best method, when a definite bleeding point is seen in a gaping wound. This is the method adopted at an operation by the surgeon, who places his finger at once upon any bleeding point, afterwards seizing the cut artery with forceps and tying a piece of silk or catgut tightly round its end. If the artery lies between the skin and a hard surface, as in the case of scalp wounds, a wedge-shaped pad and tight bandage (known as a graduated compress) may be substituted for pressure with the finger, the edges of the wound being compressed between the pad and skull.

(*b*) ELEVATION of the bleeding member is an important method, the blood running off more readily by the veins, and a smaller quantity being driven into the limb the higher it is raised. This method is applicable, of course, only in cases of bleeding from the hand or foot.

(c) PRESSURE UPON THE MAIN ARTERY of supply to the injured limb is a certain method of stopping the circulation and consequently all bleeding, much after the manner of stopping the water supply of a district by closing the main pipe. At certain points where the arteries lie close to bones and near the surface, the pulsation of the vessel may be felt, and *pressure with the finger* over the artery serves to obliterate it against the bone, the points where this may be adopted being as follows. In cases of bleeding from the upper part of the scalp, the temporal artery may be felt and compressed immediately in front of the upper part of the ear, while for wounds at the back of the head the occipital artery can be felt and compressed a short distance behind the mastoid process, the bony prominence at the back of the ear.

Bleeding from the face may be checked by pressure on the facial artery, which passes on to the face about 2·5 cm in front of the angle of the jaw, across the jaw-bone, against which it is to be pressed.

All bleeding from the head and neck may be lessened by pressure upon the common carotid artery in the neck a short distance below the prominent Adam's apple, and between it and the edge of the large sternocleidomastoid muscle. In this groove the artery is pressed straight back against the transverse processes of the spinal column.

Bleeding from the region of the shoulder and armpit is checked by pressure on the subclavian artery, the pressure being applied with the thumb directly downwards in the hollow behind the middle part of the collar-bone, so as to press the artery down upon the first rib.

Bleeding from the region of the elbow or forearm may be controlled by feeling for the brachial artery on the inner side of the upper arm, behind the biceps muscle, and pressing it against the humerus.

Bleeding from the hand is checked by pressure on the radial artery, where it lies between the skin and radius in front of the wrist, and on the ulnar artery just before it enters the hand near its inner margin.

In the lower limb the arteries lie deeply among the muscles, but bleeding from any part of the limb may be checked by pressure backwards on the femoral artery, which is to be felt pulsating in the centre of the groin, and which is compressed backwards against the head of the thigh-bone.

Bleeding from the sole of the foot may be controlled by pressure on the posterior tibial artery, which lies about 1·5 cm behind the inner ankle.

A second method for applying pressure on the main artery consists in *forced flexion* at the elbow, hip, or knee, as the case may be. A pad is placed in the bend of the joint, which is then flexed as completely as possible and firmly bound in this position, the artery being thus sharply bent upon itself.

A third method for control of the main blood supply is by the *tourniquet*, which consists of an elastic band or ligature passed round a fleshy part of any of the limbs, and pulled or twisted tight. A surgical tourniquet consists of a rubber cord or band with an arrangement for fixing the ends together, or of a strap with buckle and a screw appliance for tightening it up. A tourniquet may, however, be improvized from a piece of rope, or a handkerchief folded cravatwise, tied round the limb and then twisted up tight by a piece of wood, large key, or similar object introduced beneath it. The handle of such a tourniquet is prevented from untwisting by passing a second band round the limb and including the end of the handle within it before tying. A tourniquet may be applied to the fleshy part of the thigh, leg, upper arm, or forearm. It is most important to note on a label the time of appliction of a tourniquet. No tourniquet should ever be left on longer than an hour. It must be loosened every fifteen minutes, to be tightened again if bleeding restarts. (See TOURNIQUET.)

Occasionally, when bleeding is continuous or when it occurs from a deep-seated wound like a stab, or injury to the root of the tongue, it is impossible to get at the bleeding point, and permanent control of the bleeding is only to be achieved by the surgeon, who cuts down upon the main artery of supply and ties a ligature round it.

(d) STYPTICS are applied when the bleeding is a general ooze from a wound, or when the bleeding comes from an inaccessible position, such as the interior of the nose or a wound in the side. The most important styptics are heat and cold. Although moderate warmth greatly increases bleeding, ice-cold water and also water between 46 and 49 °C (115 and 120 °F) (i.e. a temperature which the hand can hardly bear) both favour clotting and contract the blood-vessels. Heat is much more effectual than cold, if applied directly to the wound. Various drugs, such as perchloride of iron (steel drops) and hazeline, act similarly. Cayenne pepper has a traditional reputation as a styptic in controlling superficial bleeding when applied locally: e.g. from a bleeding lip. Adrenaline has a powerful local action in contracting vessels and stopping bleeding. Russell-viper venom is most effective as a local application in cases such as bleeding from a tooth socket. Other styptics include oxidized cellulose, gelatin by-products, calcium alginate, and thrombin powder.

Control of internal haemorrhage is not to be so certainly achieved as in the case of bleeding from the vessels of the limbs. There are certain general principles to which it is most important to adhere. Chief among these is the maintenance of the recumbent position, since the heart beats less forcibly and the blood-pressure is consequently lowered as soon as the injured person lies down. For the same reason, all excitement must be avoided, and the mind of the sufferer quieted as far as possible. The patient must also be kept warm. Stimulants must be avoided. Ice-bags or compresses wrung out of cold water may be laid over the chest or stomach, according to the origin of the haemorrhage. The most valuable drug in the treatment of internal haemorrhage is morphine given hypodermically. In the haemorrhage which sometimes follows child-birth, the source of bleeding is usually the uterus. This is controlled by the injection of ergometrine, the removal of the placenta if this has not already come away, and then compression of the uterus. This may need to be supplemented by plugging of the vagina with sterile gauze. Blood transfusion may be necessary.

Treatment of bleeding from special sites:

NOSE: Keep quiet, lying or sitting; loosen collar; no blowing of nose; cold key or sponge to neck; if these are not successful, plugging of nostrils with lint soaked in tincture of perchloride of iron or adrenaline.

TONGUE: Ice to suck; pressure with the fingers; if serious, compression of carotid artery.

FACE OR SCALP: Direct pressure with fingers or bandage and pad on wound; if bleeding be severe, pressure in addition on facial, temporal, or occipital artery.

NECK: Pressure on carotid artery.

ARMPIT OR SHOULDER: Pressure on subclavian artery.

FOREARM: Pressure on brachial artery by fingers, tourniquet, or forced flexion at elbow.

HAND: Elevation and direct pressure with pad and bandage; if bleeding severe, pressure on radial and ulnar arteries, or tourniquet to forearm.

THIGH: Pressure on femoral artery at groin; tourniquet, if low down.

LEG: Tourniquet to thigh, or forced flexion at knee. In the case of ruptured varicose veins, a pad and bandage round leg extending above and below wound with elevation of limb suffice.

FOOT: Direct pressure and elevation; if bleeding severe, forced flexion at knee, or pressure on posterior tibial artery.

HAEMORRHOIDS (see PILES).

HAEMOSTASIS: The process by which bleeding stops. It involves constriction of blood vessels, the formation of a platelet plug, and blood clotting. The term is also used for surgical interventions to stop bleeding, e.g. the use of diathermy. (See HAEMORRHAGE.)

HAEMOSTATICS are any means, whether of the nature of mechanical appliances or drugs, used to control bleeding. (See FIBRIN FOAM; HAEMORRHAGE.)

HAEMOTHORAX means an effusion of blood into the pleural cavity.

HAIR (see SKIN; WHITE HAIR).

HAIR, REMOVAL OF (see DEPILATION).

HALF LIFE: The time taken for the plasma concentration of a drug to decline by half from redistribution, metabolism and excretion.

HALIBUT-LIVER OIL is the oil expressed from fresh, or suitably preserved, halibut liver. It is a particularly rich source of vitamin A (30,000 international units per gram), and also contains vitamin D (2300 to 2500 units per gram). Because of the relatively small volume required, it is often used as a means of giving vitamin D: either as drops of the oil or in capsules. Care must be taken to ensure that the child is receiving at least 700 international units of vitamin D daily. (See VITAMIN.)

HALITOSIS is another term for bad breath. (See BREATH, DISORDERS OF.)

HALLUCINATIONS are errors in perception, affecting some sense organ to such an extent that a person imagines he perceives something for which there is no foundation. For example, a person may fancy he hears himself called during perfect stillness, or may see lights in pitch darkness. *Illusions* are misinterpreted sensations: for example, a person may constantly mistake an article of furniture for the figure of some friend, or of an animal. Both these errors occur in sane people, and may indicate some slight brain derangement, due to sleeplessness, overwork, feverishness, or other cause. They are usually, however, a symptom of insanity. (See MENTAL ILLNESS.)

HALLUCINOGENS are compounds characterized by their ability to produce distortions of perception, emotional changes, depersonalization, and a variety of effects on memory and learned behaviour. They include lysergic acid diethylamide (q.v.) and mescaline (q.v.). (See also DRUG ADDICTION.)

HALLUX is the anatomical name of the great toe.

HALLUX RIGIDUS is stiffness of the joint between the great toe and the foot which induces pain on walking. It is usually due to a crush injury or stubbing of the toe. Such stubbing is liable to occur in adolescents with a congenitally long toe. If troublesome it is treated by an operation to create a false joint.

HALLUX VALGUS is outward displacement of the great toe and is always associated with a bunion. It is due to the pressure of footwear on an unduly broad foot. In adolescents this broad foot is inherited; in adults it is due to splaying of the foot as a result of loss of muscle tone. The bunion is produced by pressure of the footwear on the protruding base of the toe. In mild cases the wearing of comfortable shoes may be all that is needed. In more severe cases the bunion may need to be removed, while in the most severe the operation of arthroplasty (q.v.) may be needed. (See also CORNS AND BUNIONS.)

HALO is a coloured circle seen round a bright light in some eye conditions. When accompanied by headache it is specially likely to be caused by glaucoma (q.v.).

HALOPERIDOL is one of the butyrophenone group of drugs that is proving useful in the treatment of mania and schizophrenic excitement. It is also of value in some cases of stuttering, intractable hiccups and uncontrollable sneezing.

HALOTHANE is a non-inflammable anaesthetic, the chemical formula of which is $CF_3CHClBr$. Patients recover rapidly from its effects. (See ANAESTHESIA.)

HALOTHANE HEPATITIS: A very rare form of hepatitis following exposure to halothane during anaesthesia (1:35,000 halothane anaesthetics). Jaundice develops three to four days after exposure and will occasionally develop into a fatal massive hepatic necrosis. It is of unknown aetiology but probably has an immunological basis. It is more common following multiple exposures in a short time (less than 28 days), and in obesity, middle age and females. It is rare in children.

HAMARTOMA: These are benign tumours, usually in the lung, containing normal components of pulmonary tissue such as smooth muscle and connective tissue.

HAMMER-TOE is the deformity in which there is permanent flexion, or bending of the middle joint of the toe. The condition may affect all the toes as in claw-foot (q.v.). More commonly it affects one toe, usually the second. It is due to a relatively long toe and the pressure on it of the footwear. A painful bunion usually develops on it. In mild cases relief is obtained by protecting the toe with adhesive pads. If this does not suffice operation is necessary. (See CORNS AND BUNIONS.)

HAMSTRINGS is the name given to the tendons at the back of the knee, two on the inner side and one on the outer side, which bend this joint. They are attached to the tibia below.

HAND is the section of the upper limb below the wrist. The hand of man is more highly developed in its structure and in its nervous connections than the corresponding part in any other animal. Indeed the possession of a thumb which can be 'opposed' to the other fingers for grasping objects is one of the distinguishing features of the human race. Of all the parts of the body, the hand, which is connected with a large area on the surface of the brain, is capable of the highest degree of education, and in cases in which the brain degenerates, as in general paralysis, the uses of the hand deteriorate particularly early; while in those cases in which part of the brain is destroyed by apoplexy, the hand is apt to suffer more permanently than either face or leg.

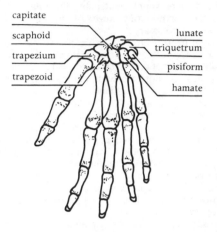

The bones of the hand and wrist, anterior view.

In structure, the hand has a bony basis of eight small carpal bones in the wrist, five metacarpal bones in the fleshy part of the hand, and three phalanges in each finger, two only in the thumb. From the muscles of the forearm twelve strong tendons or sinews run in front of the wrist. Of these, nine go to the fingers and thumb and are bound down by a strong band, the flexor retinaculum, in front of the wrist. They are enclosed in a complicated synovial sheath, and pass through the palm and down the fingers. (See FINGERS.) Behind the wrist twelve tendons likewise cross from forearm to hand.

Forming the ball of the thumb and that of the little finger, and filling up the gaps between the metacarpal bones, are other muscles, which act to separate and bring together the fingers, and to bend them at their first joints (knuckles).

Deep in the palm the ulnar artery makes an arch across the hand, giving off branches which run down the sides of the fingers; while the radial artery makes an arch across at a still deeper level, lying in close contact with the bones.

The skin of the hand is richly supplied with nerve filaments, in accordance with its highly specialized sense of touch, the outer three and a half digits being supplied in front by the median, behind by the radial nerve, whilst the inner one and a half fingers have their nerve supply both back and front from the ulnar nerve.

In addition to the diseases mentioned above, certain nervous diseases affect the hand early.

Thus in multiple sclerosis and in chorea there are tremors; in alcoholic neuritis and in lead-poisoning, drop-wrist; in progressive muscular atrophy one of the first signs is wasting of the small muscles belonging to the thumb and little finger; in syringomyelia there is loss of sensation for pain and for change of temperature in the fingers.

Deformities of the hand, in the shape of chalk-stones, may occur in gout; rheumatoid arthritis affects the joints of the hand and all too often causes crippling disabilities; and acromegaly is characterized by great enlargement of the hands. Swellings on the back or front of the wrist are usually due to collection of fluid in the tendon sheaths (see GANGLION). Deep abscesses on the front of the fingers are serious, because of the ease with which the infection spreads up the synovial sheaths of the tendons into the palm of the hand. (See WHIT-LOW.) A condition in which the fingers, especially the ring and little fingers, are gradually flexed up into the palm follows sometimes on a severe strain of the palm or long-continued pressure of a tool. (See DUPUYTREN'S CONTRAC-TURE.)

Special terms are applied to deformities of the hand. Claw hand (q.v.) or *main en griffe* is applied to a condition in which the hand is atrophied and the fingers bent in paralysis of the ulnar nerve; cleft hand (q.v.), or *lobster hand*, is a rare congenital defect characterized by the absence of one or more fingers and a deep central cleft that divides the hand into two; monkey hand or *main en singe* is applied to a condition in which the muscles of the thumb are wasted; obstetrician's hand is a condition in which the thumb and fingers are held together in a kind of cone in tetany and other conditions; and skeleton hand is a condition in which the muscles of the hand are generally wasted, as in progressive muscular atrophy. (See also DROP-WRIST.)

HAND, FOOT AND MOUTH DISEASE is a disease characterized by an eruption of blisters on the palms of the hands, on the feet (often the toes) and in the mouth. It is most common in children and is due to infection with coxsackie A16 virus. The incubation period is three to five days.

HANGING is a form of death due to suspension of the body from the neck, either suddenly, as in judicial hanging, so as to damage the spinal column and cord, or in such a way as to constrict the air passages and the blood-vessels to the brain. Death is, in any case, speedy, resulting in two or three minutes, if not instantaneous, although in bygone days criminals who were shored-up, or supported by their friends, have come round after half-an-hour's suspension. The mark of the noose on the neck is oblique in hanging, which serves to distinguish this form of death from strangling, in which the mark is circular. Apart from judicial hanging, and in the absence of any signs of a

struggle, hanging is usually due to suicide. The resuscitation of people found hanging is similar to that for drowning. (See APPENDIX: BASIC FIRST AID, cardiac/respiratory arrest.)

HANG-NAIL means a splitting of the skin at the side of the finger-nail. It is often a painful condition and difficult to heal. This is best effected by wearing constantly for several days a wet boric dressing covered by a rubber finger-stall.

HARDNESS is a term applied to water that contains a large amount of calcium and magnesium salts (lime salts) which form an insoluble curd with soap and thus interfere with the use of the water for purposes of washing. Hard water is especially found in districts where the soil is chalky. Temporary hardness, which is due mainly to the presence of bicarbonates of lime, can be remedied by boiling, when the lime is precipitated as carbonate of lime. Permanent hardness is not remedied by boiling, and is due to the presence of a large amount of sulphate of lime. It may be removed by the addition of sodium carbonate (washing soda) or by the Permutit process which involves the use of various combinations of silicate of alumina and soda. In the past hard water was often blamed for many ills – without any convincing evidence. Today medical statisticians are suggesting that the drinking of soft water may lead to heart disease.

HARE-LIP (see PALATE, MALFORMATIONS OF).

HARTMANN'S SOLUTION is a solution commonly used as a means of fluid replacement in dehydrated patients. Each litre contains 3·1 grams of sodium lactate, 6 grams of sodium chloride, 0·4 gram of potassium chloride, and 0·7 gram of calcium chloride.

HASHIMOTO'S DISEASE is a condition in which the whole of the thyroid gland is diffusely enlarged and firm. It is one of the diseases produced by auto-immunity (q.v.). The enlargement is due, not to increase of colloid, but to diffuse infiltration of lymphocytes and increase of fibrous tissue. This form of goitre appears in middle-aged women, does not give rise to symptoms of thyrotoxicosis, and tends to produce myxoedema.

HAVERSIAN CANALS are the fine canals in bone which carry the blood-vessels, lymphatics, and nerves necessary for the maintenance and repair of bone. (See BONE.)

HAY FEVER, this is caused by an allergy (q.v.) to the pollen of grasses, trees and other plants. Contact with the particular pollen that the sufferer is allergic to causes histamine (q.v.) release resulting in a blocked, runny nose and itchy watering eyes. It affects approximately 3 million people each year in the UK.

The mainstays of treatment are antihistamines (q.v.) and the use of steroid nasal spray and eyedrops. Occasionally desensitization may work if the particular allergen is known.

HAZELINE, or hamamelis water, is an extract made from the leaves or bark of *Hamamelis virginiana*, the witch-hazel. It is a useful astringent in checking bleeding and excessive mucous discharges. (See WITCH-HAZEL.)

HEAD (see BRAIN; FACE; SCALP; SKULL).

HEADACHE is very common, but its significance varies tremendously. Thus, at one extreme it may denote the presence of a tumour of the brain or meningitis, whilst at the other extreme it may only be a sign of tiredness. In spite of being such a common finding, the precise mechanism whereby it is produced is still somewhat obscure. The brain itself is insensitive to pain, but the arteries supplying it and the membranes of the brain in relationship to these arteries are sensitive to pain. The general view at the moment is that headache is usually due to dilatation of these arteries or pressure (or traction) on them. This dilatation of the intracranial arteries may be due either to a lesion in the brain or it may be caused reflexly: i.e. by a stimulus somewhere else in the body which through the nervous system (often the vagus nerve) causes such dilatation. In other cases the headache arises in the scalp or in the muscles of the back of the neck. The following are some of the more important, or more common, conditions in which headache is present.

ANXIETY: One of the most common forms of headache is that which occurs in individuals when they are worried, anxious, or overworked. In some cases it may be a manifestation of what is known as the anxiety state or of emotional instability, but quite often it occurs in individuals who are emotionally stable. On the other hand, it seldom occurs in the phlegmatic type of person. Manual workers and those who live an out-of-door life seldom complain of headache, and there can be little doubt that the stress and strain under which the modern town-dweller lives have much to do with its incidence. Aggravating factors are inadequate ventilation of offices and excessive smoking. In women it is liable to occur during or shortly before menstruation.

MIGRAINE: This is one of the most characteristic forms of headache. For further details the section on migraine should be consulted.

REFRACTIVE ERRORS OF THE EYE are not as common a cause of headache as is sometimes thought. It occurs in the region of the brow and tends to be worse in the evening, particularly if much reading or close work has been done during the course of the day. It is sometimes accompanied by a sensation of grittiness in the eye. The remedy in such cases is the wearing of spectacles which correct the faulty vision.

INFECTION OF THE SINUSES is a common cause of headache. The location of the pain depends upon which sinus is involved. If the maxillary antrum, which lies in the cheek-bone, is infected, the pain is usually over the cheek, although it may be referred elsewhere in the head. In the case of involvement of the frontal sinuses the pain is over the eyes, whilst in the case of the deeper-lying ethmoidal sinuses the pain appears to be deep-seated behind the eyes. In such cases there is usually a history of a cold in the head followed by a discharge from the nose. The pain is usually worse about midday and tends to wear off towards evening. It is usually made worse by coughing and even sometimes by change of position.

DENTAL SEPSIS: Septic teeth may sometimes be responsible for headache. Usually, of course, there is also the classical toothache, but occasionally the pain of septic teeth is referred to the head.

INDIGESTION AND CONSTIPATION: Any form of dyspepsia due to disordered function of the stomach and which is liable to be accompanied by nausea (i.e. a feeling of sickness), may be responsible for headache. On the other hand, individuals with a duodenal ulcer are not particularly liable to headache. Constipation is quite a common cause of headache, especially in children, but the old theory that the headache is due to absorption of toxic material from the gut has now been discarded. The headache is relieved so rapidly by the passing of a stool that it must be due to distension of the lower part of the bowel.

FEVER: Any infection, such as pneumonia or measles, causing a rise in temperature is liable to be accompanied by headache. This is probably due to dilatation of the blood-vessels in the brain resulting from the fever itself and from the infecting organism or its toxins.

URAEMIA: This is the terminal stage of glomerulonephritis (q.v.) and it is often accompanied by severe headache, which is due partly to the high blood-pressure which is always present and partly to the toxic substances which are retained in the body as a result of the failure of the kidneys.

HIGH BLOOD-PRESSURE: Although many people with a high blood-pressure are not unduly troubled with headache, the headache when it does occur is characteristic. It tends to occur at the back of the head and to be worse in the morning, wearing off during the course of the day.

RHEUMATIC CONDITIONS: Many rheumatic subjects are subject to aches and pains about the head. These are due to rheumatic changes in the muscles of the head and the back of the neck, and can usually be easily recognized by the fact that they are accompanied by tender spots elicited by pressure on the affected parts.

SUNSTROKE AND HEAT-STROKE: Headache is the prominent feature in these conditions, and its occurrence after undue exposure to the sun or to exceptionally hot conditions renders easy its recognition.

DISEASES OF THE BRAIN: Finally, there are the conditions in which a headache indicates the presence of some disturbance or disease of the brain. This may take the form of infections of the brain or its membranes: e.g. encephalitis, brain abscess, meningitis. There is seldom any difficulty in determining the presence of these conditions, as there are practically always other signs of involvement of the brain: e.g. rigidity of the neck and squint in meningitis. In young children meningitis must always be considered when a febrile illness is accompanied by severe headache. In tumours of the brain severe headache develops sooner or later, but here again there are other manifestations, such as giddiness and apparently causeless vomiting, which indicate the cause of the headache. In middle-aged or old people headache may be due to arteriosclerosis or thrombosis of the arteries in the brain. A relatively uncommon, but very acute, type of headache, usually in the back of the head, is caused by rupture of a small aneurysm (q.v.) in the circle of Willis, a network of arteries at the base of the brain. Headache is one of the main manifestations of concussion, whether or not this is accompanied by a fractured skull. The persistence of this headache after the individual has otherwise recovered from the concussion is sometimes most troublesome. If the concussion is due to an accident for which the victim considers he should receive compensation, this post-concussion, or post-traumatic, headache is one of the manifestations of a compensation neurosis. Once the case is settled, whether favourably or unfavourably to the claimant matters little, the headache usually clears up.

Treatment: It will be clear from this outline that in the majority of cases the treatment of headache is the treatment of the underlying cause. The main exception to this is migraine (q.v.). When the headache is associated with anxiety, worry or overwork, the same principle holds true. In these cases there may be an associated general debility, and for this the best remedy is a holiday with complete change of environment, adequate rest, and plenty of good food. If the headache is associated with sleeplessness, the administration of a mild sedative is helpful provided it is not continued indefinitely. Similarly with aspirin; this will relieve many headaches, but its continued use by an increasing number of the population is not in the interest of the health of the community. Used sensibly for short periods aspirin has its uses, but its repeated and continued use is to be deprecated. Local soothing applications to the forehead are often of value in relieving headache. For this purpose there is much to be said ·for eau-de-Cologne. If the individual is lying down, a moist handkerchief on the forehead is sometimes just as effective.

·

HEAD INJURY: Any injury to the head, whether associated with a skull fracture or not.

Patients with head injuries should be assessed for signs of neurological damage, which may not develop at once. Patients with drowsiness, vomiting, confusion, or any focal neurological signs after a head injury should be seen by a doctor.

People suffering the results of such injuries and their relatives can obtain help and advice from Headway (National Head Injuries Association), 200 Mansfield Road, Nottingham NG1 3HX (0602-622382).

HEALING (see WOUNDS).

HEALTH: The state of health implies much more than freedom from disease, and good health may be defined as the attainment and maintenance of the highest state of mental and bodily vigour of which any given individual is capable. Environment, including living and working conditions, plays an important part in determining a person's health.

HEALTH AND SAFETY EXECUTIVE: The statutory body in Britain responsible for the health and safety of workers. The HSE can be contacted at Baynards House, 1 Chepstow Place, London W2 4TE (071-221 0870).

HEALTH CENTRE: An imprecise term that may refer to a group of doctors and supporting staff operating from one building owned or leased by the doctors, or a building owned or leased by a district health authority that contains staff or services from one or more sections of the National Health Service.

HEALTH EDUCATION: The process of educating the public to adopt a healthy lifestyle and abandon dangerous or unhealthy behaviour. Information on all aspects of health education can be obtained from the Health Education Authority, Hamilton House, Mabledon Place, London WC1 (071-383 3833).

HEALTH SERVICE COMMISSIONER: An official, responsible to parliament, appointed to protect the interests of National Health Service patients in matters concerning the administration of the health service. Known colloquially as the health ombudsman, the commissioner presents regular reports on the complaints dealt with.

HEALTH VISITOR: A nurse with special training including midwifery and health education. Health visitors' main role is one of health promotion. They are responsible for children and elderly people in the community. The Health Visitors' Association is found at 50 Southwark Street, London SE1 (071-378 7255).

HEARING (see DEAFNESS; EAR).

HEARING AIDS: Nearly two-thirds of people aged over 70 have some degree of hearing impairment (see DEAFNESS). Hearing aids are no substitute for definitive treatment of the underlying cause of poor hearing, so examination by an ear, nose and throat surgeon is sensible before a hearing aid is issued (and is essential before one can be given through the NHS). The choice of aid depends on the age, manipulative skills, and degree of hearing impairment of the patient and the underlying cause of the deafness. The choice of hearing aid for a deaf child is particularly important as impaired hearing can hinder speech development.

Ear trumpets, although old fashioned, may occasionally help an elderly person who is unable to manage an electronic aid.

Electronic aids consist, essentially, of a microphone, an amplifier, and an earphone. In postaural aids the microphone and amplifier are contained in a small box worn behind the ear or attached to spectacles. The earphone is on a specially moulded earpiece. Some patients find it difficult to manipulate the controls of an aid worn behind the ear, and they may be better off with a device worn on the body. Some hearing aids are worn entirely within the ear and are very discreet. They are particularly useful for people who have to wear protective headgear such as helmets.

All types have a volume control and a special setting for use with telephone and in rooms fitted with an inductive coupler that screens out background noise.

In making a choice therefore from the large range of effective hearing aids now available, the expert advice of an ear specialist must be obtained. The Royal National Institute for the Deaf, 105 Gower Street, London, WC1E 6AH (071-387 8033, fax: 071- 388 2346, Minicom: 071-383 3154), provides a list of clinics where such a specialist can be consulted. It also gives reliable advice concerning the purchase and use of hearing aids.

HEART is a hollow muscular pump with four cavities, each provided at its outlet with a valve, whose function is to maintain the circulation of the blood. The two upper cavities are known as atria, the two lower ones as ventricles. The term auricle is applied to the ear-shaped tip of the atrium on each side.

Position: The heart lies in the chest between the two lungs, but projecting more to the left side than to the right. On the left side its apex reaches out in the adult between 8 and 9 cm (3½ and 4 inches), almost to the nipple, and lies beneath the fifth rib, while its right border extends only a short distance, at most 2·4 cm, beyond the margin of the breast-bone. Its lower border rests upon the diaphragm, by which it is separated from the liver and stomach, and this close connection has an important influence upon the heart in several disorders of the stomach. Above, the heart extends to the level of the second rib, where the great vessels, the aorta on the right side and the pulmonary

artery on the left, lie behind the breast-bone.

Shape and size: The heart of any individual was described by Laennec as, roughly, of the size and shape of the clenched fist. Its weight in the male varies from 280 to 340 grams, and in the female from 230 to 280 grams. It continues to increase in weight and size up to a ripe old age, more so in men than in women. One end of the heart is pointed (apex), the other is broad (base), and is deeply cleft at the division between the two atria. One groove running down the front and up the back shows the division between the two ventricles; a circular, deeper groove marks off the atria above from the ventricles below. The capacity of each cavity is somewhere between 90 and 180 ml.

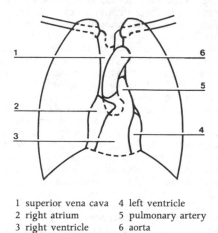

1 superior vena cava   4 left ventricle
2 right atrium   5 pulmonary artery
3 right ventricle   6 aorta

Diagram of the heart as seen using X-rays.

Structure: The heart lies within a strong fibrous bag, known as the pericardium, and since the inner surface of this bag and the outer surface of the heart are both covered with a smooth, glistening membrane faced with flat cells and lubricated by a little serous fluid (around 20 millilitres), the movements of the heart are accomplished almost without friction. The main thickness of the heart wall consists of bundles of muscle fibres, which run, some in circles right round the heart, others in loops, first round one cavity, then round the corresponding cavity of the other side. Within all the cavities is a smooth lining membrane, continuous with that lining the vessels which open into the heart. The investing smooth membrane is known as epicardium, the muscular substance as myocardium, and the smooth lining membrane as endocardium.

For the regulation of the heart's action there are important nervous connections, especially with the vagus nerve and with the sympathetic system. In the hinder part of the atria lies a collection of nerve cells and connecting fibres, known as the sinuatrial node, which forms the starting-point for the impulses that initiate the beats of the heart. Hence its alternative name of the pacemaker of the heart. In the groove between the ventricles and the atria lies another collection of similar nerve tissue, known as the atrioventricular node. From it there runs downwards into the septum between the two ventricles a band of special muscle fibres, known as the atrioventricular bundle, or the bundle of His. This splits up into a right and a left branch for the two ventricles, and the fibres of these distribute themselves throughout the muscular wall of the ventricles and control their contraction.

Openings: There is no direct communication between the cavities on the right side and those on the left; but the right atrium opens into the right ventricle by a large circular opening, and similarly the left atrium into the left ventricle. Into the right atrium open two large veins, the superior and inferior venae cavae, with some smaller veins from the wall of the heart itself, and into the left atrium open two pulmonary veins from each lung. One opening leads out of each ventricle, to the aorta in the case of the left ventricle, to the pulmonary artery from the right.

1 left atrium   4 chordae tendinae
2 left ventricle   5 mitral valve, anterior
3 papillary muscle   cusp

Interior of the left ventricle, showing structure of mitral valve.

Prior to birth there is an opening (*foramen ovale*) from the right into the left atrium through which the blood passes; but when the child first draws air into his lungs this opening closes and is represented in the adult only by a depression (*fossa ovalis*).

Valves: As stated above, there are four valves. The mitral valve consists of two triangular cusps, the tricuspid valve of three smaller cusps. The aortic and pulmonary valves each consist of three semilunar-shaped segments. The structure of a valve is a double layer of the lining membrane of the heart (endocardium) strengthened by fibrous tissue between. Two valves are placed at the openings leading from atrium into ventricle, the tricuspid valve on the right side, the mitral valve on the left, so as completely to prevent blood from running back into the atrium when the ventricle contracts. Two more, the pulmonary valve and the aortic valve, are at the entrance to these arteries, and prevent regurgitation into the ventricles of blood which has been driven from them into the arteries.

The noises made by these valves in closing constitute the greater part of what are known as the heart sounds, and can be heard by anyone who applies his ear to the front of a person's chest. Murmurs heard accompanying these sounds indicate defects in the valves, and form one of the chief signs of heart disease.

1 cavity of left ventricle
2 valve cusp

The aortic valve: (A) open, (B) closed.

Action: At each heart-beat the two atria contract and expel their contents into the ventricles, which at the same time they stimulate to contract together, so that the blood is driven into the arteries, to be returned again to the atria after having completed a circuit in about fifteen seconds through the body or lungs as the case may be. The heart beats from sixty to ninety times a minute, the rate in any given healthy person being about four times that of the respirations. The heart is to some extent regulated by a nerve centre in the medulla, closely connected with those centres which govern the lungs and stomach, and nerve fibres pass to it in the vagus nerve. By some of these fibres its rate and force can be diminished, by others increased, according to the needs of the various organs of the body. If this nerve centre is injured or poisoned, for example, by lack of oxygen, the heart stops beating in human beings, although in some of the lower animals – e.g. frogs, fishes, and reptiles – the heart may under favourable conditions go on beating for hours even after its entire removal from the body.

HEARTBURN means a burning sensation experienced in the region of the heart and up the back to the throat. It is caused by an excessive acidity of the gastric juice, and is relieved temporarily by taking alkaline substances, such as 1·2 grams of bicarbonate of soda or a similar amount of bismuth carbonate or carbonate of magnesia in water. It is also relieved by the chewing of aluminium-containing antacid tablets such as Aluminium Hydroxide Tablets, BP.

HEART DISEASES: The heart is essentially a muscle pump which receives its own nutrient supply through the coronary arteries. It contains four valves which are designed to direct blood flow and the heart itself sits in a silky sac known as the pericardium. The action of the heart is determined by a sophisticated electric circuit known as the conducting system (see HEART).

Heart disease can affect any of the structures and more than one at a time.

CONGENITAL HEART DISEASE accounts for 1–2 per cent of all cases of organic heart disease. It may be inherited, present at birth for no obvious reason or in rare cases related to German measles (q.v.) in the mother or to drugs taken in pregnancy. The commonest forms are holes in the heart (atrial septal defect, ventricular septal defect (see SEPTAL DEFECT), a patent ductus arteriosus (q.v.) and coarctation of the aorta (q.v.). Many complex forms also exist and can be diagnosed in the womb by fetal echocardiography which can lead to elective termination of pregnancy. Surgery to correct many of these abnormalities is feasible, even for the most severe abnormalities, but may only be palliative giving rise to major difficulties of management as the children become older. Heart transplantation is now increasingly employed for the uncorrectable lesions.

CORONARY ARTERY DISEASE, also known as ischaemic heart disease, is the most important cause of symptoms and death in the adult population. It may present for the first time as sudden death but more usually it causes angina pectoris (q.v.), myocardial infarction (heart attack) or heart failure. It can also lead to a disturbance of heart rhythm. Its cause is not fully known but factors associated with an increased risk of developing coronary artery disease include male sex, increasing age, diabetes, cigarette smoking, high blood pressure and a raised concentration of cholesterol in the blood. Over 150,000 people died of coronary-artery disease in England in 1989; it was the biggest single cause of death.

HEART MUSCLE DISEASE or cardiomyopathy usually indicates a weakness of the left ventricle which secondarily affects the right ventricle. The efficiency of the pump deteriorates, the heart attempts to compensate by increasing muscle thickness (hypertrophy) and by dilating (enlarged heart), but after a variable time it fails, leading to the symptoms of breathlessness due to fluid accumulation in the lungs (pulmonary oedema). With a failure to pump efficiently the output falls and fatigue becomes a problem. When more advanced, fluid distends the liver and the ankles may become swollen.

Cardiomyopathy may be secondary to coronary artery disease, present in the absence of coronary artery disease and of no obvious cause, due to an inflammation of the heart muscle (myocarditis) most commonly caused by a virus infection or due to excessive consumption of alcohol. Myocarditis may resolve, as may cardiomyopathy due to excessive alcohol consumption if drinking is stopped, but most forms of cardiomyopathy are progressive, needing regular medication to maintain quality and quantity of life.

VALVULAR HEART DISEASE primarily affects the mitral and aortic valves which can become narrowed (stenosis) or leaking (incompetence). Pulmonary valve problems are usually congenital (stenosis) and the tricuspid valve is sometimes involved when rheumatic heart disease primarily affects the mitral or aortic valves. Rheumatic fever (q.v.), usually in childhood, remains a common cause of chronic valvular heart disease causing stenosis, incompetence or both of the aortic and mitral valves, but each valve has other separate causes for malfunction.

AORTIC VALVE DISEASE is more common with increasing age. When narrowed the heart hypertrophies and may later fail. Symptoms of angina or breathlessness are common and dizziness or blackouts (syncope) also occur. Replacing the valve is a very effective treatment, even with advancing age. Aortic stenosis may be caused by degeneration (senile calcific), inheriting two leaflets instead of the usual three (bicuspid valve) or rheumatic fever. Aortic incompetence again leads to hypertrophy, but dilatation is more common as blood leaks back into the ventricle. Breathlessness is the more common complaint. The causes are the same as stenosis but also include inflammatory conditions such as syphilis (q.v.) or ankylosing spondylitis (q.v.) and other disorders of connective tissue. The valve may also leak if the aorta dilates stretching the valve ring as with hypertension (q.v.), aortic aneurysm (q.v.) and Marfans Syndrome – an inherited disorder of connective tissue that causes heart defects. Infection (endocarditis) can worsen acutely or chronically destroy the valve and sometimes lead to abnormal outgrowths on the valve (vegetations) which may break free and cause devastating damage such as a stroke or blocked circulation to the bowel or leg.

MITRAL VALVE DISEASE leading to stenosis is rheumatic in origin. Mitral incompetence may be rheumatic but in the absence of stenosis can be due to ischaemia (q.v.), infarction (q.v.), inflammation, infection and a congenital weakness (prolapse). The valve may also leak if stretched by a dilating ventricle (functional incompetence). Infection (endocarditis) may affect the valve in a similar way to aortic disease. Mitral symptoms are predominantly breathlessness which may lead to wheezing or waking at night breathless and needing to sit up or stand for relief. They are made worse when the heart rhythm changes (atrial fibrillation) which is frequent as the disease becomes more severe. This leads to a loss of efficiency of up to 25 per cent and a predisposition to clot formation as blood stagnates rather than leaves the heart efficiently. Mitral incompetence may remain mild and be of no trouble for many years but infection must be guarded against (endocarditis prophylaxis).

ENDOCARDITIS is an infection of the heart which may acutely destroy a valve or lead to chronic destruction. Bacteria settle usually on a mild lesion. Antibiotics taken at vulnerable times can prevent this happening (antibiotic prophylaxis); one of the most common occasions is before dental treatment. If established, vigorous intravenous antibiotic therapy is needed and surgery is often necessary. The mortality is

30 per cent but may be higher if the infection settles on a replaced valve (prosthetic endocarditis). Complications include heart failure, shock, embolization (generation of small clots in the blood) and cerebral (mental) confusion.

PERICARDITIS is an inflammation of the sac covering the outside of the heart. The sac becomes roughened and pain occurs as the heart and sac rub together. This is heard by stethoscope as a scratching noise (pericardial rub). Fever is often present and a virus the main cause. It may also occur with rheumatic fever, kidney failure, tuberculosis or from an adjacent lung problem such as pneumonia or cancer. The inflammation may cause fluid to accumulate between the sac and the heart (effusion) which may compress the heart causing a fall in blood pressure, a weak pulse and circulatory failure (tamponade). This can be relieved by aspirating the fluid. The treatment is then directed at the underlying cause.

DISTURBANCES OF RHYTHM are common and of several types. Many do not reflect underlying disease. Usually the patient becomes aware of his heart beat (palpitations) which may be fast or appear to miss a beat or kick. Stress or stimulants such as caffeine or alcohol are a frequent cause. Occasionally the disturbance can be troublesome, even though not dangerous, and merit treatment, but drugs should be avoided if no obvious disease exists.

Disturbances reflecting disease may lead to the heart's going fast or slow or both intermittently.

ATRIAL FIBRILLATION may occur without obvious disease but usually presents when there is coronary artery disease, cardiomyopathy, high blood pressure or mitral valve disease. The rhythm is very irregular and may lead to rapid poorly co-ordinated contractions of the ventricle leading to heart failure. It predisposes to clots' forming in the heart. Treatment may be directed to converting the heart back to normal (sinus) rhythm by drugs or electric shock treatment or to controlling the speed with drugs such as digoxin (q.v.). It is a serious irregularity. Blood-thinning medication such as warfarin (q.v.) is often prescribed.

EXTRASYSTOLES are very common and usually perceived as missed beats or extra beats (a kick or thump). They are not usually serious but they may, however, complicate coronary artery disease or heart muscle disease when certain forms need specialized therapy.

HEART BLOCK refers to a failure to conduct normally through the electric circuit of the heart. There are three types; 1st degree which can be a normal variation and does not cause slowing; 2nd degree which causes intermittent slowing and 3rd degree or complete block where there is no electrical connection and heart beats are slow and unpredictable leading to blackouts (Stokes-Adams attacks) and/or heart failure. For most 2nd degree and all complete cases a pacemaker relieves symptoms and improves life expectancy.

SINUS NODE DISEASE The main electrical control of the heart is the sinus node. If this is diseased or inherits a malfunction, the heart may develop rapid, slow or both rapid and slow rhythms. Often a tape recording for 24 hours (Holter) is used to document the irregularities. The heart itself may well be normal but these electrical disturbances can be very symptomatic. Treatment may include drugs, a cardiac pacemaker (q.v.) or both.

MISCELLANEOUS There are many infrequent causes of heart problems which for the affected individual are a cause of debility. These include a problem of heart muscle thickening (hypertrophic cardiomyopathy), which can cause angina, irregular heart beats and sudden death, and Wolf Parkinson White Syndrome which causes the heart to race due to an extra fast conducting section in the circuit. This may induce pain, dizziness and blackouts. Some electrical conditions of the heart merit specific study known as electrophysiology (EPS) which allows the abnormality to be mapped out, thus facilitating drug or intervention treatment (ablation) to stop abnormal conduction.

HEAT: (see also BURNS; HEAT-STROKE.) The curative uses of heat as applied by hot water and hot air are mentioned under BATHS. Hot-air applications are much used in the treatment of rheumatic conditions in the joints and muscles, and a more powerful application of heat for the same purpose is obtained by the use of high frequency electricity. (See DIATHERMY.) Excessive heat, in the form of the cautery, is also used in order to destroy diseased tissues. (See CAUSTICS AND CAUTERIES.)

HEAT-CRAMPS are painful cramps in the muscles occurring in workers, such as stokers, who labour in hot conditions. The cramps are the result of loss of salt in the sweat, and can be cured by giving salty water to drink. (See HEAT-STROKE.)

HEAT SPOTS is a vague term applied to small inflamed and congested areas which appear especially upon the skin of the face, neck, and chest or other parts of the body in warm weather.

HEAT-STROKE is the term applied to the effects produced on the body by exposure to excessive heat. Although most commonly observed in tropical regions, it may occur also in temperate climates during hot weather. A moist condition of the atmosphere, which interferes with cooling of the overheated body, greatly increases the liability to suffer from this ailment.

Causes: The fundamental cause of the condition is exposure of the body to amounts of radiant energy for which it cannot compensate. This inability to compensate for excessive exposure to heat results in overheating of the body and loss of fluid. In any given case one or other of these factors, or both, may come into play (see table below). In the more acute cases the condition is characterized by failure of the sweating mechanism: these are the cases which are rapidly fatal unless treatment is instituted immediately. When excessive sweating occurs, in the early stages this loss of fluid is accompanied by a corresponding loss of salt (sodium chloride), resulting in a disturbance of the electrolyte balance of the body fluids. Unless this loss of water and sodium chloride is compensated for, one of three things may occur: (i) the individual may be seized with severe cramp in the muscles: i.e. heat cramps; (ii) the blood volume is diminished and the circulation of the body is seriously disturbed, resulting in a condition analogous to surgical shock; (iii) the sweating mechanism may break down, with resultant further rise in the temperature of the body, leading to a fatal termination.

Dilatation of blood-vessels of skin
Sweating
Dilution of blood
Decreased muscle tone
Inclination to reduced activity
Stretching, or extension, of body to increase loss of heat
Decrease in volume of urine
Thirst
Loss of chloride leading to heat-cramps
Difficulty in maintaining blood supply to brain, leading
   to dizziness, nausea and heat-exhaustion
Rising body temperature
Impairment of heat-regulating centre in brain
Cessation of breathing

Effects of exposure to high temperatures.

Predisposing factors are bad living or working conditions, lack of acclimatization to tropical conditions, unsuitable clothing, poor health, and dietetic and alcoholic indiscretions.
Symptoms: The symptoms, which obviously depend upon the disorganization of the normal heat-regulating mechanism as well as of the functions of circulation and respiration, vary in their intensity and to some extent in their form. Four chief types of the disease are usually described.
(1) HEAT COLLAPSE: This is the mildest form of the condition. It is characterized by fatigue, giddiness, and temporary loss of consciousness. The blood-pressure is low and the pulse is slow. In the more severe cases there is a state of collapse, with cold, clammy skin and a subnormal temperature. Vomiting is not uncommon and there may be muscular cramps. The urine is much diminished in volume, is highly coloured and has a high specific gravity: e.g. over 1020. This type of case practically always recovers.
(2) HEAT EXHAUSTION: The mild case of heat exhaustion is similar to one of heat collapse. The more severe case tends to occur towards the end of the hot season in the tropics. The onset is characterized by increasing weakness, dizziness, and insomnia, and this is accompanied by defective sweating in the majority of cases. Cramps and vomiting seldom occur, but large volumes of urine are voided. The temperature is usually about 37·8–38·3 °C (100–101 °F), the pulse rate is within normal limits, and there are seldom signs of dehydration, the skin usually having quite a good colour.
(3) HEAT CRAMPS: These have been recognized for many years and occur in individuals who perform hard physical work in high temperatures. Hence the many different names by which they have been known: e.g. miners' cramps, stokers' cramps, bakers' cramps. The characteristic feature is agonizing cramp, usually in the legs, arms, or back. Occasionally the abdominal muscles are involved, and in these cases the intensity of the pain may suggest some acute condition of the stomach or gut. The cramps are accompanied by sweating, pallor of the skin, and a feeling of intense anxiety. There may be headache and giddiness. The temperature is seldom raised very much.
(4) HEAT HYPERPYREXIA: This is the most serious type of all. The initial manifestations are loss of energy and irritability. Then follow mental confusion and diminution or cessation of sweating. Gradually, or sometimes with startling suddenness, this passes into restlessness and then coma and the temperature rises rapidly to 41·7 °C (107 °F) or even higher. Unless treatment is instituted immediately, there is soon a fatal termination.
Prevention: Careful selection of personnel who have to perform hard physical work under tropical conditions or in high temperatures is essential. Even in the case of such selected individuals acclimatization is necessary and they should not be allowed to perform severe physical exertion at high temperatures until a period of several weeks' training has elapsed. In the tropics elderly people should move to a cool area during the hot season. Personal hygiene is important. Only light clothing should be worn, with a minimum of constrictions such as tight belts.

Diet should be light and nourishing and ample fluids should be taken. Salads and fruit should constitute an important part of the diet, and fluids should be bland: e.g. fruit drinks, tea, iced coffee. Alcoholic drinks should be taken in moderation, and only after sundown. In the case of individuals performing hard physical exertion at high temperatures, water containing salt (i.e. sodium chloride) should be drunk freely. Unless the water contains a certain amount of salt, there is an increased tendency to develop cramps. In industries where men work under such conditions, they are now provided with salt and water flavoured with lemon to disguise the salty flavour. Attention to ventilation and air-conditioning is also essential. In the tropics, when air-conditioning is not available, houses should be closed up in the early morning and opened up again at sundown. This reduces the amount of hot air entering the house during the day and allows free circulation of the cool night air. Fans are also of value, and, in hot, dry conditions, sprinkling the compound with water during the afternoon sometimes helps to keep the house cool.

Treatment: In the case of heat cramps, heat collapse, and heat exhaustion, treatment consists of removal of the affected individual to a cool place and the administration of normal saline (see ISOTONIC). In severe cases this can be given intravenously, but it can usually be given by mouth. Heat hyperpyrexia is an emergency which requires immediate attention with a view to reducing the temperature. The individual should be placed in the shade, stripped, and drenched with water. To increase the cooling property of the water the surface of the body should be fanned. The patient is then wrapped in a sheet soaked in as cool water as possible (see WET PACKS), and the fanning is continued. This treatment must be stopped when the rectal temperature falls to 38·9 °C (102 °F) and the patient is then wrapped in a dry blanket. The reason for stopping at this temperature is that the temperature continues to fall after treatment ceases and therefore if treatment was continued until the temperature became normal, the further fall in temperature might have serious consequences. As soon as the patient is conscious he should be given normal saline to drink, and this usually provokes sweating – a favourable sign. Whenever possible, further treatment should be carried out in hospital, as there is always a risk of circulatory collapse occurring. Convalescence may be prolonged, and the advisability of the affected individual returning permanently to a cooler climate must always be given careful consideration.

HEBEPHRENIA is a form of mental disorder coming on in youth and marked by depression and gradual failure of mental faculties with egotistic and self-centred delusions. It is one of the forms of schizophrenia.

HEBERDEN'S NODES are little hard knobs which appear at the sides of the last phalanges of the fingers in people who are the subject of osteoarthrosis.

HEEL is the hinder part of the foot formed by the calcaneus and the specially thick skin covering it. It is not subject to many diseases. Severe pain in the heel is sometimes a sign of gout or rheumatism.

HEIGHT (see WEIGHT AND HEIGHT).

HELIUM is the lightest gas known, with the exception of hydrogen. This property renders it of value in anaesthesia (q.v.), as its addition to the anaesthetic means that it can be inhaled with less effort by the patient. Thus it can be used in the presence of any obstruction to the entry of air to the lungs.

HELMINTHS is a name for worms.

HEMIANAESTHESIA means loss of touch-sense down one side of the body.

HEMIANOPIA, HEMIANOPSIA, and HEMIOPIA are terms meaning loss of half the usual area of vision. The affected person may see everything clearly to the left or to the right, the field of vision stopping abruptly at the middle line, or he may see things only when straight in front of him, or thirdly, he may see objects far out on both sides, although there is a wide area straight in front for which he is quite blind. The position of the blind area is important in localizing the position in the brain of the disease responsible for the condition.

HEMIATROPHY is atrophy of one side of the body, or of part of the body on one side: for example, facial hemiatrophy, in which one-half of the face is smaller than the other either in the course of development or as a result of some nervous disorder.

HEMIBALLISMUS are involuntary movements similar to choreiform movements but of much greater amplitude and force. They are violent throwing movements of the limbs which are usually unilateral. They tend to occur acutely as a result of vascular damage to the mid-brain.

HEMICOLECTOMY: An operation to remove the right or left half of the colon, usually with end-to-end anastomosis of the remaining portion of the intestine. This is often used for the treatment of malignant or inflammatory diseases of the colon.

HEMICRANIA means a headache limited to one side of the head. (See MIGRAINE.)

HEMIMELIA: This consists of defects in the distal part of the extremities such as the absence of a forearm or hands. This is a congenital defect and large numbers of cases resulted from the administration of Thalidomide during pregnancy.

HEMIPARESIS: Paralysis affecting the muscles of one side of the body. This most commonly follows a stroke and occurs when parts of the brain serving motor function on the opposite side of the body are damaged.

HEMIPLEGIA means paralysis limited to one side of the body. (See PARALYSIS.)

HENLE, LOOP OF: That part of the nephron (see KIDNEYS) between the proximal and distal convoluted tubules. It extends into the renal medulla as a hairpin-shaped loop. The ascending link of the loop actively transports sodium from the lumen of the tube to the interstitium, and this, combined with the 'counter-current' flow of fluid through the two limbs of the loop, plays a part in concentrating the urine.

HEPARIN is a substance, first obtained from the liver, which prevents coagulation of the blood. It is present chiefly in liver, muscle, and lung. It is thought to act by neutralizing thrombin. (See FIBRIN.) Heparin has a complicated chemical structure and has been prepared in crystalline form. It is carbohydrate in nature, and contains amino and sulphuric acid groups. It is used for the prevention of clot formation in the blood or to prevent the spreading of this process once it has occurred. It is not active when given by mouth and must therefore be given by injection – usually intravenously. (See also ANTICOAGULANTS.)

HEPATECTOMY is the operation for removal of the liver, or part of it.

HEPATITIS: Hepatitis, or inflammation of liver cells (see LIVER), may be acute or chronic and symptoms may be absent or non-specific. *Acute* hepatitis causes jaundice (q.v.), itching, abdominal pain and liver tenderness, malaise, anorexia (q.v.), fever and nausea. Treatment consists of bed-rest and relief of symptoms. All unnecessary drugs must be stopped and alcohol should be avoided. *Chronic* hepatitis can cause any of the symptoms above, but they tend to be more insidious in onset.

Diagnostic investigations include blood tests to assess liver function, liver biopsy to classify the type and cause of hepatitis and ultrasound scanning (see ULTRASOUND).

There are many causes; some agents can produce both acute and chronic hepatitis. Alcohol abuse is the commonest cause in Great Britain.

VIRAL HEPATITIS classically refers to infection with one of the so-called hepatitis viruses, of which there are at least five: A, B, C, D and E. Many other virus infections produce liver inflammation and these include glandular fever and HIV. Treatment with many drugs causes hepatitis as a side-effect; halothane general anaesthesia (q.v.), methyl dopa and paracetamol in overdose are examples. Autoimmune diseases such as rheumatoid arthritis (q.v.) may exhibit associated chronic hepatitis.

FULMINANT HEPATITIS is the severest form of liver inflammation; there is massive destruction of liver cells resulting in liver failure with severe jaundice, impaired consciousness, fluid retention and a bleeding tendency. Kidney failure may follow. Causes include alcohol abuse, acute viral hepatitis and paracetamol overdose. Liver transplantation has dramatically improved the outlook of this condition.

INFECTIOUS HEPATITIS is caused by hepatitis A virus. It is transmitted by eating food contaminated with faecal material from an infected individual, particularly seafood, and it is common in areas where standards of hygiene are poor. In temperate climates it tends to occur in late summer; in the tropics there is no seasonal variation. Incubation period is 15 to 45 days. Patients should not return to work until at least 7 days after complete clinical recovery, when the prognosis is good and there is no risk of chronic infection. Hepatitis E virus is similar to Hepatitis A, except that in pregnancy the mortality rate of the former may be as high as 20 per cent.

SERUM HEPATITIS is due to infection with viruses B, C or D. They share the same routes of infection – through transfusion of infected blood, sharing needles for injection of drugs, tattooing or through sexual intercourse with an infected individual – and tend to have a longer incubation period, up to 180 days in the case of virus B. These virus infections carry a much higher mortality rate (1–3 per cent in hepatitis B and C, up to 20 per cent in virus D) and the viruses may remain in the blood for many years, causing chronic carrier status (such individuals remain an infectious risk to others) and chronic hepatitis. Diagnosis of these various types of viral infection is by the demonstration of specific antibodies (q.v.) and antigens (q.v.) in the blood. Following the discovery of the responsible virus, non-A non-B hepatitis is now known as hepatitis C.

Persistence of hepatitis B virus in the blood with hepatic inflammation lasting more than 6 months after hepatitis B infection is defined as chronic type-B hepatitis. Hepatocellular carcinoma is common in areas of the world where hepatitis-B carrier status is frequent and chronic hepatitis – of any cause – may result in cirrhosis. Therefore much effort has gone into finding treatments for chronic type-B hepatitis, the most successful of which has been antiviral chemotherapy with interferon (q.v.). The response to this treatment may be disappointing with a high rate of relapse.

HEPATOLENTICULAR DEGENERATION (see WILSON'S DISEASE).

HEPATOMA: A primary malignant tumour of liver cells. It has marked geographical variation, being most common in parts of Africa and the Far East. It is more common in men and with those who have pre-existing cirrhosis (q.v.).

HEPATOMEGALY: Enlargement of the liver. This may be caused by congestion (e.g. in heart failure), infection (e.g. hepatitis), malignancy, inflammation, or early cirrhosis (q.v.).

HEREDITY is the principle on which various peculiarities of bodily form or structure, or of physical or mental activity are transmitted from parents to offspring. (See GENES.)

HERMAPHRODITE is an individual in whom both ovarian and testicular tissue is present.

Hermaphrodites may have a testis on one side and an ovary on the other, or an ovotestis on one side and an ovary or testis on the other, or there may be an ovotestis on both sides. Both gonads are usually intra-abdominal. The true hermaphrodite usually has a uterus and at least one fallopian tube on the side of the ovary. On the side of the testis there is usually a vas deferens. Most true hermaphrodites are raised as males but external virilization is not usually complete. Even when significant phallic development is present hypospadias and cryptorchism are common. At puberty gynaecomastia develops and menstruation is common, as ovarian function is usually more nearly normal than testicular function.

HERNIA means the protrusion of any organ, or part of an organ, into or through the wall of the cavity which contains it. Thus hernia of the brain may occur because of a severe injury to the skull, hernia of the lung from a wound of the chest wall, but these are uncommon, and the most common form is hernia of the bowel, the popular term for which is rupture.

Varieties: Although far the commonest organ found in a hernia is part of the bowel, any of the abdominal structures, such as stomach, kidney, ovary, womb, bladder, or omentum, may be found projecting through an opening in the wall of the abdomen and lying close beneath the skin. Probably the only two organs exempt are the liver and pancreas, by reason of their position and connections. The projecting organ carries in front of it, and is enveloped by, a sac of peritoneum, the smooth membrane lining the interior of the abdomen. It is separated from the surface at least by this sac and by the skin. A hernia is usually described according to the position at which it protrudes. There are certain natural openings in the region of the groin on either side: one, known as the inguinal canal, through which the testicle descends in early life, and which the spermatic cord keeps always more or less open; the other, known as the femoral canal, which lies to the inner side of the large femoral vessels that pass from the abdomen to the thigh. The inguinal canal ends just above the pubic bone, its exit, known as the external abdominal ring, being large enough to admit the tip of the finger. The femoral canal is smaller and is separated from the former only by the inner end of the inguinal ligament, a strong band which lies beneath the oblique groove that can be seen on the surface to separate the abdomen from the thigh. A hernia emerging from the former is known as an inguinal hernia, and tends to descend along the spermatic cord into the scrotum. A hernia emerging through the femoral canal comes forwards on the front of the thigh, and is called a femoral hernia. A weak spot exists in the centre of the abdomen at the navel, and here, not infrequently in young children of poor development, a hernia may appear, which is then known as an umbilical hernia. A hernia which protrudes at some accidental opening on the abdomen, as, for example, through the scar of an operation wound, is known as a ventral hernia. A rare form of hernia is one which passes through the gap in front of the pelvis between the ischial and pubic bones; it is known as an obturator hernia. Finally, there are various forms of internal hernia, the protruded organ passing up into the chest, or into some other region where it does not show itself on the surface. (See HIATUS HERNIA.)

A hernia may also be considered as *congenital*, that is, existing at birth, or *acquired* later on in life. The only positions in which congenital hernia is found are in the umbilical and inguinal regions. In the latter case the hernia descends along with the testicle towards the scrotum, the hernia being inside the tubular process of peritoneum which descends with the testicle in order to provide it with a smooth tunic.

An important classification of hernia is made according to the condition of the protruding organ. A *reducible hernia* is one which is so freely movable that it may be pressed back into the abdomen, although it comes down again by the same opening unless this is blocked up. An *irreducible hernia* is one which cannot be returned, either because it has become adherent to its new surroundings, because it has enlarged after emerging, because much fat has been deposited inside the abdomen, or for some similar reason. An *obstructed hernia* is one in which, a part of the bowel being protruded, some of its contents become caught inside, and cannot for a time pass on, a state of costiveness arising in fact inside the hernia. A *strangulated hernia* is by far the most important variety, because of its immediate danger to life. In this form, the circulation of blood in the protruded bowel becomes cut off by the margin of the opening through which the loop of bowel has passed; and, if an operation is not immediately performed for its relief, the bowel will become gangrenous, and the patient may die within a few days. The great danger attending all forms of hernia is that they may at any time become strangulated.

Causes: Two factors come into play in causing hernia. First, some defect or injury of the abdominal wall; and, secondly, some increase of pressure within the cavity. With regard to the hernia at the umbilicus of young children, there is usually some defect in the closure of the opening through which the navel-string passes before birth, and through this opening a loop of bowel is forced by excessive crying or the like. In inguinal hernia, which is far commoner in men than in women, the defect consists in some failure of the inguinal canal through which the testicle descends before birth to close completely. There may, in congenital hernia, be a completely open passage leading out of the abdomen, or there may be simply a small pocket in the peritoneum which, by a sudden strain or by long-continued pressure, such as coughing, gets torn or stretched in front of a protruded organ. Femoral hernia is commoner in women than in men, probably on account of the special shape and inclination of the pelvic bones, and arises in a manner similar to inguinal hernia. Both in these and in ventral hernia, the occurrence of marked changes in size of the abdomen, such as great increase in stoutness, great loss of fat, and repeated child-bearing, has the effect of greatly weakening the abdominal wall and predisposing to the formation of hernia. All laborious occupations involving great efforts, and bodily conditions involving frequently repeated strains, such as chronic cough or constipation, conduce to hernia of all sorts. Accordingly hernia is much more common in the male sex – who lead a more strenuous physical life – than among females.

Symptoms: The symptoms vary considerably, depending upon the particular organ which is protruded, upon the size of the opening, which may or may not compress the hernia, and upon the condition of the latter. In the great majority of cases the hernia consists of one or more loops of the small intestine, and, if the hernia is small and readily reducible, the symptoms are somewhat as follows. If the hernia is produced quite suddenly, as during the lifting of a heavy weight, the person affected may hear or feel a distant crack, and be conscious that something has given way, but, as a rule, suffers no sharp pain. More usually the hernia develops gradually, and the symptoms have then no definite onset, but simply increase till they attract attention. An undefinable sense of weakness, and occasionally pain, are felt in the region of the hernia. When any great effort is made, such as coughing, or straining at stool, or lifting a weight, a swelling appears with a gurgling feeling at the seat of the hernia, although this can be made to disappear by pressure when the person lies down. Even if the hernia does not come far down, a distinct impulse on coughing is communicated to the hand laid upon the swelling, which is situated usually at the inner end of the groin. When the hernia has become irreducible, the swelling does not vary in size, but the impulse on coughing is still to be felt. The presence even of a small hernia may occasion some interference with digestion, and constipation is a common accompaniment. A dragging sensation in the back is another frequent symptom.

When a hernia becomes strangulated, as the result of stoppage of its circulation by the pressure of the margin of the ring through which it comes, a marked set of symptoms ensues. The hernia first becomes inflamed, acutely painful, and then in a few hours turns gangrenous, producing general peritonitis and death if not relieved. At the same time, all passage of contents through the bowel is stopped, and as a result the bowels do not move, although some of their contents pass in the reverse direction, up to the stomach, whence they are vomited. Accordingly the onset of abdominal pain, accompanied by stoppage of the bowels and vomiting in a person possessed of a hernia, forms an ominous sign, and, even if no hernia is known to exist, the appearance of these three symptoms calls for immediate examination of the region of the groin by a medical practitioner.

Treatment: When a hernia is present, it may be treated in a palliative manner, so as to relieve unpleasant symptoms and diminish the risk of strangulation, or an attempt may be made to cure it.

PALLIATIVE TREATMENT: If the hernia is reducible, it is pushed back through the opening into the abdomen by manipulation known as taxis, and is then retained by an artificial support known as a truss. (See TRUSS.)

If the hernia is irreducible, a different type of truss designed merely to protect the hernia must be used.

CURATIVE TREATMENT: The danger of strangulation, involving an immediate operation with great risk to life, is present as long as a hernia exists, and surgical repair is the best treatment. Many operations are performed by different surgeons, but all consist briefly in this, that an opening is made over the hernia and, after the hernia has been returned into the abdomen, the sac is cut off, bunched up, turned aside, or otherwise disposed of, and the margins of the opening united by strong sutures, or by sewing together two mesh leaves. Almost all cases operated upon in this way result in complete cure, and many operations are done as day cases.

When a hernia is irreducible, some special diet or other treatment is often required before the operation, in order to diminish the amount of fat in the abdomen, reduce the size of the hernia, and so forth.

HEROIN, also known as DIAMORPHINE HYDROCHLORIDE, is a white crystalline powder of slightly bitter taste derived from morphine. It is a much more potent pain killer, or analgesic, than morphine but also a much more dangerous drug from the point of view of addiction. (See DRUG ADDICTION.)

HERPANGINA is a short febrile illness in which minute vesicles or punched-out ulcers develop in the posterior parts of the mouth. It is due to infection with the group A Coxsackie viruses (q.v.).

HERPES SIMPLEX is an acute infectious disease, characterized by the development of groups of superficial vesicles, or blebs, in the skin and mucous membrane. It is due to a virus, and infection can occur at any time from birth onwards, but the usual time for primary infection is between the second and fifteenth year. Once an individual is infected, the virus persists in the body for the rest of the individual's life. It is one of the causes of scrum-pox (q.v.).

Symptoms: The symptoms vary with the age of infection. In young infants it may cause a generalized infection which may prove fatal. In young children the infection is usually in the mouth, and this may be associated with enlargement of the glands in the neck, general irritability and fever. The condition usually settles in seven to ten days. In adults the vesicles may occur anywhere in the skin or mucous membranes. The more common sites are the lips, mouth and face where they are known as cold sores. The vesicles may also appear on the genitalia, or in the conjunctiva or cornea and the brain may be infected, causing encephalitis (q.v.) or meningitis. The first sign is the appearance of small painful swellings. These quickly develop into vesicles (q.v.), containing clear fluid, and surrounded by a reddened area of skin. Some people are particularly liable to recurrent attacks, and these often tend to be associated with some debilitating condition or infection, such as pneumonia.

Except in the case of herpes of the cornea, the eruption clears completely unless it becomes contaminated with some other organism. In the case of the cornea, there may be residual scarring, which may impair vision.

Treatment: A local treatment which may help, if the skin is involved, is idoxuridine. Should the eye be involved the patient must be referred immediately to an eye specialist. An antiviral agent such as acyclovir may be of help in treating the disease.

HERPES ZOSTER, or SHINGLES, is a skin eruption of acute nature, closely related to chickenpox, consisting in the appearance of small yellow vesicles (q.v.), which spread over an area, dry up, and heal by scabbing. It receives its name from the Greek word, for a 'circingle' or girdle, because it spreads in a zone-like manner round half the chest. Herpes of the face also occurs, particularly on the brow and round the eye.

Causes: It is due to a virus identical with that of chickenpox. This invades the ganglia of the nerves, particularly the spinal nerves of the chest and the fifth cranial nerve which supplies the face. In spite of its being due to the same virus as chickenpox, it is rare for herpes zoster to occur as a result of contact with a case of chickenpox. On the other hand, it is not unusual for a patient with herpes zoster to infect a child with chickenpox. It is a disease of adults rather than children, and the older the person the more likely is he to develop the disease. Thus in adults under 50 the incidence is around 2·5 per 1000 people a year. Between 50 and 60 it is around 5 per 1000, whilst in octogenarians it is 10 per 1000. Most adults who acquire the disease have had chickenpox in child-hood. Occasionally it may be associated with some serious underlying disease such as leukaemia, lymphadenoma, or multiple myeloma.

Symptoms: The first symptoms of herpes are much like those of any feverish attack. The person feels unwell for some days, has a slight rise of temperature, and vague pain in the side or in various other parts. The pain finally settles at a point in the side, and, two or three days after the first symptoms, the rash appears. Minute yellow blebs or vesicles as they are known are seen on the skin of the back, of the side, or of the front of the chest, or simultaneously on all three, the points corresponding to the space between one pair of ribs right round. These blebs increase in number for some days, and spread till there is often a complete half girdle round one side of the chest. The pain in this stage is severe, but it appears to vary a good deal with age, being slight in children and very severe in old people, in whom indeed herpes sometimes forms a serious illness. After one or two weeks, most of the vesicles have dried up and formed scabs, which finally drop off, leaving the skin just as it was before, or covered with small scars. Occasionally the little vesicles run together into large blebs, which leave ulcers difficult to heal, and followed by marked scars. The skin is generally healed completely in two or three weeks, but a distressing peculiarity about the pain is that, in old people especially, it may not pass off when the eruption disappears, but may remain for weeks or even months: a condition known as post-herpetic neuralgia.

Treatment: In the very early stage, before the vesicles have formed, cocaine or atropine ointment rubbed into the side eases the pain and seems to prevent to some extent the outbreak of the eruption. Later, when the vesicles have formed and are discharging, a dusting-powder of starch, zinc oxide, and bismuth subnitrate gives much relief, or the side may be painted with glycerin jelly containing menthol or with a mixture of chloral, camphor, and menthol in equal parts. Alternatively, the lesions may be dabbed with calamine lotion. In any case, the part should be kept warm by a dressing of cotton-wool. Analgesics may be required for relief of the pain.

Should post-herpetic neuralgia persist, the administration of analgesics is essential. Acupuncture is also said to be helpful.

HERTZ is the SI (International System of Units) unit of frequency. It indicates the number of cycles per second (c/s). The abbreviation for hertz is Hz.

HETEROGRAFT is a transplant from one animal to another of a different species. It is also known as a xenograft.

HETEROSEXUAL: Concerning sexual relationships between members of opposite sexes.

HETEROZYGOUS: An individual having dissimilar members of the pair of genes coding for a given characteristic (see GENES).

HEXACHLOROPHANE is a widely used antiseptic which is active against a range of microorganisms, including Gram-positive and Gram-negative organisms, *Shigella dysenteriae*, and *Salmonella typhi*. One of its advantages is that it retains its activity in the presence of soap, and it is therefore often used in soaps and creams in a concentration of 1 to 2 per cent. It must be used with caution in babies as it can be absorbed through the skin and prove harmful.

HEXAMINE is a substance which, when excreted by the kidneys, sets free formaldehyde, that has an antiseptic action. It is given in cases of cystitis when the urine decomposes within the bladder, and it exerts its beneficial action very speedily. It acts only in urine with an acid reaction, and, if the urine is alkaline, acid phosphate of soda is usually taken along with the hexamine. The dose of each of these is 0·6 to 2 grams several times daily.

HEXOESTROL (see OESTROGENS).

HIATUS HERNIA is a displacement of a portion of the stomach through the opening in the diaphragm through which the oesophagus passes from the chest to the abdominal cavity.

HICCUP An involuntary spasmodic contraction of the diaphragm (q.v.) which produces an indrawing of breath during which there is a sudden closure of the vocal cords. This results in the well-known sound and sensation.

It is usually of benign cause (e.g. indigestion) but may be a symptom of medullary brain damage, uraemia, typhoid fever or encephalitis lethargica.

There are many folk remedies for hiccups but most subside spontaneously. Prolonged hiccups due to disease may respond to treatment with chlorpromazine.

HILUM is a term applied to the depression on organs such as the lung, kidney, and spleen, at which the vessels and nerves enter it and round which the lymphatic glands cluster. The hilum of the lung is also known as its root.

HIP: That part of the body on each side of the pelvis where it articulates with the head of the femur (thigh bone).

HIP-JOINT is the joint formed by the head of the thigh-bone and the deep cup-shaped hollow on the side of the pelvis which receives it (acetabulum). The joint is of the ball-and-socket variety, is dislocated only by very great violence, and is correspondingly difficult to reduce to its natural state after dislocation. The joint is enclosed by a capsule of fibrous tissue, strengthened by several bands, of which the principal is the ilio-femoral or Y-shaped ligament placed in front of the joint. A round ligament also unites the head of the thigh-bone to the margin of the acetabulum.

For hip-joint disease see under JOINTS, DISEASES OF; DISLOCATIONS.

HIPPOCRATIC OATH: An oath traditionally taken by doctors on qualification that sets out the moral precepts of their profession and binds them to a code of behaviour and practice. It is named after Hippocrates (460–370 BC), the Greek 'father of medicine'.

HIPPUS is a tremor of the iris which produces alternating contraction and dilatation of the pupil. This is often a sign of hysteria.

HIRSCHSPRUNG'S DISEASE, or MEGACOLON, is a condition in childhood which is characterized by great hypertrophy and dilatation of the colon.

HIRSUTISM, or HYPERTRICHOSIS, is the growth of hair of the male type and distribution in women. It is either due to the excess production of androgens or to undue sensitivity of the hair follicle to normal female levels of circulating androgens. The latter is called idiopathic because the cause is unknown. The increased production of androgens in the female may come from the ovary and be due to the polycystic ovary syndrome or an ovarian tumour, or the excess androgen may come from the adrenal cortex and be the result of congenital adrenal hyperplasia, an adrenal tumour or Cushing's syndrome. However there is a wide range of normality in the distribution of female body hair. It varies with different racial groups. The Mediterranean races have more body hair than Nordic women and the Chinese and Japanese have little body hair. Many normal women, especially those with dark hair, have hair apparent on the upper lip and a few coarse hairs on the chin and around the nipples are not uncommon. Extension of the pubic hair towards the umbilicus is frequently found in normal women. Dark hair is much more apparent than fair hair and this is why bleaching is of considerable benefit in the management of hirsutism.

The treatment of hirsutism is that of the primary cause. When it is idiopathic hirsutism it must be managed by simple measures such as bleaching the hair and the use of depilatory waxes and creams. Coarse facial hairs can be removed by electrolysis, although this is time consuming. Shaving is often the most effective remedy and neither increases the rate of hair growth nor causes the hairs to become coarser.

HISTAMINE is an amine (q.v.) derived from histidine (q.v.). It is widely distributed in the tissues of plants and animals, including man. It is a powerful stimulant of gastric juice, a constrictor of smooth muscle including that of the bronchi, and a dilator of arterioles and capillaries. It is this last action which is responsible for the eruption of urticaria (q.v.).

HISTIDINE is an amino-acid from which histamine is derived by bacterial decomposition.

HISTOLOGY is the study of the minute structure of the tissues.

HISTOPLASMOSIS is a disease due to a yeast-like fungus known as *Histoplasma capsulatum*. Most cases have been reported from USA. In infants it is characterized by fever, anaemia, enlargement of the liver and spleen, and involvement of the lungs and gastrointestinal tract. In older children it may resemble pulmonary tuberculosis, whilst in adults it may be confined to involvement of the skin.

HIV: Human immunodeficiency virus: the virus that is responsible for AIDS. It is one of the family of human T-cell lymphocytotrophic viruses, others of which may cause lymphomas in man.

HIVES is a popular term applied to eruptions of the nature of urticaria (q.v.).

HLA ANTIGENS: These are inherited antigens (q.v.) first identified on the surfaces of leucocytes (q.v.) and now known to be present on the surfaces of cells throughout the body. There are five HLA gene loci (A, B, C, D, and DE) on chromosome six and the genes inherited from each parent will determine the antigens present on the cell surfaces of each individual.

These antigens are a means by which the immune system differentiates self from nonself. The rejection of transplanted material involves recognition of foreign HLAs. The more closely matched the HLAs of the donor and the recipient, the less likely the change of rejection.

It is also known that certain diseases occur more commonly in individuals with particular HLAs.

HODGKIN'S DISEASE, so called after Thomas Hodgkin (1798–1866), the Guy's Hospital pathologist who first described it, or LYMPHADENOMA, is a condition in which the lymphatic glands all over the body undergo a gradually progressive enlargement. The cause is not known. The glands affected may reach a great size. The patient often runs a characteristic form of fever (Pel-Ebstein fever), in which bouts of fever alternate with several days with no fever. Along with these changes a considerable degree of anaemia arises, and the affected person becomes gradually weaker. Treatment consists of radiotherapy when the disease is relatively localized. When it is more widespread, however, chemotherapy is the treatment of choice. This is now given in the form of a combination of drugs, rather than one single drug. The most commonly used combination at the moment is: mustine, vinblastine, procarbazine and prednisone. The results of treatment are now such that over 80 per cent treated by radiotherapy, and 78 per cent of those treated by combined chemotherapy, are still alive after five years.

HOLISTIC: A method of medical care in which patients are treated as a whole and which takes into account their physical and mental state as well as social background rather than just treating the disease alone.

HOMATROPINE is an alkaloid derived from atropine, which is used to produce dilatation of the pupil and to paralyse accommodation temporarily for the purpose of examining the interior of the eye. It is used in 1 per cent solution, and its effects pass away in the course of a few hours.

HOMOCYSTINURIA is a congenital disease due to the inability of the affected individual to metabolize, or utilize properly one of the essential amino-acids (q.v.) known as methionine. The main features of the condition are abnormality of the lens of the eye, mental retardation, fair complexion and fair hair and a high cheek colour.

HOMOEOPATHY is a system of medicine founded by Hahnemann at the end of the eighteenth century. It is based upon the theory that diseases are curable by those drugs which produce effects on the body similar to symptoms caused by the disease (*similia similibus curantur*). In administering drugs, the theory is also held that their effect is increased by giving them in minute doses obtained by diluting them to an extreme degree.

HOMOGRAFT is a piece of tissue or an organ, such as a kidney, transplanted from one animal to another of the same species: e.g. from man to man. It is also known as an allograft.

HOMOSEXUALITY is sexual activity with a member of the same sex. There has been considerable debate among psychiatrists as to whether homosexuality should be regarded as a normal sexual variant or as a psycho-pathological development or deviation. Although homosexuality is found in virtually every society and culture there is no society in which it is the predominant or preferred mode of sexual activity. Various attempts have been made to link homosexuality to hormonal factors, particularly lowered testosterone levels, or to find a genetic explanation, but there is no evidence for either. Psycho-analytic theories link homosexuality to early child-rearing influences, in particular the close binding and intimate mother.

The number of homosexual men in the UK is unknown. There has never been a representative population survey. Re-analysis of the Kinsey report suggests that only 3 per cent of adult men have exclusively homosexual leanings and a further 3 per cent have extensive homosexual and heterosexual experience. Homosexuality seems to be less common among women. Homosexual intercourse (and penetration) is a well-known means of transmission of the HIV virus.

There are still differences in the way homosexuals and heterosexuals are treated in British law. The age of consent for homosexuals is 21, while for heterosexuals it is 16.

HOMOZYGOUS: An individual having identical members of the pair of genes coding for a given characteristic, (see GENES).

HONKING is the term applied to a persistent cough of emotional origin which occurs in emotionally disturbed children. It is of an explosive brassy character and has been compared to the call of the Canada goose. When coughing the child grimaces and tends to hold the chin close to the chest. One of its major characteristics is that it never occurs at night. Quite often it follows on a cold or sore throat. No specific treatment is needed. It disappears when the cause of the emotional upset, such as, for example, difficulties at school, is dealt with and removed.

HOOKWORM (see ANCYLOSTOMIASIS).

HORDEOLUM: An outdated term meaning a stye, occasionally a chalazion.

HORMONE REPLACEMENT THERAPY (see MENOPAUSE).

HORMONES: These are 'chemical messengers' that are dispersed by the blood and act on target organs to produce effects distant from their point of release. The main organs involved in hormone production are the pituitary, pancreas, ovary, testis, thyroid, and adrenal (qq.v.). The release of many hormones is, ultimately, under the control of the central nervous system via a series of inhibiting and releasing factors from the hypothalamus (q.v.). Hormones are involved in maintaining homeostasis: e.g. insulin regulates the concentration of glucose in the blood. They also participate in growth and maturation: e.g. growth hormone promotes growth and helps to regulate fat, carbohydrate, and protein metabolism; and the sex hormones promote sexual maturation and reproduction. (See ENDOCRINE GLANDS.)

HORNER'S SYNDROME: This is the description given to a combination of changes resulting from paralysis of the sympathetic nerve in the neck. They are: small pupil, a drooping upper lid and an apparently (though not actually) sunken eye.

HORRIPILATION is another term for gooseflesh, due to contraction of the small muscles in the skin which make the hairs erect.

HORSESHOE KIDNEY (see KIDNEYS, DISEASES OF).

HOSPICE: A hospital that cares only for the terminally ill and dying. The emphasis is on providing quality of life and special care is taken in providing pain relief by whichever methods are deemed best suited to the person's needs.

HOSPITAL: An institution providing treatment for sick and injured persons. This may be done on an inpatient or outpatient basis. It provides investigative and therapeutic services which are not available on a domiciliary basis. Hospitals are broadly divided into general hospitals (available in each district in the United Kingdom) and hospitals specializing in particular ailments (e.g. ophthalmology, ear, nose and throat, neurology, etc.). In addition there are teaching hospitals which have the dual function of patient care and the education of medical staff.

HOST: An organism on which a parasite lives.

HOUR-GLASS STOMACH is the term given to the X-ray appearance of a stomach which is constricted in its middle part because of either spasm of the stomach muscle or contraction of scar tissue from a gastric ulcer.

HOUSEMAID'S KNEE is an inflammation of the bursa in front of the knee-cap, often mistaken for some disease in the joint itself (see BURSITIS).

HUMAN CHORIONIC GONADOTROPHIN: A glycoprotein hormone secreted by the placenta (see AFTERBIRTH) in early pregnancy which stimulates the corpus luteum (q.v.) within the ovary (q.v.) to secrete oestrogen (q.v.), progesterone (q.v.), and relaxin. It is essential for the maintenance of pregnancy up to about 6–8 weeks of gestation. A radio-immuno assay (q.v.) can be used to detect it and pregnancy can be diagnosed as early as six days after conception by testing for it in the urine. Some tumours also secrete human chorionic gonadotrophin, particularly hydatidiform moles (q.v.), which produce large amounts.

HUMAN IMMUNODEFICIENCY VIRUS (see HIV).

HUMAN LEUCOCYTE ANTIGEN (HLA): HLA antigens are found in most tissues of the body. They are genetically determined by genes on chromosome 6. They are the antigens that result in rejection of tissues from other individuals, such as skin, kidney, heart and liver. They are similar to the blood-group antigens that are situated on red blood cells. There are four groups of HLA antigen: A, B, C and DR.

If they are well defined, they are given a number such as HLA A1 and, if they are poorly defined, they are given a letter, for example HLA AW. If the HLA groups between two individuals are identical, graft rejection is unlikely. There are associations between HLA types and certain diseases. For example, ankylosing spondylitis tends to occur only in individuals who are HLA B27. Rheumatoid arthritis tends to occur in individuals that are HLA DR4 and thyrotoxicosis in those that are HLA B8.

HUMERUS is the bone of the upper arm. It has a rounded head, which helps to form the shoulder joint, and at its lower end presents a wide pulley-like surface for union with the radius and ulna. Its epicondyles form the prominences at the sides of the elbow.

HUMIDIFICATION of the air we breathe is essential for the efficient working of the lungs. (See RESPIRATION.) This is achieved largely by the nose (q.v.) which acts as an air-conditioner, warming, moistening, and filtering the 10,000 litres of air which we inhale daily, in the process of which, incidentally, it produces around 1·5 litres of secretion daily. Humidity is expressed as relative humidity (RH). This is the amount of moisture in the air expressed as a percentage of the maximum possible at that temperature. If the temperature of a room is raised without increasing the moisture content, the RH falls. The average outdoor RH in Britain is around 70 to 80 per cent. With central heating it may drop to 25 per cent or lower.

This is why humidification, as it is known, of the air is essential in buildings heated by modern heating systems. The aim should be to keep the RH around 30 to 50 per cent. In houses this may be achieved quite satisfactorily by having a jug or basin of water in the room, or some receptacle that can be attached to the heater. In offices some more elaborate form of humidifier is necessary. Those suffering from chronic bronchitis are particularly susceptible to dry air. (See also VENTILATION.)

HUMIDIFIER FEVER is a form of alveolitis (q.v.) caused by contamination of the water used to humidify, or moisten, the air in air-conditioning plants. The breathing of the contaminated air results in infection of the lung, which is characterized by fever, cough, shortness of breath and malaise, worse on Monday and tending to improve during the course of the week.

HUMOUR is a term applied to any fluid or semi-fluid tissue of the body: e.g. the aqueous and vitreous humours in the eye. The term, humour, is also associated with a theory regarding the causation of disease, which originated with Pythagoras and lasted in a modified form until the early part of the nineteenth century. According to this theory diseases are due to an improper mixture in the body of blood, bile, phlegm and black bile.

HUNGER is a craving for food or other substance necessary to bodily activity. Hunger for food is supposed to be directly produced by strong contractions of the stomach which occur when it is empty or nearly so. (See also THIRST.) AIR HUNGER is an instinctive craving for oxygen resulting in breathlessness, either when a person ascends to great heights where the pressure of air is low, or in some diseases such as pneumonia and diabetes mellitus.

HUNTINGTON'S CHOREA is a hereditary disease characterized by involuntary movements and dementia. Each child of a parent with the disease has a 50:50 chance of developing it. The usual time of onset is between 35 and 45, but 10 per cent of cases occur under the age of 20. Some patients show more severe mental disturbance, others more severe disturbances of movement, but in all it pursues an inexorable downward course over a period of ten to twenty years to a terminal state of physical and mental helplessness. It is estimated that there are around 6000 cases in Britain. The cause is not known and there is no effective treatment. People with Huntington's chorea and their relatives can obtain help and guidance from Huntington's Disease Association, 108 Battersea High Street, London, SW11 3HP (071- 223 7000).

HURLER'S SYNDROME (see GARGOYLISM).

HUTCHINSON'S TEETH is the term applied to the narrowed and notched permanent incisor teeth which occur in congenital syphilis. They are so named after Sir Jonathan Hutchinson (1828–1913), the London physician who first described them.

HYALINE: Tissue material that has a glass-like appearance when stained and viewed under the microscope. It occurs in a variety of tissues and diseases, particularly Respiratory Distress Syndrome (see ADULT RESPIRATORY DISTRESS SYNDROME), hyaline degeneration of arterioles and alcoholic liver disease.

HYALINE MEMBRANE DISEASE is a condition found in premature infants and infants born by Caesarean section, characterized by the onset of difficulty in breathing a few hours after birth. About half the affected babies die, death usually occurring before the third day. At post-mortem examination the alveoli and the finer bronchioles of the lungs are found to be lined with a dense membrane. The cause of the condition is obscure. (See ADULT RESPIRATORY DISTRESS SYNDROME.)

HYALURONIDASE is an enzyme (q.v.) which hydrolyses hyaluronic acid. The latter is a gel-like substance which is widely distributed throughout the body and which helps to bind together the tissue cells and also acts as a lubricant in joints. By virtue of its action in hydrolysing hyaluronic acid, hyaluronidase is now used in subcutaneous injections of fluid as it facilitates the spread of the injected fluid and therefore its absorption.

HYDATID is a cyst produced by the growth of immature forms of a tapeworm. (See TAENIASIS.)

HYDATIDIFORM MOLE, or VESICULAR MOLE as it is sometimes known, is a rare complication of pregnancy, in which there is tremendous proliferation of the epithelium of the chorion (the outer of the two fetal membranes). It seldom occurs during a first pregnancy. Treatment consists of immediate evacuation of the womb.

HYDRADENITIS SUPPURATIVA is a chronic inflammatory disease of the apocrine sweat glands (see PERSPIRATION). It is more common in women, in whom it usually occurs in the armpit, than in men in whom it is most common in the perineum of the drivers of lorries and taxis. It occurs in the form of painful, tender lumps underneath the skin, which burst often in a week or so. Treatment consists of removal by operation.

HYDRALAZINE is a hypotensive drug. (See ESSENTIAL HYPERTENSION.)

HYDRAMNIOS is the condition characterized by excess of fluid in the amniotic cavity. (See AMNION.)

HYDROCOELE is a collection of fluid connected with the testicle or spermatic cord. It is sometimes due to inflammation of the sac in which these structures are enclosed, but in many cases the cause cannot be discovered. It develops usually in middle life, although it may appear at any time, increases gradually in size, and is usually devoid of pain. The condition presents some resemblance to hernia, and there is occasionally some doubt in distinguishing between them, particularly when the hydrocoele communicates with the abdominal cavity. In infants and young children the hydrocoele disappears spontaneously. When treatment is required it takes one of three forms. It may take the form of aspirating, or withdrawing, the fluid with a needle and syringe. The fluid is liable to recur and further aspirations have to be carried out. In these cases it is more satisfactory to remove the fluid and replace it with sclerosing agent that seals off the cavity. Some surgeons prefer to operate and remove the sac.

HYDROCEPHALUS is the condition in which there is abnormal accumulation of cerebrospinal fluid within the skull. It is due to one or more of three main causes: (i) excessive production of spinal fluid (see CEREBROSPINAL FLUID); (ii) defective absorption of cerebrospinal fluid; (iii) blockage to the circulation of cerebrospinal fluid. The causes of these disturbances of circulation of cerebrospinal fluid may be congenital (most commonly associated with spina bifida (q.v.), meningitis, or a tumour.

Symptoms: In children the chief symptoms observed are the gradual increase in size of the upper part of the head, out of all proportion to the face or the rest of the body. The head is globular, with a wide anterior fontanelle and separation of the bones at the sutures. The veins in the scalp are prominent, and there is a 'crackpot' note on percussion. The normal infant's head should not grow more than 2·5 cm (1 inch) in each of the first two months of life and much more slowly subsequently. Growth beyond this rate should arouse suspicions of hydrocephalus. Another useful rule is that the circumference of the head should not exceed that of the chest. In chronic hydrocephalus, the head of an infant 3 months old has been known to measure 72·5 cm (29 inches); and in the case of the man, Cardinal, who died in Guy's Hospital, the head measured 82·5 cm (33 inches).

The cerebral ventricles are widely distended, and the convolutions of the brain flattened, while occasionally the fluid escapes into the cavity of the cranium, which it fills, pressing down the brain to the base of the skull. As a consequence of such changes, the functions of the brain are interfered with, and in general the mental condition of the patient is impaired. The child is dull and listless, irritable and sometimes suffers from severe mental subnormality. The special senses become affected as the disease advances, especially vision, and sight is often lost, as is also hearing. Towards the end paralysis is apt to occur.

The outlook for children with hydrocephalus is not as gloomy as was at one time thought to be the case. Such a child has a 50 per cent chance of survival with the disease arrested. He then has a 75 per cent chance of being educable. Almost one-third of arrested cases can be expected to enjoy normal intelligence with little or no physical disability.

Treatment: Numerous ingenious operations have been devised for the treatment of hydrocephalus. The most satisfactory of these utilize the Holter or Pudenz unidirectional valves, whereby the cerebrospinal fluid is by-passed into the right atrium of the heart or the peritoneal cavity, but it is only in a proportion of affected children that these operations produce a satisfactory result. The choice of operation and of the children likely to benefit is a highly skilled one that can only be made by an experienced surgeon.

HYDROCHLORIC ACID: A colourless, pungent, fuming liquid. Secreted by the parietal cells in the lining of the stomach, it aids in the digestion of the food.

HYDROCHLOROTHIAZIDE (see BENZO-THIADIAZINES).

HYDROCORTISONE, or compound F, has the chemical formula, 17-hydroxycorticosterone. It is closely allied to cortisone (q.v.) both in its structure (cortisone is an oxidation product of hydrocortisone) and in its action. Its anti-rheumatic potency is said to be 50 per cent greater than that of cortisone. Its main use to date in rheumatoid arthritis has been for local injection into affected joints. It is also used as a local application to the skin in the form of a cream or lotion in the treatment of certain skin diseases.

HYDROGEN PEROXIDE has the chemical formula H_2O_2 and is a thick colourless liquid. It is available in solution with water in concentrations of 3, 6 and 27 per cent and as a cream. It is readily reduced to water giving up oxygen in the process, which causes the characteristic frothing seen when used. The frothing helps to dislodge adherent discharges or dead tissue and it also has antiseptic and deodorizing properties. Thus it is used as a mouthwash, to clean wounds and ulcers and occasionally to disinfect body cavities at operation. It is also a bleach.

HYDRONEPHROSIS is a chronic disease in which the kidney becomes greatly distended with fluid. It is caused by obstruction to the flow of urine at the pelvi-ureteric junction. If the ureter is obstructed the ureter proximal to the obstruction will dilate and pressure will be transmitted back to the kidney to cause hydronephrosis. Obstruction may occur at the bladder neck or in the urethra itself. Enlarge-ment of the prostate is a common cause of bladder-neck obstruction. This would give rise to hypertrophy of the bladder muscle and both dilatation of the ureter and hydronephrosis. If the obstruction is not relieved progressive de-struction of renal tissue will occur. As a result of the stagnation of the urine infection is probable and cystitis and pyelonephritis may occur.

HYDROPHOBIA is another name for RABIES (q.v.).

HYDROPS FOETALIS (see HAEMOLYTIC DIS-EASE OF THE NEW-BORN).

HYDROTHERAPY: Treatment using water in the form baths, douches, etc.

HYDROTHORAX means a collection of fluid in the pleural cavities.

HYDROXOCOBALAMIN, or vitamin B_{12}, has now replaced cyanocobalamin (q.v.) in the treatment of pernicious anaemia. (See ANAE-MIA.) It has the practical advantage that fewer injections are required than in the case of cyanocobalamin. Like cyanocobalamin it be-longs to the group of substances known as cobalamins which have an enzyme (q.v.) action in practically every metabolic system in the body and are essential for normal growth and nutrition.

HYDROXYUREA is a drug that is proving of value in the treatment of chronic myeloid leukaemia.

HYDROXYZINE PAMOATE is a tranquil-lizer that is proving of value in the treatment of anxiety states. (See BENZODIAZEPINES.)

HYGIENE is the science of preserving health.

HYMEN is the thin membranous fold partially closing the lower end of the virginal vagina.

HYOID is a U-shaped bone at the root of the tongue. It can be felt from the front of the neck, lying about 2·5 cm above the prominence of the thyroid cartilage.

HYOSCINE: An alkaloid (q.v.) obtained from the plant henbane (hyoscyamus). It is an anticholinergic drug (q.v.) sometimes used as a premedicant in patients undergoing anaesthe-sia for its sedative and antiemetic effects and its ability to reduce saliva production. It may cause confusion in the elderly.

HYPERACUSIS means an abnormally acute sense of hearing.

HYPERAEMIA means congestion or presence of an excessive amount of blood in a part.

HYPERAESTHESIA means over-sensitiveness of a part, as found, for example, in certain nervous diseases. (See TOUCH.)

HYPERALGESIA means excessive sensitive-ness to pain. (See PAIN; TOUCH.)

HYPERCALCIURIA means an abnormally large amount of calcium in the urine. It is the most common single cause of stones in the kidneys in Britain.

HYPERCAPNIA means an abnormal increase in the amount of carbon dioxide in the blood or in the lungs (see BLOOD GASES). It may be caused by a reduced respiratory rate or effort, diseases of the chest wall and lung (affecting breathing) and cyanotic heart disease.

HYPERCHLORHYDRIA is the condition in which there is an excessive production of hydrochloric acid in the stomach. It is a characteristic finding in certain forms of dyspepsia, particularly that associated with a duodenal ulcer. It causes heartburn (q.v.) and waterbrash (q.v.). (See DUODENAL ULCER; DYSPEPSIA; STOMACH, DISEASES OF.)

HYPEREMESIS GRAVIDARUM: A rare condition (less than 0·2 per cent) of pregnancies in which there is severe vomiting. If untreated it can result in severe dehydration, ketoacidosis (an excess of ketone (q.v.) acids) and liver damage. More common in multiple pregnancy it may recur in subsequent pregnancies.

HYPERGLYCAEMIA means excess of sugar in the blood, the condition accompanying diabetes mellitus. The amount of sugar normally present in the blood is dependent upon how much sugar has been consumed, but in the fasting state it runs around 80 to 100 milligrams per 100 millilitres of blood. A fasting blood level of sugar above this is regarded as hyperglycaemia; in diabetes mellitus (q.v.) the sugar may rise to four or five times that amount.

HYPERIDROSIS, or HYPERHIDROSIS, means excessive sweating. (See PERSPIRATION.)

HYPERKALAEMIA: A serum potassium (q.v.) concentration above the normal range. Often caused by renal failure or excessive intake of potassium, perhaps in a drug. It may be complicated by cardiac dysrhythmias (abnormal rhythm of the heart).

HYPERKINETIC SYNDROME: A disorder of children characterized by excessive activity and impaired ability to learn. The child has a short attention span and may be aggressive. There is an association with mental subnormality. Treatment involves behaviour therapy (q.v.), drugs (such as amphetamines) and family therapy.

HYPERLIPIDAEMIA means an excess of fat in the blood. The two most important fats circulating in the blood are cholesterol and triglycerides. Raised blood levels of cholesterol predispose to atheroma and coronary artery disease and raised triglycerides predispose to pancreatitis. Some of the hyperlipidaemias are familial and some are secondary to other diseases such as hypothyroidism, diabetes mellitus, nephrotic syndrome and alcoholism. There is evidence that therapy which lowers the lipid concentration reduces the progression of premature atheroma, particularly in those who suffer from the familial disorder. There are a number of drugs available for lowering the lipid content of the plasma but these should be reserved for patients in whom severe hyper-lipidaemia is inadequately controlled by weight reduction. Clofibrate, bezafibrate, nicotinic acid and nicofuranose lower plasma cholesterol and plasma triglyceride concentration through their effect on reducing the hepatic production of lipoproteins. Cholestyramine and colestipol, both of which are resins, bind bile salts in the gut and so decrease the absorption of the cholesterol that these bile salts contain and hence lower plasma cholesterol concentrations. Probucol lowers plasma cholesterol concentrations by increasing the metabolism of low-density lipoproteins.

HYPERMETROPIA or HYPEROPIA, is a term applied to long-sightedness, in which the eye is too flat from front to back and rays of light are brought to a focus behind the retina. (See VISION; SPECTACLES.)

HYPERNATRAEMIA: A serum sodium concentration above normal. It is usually caused by dehydration (either from inadequate intake or excessive loss of water). Occasionally it may be caused by excessive sodium intake and rarely by a raised level of aldosterone hormone.

HYPERNEPHROMA is a term applied to a tumour resembling the tissue of the suprarenal gland and occurring in the kidney.

HYPERPARATHYROIDISM: Increased activity of the parathyroid gland. Parathyroid hormone increases serum calcium. Hyperparathyroidism may be primary (due to an adenoma or hyperplasia of the gland), secondary (in response to hypocalcaemia) or tertiary (when secondary hyperparathyroidism causes the development of an autonomous adenoma).

HYPERPITUITARISM: Overactivity of the anterior lobe of the pituitary (q.v.) causing acromegaly (q.v.) (gigantism).

HYPERPLASIA means an abnormal increase in the number of cells in a tissue.

HYPERPYREXIA means an excessive degree of fever. (See FEVER; TEMPERATURE.)

HYPERSENSITIVITY is the abnormal immunological reaction produced in certain individuals when re-exposed to antigens that are innocuous to normal individuals. An antigen or allergen stimulates an allergic response. This produces a state of altered re-activity or an allergic state. Such a state of altered re-activity may be beneficial to the host, as in establishing a state of immunity, or it may be harmful to the host and produce a state of disease. Hypersensitivity is thus an allergic reaction in an individual sensitized by previous exposure to the antigen and in whom the allergic process constitutes the disease.

HYPERTENSION is another term for high blood-pressure. (See ESSENTIAL HYPERTENSION; MALIGNANT HYPERTENSION.)

HYPERTHERMIA means abnormally high body temperature. It is also the name given to the treatment of disease by the artificial production of fever. This can be achieved by various methods, such as radiation heat cabinets boosted with radio frequency (RF); immersion in a hot wax bath; heated suits or blankets; techniques using electromagnetic waves (e.g. RF, microwaves (q.v.)); ultrasound (q.v.) of appropriate frequencies. It is sometimes of help as an adjunct to surgery, chemotherapy, or radiotherapy in the treatment of cancer.

HYPERTHYROIDISM is excessive activity of the thyroid gland: e.g. Graves' disease. (See GOITRE.)

HYPERTONIC: (1) Referring to one solution which has a greater osmotic pressure than another. Physiologically it is used to describe solutions which have a greater osmotic pressure than body fluids. (2) Muscles with abnormally increased tone (e.g. following a stroke).

HYPERTROPHY means the increase in size which takes place in an organ as the result of an increased amount of work demanded of it by the bodily economy. For example, when valvular disease of the heart is present, compensation occurs by an increase in thickness of the heart-muscle, and the organ, by beating more powerfully, is able to overtake the strain thrown upon it. Similarly, if one kidney is removed, the other hypertrophies or grows larger to overtake the double work.

HYPERVENTILATION: An abnormally rapid resting respiratory rate. If voluntary it causes lightheadedness and then unconsciousness by lowering the blood tension of carbon dioxide. It is a manifestation of chest and heart diseases which raise carbon dioxide tension or cause hypoxia (q.v.) (e.g. severe chronic obstructive pulmonary disease or pulmonary oedema). Mechanically ventilated patients may be hyperventilated to lower carbon dioxide tension in order to reduce intracranial (q.v.) pressure.

HYPERVOLAEMIA: An increase in the volume of circulating blood above the normal range.

HYPNOTICS are measures, including drugs, which produce sleep.
Varieties: As certain conditions are necessary for the onset of sleep, even a slight departure from these may be sufficient to keep people who are not in good health awake. Thus a diminution of the circulation in the brain, and freedom from pain or irritation in any bodily organ are essential, whilst quiet and darkness are desirable, though many people can adapt themselves to noise and there are not a few who can sleep equally well whether it is light or dark. Often some trivial alteration of the daily life or diet is enough to relieve habitual insomnia; in other cases the quieting of pain is alone necessary; in other cases drugs must be used which have a light dulling effect upon the brain itself. For the relief of pain the drugs known as anodynes (q.v.) are used. Of the hypnotics, which dull the brain without much other effect, there is a large variety.
Uses: Simple remedies should always receive a fair trial first of all. Thus a person may be kept awake by severe mental labour or worry just before retiring to rest. The activity of the brain continues and sleeplessness results. Some quiet employment for the latter part of the evening, or a light meal, may relieve this. In other cases sleeplessness is often due to difficulty of digestion through a meal having been taken shortly before retiring to rest, and this may be relieved by abstaining from the last meal at night. In old people insomnia may be due to cold feet, and in such cases the best hypnotic is a pair of warm sleeping socks. Should these measures fail, and a hypnotic is required, the choice of which to use can only be made satisfactorily by the family doctor.

HYPNOTISM is the process of producing a state of mind known as hypnosis. Although a process which has been known for hundreds of years, its precise nature is still unknown. One modern writer has defined hypnosis as 'a temporary condition of altered attention, the most striking feature of which is greatly increased suggestibility'. There is no evidence, as has been claimed, that women can be more easily hypnotized than men. Children and young adults are the more easily hypnotized, middle-aged people being more resistant. There are various methods of induction of hypnosis, but the basis of them is some rhythmic stimulus accompanied by the repetition of carefully worded suggestions. The most commonly used method is to ask the patient to fix his eye on a given spot, or light, and then keep on repeating to him, in a quiet soothing voice, that his eyes will gradually become tired and that he will want to close them. There are various levels of hypnosis, usually classified as light, medium, and deep, and it has been estimated that 10 per cent of people cannot be hypnotized, 35 per cent can be taken into light hypnosis, 35 per cent into medium hypnosis, and 20 per cent into deep hypnosis.

Although in the past, hypnotism has often been frowned upon by orthodox medicine, largely because of its prostitution by charlatans, at the present day it is recognized to be a most useful method of therapy. Like all effective forms of therapy, however, it is not without its dangers, and this is why it should only be practised by those who have been adequately trained. Thus, under deep hypnosis suggestion can induce the person concerned to perform some prescribed automatic action when he awakes from the hypnotic state. Although there is good evidence that no one can be hypnotized to perform acts which are fundamentally contrary to his moral or ethical principles and which he does not want to do, this is only reassuring if one has sound evidence that the hypnotized subject has conventional moral or ethical principles.

Apart from its use in psychiatry, it is of value in the treatment of many psychosomatic conditions: that is, conditions in which physical manifestations, such as skin lesions, headaches and other forms of pain, are primarily due to some psychological or emotional disturbance. It is also being used to an increasing extent in obstetrics for the relief of pain during labour, and for the relief of pain in dentistry. Asthma is another condition that sometimes responds well to it. Another condition in which it is proving most valuable is as part of the treatment of alcoholism.

HYPOCALCAEMIA: A serum concentration of calcium below the normal range (9–11 mg of calcium per 100 ml of serum). This may cause tetany (q.v.), acutely, and chronically may give rise to rickets, osteomalacia or osteoporosis (qq.v.). It may be caused by hypoparathyroidism (q.v.), vitamin D deficiency, malabsorption, renal failure or acute pancreatitis (q.v.).

HYPOCAPNIA: A blood tension of carbon dioxide below normal. It is produced by hyperventilation which may be voluntary, mechanical (if the patient is on a ventilator) or in response to a physiological insult such as metabolic acidosis or brain injury.

HYPOCHLORHYDRIA means an insufficient secretion of hydrochloric acid from the digestive cells of the stomach lining.

HYPOCHONDRIASIS is a chronic mental condition in which the affected person's mind is constantly occupied with a delusion that he is seriously ill. As a rule, the ailments are referred to the stomach or the liver, and very often some trivial derangement of these exists to give colour to the person's views. Along with these complaints, there is a self-centred and gloomy turn of mind that prevents the patient from doing much of his proper work. Not uncommonly this mental trouble is hereditary, and passes gradually at a later stage into melancholia. The condition, apart from the affected person's making a strong effort of will and taking up some active work which may distract his thoughts, is very difficult to treat.

HYPODERMIC means of, or pertaining to, the region immediately under the skin. Thus, a hypodermic injection means an injection given underneath the skin. A hypodermic syringe is a small syringe which, fitted with a fine needle, is used to give such injections. A hypodermic injection is given for one of three main reasons: (1) because the substance administered cannot be given by mouth on account of its being destroyed in the stomach before it can be absorbed, e.g. insulin; (2) because it is not possible or it is inadvisable to give anything by mouth to the patient, e.g. because of vomiting; (3) because a quick action is necessary, e.g. morphine in cases of severe pain.

HYPOGASTRIC means pertaining to the lower middle part of the abdomen just above the pubis.

HYPOGLOSSAL NERVE is the twelfth cranial nerve, and supplies the muscles of the tongue, together with some others lying near it.

HYPOGLYCAEMIA is a deficiency of sugar in the blood. It may occur in states of starvation, or after the administration of insulin in too large doses, causing symptoms of weakness, tremors, nervousness, breathlessness and excitement, followed sometimes by unconsciousness. These symptoms are relieved by taking sugar or by an injection of adrenaline, which antagonizes the action of insulin.

HYPOGLYCAEMIC AGENTS: There are two groups of oral hypoglycaemic drugs, the sulphonylureas and the biguanides. Both have been used in the treatment of diabetes for about 30 years. The sulphonylureas act on the beta cell to stimulate insulin release and on peripheral tissues to increase sensitivity, though the latter is a less important action. Chlorpropamide and glibenclamide have a higher ceiling of potency than tolbutamide and this is associated with a considerably longer half life in the body. A newer arrival, gliquidone, claims to have the hypoglycaemic power of the second generation and the short biological half life of tolbutamide and may therefore be more suitable for those who require protection from nocturnal hypoglycaemia. The biguanides reduce carbohydrate absorption and facilitate the action of insulin on peripheral tissues. In the obese diabetic in whom increased insulin production is better avoided metformin alone may be used to reinforce the dietary treatment.

HYPOGONADISM is the condition characterized by deficient production of the hormones secreted by the gonads: that is, the ovaries and testes.

HYPOMANIA is a slight degree of mania.

HYPONATRAEMIA: A serum concentration below the normal range. It may be produced by dilution of blood (giving large volumes of salt-poor solutions intravenously), excessive water retention (inappropriate secretion of antidiuretic hormone), excessive sodium loss, and, rarely, by inadequate salt intake.

HYPOPARATHYROIDISM: Underactivity of the parathyroid glands (q.v.). Thus there is a lack of parathyroid hormone resulting in hypocalcaemia (q.v.). It may be caused by inadvertent removal of the glands when the thyroid gland is surgically removed or by failure of the glands because of autoimmune disease.

HYPOPHOSPHITES of lime, iron, etc., are administered in combination as 'a tonic'.

HYPOPHYSECTOMY means surgical excision of the pituitary gland.

HYPOPHYSIS is another name for the pituitary gland.

HYPOPIESIS is the condition, or state, characterized by abnormally low blood-pressure.

HYPOPITUITARISM: Underactivity of the pituitary gland. It can cause dwarfism (see DWARF), delayed puberty, impotence, infertility, amenorrhoea, hypothyroidism (q.v.), and hypoadrenalism. Causes include tumours, irradiation of the gland, sarcoidosis, and necrosis associated with postpartum haemorrhage (Sheehan's syndrome).

HYPOPLASIA means excessive smallness of an organ or part, arising from imperfect development.

HYPOSPADIAS is a developmental abnormality in the male, in which the urethra opens on the under-surface of the penis or in the perineum (q.v.).

HYPOSTASIS is the term applied to the condition in which blood accumulates in a dependent part as a result of a feeble circulation. Congestion of the base of the lungs in old people from this cause, and infection, is called hypostatic pneumonia.

HYPOTENSION means abnormally low blood-pressure. *Postural hypotension* is the abnormal fall in blood-pressure which may occur on suddenly standing up. It is more liable to occur in old folk.

HYPOTHALAMUS is that part of the forebrain situated beneath the thalamus on each side and forming the floor of the third ventricle. The hypothalamus contains collections of nerve cells believed to form the controlling centres of (1) the sympathetic and (2) the parasympathetic nervous systems. The hypothalamus is the nervous centre for primitive physical and emotional behaviour. It contains nerve centres for the regulation of certain vital processes: the metabolism of fat, carbohydrate and water; sleep; body temperature and genital functions.

HYPOTHERMIA: A core body temperature of less than 35 °C. As the temperature of the body falls, there is increasing dysfunction of all the organs, particularly the central nervous and cardiovascular systems. The patient becomes listless and confused, with onset of unconsciousness between 33–28 °C. Cardiac output at first rises with shivering but then falls progressively, as do the oxygen requirements of the tissues. Below 17–26 °C cardiac output is insufficient even to supply this reduced demand for oxygen by the tissues. The heart is susceptible to spontaneous ventricular fibrillation below 28 °C. Metabolism is disturbed and the concentration of blood glucose (q.v.) and potassium (q.v.) rise as the temperature falls. Cooling of the kidneys produces a diuresis (q.v.) and further fluid loss from the circulation to the tissues causes hypovolaemia (q.v.).

Severe hypothermia is sometimes complicated by gastric erosions and haemorrhage and pancreatitis. Infants and the elderly are less efficient at regulating temperature and conserving heat than other age groups and are therefore more at risk from accidental hypothermia during cold weather, if their accommodation is not warm enough. Approximately half a million elderly people are at risk in Britain each winter from hypothermia. The other major cause of accidental hypothermia is near drowning in icy water. Deliberate hypothermia is sometimes used to reduce metabolic rate so that prolonged periods of cardiac arrest may occur without tissue hypoxia developing. This technique is used for some cardiac and neurosurgical operations and is produced by immersion of the anaesthetized patient in iced water or by cooling an extracorporeal circulation.

Treatment of hypothermia is by warming the patient and treating any complications that arise. Passive warming is usual with conservation of the patient's own body heat with insulating blankets. If the core temperature is below 28 °C, then active rewarming should be instituted by means of warm peritoneal, gastric or bladder lavage or using an extracorporeal circulation. Care must be taken in moving hypothermic patients as a sudden rush of cold peripheral blood to the heart can precipitate ventricular fibrillation. Prevention of hypothermia in the elderly is important. Special attention must be paid to diet, heating the home and adequate clothing in several layers to limit heat loss.

HYPOTHYROIDISM means the condition produced by defective action of the thyroid gland. (See MYXOEDEMA.)

HYPOTONIC: (1) Referring to a solution which has a lower osmotic pressure (see OSMOSIS) than another. Physiologically it describes a solution with a lower osmotic pressure than body fluids. (2) Muscles with abnormally reduced tone.

HYPOVENTILATION: Shallow and/or slow breathing, often caused by the effects of injury or drugs on the respiratory centre. It causes hypercapnia and hypoxia (qq.v.).

HYPOVOLAEMIA: A reduced circulating blood volume. Acutely it is caused by unreplaced losses from bleeding, sweating, diarrhoea, vomiting or diuresis. Chronically it may be caused by inadequate fluid intake.

HYPOXIA: A low blood tension of oxygen. It may be caused by low inspired concentration of oxygen, an abnormal breathing pattern, lung disease or heart disease. If severe and prolonged it will cause organ damage and death as cellular function is dependent on oxygen.

HYSTERECTOMY is the operation of removing the uterus. HYSTERO-OOPHORECTOMY is the term applied to removal of the uterus and ovaries.

HYSTERIA is a condition or set of conditions which it is difficult to define. The condition is also known as PITHIATISM because many of its symptoms appear to be due to auto-suggestion and are readily relieved by suggestion from another person. Hysteria manifests itself by over-action of some parts of the nervous system, or by failure of other parts to perform their necessary work. In consequence, there follow mental changes, convulsive seizures, spasms and contractions of limbs, paralyses, loss of sensation over areas of the body, affections of various internal organs, derangements of joints and combinations of these which closely mimic various organic diseases. Hysterical manifestations are among the most difficult affections upon which the specialist is called to give an opinion.

Causes: The condition is far more common in women than in men. It used to be supposed that the origin of the disease, as its name indicates, lay in trouble of the womb, but, though sexual disturbances often occur in the condition, they should more probably be classed as symptoms. Heredity is of importance, as is upbringing.

Symptoms: MENTAL CHANGES are almost always observable in hysterical cases, although the other symptoms in different cases may differ widely from one another. The affected person becomes whimsical, dominated by ideas, and incapable of the same work and concentration as before. She becomes easily excitable, and is either morbidly sensitive, feeling slight rebuffs keenly, or unusually demonstrative, bursting into fits of laughter or paroxysms of weeping upon slight provocation. In marked cases, hysterical subjects become morally unhinged, deceiving everyone around them, so that little credence can be given to their statements.

CONVULSIVE HYSTERIA is the most marked form. An attack may begin upon some excitement, with laughter or weeping, or may give no warning sign. The person falls in an unconscious or half-conscious condition, but whereas the fall in epilepsy is downright, the hysterical person subsides gently in general upon a couch or chair, and rarely or never so as to hurt herself, and seldom without an audience. She may then lie still, or more generally moans or talks incoherently, rolls the head from side to side, and tosses the hands and feet about. In serious attacks, known as hystero-epilepsy, the onset resembles epilepsy and may be followed by curious posturing, the sufferer placing herself in attitudes which suggest powerful emotions of fear, ecstasy or joy. In this state visions are seen, voices heard, and conversations held with imaginary persons. This forms one of the most perverted types of hysteria and one of the least hopeful as regards a cure.

LOSS OF SENSATION over some part of the body is one of the commonest symptoms. This loss may affect a limb, or may be irregularly distributed in patches, or may affect some special sense organ, causing, for example, failure of taste, blindness for all objects to one side of the field of vision, or for objects of some special type repugnant to the patient, or deafness in one ear. Sometimes there is complete loss of the sense of pain, so that pricks, pinches, and other painful stimuli are borne without wincing.

SPASMS AND CONTRACTIONS of muscles also form a common manifestation of hysteria without any other sign save mental lethargy. If this contraction exists in the muscles of the body wall, it may, and often does, give rise to the idea that the person is the subject of a tumour. Such spasms may also lead to the drawing up of an arm or foot, so that the limb in time becomes permanently deformed. Or when the mind becomes powerfully impressed by some person or idea, the spasm may pass off, and gradual or sudden recovery takes place.

PARALYSIS is perhaps the most troublesome symptom of all to overcome. It may extend over one-half of the body, and is then very difficult to differentiate from the effects of apoplexy. Most commonly the foot is affected and the person declares herself unable to walk. As the paralysis sometimes lasts for years unimproved, and then suddenly vanishes, these cases are eminently suited for successful ministration by the faith-healer or by wonder-working shrines. Such people, when the paralysis affects both legs, and is accompanied by pain in the back, have again and again been confined for years to bed or couch as cases of spinal disease, only to recover suddenly when some new interest has come into their lives, or force of circumstances has rendered an active life imperative. The muscles of the larynx are often affected, and the person may be deprived of speech for years, till some powerful influence forces her to exert her will and the organ of voice again comes into play.

CHANGES IN INTERNAL ORGANS take place in some cases and produce such signs as constant hiccup, barking noises, excessive vomiting, diarrhoea, absolute loss of appetite, and profound changes in the circulation.

JOINT AFFECTIONS are among the most remarkable physical changes. A joint, especially the hip or knee, becomes swollen, stiff, and painful, and may remain so for months. (See PAIN.)

MASS HYSTERIA is a phenomenon characterized by extreme suggestibility. It most commonly occurs when large numbers of girls are massed together under conditions, such as fêtes and competitions, which induce emotional tension and excitement. Under such conditions the girls often feel faint or giddy, or sick. If one of them actually faints or is sick in the presence of the others, then they may start following her example, and faint or vomit. In this way a chain reaction is started, and large numbers may be affected. It is a well-recognized hazard in girls' schools, particularly among the older girls. Recovery quickly ensues when the affected girls are separated from each other.

Treatment: In acute hysterical attacks rest and quiet are chiefly necessary. For symptoms such as vomiting, joint affections, loss of sensation, and spasms, removal from home and from the attention of sympathetic friends to strict isolation, where the patient sees nobody but a nurse and eats only the simplest of food, is a useful form of treatment. For the severest forms of hysteria isolation and absolute rest in bed are employed. In all cases of hysteria psychotherapy forms an important element in treatment. This is carried out especially by suggestion, but in other cases it may take the form of persuasion, psycho-analysis, or education and employment.

HYSTEROTOMY: An operation in which the uterus (q.v.) is opened to remove a fetus (q.v.) before 28 weeks' gestation. After 28 weeks it would be called a Caesarean section (q.v.). It is now seldom used as a means of abortion.

I

IATRIC means anything pertaining to a physician.

IATROGENIC DISEASE is disease induced by a physician: essentially a drug-induced disease.

IBUPROFEN is a drug which is of value as an anti-inflammatory agent and as an analgesic in the treatment of rheumatoid arthritis and other forms of rheumatism. (See NON-STEROIDAL ANTI-INFLAMMATORY DRUGS.)

ICD: See INTERNATIONAL CLASSIFICATION OF DISEASE.

ICHTHAMMOL, ICHTHYOL, is ammonium ichthosulphonate, an almost black, thick liquid of fishy smell, prepared from a bituminous shale. It is used in several chronic skin diseases.

ICHTHYOSIS is a skin disease in which the surface is very rough and presents a dry, cracked appearance, resembling fish-scales. The peculiarity is generally hereditary, and persists through life, the skin being permanently hard, and deficient in oily material. The appearances differ considerably according to the part affected and the surrounding conditions. Thus the knees and elbows when affected become black from the collection of dirt in the deep crevices, and in winter the skin becomes specially hard and the condition still more marked.

Treatment: There is no specific internal treatment, but improvement sometimes follows the administration of vitamin A. Those who suffer from the disease should live, if possible, in a warm sunny climate. External treatment is most important and consists of daily warm baths with bran or starch, followed by the application of 20 to 50 per cent glycerin in water, olive oil, or equal parts of salicylic acid ointment (2 per cent) and glycerin. An alternative form of treatment is to add the *British Pharmacopoeia* Emulsifying Ointment to the bath: 28·5 grams (1 ounce) is added after preliminary creaming in a jug of hot water. This is followed by the application to the skin of the *British Pharmacopoeia* Hydrous Ointment as often as is required. Another promising line of treatment is the use of a urea cream. (See UREA.)

ICTERUS is another name for jaundice (q.v.).

ICTUS is another term for a stroke.

IDIOCY is a term no longer used. Those who were described as idiots are now included in the category of 'severe subnormality' as defined in the Mental Health Act, 1983. (See MENTAL HANDICAP.)

IDIOPATHIC is a term applied to diseases to indicate that their cause is unknown.

IDIOSYNCRASY implies an inherent abnormal qualitative reaction to a drug that is primarily the result of a constitutional defect in the patient. The abnormal sensitivity of patients with porphyria to barbiturates and sulphonamides is an example. Hereditary biochemical defects of red blood cells are responsible for many drug-induced haemolytic anaemias and for favism. Drug-sensitive red cells are deficient in the enzyme glucose phosphate dehydrogenase which plays an important part in the metabolism of glucose and is necessary for the continued integrity of the cell. When patients with porphyria are given certain drugs, particularly barbiturates and sulphonamides, they are liable to develop acute neurological episodes with peripheral and respiratory paralysis which may result in death. Porphyria variegata, the South African variety of porphyria, is an example of an inborn error of metabolism which was without serious symptoms until the advent of barbiturate drugs. Taking these drugs can precipitate total paralysis and death. A metabolic error is inherited as a dominant characteristic and there are now 8,000 affected people in South Africa, all of whom can be traced to a single couple who married in the seventeeth century.

IDOXURIDINE: An antiviral agent still widely used in the treatment of cases of herpes simplex involvement of the cornea of the eye (see EYE DISEASE AND INJURIES).

IFOSFAMIDE (see CYTOTOXIC).

ILEITIS means inflammation of the ileum. REGIONAL ILEITIS, or CROHN'S DISEASE, is the term applied to a condition in which there is an inflammation of an area of the small intestine. This is accompanied by colicky abdominal pain, irregularity of the bowels, loss of weight and slight fever. The abdomen is distended and the thickened intestine may be felt. The narrowed intestinal canal may become obstructed, necessitating immediate operation. The cause is unknown. The primary lesion is hyperplasia (q.v.) of the lymph tissue in the submucosa of the intestine and in the lymph glands.

As the cause is not known, there is no specific treatment. In the early stages, treatment is medical, including a high- vitamin, low-residue diet, sulphonamides and antibiotics. Promising results have been reported from the use of corticosteroids in some cases. Operation, consisting of removal of the damaged section of gut, is reserved for cases which do not respond to medical treatment. Even in cases apparently successfully operated on, recurrence tends to occur in 15 per cent or more of cases.

Patients and their relatives can obtain help and guidance from the National Association for Colitis and Crohn's Disease, 98a London Road, St. Albans, Hertfordshire AL1 1NX (0727-44296).

ILEO-CAECAL is the term applied to the region of the junction between the small and large intestines in the right lower corner of the abdomen. The ileo-caecal valve is a structure which allows the contents of the intestine to pass onwards from the small to the large intestine, but, in the great majority of cases, prevents their passage in the opposite direction.

ILEOSTOMY is the operation by which an artificial opening is made into the ileum. It is most often performed as part of the operation for cancer of the rectum, in which the rectum has usually to be removed. An ileostomy is then performed which acts as an artificial anus. Distressing though this may at first be, the vast majority of people with an ileostomy learn to lead a fully active and normal life. Help and advice in adjusting to what can be described as an 'ileostomy life' can be obtained from the Ileostomy Association of Great Britain and Ireland, Amblehurst House, Black Scotch Lane, Mansfield, Notts. NG18 4PF (tel. and fax: 0623-28099). (See STOMA.)

ILEUM is the lower part of the small intestine. (See INTESTINE.)

ILEUS is a paralysis of the bowel muscle. (See INTESTINE, DISEASES OF.)

ILIUM is the uppermost of the three bones forming each side of the pelvis. (See BONE; PELVIS.)

ILLUSIONS (see HALLUCINATIONS).

IMIPRAMINE is one of the so-called tricyclic antidepressants which is proving of value in the treatment of depression. (See ANTIDEPRESSANTS.)

IMMERSION FOOT is the term applied to a condition which develops as a result of prolonged immersion of the feet in cold or cool water. It was a condition commonly seen during the 1939–45 War in shipwrecked sailors and airmen who had crashed in the sea and spent long periods before being rescued. Such prolonged exposure results in vasoconstriction of the smaller arteries in the feet, leading to coldness and blueness of the feet, and finally, in severe cases, to ulceration and gangrene.

IMMUNITY (from *immunus*, Latin for exempt) is a principle by which the body is protected from the invasion of certain diseases, or the action of certain poisons. Some people can expose themselves again and again to the risk of infection and are not affected, whilst others seem prone to contract any disease with which they are brought into contact. The immunity so enjoyed is of several types. Natural immunity is one which is inborn; but immunity may also be acquired in the course of life, or it may be produced artificially by inoculation, or by injection of the blood serum of immune individuals.

Natural immunity: Certain animals seem to be little affected by poisons which to others are very deadly. Thus the snake-killing mongoose of India is said to be highly immune to cobra poison. The rat is little affected by tuberculosis, to which other creatures, including particularly man and the guinea-pig, are very susceptible. Man, on the other hand, is unaffected by swine fever, and some other diseases which are very infectious and fatal among the lower animals. **Acquired immunity** is that which is gained by surviving an attack of some disease. Protection is probably given by all infectious diseases for a longer or shorter period against a second attack of the same disease. In the case of some, such as smallpox, typhoid fever, scarlet fever, the protection seems to be lifelong. Recovery from a disease is in fact a process of immunity, the poison of the disease being destroyed by antagonizing substances, known as antibodies, produced in the tissues of the body. Some individuals acquire these antibodies by coming in contact with the infecting organisms without ever actually showing signs of the disease or possibly by having it in a mild unrecognized form.

Artificial immunity is of two kinds: active and passive immunity.

(*a*) ACTIVE IMMUNITY is produced by injecting beneath an animal's skin, or administering by the mouth in some cases, a small dose of some particular poison insufficient to produce death. This has the effect of stimulating the animal's powers of resistance, so that next time it can withstand a larger dose. The process is repeated over and over, the dose each time increasing, till finally the animal is unaffected by many times the dose which would have originally killed it. This applies to snake poisons also, and the snake-charmers of India appear to render themselves indifferent to cobra-bites by a similar process.

With regard to disease-producing bacteria and the toxins or poisons which they form, immunity is reached by injecting small quantities of bacteria, or of their toxins, which have been weakened by mixing with antiseptics, by drying in air, by passing through the bodies of partially immune animals, or by other technical processes. The best-known practical example of this treatment is vaccination against smallpox, in which cowpox, a modified form of the

disease, is produced in persons so as to render them immune to the far severer smallpox. Another is Pasteur's preventive treatment for rabies, in which, during the long incubation period before the disease has had time to appear, the person is treated by increasing doses of the poison, taken from rabbits that have been killed by the disease. (See RABIES.)

The principle of this method, then, consists in stimulating the power of the body to resist the action of poisons. Great success in preventing diphtheria has been achieved by injecting one to three doses of diphtheria toxoid (inactivated toxin). Other common diseases against which protection can be provided in this way include typhoid fever, whooping-cough, tetanus, measles, rubella, mumps and poliomyelitis. For a summary of current practice of immunization for children see the table in IMMUNIZATION. (See also VACCINE.)

(*b*) PASSIVE IMMUNITY is that form of artificial immunity obtained by injecting into the body blood serum drawn from an individual already rendered immune by the active method. (See SERUM THERAPY.)

IMMUNIZATION: The introduction of antigens (q.v.) into a body to produce immunity (q.v.). See table below.

IMMUNO-ASSAY: Procedures by which the amounts of antigen and antibody (qq.v.) in the serum (q.v.) can be identified.

IMMUNOGLOBULINS: Antibody globulin is now called immunoglobulin. In man there are five different types of immunoglobulin and differences in structure between these groups coincide with variations in biological behaviour. Most antibodies have a molecular weight of about 160,000 and when their rate of sedimentation is measured they have a sedimenta-

Recommended immunization schedules in the United Kingdom

Age	Disease and mode of administration
3 months	Poliomyelitis (oral); diphtheria, whooping-cough (pertussis)[1] and tetanus[2] (given together by injection)
5 months	Poliomyelitis (oral); diphtheria, whooping-cough (pertussis)[1] and tetanus[2] (given together by injection)
9–12 months	Poliomyelitis (oral); diphtheria, whooping-cough (pertussis)[1] and tetanus[2] (given together by injection)
1–2 years	Measles, mumps, and rubella (German measles) (given together by injection)
School entry	
4–5 years	Poliomyelitis (oral); diphtheria and tetanus (given together by injection)
10–14 (females)	Rubella (by injection)
10–14	BCG (Bacille Calmette-Guerin) by injection to tuberculin negative children to prevent tuberculosis
15–18	Poliomyelitis (oral); tetanus (by injection)

[1] Pertussis may be excluded in certain susceptible individuals
[2] Known as DPT or triple vaccine

tion constant of about 7 Svenberg units (7s). There is, however, another group of antibodies which move faster on electrophoresis, have a greater molecular weight (900,000) and have a sedimentation constant of 19 Svenberg units (19s). Immunoglobulin G, or IgG, constitutes three-quarters of the protein within the electrophetically defined gamma area of serum. It is a 7s antibody and constitutes the majority of the acquired antibacterial and antiviral antibodies. It is distributed equally between the blood and interstitial tissues and it is the only immunoglobulin which passes across the placenta to reach the fetal circulation. This transfer is not due to simple filtration but to an active cellular process. IgM on macroglobulin is so named because of its high molecular weight (900,000), and is predominantly intra-vascular. It is a 19s globulin and includes the blood-group antibodies.

IgG and IgM antibodies combine with antigen to form either soluble complexes or precipitates, depending on the relative proportion of antigen to antibodies. They activate complement and this enables them to neutralize toxins, bacteria and viruses and to promote phagocytosis. If the reaction occurs across a vascular membrane the result will be an Arthus reaction consisting of oedema and haemorrhage. Complement consists of nine different substances which act as a cascade analogous to the clotting mechanism. Some of the substances making up the complement are only present in trace quantities; others can be measured in milligrams. Two of these substances (C3 and C5) release histamine from mast cells, another (C5) is chemotactic to polymorphs, and others cause damage to cells by forming micelles in the surface layer of cells (C8 and C9).

IgA is a 7s gamma globulin synthesized by plasma cells at mucosal surfaces and appearing in secretions in which its concentration is often much higher than that of IgG. IgA antibodies do not activate the complement system: they are mainly protective and are not involved in hypersensitivity reactions. They have been aptly described as an antiseptic paint. The immunological function of the IgD group of antibodies is unknown. IgE possesses reagin activity and is the anaphylactic antibody in man.

Each immunoglobulin consists of four polypeptide chains. Each has a basic molecular unit of two heavy chains (molecular weight 50,000) joined to light chains (molecular weight 25,000). The heavy chains are specific to the type of immunoglobulin but there are two light chains (k and) which are common to all classes of immunoglobulin. The specificity of different antibodies is due to differences in the sequence of amino acids in those parts of the polypeptide chains which form the antibody-combining sites. In normal antibody-forming cells immunoglobulin synthesis is so well balanced that none of these peptide chains escapes from the cells. In myelomatosis, however, the malignant proliferation of plasma cells results in an imbalanced production of the heavy and light chains of immunoglobulin molecules and the

excess of free light chains escapes into the circulation and is filtered through the renal glomeruli as Bence-Jones protein. Such incoordinate production of immunoglobulin is a manifestation of the greater malignancy of the cell and hence augurs a worse prognosis for the disease. It must however be realized that rarely are humoral factors solely responsible for protection against infection, as the scavenger action of cells such as polymorphs and macrophages is also necessary.

IMMUNOLOGY: The study of immunity and an individual's response to antigens. Specialists in immunology – immunologists – investigate and treat disorders of the immme system and explore ways in which it can be provoked to provide immunity to particular diseases.

SERUM THERAPY Human immunoglobulin is now used to provide passive immunity. Serum is collected from hyperimmunized human individuals, such as those convalescing from the specific infection, and the relevant immunoglobulin is isolated and used parenterally to provide passive immunity. Horse serum is still used to provide passive immunity for diphtheria but human tetanus antitoxin is now available and has largely replaced the horse serum antitoxin. Passive immunity for hepatitis, both hepatitis A and hepatitis B, can be provided by immunoglobulin obtained from convalescent serum. Snake venom antiserum (antivene) is still prepared from horse serum so that there is always a risk of producing serum sickness of anaphylactic shock. Snake venom antiserum must be specific for the species of snake involved if it is to be effective.

Passive immunization against viruses is also available and passive immunization against measles can be achieved by the administration of pooled human immunoglobulin. Similarly passive protection by normal human immunoglobulin can be given to women during the first four months of pregnancy who have been in contact with rubella and whose serum does not contain rubella antibody. After exposure to rabies the course of active immunization is proceeded by a single injection of hyperimmune anti-rabies serum. Normal human immunoglobulin is used for protection against hepatitis A virus in travellers and occasionally for patients and staff in residential institutions to control outbreaks. Specific antibody preparations of known high titres against particular antigens, such as tetanus, rabies, vaccinia and hepatitis B, are now available. Zoster-immune globulin is also available for contacts with diseases in which varicella would present a special danger. These preparations are available through the Public Health Laboratory service.

IMMUNOSUPPRESSION: Any treatment that curtails the body's immunological responses. Drugs which do this are called immunosuppressants and they are prescribed after transplant surgery to prevent the rejection of foreign tissues. Immunosuppressants are also used to check the development of auto-immune disorders.

IMMUNOTHERAPY: Stimulation of the body's immune system as a means of treating cancer. This method is still experimental but is useful as a supportive treatment for anticancer drugs. Certain drugs will stimulate the body's immune system, as will an inoculation of the patient with tumour cells, from another person with a similar disease, that have been irradiated to make them harmless.

IMPACTION is a term applied to a condition in which two things are firmly lodged together. For example, when after a fracture one piece of bone is driven within the other, this is known as an impacted fracture; when a tooth is firmly lodged in its socket so that its eruption is prevented, this is known as dental impaction.

IMPETIGO is an infectious skin disease often found in schools and also in rugby football players (see SCRUM-POX), and caused usually by the *Staphylococcus aureus*. It consists of vesicles which appear here and there, on the face particularly, and dry up, leaving yellowish-brown scabs from which the discharge is infectious. These scabs fall off, leaving no scars, but the disease spreads from place to place over the skin, and may last for months if untreated. When it occurs in very young children, it is liable to run a severe course unless treatment is initiated immediately. This form of the disease is known as pemphigus neonatorum (see PEMPHIGUS) because of the marked blistering of the skin that tends to occur.
Treatment: Affected children should be off school and use separate washing and eating utensils. Infected crusts are removed by washing with saline or cetrimide lotion. Starch poultices may be necessary where the crusts are extensive. Infection can be caused by *Staphylococcus aureus* or *Streptococcus* and both are sensitive to synthetic penicillins.
    When nits are present on the hair, treatment is ineffective until these have been removed. (See PEDICULOSIS.)

IMPOTENCE is the inability to perform the sexual act. It may be partial or complete, temporary or permanent. Of the many classifications of this quite common condition, the most satisfactory is probably that which divides it into two main groups: *organic* and *psychological*. Among organic causes are lesions of the external genitalia, e.g. a tight foreskin; disturbances of the endocrine glands, such as diminished activity of the gonads, thyroid gland or pituitary gland; diseases of the central nervous system, e.g. tabes dorsalis; any severe disturbance of health, such as diabetes mellitus, addiction to alcohol and the like. Psychological factors are the commonest cause and these are anxiety, ignorance, fear, guilt, weakness of

sexual desire or abnormality of such desire. Counselling or sex therapy, preferably with the partner, has a 50-per-cent chance of helping to cure long-term impotence of psychological origin.

INCIDENCE: One of the main ways to measure the frequency of a disease in a particular population; the incidence of a disease is the number of new cases that occur during a particular time. Prevalence, the other measure, is the total number of cases of disease present at any one time and covers both old and new cases.

INCISION means a cut or wound and is a term specially applied to surgical openings.

INCISOR is the name applied to the four front teeth of each jaw. (See TEETH.)

INCOMPATIBILITY is a term applied to unsuitability in a prescription owing to the fact that its different contents either cannot be mixed, or that when mixed they undergo chemical changes, or that their actions are opposed to one another.

INCOMPETENCE is a term applied to the valves of the heart when, as a result of disease in the valves or alterations in size of the chambers of the heart, the valves become unable to close the orifices which they should protect. (See HEART DISEASES.)

INCONTINENCE is a term applied to the inability to retain the evacuations of the bowels and bladder. It occurs in diseases of these organs, injuries and diseases of the spinal cord, etc.

INCOORDINATION is a term applied to irregularity of movements produced either by loss of the sensations by which they are governed or by defects in the muscles themselves or their nerves.

INCUBATION means the period elapsing between the time when a person becomes infected by some agent and the first appearance of the symptoms of the disease. Most acute infectious diseases have fairly definite periods of incubation, and it is of great importance that people who have run the risk of infection should know the length of time which must elapse before they can be sure whether or not they are to contract the disease in question. A person who has been exposed to infection is, during the incubation period, technically known as a contact. By isolating and watching contact cases medical officers can often successfully check a threatened epidemic. It must be noted that diseases are not communicated to others by a person while passing through the stage of incubation. Some diseases, however, such as measles, become infectious as soon as the first symptoms set in after the incubation period is over; others, like scarlet fever and smallpox, are not so infectious then as in their later stages. The incubation period for any given disease is remarkably constant, although in the case of a severe attack the incubation is usually slightly shortened, and if the oncoming attack be a mild one, the period may be lengthened. So far as schools are concerned, children who have been contacts should not be allowed to return to school till several days beyond the maximum incubation period has elapsed since exposure to infection. All of these may, however, take a few days longer than the time stated to show themselves. (See INFECTION.) Several also, and especially whooping-cough, may be difficult to recognize in their early stages.

	days
Chickenpox	14–21
Diphtheria	2–5
German measles	14–21
Measles	10–15
Mumps	18–21
Poliomyelitis	3–21
Smallpox	10–16
Typhoid fever	7–21
Whooping-cough	7–10

Incubation periods of the commoner infectious diseases.

INDIAN HEMP (see CANNABIS INDICA).

INDIGESTION (see DYSPEPSIA).

INDOMETHACIN is a drug that is used in the treatment of gout and rheumatoid arthritis. It is said to be of particular value in the relief of night pain and morning stiffness. It is also proving of value in the treatment of the congenital abnormality of the heart known as patent ductus arteriosus. (See DUCTUS ARTERIOSUS.)

INDOPROFEN (see NON-STEROIDAL ANTI-INFLAMMATORY DRUGS).

INDORAMIN is an alpha-adreno-receptor-blocking drug which is proving of value in the treatment of high-blood-pressure. (See ADRENERGIC RECEPTORS.)

INDUCTION: Bringing about a particular event, for example, the induction or starting of labour; the induction of anaesthesia.

INDURATION: The pathological hardening of a tissue or organ. This may occur when a tissue is infected or when it is invaded by cancer.

INDUSTRIAL DISEASES (see OCCUPATIONAL DISEASES).

INFANT: A baby who is under 1 year old.

INFANT FEEDING: The new-born infant may be fed naturally from the breast or artificially from a bottle.
BREAST-FEEDING: Unless there is a genuine contra-indication, every baby should be breast-fed. The nutritional components of human milk are in the ideal proportions to promote the healthy growth of the human new-born. The mother's milk, especially colostrum (the fluid secreted before full lactation is established) contains immune cells and antibodies that increase the baby's resistance to infection. In addition, breast milk does not require elaborate and expensive preparation rituals. From the mother's point of view, breast-feeding helps the womb to return to its normal size and helps her to lose excess body fat gained during pregnancy. Most importantly, breast-feeding promotes intimate contact between mother and baby. A final point to be borne in mind, however, is that drugs taken by a mother can be excreted in her milk. These include antibiotics, sedatives, tranquillizers, alcohol, nicotine and high-dose steroids or vitamins.
ARTIFICIAL FEEDING: Unmodified cows' milk is not a satisfactory food for the human new-born and may cause dangerous metabolic imbalance. If breast-feeding is not feasible, one of the many commerciallly available formula milks should be used. Most of these are made from cows' milk which has been modified to reflect the composition of human milk as nearly as possible. For the rare infant who develops cows'-milk-protein intolerance, a milk based on soya-bean protein is indicated.
FEEDING AND WEIGHT GAIN: The main guide as to whether an infant is being adequately fed is the weight. During the first days of life a healthy infant loses weight, but, however, by the end of the second week, should return to birth weight. From then on, weight gain should be approximately 6oz. (170g) each week.
The timing of feeds reflects social convention rather than natural feeding patterns. Among the most primitive hunter-gatherer tribes of South America, babies are carried next to the breast and allowed to suckle at will. Fortunately for developed society, however, babies can be conditioned to intermittent feedings. As each bottle feed requires considerable preparation, it has been expedient to define rigid feeding guidelines. Whilst these are a useful starting point, they should not be viewed in the same light as the Ten Commandments, and allowance should be made for each baby's individual temperament.
As the timing of breast-feeding is more flexible, little or no preparation time being required, mothers can feed their babies on demand. Far from spoiling the baby, demand feeding is likely to lead to a contented infant. The only necessary caution being that a crying baby is not always a hungry baby.
In general, a new-born will require feeding every two to four hours and, if well, is unlikely

to sleep for more than six hours. After the first months, a few lucky parents will find their infant sleeping through the night.

WEANING: Weaning on to solid foods is again a matter of some individuality. Most babies will become dissatisfied with a milk-only diet round about six months and develop enthusiasm for cereal-based weaning foods. Introduction of solids before the age of four months is unusual and, unless really necessary to quell an apparently insatiable appetite, should be avoided. Similarly, delaying the commencement of weaning beyond nine months is nutritionally undesirable. As weaning progresses, the infant's diet requires less milk. Once established on a varied solid diet, breast and formula milks can be safely replaced with cows' milk. There is, however, no nutritional contra-indication to continued breast-feeding until the mother wishes to stop.

It is during weaning that infants realize that they can arouse extreme maternal anxiety by refusing to eat. This can lead to force-feeding and battles of will which may culminate in a breakdown of the mother–child relationship. To avoid this, parents must resist the temptation to coax the child to eat. If the child refuses solid food, the meal should be taken away with a minimum of fuss. Children's appetites reflect their individual genetic structure and a well child will eat enough to grow and maintain satisfactory weight gain. If a child is not eating properly, weight gain will be inadequate over a prolonged period and an underlying illness is the most likely cause. Indeed, failure to thrive is the paediatrician's best clue to chronic illness. ADVICE ON FEEDING: Many sources of conflicting advice are available to new parents. It is impossible to satisfy everyone and ultimately it is the well-being of the mother and infant and the closeness of their relationship that matter. In general, mothers should be wary of people who give rigid advice, as this suggests that their understanding of infant nutrition may be rather limited. An experienced midwife, health visitor or well- baby-clinic nursing sister are among the most reliable sources of information.

	Protein per cent	Fat per cent	Sugar per cent	Calories per cent
Human milk	1·1	4·2	7·0	70
Cow's milk	3·5	3·9	4·6	66

Composition of human and cow's milk

INFANTILE PARALYSIS is an old name for POLIOMYELITIS (q.v.).

INFANTILISM is the condition characterized by imperfect sexual development at puberty. It may or may not be associated with small stature. It may be due to lack of development of certain of the endocrine glands: i.e. the gonads (q.v.), pituitary gland or the adrenal glands. In other cases it may be associated with a generalized disease such as diabetes mellitus,

asthma, ulcerative colitis and rheumatoid arthritis.

INFANT MORTALITY is the number of deaths of infants under one year of age. The infant mortality rate in any given year is calculated as the number of deaths in the first year of life in proportion to every 1000 registered live births in that year. Along with perinatal mortality (q.v.), it is accepted as one of the most important criteria for assessing the health of the community and the standard of the social conditions of a country.

The improvement in the infant mortality rate has occurred mainly in the period from the second month of life. There has been much less improvement in the neonatal mortality rate: i.e. the number of infants dying during the first four weeks of life, expressed as a proportion of every 1000 live births. During the first week of life the main causes of death are asphyxia, prematurity, birth injuries and congenital abnormalities. After the first week the main cause of death is infection.

Social conditions also play an important rôle in infant mortality. In England and Wales the infant mortality rate in 1930–32 was: Social Class I (professional), 32·7; Social Class III (skilled workers), 57·6; Social Class V (unskilled workers), 77·1. The comparable figures for Scotland for 1939–45 were: Class I, 30·9; Class III, 53·4; Class V, 78·6. Many factors come into play in producing these social variations, but overcrowding is undoubtedly one of the most important. For instance, in 1936 the infant mortality rate in Bournemouth, where only 0·3 per cent of working-class families were overcrowded, was 78 per cent of that for the entire country, compared with 145 per cent in Newcastle-upon-Tyne where 10·7 per cent of working-class families were overcrowded. The same discrepancy persists to the present day as shown by a comparison of the Standardized Mortality Ratios in the areas covered by the North Western (which includes Lancashire) and the East Anglian Regional Health Authorities. In 1976–78 for children under the age of 1

1838–39	146	1951–55	26·9
1841–50	153	1956–60	22·6
1851–60	154	1961–65	20·6
1861–70	154	1968	18·3
1871–80	149	1970	18·2
1881–90	142	1971	17·5
1891–1900	153	1972	17·2
1901–05	138	1973	16·9
1906–10	117·1	1974	16·3
1911–15	108·1	1975	15·7
1916–20	90·9	1976	14·2
1921–25	74·9	1977	13·7
1926–30	67·9	1978	13·1
1931–35	62·2	1979	12·7
1936–40	55·3	1980	12·0
1941–45	49·8	1990	7·9
1946–50	36·4		

Infant mortality rate in England and Wales (1838–1968) and England 1970–90.

year these were 110·2 for boys and 110·7 for girls in the former and 86 for boys, and 69·5 for girls in East Anglia.

It is thus evident that for a reduction of the infant mortality rate to the minimum figure the following conditions must be met. The mothers and potential mothers of the country must be housed adequately amid surroundings which permit adequate fresh air and healthy exercise. The pregnant and nursing mother must be ensured an adequate diet. Effective antenatal supervision must be available to every mother, as well as skilled supervision during labour. The new-born infant must be adequately nursed and adequately fed. This means that all possible steps must be taken to encourage breast feeding. Mothers must be instructed in the proper care and feeding of their children, particularly during the first year of life. This in itself would reduce the mortality rate, but adequate environmental and public-health measures must be taken to ensure adequate housing, a clean milk supply and full availability of such protective measures as immunization against diphtheria, measles, poliomyelitis and whooping-cough. (See also PERINATAL MORTALITY.)

INFARCTION means the changes which take place in an organ when an artery is suddenly blocked, leading to the formation of a dense, wedge-shaped mass in the part of the organ supplied by the artery. It occurs as the result of embolism or of thrombosis. (See EMBOLISM.)

INFECTION is the process by which a disease is communicated from one person to another. All diseases so communicable are called infectious. There is, in the case of all such diseases, some micro-organism produced in the body of the diseased person which, on being transmitted to a second person, is capable of reproducing itself in larger quantity and causing a particular disease.

This micro-organism may be a bacterium, a Rickettsia, a virus, a protozoon, or a metazoon. Invasion of the body by a metazoon (e.g. by an intestinal worm) is more often known as an infestation.

The germs of disease may be grouped into those which will not flourish except about the temperature of the body, and those which are capable of maintaining their existence in decaying animal or vegetable matter, making only occasional migrations into the body and setting up disease. Speaking generally, bacteria of the first group are consistently much more deadly in their action, whilst those in the second group vary much in the severity of the disease they produce, causing a severer type if they have come direct from an infected person than if they have been germinating in drains, in the soil or floating on dust particles in the air. This principle is of immense practical importance. In the course of a surgical operation many bacteria must fall from the air into the wound, but this does not appear to be any drawback, unless the bacteria are derived direct from suppurat-

ing wounds or like virulent source. Similarly diphtheria or pneumonia bacteria of a mild type may be found in the mouth of people who are, nevertheless, quite healthy, if certain conditions, necessary to render the bacterium virulent, are not present.

The same bacterium may produce very different types of disease, not only on account of its previous life-history, but even according to the channel by which it enters the body. The *Mycobacterium tuberculosis*, for instance, produces a very different picture, depending upon whether it invades the lungs, the intestines, the joints, the glands or the skin. A certain amount of protection against the entrance of infective matter into the tissues of the body is afforded by the horny layer of the skin, by the acid of the gastric juice, and by the movements of the intestine, and a still greater measure of protection is afforded by the factors which ensure immunity against diseases. (See IMMUNITY.)

Modes of infection: The infective material may be transmitted to the person by direct contact with a sick person, when the disease is said to be contagious, although such a distinction is purely artificial. Different diseases are specially infectious at different periods of their course; and the practical question of guarding against infection is rendered much more difficult by the fact that some diseases are infectious at a stage even before they are clearly recognizable. This applies particularly to the early stage of measles before the rash appears, when the infected child is showing symptoms merely resembling those of catarrh or a cold in the head.

Infection may be conveyed on dust driven by the wind, in drinking-water, food, particularly milk, evacuations with which the healthy person's hands have become contaminated, crusts and scabs from the infected person's body, or even clothes and linen which have been in contact with him.

In this connection what are termed carriers are of great importance. Some people who have suffered from a disease, or who have simply been in contact with an infectious case, harbour the germ of the disease. This is particularly the case in typhoid fever, the bacillus continuing to develop in the gall-bladder of some people, who have had the disease, maybe for years after the symptoms have passed away; it is estimated that 2 to 5 per cent of patients with typhoid fever become permanent typhoid carriers and where a cook or food purveyor is affected, he is apt to start an epidemic unless he exercises the most scrupulous cleanliness. In the case of cholera, which is endemic in some localities of the East, 80 per cent or more of the population may harbour the bacillus and spread infection when other circumstances favour this. Similarly in the case of dysentery, people who have completely recovered may still be capable of infecting dust and drinking-water by their stools. Diphtheria is similarly liable to be carried by people in whose throat the germ remains after recovery from the disease. Cerebrospinal meningitis, which is particularly liable to infect children, appears to be transmitted through the germ being carried in the nose of people who may not develop any symptoms.

Flies pass from garbage heaps to unprotected food, and are especially dangerous as regards the infection of milk and other food with the organisms causing typhoid fever and food poisoning. Mosquitoes convey from sick to healthy the germs of malaria and yellow fever, these undergoing part of their development in the body of the mosquito. Fleas convey the germ of plague from rat to man, lice are responsible for inoculating typhus fever and one form of relapsing fever by their bite. A tick is responsible for spreading another form of relapsing fever, and kala-azar (or leishmaniasis) is spread by the bites of sandflies.

Notifiable diseases: Certain of the common and most serious infectious diseases were scheduled in the Infectious Diseases Act of 1889 as notifiable in Great Britain. That is to say that any medical practitioner, attending or called in to visit a person suffering from one of these, must immediately, on becoming aware that the patient is suffering from it, send a notice to the local medical officer for environmental health as he is now known. For the current list of notifiable infectious diseases in the UK see NOTIFIABLE DISEASES.

Prevention of infection: The various channels of infection are mentioned under the heading of the different infectious diseases. As children are much more liable to contract infectious diseases than adults, attempts to prevent the spread of these diseases are specially directed towards separating affected people from healthy children. The measures taken apply particularly to schools, which form the places of dissemination in a large proportion of cases, but the rules applicable to children may well be practised with regard to people of any age and in respect of any public institution. If, in opposition to medical advice, a patient with a communicable disease refuses to go to an infectious disease hospital, the local authority has compulsory powers to insist on such transfer provided the medical officer for environmental health certifies that there is a risk of infection, and that the sufferer should be detained in an isolation unit until he is certified as no longer likely to spread the disease in question. (See also IMMUNITY; INCUBATION.)

INFECTIOUS MONONUCLEOSIS (see MONONUCLEOSIS).

INFERTILITY

INFERTILITY is present when a couple have not achieved a pregnancy after one year of regular unprotected sexual intercourse. Between 15–20 per cent of couples have difficulties in conceiving. The 'fault' lies with the male partner in about a third of cases, with the female partner in about a third and with both partners in about a third. Couples should be investigated together efficiently and as quickly as possible to decrease the distress which is invariably associated with the diagnosis of infertility. In about 10–15 per cent of women

suffering from infertility ovulation is disturbed. Mostly they will have either irregular periods or no periods at all.

Checking a hormone profile in the woman's blood will help in the diagnosis of ovulatory disorders like polycystic ovaries, an early menopause, anorexia or other endocrine illnesses. Ovulation itself is best assessed by ultrasound scan at mid-cycle or by a blood hormone progesterone level in the second half of the cycle.

The fallopian tubes may be damaged or blocked in 20–30 per cent of infertile women. This is usually caused by previous pelvic infection or endometriosis, where menstrual blood is thought to flow backwards through the fallopian tubes into the pelvis and seed with cells from the lining of the uterus in the pelvis. This process often leads to scarring of the pelvic tissues; 5–10 per cent of infertility is associated with endometriosis.

To assess the fallopian tubes adequately a procedure called laparoscopy is performed. A telescope is inserted through the umbilicus and at the same time a dye is pushed through the tubes to assess their patency. The procedure is performed under a general anaesthetic.

In a few cases the mucus around the cervix may be hostile to the partner's sperm and therefore prevents fertilization.

Defective sperm production is responsible for up to a quarter of infertility. It may result from the failure of the testes to descend in early life, from infections of the testes or previous surgery for testicular torsion. The semen is analysed to assess the numbers of sperm and their motility and to check for abnormal forms.

In a few cases the genetic make-up of one partner does not allow the couple ever to achieve a pregnancy naturally.

In about 25 per cent of couples no obvious cause can be found for their infertility.

Ovulation may be induced with drugs.

In some cases damaged fallopian tubes may be repaired by tubal surgery. If the tubes are destroyed beyond repair a pregnancy may be achieved with in vitro fertilization (q.v.).

Endometriosis may be treated either with drugs or laser therapy and pregnancy rates after both forms of treatment are between 40–50 per cent, depending on the severity of the disease.

Few options exist for treating male-factor infertility. These are artificial insemination by husband or donor and more recently in vitro fertilization. Drug treatment and surgical repair of varicoceles have disappointing results.

Following investigations between 30 and 40 per cent of infertile couples will achieve a pregnancy usually within two years.

INFESTATION is a term applied to the occurrence of animal parasites in the intestine, hair or clothing. (See INSECTS IN RELATION TO DISEASE.)

INFILTRATION: The invasion of tissues or organs by cells or fluid that are not normally present. Local anaesthetic is infiltrated into an area of tissue to produce analgesia (q.v.) in a defined area.

INFLAMMATION is the reaction of the tissues to any injury, short of one sufficiently severe to cause their immediate death. The term is limited sometimes to the changes which take place when bacteria enter the body, but the changes in the latter case, though specially severe, are essentially the same as those produced by any other source of irritation. There are four cardinal symptoms of inflammation: redness, heat, pain and swelling, all of which, and particularly the last, are present in greater or less degree, so that these are also made a basis for defining the condition.

The first sign of inflammation consists in a dilatation of the arteries and veins of the affected part, so that the blood circulates in it more quickly and in larger quantity than before, thus causing heat and redness. Very soon, however, and apparently as the result of some change in the walls of the smaller blood-vessels, the circulation becomes gradually slower, and the white corpuscles of the blood are seen to adhere to the inner surface of these vessels. Later, these corpuscles push their way in great numbers through the walls of the smaller veins and capillaries, migrating into the surrounding tissues along with large quantities of the fluid material of the blood and a few red corpuscles, a process known as DIAPEDESIS. Hence the swelling, which is the most characteristic sign of inflammation. These white corpuscles subserve many functions. In the first place, they have been shown to attack the bacteria which have invaded the tissues, to envelop them in their own substance, and, apparently by a process of digestion, to break them up. They also remove tissues which are dead or useless. Other corpuscles, at a later stage, when the source of irritation has been removed, play a part in producing the new tissues to repair the damage done, although the greater part of this repair is effected by cells from the surrounding tissues.

One of two results may follow inflammation. Either *resolution* may take place, when the white corpuscles, having played their part, find their way back into the circulation after the process of repair has been started at the site of injury, and the circulation proceeds as before, or *abscess-formation* results, the circulation comes to a complete standstill in the affected part, an excessive number of white corpuscles migrate from the vessels, an area of tissue becomes destroyed, and the process ends by a discharge of pus through the surface of the body, after which repair proceeds. (See ABSCESS, ACUTE.)

Symptoms: As already mentioned, redness, heat, pain and swelling are the classical symptoms of inflammation, and there are usually general symptoms of feverishness, varying with the severity of the inflammation. Various special symptoms are set up in special localities: for example, inflammation of the mucous membranes of the stomach and bowels leads to a copious excretion of mucus; inflammation of outlying parts, if very severe, may cause death of these parts, and are then called gangrenous inflammation; intense inflammation limited to a surface may destroy patches of the surface and convert them into a leather-like membrane, such types being known as croupous inflammations. Inflammation may become chronic, and in this case not only does the process described proceed in a minor degree, but there is an exaggerated process of repair leading to the formation of much fibrous or scar tissue, which may come to replace almost entirely the organ in which the chronic inflammation is proceeding, thus rendering the organ small, hard and irregular in outline.

Treatment: This depends upon different factors, such as the type of organism responsible, the site of infection and the severity of the infection. Thus, if the inflammation is due to tuberculosis, treatment will be by means of a combination of two, or more, anti-tuberculosis drugs. If, on the other hand, it is in the appendix, immediate removal of the appendix is called for, whilst in the case of superficial inflammation of the skin, all that may be required is careful cleansing of the skin and the application of some antiseptic preparation.

Two general principles, however, apply to the treatment of all forms of inflammation: rest and the maintenance of the general health of the patient.

INFLUENZA is an acute infectious disease, characterized by a sudden onset, fever and generalized aches and pains, which usually occurs in epidemics and pandemics.

Cause: The disease is caused by a virus of the influenza group. There are at least three types of influenza virus, known respectively as A, B and C. One of their most characteristic features is that infection with one type provides no protection against another type. Equally important is the ease with which the influenza virus can change its character. It is these two characteristics which explain why one attack of influenza provides little, if any, protection against a subsequent attack, and why it is so difficult to prepare an effective vaccine against the disease.

Epidemics of influenza due to virus A occur in Britain at two- to four-year intervals, and outbreaks of virus B influenza in less frequent cycles. Virus A influenza, for instance, was the prevalent infection in 1949, 1951, 1955 and 1956, whilst virus B influenza was epidemic in 1946, 1950, 1954 and, along with virus A, in 1958–59. The pandemic of 1957, which swept most of the world, though fortunately not in a severe form, was due to a new variant of virus A – the so-called Asian virus – and it has been suggested that it was this variant that was responsible for the pandemics of 1889 and 1918. Since 1957, variants of virus A have been the predominating causes of influenza accompanied on occasions by virus B.

Symptoms: The incubation period of influenza A and B is two to three days and the disease is characterized by a sudden onset. In most cases this is followed by a short, sharp febrile illness of two to four days' duration, associated with headache, prostration, generalized aching and respiratory symptoms. In many cases the respiratory symptoms are restricted to the upper respiratory tract, and consist of signs of irritation of the nose, pharynx and larynx. There may be nose-bleeds, and a dry hacking cough is often a prominent and troublesome symptom. The fever is usually remittent and the temperature seldom exceeds 39·4 °C (103 °F), tending to fluctuate between 38·3 and 39·4 °C (101 and 103 °F).

The most serious complication is infection of the lungs. This infection is usually due to organisms other than the influenza virus. It is a complication which can have serious results in elderly people.

The very severe form which tends to occur during pandemics – and which was so common during the 1918–19 pandemic – is characterized by the rapid onset of broncho-pneumonia and severe prostration. Because of the toxic effect on the heart there is a particularly marked form of cyanosis, known as heliotrope cyanosis.

Convalescence following influenza tends to be prolonged. Even after an attack of average severity there tends to be a period of weakness and depression.

Treatment: Expert opinion is still divided as to the real value of influenza vaccine in preventing the disease. Part of the trouble is that, as already pointed out, there is no value in giving any vaccine until it is known which particular virus is causing the infection. As this varies from winter to winter, and as the protection given by vaccine does not exceed one year, it is obviously not worth while attempting to vaccinate the whole community. The general rule therefore is that, unless there is any evidence that a particularly virulent type of virus is responsible, only those should be vaccinated who are particularly vulnerable, such as children in boarding schools, elderly people, pregnant women, and people who suffer from chronic bronchitis. In the face of an epidemic, people in key positions, such as doctors, nurses and those concerned with public safety, transport and other public utilities should be vaccinated.

For an uncomplicated attack of influenza, treatment is symptomatic: that is, rest in bed, analgesics to relieve the pain, sedatives, and a light diet. A linctus is useful to sooth a troublesome cough. The best analgesic is aspirin – either alone, or combined with paracetamol and codeine. None of the sulphonamides or the known antibiotics has any effect on the influenza virus. On the other hand, should the lungs become infected, antibiotics should be given immediately, because, as has already been pointed out, such an infection is usually due to other organisms. If possible, a sample of sputum should be examined to determine which organisms are responsible for the lung infec-

tion. The choice of antibiotic then depends upon which antibiotic the organism is most sensitive to.

INFUNDIBULUM: A funnel-shaped passage. The word is used specifically to describe the hollow conical stalk that links the hypothalmus (q.v.) to the posterior lobe of the pituitary gland (q.v.).

INFUSIONS are preparations of vegetable drugs made by steeping them for some time in water and straining. In order that an infusion may keep well it is usually concentrated and mixed with spirit, being diluted just before it is dispensed.

Infusion is also the term applied to the injection into blood-vessels or subcutaneous tissues of warm normal salt solution, glucose solution or gum acacia solution, in the case of persons who are in a feeble state from loss of blood, loss of fluid by diarrhoea, etc. The infusion is sometimes administered in an amount of about 570 ml (1 pint) at a time, or is often used by a drip method in which the warm fluid is suspended at a height and allowed to pass drop by drop for several hours into a vein.

INGESTION: The act of taking fluid, food, or medicine into the stomach. The way in which a phagocytic cell surrounds and absorbs foreign substances such as bacteria in the blood.

INGUINAL REGION (see ABDOMEN, REGIONS OF).

INHALANTS: Substances that can be inhaled into the body through the lungs. They may be delivered in traditional form dissolved in hot water and inhaled in the steam or as an aerosol, a suspension of very small liquid or solid particles in the air. The latter are now usually delivered by devices in which the aerosol is kept under pressure in a small hand-held cylinder and delivered in required doses by a release mechanism.

AEROSOLS Asthmatic patients find aerosol devices of value in controlling their attacks. They provide an effective and convenient way of applying drugs directly to the bronchi, thus reducing the risks of unwanted effects accompanying systemic therapy. They are of particular use in asthma. Broncho-dilator aerosols contain either a beta-sympathomimetic agent or ipratropium bromide which is an anticholinergic drug. Of the beta-adrenoceptor agonists isoprenaline was the first compound to be widely used as an aerosol. It did however stimulate beta$_1$ receptors in the heart as well as beta$_2$ receptors in the bronchi and so produced palpitations and even dangerous cardiac arrhythmias. Newer beta-adrenoceptor agonists are specific for the beta$_2$ receptors and thus have a greater safety margin. They include salbutamol, terbutaline, rimiterol, fenoterol and reproterol. Unwanted effects such as palpitations, tremor and restlessness are uncommon with these more specific preparations. In patients who get insufficient relief from the beta-adrenoreceptor agonist the drug ipratropium bromide is worth adding.

Patients must be taught carefully and observed while using their inhalers. It is important that patients should realize that if the aerosol no longer gives more than slight intransient relief they should not increase the dose but seek medical help.

INHALATION is a method of applying drugs in a finely divided or gaseous state, so that, when breathed in, they may come in contact with the nose, throat and lungs. There are two chief means by which drugs are mingled with the air and so taken in by breathing. These are traditional steam inhalations and modern aerosol devices which deliver a fine spray direct into the mouth.

INHIBITION means arrest or restraint of some process effected by nervous influence. The term is applied to the action of certain inhibitory nerves: e.g. the vagus nerve which contains fibres that inhibit or control the action of the heart. It is also applied generally to the mental processes by which instinctive but undesirable actions are checked by a process of self-control.

INJECTIONS (see ENEMA; HYPODERMIC).

INNER EAR: This comprises three fluid-filled chambers or labyrinths situated in the bony temporal area that are concerned with identifying a person's position in space. Each chamber lies in a different plane and movement of fluid in it is picked up by sensory cells that transmit the information to the brain. Disease or damage to the inner ear upsets the sense of balance and causes vertigo. Motion sickness (q.v.) is caused by the inner ear's being unable to accommodate to the changes in position resulting from motion.

INNERVATION: The nerve supply to a tissue, organ or part of the body. It carries motor impulses to and sensory impulses away from the part.

INOCULATION is the process by which infective material is brought into the system through a small wound in the skin or in a mucous membrane. Many infectious diseases and blood-poisoning are contracted by accidental inoculation of microbes. Inoculation is now used as a preventive measure against many infectious diseases. (See VACCINE.)

INOTROPIC: Adjective describing anything that affects the force of muscle contraction. It is usually applied to the heart muscle and an inotrope is a drug that improves its contraction.

INPATIENT: A person who stays in a bed in hospital for investigation or treatment.

INSANITY (see MENTAL ILLNESS).

INSECT REPELLENTS (See DIBUTYL PHTHALATE; DIMETHYL PHTHALATE.)

INSECTICIDES are substances which kill insects. Since the discovery of the insecticidal properties of DDT in 1940, a steady stream of new ones has been introduced, and their combined use has played an outstanding part in international public health campaigns, such as that of the World Health Organization for the eradication of malaria.

Unfortunately, insects are liable to become resistant to insecticides, just as bacteria are liable to become resistant to antibiotics, and it is for this reason that so much research work is being devoted to the discovery of new ones.

It is against this beneficial background that must be viewed the increasing evidence that the indiscriminate use of some of these potent preparations is having an adverse effect, not only upon human beings, but also upon the balance of nature.

Some such as DDT, the use of which is now banned in the UK, are very stable compounds that enter the food chain and may ultimately be lethal to many animals, including birds and fishes.

INSECTS IN RELATION TO DISEASE: Many insects play an important part in the transmission of infectious diseases. Thus, flies by their feet and their feeding habits carry the organisms which cause typhoid fever, the tsetse fly spreads sleeping sickness, mosquitoes transmit the germs of malaria and yellow fever, fleas convey plague germs and lice convey typhus fever and one form of relapsing fever. In addition, these creatures are nuisances as well as dangers.

HOUSE-FLY (*Musca domestica*): This fly lays its eggs in manure, or in moist, fermenting vegetable matter. The maggot is hatched in eight hours to two days, feeds on the manure, passes through the pupa stage in anything from a few days to four weeks, and, becoming a fly, is capable of egg-laying about three weeks from its own appearance as an egg. As 120 to 150 eggs are laid in a batch by each female fly, this fly is capable, under the most favourable conditions, of producing over half-a-million progeny within her life of three months. The fly gorges on fluid food which it sucks up by means of its proboscis, and it has the habit of repeatedly vomiting and re-swallowing the contents of its crop as it feeds. It walks in filth habitually, and being provided with hairy legs and body it is apt to carry off portions of this, in which are entangled numbers of bacteria. The fly has been well described as a 'winged sponge', and its immense power to distribute disease germs over the surface of uncovered food is evident.

BLOW-FLY, or BLUE-BOTTLE (*Calliphora erythrocephala*), lays its eggs (450 to 600 in number) on meat, fish or decaying animal matter. The maggot hatches out within a day, passes through the pupa stage and becomes a full-grown fly in about three weeks. Its habits are similar to those of the house-fly, though in numbers it is much less plentiful.

Treatment of flies: The most important measure is to destroy their breeding grounds near human dwellings. No kitchen refuse should be left exposed so that flies may deposit their eggs in it. Stable litter and manure must be disposed of, or kept covered and shut up in outhouses, not allowed to accumulate in the open air and sunshine near houses. Adult flies may be destroyed in a great extent by proper protection and storage of all food. An insecticide may be used as a powder, a spray or a paint, but care must be exercised that it does not come in contact with food or with surfaces on which food is prepared.

LICE: There are three lice which infest man: the body louse (*Pediculus corporis*), the head louse (*Pediculus capitis*) and the crab louse (*Pediculus pubis*). The head louse is by far the most common in Britain. Infestation is most common in children under school age, but it is not unusual in adults. In schoolchildren it seems to be ineradicable: one large survey in England showed that 9 per cent of 12,000 schoolchildren were infested. It used to be much commoner in girls than boys, but this sex difference is disappearing. Head lice spread by close human contact. (See also PEDICULOSIS.)

As already noted, lice convey the causative micro-organisms of typhus fever, one form of relapsing fever, and trench fever, and it has been estimated that in this way the louse is responsible for more human deaths than any other insect barring the malaria mosquito (see RELAPSING FEVER; TRENCH FEVER; TYPHUS FEVER).

Treatment of lice: In individuals infested with the body louse the clothing should be dusted with an insecticide, packed in a bag and then sent for washing or storing. A temperature of 54 °C (129 °F) is rapidly lethal to both lice and their eggs. At a temperature of −20 °C (−4 °F) lice are killed in half-an-hour and eggs are killed in five hours. As the lice tend to congregate into the seams, hot ironing these is a useful measure.

For body lice, the body should be coated with malathion cream or 1 per cent dusting powder. This may need to be repeated for several days. Calamine lotion containing 1 per cent phenol eases the itching. For crab, or pubic, lice, the affected area is rubbed with either Dicophane Application BPC, or Malathion dusting powder which is left on for two days, and the process then repeated. Alternatively, carbaryl or malathion may be used.

For head lice, a lotion containing 0·5 per cent Malathion in 10 ml should be rubbed with the fingers into the hair and its roots and left for twenty-four hours. The hair is then washed. This may need to be repeated twice or three times. The hair is then carefully combed with a fine comb to remove the nits. Removal may be easier if the hairs are rubbed previously with a swab soaked in vinegar. Unfortunately the head louse is becoming resistant to gamma benzene hexachloride, which is therefore being replaced by malathion (q.v.) or carbaryl. Malathion is applied in a 0·5-per-cent solution in spirit until the scalp is thoroughly moist. The hair is then allowed to dry naturally without the use of any heat. After twelve hours the hair is shampooed and combed with a fine metal comb while wet to remove the dead nits. Only one such treatment is usually necessary, but all close contacts including the parents of the infested child should be examined and treated forthwith with malathion if infested. Only in this way can the infestation be eradicated from the family. Carbaryl is available as a shampoo and a lotion. The lotion is the preparation of choice. It is rubbed gently into the hair. The hair is then left to dry naturally and washed with a shampoo the next day. After the shampoo, the hair, while still wet, is combed with a fine metal comb to remove the dead lice and eggs (nits).

FLEAS: *Pulex irritans* is the common flea that afflicts mankind. *Xenopsylla cheopis* is the rat flea that conveys *Pasteurella pestis*, the causative organism of plague, from rat to man. The flea lays its eggs singly. They take two to four days in summer, two weeks in winter, to hatch into larvae which are fully grown in a fortnight. The larva then becomes a pupa from which the adult emerges two weeks later. The flea can survive for a long time without food.

Treatment of fleas: Human beings vary tremendously in their susceptibility to flea bites. For those who are susceptible the best preventive is dimethyl phthallate sprayed on the trousers or socks where it is effective for several days. In the absence of dimethyl phthallate, alternative methods of prevention are the smearing of the skin with oil of pennyroyal, oil of lavender, or 10 per cent crotamiton cream or lotion, or dusting the socks and underclothing with pyrethrum powder, menthol or camphor. For disinfestation of buildings, a solution of insecticide in kerosene is effective. For bedding a powder containing 0·5-per-cent gamma benzene hexachloride is effective. Other anti-flea agents are pyrethrum, flaked naphthalene, or parachlorbenzene.

BED BUGS (*Cimex lectularius*) are best got rid of by a solution of insecticide in kerosene, with or without the addition of pyrethrum. (See BED BUG.)

MOSQUITOES: One of these (*Anopheles gambiae*) is responsible for conveying the parasite of malaria, another (*Aedes aegypti*) for distributing the infection of yellow fever.

Treatment of mosquitoes: See under MALARIA; YELLOW FEVER.

INSEMINATION: The ejaculation of semen in the vagina in the act of sexual intercourse. In artificial insemination the semen is placed there by the use of an instrument.

INSOLATION is a term applied both to treatment by exposure to the sun's rays (see LIGHT TREATMENT) and to fever caused by excessive heat (see HEAT-STROKE).

INSOMNIA (see SLEEP; HYPNOTICS).

INSPISSATION is the process of the drying or thickening of fluids or excretions by evaporation.

INSTITUTIONALIZATION: A condition brought about by a prolonged stay in an impersonal institution. The individual becomes apathetic and listless as a result of inadequate stimulation in an uninteresting environment. The condition can occur in mental institutions or long-stay nursing homes; the affected person loses the ability to make any decisions.

INSUFFLATION means the blowing of powder or vapour into a cavity, especially through the air passages, for the treatment of disease.

INSULIN is the internal secretion of the pancreas formed by groups of cells called the islets of Langerhans in this organ. Its existence was indicated by Sharpey-Schafer in 1909, and it was successfully isolated in a pure form by McLeod, Banting and Best in 1921. It acts by enabling the muscles and other tissues which require sugar for their activity to take up this substance from the blood. When it is deficient, the sugar derived from the food accumulates in the blood and is wastefully excreted in the urine. Insulin is administered by hypodermic (subcutaneous) injection in cases of diabetes mellitus (q.v.), and thus enables the sugar in the circulation to be utilized so that its excretion in the urine ceases. Each unit of insulin administered to a diabetic patient enables him to utilize somewhere between one and two grams of additional carbohydrate material. The appropriate dose of insulin in any given case depends upon its severity.

Over 40 insulin preparations are listed in the British National Formulary. These differ in their speed of onset, and duration, of action.

Hitherto insulin has been obtained from the pancreas of oxen and pigs. Human insulin is now available. This is made either by genetic manipulation of the micro-organism, Escherichia coli, or by enzymatic manipulation (see ENZYME) of pig insulin. Beef, pig, and human insulin differ in the number of amino-acids (q.v.) they contain. Hitherto insulin was available in three strengths: of 20, 40 and 80 units per millilitre. These have now been replaced by one strength of 100 units per millilitre, known as U100 insulin.

INTELLIGENCE QUOTIENT, or IQ as it is usually known, is the ratio between the mental age and chronological age multiplied by 100. Thus, if a boy of 10 years of age is found to have a mental age of 12 years, his IQ will be: 120.

On the other hand, if he is found to have a mental age of 8 years his IQ will be: 80.

The mental age is established by various tests, the most widely used of which are the Stanford-Binet Scale, the Wechsler Adult Intelligence Scale, and the Mill Hill Vocabulary Test.

Average intelligence is represented by an IQ of 100, with a range of 85 to 115. For practical purposes it is taken that the intellectual level reached by the average 15-year-old is indistinguishable from that of an adult.

INTENSIVE THERAPY UNIT (ITU): A hospital unit in which patients undero specialized resuscitation, monitoring and treatment procedures. People who have had severe injuries, heart attacks, or major operations – for example, cardiac surgery – are admitted to ITUs, which are staffed 24 hours a day with highly trained nurses, technicians and doctors and equipped with electronic monitoring devices that allow continuous assessment of vital body functions such as heart rate, blood pressure and blood chemistry.

INTERCOSTAL is the term applied to the nerves, vessels and muscles that lie between the ribs, as well as to diseases affecting these structures.

INTERFERON: It has been known for many years that one virus will interfere with the growth of another. In 1957, workers at the National Institute for Medical Research in London isolated the factor that was responsible for the phenomenon. They gave it the name of interferon. There are now known to be three human interferons. They are glycoproteins and are released from cells infected with virus or exposed to stimuli which mimic virus infection. They not only inhibit the growth of viruses. They also inhibit the growth and reduplication of cells. This is the basis for their investigation as a means of treating cancer. Hitherto the major difficulty has been obtaining sufficient supplies, but methods have now been evolved which promise to provide adequate amounts of it. The most promising of these is by means of what is known as genetic engineering, or manipulation, whereby a portion of DNA (q.v.) from interferon is inserted into the micro-organism known as Escherichia coli (see ESCHERICHIA) which thus becomes a source of almost unlimited amounts of interferon as it can be grown so easily. The evidence to date indicates that interferon is of value in treating certain virus infections, particularly different forms of herpes. The case for its value in the treatment of cancer is still not proven.

INTERLEUKINS: Interleukins are lympho-kines, that is polypeptides produced by acti-vated lymphocytes. They are involved in signalling between cells of the immune system and are released by several cell types, including lymphocytes. They interact to control the im-mune response of cells and also participate in haemopoiesis. There are seven varieties, interleukins 1 to 7. For example, interleukin 1 is produced as a result of inflammation and it stimulates the proliferation of T and B lymphocytes. They enhance the immune re-sponse by stimulating other lymphocytes and activating dormant T cells. Interleukin 2 has anti-cancer effects as it is able to activate T lymphocytes to become killer cells which de-stroy foreign antigens such as cancer cells, and this anti-cancer effect is being developed for clinical use. The remaining interleukins have a range of properties in cell growth and differen-tiation.

INTERMITTENT is a term applied to fevers which continue for a time, subside completely and then return again. The name is also used in connection with a pulse in which occasional heart-beats are not felt, in consequence of irregular action of the heart.

INTERMITTENT CLAUDICATION is a con-dition occurring in middle-aged and elderly people, which is characterized by pain in the legs after walking a certain distance. The pain is relieved by resting for a short time. It is due to arteriosclerosis (see ARTERIES, DISEASES OF) of the arteries to the leg, which results in inad-equate blood supply to the muscles. Drugs have little effect in easing the pain, but useful preventive measures are to stop smoking, re-duce weight (if overweight) and to take as much exercise as possible within the limits imposed by the pain.

INTERN: A doctor in training who carries out his duties and training in hospital and usually spends some of his time living in the hospital. The description is used mainly in North America. Alternative terms are house officer or resident which are used in the United Kingdom.

INTERNATIONAL CLASSIFICATION OF DISEASE: A World Health Organization classification of all known diseases and syn-dromes. The diseases are divided according to system (respiratory, renal, cardiac, etc.) or type (accidents, malignant growth, etc.). Each of them is given a three-digit number to facilitate computerization. This classification allows mortality and morbidity rates to be compared nationally and regionally.

INTERSEXUALITY is the condition resulting from faulty sex differentiation during the devel-opment of the fetus. Although not a common condition, it is one that, it is now recognized, should be diagnosed as early as possible in life in order that an early decision may be reached as to the sex of the child, or at least the sex he (or she) is to be brought up as. Equally important is it that any treatment that may be possible should be instituted at the optimum moment.

INTERSTITIAL is a term applied to indiffer-ent tissue set among the proper active tissue of an organ. It is generally of a supporting char-acter and formed of fibrous tissue. The term is also applied to the fluid always present in this in a small amount, and to diseases which specially affect this tissue, such as interstitial keratitis. (See EYE, DISEASES OF.)

INTERTRIGO is a term applied to a chafed or abraded condition between two surfaces of skin that rub together: e.g. under the breast, be-tween the toes, or the armpit. (See ATHLETE'S FOOT; CHAFING OF THE SKIN.)

INTERVERTEBRAL DISC: The fibrous disc that acts as a cushion between the bony verte-brae, enabling them to rotate and bend one on another. The disc tends to degenerate with age and may get ruptured and displaced – prolapsed or slipped disc – as a result of sudden strenuous action. Prolapsed disc occurs mainly in the lower back and is more common in men than women and in the 30–40 age group.

INTESTINE is the whole of the alimentary canal situated below the stomach. In it most digestion is carried on, and through its walls all the food material is absorbed into the blood and lymph streams. (See DIGESTION.) The length of the intestine in man is about 8·5 to 9 metres (28 to 30 feet), and it takes the form of one continuous tube suspended in loops in the abdominal cavity.

Divisions: The intestine is divided into small intestine and large intestine. The former com-prises that part of the tube which extends from the stomach onwards for 6·5 metres (22 feet) or thereabout, and at its broadest point is about 35 mm (1½ inches) in width. The large intestine is the second part of the tube, and though shorter (about 1·8 metres (6 feet) long) is much wider than the small intestine, reaching in places a width of 65 mm (2½ inches). The *small intestine* is divided rather arbitrarily into three parts: the *duodenum*, consisting of the first 25 or 30 cm (10 or 12 inches), into which the ducts of the liver and pancreas open; the *jejunum*, which is gen-erally found empty after death, and comprises the next 2·4 or 2·7 metres (8 or 9 feet); and finally the *ileum*, which at its lower end opens into the large intestine.

The large intestine begins in the lower part of the abdomen on the right side. The first part is known as the caecum, and into this opens the appendix vermiformis. The appendix is a small tube, about the thickness of a quill, from 2 to 20 cm (average 9 cm) in length, which has much the same structure as the rest of the intestine. At one end it is closed, at the other it opens into the caecum, and although it appears to play little or no part in digestion, it is of great importance because of the frequency with which serious inflammation takes place in it. (See APPENDICITIS.) The caecum is continued into the colon. This is subdivided into: the ascending colon which ascends through the right flank to beneath the liver; the transverse colon which crosses the upper part of the abdomen transversely to the left side; the descending colon which bends downwards and descends through the left flank into the pelvis where it becomes the sigmoid colon. The last part of the large intestine is known as the rectum, which passes straight down through the back part of the pelvis, to open to the exterior through the anus.

Structure: The intestine, both small and large, consists of four coats, which vary slightly in structure and arrangement at different points, but are of the same general nature throughout the entire length of the bowel. On the inner surface there is a mucous membrane; outside this is a loose submucous coat, in which blood-vessels run; next comes a muscular coat in two layers; and finally a tough, thin peritoneal membrane. The total thickness of all four coats amounts to about 3 mm.

MUCOUS COAT: The interior of the bowel is completely lined by a single layer of pillar-like cells placed side by side. These rest upon a smooth, fine membrane, beneath which is a loose network of connective tissue and muscular fibres, richly supplied with blood-vessels and lymphatic-vessels. There are two arrangements by which the surface in the small intestine is much increased for the purposes of digestion and absorption. Countless ridges with deep furrows between them run across the upper part, and the whole surface is thickly studded with short hair-like processes called villi. As blood- and lymph-vessels run up to the end of these villi, the digested food passing slowly down the intestine is brought into very close relation with the circulation. Between the bases of the villi are set little openings, each of which leads into a simple, tubular gland lined by cells, which are similar to those covering the surface, and which produce a fluid with digestive powers. In the small intestine, cells here and there produce mucus, and, in the large intestine, a great number of cells are devoted to the production of this substance for lubricating the passage of the food through the bowel. A large number of minute masses, called lymph follicles, similar in structure to the tonsils and lymphatic glands, are scattered over the inner surface of the intestine. In the lower part of the small intestine these are grouped into patches of 2·5 square centimetres or thereabout in size, known as Peyer's patches, which are of special interest, because the inflammation and ulceration of the bowels that occur in typhoid fever are limited to them and to the scattered follicles. The large intestine is bare both of ridges and of villi, and, as already stated, its mucous membrane produces mucus in large amount.

SUBMUCOUS COAT: This consists of a loose connective tissue which allows the mucous membrane to play freely over the muscular coat. The blood-vessels and lymphatic-vessels which absorb the food in the villi pour their contents into a network of large vessels lying in this coat.

MUSCULAR COAT: The muscle in the small intestine is arranged in two definite layers, in the outer of which all the fibres run lengthwise with this coat.

1 small intestine	5 intestinal gland	9 longitudinal muscles
2 duodenum	6 muscularis mucosae	10 peritoneum
3 lymph follicle	7 submucous coat	11 duodenal gland
4 villi	8 circular muscles	

Diagram of intestine.

the bowel, whilst in the inner they pass circularly round it. The muscular coat is of immense importance, because by its contraction and relaxation the food is slowly squeezed down the bowel, the process being known as peristalsis. In the large intestine the only departure from this arrangement is that the fibres which are placed lengthwise are collected into three thick bands upon the outward surface of the bowel, and these bands, being slightly shorter than the other coats of the bowel, cause it to present a puckered appearance.

PERITONEAL COAT forms the outer covering for almost the whole intestine except parts of the duodenum and of the large intestine. It is a tough, fibrous membrane, covered upon its outer surface with a smooth layer of cells, which in the movements of the bowel rub against a similar surface upon the peritoneum lining the general cavity of the abdomen, and so cause a minimum of friction. From the peritoneal coat of the intestine of animals catgut is prepared.

Support: The duodenum and greater part of the large intestine are covered only in front by the peritoneum which lines the abdominal cavity, and this tough membrane serves to bind these parts of the intestine firmly against the back wall of the abdomen. The jejunum and ileum, the transverse colon, and the first part of the rectum are not only completely surrounded by peritoneum, but a double layer of this membrane suspends these parts of the bowel at a distance of several inches from the lines on the back of the abdomen, where the two layers become continuous with the rest of the peritoneum. In this way freedom is given to the movements of these parts of the bowels. These suspending structures are known as mesenteries. That of the small intestine is the largest, being shaped like a fan, 200 mm (8 inches) long at its attached margin, and spreading out to 6·5 metres (22 feet) at its frilled border, where it meets the intestine. The vessels and nerves which supply the intestine run between the two layers of the mesentery.

INTESTINE, DISEASES OF: The principal signs of trouble which has its origin in the intestines consist of pain somewhere about the abdomen, sometimes vomiting, and irregularity in movement of the bowels in the direction either of stoppage or of excessive action.

Several diseases are treated under separate headings. (See APPENDICITIS; CHOLERA; COLITIS; CONCRETIONS; CONSTIPATION; DIARRHOEA; DYSENTERY; ENTERIC FEVERS; HERNIA; ILEITIS; INTUSSUSCEPTION; IRRITABLE BOWEL SYNDROME; PERITONITIS; PILES; RECTUM, DISEASES OF.)

INFLAMMATION of the bowel may affect either its outer or its inner surface. The outer surface is covered by peritoneum, and peritonitis is a serious disease. (See PERITONITIS.) Inflammation of the inner surface is known generally as enteritis, inflammation of special parts receiving the names of colitis, appendicitis, and the like. Enteritis may form the chief symptom of certain infective diseases due to special organisms: for example in typhoid fever, cholera, dysentery. Again, it may be acute, though not connected with any definite organism, when, if severe, it is a very serious condition, particularly in young children. Or it may be chronic, especially as the result of dysentery, and then constitutes a less serious though very troublesome complaint. Indiscretions in diet, such as the eating of unripe fruit, are a not uncommon cause. A very serious type results from the action of irritant poisons. In some people inflammation of the stomach and bowels is liable to result from exposure to cold and damp.

Symptoms: Diarrhoea is the most common and most marked symptom, and in chronic cases usually the only symptom, although, when the small intestine alone is affected, constipation is a more usual result than diarrhoea. Pain, particularly of a griping nature, which comes and goes, is also common. The temperature in acute cases is raised, and there is restlessness, even delirium. If the diarrhoea is very profuse, collapse speedily comes on.

Treatment: Each case requires special handling, according to the cause and the severity. Where diarrhoea is very severe this requires special treatment. (See DIARRHOEA.) There are a few general principles which are applicable to all cases. The diet should be light, bland, non-irritating and containing a minimum of roughage. In more acute cases only milk and glucose drinks should be given for the first twenty-four hours. If there is much diarrhoea ample fluids should be given to prevent dehydration. Rest in bed is essential. Considerable quantities of warm water, containing bicarbonate of soda, have a beneficial action by flushing out the bowel and removing irritating substances. In general, water is given by the mouth, but in some cases it is introduced by an enema to irrigate the lower bowel. Various drugs which have a mildly astringent and soothing action, of which the chief are bismuth carbonate and kaolin, are given by the mouth. When the inflammation is not the result of a chemical or physical irritant, but the result of an infection, as in dysentery, treatment with a sulphonamide drug absorbed only slowly from the intestine is indicated. Phthalylsulphathiazole, succinylsulphathiazole and sulphadimidine have proved particularly useful in the treatment of dysentery.

ULCERATION of the bowels arises in a manner similar to the production of ulcers on the skin surface, although probably these internal ulcers heal much more rapidly than others. Typhoid fever regularly produces ulcers in the lower part of the small intestine, this variety arising in the patches of lymphatic tissue found in this region. Tuberculous ulcers arise late in the course of tuberculosis, and produce a diarrhoea which is always a serious sign. Ulceration also occurs in amoebic dysentery.

Symptoms of ulceration are much the same as those of enteritis, and the formation of ulcers is simply an advanced stage of this condition. In addition, the ulcerated surface is apt to bleed, and, if the ulcer is situated high up in the bowel, this blood is voided as black or brown material; if it comes from near the lower end of the bowel the blood is red and unchanged. The healing of these ulcers leads, in the case of all save those of typhoid fever, to the formation of scars, and, as these scars contract there is a tendency to narrowing of the bowel and obstruction. This is particularly apt to follow tuberculous ulcers, if these should heal, because they often run circularly round the inside of the bowel.

Treatment in cases of ulceration is similar to that for inflammation.

PERFORATION of the bowel may take place as the result either of injury or of disease. Stabs and other wounds which penetrate the abdomen may damage the bowel, and severe blows or crushes may tear it without any external wound. Ulceration, as in typhoid fever, or, more rarely, in tuberculosis, may cause an opening in the bowel-wall also. Again, when the bowel is greatly distended above an obstruction, faecal material may accumulate and produce ulcers, which rupture with the ordinary movements of the bowels. Whatever the cause, the symptoms are much the same.

Symptoms: The contents of the bowel pass out through the perforation into the peritoneal cavity, and, making their way between the coils of intestine, set up a general peritonitis. In consequence, the abdomen is painful, and after a few hours becomes extremely tender to the touch, as a result of the peritonitis. The abdomen swells, particularly in its upper part, owing to gas having passed also into the cavity. Vomiting is a symptom, and the person passes into a state of collapse. Such a condition is almost invariably fatal in two, or at most three, days, if not promptly treated. Occasionally, however, the perforation is preceded by a certain amount of peritonitis, which forms adhesions in the neighbourhood of the ulcerated part, so that when perforation finally takes place a localized abscess, instead of general peritonitis, may result, and the person may recover.

Treatment: All food should be withheld, because whatever is taken into the stomach is either vomited or is liable to pass out of the perforation into the peritoneal cavity. An operation is urgently necessary, the abdomen being opened in the middle line, the perforated portion of bowel found, and the perforation stitched up. If the bowel is damaged badly, a part is often cut out and the divided ends joined together. Finally, the peritoneal cavity is thoroughly washed out, and a drainage tube left for some days in the abdominal wound. The local application of penicillin or sulphonamides to the peritoneum during operation has effected a marked reduction in the mortality rate.

OBSTRUCTION of the bowels means a stoppage to the passage down the intestine of the partially digested food. Obstruction may be due either to some cause within the abdomen or to the thrusting of a loop of bowel through an opening in the wall of this cavity. The latter class of cases has been referred to under HERNIA. Obstruction may be acute when it comes on suddenly with intense symptoms, or it may be chronic, when the obstructing cause gradually increases and the bowel becomes slowly more narrow till it closes altogether, or when slight obstruction comes and goes till it ends in an acute attack. In chronic cases the symptoms are much the same as those of the acute variety, although they are milder in degree and more prolonged.

Causes: Obstruction may be due to causes outside the bowel altogether, for example, the pressure of tumours in neighbouring organs, the twisting round the bowel of bands produced by former peritonitis, or even the twisting of a coil of intestine round itself so as to cause a kink in its wall. Chronic and partial forms of obstruction are sometimes due to such kinks near the end of the small intestine, sometimes to the pressure of the mesentery on the upper end of the small intestine. Chronic causes of the obstruction may exist in the wall of the bowel itself: for example, a tumour, or the contracting scar of an old ulcer. The condition of intussusception (q.v.), where part of the bowel passes inside of the part beneath it, in the same way as one turns the finger of a glove outside in, causes obstruction and other symptoms. Finally some body, such as a concretion, or the stone of some large fruit, or even a mass of hardened faeces, may become jammed within the bowel and stop up its passage.

Symptoms: There are four chief symptoms of this condition, and any case in which these are combined demands immediate treatment. These are pain, vomiting, constipation and swelling of the abdomen. The *pain* is of a griping character, and may be very severe although it comes and goes, getting now stronger and again for a time less marked. When the small intestine is the seat of obstruction the pain is almost always referred to the region round the navel; when the large intestine is affected the pain may be more accurately referred to the part from which it arises. In addition to this, acute cases are marked by great tenderness of the abdomen to touch. The *vomiting* is peculiar in character. It begins with the first onset of pain, and consists of the contents of the stomach. Later it is yellow or green, bitter, and contains much bile, while, after several hours have elapsed, it becomes brown and ill-smelling, and is then known as faecal vomiting. The *constipation* in acute cases comes on suddenly, whilst in chronic cases it may be preceded by a state in which constipation and diarrhoea alternate, or by one in which the stools gradually get smaller and smaller in size, possibly over a period lasting for several months. In chronic cases of obstruction to the large intestine, it is not uncommon for the sufferer to possess a constant desire to go to stool with straining pain, although he can pass nothing (tenesmus). In some conditions, particularly that due to intussusception, though there is constipation in the ordinary sense, the excessive straining produces a copious discharge of blood-stained mucus. The *swelling of* *the abdomen* varies in different cases. In acute cases the whole belly is blown up with gas, much increasing the pain of the condition. The constipation is so complete as to prevent even flatus from being passed – a very important sign of its gravity. Another grave sign is the absence of the sounds of intestinal movement which can be heard on auscultation over the normal abdomen. In chronic cases, in which the wall of the intestine is thickened, individual loops stand out now and then and become visible on the surface in their attempts to force their contents past the obstruction. When the small intestine is affected, its loops stand out one over the other, resembling the rungs of a ladder; whilst obstruction low down in the large intestine causes a bulging in the flanks and across the upper part of the abdomen.

In addition to these abdominal symptoms, in the later stages there is generally collapse, although consciousness is retained till the end. If the condition is not relieved by operation, death almost always results: in acute cases, in the course of three to six days.

Treatment: As a rule the surgeon opens the abdomen, finds the obstruction and relieves it or if possible removes it altogether. The task of the surgeon is rendered specially hard by the difficulty of determining, before he opens the abdomen, where the obstruction is, by the fact that the intestine is inflamed, and by its distension with gas and faeces. He has generally to open the abdomen in the middle line, examine the usual sites of obstruction, and, failing to find any cause at these points, to pass the whole length of intestine carefully through his hands till he finds the obstruction. Even after this is found, if it is of the nature of a tumour, it may be impossible to remove. If the obstruction is successfully removed, something must next be done, by puncturing the bowel or other means, to relieve the collection of gas and faeces, and this adds to the operation the great risk of sepsis. The introduction of the sulphonamides and antibiotics, however, has diminished this risk considerably. In all these manipulations care must be taken, by warm towels and the like, to prevent unnecessary exposure and chilling of the bowel.

TUBERCULOSIS of the intestine is a relatively uncommon disease in the United Kingdom today, where it is encountered predominantly in Asian immigrants. Treatment consists of the administration of ethambutol, rifampicin and isoniazid, as in the case of pulmonary tuberculosis, but for a longer period: 18 months. In order to prevent the risk of obstruction occurring, the use of corticosteroids (q.v.) has also been recommended for two months. As these patients are often debilitated and anaemic, they must be put on a high-protein diet with ample vitamins, and the anaemia must be energetically treated. This may require a blood transfusion in the initial stages.

TUMOURS are relatively uncommon in the small intestine and, when they do occur, they are usually benign. Conversely, they are relatively common in the large intestine where they are usually cancerous. The most common site for cancer of the large intestine is the rectum, with the sigmoid, caecum and ascending colon next in order of frequency. It is a disease of the older age-groups, and occurs with equal frequency in men and women. A history of altered bowel habit, in the form of increasing constipation or diarrhoea, or an alternation of these, or of bleeding from the anus, in a middle-aged person is an indication for taking medical advice. If the condition is cancer, then the sooner it is operated on, the better the result.

INTIMA is the innermost coat lining the arteries and the veins.

INTOLERANCE: An adverse reaction of a patient to a drug or treatment.

INTOXICATION is a term applied to states of poisoning. The poison may be some chemical substance introduced from outside, e.g. alcohol (see ALCOHOLISM), or it may be due to the products of bacterial action, the bacteria either being introduced from outside or developing within the body. The term auto-intoxication is applied in the latter case.

INTRACRANIAL is the term applied to structures, diseases, and the like, contained in or rising within the head.

INTRACRANIAL PRESSURE: This is the pressure that is maintained by the brain tissue, intracellular and extracellular fluid, cerebrospinal fluid and blood. An increase in intracranial pressure may occur as a result of inflammation, injury, haemorrhage, or tumour in the brain tissue as well as of some congenital conditions. The pressure is measured by lumbar puncture in which a syringe attached to a mamometer (pressure-measuring device) is inserted into the cerebrospinal fluid surrounding the lower part of the spinal cord.

INTRATHECAL means within the membranes or meninges which envelop the spinal cord. The intrathecal space, between the arachnoid and the pia mater, contains the cerebrospinal fluid.

INTRAUTERINE CONTRACEPTIVE DEVICE (IUD): A mechanical device, commonly a coil, inserted into the uterus to prevent conception. For many, though not all, women IUDs are an effective and acceptable form of contraception, though only about 10 per cent of women in the UK use them. The devices are of various shapes and made of plastic or copper; most have a string that passes through the cervix and rests in the vagina. (See CONTRACEPTION.)

INTRAVENOUS: A term which means inside a vein. An intravenous injection is one that is given into a vein. Blood transfusions are given intravenously, as are other infusions of fluid.

INTRAVENOUS UROGRAM: A procedure for getting X-ray pictures of the urinary tract. A radio-opaque medium is injected into a vein and, when it is excreted by the kidneys, the substance can be identified on X-rays. Any abnormalities in structure or foreign bodies such as calculi are outlined by the dye.

INTROSPECTION is the observation of one's own thoughts or feelings. It is generally applied to this process when it occurs to an abnormal extent in association with melancholia.

INTUBATION is a simple operation consisting in the introduction, through the mouth into the larynx, of a tube designed to keep the air passage open at this point.

INTUSSUSCEPTION is a form of obstruction of the bowels in which part of the intestine enters within that part immediately beneath it. This can best be understood by observing what takes place in the fingers of a tightly fitting glove as they turn outside in when the glove is pulled off the hand. The people affected are almost always infants. The cause is not known. The point at which it most often occurs is the junction between the small and the large intestines, the former passing within the latter. The symptoms are those of intestinal obstruction in general, and in addition there is often a discharge of blood-stained mucus from the bowel. The treatment consists – unless the symptoms rapidly subside, when it may be assumed that the bowel has righted itself – of either hydrostatic reduction by means of a barium enema, or an operation. At operation the intussusception is either reduced or, if this not possible, the obstructed part is cut out and the ends of the intestine then stitched together. If treated adequately and in time, the mortality is now reduced to around 1 per cent.

INVASION: The entry of bacteria into the body. The spread of cancer into normal, nearby tissues or organs.

IN VITRO is a term commonly used in medical research and experimental biology. Literally 'in a glass', it refers to observations made outside the body: e.g. on the action of drugs on bacteria. The opposite term is IN VIVO, which refers to observations of processes in the body.

IN VITRO FERTILIZATION (IVF): Fertilization of the egg outside the body. The fertilized ovum is then incubated until the blastocyst stage develops when it is implanted into the uterus. The procedure was developed in Britain and the first successful in vitro baby, a girl, was born in 1978. IVF is used when a woman has blocked fallopian tubes or when the sperm and ovum are unable to fuse in the reproductive tract. Hormone treatment results in the potential mother's producing several mature ova, some of which are removed from the ovary using a laparoscope and fertilized with her partner's semen.

IN VIVO: A Latin term to describe biological events that take place inside the bodies of living organisms.

INVOLUCRUM is the term applied to the sheath of new bone which is formed round a piece of dead bone in, for example, osteomyelitis.

INVOLUNTARY MUSCLE: Muscle that does not operate under a person's conscious control. Involuntary muscle, also called smooth muscle because the cells do not contain the striations that occur in voluntary muscle (q.v.), is found in blood vessels, the heart, stomach, and intestines.

INVOLUTION is the process of change whereby the uterus returns to its resting size after parturition. The term is also applied to any retrograde biological change, as in senility.

IODIDES are salts of iodine, those which are especially used in medicine being the iodide of potassium and iodide of sodium. Iodides are excreted in the mucus secretions, as well as in the urine, saliva and sweat, and have an action in liquefying the mucus secretion of the bronchial tree. They are therefore used in expectorant mixtures. They are also used to assist in providing a supply of iodine in patients with goitre, or in individuals who live in an area where goitre is liable to occur because of a deficiency of iodine in the drinking water. They may be given in the form of iodized salt. (See GOITRE.)

Over-dosage of iodides results in iodism (q.v.).

IODINE is a non-metallic element which is found largely in seaweed. The body contains about 30 mg, largely concentrated in the thryoid gland where it is used to synthesize thyroid hormones. Iodine has a highly irritating action and when applied to the skin, stains the latter dark brown and causes it to peel off in flakes, while internally it is a violent irritant poison in large doses.

Externally iodine is used as an antiseptic. Its drawback is that it is fixed by protein, which reduces its antiseptic efficiency in open wounds. Its main use in this sphere therefore is for sterilizing the unbroken skin, as before an operation. Radioactive iodine is used for diagnosing and treating disease of the thyroid gland.

IODISM is the condition which is produced by an over-dose of iodides, but in some susceptible individuals iodism may be produced by very small amounts of iodides. It is characterized by running of the eyes and nose, sore throat, a heavy, dull feeling over the eyes, increased secretion of saliva and a typical skin eruption. These manifestations usually disappear rapidly upon the drugs being withdrawn.

ION EXCHANGE RESINS are synthetic organic substances which have the power of exchanging ions. Chemically, they are closely related to plastics. They are divided into two groups: *cation exchange resins*, which take up and liberate cations, e.g. sodium, potassium, hydrogen ions; *anion exchange resins*, which take up and liberate anion, e.g. chloride, hydroxyl ions. The former are used in the treatment of oedema, and the latter in the treatment of peptic ulcers.

IONIZATION means the breaking up of a substance in solution into its constituent ions.

IPECACUANHA, IPECAC, or HIPPO, is the root of *Cephaëlis ipecacuanha*, a Brazilian shrub. It contains an alkaloid, emetine, which acts as an irritant when brought in contact with the interior of the stomach, producing vomiting. This effect is also brought about after its absorption into the blood by its action on the vomiting centre in the brain. In small doses it acts, not as an irritant, but as a gentle stimulant to the mucous membrane of the stomach, bowels and respiratory passages. Emetine was for long the great stand-by in the treatment of amoebic dysentery.
Uses: Ipecacuanha is a constituent of many expectorant mixtures given in the treatment of bronchitis. It is of value in this connection because of its action in liquefying the thick mucous secretion which occurs in bronchitis. Syrup of ipecacuanha is the treatment of choice for evacuating the stomach in young children who have swallowed a poison.

IPRATROPIUM is a bronchodilator drug of value in the treatment of asthma, bronchitis and rhinitis.

IPRONIAZID is a drug which inhibits monoamine oxidase (q.v.), an enzyme which plays an important part in the metabolism of the brain. Originally introduced into medicine for the treatment of tuberculosis, it proved too toxic for this purpose, but is now used in the treatment of depressive states. (See ANTIDEPRESSANTS.)

IRIDECTOMY: The operation by which a hole is made in the iris, as, for example, in the treatment of glaucoma (q.v.) or as part of cataract surgery (q.v.).

IRIDENCLEISIS was an operation formerly used in the treatment of glaucoma. It has now been replaced by trabeculectomy (see GLAUCOMA).

IRIDOLOGY is the study of the iris (see EYE). It is an old practice dating back to the days of Aristotle, which has been revived in recent days as one of the more exotic branches of what is popularly known as 'fringe medicine'. By its exponents it is defined as 'diagnosis through photography of the iris', and extravagant, as yet unsupported, claims are made for its validity.

IRIS (see EYE).

IRITIS (see UVEITIS).

IRON is a metal which is an essential constituent of the red blood corpuscles, where it is present in the form of haemoglobin. It is also present in muscle, myoglobin, and in certain respiratory pigments which are essential to the life of many tissues in the body. Iron is absorbed principally in the upper part of the small intestine. It is then stored: mainly in the liver; to a lesser extent in the spleen and kidneys, where it is available, when required, for use in the bone marrow to form the haemoglobin in red blood corpuscles. The daily iron requirement of an adult is 15 to 20 milligrams. This requirement is increased during pregnancy. Iron salts also have an astringent action, especially the chloride, and this property is sometimes made use of when it is used as a styptic to check bleeding.
Uses: The main use of iron is in the treatment of iron-deficiency anaemias. (See ANAEMIA.) The main form in which it is used is ferrous sulphate. Iron preparations sometimes cause irritation of the gastro-intestinal tract, and should therefore always be taken after meals. They sometimes produce a tendency towards constipation. Whenever possible, iron preparations should be given by mouth. It is a very small proportion indeed of cases of iron-deficiency anaemia which will not respond satisfactorily to iron given by mouth. For the occasional cases in which oral administration is not suitable, a preparation of iron is now available which can be given intravenously.

IRRADIATION is treatment by various forms of light and radiant activity.

IRRIGATION is the method of washing out wounds, or cavities of the body, like the bladder and bowels. (See DOUCHE; ENEMA.)

IRRITABLE BOWEL SYNDROME is a motility disorder of the gut. It is not confined to the large intestine so that the terms spastic colon or irritable colon are inaccurate. Some of the symptoms of the irritable bowel syndrome affect more than 10 per cent of the normal adult population, but most people accept these symptoms as a minor nuisance. Only those with severe symptoms or those who worry about their symptoms consult a doctor.

Symptoms: Abdominal pain is the commonest symptom and it frequently moves from one area of the abdomen into another. A disturbed bowel habit is also common and this may alternate between diarrhoea and constipation. A feeling of abdominal distension is common, as is heartburn. Some patients suffer from painless, watery diarrhoea. The symptoms are either due to abnormal motility of the gut or to increased intestinal sensitivity to distension. The pain can, in fact, often be produced in patients by balloon inflation within the colon or other parts of the gut. The symptoms frequently start after an acute intestinal infection, and acute psychological stresses can also influence the activity of the bowel.

Treatment requires reassurance and explanation of the functional nature of the disorder. Anticholinergic drugs inhibit colonic motor activity and mebeverine has a direct relaxant effect on intestinal smooth muscle. Antidiarrhoeal drugs such as codeine phosphate reduce the frequency and urgency of defaecation. Lomotil is an effective alternative. Bulking agents speed colonic transit and allow the passage of softer, bulkier motions. High-fibre diets are beneficial.

ISCHAEMIA means bloodlessness of a part of the body, due to contraction, spasm, constriction or blocking (by embolus or by thrombus) of the arteries: for example, of the heart.

ISCHAEMIC HEART DISEASE (see CORONARY THROMBOSIS).

ISCHIO-RECTAL ABSCESS is an abscess arising in the space between the rectum and ischial bone and often resulting in a fistula.

ISCHIUM is the bone which forms the lower and hinder part of the pelvis. It bears the weight of the body in sitting.

ISHIHARA TEST (see VISION).

ISLETS OF LANGERHANS: Groups of specialized cells distributed throughout the pancreas (q.v.), that produce three hormones, insulin (q.v.), glucagon, and somatostatin.

ISOCARBOXAZID (see ANTIDEPRESSANTS).

ISO-IMMUNIZATION is the immunization of one member of a species by an antigen lacking in himself but present naturally in other members of the species, as, for example, the immunization of an Rh-negative mother by an Rh-positive fetus, the mother as a result producing anti-Rh agglutinins which injure the fetus. (See also HAEMOLYTIC DISEASE OF THE NEW-BORN; BLOOD GROUPS.)

ISOLATION in infectious diseases is an important procedure, applied both to people who are themselves sick and to those who have come in contact with them, technically known as contacts or suspects, and who may later develop the disease. (See INCUBATION; INFECTION; QUARANTINE.)

ISOMETRIC: Of similar measurement. Isometric exercises are based on the isometric contraction of the muscles. Fibres are provoked into working by pushing or pulling an immovable object but this technique prevents them from shortening in length. These exercises improve a person's fitness and builds up his or her muscle strength.

ISONIAZID is one of the anti-tuberculous drugs. It has the advantages of being relatively non-toxic and of being active when taken by mouth. Unfortunately, like streptomycin, it may render the *Mycobacterium tuberculosis* resistant to its action. This tendency to produce resistance is considerably reduced if it is given in conjunction with streptomycin and/or para-aminosalicylic acid.

ISOPRENALINE is a bronchodilator drug that is widely and successfully used in the treatment of asthma, mainly as an aerosol for inhalation. In view of its action on the heart it must be used with caution.

ISOTONIC is a term applied to solutions which have the same power of diffusion as one another. An isotonic solution used in medicine is one which can be mixed with body fluids without causing any disturbance. An isotonic *saline solution* for injection into the blood, so that it may possess the same osmotic pressure as the blood serum, is one of 0·9-per-cent strength or containing 9 grams of sodium chloride to 1 litre of water. This is also known as *normal* or *physiological salt solution*. An isotonic solution of *bicarbonate of soda* for injection into the blood is one of 1·35-per-cent strength in water. An isotonic solution of *glucose* for injection into the blood is one of 5-per-cent strength in water.

Solutions which are weaker, or stronger than, the fluids of the body with which they are intended to be mixed are known as hypotonic and hypertonic, respectively.

ISOTOPES: There are four fundamental atomic particles: the proton, the neutron, the electron and the positron. The proton has mass and a unit positive electrical charge. The neutron has mass and no charge. The electron has very small mass compared with the proton and neutron, and has unit negative electrical charge. The positron is the positively charged counterpart of the electron, having equal mass and unit positive charge.

The atom is composed of a positively charged central nucleus surrounded by a number of electrons. The nucleus is made up of protons and neutrons. The number of protons determines the positive charge and is known as the atomic number. The number of protons plus the neutrons is the atomic mass number and determines the atomic weight. The number of orbital electrons surrounding the nucleus of an atom is equal to the number of protons in the nucleus. Hence the atom is electrically neutral. Since chemical reactions concern only interactions between the outer electrons the chemical properties of an atom are determined by the number of orbital electrons – that is, they are characterized by the atomic number.

An element is matter consisting of atoms having the same atomic number. The number of neutrons in the atom of an element may vary and therefore its atomic mass number may vary. A nuclide is a species of atom characterized by its atomic number, atomic mass number and nuclear energy state. Isotopes are nuclides having the same atomic number but different mass number. For example hydrogen with atomic number one occurs in nature as a mixture of the nuclides hydrogen-1 with mass number one (that is, one proton in its nucleus), and hydrogen-2 (deuterium or heavy hydrogen) with mass number two – that is, one proton and one neutron is its nucleus.

Hydrogen-1 and hydrogen-2 are both isotopes of hydrogen and are chemically indistinguishable. The terms isotope and radioactive isotope are frequently used when nuclide and radioactive nuclide would be more accurate. Atomic weight is not quite synonymous with atomic mass number. The atomic weight for a given specimen of an element is the mean weight of its atoms expressed in atomic mass units, for many elements consist of a mixture of different nuclides of that element.

Isotopes may be stable or radioactive. In stable isotopes the relative number of protons and neutrons are found to lie within quite close limits. In radioactive isotopes this balance is upset owing to an excess or deficiency of neutrons, with the result that the nuclei become unstable. They tend to change into stable configurations by processes known collectively as radioactive decay. This involves spontaneous disintegration with emission of radiation.

The artificially produced radioactive isotopes may be grouped roughly in two categories: those produced in a nuclear reactor and those produced in a cyclotron. In nuclear reactors the target elements are bombarded with neutrons. The nuclides produced, therefore, are usually isotopic with the stable target elements, and have more neutrons in their nuclei. The radioactive isotope of hydrogen, tritium, has a mass number of 3 and the ratio of neutrons to protons is 2:1. Isotopes with excess neutrons in the nuclei tend to decay by

the emission of beta rays. In the process of producing isotopes in a cyclotron the target material in bombarded with protons, deuterons, or alpha particles. The radioactive products are thus isotopes of a different element from the target. They are deficient in neutrons, and therefore tend to decay by emission of positrons.

Each radioactive substance, whether naturally occurring, produced in a nuclear reactor, or in a cyclotron, is characterized not only by the type and energy of radiation given off but also by the rate of disintegration. The half-life is the time taken for one-half of the original number of unstable atoms to disintegrate. Half-lives of different isotopes vary enormously. For example, carbon-14 has a half-life of over 5,000 years, while silver-109 has a half-life of only 39 seconds. The unit of radioactivity is the curie, which may be defined as that activity in which the number of disintegrations per second is 3.7×10^{10}.

Within the atomic nucleus the particles are in constant motion, and therefore they collide frequently. In these collisions energy transfers take place, so that all particles do not have the same kinetic energy. In a stable nucleus no particle ever acquires sufficient energy to overcome the potential barrier and to escape from the nucleus. In an unstable nucleus, owing to the presence of an excess number of neutrons, there is an excess of energy among the particles, so that there is a probability that one particle will acquire sufficient kinetic energy to overcome the barrier and to escape from the nucleus.

Types of Radiation: The type and energy of radiation given off by radioactive substances are the same for any one nuclide. The primary radioactive decay process is always either the emission of a charged particle (alpha particle, beta particle, or positron) or the capture by the nucleus of an orbital electron. These processes alter the charge on the nucleus, giving rise to a chemically different element. Any one of these may be accompanied by gamma rays or X-rays. In medical diagnosis the beta particles and gamma rays are the most commonly encountered forms of radioactivity.

Beta particles are electrons and have limited tissue penetration dependent on their energy. Even energetic beta particles are only able to penetrate about 1 cm of tissue, so they are not suitable for the study of deep organs. Gamma rays are not particulate, but are electromagnetic radiations of the same nature as light, though of much shorter wavelength, and therefore of much higher energy. They may be considered as being made up of discrete amounts of energy or photons. They have a much greater power of penetration than beta particles and this power is dependent on their energy.

Isotopes having an excess of neutrons usually decay by emission of negative beta particles. Decay of an isotope by emission of a beta particle may be thought of as the conversion of a neutron into a proton and electron, with the immediate ejection of the electron from the nucleus. The loss of a unit of negative charge means that the nucleus has effectively gained a proton in place of a neutron, and the resulting nucleus is that of the next higher element in the periodic system. To maintain electrical neutrality the atom must acquire an extra orbital electron. The decay of radioactive isotopes has thus fulfilled the dream of the alchemist. Radioactive carbon decays by emission of a beta particle and become stable nitrogen. Similarly phosphorus-32 disintegrates with the emission of a beta particle, and thereupon becomes stable sulphur.

The beta particles from a particular isotope have varying energies up to a maximum characteristic of that isotope. Phosphorus-32, sulphur-35, carbon-14 and hydrogen-3 are beta emitters. In some isotopes the available energy in the radioactive nucleus is not accounted for completely by beta decay. The excess energy is then emitted as a gamma ray. This occurs with such isotopes as iodine-131, iodine- 132, sodium-24 and potassium-42.

Measurement of Radioactivity: Radioactive substances are detected by virtue of the radiation they emit. Ionization and excitation of the atoms are produced in the absorbing medium through which they pass. The beta rays produce ionization directly by their electrical charge. The gamma rays, by interaction with the atoms in the absorbing medium, produce so-called secondary electrons which behave in the same way as beta particles. Some radiation detectors – namely the ionization chamber, the proportional counter and the Geiger counter – depend on the ionization produced in a gas. Essentially each of these instruments consists of two electrodes in a chamber filled with gas, across which a potential difference is maintained. The passage of ions between the electrodes gives rise to an electric current or a series of pulses, both of which may be measured.

The scintillation detector consists of a phosphor, such as a sodium iodide crystal, photomultiplier tube and associated electronic equipment. When radiation energy is absorbed in the phosphor each quantum absorbed gives rise to a number of light quanta (photons). These cause emission of electrons from the photocathode of the photo-multiplier tube, which in turn gives rise to a pulse at its output. The size of these pulses is proportional to the energy of the absorbed radiation and the number of pulses to the intensity of the absorbed radiation. The pulses are measured and counted by the associated electronic equipment.

Ionization chambers are the least sensitive of detectors. The Geiger counter and the scintillation counter are equally sensitive to beta radiations, but the scintillation counter has much greater sensitivity to gamma radiation than the Geiger counter.

Applications of Radioactive Isotopes to Diagnosis: The use of radioactive isotopes in diagnosis is based on the fact that it is possible to tag many of the substances normally present in the body with a radioactive label. Because it is possible to detect minute quantities of radioactive material, only very small doses may be given. The body pool of the material is therefore not appreciably altered, and metabolism is not disturbed. Thus in studies of iodine metabolism the ratio of radioactive atoms administered to stable atoms in the body pool is of the order of 1 to 1,000 million. By measuring radioactivity in the body, in blood samples, or in the excreta it is possible to gain information about the fate of the labelled substance, and hence of the chemically identical inactive material. Hence it is theoretically possible to trace the absorption, distribution and the excretion of any substance normally present in the body, provided that it can be tagged with a suitable radioactive label.

If the investigation necessitates tracing the path of the material through the body by means of external counting over the body surface it is obviously essential to use an isotope that emits gamma radiation or positrons. If, however, only measurements on blood sample or excreta are required it is possible to use pure beta emitters. Recently whole-body counters have been introduced which measure the total radioactivity in the body, and these are of great value in absorption studies. Another development has been that of more sensitive scanning devices, which are used in studying the distribution of radioactive isotopes in various organs and tissues. Furthermore, the recent production of isotopes with shorter lives has made it possible to give higher radioactive doses without increasing the radiation hazard. This is of particular advantage to the scanning techniques which now enable most organs of the body to be visualized.

Five main groups of diagnostic uses may be defined:

(1) METABOLIC STUDIES: The use of radioactive materials in metabolic studies is based on the fundamental property that all isotopes of an element are chemically identical. The radioactive isotope is used as a true isotope tracer – that is, when introduced into the body (in whatever form) it behaves in the same way as the inactive element. Thus isotopes of iodine are used to measure thyroid function, and isotopes of calcium enable kinetic studies of bone formation and destruction to be performed. The distribution of iron-59 from the serum to the bone marrow, liver and spleen may be followed and its incorporation into the haemoglobin of the red cell used as a measure of bone marrow function. Orthoiodohippurate (Hippuran) labelled with iodine-131 may be used to assess renal vascularity and to detect differences in renal blood supply due to such conditions as renal artery stenosis.

(2) ABSORPTION AND DISTRIBUTION STUDIES: The fate of labelled substances given by mouth can be followed to assess their absorption, utilization and excretion. In most of these studies the isotope is a true isotope tracer. For example, iron absorption can be measured with radioactive iron; vitamin-B_{12} absorption may be investigated with vitamin B_{12} tagged with radioactive

cobalt. In studies of fat absorption, on the other hand, triolein labelled with iodine-131 may be used, but this is not a true isotopic tracer.

(3) BODY COMPOSITION BY DILUTION STUDIES: By introducing an isotope into a compartment, such as the blood or extracellular space, it is possible to measure the volume of that compartment by determining the dilution of radioactivity when equilibrium has been reached. In this way iodine-131-labelled human serum albumin is used to estimate the plasma volume; chromium-51-labelled red cells to measure the red-cell volume; and bromine-82 to determine the extracellular water. The total body exchangeable potassium can be measured with potassium-42 and total exchangeable sodium with sodium-24 or sodium-22.

(4) PHYSICAL TRACING STUDIES: In this type of study the isotope is not necessarily used as a true isotopic tracer. In other words, it does not trace the path of the corresponding inactive isotope. For example, xenon-133 is used in measurements of blood flow in muscles, and in lung-function studies; krypton-85 is used to detect intracardiac shunts. Neither of these elements is normally present in the body. The survival of red cells may be followed and the organ of sequestration revealed by labelling red cells with radioactive chromium. Though chromium is normally present in the body, it does not take part in the metabolic process of the red cell, and the labelling of cells with chromium-51 is simply used as a convenient tag to trace their fate.

(5) SCANNING OF ORGANS AND TISSUES: Scanning is a technique which is used to determine the distribution of radioactive isotopes within the body or within one particular organ. In the conventional scanner the radiation detector, which is a scintillation counter, 'sees' only a small cross-sectional area of the body at a time. The activity 'seen' at each point is registered, and a 'map' of the activity seen over the scanned area is recorded. Various methods of presentation have been used, and the recently improved display systems present the information gathered by the scanner more effectively. Mechanical printing of blacks, which are closer together for higher count rates, has been followed by photoscanning and by 'colour printouts', where the colour of the mark is selected by the count rate. A pictorial representation of the degree of radioactivity is thus achieved. This is advantageous, as the eye can detect quite small variations in colour pattern from point to point much more easily than in monochrome. More recent developments are stationary detectors such as the gamma camera, auto-fluoroscope, and other devices which can view the whole of the area simultaneously. Thus when selective concentration of an isotope in a tissue occurs it is possible to examine the distribution of that isotope by means of scanning. A toxic nodule in the thyroid may be identified by its selective concentration of iodine-131. Areas of absent function on the radioactive scan ('cold' areas) suggest the presence of tumours, abscesses, and similar lesions. Iodine-131 may be used to localize tumours of the thyroid, and chlormerodrin labelled with mercury-197 to delineate tumours of the kidneys. Of even greater practical application is the localizing of brain tumours with human serum albumin labelled with iodine-131 or with radioactive technetium.

Treatment: Radioactive isotopes are also used in medical treatment. The overactivity of the thyroid gland in thyrotoxicosis can be treated by the ingestion of radioactive iodine. The ingested iodine is taken up by the thyroid gland where local irradiation of the gland takes place, reducing its activity. Radioactive phosphorus is used in the treatment of polycythemia rubra vera. It is largely taken up in bone as this is the main source of body phosphate and irradiation of the bone marrow results, controlling the overactivity that is characteristic of polycythemia rubra vera. In cobalt teletherapy the isotope cobalt 60 is used to deliver 1·2–1·3-million-volt radiation which is equivalent to X-rays generated at a peak voltage of 3–4-million-volts. (See RADIOTHERAPY.)

ISSUE is an old term for a suppurating sore.

ITCH is a popular name for scabies (q.v.).

ITCHING, or PRURITUS, is an unpleasant condition of the skin surface which in some cases is so constant as to become unbearable.

Causes: It is due to many different conditions, some of which are local and can be easily removed. Some are general, while occasionally the condition becomes so chronic and the skin so changed by scratching, that it is incurable. Itching is produced by slight mechanical irritation, such as contact with rough woollen underclothing, also by parasites such as lice, or scabies ('the itch'), and these mechanical causes being removed the itching speedily vanishes. There is often a large psychological factor and this must always be borne in mind. (See NEURODERMATOSES.)

Various skin diseases, of which eczema is the chief, have itchiness as one of their main symptoms. In old age, when the skin is becoming thin and inelastic, itching sometimes becomes a troublesome complaint. In these and other conditions, a habit of scratching, which in course of time renders the skin rough and thickened, is apt to be acquired and this of itself aggravates and keeps up the itchiness. Among the general diseases which set up itchiness, the chief is diabetes mellitus. In fact, any one who is much troubled by itchiness, especially if this is situated about the genital organs, should have his urine examined for the presence of sugar. Jaundice caused by various liver derangements, and glomerulonephritis are often accompanied by itchiness in a milder degree. Food allergy is not uncommonly the cause of nettle-rash, which may be of an itching type and appear soon after the food has been taken. Some people are much troubled by itching of the body when changes in size of the blood-vessels in the skin take place, as occur upon getting warm in bed or at the start of spring and autumn. A similar condition, which affects people on going to the tropics, is known as prickly heat (q.v.).

Cold weather itch is a common form of itching in cold weather when the skin tends to become dry. It is commonest and most marked on the legs of old people.

A special and often very aggravated form of itching occurs sometimes at the anus, known as pruritus ani. In all cases of irritation in or around the anus, a careful search should be made for threadworms. (See RECTUM, DISEASES OF.) An equally troublesome form of itching occurs round the vagina, known as pruritus vulvae. It may be associated with excessive vaginal discharge. (See LEUCORRHEA.)

Treatment: The use of detergents should be avoided, and as little soap as possible should be used for cleansing purposes. Warm baths, alkaline or containing bran, are among the most soothing applications for general itching. The addition of an ounce or two (30 to 60 grams) of the *British Pharmacopoeia* Emulsifying Ointment is often beneficial. Calamine lotion is the most efficient local application, but talcum powder is often useful. In the treatment of cold weather itch some such preparation as E45 Cream or *British Pharmacopoeia* Emulsifying Ointment should be applied regularly, especially after a bath. Overwashing with soap should be avoided, and a non-alkaline substitute such as *British Pharmacopoeia* Aqueous Cream used instead of soap. Rough winter underclothing should not be used next the skin. It is essential that a proper examination should be made as to the functions of the internal organs in cases in which itching is a chronic complaint. In diabetic cases the surest remedy to prevent the itching is to treat the diabetes. In pruritus ani attention to anal hygiene is important, and the anal region should be washed twice a day, using a soft sponge, and, if possible, every time the bowels move. Talcum powder should be applied after the washing and careful drying. In persistent cases of pruritus ani and pruritus vulvae the application of a corticosteroid (q.v.) ointment is often helpful. If there is a psychological cause, this must always be dealt with.

-ITIS is a suffix added to the name of an organ to signify any diseased condition of that organ.

IVORY, or DENTINE, is the hard material which forms the chief bulk of the teeth. (See TEETH.)

J

JACKSONIAN EPILEPSY (see EPILEPSY).

JAUNDICE is a yellow discoloration of the skin due to the deposition of bile pigment in its deeper layers. (See also HEPATITIS.)

Causes: Jaundice is divided into two main classes: *hepatogenous jaundice*, arising from the absorption of bile formed by the liver, and *haemolytic jaundice*, arising from the formation of a yellow pigment in the blood, derived from the breaking down of red blood corpuscles. The former is the usual type, and is described below; the latter is found in such conditions as pernicious anaemia, haemolytic anaemia, acholuric jaundice and snake poisoning.

When the bile cannot escape into the intestine in the usual way, it is absorbed by the blood- and lymph-vessels, and some of its constituents are deposited in the various tissues throughout the body. Some obstruction to the outflow of bile is therefore a necessary condition, and this obstruction may either exist in the bile-ducts, which convey the bile from liver to intestine, or it may be caused by some disorganization in the liver (e.g. hepatitis) which prevents the bile, formed by the liver-cells, from finding its way to the bile-ducts at all. The tint of the jaundice has not necessarily any direct relation to the severity of the cause. Obstruction may be due to gall-stones, and the resulting jaundice is then a symptom of this condition. (See GALL-BLADDER, DISEASES OF.) Obstruction may be due to some cause quite outside the liver and bile-ducts, for example, enlarged glands lying near the liver or cancer of the pancreas, the seriousness of the jaundice depending then upon the seriousness of the disease responsible for the pressure. In elderly people, who are likely to be the subject of cancer, long-continued jaundice is for this reason a serious symptom. Cirrhosis of the liver, in which the small branches of the bile-duct become compressed by the formation of fibrous tissue, may also be a cause of chronic jaundice. (See CIRRHOSIS.)

Among the causes which disorganize the liver, one finds many poisons which are carried to it in the blood – for example, phosphorus, mercury, and snake poison, as well as a number of widely used drugs. Much more common as a cause of jaundice are two inflammatory conditions of the liver, known as infective hepatitis and serum hepatitis (q.v.). They are both due to viruses but they differ in that the former has a shorter incubation period. Infective hepatitis, which is much the more common of the two, is the condition which used to be known as catarrhal jaundice. Certain infective diseases are also prone to produce this effect: e.g. yellow fever, malaria, typhoid fever and pyaemia. A serious but uncommon condition, accompanied by rapid and often fatal jaundice, is that known as acute yellow atrophy of the liver. Another form of jaundice is known as spirochaetal jaundice or *spirochaetosis ictero-haemorrhagica* (see LEPTOSPIROSIS). These conditions cause such changes in the liver that the bile is unable to escape except by reabsorption into the blood.

Neonatal jaundice is a form of jaundice not uncommon in the newborn infant. It is due to temporary inability to deal with the normal metabolism of bilirubin and usually passes off in a few days. If it should persist, however, or become severe, it requires treatment. The most effective form of treatment is exposure of the infant to blue light. This converts bilirubin into the harmless bile pigment known as biliverdin (q.v.). (See also BILIRUBIN; HAEMOLYTIC DISEASE OF THE NEW-BORN; KERNICTERUS.)

Symptoms: Yellowness, appearing first in the whites of the eyes and later over the whole skin, is the symptom that attracts notice. This tint varies from a pale sulphur-yellow through all gradations to a deep olive or bronze colour, according to the completeness of the obstruction and the length of time the jaundice has lasted. The urine passed during the time the jaundice lasts is of a dark greenish-brown colour, owing to the excretion of bile by the kidneys. Various digestive disturbances are present: the tongue is furred, the appetite poor, and a feeling of sickness is often felt, and is aggravated by eating fats. The stools are of a grey or white colour, owing to the want of bile in the intestine, and for the same reason constipation, relieved occasionally by diarrhoea, is present, and the stools have an excessively offensive smell. A bitter taste in the mouth is generally felt by the jaundiced person, due, as it is supposed, to the presence in the saliva of salts of the bile-acids; and the same or other substances in the sweat lead to itching of the skin. Slowness of the pulse, and, in long-continued cases, mental confusion and dullness, are other less evident accompaniments of jaundice.

Treatment: The first essential is to treat the underlying cause if possible: for instance, gallstones, if these be the cause of the jaundice. For the actual treatment of the jaundice the patient must be kept in bed. The diet should contain as much protein and carbohydrate as possible and a minimum of fat. The diet to be aimed at should contain 3000 Calories daily, including 100 to 120 grams of protein and supplemented with vitamins. Such a diet should not be forced in its entirety in the early days of treatment when the appetite is poor and the mere thought of food nauseating. For the pruritus, or itching, which may be very severe, calamine lotion containing 2 per cent phenol should be used. This may need to be supplemented with analgesics: e.g. aspirin or a tablet containing aspirin, paracetamol and codeine. Sedatives may also be required.

As the jaundice clears, the amount of protein may be reduced, and if there is much residual indigestion this is best treated by a modified peptic ulcer diet.

JAW is the name applied to the bones that carry the teeth. The two upper jaw-bones, the maxillae, are firmly fixed to the other bones of the face. The lower jaw, the mandible, is shaped somewhat like a horseshoe, and, after the first year of life, consists of a single bone. It forms a hinge-joint with the squamous part of the temporal bone, immediately in front of the ear. Both upper and lower jaw-bones possess deep sockets, known as alveoli, which contain the roots of the teeth. (See DISLOCATIONS; FRACTURES; GUMBOIL; MOUTH; TEETH.)

JEJUNUM is part of the small intestine. (See INTESTINE.)

JELLY (see GELATIN).

JERK: A sudden involuntary movement. The term is often used to describe the tendon reflexes.

JOINT-MOUSE is a popular term for a loose body in a joint. It is found especially in the knee. (See JOINTS, DISEASES OF.)

JOINTS: A joint or articulation is the meeting-place between different parts of the skeleton, whether bones or cartilages.

Structure: The great division of joints is into those which are fixed or relatively fixed (*fibrous* and *cartilaginous joints*), and those at which free movement can take place (*synovial joints*). In the former, a layer of cartilage or of fibrous tissue intervenes between the bones and binds them firmly together. This type of joint is exemplified by the sutures between the bones that make up the skull. Among these fixed joints, some have a thick disc of fibro-cartilage between the bones, so that, although the individual joint is really capable of very little movement, a series of these, like the joints between the bodies of the vertebrae, gives to the spinal column, as a whole, a flexible character (amphiarthrodial joint).

Into the formation of every *movable joint* four structures enter. These are the bones whose junction forms the joint; a layer of cartilage covering the end of each of these and rendering the ends smooth; a sheath of fibrous tissue known as the capsule, thickened at various points into bands or ligaments, which hold the bones together; and, finally, a membrane known as synovial membrane, which lines this capsule and produces a synovial fluid to lubricate the movements of the joint. Further, the bones are kept in position at the joints by the various muscles passing over them and by atmospheric pressure. This type of joint is known as a synovial joint.

Some joints possess subsidiary structures, such as discs of fibro-cartilage, which adapt the ends of the bones more perfectly to one another in places where these do not quite correspond. In others, movable pads of fat under the synovial membrane fill up larger cavities and afford additional protection to the joint.

Varieties: Apart from the main division of joints into those which are fixed and those which are movable, the movable joints fall into several groups. Gliding joints are those in which, like the wrist and ankle, the bones have

| 1 synovial membrane | 3 articular disc |
| 2 articular cartilage | 4 capsule |

(A) diagram of a simple synovial joint. (B) diagram
of a synovial joint with an articular disc.

flat surfaces capable of only a limited amount of movement. In hinge-joints, like the elbow and knee, the chief movement takes place round one axis. The ball-and-socket type is exemplified by the shoulder and hip, in which free movement is possible in any direction. There are other subsidiary varieties, named according to the shape of the bones which enter into the joint.

JOINTS, DISEASES OF: The larger joints, on account of their exposed position, are subject to constant injuries, and this, together with the wear they suffer and the richness of their blood supply, renders them liable to a number of serious diseases. The knee is the joint most often diseased, and after it, in order, the hip, ankle, and elbow. Although minor injuries may be followed by serious diseases, it is an important fact that very severe injuries, in which the skin remains unbroken, such as dislocations of, and fractures into, the joints rarely occasion any serious disease beyond stiffness and other direct results of the injury. On the other hand, penetrating wounds of joints are among the most serious injuries, and require immediate and expert treatment. The following are some of the conditions from which joints suffer.

SYNOVITIS is the name given to any inflammation of the membrane lining the joint cavity. It may be acute, subacute or chronic.

Causes: The joints being much exposed to blows, wounds and strains, some injury often precedes the onset of inflammation. In many cases, the condition is due to some rheumatic condition such as rheumatoid arthritis, osteoarthrosis, gout, or tuberculosis (qq.v.).

Symptoms: In acute synovitis, following usually upon some injury, the synovial membrane becomes inflamed, thickened, and secretes an excessive amount of fluid into the joint. As a result, the joint becomes painful, red, swollen and hot to touch. It is usually kept more or less bent, and is painful to straighten and to handle. If the synovitis remains of a simple nature, these symptoms last some days and then gradually subside. Or the condition may persist for a long time, getting better for a little and then relapsing; or it may become chronic, and, whilst

the heat and redness disappear, the joint remains stiff and distended with fluid. This condition most frequently affects the knee, and is then popularly known as water on the knee. On the other hand, in occasional cases which have begun in the simple form, and in cases due to a penetrating wound of the joint to which bacteria have gained entrance, a very serious inflammation occurs. Suppuration then takes place in the joint, an abscess forms with fever, great pain and other aggravated symptoms of abscess. A joint cavity is very difficult to render free from suppuration, and may even necessitate amputation of the limb in order to save life.

Treatment: In the early stages, complete rest of the joint, the limb being placed on a splint, together with the application of cold or of warm fomentations to soothe the pain, is alone necessary. Later, massage and compression of the joint by a bandage aid the absorption of the fluid and dispel the stiffness. When the condition becomes chronic, counter-irritation by iodine, blisters, etc., is necessary, and the joint is often punctured to draw off the fluid. Suppuration is, as already stated, a serious matter, and is treated like an abscess elsewhere by opening, irrigation with antiseptics, drainage and the administration of antibiotics.

SYNOVITIS OF THE HIP in a transient form is not uncommon in children. The precise cause is not known, but it tends to follow a cold or sore throat or an injury, and is more common in fat children. It occurs more often in boys than girls, and the commonest age is around six. The child suddenly complains of pain in the hip or is seen to be limping. No treatment is required except to prevent weight-bearing during the acute phase. The condition usually lasts for about a fortnight, and recovery is complete within a couple of months.

EPIPHYSITIS is an inflammation situated at the end of a long bone just outside the joint. An important point regarding this type of inflammation in children is that if the inflammation is severe it may permanently damage the plate of cartilage, situated close to the end of the bone, from which increase in length takes place, so that the child's limb may be seriously impaired in growth.

TUBERCULOUS DISEASE of a joint begins in the

synovial membrane or in the end of the bone, and is popularly known as white swelling, on account of the characteristic appearance of the affected joint, particularly when the knee is involved. In many cases there are other manifestations of the disease, the lungs, for example, being affected, or the glands of the neck enlarged. Tuberculosis of the joints is commoner in children than in older persons. A proportion of cases, especially in children, are due to the drinking of tuberculous milk.

Symptoms: The condition is usually chronic, begins insidiously, sometimes being dated from a slight accident, and progresses slowly. Slight stiffness, wasting of the muscles in the affected limb, and pain and tiredness brought on by slight exertion, are the earliest symptoms. The joint later on assumes its characteristic appearance, becoming enlarged, losing the natural hollows about it, and appearing white and glistening, with large veins showing through the skin. The wasting of muscle above and below the joint causes it to look still more enlarged than it really is. Gradually the use of the limb is lost, and the general health deteriorates. Later in the disease, when the joint is becoming thoroughly disorganized, starting-pains at night, which waken the sufferer as he is dropping off to sleep, become troublesome. If the condition remains untreated after this stage is reached, an abscess forms in the joint and bursts through the skin, and hectic fever develops.

Treatment: As in all other forms of tuberculosis the outlook has been revolutionized by the excellent results which have been obtained from the use of chemotherapy, giving combined therapy for at least six months. The use of chemotherapy has not only reduced the time of treatment by one-half, but has resulted in a much larger number of patients being left with almost full range of movement of the diseased joints.

STIFFNESS OF JOINTS may be due to various causes. It may result from spasm of the muscles around the joint in cases of early tuberculous disease and of hysterical joints, or it may be due to permanent shortening in these muscles or contraction of the skin, due, for example, to a burn. Often a severe injury to the joint itself, such as a fracture of one of the bones that form it, or a dislocation, is followed by some stiffness. A large number of slight injuries, which set up a mild degree of inflammation, are followed by some adhesions in the joint, often of a painful nature. These limit the use of the joint considerably, but, when they are broken by forcible movements of the limb, recovery and relief are immediate.

LOOSE BODIES IN JOINTS result from inflammation of various types, the bodies being developed as projections on the synovial membrane or on the cartilages of the joint, and later pulled off by its movements. They bring on repeated attacks of synovitis, and often cause sudden locking of the joint, so that for a time it is immovable. They are removed by operation.

GOUT, RHEUMATISM AND RHEUMATOID ARTHRITIS are diseases of a constitutional nature which affect joints. (See under these headings.)

SPRAIN is a vague popular term indicating the result of any slight wrench to a joint. A sprain consists generally of a mild attack of synovitis, or of tearing of ligaments with effusion of fluid into or round the joint. At the ankle, a twist of the foot inwards is followed by some tearing of the outer lateral ligament of the joint constituting a severe sprain, but a more serious accident, consisting of fracture at the lower end of the fibula, is apt to follow a wrench or twist of the foot outwards. (See FRACTURES.) In the knee, a sudden twist is occasionally responsible for loosening and rumpling up the inner of the two fibro-cartilages found in that joint. This accident has the awkward consequence of producing at subsequent times attacks of synovitis, or of sudden locking of the knee-joint. Behind the wrist and at the ankle, a sprain results sometimes in the displacement of some of the tendons which should be bound firmly to the bone, leading to occasional pain and a sense of weakness till the tendon happens to get replaced by another twist.

Treatment: When a sprain is of inflammatory character, the treatment is of the nature described under synovitis, and in the case of a bad sprain rest for a week or two may be essential. A sprain consisting in tearing of the ligaments round a joint, accompanied by effusion of blood beneath the skin, may be treated at the very beginning by applying wet compresses, or by holding the joint in a stream of cold water, which materially checks the effusion. After some time has elapsed, this form of treatment is of little use, and compression by a moderately tight, or by an elastic, bandage over the injured joint, together with elevation of the limb, forms a better line of treatment. The immediate application of an ointment containing heparinoid may also be of value. Massage is of great assistance in cases of sprain to prevent stiffness of the affected joint and to aid repair of injured tissues. Strapping (q.v.) of the affected joint is of use in the later stages of treatment and, in the case of sportsmen, may be retained during training, but should never be used, it has been said, 'as an excuse to allow an unfit joint back to competitive activity. Joints which are not strong enough to stand competition without strapping are not strong enough to stand competition at all.'

DISLOCATION (see DISLOCATIONS).

BURSITIS often occurs over the region of a joint. The prominences of several joints are protected by large bursae, and inflammation of these structures is sometimes mistaken for inflammation of the joint. (See BURSITIS.)

JOULE is the unit of energy in the International System of Units. The official abbreviation is J. 4186·8 J = 1 Calorie (or kilocalorie). (See also CALORIE; WEIGHTS AND MEASURES.)

JUGULAR is a general name for any structure in the neck, but is especially applied to three large veins, the anterior, external and internal jugular veins, which convey blood from the head and neck regions to the interior of the chest.

K

KALA-AZAR is another name for visceral leishmaniasis. (See LEISHMANIASIS.)

KANAMYCIN is an antibiotic derived from *Streptomyces kanamyceticus*. It is active against a wide range of organisms, including *Staphylococcus aureus* and *Mycobacterium tuberculosis*.

KAOLIN or CHINA CLAY, is a smooth white powder consisting of natural white aluminium silicate resulting from the decomposition of minerals containing felspar. It is used as a dusting powder for eczema and other forms of irritation in the skin. It is also used internally in cases of diarrhoea. The dose is 10 ml of Kaolin Mixture, BPC, best taken in water or milk before meals. Talc, French chalk and Fuller's earth are similar silicates.

Kaolin poultice contains kaolin, boric acid, glycerin and various aromatic substances.

KAOLINOSIS is a form of pneumoconiosis (q.v.) caused by the inhaling of clay dust.

KAPOSI'S SARCOMA: Once a very rare disease in Western countries, though more common in Africa, it is now a feature of AIDS (q.v.). It is a condition in which malignant skin tumours develop, originating from the blood vessels. The tumours form purple lumps which customarily start on the feet and ankles, then spread up the legs and develop on the arm and hands. In AIDS the sarcoma appears in the respiratory tract and gut and it causes serious bleeding. Radiotherapy normally cures mild cases of Kaposi's sarcoma but severely affected patients will need anti-cancer drugs to check the tumour's growth.

KAWASAKI DISEASE is a disease of childhood of unknown origin, which was first described in Japan but has now spread to Europe. It most commonly occurs between the ages of 6 months and 2 years, and is characterized by high fever, conjunctivitis (see EYE, DISEASE AND INJURIES), skin rashes, and swelling of the glands in the neck. In most cases there is complete and spontaneous recovery. Arteritis is however a common complication and results in the development of coronary artery aneurysms in 20 to 60 per cent of cases. These aneurysms and myocardial infarction are commonly detected after the second week of the illness.

KELOID is an overgrowth of fibrous tissue, usually on the site or scar of a previous injury. It gets its name from its claw-like off-shoots which pucker up the surrounding skin. It is sometimes painful, sometimes painless. It is much commoner in coloured than in white people. The most effective form of treatment is by injection of corticosteroids (q.v.) directly into the abnormal tissue. If this fails, surgical excision is performed.

KERATIN is the substance of which horn and the surface layer of the skin are composed.

KERATITIS (see EYE, DISEASE AND INJURIES OF).

KERATOMALACIA: Softening of the cornea due to a severe vitamin A deficiency (see EYE, DISEASE AND INJURIES OF).

KERATOPLASTY: Technical term for corneal graft.

KERATOSIS is a disease of the skin characterized by overgrowth of the horny layer of the skin (q.v.). It is induced by exposure to sunshine and in temperate climates usually develops in older people. In sunnier areas it may develop much earlier particularly in sun-bathing enthusiasts who repeatedly over-expose their skin to the sun. It takes the form of firm, dry adherent scales with redness of the surrounding skin and patchy pigmentation of the skin exposed to sunlight. Treatment, and prevention, consist of avoiding over-exposure to the sun.

KERION is a suppurating form of ringworm (q.v.).

KERNICTERUS is the staining with bile of the basal nuclei of the brain, with toxic degeneration of the nerve cells, which sometimes occurs in HAEMOLYTIC DISEASE OF THE NEWBORN (q.v.).

KERNIG'S SIGN is a sign found in cases of meningitis, consisting in the fact that, whereas a healthy person's thigh can be bent to a right angle with the body when the knee is straight, in cases of meningitis the knee cannot be straightened when the thigh is thus bent, or intense pain is caused to the patient by doing so.

KETOCONAZOLE is an imidazole antifungal drug available for both oral and topical use. It also has an anti-androgen effect which may give rise to gynaecomastia and impotence in men. In view of its potential hepatotoxicity it should not be given orally for trivial infections but reserved for systemic fungal infections.

KETOGENESIS: The production of ketones (q.v.) in the body. Abnormal ketogenesis may result in ketosis (q.v.).

KETOGENIC DIET is one containing such an excess of fats that acetone and other *ketone bodies* appear in the urine. It is sometimes used in the treatment of epilepsy and chronic infections of the urinary tract by *Escherichia coli*. In this diet, butter, cream, eggs and fat meat are allowed, whilst sugar, bread and other carbohydrates are cut out as far as possible.

KETONE is another name for acetone or dimethyl ketone. The term, ketone bodies, is applied to a group of substances closely allied to acetone, especially beta-hydroxybutyric acid and acetoacetic acid. These are produced in the body from imperfect oxidation of fats and protein foods, and are found in specially large amount in severe cases of diabetes mellitus. KETONURIA is the term applied to the presence of these bodies in the urine.

KETOPROFEN (see NON-STEROIDAL ANTI-IN-FLAMMATORY DRUGS).

KETOSIS: A condition in which an excessive amount of ketones (q.v.) are produced by the body and these accumulate in the blood stream. The affected person becomes drowsy, suffers a headache, breathes deeply, and may lapse into a coma. The condition results from an unbalanced metabolism of fat, which may occur in diabetes mellitus (q.v.) or starvation.

KIDNEY, ARTIFICIAL, is the term applied to a device designed to take over the function of the kidneys in cases of renal (kidney) failure. Such failure of the kidneys may be acute or chronic. In the acute form it may occur in a number of circumstances, including severe accidents such as the crush syndrome (q.v.), incompatible blood transfusions, mercury poisoning and severe haemorrhage in the later stages of pregnancy. It is also used in the treatment of chronic renal failure, and with increasingly satisfactory results. Thirty years ago, patients with chronic renal failure were not expected to survive. Today, as a result of progress in dialysis and kidney transplantation, a young patient with chronic renal failure and no complicating features has a better than 90-per-cent chance of living ten years and more. In most patients accepted for such treatment, the survival rate over five years exceeds 50 per cent.

The principle of the artificial kidney is that the patient's blood circulates through it and there comes in contact with a dialysing membrane, on the other side of which is a specially prepared dialysing fluid. In this way the biochemical balance of the blood is restored to normal, just as it would have been had the kidneys been functioning normally. (See DIALYSIS; HAEMODIALYSIS; TRANSPLANTATION.)

KIDNEYS are a pair of glands situated close to the spine in the upper part of the abdomen. They are on a level with the last dorsal and upper two lumbar vertebrae, and each is, to a great extent, covered behind by the twelfth rib of its own side. They are kept in this position by a quantity of fat and loose connective tissue, in which they are embedded, by the large vessels which supply them with blood, and by the peritoneal membrane stretched over their front surface.

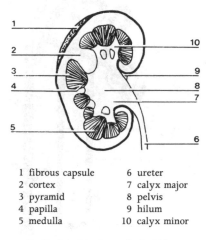

1	fibrous capsule	6	ureter
2	cortex	7	calyx major
3	pyramid	8	pelvis
4	papilla	9	hilum
5	medulla	10	calyx minor

Vertical section through the kidney

Structure: In size each is about 10 cm (4 inches) long, 6·5 cm (2½ inches) wide, 5 cm (1½ inches) thick and weighs around 140 grams (5 ounces). The size, however, varies a good deal with the development, and probably with the habits of the individual. Kidney mass maintains a remarkably constant ratio to body weight. The left kidney is slightly longer and narrower, and lies a trifle higher in the abdomen than the right.

The kidney in adults presents a smooth exterior, although in early life (as in many animals) it is divided up into distinct lobes, corresponding to the pyramids found in the interior. Enveloping it is a tough fibrous coat, which, in the healthy state, is bound to the kidney only by loose fibrous tissue and by a few blood-vessels that pass between it and the kidney. The outer margin of the kidney is convex, the inner is concave, presenting a deep depression, known as the hilum, where the vessels enter its substance. At the hilum the renal vein lies in front of the renal artery, the former joining the inferior vena cava, and the latter springing from the aorta almost at a right angle. Here, too, is attached the ureter, which conveys urine down to the bladder. The ureter is spread out into an expanded, funnel-like end, known as the pelvis, to which the capsule of the kidney is firmly attached, and which further divides into little funnels known as the calyces. On splitting open a kidney, one finds it to consist of two distinct parts: a layer on the surface, about 4 mm thick, known as the cortex, and a part towards the hilum known as the medulla. The latter consists of pyramids, arranged side by side, with their base on the cortex and their apex projecting into the calyces of the ureter. The apex of each pyramid, of which there are about twelve, is studded with minute holes, which are the openings of the microscopic uriniferous tubes.

1 glomerulus
2 proximal tubule
3 distal tubule

Diagram of a nephron.

Each pyramid is, in effect, taken together with the portion of cortex lying along its base, an independent little kidney. About a score of small tubes open on the surface of each pyramid, and these, if traced up into its substance, divide again and again so as to form bundles of convoluted tubules, known as medullary rays, passing up towards the cortex. If one of these is traced still further back, it is found, after a very tortuous course, to end in a small rounded body: the Malpighian corpuscle or glomerulus. Each glomerulus and its convoluted tubule is known as a nephron, which constitutes the functional unit of the kidney. Each kidney contains around one million nephrons.

If the blood-vessels are now traced through the kidney their course is found to be as follows. The renal artery splits up into branches, which form arches at the line of junction of cortex and medulla, and from these again spring vessels that run up through the cortex, giving off small branches in every direction. Each of these last ends in a little tuft of capillaries enclosed in a capsule (Bowman's capsule) that forms the end of the uriniferous tubule just described, and capillaries with capsule are known as a glomerulus. After circulating in the glomerulus, the blood emerges by a small vein, which again splits up into capillaries on the walls of the uriniferous tubules. From these it is collected

finally into the renal veins and by them leaves the kidney. By means of the double circulation, first through the glomerulus and then around the tubule, a large amount of fluid is removed from the blood in the glomerulus, and then the concentrated blood passes on to the uriniferous tubule for removal of parts of its solid contents. Other straight arteries come off from the arches mentioned above and supply the medulla direct, the blood from these passing through another set of capillaries and also finally into the renal veins. Although the circulation just described is confined entirely to the kidney, it has certain small connections both by arteries and veins which pass through the capsule and, joining the lumbar vessels, communicate direct with the aorta.

1 capillary tuft   4 glomerular capsule
2 tubule   5 efferent vessel
3 capsule   6 afferent vessel

Diagram of glomerulus.

Function: The chief function of the kidneys is to separate fluid and certain solids from the blood. Briefly, the glomeruli filter from the blood the non-protein portion of the plasma. As this filtrate passes through the convoluted tubules, varying parts of it are reabsorbed. It is estimated that in 24 hours the total human glomeruli will filter between 150 and 200 litres, 99 per cent of which is reabsorbed by the tubules. The constituents of the filtrate may be grouped according to the extent to which they are reabsorbed by the tubules: (1) substances actively reabsorbed, such as amino-acids, glucose, sodium, potassium, calcium, magnesium and chlorine; (2) substances passing through the tubular epithelium by a simple process of diffusion when their concentration in the filtrate exceeds that in the plasma, such as urea, uric acid, phosphates; (3) substances not returned to the blood from the tubular fluid: e.g. creatine.

When the kidneys are diseased and the number of glomeruli and tubules decreased in consequence, this alternating action is not so readily carried out, and therefore the work

1 interlobular artery
2 arcuate artery
3 interlobular vein
4 arcuate vein
5 ascending limb of Henle's loop
6 descending limb of Henle's loop
7 collecting tubule
8 distal convoluted tubule
9 proximal convoluted tubule
10 efferent arteriole
11 afferent arteriole

Diagram of renal tubules and blood supply of the kidney.

of the diseased kidney becomes increasingly embarrassed. When the blood-vessels of the kidney are partially closed by disease (arteriosclerosis), the general blood-pressure rises with the object of forcing more blood through the kidneys; in consequence, marked changes are produced upon the heart in this type of renal disease.

When the kidneys fail to act, these solid waste substances accumulate in the blood. The general 'poisoning' resulting from failure of renal functions produces the clinical condition known as uraemia (q.v.).

KIDNEYS, DISEASES OF: The kidneys, being deeply buried in the abdomen, give little direct sign even when seriously diseased, although many of the effects upon the general constitution are sufficiently marked and serious. Renal failure may be caused by a wide range of systemic disorders or by disease in the kidney itself. It can be treated by dialysis or by transplantation of a kidney (see KIDNEY, ARTIFICIAL).
General symptoms: The following are some of the general symptoms common to various types of kidney disease.

PAIN, of an aching nature, situated high up in the loins, is occasionally a symptom of inflammation of the kidneys, but pain in the lower part of the back is found in so many other diseases, and is so generally absent in serious kidney affections, that it is of little importance as a symptom. When a stone lodges in the ureter, however, there is a very definite type of pain known as renal colic. This pain is of an agonizing nature, shoots down from the kidney region to the groin, and usually appears with great suddenness.

URINE almost invariably shows changes in kidney diseases. In acute conditions it is diminished, generally contains albumin, and may be bloody. When unusual material is present in the kidney, careful examination of the urine generally reveals evidence of it: for example, pus in the urine points to an infection somewhere in the urinary tract; and when a stone is present in the kidney, its nature may often be shown by an examination of the crystalline deposit in the urine. In chronic glomerulonephritis the urine is generally increased in amount, pale and, as a rule, contains greater or less amounts of albumin. (See PROTEINURIA.)

OEDEMA, though due to many other conditions than glomerulonephritis, is an important symptom of this and other kidney troubles. When dependent upon some defect in the kidneys, it appears generally in the morning after sleep, and affects the loose tissues of the body, such as the skin beneath the eyes and that on the back of the hands, which become swollen and puffy.

URAEMIA is a condition which is present in all cases in which the function of the kidneys is seriously impaired. It is a general poisoning of the system by waste products which the kidneys have failed to excrete, and may be acute or chronic in type. (See URAEMIA.)

The most important class of diseases affecting the kidneys is that comprising the changes grouped together as glomerulonephritis, in which albumin is excreted in the urine and oedema is often present. (See GLOMERULONEPHRITIS.) The following are some of the other important affections of the kidney. (See also PYELITIS.)

GRAVEL and STONE are produced by the deposit in the urinary passages of solid substances which are naturally present in the urine, and whose deposition depends upon their presence in excessive amount, or upon the failure of some condition which in general keeps them in solution. The most common constituents of such stones or calculi are ammonium phosphate, calcium phosphate and calcium carbonate, calcium oxalate, and uric acid and urates.

Among many factors responsible for the formation of stones in the kidneys is alteration in the acidity or alkalinity of the urine. Thus an excessive acid reaction may be accompanied by the formation of uric-acid stones, whilst phosphate stones form in alkaline urine. Other factors which are associated with the formation of stones in the kidneys are prolonged recumbency; infection of the kidney; lack of vitamin A in the diet; over-action of the parathyroid glands (q.v.); a high level of calcium in the urine; excessive sweating, as in hot climates, leading to a persistently concentrated urine; gout; and leukaemia. The most common cause in Britain is an abnormally high level of calcium in the urine: the condition known as hypercalciuria. Stones are more common in men than in women, and may occur at any age and particularly among sedentary workers. Around 2 per cent of the population in the United Kingdom may have calculi, but a much higher incidence has been reported from other parts of the world, particularly the Middle East. In cases in which the presence of a stone is suspected, X-ray examination is an important procedure in diagnosis.

Treatment: This depends upon the size of the stone. If it is large, it has usually to be removed by operation. If it is small – less than 0·5 cm, it may be passed out in the urine spontaneously or following medical treatment. Stones larger than 1 cm require surgery. The drinking of large amounts of fluid may help. It is also helpful to alter the reaction of the urine. Thus, in the case of a uric-acid stone, the excessively acid urine is made alkaline by giving large doses of alkali: e.g. 2 grams of sodium bicarbonate four times daily. In the case of stones associated with a high level of calcium in the urine, promising results are being obtained from the administration of: bendrofluazide, one of the benzothiazines (q.v.); cellulose phosphate; a combination of the two; unprocessed bran. In the case of phosphate stones the excessively alkaline urine is made acid by the taking of 1 gram of ammonium chloride four times daily. If there is any infection of the kidney, this must be fully treated. The latest development is the use of ultrasonics to smash the stone into minute pieces which can then be passed in the urine. (See LITHOTRIPSY.)

RENAL CARBUNCLE is an abscess within the kidney. At one time the commonest cause was *Staphylococcus aureus* which reached the kidney via the blood-stream from staphylococcal infection elsewhere in the body. It is now more commonly due to infection spreading from the ureter or bladder. Patients debilitated by drug addiction and diabetes mellitus are especially at risk. The condition is characterized by pain in the loin and fever. The onset may be sudden with all the manifestations of septicaemia, or more gradual. Treatment consists of withdrawal of the pus and injection of the appropriate antibiotic into the abscess cavity.

TUBERCULOSIS of the kidneys is more common in adults than in children, and more common in men than in women. For a long time it may give rise to no symptoms or signs. It must therefore always be considered a possible diagnosis in cases in which urinary symptoms arise for which no cause can be found. Diagnosis partly depends upon the finding of *Mycobacterium tuberculosis* in the urine. As in other forms of tuberculosis, treatment is by anti-tuberculosis drugs: e.g. rifampicin, ethambutol and isoniazid. It is only in a minority of cases that surgical removal of the kidney is required.

INJURIES OF THE KIDNEY are very serious, although one of these organs may be completely shattered without a necessarily fatal result if the other kidney is healthy and uninjured. The kidney may be ruptured by a blow in the small of the back or when a person is run over, and death may result from the consequent loss of blood, which may appear in the urine.

TUMOURS of the kidney are not common. As a rule, they give little or no trouble till they have reached a large size. If growing in the pelvis of the kidney, large quantities of blood may be passed now and then in the urine with, however, no pain or other symptom referable to the kidney. *Congenital cystic kidney* is a form of tumour in the kidney which may last for many years with little trouble to the person in whom it occurs. *Hypernephroma* is a tumour that occasionally develops in the kidney, being composed of cells resembling the suprarenal gland in appearance. *Nephroblastoma* (or *Wilms' tumour*) is the commonest kidney tumour in infancy. It is a malignant tumour, which occurs in around 1 per 10,000 live births. The survival rate with modern treatment (removal of the kidney followed by radiotherapy and chemotherapy) is now around 80 per cent.

HORSESHOE KIDNEY: Around 10 per cent of all live-born infants are born with malformations of the kidneys. Horseshoe kidney, so called because of its shape, is among the commonest of these. It results from a partial fusion of the two kidneys, and is more common in males than females. In quite a number of cases, ranging from one-quarter to one-half according to different reports, the kidneys function normally. In the others the complications that are liable to occur are hydronephrosis (q.v.), pyelonephritis (see PYELITIS) and stones. Such kidneys are also more liable to develop cancer than normal kidneys. (See also TRANSPLANTATION.)

KINAESTHETIC SENSATIONS is a term used to describe those sensations which underlie muscle tension and position of joint and muscle. These sensations send impulses along nerves to the brain, and thus inform it of the position of the limb in space and of the relative position to each other of individual muscles and muscle-groups and of joints.

KININS are substances present in the body which are powerful vasodilators (q.v.). They also induce pain and are probably involved in the production of the headache of migraine. In addition, they play a part in the production of allergy (q.v.) and anaphylaxis (q.v.).

KINO is the dried juice of *Pterocarpus marsupium*, an Indian tree. It contains an astringent principle, and its powder is useful in the treatment of diarrhoea, the tincture being also used as a gargle for relaxed throat.

KISS OF LIFE (see RESUSCITATION).

KLEBSIELLA: A Gram-negative bacteria found in the intestinal, respiratory, and urogenital tracts of man and animals. Varieties of the bacteria, which are rod shaped and non-motile, can cause pneumonia and urinary infections.

KLEPTOMANIA is a psychological disorder in which the person afflicted has an irresistible compulsion to steal things, without necessarily having any need for the object stolen.

KLINEFELTER'S SYNDROME: The original syndrome described by Klinefelter consisted of gynaecomastia, testicular atrophy and infertility. Intelligence was unimpaired. Cases have been described with associated mental defects and striking tallness of stature but the only constant feature of the syndrome is testicular atrophy with resulting azoospermia and infertility. The atrophy of the testis is the result of a peritubular fibrosis which begins to appear in childhood and progresses until all the seminiferous tubules are replaced by fibrous tissue. Gynaecomastia, mental retardation and eunuchoidism may be associated but the first is inconstant and the two last are infrequent. Most patients with Klinefelter's syndrome have 47 chromosomes instead of the normal 46. The extra chromosome is an X chromosome so that the sex chromosome constitution is XXY instead of XY. Klinefelter's syndrome is one of the most common chromosome abnormalities and occurs in 1 in 300 of the male population. Patients with this syndrome show that the Y chromosome is strongly sex determining. Thus a patient who has an XXY chromosome constitution may have the appearance of a normal male and the only incapacity is infertility. However the loss of a Y chromosome leads to the development of a bodily form which is essentially feminine (see TURNER'S SYNDROME).

KLUMPKE'S PARALYSIS: Injury as a result of the stretching of a baby's brachial plexus during its birth may cause partial paralysis of the arm with atrophy of the muscles of the forearm and hand.

KNEE is the joint formed by the femur, tibia and patella (knee-cap). It belongs to the class of hinge-joints, although movements are much more complex than the simple motion of a hinge, the condyles of the femur partly rolling, partly sliding over the flat surfaces on the upper end of the tibia, and the acts of straightening and of bending the limb being finished and begun, respectively, by a certain amount of rotation. The cavity of the joint is very intricate: it consists really of three joints fused into one, but separated in part by ligaments and folds of the synovial membrane. The ligaments which bind the bones together are extremely strong, and include the popliteal and the collateral ligaments, a very strong patellar ligament uniting the patella to the front of the tibia, two cruciate ligaments in the interior of the joint, and two fibro-cartilages which are interposed between the surfaces of tibia and femur at their edge.

All these structures give to the knee-joint great strength, so that it is seldom dislocated. Its exposed position and the intricacy and consequent difficulty in cleansing its cavity, render this joint liable to be wounded, and make wounds of it very serious. The knee may also be affected by tuberculous disease.

A troublesome condition often found in the knee consists of the loosening of one of the fibro-cartilages lying at the head of the tibia, especially of that on the inner side of the joint. The cartilage may either be loosened from its attachment and tend to slip beyond the edges of the bones, or it may become folded on itself. In either case, it tends to cause locking of the joint when sudden movements are made. This causes temporary inability to use the joint until the cartilage is replaced by forcible straightening, and the accident is apt to be followed by an attack of synovitis, which may last some weeks, causing a certain amount of lameness with pain and tenderness especially felt at a point on the inner side of the knee. This condition can be relieved by wearing for a prolonged period of some months a bandage with pad or knee-truss which presses upon the inner side of the joint, or it may be more quickly remedied by an operation to remove the loose portion of the cartilage. Patients whose knees are severely affected by osteoarthritis or rheumatoid arthritis which cause pain and stiffness can now have the joint replaced with an artificial one. (See also JOINTS, DISEASES OF.)

KNEE JERK (See REFLEX ACTION).

KNOCK-KNEE, or GENU VALGUM, is a deformity of the lower limbs in such a direction that when the limbs are straightened the legs diverge from one another. As a result, in walking the knees knock against each other. The amount of knock-knee is measured by the distance between the medial malleoli of the ankles, with the inner surfaces of the knee touching and the knee-caps facing forwards.

Causes: The condition is so common in children between the ages of 2 to 6 years that it may almost be regarded as a normal phase in childhood. When marked, or persisting into later childhood, it is usually due to faulty muscular tone. The condition is aggravated in children who are overweight or debilitated. At one time rickets was a common cause, but this is seldom the cause today in Great Britain.

Treatment: If rickets is the cause this must be treated. If, as is usually the case, there is no obvious cause, no treatment is required for knock-knee up to 75 mm (3 inches) in a child under 7 years of age. In the vast majority of cases it will have righted itself by this age. If the degree of knock-knee is more severe than this splints may be necessary, or even operation. When there is established bony deformity with over 100 mm (4 inches) of separation at the age of 4 years, or when there is still a considerable degree of knock-knee at the age of 9 years, operation should be performed. This may consist of cutting away the prominent part of the inner side of the lower end of the femora.

KOCH'S BACILLUS: The original name for *Mycobacterium tuberculosis*, which causes tuberculosis (q.v.) It stems from the name of the German doctor who first identified the bacillus.

KOILONYCHIA is the term applied to nails that are hollow and depressed like a spoon, a condition sometimes associated with chronic iron deficiency.

KOPLIK SPOTS are bluish-white spots appearing on the mucous membrane of the mouth in cases of measles about the third day, and forming the first part of the rash in this disease.

KORSAKOW'S SYNDROME is a form of mental disturbance occurring in chronic alcoholism and other toxic states, such as uraemia, lead poisoning and cerebral syphilis. Its special features are talkativeness with delusions in regard to time and place, the patient, although clear in other matters, imagining that he has recently made journeys or been in distant places.

KREBS CYCLE: A series of cellular reactions starting and ending with oxaloacetic acid. Also called the citric acid or tricarboxylic acid cycle, it produces energy in the form of adenosine triphosphate and is the last stage in the biological oxidation of fats, proteins, and carbohydrates. Named after Sir Hans Kreb, a German biochemist working in England in 1900, who won the Nobel Prize for his discovery.

KUPFFER CELLS are the star-shaped cells present in the blood- sinuses of the liver (q.v.). They form part of the reticulo-endothelial system (q.v.) and are to a large extent responsible for the breakdown of haemoglobin into the bile pigments.

KURU is a slowly progressive fatal disease due to degeneration in the central nervous system, particularly the cerebellum (see BRAIN). It is confined to the Fore people in the Eastern Highlands of New Guinea. It is believed to be due to a slow virus infection acquired from the cannibalistic rite of eating the organs, particularly the brains, of deceased relatives (out of respect). This origin of the disease was suggested by the fact that originally it was a disease of women and children, and it was they who practised this rite. Since the rite was given up, the disease has largely disappeared in children, but still occurs in women as it has an incubation period of up to 20 years.

KWASHIORKOR is one of the most important causes of ill health and death among children in the tropics. It is predominantly a deficiency disease due to a diet deficient in protein. There is also some evidence that there may also be a lack of the so-called essential fatty acids. It affects typically the small child weaned from the breast and not yet able to cope with an adult diet, or for whom an adequate amount of first-class protein is not available, and it is mainly found in the less well-developed countries.

The onset of the disease is characterized by loss of appetite, often with diarrhoea and loss of weight. The child is flabby, the skin is dry, and the hair is depigmented, dry, sparse and brittle. At a later stage oedema develops and the liver is often enlarged. In the early stages the condition responds rapidly to a diet containing adequate first-class protein, but in the later stages this must be supplemented by careful nursing, especially as the child is very liable to infection.

KYPHOSCOLIOSIS: A combination of scoliosis and kyphosis (qq.v.) in which the spine is abnormally curved sideways and forwards. The condition may be the result of several diseases affecting the spinal muscles and vertebrae or it may happen during development for no obvious reason. Although braces may reduce the deformity, an operation may be necessary to correct it.

KYPHOSIS is the term applied to curvature of the spine in which the concavity of the curve is directed forwards. (See SPINE AND SPINAL CORD, DISEASES AND INJURIES OF.)

L

LABETALOL is an alpha- and beta-adrenoceptor blocker (see ADRENERGIC RECEPTORS) which is proving of value in the treatment of high blood-pressure.

LABIA: Lips. The labia majora and labia minora are the outer and inner lip-like folds of skin surrounding the entrance to the vagina.

LABIUM is the Latin word for a lip or lip-shaped organ.

LABORATORY ANIMAL ALLERGY (see ALLERGY).

LABOUR, or PARTURITION is the act of bringing forth young, and forms the end of pregnancy. Generally speaking, a normal labour is one in which the vertex of the child's head is born first, and the whole process ends favourably to mother and child within twenty-four hours, and without any operative interference. A first labour usually lasts from eight to sixteen hours, whilst the births of second and subsequent children tend to become progressively shorter. In 96 per cent of all cases the vertex of the child's head presents (that is, leaves the womb and descends through the vagina to the exterior first). In some cases, owing to a faulty position of the head or to the presentation of the child's face, the labour is considerably delayed, while for various reasons operative assistance may be necessary, in which case the labour is known as an instrumental one. The second most common presentation is the breech or buttocks. A rarer and more serious presentation is a transverse presentation, where the child lies obliquely across the womb. Various complications, such as deformities of the mother and child, an excessive amount of bleeding, the birth of twins, and various general conditions of the mother, such as heart or kidney disease or convulsions, may influence the progress of the labour.

Stages of labour: The process of labour is naturally divided into three stages. The *first stage* is that of dilatation of the cervix to permit the subsequent descent of the child. This is ushered in by the onset of the pains caused by the powerful intermittent contractions of the muscular wall of the womb. As time passes, these become more frequent and stronger. This stage is much the longest. The full dilatation of the cervix is usually accompanied by the rupture of the amnion, the membrane containing the fluid in which the fetus moves, and the sudden escape of the amniotic fluid or 'waters'. The two events, however, do not necessarily take place at the same time, and sometimes the amnion ruptures at a much earlier, and sometimes at a later, period.

The *second stage* is the stage of expulsion of the child, which descends through the bony girdle of the pelvis and passes down through the vagina to the exterior. During this passage through the pelvis, the child's head goes through certain movements by which it adapts itself to the alterations in the shape of the pelvic canal as it passes down. The size of the head of an average child is such that there is just room for it to pass through the pelvis and no more. Accordingly the head is liable to be considerably pressed upon during this stage of labour, and this pressure manifests itself in the moulding of the child's skull. This moulding, which is rendered possible by the softness of the bones and by the presence of spaces between the bones enables the head to pass down with the minimum of damage to the child and to the mother. In most cases the moulding disappears in the first day or two after birth. The second stage is one of strenuous muscular exertion, as not only the muscular wall of the womb, but the abdominal muscles and the diaphragm are all involuntarily called into play to aid the expulsion of the child. Pains are more severe, but at the same time the patient has a consciousness that she is making progress and this sometimes makes them more easily tolerated than the

pains of the first stage. The tying and cutting of the umbilical cord (see AFTERBIRTH) finally sever the child's vital connection with the mother.

The *third stage* is the stage of delivery of the placenta. It begins immediately the child is born and rarely lasts more than half an hour. It is associated with the loss of a certain amount of blood: on average about 280 ml (10 fluid ounces).

Many women find that moving about and changing position during the first stage eases the pain of the contraction. During the second stage the mother will tend involuntarily to hold her breath and press down during the pains, and this down-bearing, as it is called, is helpful and should be encouraged, as it will expedite delivery. It is a mistake to urge a woman to bear down during the first stage, as it does no good and merely exhausts her strength. After the child is born the cord is clamped in two places and cut between the clamps. After the delivery of the child there will be an interval of some minutes before the uterine contractions start once more, and as a rule only a few contractions are needed to bring about the expulsion of the placenta.

Abnormalities and dangers of labour: These may arise in connection with the presentation or position of the child, with the uterus or maternal pelvis, or from the mother's health. Although they are rare, they carry a significantly increased risk to mother and child, and expert help should be available during the delivery.

Complications of labour include bleeding during the third stage and puerperal infection. Expert help should be sought if any complication occurs.

Since 1955 maternal mortality in the United Kingdom has fallen by 50 per cent each decade. In the 1980s maternal deaths were well under 10 per 100,000 births. The main causes are thromboembolism, eclampsia and pre-eclampsia, ectopic pregnancy, and haemorrhage (qq.v.).

LABYRINTH: A convoluted system of structures forming the inner ear and involved in hearing and balance.

LACERATION: A wound to the skin or surface of an organ which results in a cut with irregular edges (cf. an incision produced with a knife which has smooth, regular edges).

LACHESINE is a mydriatic: i.e. it dilates the pupil of the eye. It is sometimes used for this purpose instead of atropine, as its action is of shorter duration.

LACRIMAL: Gland, duct, apparatus (see EYE, DISEASE AND INJURIES OF).

LACTATION is the period during which an infant is suckled on the mother's breast. (See BREASTS, DISEASES OF; INFANT FEEDING.)

LACTEAL is a lymphatic vessel that transmits chyle (q.v.) from the intestine. (See LYMPH.)

LACTIC ACID is a colourless, syrupy, sour liquid, which is produced by the action of a bacterium upon lactose. The growth of this organism and consequent formation of lactic acid cause the souring of milk, and the same change takes place to a limited extent when food is long retained in the stomach.

Lactic acid ($CH_3.CHOH.COOH$) is produced in the body during muscular activity, the lactic acid being derived from the breakdown of glycogen. Muscle fatigue is associated with an accumulation of lactic acid in the muscle. Recovery follows when enough oxygen gets to the muscle, part of the lactic acid being oxidized and most of it then being built up once more into glycogen.

LACTIC ACID BACILLI were introduced by Metchnikoff to prepare milk as a special article of diet. The bacilli, which are issued in various forms, are added to fresh milk, allowed to act on it in a warm place for several hours (according to the degree of sourness desired), and the milk is then consumed with the active bacilli. These, after a course of such treatment, come to replace the bacteria naturally found in the intestines, and are supposed to be less injurious to the system. The bacilli, which are harmless, have, in some cases of intestinal disease or of rheumatism, a beneficial action. Buttermilk has a similar effect. (See YOGHURT.)

LACTOSE is the official name for sugar of milk. (See SUGAR.)

LACTOSE INTOLERANCE is a form of indigestion which is much more common in certain coloured races than in white races. It is due to lack in the intestine of the enzyme (q.v.) known as lactase which is responsible for the digestion of lactose, the sugar in milk. In individuals the taking of milk is followed by nausea, a sensation of bloating, or distension, in the gut, abdominal pain and diarrhoea. Such disturbances after taking milk may also be due to the individual's being allergic to milk. Treatment is by means of a low-lactose diet. Foodstuffs high in lactose, such as fresh or powdered milk, and milk puddings should be avoided. Most people subject to it can tolerate fermented milk products and the small amounts of milk used in baking and added to margarine and sausages. In Britain it is said to occur in up to 80 per cent of non-white adults but only 5 per cent of white adults.

LACUNA means a small pit or depression.

LAEVULOSE is a sugar which forms one of the constituents of invert sugar. (See SUGAR.)

LAMBLIA (see GIARDIASIS).

LAMELLA is a small disc of glycerin jelly, 3 mm (⅛ inch) in diameter, containing an active drug for application to the eye. It is applied by insertion behind the lower lid.

LAMINECTOMY is an operation in which the arches of one or more vertebrae are removed so as to expose a portion of the spinal cord for removal of a tumour, relief of pressure due to a fracture, or disc protrusion.

LANOLIN is a fat derived from the wool of the common sheep. It is much used for ointments because it does not become rancid, and because it is supposed to have a special power of penetrating the skin. It is very sticky, and for use is mixed generally with an equal quantity of petroleum jelly to make it softer. Lanolin also possesses the valuable property of being able to mix with and absorb water to a considerable extent.

LANUGO: Soft fine hair covering the fetus. It disappears by the ninth month of gestation and is therefore only seen on premature babies.

LAPAROSCOPE: An instrument, consisting, essentially, of a metal cylinder, an eyepiece and a light source, which is inserted through a small incision into the abdominal cavity (which has already been distended with carbon dioxode gas). The laparoscope allows the contents of the abdominal cavity to be examined without performing a laparotomy (q.v.). Some operations may be performed using the laparoscope to guide the manipulation of instruments inserted through another small incision (e.g. sterilization, cholecystectomy). (See ENDOSCOPE.)

LAPAROTOMY is a general term applied to any operation in which the abdominal cavity is opened.

LARVA: The pre-adult stage in insects and nematodes occurring between the egg and the sexually mature adult.

LARYNGECTOMY is the operation for removal of the larynx.

LARYNGITIS, or inflammation of the mucous membrane of the larynx, may be either acute or chronic. This may be due to an infectious cause most commonly viral but also bacterial, or may be due to voice abuse.

ACUTE LARYNGITIS: **Causes**: This complaint is usually a concommitant feature of an upper respiratory-tract infection, usually viral in ori gin. It may accompany any form of infection of the upper respiratory tract. Excessive use of the voice, as in loud and prolonged speaking, singing or shouting, may also produce an acute laryngitis. Inhalation of irritating particles in vapours may also lead to acute laryngitis.

Symptoms: The main symptom is of hoarseness but there may also be pain in the throat. If there is marked swelling this may narrow the channel for the entrance of air leading to a noisy form of breathing called stridor. There may be some constitutional disturbance in the form of fever, malaise, generalized aches and pains and there may also be some difficulty in swallowing. A cough is a common accompanying symptom. The cough may be dry or may be productive of purulent sputum. The voice is hoarse and the breathing stridulous. The majority of cases of acute laryngitis require early voice rest, perhaps some steam inhalation and symptomatic treatment. Antibiotics are seldom necessary, although these would be prescribed if a bacterial infection were thought to supervene. Acute airway obstruction is an unusual event following laryngitis but, if the airway becomes threatened in any way, immediate specialist referral should be sought.

Treatment: Bed rest may be indicated if severe constitutional symptoms are present. The voice should be rested and smoking forbidden. Steam inhalations and warm gargles are often soothing and help reduce mucosal oedema or swelling. Antibiotics should be prescribed if indicated. Some form of airway intervention, either endotracheal intubation or tracheostomy may have to be performed on rare occasions if severe obstruction results.

CHRONIC LARYNGITIS: This may occur as a result of repeated attacks of acute laryngitis or may arise independently due to such causes as habitual exposure, especially when, along with this, there is an over-indulgence in alcohol and the habitual over-use of the vocal cords. Patients are often smokers. Chronic laryngitis may be caused, or exacerbated, by nasal obstruction, leading to excessive mouth breathing. The changes taking place in the vocal cords are more permanent than in the acute form, consisting mainly in thickening of the mucous membrane of the vocal cords. Rarely, chronic laryngitis is due to tuberculosis, syphilis or other chronic inflammatory diseases. These are apt also to produce ulceration of the vocal cords and other parts of the larynx with gradual destruction of its cartilages. The symptoms are similar to those of acute laryngitis except more prolonged. Any doubts as to diagnosis on initial examination would require examination under anaesthetic using a direct laryngoscope by which a view of the affected parts can be obtained and the proper treatment instituted.

Treatment: Voice rest is essential. Any aggravating factors should be removed. Antibiotics are indicated if bacterial infection has supervened. The assistance of a speech therapist is of immense value. Smoking should be forbidden and alcohol preferably avoided. In resistant cases of chronic laryngitis a surgical procedure may be required in which the mucous membrane of the vocal cords is stripped in the hope that a more normal mucous membrane may be generated.

TUBERCULOUS LARYNGITIS practically always occurs as the result of infection spreading from the lungs. This is fortunately a rare disease in developed countries and the treatment involves the administration of anti-tuberculous drugs. It is always necessary to distinguish tuberculous laryngitis from carcinoma of the larynx.

TUMOURS and various inflammatory growths are often met with in the larynx and may give rise to hoarseness. Such growths may be benign or malignant. Benign tumours or small nodules, such as singer's nodules, may be dealt with by speech therapy or may be removed at the operation of direct laryngoscopy. This is usually performed under general anaesthetic. Cancer of the larynx may be treated either by radiotherapy or by surgery, depending on the extent of the disease. Hoarseness may indeed be the only symptom of vocal cord disturbance or of carcinoma of the larynx and any case of hoarseness which has lasted for 6 weeks should be referred for a specialist opinion, so that the larynx can be viewed to exclude the presence of carcinoma. The earlier the diagnosis is made, the more successful the results of treatment are. Laryngectomy clubs are now being established throughout the country to advise and help patients who have had laryngectomy. Details of these can be obtained from the National Association of Laryngectomee Clubs, Ground Floor, 6 Rickett Street, Fulham, London SW6 1RU (071-381 9993). An important feature of patients who have undergone laryngectomy is the rehabilitation of their speech and the assistance of a speech therapist is fundamental to performing such surgery with the aim of the patient's producing some form of voice following surgery.

Other abnormalities of voice may be caused by paralysis of either of the vocal cords. This may be a congenital problem or may be the result of pressure upon the recurrent laryngeal nerve by aneurysm or tumour or the nerve may be damaged in operations on the chest and neck. The symptom in this condition is one of weakness of the voice rather than actual hoarseness. *Aphonia* is a condition in which there is no voice at all. This is usually of psychological origin and the diagnosis is made after excluding any local pathology. Once again, the assistance of a speech therapist is invaluable.

LARYNGOLOGY is that branch of medical science concerned with disorders and diseases of the larynx.

LARYNGOSCOPE: Examination of the larynx may be performed indirectly with use of a laryngeal mirror, or directly by use of a laryngoscope. The direct examination is usually performed under general anaesthetic.

LARYNGO-TRACHEO-BRONCHITIS

(CROUP) is an acute infection of the respiratory tract in infants and young children. It is usually a virus infection or may be caused by *Haemophilus influenzae*. The onset is variable but the croupy cough and stridulous breathing usually occur a few days after the onset of a viral upper-respiratory-tract infection. The harsh barking cough is typical of the condition. The majority of children with this condition can be treated with humidification and antibiotics if necessary, but they should always be referred for specialist assessment and hospitalization is preferable in all cases. Rarely, some form of intervention is necessary and this will either be in the form of endotracheal intubation or of a tracheostomy.

LARYNX is the organ of voice and also forms one of the higher parts of the air passages. It is placed high up in the front of the neck and there forms a considerable prominence on the surface. It is covered in front by the skin, a layer of fibrous tissue and a thin layer of muscles, whilst its sides are protected by the lateral lobes of the thyroid gland and by the large sterno-cleidomastoid muscles.

The larynx is almost 5 cm or 2 inches in height and forms a sort of box, well protected in front by cartilages, rather more open behind and communicating above with the pharynx at the root of the tongue and below the windpipe or trachea. The larynx is enclosed by five large cartilages: the thyroid cartilage, whose prominent pointed front forms the Adam's apple; the cricoid cartilage, a ring placed below it; the epiglottis, a leaf-like cartilage projecting above the thyroid cartilage into the interior of the throat at the root of the tongue; and a pair of arytenoid cartilages jointed to the top edge of the cricoid cartilage behind, where the thyroid cartilage is deficient. There are also four small nodules of cartilage above the arytenoids. The edges of the laryngeal cartilages do not fit closely together, and the spaces between are filled up by membranes. Certain of the ligaments which bind the cartilages together are of great importance. These pass along each side of the larynx, from the arytenoid cartilage behind to the thyroid cartilage in front, two bands of elastic fibres covered by the mucous membrane which lines the whole larynx. One pair of these bands lies directly above the other, the upper pair being known as the false vocal cords; the lower pair are the true vocal cords. The latter are capable of various degrees of tenseness and slackness and of approximation and separation, these results being achieved by several small muscles, which are attached to the arytenoid cartilages and governed in their movements through branches of the vagus nerves. Between the true and false cord is a deep depression on each side known as the ventricle of the larynx. The larynx is lined throughout by mucous membrane, which generally is covered by ciliated cells; but over the true cords, which are subject to much friction in the production of the voice, the surface consists of flattened cells similar to those of the skin.

The vocal cords vibrating in different notes, according to their tenseness and the like, produce the sounds of voice and speech (q.v.).

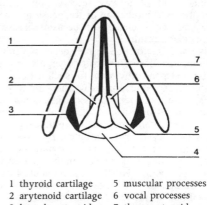

1 thyroid cartilage 5 muscular processes
2 arytenoid cartilage 6 vocal processes
3 lateral arytenoid 7 thyroarytenoid
4 arytenoid muscles

Diagram of the opening of the larynx to show the action of the muscles. The cords are now held together by the action of 3, 4 and 7.

1 thyroid cartilage
2 arytenoid cartilage
3 upper border of cricoid cartilage
4 posterior crico-arytenoid muscles
5 muscular processes
6 vocal processes

Diagram of the opening of the larynx to show the action of the muscles. A horizontal section has been made at the level of the true vocal cords. The two cords are widely separated by the action of 4.

LASER stands for Light Amplification by Stimulated Emission of Radiation. The light produced by a laser is of a single wavelength and all the waves are in phase with each other, allowing a very high level of energy to be projected as a parallel beam or focused on to a small spot. Various gases, liquids and solids will emit light when they are suitably stimulated. A gassed laser is pumped by the ionizing effect of a high voltage current. This is the same process

1 epiglottis 5 corniculate cartilage 8 vocal fold
2 vallecula 6 aryepiglottic fold 9 tubercle of epiglottis
3 trachea 7 vestibular fold 10 glossoepiglottic fold

A laryngoscopic view of the interior of the larynx.

1 epiglottis 9 ventricle of larynx 16 cricoid cartilage
2 aryepiglottic fold 10 thyroid cartilage 17 vocal cord
3 tubercle 11 epiglottis 18 respiratory glottis
4 ventricular fold 12 adipose tissue 19 artyenoideus muscle
5 vocal fold 13 ventricle 20 corniculate cartilage
6 interior thyro-arytenoid muscle 14 thyroid cartilage 21 cuneiform cartilage
7 cricoid membrane 15 cricothyroid membrane 22 false vocal cord
8 cricothyroid membrane

Vertical section of larynx: (A) from behind, (B) from left side.

as that used in a fluorescent tube. Each type of laser has a different effect on biological tissues and this is related to the wavelength of the light produced. The wavelength determines the degree of energy absorption by different tissues and because of this different lasers are needed for different tasks. The argon laser produces light in the visible green wavelength which is selectively absorbed by haemoglobin. It heats and coagulates tissues and it is thus possible to seal bleeding blood vessels and to selectively destroy pigmented lesions. The carbon-dioxide laser is the standard laser for cutting tissue. The infra-red beam it produces is strongly absorbed by water and so vaporizes cells. Thus by moving a finely focused beam across the tissue it is possible to make an incision.

The two main uses of the laser in surgery are the endoscopic photocoagulation of bleeding vessels and the incision of tissue. Lasers have important applications in ophthalmology in the treatment of such disorders of detachment of the retina and the diabetic complication of proliferative retinopathy. Lasers have three great advantages. They are potent, they act speedily and they can be focused on a small area, even an area as small as one micrometre.

LASSA FEVER, which derives its name from the fact that it was first reported in Lassa in Nigeria, is a disease due to an arenavirus (q.v.). This may be transmitted by rodents or direct from an infected person to those around him. The incubation period is three to twenty-one days. It is characterized by headache, lethargy and severe muscular pains, and there is often a rash due to bleeding into the skin and mucous membranes. Sore throat is often present. It may carry a high mortality rate, particularly in pregnant women. As it is a virus infection, there is no specific treatment, and all that can be done is careful nursing, with rest in bed.

LASSAR'S PASTE, officially known as Zinc and Salicylic Acid Paste, BP, is a preparation used as a remedy for eczema. It has a combined softening, antiseptic, astringent, and soothing action. It is made up of zinc oxide 24 grams; salicylic acid 2 grams; starch 24 grams; white soft paraffin 100 grams.

LATERAL Referring to the sides of an organ or the body or that part furthest from the midline or median plane.

LAUDANUM is the popular name for tincture of opium. (See OPIUM.)

LAUGHING-GAS is a popular name for nitrous oxide gas (q.v.).

LAVAGE is the name applied to the washing out of the stomach.

LAXATIVES (see PURGATIVES).

LEAD has no action itself upon the system, but its salts, when absorbed in any quantity, or for any length of time, have very important effects. When a lead salt comes in contact with a wound or with any mucous surface, it combines with the albuminous material of the discharge or secretion to form a whitish glaze, which affords a degree of protection to the surface. Further, the lead salt has an astringent action upon the blood-vessels, and therefore helps to stop bleeding or relieve the congestion of inflammation. If one of the soluble lead salts is taken internally, in large amount, it has an irritant action, and the acetate (sugar of lead), subacetate, and nitrate of lead are irritant poisons when taken into the stomach, although their action is comparatively feeble.

LEAD POISONING: Acute poisoning by lead acetate (sugar of lead) is an accident which sometimes, though rarely, happens to a child, and is treated, like cases of irritant poisoning generally, by administering diluents such as milk together with Epsom salts, which form an antidote, followed by emetics.

Chronic poisoning is apt to affect those who come in contact with lead or its salts, either in the production of these or in the course of their use. In Great Britain in 1978–79 there were 24 cases of certified incapacity due to lead poisoning arising out of the victim's work but only one case in 1984. Thus lead-smelters, plumbers, file-makers, pottery workers who use lead in glaze, painters, dyers, above all, those who make white-lead, are liable to suffer. Another industrial lead health hazard is tetra-ethyl lead which is added to petrol as an 'anti-knocking' agent. The risk here is to workers cleaning petrol storage tanks. Whether it has any effect on the general population in this automobile-ridden age is still a moot point, but the lead content of petrol is being reduced. Lead-containing paint was a common cause of lead poisoning in children in the form of pica (q.v.) which manifests itself by the chewing of painted woodwork. Lead may also be introduced into the system through food and water, in those who have nothing to do with the metal in their work. For example, drinking-water is sometimes contaminated by lead which it has dissolved off the pipes through which it passes. Cider, made in leaden presses, may so readily take up lead that 'Devonshire colic' was once a name given to lead-poisoning occurring in this part of the country, where cider forms a favourite beverage. The experts differ as to the critical level of lead in the blood. For many years it has been accepted that blood lead concentrations of over 80 micrograms per decilitre are likely to pose health risks, with clear evidence of the risk of mental and behavioural impairment above this level. Conversely the general view has been that blood lead levels of under 35 micrograms per decilitre will not normally produce a health hazard. The current view is that it would be a wise precaution to accept this lower level and to investigate any individual in whom the blood lead level exceeds 35 micrograms per decilitre.

Control over lead in food in England and Wales is exercised by the Lead in Food Regulations 1961 (revised in 1979). These Regulations lay down a limit of 1 mg per kg for most foods, with different levels for certain specified foods including canned meat and meat pastes, fish and fish pastes, for which a maximum of 5 p.p.m. is permitted. There are similar regulations for Scotland and Northern Ireland. Subsequent Regulations created a new category for foods specially prepared for infants and young children, and set a limit of 0·5 p.p.m. for this category. The upper allowable limit for lead in potable water is 0·1 mg per litre. Under an EEC directive the permitted quantity is 0·05 mg per litre. As regards drinking-water there is, in general, no danger, because the minerals in the water form, with the lead, insoluble compounds which are deposited in a thin coat upon the inside of the pipes. A greater danger exists in peaty or soft water, or in water contaminated by organic impurities, both of which give the water a high power of dissolving lead. Not only may the lead be introduced into the system through the skin of those who constantly handle lead-containing materials, and by way of the stomach, but in some of the most rapidly produced and serious cases – for example, among white-lead workers, and glazers of pottery – the lead is inhaled as dry dust. Lead is often similarly inhaled by men engaged in cutting up iron plates which have been fitted by the aid of red lead; this, being driven off by the heat of the blow-pipe employed, is apt to be inhaled.

Symptoms: Among the early symptoms of a chronic and insidious case are constipation, muscular weakness, and pallor of the skin. A blue line on the margin of the gums, due to deposit of lead sulphide in this locality, is also an important sign of the condition. Colic of a very painful nature, affecting the centre of the abdomen and lasting often for several days at a time, appears and forms one of the most prominent symptoms in almost every case. Lead has a specially damaging action upon the nervous system, causing an inflammatory process in the nerves, which results in tremors and paralysis, usually affecting the muscles on the back of the wrist first of all, and later those on the front and outer side of the leg, and causing wrist-drop and foot-drop. Convulsions, which may develop rapidly and may end in death, are also produced by poisoning of the nervous system, leading to a brain disorder known as lead encephalopathy. Occasionally, though fortunately rarely, affection of the optic nerve leads to blindness, which is either temporary or permanent. Owing to interference with the kidney functions, the urine becomes scanty, while a destructive action on the blood leads to anaemia.

Treatment: With regard to workers in lead and its salts, government regulations have been introduced which very effectively protect them. Among these preventive measures are included: personal cleanliness in washing the hands and changing the clothes before partaking of meals, the use of respirators by those who come in contact with white-lead dust, the provision of exhaust flues and electric fans beneath the tables at which pottery glazers work, and the drinking of at least a glass of milk daily. These and other measures confer a great degree of protection upon those engaging in these otherwise dangerous trades. Workers who begin to show symptoms of lead poisoning should at once undergo treatment. A frequent recurrence of symptoms shows a special liability to this form of poisoning, and indicates that the worker should seek some totally different employment. In the case of drinking-water the source of contamination must, of course, be removed. The drug which is of special use in treatment of lead-poisoning is sodium calcium-edetate, by which lead salts deposited in the tissues are dissolved, to be afterwards excreted from the body. Colic is treated by hot fomentations, magnesium sulphate, and belladonna, and a high calcium diet.

In acute cases of lead colic the intravenous administration of calcium gluconate or calcium chloride gives immediate relief.

LEBER'S DISEASE, or HEREDITARY OPTIC ATROPHY, is a hereditary disease in which blindness comes on at about the age of twenty.

LECITHIN is a very complex fat found in various tissues of the body, but particularly in the brain and nerves, of which it forms a large part. It is also found in large quantities in the yolk of an egg.

LEECHES are animals belonging to the class Vermes, provided with suckers and living a semi-parasitic life, their food being mainly derived from the blood of other animals. They abstract blood by means of a sucker surrounding the mouth, which is provided with several large sharp teeth. The medicinal leech, *Hirudo medicinalis*, was formerly employed for the abstraction of small quantities of blood in inflammatory and other conditions.

LEG: This term is generally applied to the whole lower extremity but, properly speaking, includes that part between the knee and ankle joints. The lower limb is attached to the pelvic bones by strong muscles, especially the gluteal and hamstring muscles behind and the abductor muscles on the inner side of the thigh. The head of the femur, or thigh bone, lies in a deep cup-shaped hollow, the acetabulum, on the outer side of the pelvis. The femur, which is the longest and strongest bone in the body, forms at its lower end the joint of the knee with the tibia. The knee-joint is protected in front by the patella or knee-cap. Along the outer side of the tibia lies the smaller fibula, which does not extend up to the knee but which, along with the tibia, forms the ankle joint. The two prominences on the ankle (*malleoli*) are formed by the tibia on the inner side and the fibula on the outer side. Seven tarsal bones comprise the hinder part of the foot, of which the talus takes the weight of the body from the tibia and fibula. There are five metatarsal bones in the front portion of the foot and each toe has three phalangeal bones, excepting the great toe which has two. The powerful quadriceps extensor muscle in front of the thigh is attached to the knee-cap, which in turn is attached to the front of the tibia by the patellar ligament. This muscle straightens the knee and keeps the body in an erect posture. Below the knee the muscles of the calf, attached to the heel through the tendo calcaneus, or tendon of Achilles, raise the heel off the ground in walking. In front of and to the outside of the leg lie the tibial and peroneal muscles, which bend the ankle upwards and raise the toes. In the sole of the foot are a number of small muscles which bend the toes downwards. The arch of the foot is a very important structure. (See FOOT.)

Most of the blood supply to the lower limb is carried by the femoral artery, which issues from the abdomen in the middle of the groin where its pulse can be felt. This passes down the inner side of the thigh to reach the middle of the back of the knee where it is known as the popliteal artery. Below the knee it divides into anterior and posterior tibial vessels. The former of these runs down the front of the leg and upper surface of the foot, and the latter, which is the larger, passes behind the inner ankle where its pulse can be felt about a finger's breadth behind the bony prominence. The blood returns from the leg partly by deep veins lying alongside the arteries, but to a large extent by the great saphenous vein, which can be seen or felt under the skin for most of the distance from the ankle up the inside of the leg and thigh to the inner side of the groin, where it joins the femoral vein.

The chief nerve in the lower limb is the sciatic nerve which runs down the middle of the back of the thigh deeply embedded in muscles. Above the knee it divides into two parts: the tibial and common peroneal nerves. The former of these runs down the back of the leg, deeply embedded in muscles, to the foot, and the latter passes round the upper end of the fibula on the outer side of the leg, where it can be felt and is liable to be damaged.

The arch of the foot is liable to give way, especially in debilitated or overworked people, thus producing flat foot. The ankle joint is liable to sprains which consist of tearing of the ligaments, especially on the inner side. The fibula is liable to be fractured near its lower end (a common accident in professional soccer players), either by twists of the foot or by a blow on the outer side of the leg. Fracture of the tibia is also a common accident and, as the tibia lies immediately beneath the skin, this fracture is in danger of becoming compound. The knee-joint, by reason of its great strength, is seldom dislocated, but the partial displacement of a cartilage in the knee is a common occurrence. Fracture of the femur is a serious accident, requiring a period of several months for complete union of the bone. The long and poorly supported vein on the inner side of the leg and thigh is very apt to become distended along with its branches, producing the condition known as varicose veins with resultant eczema and ulcer. The bursa in front of the knee-cap, in people who kneel a lot, readily becomes inflamed and thickened in the condition known as 'housemaid's knee'. (See also FOOT; FRACTURES; JOINTS; KNEE; LIMBS; VEINS.)

LEGIONNAIRE'S DISEASE is a form of pneumonia due to a bacterium known as *Legionella pneumophila*. The bacterium is widely distributed in nature and is commonly found in surface water and soil. Legionnellae are ubi-quitous in water. Stationary water and sludge in water tanks provide favourable conditions for primary multiplication. Inhalation of water aerosols seems the most likely way that people acquire the disease. The organism is able to multiply at water outlets. Some rubber outlets in showers and taps are able to support the growth of legionnellae so that high concentrations of the organism are released when the tap is first used in the morning. In the presence of the disease the treatment of infected water systems is essential by cleaning, chlorination or heating or a combination of all three.

The pneumonia caused by legionnellae has no distinctive clinical or radiological features, so that the diagnosis is based on laboratory findings. This depends on the detection of antibodies by the indirect fluorescent antibody test. There is no evidence that the disease is transmitted directly from person to person. The predominant root of infection is by inhalation. The incubation period is two to ten days. The disease starts with aches and pains followed rapidly by a rise in temperature, shivering attacks, cough and shortness of breath. The X-ray tends to show patchy areas of consolidation in the lungs. The assessment of treatment is still hampered by the lack of proper clinical trials but it does seem that erythromycin and rifampicin are the most useful antibiotics. Rifampicin, however, should never be given alone because of the rapid development of drug resistance. In England in 1984 there were 151 cases reported to the Public Health Surveillance unit. Between 1985 and 1987 200 cases were reported each year and in 1990 the total in England and Wales had fallen to 179, with a ratio of three men to one woman's being affected.

LEIOMYOMA is a tumour made up of unstriped or involuntary muscle fibres.

LEISHMANIASIS is a group of diseases due to infection with a number of parasites, of the genus known as Leishmania. The parasite is transmitted to man by the bite of certain sandflies. It is estimated that there are 400,000 new cases every year.

VISCERAL LEISHMANIASIS or KALA-AZAR, also known as DUM-DUM FEVER, occurs in tropical and sub-tropical Africa and Asia, the Mediterranean area and in tropical South America. It is caused by a parasite known as *Leishmania donovani*. The source of the infection, the type of sandfly that transmits it to man, and the common age of infection vary from one area to another. Thus, in the Mediterranean region it is predominantly a disease of infants, whereas in Africa it tends more to occur in adolescents and young adults. The onset may be sudden or gradual. In the well-established case there is enlargement of the spleen and of the liver, accompanied by fever and generalized glandular enlargement. The diagnosis is established by removing a piece of bone marrow, spleen or liver, and examining it for the presence of the cutaneous   visceral

Distribution of cutaneous and visceral leishmaniasis.

causative parasite. Untreated the disease is usually fatal in at least 70 per cent of cases either in the acute stage or after two years or so.
Treatment: Sodium stibogluconate, a pentavalent antimonial compound, is the drug of choice. The response to treatment varies with the area in which the infection occurs. Thus, in India, the disease usually responds to one ten-day course of injections, whereas in the Mediterranean region two or three such courses may be needed. A high proportion of cases are cured in this way.
CUTANEOUS and MUCO-CUTANEOUS LEISHMANIASIS is the form of the disease in which the parasite involves predominantly the skin and mucous membranes, and sometimes also cartilage. It is caused by a variety of species of Leishmania, and is known by different names in different geographical areas. Thus, in South America it is known as espundia, whereas in Asia it is known variously as oriental sore, Delhi boil, Aleppo boil, Baghdad boil, Biskra boil (or button). In the Old World it tends to be restricted to the skin, producing a chronic ulcer, whereas in the New World it tends to be more diffuse, involving the nose and throat, and leading to widespread erosion of the nasal cartilage; it may well terminate in a fatal broncho-pneumonia.
Treatment is by sodium stibogluconate, but most of the cases in the Old World heal spontaneously, though slowly, and the affected area merely needs to be protected and kept clean.

LEMON is used in the form of the fresh peel, tincture, syrup, and oil. Its main value, however, is as a source of vitamin C (or ascorbic acid), the average content of ascorbic acid in the juice being 45 mg per 100 grams. (See also CITRIC ACID; VITAMIN.)

LENS OF THE EYE (see EYE).

LENTIGO is another name for freckles (q.v.).

LEPROSY is a chronic disease which affects particularly the skin, mucous membranes, and nerves.
Causes: The causative organism of leprosy is the *Mycobacterium leprae* which was discovered by Hansen in 1872. It is a straight or slightly curved rod which closely resembles the *Mycobacterium tuberculosis* in its size and acid-fast staining reaction.
The World Health Organization estimates that there are between 10 and 15 million people world-wide affected by leprosy, about half of them in Africa and India. The incubation period, or latent period between the infection's being acquired and the disease's manifesting itself is considered to be between 3 and 5 years or even longer. Males are more commonly infected than females. It is uncommon below the age of 4 years, and no case has yet been reported before the age of 18 months. The variation of incidence among different races is due to contact rather than racial susceptibility, but the type of the disease varies in different races. Thus, the European and Mongol races appear to be more likely to acquire the serious lepromatous type of leprosy than the Indian and African races. There is some evidence that malnutrition may increase susceptibility to the disease. The disease is transmitted by contact with open cases of leprosy. The nasal secretion of such open cases is swarming with leprosy bacilli, and this is the likeliest source of infection for people in contact with open cases. The bacillus can also be present in the breast milk of infected mothers. Only a few of the people exposed to infection develop the disease, and those in contact with tuberculoid cases are much less likely to develop the disease than those in contact with lepromatous cases.
Symptoms: There are two distinct types of leprosy: tuberculoid and lepromatous. The differentiation is important because the former

runs a relatively benign course and is often self-healing, whereas the latter is a steadily progressive form of the disease. The differentiation, however, is not always clear cut, and there is a group of 'indeterminate' or 'dimorphous' cases in which lesions similar to tuberculoid and lepromatous leprosy are seen in the same patient. The differentiation of those three types is a matter for the expert, and no attempt will be made here to go into the details of the different types.

Whatever form of leprosy may be present, the symptoms and signs can be divided into two main groups: those involving the skin and those arising from involvement of the nerves. The skin manifestations range from areas of whitening of the skin to massive nodules. The nerve manifestations range from localized swellings of the nerve to extensive areas of anaesthesia in the skin. The ultimate destruction of the nerves leads to the deformities which used to be such a marked feature of leprosy before adequate means of treatment became available. These included foot-drop, wrist-drop, claw-foot, extensive ulceration of the extremities leading to loss of the fingers and toes, and absorption of bone. The eyes may also be infected, leading to blindness, and ulcers may occur in the mouth and in the larynx. In the larynx they may cause hoarseness or even go on to the stage of producing complete blockage of it. These tragic cases of gross deformity, which in the past have made leprosy such a terrifying disease, should no longer occur. As Cochrane has pointed out: 'With the introduction of modern therapy the vast majority of cases, if treated adequately before extensive deformity has set in, should recover without any disability. Nevertheless, until adequate treatment and properly administered therapy are within the reach of all, the shadow of tragic deformity will remain, particularly where there is a failure to understand the importance of physiotherapy in preventing this.'

Treatment: Widespread use of the sulphones has gone far to bringing leprosy under control. The most widely used sulphone is dapsone, which is given by mouth. Given over long periods of time, most cases of leprosy respond satisfactorily. Various other drugs have been introduced during recent years for the treatment of leprosy. The most promising are rifampicin, clofazimine, and ethionamide. Unfortunately the *Mycobacterium leprae* is developing resistance to dapsone when this is given alone. To reduce this risk to a minimum, it is necessary to give it along with some other anti-leprosy drug.

Chemotherapy, however, has not diminished the importance of physiotherapy in the treatment and prevention of deformity in leprosy. Equally important is the role of plastic and orthopaedic surgery in treating these deformities when they have reached a stage in which physiotherapy is of little use. Many patients with advanced leprosy, hitherto condemned to a life of chronic invalidism as a result of their deformities, are now being returned to the community as useful members who are able to use their hands and feet sufficiently to be able to earn a living and lead a reasonably active life.

LEPTOMENINGITIS means inflammation of the inner and more delicate membranes of the brain or spinal cord.

LEPTOSPIRA is a group, or genus, of spiral micro-organisms, normally found in rodents and other small mammals in which they cause no harm. When transmitted to man by these animals, either directly or indirectly as through cows, they give rise to various forms of illness.

LEPTOSPIROSIS is the disease caused by infection with Leptospira. The three most common members of this group in the United Kingdom are *L. icterohaemorrhagiae*, *L. canicola*, and *L. hebiomadis*. It is an occupational hazard of farmers, sewage and abattoir workers, fish cutters and veterinary surgeons, but the infection can also be acquired from bathing in contaminated water. There were 72 cases, seven of them fatal, in the British Isles in 1981. Nine of them were due to immersion in polluted water. The figures for 1984 show a reduction in the incidence in sewage workers but a rise in the incidence in farmers. The disease varies in intensity from a mild influenza-like illness to a fatal form of jaundice due to severe liver disease. The kidneys are often involved and there may be meningitis. Penicillin or tetracycline are the usual treatment but unless they are given early in the disease their effect is limited. SPIROCHAETOSIS ICTEROHAEMORRHAGICA, or WEIL'S DISEASE, is the term applied to infection with the *Leptospira icterohaemorrhagiae* which is transmitted to man by rats, these animals excreting the organism in their urine; hence the liability of sewer workers to the disease. The condition is characterized by fever, jaundice, enlarged liver, nephritis, and bleeding from mucous membranes. There were 39 cases in the British Isles in 1981.

LESBIAN: A female homosexual (q.v.)

LESION meant originally an injury, but is now applied generally to all disease changes in organs and tissues.

LETHARGY or LASSITUDE means a loss of energy. It is a common presenting complaint to both the general practitioner and hospital consultant. It may have a physical cause or a psychological cause. It may be the result of inadequate rest, environmental noise, boredom, insomnia or recent illness. It may be the result of drugs, the most common of which are beta-blockers and diuretics. The common psycho-social problems producing lethargy are depression and anxiety. If the patient with lethargy runs a fever the differential diagnosis is that of a PUO (Pyrexia of unknown origin).

Many patients with fatigue can establish the onset of the symptom to a febrile illness even though they no longer run a fever. The lethargy that follows glandular fever and other viral infections is well recognized. Some of these patients have a true depressive illness and their presentation and response to treatment is little different to sufferers from any other depressive illness. Organic causes of lethargy include anaemia, malnutrition, hypothyroidism, uraemia, alcoholism and diabetes mellitus.

LETTUCE is a green vegetable consisting of leaves of *Lactuca sativa*. It is a relatively rich source of vitamin A. The content of vitamin C is variable, ranging from 1 to 17 mg per 100 grams.

LEUCINE is one of the essential, or indispensable, amino-acids (q.v.). They are so called because they cannot be synthesized, or manufactured, in the body, and are therefore essential constituents of the diet.

LEUCO- (or LEUKO-) is a prefix meaning white.

LEUCOCYTE is the term applied to the white blood cells. Leucocytes differ from erythrocytes in that they contain no haemoglobin and are therefore colourless, and contain a well- formed nucleus. Most of them are larger than erythrocytes, being 8 to 15 micrometres in diameter, and there are many fewer in the blood – usually about 8000 per cubic millimetre of blood. There are three main classes of white cells: granulocytes, lymphocytes, and monocytes. *Granulocytes*, or polymorphonuclear leucocytes as they are sometimes termed, which normally constitute 70 per cent of the white blood cells, have a lobed nucleus and a granular cytoplasm. They are divided into three groups according to the staining reactions of these granules: neutrophils, which stain with neutral dyes and constitute 65 to 70 per cent of all the white blood cells; eosinophils, which stain with acid dyes (e.g. eosin) and constitute 3 to 4 per cent of the total white blood cells; and basophils, which stain with basic dyes (e.g. methylene blue) and constitute about 0·5 per cent of the total white blood cells. *Lymphocytes*, which constitute 25 to 30 per cent of the white blood cells, have a clear non-granular cytoplasm and a relatively large nucleus which is only slightly indented. They are divided into two groups: small lymphocytes which are slightly larger than erythrocytes (about 8 micrometres in diameter); large lymphocytes, which are about 12 micrometres in diameter. *Monocytes*, which constitute about 5 per cent of the white blood cells, are 10 to 15 micrometres in diameter and differ from lymphocytes in having a rather smaller nucleus which tends to be more indented and to be placed more eccentrically. Monocytes are motile phagocytic cells that circulate in the blood and migrate into the tissues where they develop into various forms of macrophages such as tissue macrophages and Kupffer cells. They remove micro-organisms from the body and identify and present antigenic material to lymphocytes. The cytoplasm is non-granular.

Site of origin: The granulocytes are formed in the red bone marrow. The lymphocytes are formed predominantly in lymphoid tissue. There is some controversy as to the site of origin of monocytes: some say they arise from lymphocytes, whilst others contend that they are derived from histiocytes: i.e. the reticuloendothelial system (q.v.).

Function: The leucocytes constitute one of the most important of the defence mechanisms against infection. This applies particularly to the neutrophil leucocytes. (See LEUCOCYTOSIS.) (See also ABSCESS; BLOOD; INFLAMMATION; PHAGOCYTOSIS; WOUNDS.)

LEUCOCYTOSIS means a temporary condition in which the polymorphonuclear leucocytes in the blood are increased in number. It occurs in many different circumstances, and forms a valuable means of diagnosis in certain diseases. It may occur, however, as a normal reaction in certain conditions: e.g. pregnancy, menstruation, and during muscular exercise. Apart from these conditions, leucocytosis is usually due to the presence of inflammatory processes. It is part of the body's defence mechanism against infection with micro-organisms, the purpose of the increase in the number of leucocytes being to help to destroy the invading bacteria. Thus, during many acute infective diseases, such as pneumonia, the number is greatly increased. In all suppurative conditions there is also a leucocytosis, and if it seems that an abscess is forming deep in the abdomen, or in some other site where it cannot be readily examined, as, for example, an abscess resulting from appendicitis, the examination of a drop of blood gives a valuable aid in the diagnosis, and may be sufficient, in the absence of other signs, to point out the urgent need of an operation. Typhoid fever constitutes the major exception to the statement that acute infective diseases show this increase of white corpuscles in the blood, and, accordingly, in the case of this disease, the presence of an increase is a specially reliable sign of abscess formation, or other severe complication.

Other infective conditions in which a leucocytosis does not occur include measles and influenza.

LEUCODERMA, or LEUCODERMIA, is a condition of the skin in which areas of it become white, as the result of various skin diseases.

LEUCOPENIA is a condition in which the white corpuscles of the blood are greatly reduced in numbers.

LEUCOPLAKIA is a chronic condition of the tongue in which, as the result of various forms of irritation, hard, smooth, whitish patches develop on its surface.

LEUCORRHOEA is a vaginal discharge that may be acute, when the discharge is thick and white, consisting mainly of pus, or more often chronic and catarrhal, when the discharge is usually thinner, sometimes of a clear mucous nature; in other cases acrid and offensive. The discharge may precede or follow the menstrual flow; in severer cases it continues throughout the whole intervening periods.

Causes: Leucorrhoea may arise as a result of infection anywhere in the genital tract in women: i.e. in the uterus, cervix, or vagina. The commonest cause is some chronic inflammation of the womb following on childbirth, and associated with some laceration of its neck. Another important cause is gonorrhoea. In other cases is is due to infection of the vagina with the *Trichomonas vaginalis* (q.v.). A not uncommon cause is infection with *Candida albicans* resulting in the condition known as thrush. The condition may occur as a symptom of general debility. It may also be due to a tumour in the uterus or the cervix. An occasional cause of very offensive discharge is found in the irritation set up by the presence of a foreign body, such as a pessary that has been introduced for the support of a displaced womb, and then forgotten.

Treatment: This depends upon the cause of the discharge. Thus, if it is due to infection with *Trichomonas vaginalis* (q.v.) metronidazole should be given. If it is due to gonorrhoea it is this that must be treated. (See GONORRHOEA.) If it is due to *Candida albicans* nystatin should be given. If it is due to an erosion of the cervix, or neck of the womb, this must be treated. In women past the menopause, or the change of life, the most effective treatment may be administration of an oestrogen (q.v.). (See also UTERUS, DISEASES OF.)

LEUCOTOMY (see PSYCHOSURGERY).

LEUKAEMIA, or LEUCOCYTHAEMIA, is a disease in which the number of white corpuscles in the blood is permanently increased. The disease is also characterized by great enlargement of the spleen, changes in the marrow of the bones, and by enlargement of the lymph glands all over the body. The condition may be either acute or chronic. According to the type of corpuscles chiefly present the acute form is called acute lymphoblastic leukaemia, or acute myeloblastic leukaemia. The names for the corresponding chronic forms of the disease are chronic lymphatic leukaemia, and chronic myeloid leukaemia. Acute lymphoblastic leukaemia is most common in the first five years of life, and rare after the age of 25. Acute myeloblastic leukaemia is most common in children and young adults, but may occur at any age. Chronic lymphatic leukaemia occurs at any age between 35 and 80, most commonly in the 60s, and is twice as common in men as in women. Chronic myeloid leukaemia is rare before the age of 25, and most common between 30 and 65. Men and women are equally affected. Each year over 5,000 new cases of leukaemia are diagnosed in the UK: around 4,000 people die from it.

Cause: The cause of the disease is unknown. In many ways it resembles a form of malignant disease characterized by uncontrolled overproduction of the white blood corpuscles.

Symptoms: In the acute cases the patient shows pallor, occasional purpuric rash, and enlargement of the lymphatic glands and spleen. The temperature is raised, and the condition may be mistaken for an acute infection. Such cases usually run a rapid course, lasting a few weeks or months. In the chronic type of the disease the onset is gradual, and the first symptoms which occasion discomfort are either swelling of the abdomen and shortness of breath, due to painless enlargement of the spleen, or the enlargement of glands in the neck, armpits and elsewhere, or the pallor, palpitation, and other symptoms of anaemia which often accompany the malady. Occasional haemorrhages from the nose, stomach, gums, or bowels may occur, and may be severe. Generally, there is a slight degree of fever. When the blood is examined microscopically, not only is there an enormous increase of the white corpuscles, which may be multiplied thirty- or sixty-fold, but various immature forms of corpuscles are found. In the lymphatic form of the disease the white corpuscles consist chiefly of corpuscles resembling in some measure the lymphocytes, which, in healthy blood, are present only in small numbers. In the myeloid form, myelocytes, or large immature corpuscles out of the bone-marrow, which are never present in healthy blood, appear in large numbers, and there may also be large numbers of immature, nucleated, red blood corpuscles.

Although there is still no cure, the outlook in both acute and chronic leukaemia has changed considerably for the better; particularly is this the case in the acute form of the disease. Thus, in the case of acute lymphoblastic leukaemia, which accounts for around 85 per cent of all childhood leukaemias, the overall survival rate may be as high as 60 per cent, with the chance of inducing a remission reaching 90 per cent. The results in acute myeloblastic leukaemia are not nearly so satisfactory. In the case of chronic lymphatic leukaemia the average period from the time of diagnosis to death is around six years, although quite a number of cases, particularly the elderly, survive for ten years or more. In chronic myeloid leukaemia the average survival time is around three to four years, with 20 per cent surviving for more than five years.

Treatment: Unfortunately, there is no certain cure for either the acute or the chronic forms of leukaemia but, as has been noted, promising results are being obtained in the control of the disease, especially by means of chemotherapy and bone-marrow transplantation. In the case of acute leukaemia the drugs now being used include mercaptopurine, methotrexate, cyclophosphamide, and vincristine. But cortisone and its derivatives sometimes produce dramatic temporary improvement. Blood transfusion plays an important part in controlling the condition during the period before the response to chemotherapy or hormone therapy can be expected. Chemotherapy has almost completely replaced radiotherapy in the treatment of chronic leukaemia. For the myeloid form busulphan is the most widely used drug, replaced by hydroxyurea, mercaptopurine, or one of the nitrogen mustard derivatives (q.v.) in the later stages of the disease. For the lymphatic form the drugs used are chlorambucil, cyclophosphamide, and the nitrogen mustard derivatives.

LEUKOPLAKIA: A white plaque on mucous membranes caused by overgrowth of the tissues. It is occasionally a precancerous condition.

LEUKOTRIENES are a group of slow-reacting substances (SRSS) which have powerful smooth-muscle stimulating properties.

LEVALLORPHAN TARTRATE is an antidote to morphine. It is usually given intravenously. In opium poisoning the dose is 1 to 2 mg, repeated if necessary.

LEVAMISOLE is a drug that is proving of value in the treatment of ascariasis (q.v.). Its main advantage seems to be in mass treatment as one dose may prove effective. It is also being used in the treatment of a group of diseases of obscure origin including Crohn's disease (q.v.) and rheumatoid arthritis.

LEVODOPA: A drug used in the treatment of Parkinson's disease (q.v.). It is converted to dopamine in the brain, correcting the deficiency which causes the disorder. Carbidopa is often given with it to prevent its conversion to dopamine in the body before it reaches the brain. It may cause nausea, hypotension (q.v.) or cardiac dysrhythmias.

LEVORPHANOL is a synthetic derivative of morphine. It is an effective analgesic but, like morphine, is a drug of addiction.

LIBIDO is the desire for sexual intercourse. Lack of desire or diminished libido may occur in any general medical illness as well as in endocrine diseases when there is a lack of production of the sex hormones. It is frequently associated with psychiatric diseases and may be the result of certain drugs. It must be distinguished from impotence where the desire for intercourse is normal but the performance is defective due to the inability to achieve or maintain an erection.

LICE (see INSECTS IN RELATION TO DISEASE; PEDICULOSIS).

LICHEN is a term applied to a group of chronic skin diseases characterized by thickening and hardening of the skin, with the formation of papules (q.v.). *Lichen simplex* develops as a result of persistent scratching. The cause of the itching is often obscure. The disease is more common in women than in men. In women it occurs most commonly in the nape of the neck. It also occurs on the back of the forearm, the inner part of the thigh, the back of the knee and around the ankle. The skin becomes thickened, and has been compared in appearance to that of morocco leather, but there are no papules. Treatment consists of that of the underlying condition if this can be recognized, and the application of corticosteroid cream and emollients. *Lichen planus* begins on the wrists and then spreads to the body and legs. The eruption is characteristic, consisting of purplish, shiny papules with thickening of the surrounding skin. The papules are often found as well in the mouth. The cause is obscure. In some it is apparently nervous or emotional in origin. In some it is due to drugs, including the organic arsenical drugs, gold, mepacrine, chloroquine, and para-aminosalicylic acid (PAS). It usually persists for some three months, but occasionally it may last for years. Treatment consists of the corticosteroids (q.v.) given by mouth and applied locally.

LIGAMENTS are strong bands of fibrous tissue which serve to bind together the bones entering into a joint. They are, in some cases, cord-like, in others flattened bands, whilst most joints are surrounded by a fibrous capsule or capsular ligament. (See JOINTS.)

LIGATION: Tying off – for example, a blood vessel – by completely encircling it with a tight band usually of catgut or some other suture material.

LIGATURE means a cord or thread used to tie round arteries in order to stop the circulation through them, or to prevent escape of blood from their cut ends. Ligatures are generally made of catgut or silk, and are tied with a reef-knot.

LIGHT REFLEX: Pupillary constriction in the eye in response to light. The direct light reflex involves pupillary constriction in the eye into which a light is shone; the consensual light reflex is the pupillary constriction that occurs in the other eye. The afferent or inward pathway of the reflex is via the optic nerve (see EYE) and the efferent or outward pathway is via the occulomotor nerve.

LIGHTNING INJURIES are not uncommon – it is estimated that lightning strikes somewhere on the earth an average of 100 times a second, but the majority of those struck by lightning recover. A direct hit, however, means instantaneous death, with the clothes torn off, and the victim may be hurled quite a long distance. Even the individual who recovers falls unconscious the moment he is struck. Those who are a little farther away experience tingling of the skin and their hair may stand on end.

Preventive measures indoors during a lightning storm consist of keeping away from the fireplace, the main electrical switch, the bathroom, the kitchen sink and the television aerial. It is perfectly safe to use the telephone. There is no point in drawing the curtains, pulling down the blinds, covering mirrors or taking off metal-frame spectacles. Out of doors, solitary trees, walls, wire fences and other metallic structures such as sheds, park seats and tent-poles, ponds and river banks should be avoided. So also should flat open spaces, such as golf courses, where an individual may form the highest point. To use a metal-tipped umbrella or a golf club is asking for trouble. There is no risk inside a motor car, but it is wise to avoid moors or hills and make for the nearest low ground. If the storm is really severe, the safest thing is to lie down in a ditch. In Britain, there are around 10 deaths a year from being struck by lightning.

Treatment of an individual struck by lightning consists of artificial respiration, which may need to be prolonged for several hours. (See APPENDIX: BASIC FIRST AID.)

LIGHT TREATMENT: The visible spectrum of white light, extending from red to violet, gives waves of different character. Beyond these, in the infra-red and ultra-violet regions, are numerous varieties of waves.

SUNLIGHT TREATMENT: Much of the benefit of sunshine is derived from its ultra-violet rays, and natural sunshine is preferable to ultra-violet rays produced by an ultra-violet lamp as it contains the complete spectrum of rays as well as those of light and heat. It is essential for the formation of 1–25 dihydrocholecalciferol, and children who do not get enough exposure to sunlight are at risk of developing rickets. Too much ultraviolet light predisposes to malignant melanoma.

INFRA-RED RADIATIONS employed in treatment are those with wave-lengths immediately below those of luminous rays. Infra-red rays are given out by bodies at a dull red or glowing temperature. The best source of these is sunshine, and they are also derived from incandescent light bulbs with tungsten filament, carbon arc lamps, and ordinary electric radiators at a red heat. These infra-red rays penetrate through the skin to a depth of 6 to 25 mm (¼ to 1 inch), and their action in moderate dosage is to dilate blood vessels and so produce an increased blood supply to the exposed part, and to exert a soothing action on its sensory nerves. They are useful therefore in rheumatic conditions, injury near the surface, to promote absorption and relieve pain, and in certain septic skin conditions such as boils and carbuncles. Apparatus is obtainable which supplies infra-red rays without luminous rays, but this has no advantage over sunshine or electric bulbs, which supply both infra-red and luminous rays, except in cases in which strong light is objectionable, as for example in treatment of conditions near the eyes. When deep penetration of heat is required, diathermy apparatus is used. (See DIATHERMY.)

LIGNOCAINE is a local anaesthetic. It is also used in the treatment of certain disorders of cardiac rhythm known as ventricular arrhythmias which may be particularly dangerous following a coronary thrombosis (q.v.).

LIMBS are outgrowths from the sides of the body, which, in man as in all the higher animals, number four. The limbs of all the higher animals, though differing much in outward appearance, are constructed on a similar plan, modified to suit the requirements of the owner, the fore-limb, for example, developing in birds into a wing, in seals into a flipper. In all, however, the various muscles, bones, and blood-vessels, though differing in size and shape, correspond in arrangement. Also, between the upper and lower limb, a strict comparison is possible, and the bones, muscles, and main arteries of the arm, forearm, and hand have all representatives in the thigh, leg, and foot. (See ARM; LEG.)

The union of the lower limb with the body is, however, more intimate than that of the upper limb. For, whilst the shoulder-blade and collar-bone of the upper limb are separated from the organs of the chest by the ribs and their muscles, the haunch-bone is applied on each side directly to the spine and forms the side of the pelvis.

In structure, each limb consists of four segments, the shoulder, arm, forearm, and hand in the case of the upper limb, corresponding to the haunch, thigh, leg, and foot in the lower limb. Upon the surface, the limb is enveloped by skin which, over the hand, is specially rich in its supply of sensory nerves. Beneath the skin is a layer of loose cellular tissue containing an amount of fat which varies with the corpulence of the individual. Next comes a strong layer of fibrous tissue, known as fascia, which provides a complete investment for the limb, and supplies a separate sheath for each muscle. The chief bulk of the limb is made up by the muscles or flesh. Finally, in the centre of the limb lie the bones which give it rigidity; and in general the large arteries and nerves are embedded among the muscles close to the bones.

The diseases affecting the limbs are those of the skin, muscles, bones, etc., forming them. (For injuries of the limbs see FRACTURES; HAEMORRHAGE; JOINTS, DISEASES AND INJURIES OF; WOUNDS.)

LIME-JUICE is a yellow liquid obtained by squeezing lime-fruit, *Citrus limetta*. In common with lemon-juice, it is a rich source of vitamin C (16·8 to 62·5 mg per 100 ml) and contains a large quantity of citric acid. It is used as a refreshing drink and as a preventive of, and remedy for, scurvy (q.v.). Lime-juice which has been boiled, or preserved for a prolonged period, loses its anti-scorbutic properties.

LINCOMYCIN is an antibiotic derived from *Streptomyces lincolnensis*. It is active against a relatively limited number of bacteria, including staphylococci, streptococci, pneumococci and *B. anthracis*.

LINCTUS is a term applied to any thick syrupy medicine. Most of these are remedies for excessive coughing.

LINEA ALBA is the line of fibrous tissue stretching down the mid-line of the belly from the lower end of the sternum to the pubic bone. The linea alba gives attachment to the muscles of the belly wall.

LINEA NIGRA: During pregnancy the linea alba (q.v.) becomes pigmented and appears as a dark line down the middle of the belly, and is called the linea nigra.

LINEAR ACCELERATOR (see RADIO-THERAPY).

LINGUAL: Referring or related to the tongue: e.g. the lingual nerve supplied sensation to the tongue.

LINIMENTS, or EMBROCATIONS, are preparations intended for external application, generally with rubbing. Almost all are of an oily nature, and are highly poisonous, being dispensed therefore in green or blue bottles. Liniments should never be kept alongside medicines intended for internal use, because many fatalities occur through careless administration, a dose being poured out of the wrong bottle. Among the chief liniments are: aconite, belladonna, and camphor liniments, often mixed together in equal parts to form ABC liniment, which is used for neuralgia, rheumatism, and other painful conditions; iodine liniment, used to paint over enlarged glands, and swollen joints; methyl salicylate liniment, used to apply in various painful rheumatic conditions; white liniment, which contains turpentine, used especially for sprains, bruises, and rheumatic conditions; liniment of ammonia, popularly known as 'hartshorn and oil', used for the same purpose; and soap liniment, known also as 'opodeldoc', of like application.

LINT was originally made of teased-out linen; now it consists of a loose cotton fabric, one side of which is fluffy, the other being smooth and applied next to the skin when the surface is broken. Marine lint consists of tow impregnated with tar, and is used where large quantities of some absorbent and deodorizing dressing are required. Cotton lint is impregnated with various substances, the most common being boracic lint. Lint containing perchloride of iron (15 per cent) is valuable as a styptic.

LIPAEMIA means the presence of an excessive amount of fat in the blood.

LIPASE is an enzyme widely distributed in plants, and present also in the liver and gastric and pancreatic juices, which breaks down fats to the constituent fatty acids and glycerol.

LIPID is a term which is used rather loosely. Strictly speaking, it means a substance which is insoluble in water but soluble in fat solvents such as alcohol and ether. The important lipids, so far as medicine is concerned, are the fats (or triglycerides), and the phospholipids which play an important part in the functioning of the membranes of the cells of the body.

LIPODYSTROPHY is a congenital maldistribution of fat tissue. Subcutaneous fat is totally absent from a portion of the body and hypertrophied in the remainder. Another form of lipodystrophy occurs at the site of insulin injections. These are much less frequently seen nowadays as the new synthetic preparations of insulin are pure and unlikely to cause this reaction which was not uncommon with the older preparations. Occasionally the converse occurs at the site of insulin injections where the lipogenic action of insulin stimulates the fat cells to hypertrophy. This can also be disfiguring and usually results from using the same site for injections too frequently.

LIPOLYSIS: The enzymatic breaking down of fat.

LIPOMA is a tumour mainly composed of fat. Such tumours arise in almost any part of the body, developing in fibrous tissues, particularly in that beneath the skin. They are simple in nature, and seldom give any trouble beyond that connected with their size and position. (See TUMOUR.)

LIPOSARCOMA: A malignant tumour of adipose or fatty tissue. It occurs most frequently in the thighs, buttocks or retroperitoneum. The four main types are: well differentiated, myxoid, round cell and pleomorphic.

LIPOSOMES are essentially tiny oil droplets consisting of layers of fatty material known as phospholipid separated by aqueous compartments. Drugs can be incorporated into the liposomes, which are then injected into the bloodstream or into the muscles, or given by mouth. Using this method of giving drugs, it is possible to protect them from being broken down in the body before they reach the part of the body where their curative effect is required: for example, in the liver or in a tumour.

LIPS form a pair of curtains before the mouth, each composed of a layer of skin and of mucous membrane, between which lies a considerable amount of fat and of muscle fibres.

The diseases to which the lips are liable are not numerous. *Fissures*, coming on in cold weather, form a troublesome condition often difficult to get rid of. Such peeling and cracking of the vermilion of the lips is common in those exposed for long periods to wind and sunlight. Treatment consists of the application of aqueous cream BP. If the main cause is excessive exposure to sunlight, in which case the lower lip is mainly affected, the best application is mexenone cream BPC. Mexenone is also available as a proprietary lipstick (Uvistat). *Herpes*, in the form of what are known as 'cold sores', often develops on the lip as a result of a cold or other feverish condition, but quickly passes off. (See HERPES.) *Ulcers* may form on the inner surface of the lip, usually in consequence of bad teeth or of dyspepsia, while in infants ulceration on the lips may be a sign of inherited syphilis. *Boils* sometimes form on the upper lip; if large they produce a serious condition. (See BOILS.) Small *cysts* sometimes form on the inner surface of the lip, and are seen as little bluish swellings filled with mucus; they are of no importance. *Hare-lip* is a deformity sometimes present at birth. (See PALATE, MALFORMATIONS OF.) *Cancer* of the lip sometimes occurs, almost always in men, and usually on the lower lip. (See also MOUTH, DISEASES OF.)

LIQUOR (see SOLUTION).

LIQUORICE is the root of *Glycyrrhiza glabra*, a plant of southern Europe and Asia. It is a mild expectorant, but is mainly used to cover the taste of disagreeable and more powerful drugs. Solid and liquid extracts are made from it, but the most commonly used preparation is compound liquorice powder, which contains also senna and sulphur.

LISTERIOSIS is an infectious, contagious disease of animals which is sometimes transmitted to man, in whom it usually affects the central nervous system, causing meningitis and encephalitis. It sometimes occurs in new-born babies as a result of infection through the placenta from the mother. The causative micro-organism is *Listeria monocytogenes*. The infection responds well to penicillin and other antibiotics. There were 32 cases of meningitis and 54 of septicaemia reported in 1984. In 1987, 200 cases were reported.

LITHIASIS is a general name applied to the formation of calculi and concretions in tissues or organs: e.g. cholelithiasis means the formation of calculi in the gall-bladder.

LITHIUM CARBONATE is a drug widely used in the treatment of certain forms of mental illness. About one person in two thousand in Britain is said to be prescribed it. The major indication for its use is acute mania. It induces improvement or remission in over 70 per cent of such patients. In addition, it is effective in the treatment of manic-depressive patients, preventing both the manic and the depressive episodes. There is also evidence that it lessens aggression in prisoners who behave antisocially and in mentally retarded patients who mutilate themselves and have temper tantrums. It is not recommended for children. Because of its possible toxic effects it is a drug that must only be administered under medical supervision and with monitoring of the blood levels. Because of the risk of its damaging the unborn child, it should not be prescribed, unless absolutely necessary, during pregnancy, particularly in the first three months. Neither should mothers take it while breast feeding as it is excreted in the milk in high concentrations.

LITHOTOMY is the operation of cutting for stone in the bladder. The operation is of great historic interest, because more has probably been written about it in early times than about any other department of surgery, and because, for long, it formed almost the only operation in which the surgeon dared to attack diseases of the internal organs. It seems, from the fact that large numbers of people were cut for stone, and also from the fact that this operation remained, in France at least, in the hands of a special class of surgeons, referred to as lithotomists, that stone in the bladder must have been far commoner two or three centuries ago than it is today.

LITHOTRIPSY: Extracorporeal shock-wave lithotripsy (ESWL) causes disintegration of renal stones without contact and is therefore an attractive procedure both for patients with renal stones and for their surgeons. Urolithiasis of the upper urinary tract is a common condition in the United Kingdom causing considerable morbidity and requiring large and lengthy operations with an extensive convalescent period. Percutaneous renal surgery has changed this picture but it requires at least puncture of the kidney and possibly open nephrolithotomy for large branched calculi. Extracorporeal shock-wave lithotripsy causes disintegration of the stone without contact and is therefore a far more attractive procedure.

The generation of shock waves as a form of treatment for urinary calculi was first described in 1955 by the Russian engineer Yutkin. Shock waves generated outside the body can be accurately focused with a reflector whilst the patient is suspended in water to facilitate transmission of the waves. These are focused on the calculus. The resultant fine fragments are passed spontaneously in the urine with minimal, if any, discomfort. The procedure has been shown to be safe and effective and is most acceptable to patients. It is clearly a specialized urological procedure. There is an extremely brief convalescent period after discharge which affects large savings to the hospital, patient and community. A report of the first 50 patients treated for upper tract urinary calculi by ESWL has showed that the average stay for an in-patient was 3·7 days. All patients suffered minimal post-operative discomfort and nearly all resumed normal activity within one day after discharge.

LITHOTRITY, or LITHOLAPAXY, is the term applied to the operation in which a stone in the bladder is crushed by an instrument introduced along the urethra, and the fragments washed out through a catheter.

LITMUS, which is prepared from several lichens, is a vegetable dye-substance, which on contact with alkaline fluids becomes blue, and on contact with acid fluids, red. Slips of paper, impregnated with litmus, form a valuable test for the acidity of the secretions and discharges.

LITTLE'S DISEASE is a form of cerebral palsy. (See CEREBRAL PALSY.)

LIVER: The liver is a solid organ of dark-brown colour and the largest gland in the body. It discharges several functions, acting both as an excreting organ and as an elaborator and storehouse of nourishment.
Form: The shape of the liver is generally described as that of a right-angled triangular prism, with the right angle rounded off. It has five surfaces, superior, anterior, right, posterior, and inferior, of which the anterior and posterior surfaces are triangular, with the base towards the right side and tapering off to the left. The surfaces are separated from one another by rounded margins, except in the case of the lower surface, which is divided from the right, front, and upper surfaces by a sharp edge. The organ is divided also into four lobes. The great bulk of it constitutes the right lobe; the left lobe is small and extends a little way into the left half of the abdomen, to end in a sharp left border, whilst the quadrate and caudate lobes are two small divisions upon the back and under surface. About the middle of the under surface, towards the back, is placed the porta hepatis, a transverse fissure, by which the hepatic artery and portal vein carry blood into the liver, and by which the right and left hepatic ducts emerge, carrying off the bile formed in the liver. The *gall-bladder* is attached to the under surface of the right lobe and projects from beneath the lower margin, where, if distended, it may be felt as a rounded swelling immediately

beneath the end of the ninth rib. The connection of the gall-bladder – in which bile is stored – with the liver is rather complicated. The hepatic ducts emerge at the porta hepatis, one coming from the right and one from the left lobe. They immediately join to form the common hepatic duct, which is about 3 cm (1¼ inches) long, and joins the cystic duct, coming from the gall-bladder, at an acute angle. The hepatic and cystic ducts by their union form the bile duct, which is about 75 mm (3 inches) in length, and opens into the small intestine. Bile, which passes down from the liver by the hepatic duct, may either pass directly into the bile duct and so into the intestine, or it may pass upwards through the cystic duct into the gall-bladder, to be stored there, and later retraces its way through the cystic duct to the bile duct, and so to the intestine. The cystic duct and gall-bladder therefore together form a cul-de-sac in the bile passages.
Position: The liver occupies the right-hand upper portion of the abdominal cavity. Its upper surface is in contact with the diaphragm, which also separates its right surface from the right lower ribs. About four-fifths of the organ lies to the right of the middle line of the body. As it is of a rounded shape it fills up the dome of the diaphragm, the lower part of the right lung being hollowed out to receive the liver, from which it is separated only by the diaphragm and pleural membrane. The liver, in turn, rests upon various abdominal organs, the right kidney and suprarenal gland, the large intestine, the duodenum, and the stomach all making impressions upon it. In addition, the liver is swung from the walls of the abdomen by five ligaments, four of which consist of thickened parts of the peritoneal membrane lining the whole abdominal cavity, and reflected from the upper part of the liver to its walls. These are the coronary ligament, right and left triangular ligaments, falciform ligament, and a dense fibrous cord, the round ligament, or ligamentum teres.
Dimensions: The vertical thickness of the liver amounts, towards the right side, to over 12 cm (5 inches), and its extent from side to side is considerably more. Its weight is over 1·5 kg (50 ounces), varying with the size of the person, but making up about 1/40 or thereabout of the whole body weight. In young children it is relatively larger, accounting, to a large extent, for their protuberant abdomen, and making up about 1/18 of the weight of the whole body.
Vessels: The blood supply of the organ differs from that of any other part of the body, in that the blood collected from the stomach and bowels into the portal vein does not pass directly to the heart, but is distributed to the liver, in the substance of which the portal vein breaks up into capillary vessels. The effect of this is that some harmful substances, absorbed from the stomach and bowels, are abstracted from the blood-stream and destroyed, while various constituents of the food are stored up in the liver for gradual use. In addition, the liver receives a large hepatic artery from the coeliac

axis, which also distributes branches to the stomach and pancreas, this blood supply serving to nourish the organ. After the blood has circulated through capillaries, it is collected together from both sources and emptied into the hepatic veins, which pass directly from the back surface of the liver into the inferior vena cava.

Minute structure: The liver is enveloped in a capsule of fibrous tissue, Glisson's capsule, from which strands run along the vessels, and, penetrating to the furthest recesses of the organ, bind its structure together. The hepatic artery, portal vein, and bile-duct divide and sub-divide, the branches of each lying alongside corresponding divisions of the other two, till the finest divisions of artery, vein, and bile-duct, known as interlobular vessels, lie between the lobules, of which the whole gland is built up. These lobules, each about the size of a pin's head, form each in itself a complete secreting unit, and the liver is built up of many hundred thousands of such exactly similar lobules.

A lobule has the following structure: from the small vessels lying round its margin capillaries, or sinusoids, lined with stellate Kupffer cells (q.v.), are given off which run in towards the centre of the lobule, where they empty into a small central vein. These central veins from neighbouring lobules collect together, and ultimately the blood passes into the hepatic veins, and so leaves the liver. Between the capillaries, which radiate from the central vein to the edge of the lobule, lie rows of large liver cells, these forming the distinctive tissue of the organ, upon which its activity depends. Between the rows of cells also lie fine bile capillaries, which collect the bile produced by the cells and discharge it into the bile-ducts lying along the margins of the lobules. The liver cells are among the largest cells in the body, and each contains one or two large, round nuclei. In the cells can often be seen droplets of fat or granules of glycogen, i.e. animal starch.

Functions: The liver is a vast chemical factory. The heat produced by the chemical changes taking place in it forms an important contribution to the general warming of the body. The liver secretes bile, the chief constituents of which are the bile salts (sodium glycocholate and taurocholate), the bile pigments (bilirubin and biliverdin), cholesterol, and lecithin. The

1 central vein connected by network of sinusoids with 2
2 interlobular bile-duct commencing in network of intercellular bile-canaliculi within the lobule
3 peripheral or interlobular veins

Diagram of liver lobule.

bile acids from which the salts are obtained are formed in the liver by the union of glycine and taurine with cholic acid. The bile salts are absorbed from the intestine and so find their way back to the liver again. The bile pigments are the iron-free and globin-free remnant of haemoglobin, being formed in the Kupffer cells of the liver. Bile pigments can, however, be formed in many other parts of the body: in the spleen, the lymph glands, bone-marrow, connective tissues (giving the colour to a bruise). Bile, then, serves to excrete pigment, the result of breakdown of old red blood corpuscles, and to aid the digestion of fat. Bile salts aid digestion of fat by emulsifying the fat, by activating pancreatic lipase, and by promoting fat absorption. Bile is necessary for the absorption of vitamins D and E.

In addition to forming bile the liver has a number of important functions. These are enumerated briefly: (1) In the embryo it forms red blood corpuscles, and in the adult stores vitamin B_{12}, a substance necessary for the proper functioning of the bone-marrow in the manufacture of red corpuscles. (2) It manufactures the fibrinogen of the blood, and also the albumin and globulin. (3) It stores iron and copper necessary for the manufacture of red corpuscles. (4) It produces heparin and, with the aid of vitamin K, prothrombin. (5) Its Kupffer cells in the liver blood-sinusoids are an important element in the reticulo-endothelial system, which breaks down red corpuscles, and probably manufactures antibodies. (6) It detoxicates noxious products made in the intestine and absorbed into the blood. (7) It stores carbohydrate in the form of glycogen, and maintains the two-way process: glucose $\rightleftarrows$ glycogen. (8) It forms vitamin A from carotene and stores the B vitamins. (9) It splits up amino-acids and manufactures urea and uric acids. (10) It plays an essential part in the storage and metabolism of fat.

LIVER DISEASES: The liver may be extensively diseased without any very urgent symptoms, unless the circulation through it is impeded, the outflow of bile checked, or neighbouring organs implicated. Jaundice, which is a symptom of several liver disorders, is dealt with elsewhere. Ascites, which may be caused by interference with the circulation through the portal vein of the liver, as well as by other causes, is also considered separately. The presence of gall-stones is a complication of some diseases connected with the liver, and is treated under GALL-BLADDER, DISEASES OF. For hydatid cyst of the liver see TAENIASIS.

INFLAMMATION OF THE LIVER, or HEPATITIS, may occur as part of a generalized infection or may be a localized condition. Infectious hepatitis, which is the result of infection with a virus, is one of the most common forms of hepatitis. (See HEPATITIS, ACUTE INFECTIVE.) There are many other viruses that can cause hepatitis, including that responsible for glandular fever (q.v.). Certain spirochaetes may also be the cause, particularly that responsible for leptospirosis (q.v.), as can many drugs. In tropical countries amoebic hepatitis, which often goes on to abscess formation, is an important complication of amoebic dysentery. (See ABSCESS, CHRONIC; DYSENTERY.) Other tropical conditions in which the liver is always involved include malaria and yellow fever. Hepatitis may also occur if there is obstruction of the bile duct, as by a gall-stone.

CIRRHOSIS OF THE LIVER: The cause of cirrhosis (q.v.) of the liver is still obscure. Experimentally it has been shown that the condition can be produced by a deficiency of certain of the amino-acids found in protein, but this only explains a small proportion of the cases found in man. It is probable that in most cases three factors are involved in varying degrees: a nutritional deficiency, a toxic factor, and an infective factor. Alcohol is the most common cause of cirrhosis in the United Kingdom and the USA. In Africa and many parts of Asia, infection with hepatitis B virus is a common cause.

Symptoms: In one form of cirrhosis the liver is much contracted (atrophic or coarse cirrhosis), its blood-vessels are pressed upon, and ascites results. In another form there is great enlargement of the organ (hypertrophic or biliary cirrhosis) and jaundice appears. In all cases there is loss of appetite and other signs of dyspepsia. There is a variable degree of anaemia. There may be a low-grade fever. In a certain number of cases, two characteristic signs may appear. One is so-called spider naevi (see NAEVUS). Each has a central red spot and may measure up to a centimetre in diameter. They rarely appear below the waist. The nose-bleeds which occur in around 20 per cent of cases may be due to naevi in the nose. The other is so-called liver palms, or reddening of the palms of the hands, most marked on the ball of the thumb and the outer edge of the hand.

Treatment: Nothing can be done to repair a cirrhosed organ, but the cause, if known, must be removed and further advance of the process thus prevented. In the case of the liver a high-protein, high-carbohydrate, low-fat diet is given, supplemented by liver extract and vitamins B and K. The consumption of alcohol should be banned.

ABSCESS OF THE LIVER: When an abscess develops in the liver, it is usually a manifestation of amoebic dysentery, appearing sometimes late in the disease, even after the diarrhoea is cured. It may also follow upon inflammation of the liver due to other causes; and abscesses may form in this organ as in other sites in cases of blood-poisoning. The symptoms of abscess are much the same as in other types of inflammation, only they are more pronounced, and accompanied often by rigors, severe pain over the liver which may also be referred to the right shoulder, and by great enlargement of the liver. In the case of an amoebic abscess treatment consists of oral metronidazole. Aspiration of the contents of the abscess is now rarely necessary.

ACUTE YELLOW ATROPHY, or ACUTE HEPATIC NECROSIS as it is now known, is a destructive and often fatal disease of the liver which is very rare. It may be due to chemical poisons, such as carbon tetrachloride, chloroform, phosphorus and industrial solvents derived from benzene. It may also be the cause of death in cases of poisoning with fungi. Very occasionally it may be a complication of acute infectious hepatitis. It is also a rare complication of pregnancy. It sets in with a slight degree of jaundice, which cannot be distinguished from simple jaundice, and lasts several days. Then the jaundice suddenly deepens, there is pain in the region of the liver, convulsions and delirium appear, the heart grows very weak, and death ensues in a day or two. Crystals of leucine and tyrosine are found in the urine. The destruction of the liver as a secreting organ may be complete, but occasionally areas here and there only are affected, and recovery may then take place with restoration of the damaged areas after a prolonged illness.

CANCER OF THE LIVER is not uncommon, although it is rare for the disease to begin in the liver, the involvement of this organ being usually secondary to disease situated somewhere in the stomach or bowels. Cancer originating in the liver is more common in Asia and Africa. It usually arises in a fibrotic (or cirrhotic) liver and in carriers of the hepatitis B virus. There is great emaciation, which increases as the disease progresses. The liver is much enlarged, and its margin and surface are rough, being studded with hard cancer masses of varying size, which can often be felt through the abdominal wall. Pain may be present. Jaundice and oedema often appear. (See also TRANSPLANTATION.)

LIVER-FLUKE is the popular name of *Fasciola hepatica*, a parasite which infests sheep, and which is occasionally found in the bile-passages and liver of man. (See FASCIOLIASIS.)

LIVER PILLS (see CHOLAGOGUES).

LIVER SPOT is a popular term applied to brownish marks which appear on the skin, especially of the face. This is sometimes caused by the growth of a parasite (*Tinea versicolor*) in the surface layers of the epidermis. It also frequently accompanies pregnancy or the presence of abdominal tumours. It may also be due simply to some long-continued form of local irritation.

LOBE is the term applied to the larger divisions of various organs, such as to the four lobes of the liver, the three lobes of the right and the two lobes of the left lung, which are separated by fissures from one another, and to the lobes or superficial areas into which the brain is divided. The term lobar is applied to structures which are connected with lobes of organs, or to diseases which have a tendency to be limited by the boundaries of lobes, such as lobar pneumonia.

LOBECTOMY is the operation of cutting out a lobe of the lung in such diseases as abscess of the lung and bronchiectasis.

LOBELIA, or INDIAN TOBACCO, is a remedy used for asthma. It consists of the leaves and tops of *Lobelia inflata*, a common weed in the United States. In large doses, it causes vomiting and paralyses the heart's action, being a dangerous poison, but in moderate doses it relieves the spasm to which asthma is due. It is a constituent of many burning powders made for smoking by asthmatics, but it is more commonly used in the form of tincture of lobelia combined with other drugs.

LOBOTOMY is the cutting of a lobe.

LOBULE is the term applied to a division of an organ smaller than a lobe: for example, the lobules of the lung are of the size of millet seeds, those of the liver slightly larger. Lobules form the smallest subdivisions or units of an organ, each lobule being similar to the others, of which there may be perhaps several hundred thousand in the organ.

LOCHIA is the discharge which takes place during the first week or two after child-birth. During the first four days it consists chiefly of blood; after the fifth day the colour should become paler, and after the first week the quantity should diminish and the appearance be creamy. There should at no time be any putrid odour, the presence of this being an indication of dangerous septic infection. The presence of blood after the second week indicates that the patient has been too active or that the natural absorptive changes are not duly taking place. (See PUERPERIUM.)

LOCKJAW is a prominent symptom of tetanus (q.v.) and is the popular name for this condition.

LOCOMOTOR ATAXIA: The uncoordinated movements and unsteady lurching gait that occurs in the tertiary stage of untreated syphilis.

LOCUM TENENS: A doctor who stands in for another.

LOFEPRAMINE (see ANTIDEPRESSANTS).

LOGORRHOEA is the technical term for garrulousness, a feature which may be exaggerated in certain states of mental instability.

LOIASIS is the disease caused by the filarial worm *Loa loa*, a thread-like worm which differs from *W. bancrofti* in that it is shorter and thicker, and it is found in the blood-stream during the day, not at night. It is transmitted by the mango fly, *Chrysops dimidiata*, but other flies of this genus can also transmit it. It is confined to West and Central Africa. The characteristic feature of the disease is the appearance of fugitive swellings which may arise anywhere in the body in the course of the worm's migration through the body. These are known as Calabar swellings. The worm is often found in the eye, hence the old name of the worm in Africa – the eye worm. Satisfactory results are being reported from the use of diethylcarbamazine in the treatment of this form of filariasis (q.v.).

LOIN is the name applied to the part of the back between the lower ribs and the pelvis. (For pain in the loins see BACKACHE; LUMBAGO.)

LONG-SIGHT (see REFRACTION).

LOPERAMIDE is a drug that is proving of value in the treatment of diarrhoea.

LORAZEPAM is a tranquillizer that is proving of value as a sedative for administration before operation. Its advantage, compared with other similar drugs, is that it stimulates, rather than depresses, breathing. It is used in the treatment of pre-eclampsia (q.v.) on the grounds that it has less of a depressant effect on the new-born child than other tranquillizers.

LORDOSIS means an unnatural curvature of the spine forwards. It occurs chiefly in the lumbar region, where the natural curve is forwards, as the result of muscular weakness, spinal disease, etc. (See SPINAL COLUMN.)

LOSS OF BLOOD (see HAEMORRHAGE).

LOTIONS are fluid preparations intended for bringing in contact with, or for washing, the external surface of the body. Lotions are generally of a watery or alcoholic composition, and many of them are known as 'liquors'. Those external applications which are of an oily nature, and intended to be rubbed into the surface, are known as liniments.

LOUSE (see INSECTS IN RELATION TO DISEASE).

LOZENGES, also known as TROCHES, or TROCHISCI, consist of small tablets containing drugs mixed with sugar, gum, glycerin-jelly, or fruit-paste. They are used in various affections of the mouth and throat, being sucked and slowly dissolved by the saliva, which brings the drugs they contain in contact with the affected surface. Some of the substances used in lozenges are benzalkonium, benzocaine, betamethasone, bismuth, formaldehyde, hydrocortisone, liquorice, penicillin.

LSD (see LYSERGIC ACID).

LUGOL'S SOLUTION is a compound solution of iodine and potassium iodide.

LUMBAGO: Pain in the lower (lumbar) region of the back. It may be muscular, skeletal or neurological in origin. A severe form associated with sciatica (c.v.) may be due to a prolapsed intervertebral disc. Less severe forms may be caused by osteoarthritis (q.v.) of the spine, a trapped nerve, inflammation of connective tissue or may follow an old injury.

The treatment will depend on the cause but mild lumbago will usually respond to non-steroidal anti-inflammatory drugs and the application of warmth.

LUMBAR is a term used to denote structures in, or diseases affecting, the region of the loins, as, for example, the lumbar vertebrae, lumbar abscess.

LUMBAR PUNCTURE is a procedure for removing cerebrospinal fluid from the spinal canal in the lumbar region in order: (1) to diagnose disease of the nervous system; (2) to introduce medicaments: spinal anaesthetics, or drugs, or serum.

LUMBAR SYMPATHECTOMY: Destruction of the lumbar chain of sympathetic nerves by means of surgery, diathermy or injection of chemicals (phenol or alcohol). The technique is used to improve the blood flow to the leg in patients with peripheral vascular disease and to treat some types of chronic leg pain.

LUMBAR VERTEBRA: There are five lumbar vertabrae in the lower spinal column between the thoracic vertebrae and the sacrum (q.v. SPINAL COLUMN).

LUMBRICUS is a name sometimes applied to the roundworm or *Ascaris lumbricoides*. (See ASCARIASIS.)

LUMEN: (1) The space enclosed by a tubular structure or hollow organ (e.g. the gastro-intestinal tract or bladder). (2) The SI unit of luminous flux (1 lumen (1m) = the amount of light emitted per second in a unit solid angle of 1 steradian by a 1-candela point source).

LUMPECTOMY: An operation for breast cancer in which the tumour is removed from the breast rather than with it (see MASTECTOMY).

LUNAR CAUSTIC is another name for nitrate of silver.

LUNATIC is a general term applied to people of disordered mind, because lunacy was supposed at one time to be largely influenced by the moon. (See MENTAL ILLNESS.)

LUNGS: The lungs form a pair of organs situated in the chest, and discharge the function of respiration. (See RESPIRATION.) Whilst this is their primary function, they also act as a filter for the blood. The air, which enters through the nose and passes down the throat, larynx, and windpipe in succession (see AIR PASSAGES), reaches the lungs by the right and left bronchial tubes, into which the windpipe divides within the chest, at the level of the second rib. The texture of the lungs is very highly elastic, so that when the chest is opened each lung collapses to about one-third of its natural bulk.

Form and position: Each lung is roughly conical in shape, with an apex projecting into the neck, and a base resting upon the diaphragm. The rounded outer surface of each is in contact with the ribs of its own side, while the heart, lying between the lungs, hollows out the inner surface of each to some extent. There is an anterior border, along which the outer and inner surfaces meet, and the borders of the two lungs touch one another for a short distance behind the middle of the breast-bone. The apex, which is blunt, extends 35 mm (1½ inches) or more into the neck above the line of the collar-bone, being covered here by the muscles of the neck. The base is deeply hollowed, in correspondence with the domed shape of the diaphragm, which is pushed up by the liver on the right side, and by the stomach and spleen on the left. The right lung is split by two deep fissures into three lobes; the left has two lobes divided by a single fissure. The weight of the two lungs together is about 1·1 kg, the right being rather heavier than the left. The lungs of men are heavier than those of women. There is a tendency for lung mass to increase throughout life. Each lung is enveloped in a membrane, the pleura or pleural membrane, in such a way that one layer of the membrane is closely adherent to the lung, from which indeed it cannot be separated, while the other layer lines the inner surface of one half of the chest. These two layers form a closed cavity, the pleural cavity, which everywhere surrounds the lung except at the point where the bronchi and vessels enter it. This cavity is, in the natural state, a merely potential space, the two layers of pleural membrane being separated only by a thin layer of fluid, which enables them to glide with very little friction over one another as the lung expands and retracts in breathing; but, in certain states, fluid collects in the pleural cavity, so that several pints of fluid may be effused there, compressing the lung. In some circumstances air escapes into the pleural cavity, and the lung then collapses temporarily upon its root, but air in the pleural cavity is usually

absorbed, and the lung comes to occupy its original volume.

Colour: In children, the colour of the lungs is rose-pink but, as life advances, they become more and more of a slaty hue, mottled with streaks and patches of dark grey and black, which are due to deposits in the lymph spaces of dust inhaled on the breath. Eskimos and others who live in an atmosphere free from dust retain the colour of childhood; on the other hand, the lungs of coal-miners become often of an almost uniform jet-black shade.

Changes at birth: Before birth, and in stillborn children, the lungs are of a yellowish colour, of solid gland-like appearance, and packed away in the back of the chest. Further, such lungs do not float in water, and their weight amounts to about ¹/₇₀ of the whole body-weight. Immediately upon birth a remarkable change takes place: the tissue of the lungs expands, like the petals of an opening flower; the colour changes to rose-red, and the weight is suddenly doubled from the inrush of blood; the consistency becomes spongy, as air is drawn into the lungs, and if the child should die after drawing a few breaths, any portion of the lung which may be cut off floats in water. These changes are of importance, from the medico-legal point of view, in determining whether a dead infant was born alive or not.

Connections with heart: Not only does the heart lie in contact with the two lungs, so that changes in the volume of the lungs cannot fail to have an effect upon the heart's action, but the heart is also connected by vessels with both lungs. The pulmonary artery passes from the right ventricle and divides into two branches, one of which runs straight outwards to each lung, entering its substance along with the bronchial tube at the hilum or root of the lung. From this point also emerge the pulmonary veins, which carry the blood purified in the lungs back to the left atrium.

Minute structure: Each main bronchial tube, entering the lung at the root, divides into branches, which subdivide again and again, to

1 respiratory bronchiole	4 air saccule
2 alveolar duct	5 alveolus
3 atrium	

Diagram of the internal division of the air tubes.

be distributed all through the substance of the lung, till the finest tubes, known as respiratory bronchioles, have a width of only 0·25 mm (¹/₁₀₀ inch). In structure, all these tubes consist of a mucous membrane surrounded by a fibrous sheath. The windpipe as well as the larger and medium bronchi have in the fibrous layer large pieces of cartilage, which in the windpipe and largest bronchial tubes form regular hoops, in the medium-sized tubes are disposed as irregular plates. These pieces of cartilage have the function of preventing the tubes from closing or being compressed, and so obstructing the passage of air. The larger and medium bronchi are richly supplied with glands secreting mucus, which is poured out upon the surface of the membrane. This surface is composed of columnar epithelial cells, which are provided with cilia. These have a co-ordinated beating action which sweeps mucus and bacteria upwards towards the throat. The wall of the bronchial tubes is rich in fibres of elastic tissue, and immediately beneath the mucous membrane is a layer of circularly placed unstriped muscle fibres, which is specially well developed in the smaller bronchi. This muscular layer plays an important role in the removal of mucus by coughing; it is also of great importance in connection with the causation of asthma. (See ASTHMA.)

The smallest divisions of the bronchial tubes, or bronchioles, divide into a number of tortuous tubes known as alveolar ducts and these branch into expanded passages known as atria, each of which leads into a terminal air saccule. The walls of the alveolar ducts, atria and air saccules are covered with minute sacs, known as alveoli, of which there are around 300 million. Each alveolus consists of a delicate membrane composed of flattened, plate-like cells, strengthened by a wide network of elastic fibres, to which the great elasticity of the lung is due; and in these thin-walled air-cells the important function of the lungs is carried on.

The branches of the pulmonary artery accompany the bronchial tubes to the furthest recesses of the lung, dividing like the latter into finer and finer branches, and ending in a dense network of capillaries, which lies everywhere between the air-vesicles, the capillaries being so closely placed that they occupy a much greater area than the spaces between them. The air in the air-vesicles is separated therefore from the blood only by two delicate membranes: the wall of the air-vesicle and the capillary wall, through which an exchange of gases readily takes place. The blood from the capillaries is collected by the pulmonary veins, which also accompany the bronchi to the root of the lung.

Another and much smaller set of bronchial blood-vessels runs actually upon the walls of the bronchial tubes, and these serve the purpose of nourishing the lung tissue.

There is in the lung also an important system of lymph vessels, which start in spaces situated between the air-vesicles, under the pleural membrane and in the walls of the bronchial tubes. These vessels leave the lung along with the blood-vessels, and are connected with a chain of bronchial glands lying near the end of the windpipe.

LUNGS, DISEASES OF: The general symptoms and signs produced by disease of the lungs are mentioned under CHEST DISEASES and the chief affections to which these organs are liable are also treated under special headings. (See BRONCHIECTASIS; BRONCHITIS; CHEST, DEFORMITIES OF; CHILLS AND COLDS; EMPHYSEMA; EXPECTORATION; HAEMOPTYSIS; HAEMORRHAGE; OCCUPATIONAL DISEASES; PLEURISY; PNEUMONIA; PULMONARY EMBOLISM; TUBERCULOSIS.)

INFLAMMATION OF THE LUNGS is generally known as pneumonia when it is due to infection, as alveolitis when the inflammation is immunological and as pneumonitis when it is due to physical or chemical agents. (See PNEUMONIA.)

ABSCESS OF THE LUNG is a comparatively rare condition, and consists, like abscesses elsewhere, of a collection of pus in one or more areas of the lung. It may result from an acute pneumonia which does not clear up properly, or it may be due to a wound of the lung from without, or to the presence of foreign bodies, such as buttons, pins, or fragments of food, which have been sucked down the air passages. An abscess may also occur in the lung, as in other organs, during the course of blood poisoning (pyaemia), or may be produced by the bursting of an abscess into the lung after its formation in some neighbouring organ. The condition may be difficult to differentiate from cavity formation due to tuberculosis, although the failure to find tubercle bacilli in the expectoration, after repeated examination, is an important point against the latter condition.

An abscess in the lung may burst into one of the bronchial tubes, and, after the pus is spat up, healing and recovery may take place. Most cases respond to appropriate antibiotics and postural drainage (q.v.) but occasionally it may be necessary to resort to surgery and drain the abscess through the chest wall.

GANGRENE OF THE LUNG may also follow pneumonia in those of poor constitution or debilitated by serious illness. Just as in the case of gangrene of the limbs, a portion of lung dies and putrefies, giving rise to a most offensive smell, as the dead and broken-down lung tissue is spat up. The prospect of recovery is small, even when the portion of lung involved is very limited.

CONGESTION OF THE LUNGS is a term which is used in two quite different senses. The term is popularly used for acute inflammation of the lung in its early stages. When the patient recovers after a few days, the illness is often described as an attack of acute congestion.

In a strict medical sense, the term is used to mean quite a different condition of a more chronic nature: passive or mechanical congestion of the blood-vessels in the lungs due to some defect in the pumping action of the heart. Passive congestion arises under two sets of conditions. A very serious form, known as hypostatic congestion, arises when the heart is failing, towards the end of severe and long-continued fevers, such as typhoid fever; after severe surgical operations; and in old people who, for any reason, such as the occurrence of a broken leg, are confined for some weeks to bed. It occurs in the back parts of the lungs, as the feeble heart is unable to drive out the blood which gravitates into these dependent parts. Inflammation is very apt to arise in these congested parts, and hypostatic pneumonia often ends the life of old or feeble people confined to bed. The other form of passive congestion is due, not so much to weakness in the pumping action of the heart, as to some obstruction which hinders the escape of blood from the lungs into the left atrium of the heart. Narrowing of the opening which leads from the left atrium to the left ventricle (mitral stenosis) is the chief cause of this, and, although the condition is by no means so serious as the hypostatic form of congestion, it predisposes the people affected by this form of heart disease to sharp attacks of blood-spitting on exertion, to bronchitis, and to pneumonia. The treatment, in both cases, must be directed towards the heart.

OEDEMA OF THE LUNGS results when the left ventricle myocardium is unable to handle the blood delivered to it. There is an abrupt increase in the venous and capillary pressure in the pulmonary vessels followed by flooding of fluid into the interstitial spaces and alveoli. The commonest cause of acute pulmonary oedema is myocardial infarction which reduces the ability of the left ventricular myocardial muscle to handle the blood delivered to it. Pulmonary oedema may result from other causes of left ventricular failure such as hypertension or valvular disease of the mitral and aortic valves. The initial symptoms are cough with breathlessness and occasionally with wheezing. The patient becomes extremely short of breath with a sensation of imminent death. In a severe attack the patient is pale, sweating and cyanosed and obviously gasping for breath. Frequently frothy sputum is produced which may be blood stained.

COLLAPSE OF THE LUNG occurs under several conditions. The lungs are so resilient in consequence of the elastic fibres with which they are everywhere interspersed that, if air is admitted to the pleural cavities, the lungs immediately collapse to a third of their natural bulk. Accordingly, if one side of the chest is wounded and air is admitted (pneumothorax), the lung collapses, although, after the wound is healed, the air is absorbed from the pleural cavity and the lung quickly regains its size. Also, when fluid is effused into the pleural cavity the lung is compressed and collapses, and if the fluid is not absorbed or drawn off within some weeks, the collapse is apt to be permanent through the formation of adhesions round the lung. Again, if anything blocks a bronchial tube, the part of the lung to which it leads collapses, since these tubes do not communicate with one another. Thus, in children suffering from bronchitis or

pneumonia areas of the lung may collapse through a plug of mucus sticking in a bronchus which the child is not sufficiently strong to free by coughing. A similar result is brought about by foreign bodies drawn into the air passages. It also occurs when the chest is opened on one side to drain away a collection of pus. The second lung, being healthy, is sufficient to overtake the needs of respiration, expanding as a rule somewhat in the process. The lungs of an infant at birth are collapsed in the sense that they have never been expanded, and any signs of expansion in the lungs of a dead infant form a sure token that he has been born alive. (See LUNGS.)

TUMOURS OF THE LUNG: Since the beginning of the twentieth century cancer of the lung has become increasingly frequent, particularly so in the last decade, and in 1984 was responsible for 35,739 deaths in England, compared with 10,360 deaths from carcinoma of the stomach and 13,409 deaths from carcinoma of the breast. It was the commonest form of cancer among cancer deaths in men, accounting for 39 per cent of all cancer deaths, and the second commonest among women (14 per cent), the commonest site for whom is the breast (20 per cent). Tumours may arise in the mediastinum or in connection with the pleura. Hydatid cysts are found from time to time in the lungs. (See TAENIASIS.)

WOUNDS OF THE LUNG are serious both by reason of the damage they may do to this organ and by admitting air into the pleural cavity, so that the lung collapses. The lung may be wounded by the end of a fractured rib, or by some sharp body pushed between the ribs, and it may also be torn as the result of disease: for example, a tuberculous and excavated lung may be perforated during a fit of coughing. If by any cause a free opening is made between the pleural cavity and air passages, immediate difficulty of breathing, due to collapse of the lung, ensues. Generally, however, the person recovers from the immediate symptoms, and, if the perforation is caused by an external wound, the wound may heal without leaving any permanent damage. Frequently, in such cases, blood is effused into the pleural cavity (haemothorax). This is gradually absorbed, leaving usually some thickening of the pleural membrane and adhesions between the lung and chest wall. Such a wound is liable, at the time of infliction, to become infected by organisms, and empyema (q.v.) may then result, with a tedious illness.

Wounds of the lung are chiefly dangerous on account of the risk of wounding large blood-vessels. Spitting of blood in any quantity after a wound of the chest has been received is a sign that the lung has been injured. A stab or bullet wound, which does not injure any large vessel, may traverse the lung without any serious consequences, but if one of the main veins or arteries is torn, death is likely to ensue.

LUNG VOLUMES: The volume of air within the lungs changes with the respiratory cycle.

The volumes defined below can be measured and may be useful indicators of some pulmonary diseases.

Total lung capacity (TLC): The volume of air that can be held in the lungs at maximum inspiration.

Tidal volume (TV): The volume of air taken into and out of the lungs with each breath.

Inspiratory reserve volume (IRV): The volume of air that can still be inspired at the end of a normal quiet inspiration.

Expiratory reserve volume (ERV): The volume of air that can still be expired at the end of a normal quiet expiration.

Residual volume (RV): The volume of air remaining in the lungs after a maximal expiration.

Vital capacity (VC): The maximum amount of air that can be expired after a maximal inspiration.

Functional residual capacity (FRC): The volume of air left in the lungs at the end of a normal quiet expiration.

Normal values for a 60-kg man are:

	ml
TLC	5000–6000
TV	400–600
IRV	3300–3750
ERV	950–1200
RV	1200–1700
VC	3400–4800
FRC	2300–2600

LUPUS is a term used to designate a group of skin diseases of intractable character. There are two chief types of the disease: *Lupus vulgaris*, which is due to the *Mycobacterium tuberculosis*; and *Lupus erythematosus*, which is of unknown origin.

LUPUS VULGARIS begins most commonly before the age of 20, and, not infrequently, persists all through life, healing in one place to break out a short distance off. The nose, cheeks, brow, and sides of the neck are most commonly attacked, although the hands and the mucous membrane inside the nose and mouth are also common seats of the malady. The first sign of the disease is a small, soft nodule of yellowish transparent appearance, on this account often called an 'apple-jelly' nodule. No pain or itching accompanies the disease, but the skin gradually becomes thickened and discoloured, other nodules appear, and finally ulcers or small abscesses form. The disease progresses very slowly, but, after it has been in existence some years, the deformity produced may be very great. The nose may be partly or wholly eaten away; the lower eyelids, if attacked, become drawn down, showing the red inner surface. The condition is of little infective power.

Treatment: These horrors have now been removed by the excellent results obtained from the use of anti-tuberculous drugs. In certain cases it is still sometimes helpful to remove individual nodules by excision or by curettage, followed by the application of trichloracetic acid. The local application of intensive ultra-violet light is also sometimes of value.

LUPUS ERYTHEMATOSUS is a disease of unknown etiology. It occurs in two forms. The more common form, *discoid lupus erythematosus*, which is more common in women, involves only the skin and consists of rounded, red, and slightly raised patches, which are distributed most commonly on the nose and cheeks. These patches, by fusing together at their edges, sometimes give a characteristic butterfly-like appearance to the reddened nose and cheeks. There is no tendency to the formation of ulcers, as in lupus vulgaris, and deformity in consequence does not result, although the patches of red alternating with white and atrophied skin can render the complexion quite unsightly.

The second form, *systemic lupus erythematosus*, occurs predominantly in women in the proportion of nine women to one man. It is an auto-immune disease. There is some evidence that people who possess certain antigens (q.v.) are more vulnerable to it. It may be precipitated by a virus, exposure to sunlight, infection or the administration of sulphonamide drugs. Its manifestations vary considerably and include eruptions on the skin as in the discoid form, painful joints, involvement of the kidneys, alveolitis (q.v.), enlargement of the spleen, and fever. With adequate supervision the outlook is much better than was at one time thought to be the case, particularly if detected at an early stage. The disease usually responds dramatically to treatment with corticosteroids. Patients with systemic lupus erythematosus can obtain help and advice from Lupus U.K., Queen's Court, 9–17 Eastern Road, Romford, Essex RM1 3NG (0708-731251, fax: 0708-731252).

LUTEINIZING HORMONE: A hormone secreted by the anterior pituitary which stimulates ovulation, maturation of the corpus luteum and the synthesis of progesterone by the ovary and testosterone by the testis.

LUX is the unit of illumination. The abbreviation is lx.

LUXATION is another word for dislocation. (See DISLOCATIONS.)

LYING-IN (see LABOUR).

LYME DISEASE: This comprises arthritis associated with skin rashes, fever and sometimes encephalitis (q.v.) or carditis (inflammation of the heart). It is caused by a spirochaete (q.v.) which is transmitted by tick bite. Treatment is with antibiotics.

LYMPH is the fluid which circulates in the lymphatic vessels of the body. It is a colourless fluid, like blood plasma in composition, only rather more watery. It contains salts similar to those of blood plasma, and the same proteins, though in smaller amount: fibrinogen, serum albumin, and serum globulin. It also contains colourless lymph corpuscles, or lymphocytes as they are known, derived from the glands. In certain of the lymphatic vessels, the lymph contains, after meals, a great amount of fat in the form of a fine milky emulsion. These are the vessels which absorb fat from the food passing down the intestine, and convey it to the thoracic duct; they are called lacteals on account of the milky appearance of their contents. (See CHYLE.)

1 vein   4 lymph capillaries
2 lymphatic vessel   5 small artery
3 blood capillaries

Diagram showing the relation of the blood and lymph streams along the tissues.

The lymph is derived, in the first place, from the blood, the watery constituents of which exude through the walls of the capillaries into the tissues, conveying material for the nourishment of the tissues and absorbing waste products.

The various gaps and chinks in the tissues communicate with lymph capillaries, which have a structure similar to that of the capillaries of the blood-vessel system, being composed of delicate flat cells joined edge to edge. These unite to form fine vessels, resembling minute veins in structure, to which the name of lymphatics is applied. These ramify all through the body, passing here and there through lymphatic glands, and ultimately discharge their contents into the blood circulation once more, by opening into the jugular veins in the root of the neck. Other lymph vessels commence in great numbers as minute openings on the surface of the pleura and peritoneum, and act as drains for these otherwise closed cavities. When fluid is effused into these cavities, as in a pleural effusion, for example, its absorption takes place through the lymphatic vessels. The course of these vessels is described under GLANDS. The circulation of the lymph is effected in some of the lower animals by lymph-hearts, which pump the lymph, just as the heart belonging to the blood-vessels keeps the blood in circulation. In man and most of the higher animals there is no heart for the lymph, which circulates partly by reason of the pressure at which it is driven through the walls of the blood capillaries, but mainly in consequence of incidental forces. The lymph capillaries and vessels are copiously provided with valves, which prevent any back flow of lymph, and every time these vessels are squeezed, as by the contraction of a muscle, or movement of a limb, the lymph moves on a little, leaving room for the exudation of fresh lymph. From this fact one can perceive the immense importance of regular exercise in maintaining the free circulation of lymph.

Lymph, like blood, possesses, in virtue of the fibrinogen which it contains, the power of clotting, forming, when it does so, a faintly yellow or colourless coagulum. This can be seen in the case of small wounds, after the blood has ceased to flow.

The term lymph is also applied to the serous fluid contained in the vesicles which develop as the result of vaccination, and used for the purpose of vaccinating other individuals. (See VACCINATION.)

The term lymph is also loosely applied to the layers and flakes of fibrin which are derived from the lymph and are found on the pleura and other serous membranes as the result of inflammation.

LYMPHADENITIS means inflammation of lymphatic glands. (See GLANDS, DISEASES OF.)

LYMPHADENOMA is another name for Hodgkin's disease (q.v.).

LYMPHANGIECTASIS means an abnormal dilatation of the lymph vessels, as in filariasis (q.v.).

LYMPHANGIOGRAPHY, or LYMPHOGRAPHY, is the procedure whereby the lymphatics (q.v.) and lymphatic glands can be rendered visible on X-ray films by means of the injection of radio-opaque substances.

LYMPHANGITIS means inflammation situated in the lymphatic vessels.

LYMPHATICS is the term applied to the vessels which convey the lymph (q.v.). (For an account of their arrangement, see GLANDS.)

LYMPH NODE: Swellings which occur at various points in the lymphatic system through which lymph drains. They consist of a cortex, medulla and lymph sinuses and have two main functions: (1) The interception and removal of abnormal or foreign material from the lymph. (2) The production of immune responses. The lymph nodes become enlarged when the area of the body which they drain is the site of infection or as a manifestation of some systemic diseases.

Occasionally they are the site of primary or metastatic malignant disease.

LYMPHOCYTE is a variety of white blood corpuscle produced in the lymphoid tissues and lymphatic glands of the body. It contains a simple rounded nucleus surrounded by protoplasm generally described as non-granular. Two varieties of lymphocyte are described, small lymphocytes and large lymphocytes, and together they form over 20 per cent of the white corpuscles of the blood. They play an important part in the production of antibodies (q.v.), and in the rejection of transplanted organs such as the heart. (See TRANSPLANTATION.) This they do in two different ways. What are known as **B** lymphocytes produce antibodies, while **T** lymphocytes attack and destroy antigens (q.v.) directly. They are known as T lymphocytes because they are produced by the thymus gland. Their numbers are increased in tuberculosis and certain other diseases. Such an increase is known as lymphocytosis.

LYMPHOCYTOSIS: An increase in the number of lymphocytes (q.v.) in the blood, e.g. in response to infection or in chronic lymphocytic leukaemia (q.v.).

LYMPHOEDEMA means dropsical swelling of a part or organ due to obstruction to the lymph-vessels draining it.

LYMPHOGRANULOMA INGUINALE, LYMPHOGRANULOMA VENEREUM; PORADENITIS VENEREA; LYMPHOPATHIA VENEREUM, is a venereal disease in which the chief characteristic is enlargement of glands in the groin, the infecting agent being a virus. There were 17 cases in England in 1985.

LYMPHOID TISSUE: Tissue involved in the formation of lymph, lymphocytes, and antibodies. It consists of the lymph nodes, thymus, tonsils and spleen.

LYMPHOKINES: Lymphokines are polypeptides that are produced by lymphocytes as part of their immune response to an antigen and their function is to communicate with other cells of the immune system. Some lymphokines stimulate B cells to differentiate into antibody-producing plasma cells; others stimulate T lymphocytes to proliferate and other lymphokines become interferons.

LYMPHOMA is a tumour of lymphoid tissue, one variety of which is found in children in Africa; sometimes called Burkitt's lymphoma after the surgeon who first described it. Because of its geographical distribution it is thought to be due to a virus which is transmitted by mosquitoes, but no virus has yet been definitely isolated from the tumour.

LYMPHOSARCOMA is a malignant growth of the lymphoid elements of the body, and is characterized by generalized enlargement of the lymphatic glands, spleen, and liver. The majority of cases – about 55 per cent – occur in the 60 to 70 age-group, but it may occur at any age. The prognosis is poor, 80 per cent of cases dying within six years. Treatment is by means of irradiation or chemotherapy.

LYSERGIC ACID, or LYSERGIC ACID DIETHYLAMIDE, popularly known as LSD, belongs to the ergonovine group of alkaloids. In minute doses it induces psychic states in which the individual becomes aware of repressed memories. Under the influence of the drug he feels he is watching himself and relives feelings from his childhood and infancy. It is proving of value in the treatment of certain anxiety states, but is a drug that must only be used under skilled supervision. (See DRUG ADDICTION.)

LYSIS means the gradual ending of a fever, and is opposed to crisis, which signifies the sudden ending of a fever. (See CRISIS.) It is also used to describe the process of dissolution of a blood-clot, or the loosening of adhesions.

LYSOFORM is a liquid soap containing formalin, which gives it a strong antiseptic power.

LYSOL is a brown, clear, oily fluid with antiseptic properties, made from coal-tar and containing 50 per cent cresol. When mixed with water it forms a clear soapy fluid. (See CRESOL.)

LYSOL POISONING: When lysol is swallowed there is a sense of burning about the mouth and throat. There are signs of corrosion around and in the mouth, with brown discoloration, and the characteristic smell of lysol is very evident in the breath. If the lysol is not speedily removed, unconsciousness and stupor gradually come on and death may occur within 24 hours. Septic pneumonia is also liable to supervene, and may produce death at a later period.
Treatment: If the skin has been contaminated with the lysol, it must be washed with water, and any lysol-contaminated clothing must be taken off. Large quantities of tepid water and salt may be given at once to dilute the lysol if it has been swallowed, and produce vomiting.

LYSOZYME is a bactericidal substance present in tears.

LYSSA is another term for rabies or hydrophobia.

M

McBURNEY'S POINT is an area of small size on the front of the abdomen, at which the tenderness experienced in appendicitis is felt with special keenness. It is situated between the navel and the prominent anterior superior spine of the right iliac bone, about 50 mm (2 inches) from the latter.

MACERATION is the softening of a solid by soaking in fluid.

MACROCYTE is an unusually large red blood corpuscle especially characteristic of the blood in pernicious anaemia.

MACROCYTOSIS: This condition, present in certain anaemias, is characterized by the existence of abnormally large red cells in the blood. It is particularly associated with pernicious anaemia (q.v.).

MACROGLOSSIA means an abnormally large tongue.

MACROPHAGE: A large phagocyte (q.v.) that forms part of the reticuloendothelial system. It is found in many organs and tissues, including connective tissues, bone marrow, lymph nodes, spleen, liver and central nervous system. Free macrophages move between cells and, using their scavenger properties, collect at infection sites to remove foreign bodies, including bacteria. Fixed macrophages are found in connective tissue.

MACROPSIA: Condition in which objects appear larger than normal. It can be due to disease of the macula.

MACULA: A spot or area of tissue that is different from surrounding tissue. An example is the macula letea, the yellow spot in the retina of the eye (see EYE).

MACULES are spots or stained areas of brown or purplish-brown colour in the skin. They may be due to old haemorrhages, sunburn, disease of internal organs, pregnancy, skin diseases such as eczema and psoriasis, syphilis, and burns.

MACULOPAPULAR: A skin rash that is made up of macules (discoloration of the skin) and papules (raised abnormality of the skin).

MADURA FOOT is the name given to a disease found in the Tropics in which the foot becomes swollen and its bones and other tissues riddled by sinuses. It is caused by the presence of a fungus.

MAGNESIUM is a light metallic element. Magnesium is one of the essential mineral elements of the body, without which it cannot function properly. The adult body contains around 25 grams, the greater part of which is in the bones. More than two-thirds of our daily supply come from cereals and vegetables. As most other foods also contain useful amounts, there is thus seldom any difficulty in maintaining an adequate amount in the body. It is an essential constituent of several vital enzymes (q.v.). Deficiency leads to muscular weakness and interferes with the efficient working of the heart. The salts of magnesium used as drugs are the hydroxide of magnesium, the oxide of magnesium, generally known as 'magnesia', and the carbonate of magnesium, all of which have an antacid action; also the sulphate of magnesium generally known as 'Epsom salts', which acts as a purgative.
Uses: Light and heavy carbonates of magnesia are used to correct hyperacidity of the stomach, as are the hydroxide and the light oxide. They are also used as feeble laxatives. Cream of magnesia, the official *British Pharmacopoeia* name of which is Magnesium Hydroxide Mixture, is a widely used, effective antacid. In large doses it is a useful safe laxative.

Magnesium sulphate is the most commonly used saline purge. (See EPSOM SALTS.)

MAGNESIUM TRISILICATE: A white powder with antacid properties. A mild antacid with prolonged action, it is used for treating peptic ulceration, commonly combined with quickly acting antacids. It has no side-effects so can be used in large doses.

MALABSORPTION SYNDROME includes a multiplicity of diseases, all of which are characterized by faulty absorption from the intestine of essential foodstuffs, such as fat, vitamins and mineral salts. Among the conditions in this syndrome are coeliac disease (q.v.), sprue (q.v.), cystic fibrosis and pancreatis. Surgical removal of the small intestine also causes the syndrome. Symptoms include anaemia, diarrhoea, oedema, vitamin deficiencies, weight loss and, in severe cases, malnutrition.

MALACIA is a term applied to softening of a part or tissue in disease: e.g. osteomalacia or softening of the bones.

MALAISE means a vague feeling of feverishness, listlessness, and languor, which often precedes the onset of serious acute diseases, or accompanies passing derangements, such as dyspepsia, chills, and colds.

MALAR: Anything relating to the cheek. For example, the malar (zygomatic) bone is also known as the cheek bone, and a malar flush is reddening of the cheeks.

MALARIA, which derives its name from *mala aria* – the Italian for bad air – and also known as AGUE, PALUDISM, JUNGLE FEVER, MARSH FEVER, PERIODIC FEVER, is a disease caused by the presence of certain parasites in the blood. It consists at first of a series of febrile attacks, which may come on every day, every second day, or every third day; later it assumes a chronic form, in which a poor state of health known as chronic malaria or malarial cachexia is developed, and there is a tendency towards frequent relapses.

History: It has been known from the earliest times, having been recorded as far back as 1500 BC. Devastating malarial epidemics contributed significantly to the fall of the Roman Empire. Not only is it described by many of the medical writers of antiquity, but numerous references to it exist in general literature, such as the works of Horace. From these it appears that its connection with swampy ground was recognized even in ancient times.

The first important advance was made in 1640, when the Countess of Chinchon, wife of the Viceroy of Peru, brought home to Europe the bark by which the South American Indians had learned to treat the disease successfully. From this bark, named after her Cinchona bark (by Linnaeus who made a mistake in her name), and also known as Jesuit's bark, since the secret had been learned by priests from the Indians, quinine is derived. By this drug a means of treating the paroxysms of fever, as well as an aid in warding off the disease, was obtained. From the fact that quinine is an antiseptic it was assumed that the disease must be due to some poison circulating in the blood which the quinine could destroy.

In 1880 Laveran, a French military surgeon, discovered the presence of minute parasites in the corpuscles of blood drawn from malarious persons and examined them under the microscope. He described more than one form of the parasites, and subsequent observers demonstrated that the parasites go through a process of development, leading up to the production of spores, which are formed all through the blood of the affected person at one time, and from which a new set of parasites develops.

It had long been noticed, even by West African natives, that mosquitoes seem to flourish together with malaria, and several scientists endeavoured to establish a connection between the two. This was successfully proved by Manson in 1894, through bringing from Italy live mosquitoes which had been allowed to suck blood from malarious persons in that country, and allowing the insects to bite healthy people in London, who had no other possible connection with the disease. The experiment was successful, and those people who had offered themselves for the experiment proved conclusively that malaria is carried by mosquitoes. Others proved the converse of this proposition, and

showed, by living for some months in a malarious district, such as the Roman Campagna, that infection does not take place if mosquitoes are kept off by gauze and other means.

From the examination of the blood in malarious people, Manson reasoned that the parasites go through a stage of their development in the bodies of the mosquitoes, passing, in the tissues of those insects, through a sexual stage, in which male and female forms unite in the production of masses of new parasites. The arduous work of demonstrating this was undertaken by Ross, then a military surgeon in India. The difficulty of this work is understood when one considers that the dissection of a great number of mosquitoes and their examination under the microscope were necessary before Ross was able in 1898 to confirm the truth of Manson's theory, by demonstrating the genus Anopheles as the insect in which the development of the malaria parasite takes place. Other observers confirmed his observations, and traced out in detail the changes which the parasites undergo while in the mosquito.

Causes: As shown by these discoveries, the presence of people infected by the malarial parasite and the access of the Anopheles mosquito to these and to healthy people form two of the conditions producing infection of fresh cases. But there are various factors which aid or retard the development of the parasite and of the mosquito. The disease is known all round the world, but is chiefly found in tropical climates, spreading here and there into temperate regions, where it occurs in summer and autumn, if the other conditions are suitable. The presence of swamps, pools of surface water, rank vegetation, and a poorly fed population are also important factors. Its chief seats are Africa, India, South East Asia and Central America. The estimated world incidence is 150 million. There is a growing incidence of it in the United Kingdom in people who have acquired the disease abroad. In 1986, 1663 cases were reported in the United Kingdom.

The parasites of malaria are three in number, corresponding to the tertian fever, the quartan fever, and the malignant tertian malaria. The parasites are protozoa, belonging to the order *Sporozoa*, and to the genus *Plasmodium*. The specific names for benign tertian, quartan, and malignant malaria are, respectively, *Plasmodium vivax, P. malariae*, and *P. falciparum*. As has been stated, the malarial parasite passes one phase of its life-cycle in man and the other in the stomach and tissues of the mosquito (the sexual phase). After sexual union of male and female forms in the mosquito's stomach, the resulting offspring – the asexual sporozoites – eventually find their way into the mosquito's salivary gland. Once a mosquito has become infected it remains infective for life.

When the infected female mosquito bites a human being, these filamentous sporozoites are injected into the blood. They then find their way into the liver where they develop into what are known as schizonts. After a period ranging from six to sixteen days (depending on the species of plasmodium) these schizonts have reached maturity, and in the course of maturation each one has produced up to 40,000 merozoites. These merozoites are then released into the blood stream where they penetrate the red blood cells and form trophozoites or rings. These in turn enlarge, each to the capacity of the red corpuscle. The large trophozoite thus formed finally splits into numerous small parasites now called merozoites. These burst out of the red blood corpuscle into the blood stream and then attack other red corpuscles, the whole asexual cycle repeating itself once more. The paroxysm of malarial fever coincides with the bursting of the red blood corpuscles and the setting free of the merozoites into the bloodstream. Sexual forms – male and female gametocytes – also develop in the blood, but they undergo no further change until a mosquito bite sucks them into the mosquito's stomach.

Symptoms: For a day or two before the actual fever sets in, there may be headache, vague pains about the body and limbs, chilliness, and slight rises of temperature. When the parasites have multiplied up to the stage already mentioned, the attack suddenly comes on.

The acute malarial attack has, in general, three stages, although in occasional cases one of the stages may be excessively marked or may be wanting. These are the cold stage, the hot stage, and the sweating stage.

The cold stage begins with a feeling of chilliness even in the hottest weather. This increases till the person has to betake himself to bed and heap himself with clothes, face and nails being blue with cold, and the whole body shaken with shivering (rigors). Nevertheless, if the temperature is measured, it is found to be considerably raised. This stage lasts an hour or less.

The hot stage comes on as the temperature of the body rises, beginning with hot flushes, which lengthen till the body feels burning hot, the temperature rising to 40·5 to 41·1 °C (105 or 106 °F). There are also headache, dizziness, sickness, pain throughout the body, and sometimes even delirium. This stage may last several hours.

The sweating stage comes on after the fever reaches its height, as the temperature begins to fall. Profuse perspiration breaks out, the person begins to feel decidedly better, and the headache and pains at the same time pass off. Finally, after two or three hours the patient feels quite well, though much weakened, and remains so till the next attack begins.

If the parasite present is that of *quartan fever* there is an intermission of two days before the next attack: that is to say, if the first attack is on the 1st day of the month the succeeding ones are on the 4th, 7th, and so on. If the parasite is that of *tertian fever*, the attacks are on the 1st, 3rd, 5th, and so on; whilst in the severe *malignant tertian fever*, each attack may last considerably over a day, so that there may not be time for one to pass off completely before the next begins. The patient then is in a continued

state of fever, known as *subtertian fever*. A person may get a double or treble infection of the malarial parasites, and then the fever may also occur every day. When the fever occurs every day, whatever the cause, it is sometimes called a *quotidian fever*.

As a rule people, after passing through an ague, feel completely recovered till the next attack is due, but now and then the attack may develop seriously. Thus hyperpyrexia (q.v.) may develop, the temperature continuing to rise till death occurs before the sweating stage sets in. Insensibility may set in and the person die owing to blockage of the small vessels in the brain by immense numbers of the parasites; this is known as cerebral malaria. Severe vomiting or diarrhoea may also endanger the patient's life, or he may become very collapsed during the sweating stage. One of the most dread complications is blackwater fever (q.v.).

If treatment is adopted between two attacks, the succeeding attack or the next after that is generally checked. Even when no treatment takes place, after a few weeks of the attacks these gradually get less and less marked and finally disappear. The parasites become so diminished that they are unable to cause fever, but they are not entirely destroyed in the blood, and so the affected person is subject after some weeks or months to a relapse, when the attacks of ague are repeated as in the first seizure. These rallies and relapses may go on for several years, especially if the person leads an exposed, laborious life, or is poorly nourished. Anything which depresses the vitality, such as a chill, is apt to lead to a fresh relapse. On the other hand, under efficient treatment complete recovery occurs.

If the disease becomes chronic, various symptoms set in. The person becomes very anaemic in consequence of the large number of blood corpuscles destroyed by the parasites in each paroxysm of fever. A feeble state of health, accompanied by bodily wasting and yellow discoloration of the skin, ensues, and the spleen and liver, particularly the former, become enlarged.

Treatment: This falls into two important sections, preventive and curative.

PREVENTIVE TREATMENT may be directed either against the parasites or against the mosquitoes which convey them. Recommendations for drugs to use in the prevention of malaria are regularly updated and travellers should consult a doctor for up-to-the-minute advice. Among those used are chloroguine, Maloprim (pyrimethamine and dapsone) or Fansidar (pyrimethamine and sulfadoxine). Fansidar should not be taken by pregnant women or by those sensitive to sulphonamides. There is a geographical variation in the choice of recommended drugs because of increasing evidence of resistance to drugs being acquired by the causative organism, particularly *P. falciparum* to chloroquine in South Asia. Travellers should start taking antimalarial drugs one week before setting out and should continue taking them for at least six weeks after their return to the United

Kingdom. People may catch malaria despite preventive measures and anyone returning from a malarial zone who develops headache, fever and malaise should see a doctor. About 1500 cases occur annually in the United Kingdom. Full details of which drugs to take and when, are given in two leaflets – *Notice to Travellers* published by the Department of Health, and *Advice to Travellers* published by the Health Education Council – which are available from travel agencies, as well as in *Preservation of Personal Health in Warm Climates* published by the Ross Institute of Tropical Hygiene, Keppel Street, London WC1E 7HT, price £2.50, including postage and packing.

It is still more important to attack the mosquitoes in their developing stage. The eggs are laid on or near pools of stagnant water in which the larvae and pupae swim just below the surface, breathing through a tube which projects above the surface of the water. These larvae may be destroyed by pouring on the surface of these pools some fluid through which the breathing-tube of the larva cannot be protruded. Crude petroleum and a special oil known as 'malariol' are used for this purpose. Stagnant water should be drained.

Although these methods are still of value, they have largely been replaced or supplemented by the use of insecticides such as DDT, benzene hexachloride (BHC) and dieldrin which have proved most effective in destroying mosquitoes. Wire-gauze screens to all the windows of a house and muslin mosquito netting over the beds also form an efficient protection.

CURATIVE TREATMENT depends upon a wide range of drugs, including chloroquine, primaquine, pyrimethamine, and quinine. In cases in which the malaria organism has become resistant to these the World Health Organization recommends amodiaquine or sulfadoxine. (See also BLACKWATER FEVER.)

MALATHION is one of the less toxic organophosphorus insecticides (q.v.).

MALFORMATION (see DEFORMITIES).

MALIGNANT is a term applied in several ways to serious disorders. Tumours are called malignant when they grow rapidly, tend to infiltrate surrounding healthy tissues, and to spread to distant parts of the body, leading eventually to death. (See CANCER.) The term is also applied to types of disease which are much more serious than the usual form, such as malignant hypertension, malignant smallpox. Malignant pustule is another name for anthrax (q.v.).

MALIGNANT FEVER, also known as MALIGNANT HYPERPYREXIA and MALIGNANT HYPERTHERMIA, is a rare, but dangerous, complication of general anaesthesia, commoner in children and adolescents than adults. The over-all frequency is 1 in 15,000 anaesthetics in children and 1 in 50,000 in adults. It is characterized by a sudden rise in the temperature of the patient during anaesthesia. This may occur after a few minutes or several hours, and the temperature may rise as high as 44 °C (112 °F). It is associated with an abnormality of the muscles which tends to run in families. This may be detected by estimating the level of creatine phosphokinase in the blood, which is raised in those liable to develop this condition. The shorter the duration of the anaesthesia and the smaller the rise in temperature, the greater are the chances of recovery; this is one reason why a careful check is kept of the patient's temperature during general anaesthesia. In those liable to develop this complication, operations are carried out under regional or local anaesthesia whenever possible. (See ANAESTHESIA.)

MALIGNANT HYPERPYREXIA: A rare condition of widespread rigidity of the skeletal muscles accompanied by a high temperature developing after general anaesthetic. It is caused by an unknown muscle membrane defect and has a genetic link.

MALIGNANT HYPERTENSION has nothing to do with cancer. It derives its name from the fact that, if untreated, it runs a rapidly fatal course. It is still undecided whether it is a disease entity in itself or is merely a terminal stage in certain cases of essential hypertension (q.v.). Its characteristic features are that it occurs in a younger age-group than essential hypertension, and that there is a very high diastolic blood-pressure, with papilloedema (q.v.) and kidney failure. This is the type of hypertension in which the antihypertensive drugs (see ESSENTIAL HYPERTENSION) have proved so successful. Indeed, the introduction of these drugs has revolutionized the outlook. At one time an invariably fatal disease within two years, many patients with this condition can now enjoy many years of comparatively good health.

MALINGERING is a term applied to the feigning of illness. In the great majority of cases a person who feigns illness has a certain amount of disability, but exaggerates the illness or discomfort for some ulterior motive.

MALLEOLUS is the term applied to either of the two bony prominences at the ankle. (See LEG.)

MALLET FINGER is due to sudden forced flexion of the terminal joint of a finger, resulting in rupture of the tendon. As a result the individual is unable to extend the terminal part of the finger which remains bent forward. The middle, ring and little fingers are most commonly involved. Treatment is by splinting the finger. The end result is satisfactory provided the victim has sufficient patience.

MALLET TOE is the condition in which it is not possible to extend the terminal part of the toe. It is usually due to muscular imbalance but may be due to congenital absence of the extensor muscle. A callosity (q.v.) often forms on it which may be painful. Should this be troublesome, treatment consists of removal of the terminal phalanx.

MALLEUS: The hammer-shaped lateral bone of the group of three that form the sound-transmitting ossicles in the middle ear. (See EAR.)

MALNUTRITION: The condition arising from an inadequate or unbalanced diet. The causes may be a lack of one or more essential nutrients or inadequate absorption from the intestinal tracts. A diet that is deficient in carbohydrate usually contains inadequate protein, and this type of malnutrition occurs in Africa and Asia as a result of poverty, famine or war.

MALOPRIM is a combination of pyrimethamine (q.v.) and dapsone (q.v.) which is used for the prevention of malaria (q.v.). It has the advantage of only needing to be taken once weekly. It should not be taken by anyone hypersensitive to sulphonamides, and should not be used for the treatment of an acute attack.

MALPRACTICE: Improper or inadequate medical treatment that fails to match the standards of skill and care that is reasonably expected from a qualified health care practitioner – usually a doctor or dentist.

MALPRESENTATION: A situation during childbirth in which a baby is not in the customary head-first position before delivery. The result is usually a complicated labour in which a caesarean operation may be necessary to effect the birth.

MALT is a substance derived from barley by allowing a certain amount of growth to take place in the moistened grain, which is then dried and crushed. It contains a ferment named diastase, together with a large amount of malt-sugar and dextrin, the latter constituents being still further developed from the starch of the barley by the action of the ferment, when the malt is allowed to digest in water at a temperature approaching 40 °C (104 °F). Similarly, the ferment will convert into sugar a large amount of the starch in flour mixed with malt, and so perform some of the functions of the saliva and pancreatic juice.

For these reasons malt is mixed with various proportions of flour to form some of the popular foods for children. It is also used in the form of malt extracts, 28 grams of which is equivalent to 80 Calories.

MALTA FEVER (see BRUCELLOSIS).

MAMMARY GLAND (see BREAST).

MAMMILLA is the Latin term for the nipple.

MAMMOGRAPHY is the special technique whereby X-rays can be taken that reveal the structure of the breast. It is an effective way of distinguishing benign from malignant tumours. It can detect tumours that are not palpable. In a multi-centre study in the USA, called The Breast Cancer Detection Demonstration Project, which involved nearly 300,000 women in the 40–49 age group, 35 per cent of the tumours were found by mammography alone, 13 per cent by physical examination and 50 per cent by both methods. Two Dutch studies published in 1984 confirmed the benefits of breast screening with a reduction in mortality of 50 to 70 per cent in screened women. The optimum frequency of screening is debatable. The American College of Radiologists recommends a baseline mammogram at the age of 40 years with subsequent mammography at one to two year intervals up to the age of 50. Thereafter, annual mammography is recommended. As breast cancer is the commonest malignancy in Western women and is increasing in frequency, the importance of screening for this form of cancer is obvious.

MANDELIC ACID is a non-toxic keto-acid used in the treatment of infections of the urinary tract, especially those due to the *Escherichia coli* and the *Streptococcus faecalis* or *Enterococcus*. It is administered in doses of 3 grams several times daily. As it is only effective in an acid urine, ammonium chloride must be taken at the same time.

MANDIBLE is the bone of the lower jaw.

MANDL'S PAINT consists of iodine 1·25 grams, potassium iodide 2·5 grams, water 2·5 ml, oil of peppermint 0·4 ml, alcohol (90 per cent) 4 ml, glycerin to 100 ml. It is used as a throat paint in pharyngitis and tonsillitis. It should be well shaken before use.

MANGANESE is a metal, oxides of which are found abundantly in nature. Permanganate of potassium is a well-known disinfectant.

MANIA is a form of mental disorder characterized by great excitement. (See MENTAL ILLNESS.)

MANIC-DEPRESSIVE INSANITY, or CYCLOTHYMIA, is a form of madness characterized by alternate attacks of mania and depression. (See MENTAL ILLNESS.)

MANIPULATION is the term applied to the forceful passive movement of joints. In skilled hands it is a most effective means of treatment of stiff joints or of pain in the back due to a prolapsed intervertebral disc (q.v.).

MANNITOL is an osmotic diuretic (q.v.) given intravenously. (See DIURETICS.)

MANOMETER is an instrument for measuring the pressure or tension of liquids or gases. (See BLOOD-PRESSURE.)

MANTOUX TEST, also known as MENDEL'S TEST, is a test for tuberculosis. It consists in injecting into the superficial layers of the skin (i.e. intradermally) a very small quantity of old tuberculin. A positive reaction of the skin – swelling and redness – shows that the person so reacting has been infected with the *Mycobacterium tuberculosis*. But it does not mean that such a person is suffering from active tuberculosis. (See TUBERCULIN.)

MANUBRIUM is the uppermost part of the breast-bone.

MAPLE-SYRUP URINE DISEASE is a condition in which there is an association between mental defect and a disorder of amino-acid metabolism. It is so named because the urine has the odour of maple-syrup.

MARASMUS means progressive wasting, especially in young children, when there is no ascertainable cause. It is generally associated with defective feeding. (See ATROPHY; INFANT FEEDING.)

MARBURG DISEASE, also known as GREEN MONKEY DISEASE and VERVET MONKEY DISEASE because the first recorded cases acquired their infection from monkeys of this genus, is a viral infection with a high mortality rate. The incubation period is 4 to 9 days. The onset is sudden with marked nausea and severe headache. This is followed by rising temperature, diarrhoea, and vomiting. Towards the end of the first week a rash appears which persists for a week and is accompanied by internal bleeding. In those who recover convalescence is slow and prolonged. The world distribution of the causative virus is unknown, but apart from laboratory infections acquired through working with vervet monkeys, all the cases so far reported have occurred in Africa.

MARCH FRACTURE is a curious condition in which a fracture occurs of the second (rarely the third) metatarsal bone in the foot without any obvious cause. The usual story is that a pain suddenly developed in the foot while walking (hence the name) and that it has persisted ever since. The only treatment needed is immobili-

zation of the foot and rest, and the fracture heals satisfactorily.

MARCH HAEMOGLOBINURIA is a complication of walking and running over long distances. It is due to damage to red blood cells in the blood-vessels of the sole of the feet. This results in haemoglobin (q.v.) being released into the bloodstream, which is then voided in the urine, the condition known as haemoglobinuria (q.v.). No treatment is required, but the complaint may be minimized by wearing shoes with resilient soles and, so far as possible, avoiding running on hard surfaces.

MARFAN'S SYNDROME: An inherited disorder affecting about one person in 50,000 in which the connective tissue is abnormal. The result is defects of the heart, skeleton and eyes. The victims are unusually tall and thin with deformities of the chest and spine. They have spider-like hands and their joints and ligaments are weak. Orthopaedic intervention may help, as will drugs to control the heart problems. As affected individuals have a 50-per-cent chance of passing on the disease to their children, they should receive genetic counselling.

MARIHUANA is another term for CANNABIS INDICA, or hemp, or hashish. (See DRUG ADDICTION.)

MARRIAGE GUIDANCE (see RELATE MARRIAGE GUIDANCE).

MARROW (see BONE MARROW).

MARSH FEVER (see MALARIA).

MASOCHISM: A condition in which a person gets pleasure from physical or emotional pain inflicted by others. The term is often used in the context of achieving sexual excitement through inflicted pain. Masochism may be a conscious or subconscious activity.

MASSAGE, or RUBBING, is a method of treatment in which the operator uses his hands, or occasionally other appliances, to rub, knead, or press the skin and deeper tissues of the person under treatment. It is often combined with (*a*) passive movements, in which the masseur moves the limbs in various ways, the person treated making no effort; or (*b*) active movements, which are performed with the combined assistance of masseur and patient. Massage is also often combined with baths and gymnastics in order to strengthen various muscles. The beneficial effects of massage are exerted in different ways. Applied gently, it has a soothing action; applied more vigorously, certain methods have the effect of quickening the circulation of lymph and blood, and so leading to the rapid absorption of waste products in the muscles.

Other forms of massage cause muscular contractions and so provide exercise for the muscles in cases in which movements of the whole body are not desired.

Varieties: STROKING, or *effleurage*, consists of gentle pressure with the hand moved in one direction. It soothes the nerves of the part treated and empties the main lymph-vessels and veins, thus increasing the circulation locally. It is carried out either with the flat of the hand or with the edges of thumb and first finger widely separated.

KNEADING, or *pétrissage*, is the most commonly employed form, and consists of squeezing, kneading, rolling, or rubbing movements coupled with a considerable amount of pressure, effected, it may be, with the fingers or knuckles, but generally with the pulp or the ball of the thumb. It has a still greater effect than stroking in moving on the lymph and blood circulation of deep-seated parts, and so leading to the absorption of inflammatory thickenings in and around joints, tendon-sheaths, and muscles. (See LYMPH.)

STABILE MOVEMENTS include such applications as the following. *Pressing* may be done with the finger-tips or with the knuckles; it is usually combined with rubbing. *Tapping* is done with the points of the fingers from the wrist, and, when applied gently, has a soothing effect. *Thrusting*, which consists in poking up the deeper parts with the points of the fingers, and *hacking*, in which the muscles are struck with the inner edge of the hand, the arms moving from the elbows, are employed to cause muscular contractions.

VIBRATORY MOVEMENTS are made either by tapping (as above) or by special pads, to which a very rapid oscillation is communicated from an electric motor. This form of massage has been used in order to exert a soothing influence, for example, in cases of headache.

PASSIVE MOVEMENTS are made chiefly for their effect upon the joints. The synovial fluid is increased if scanty, and tends to be absorbed if excessive, while adhesions, which limit the motions of the joint or render these painful, are broken down by passive movements of a more forcible type. This type of massage is the form chiefly employed in the treatment of stiff joints by bone-setters.

ACTIVE MOVEMENTS of a carefully regulated type, in which the person's will is concentrated upon the movement made, are specially useful for developing the muscles brought into play thereby. The amount of muscular force required is graduated and increased by the masseur resisting the movements with varying degrees of force.

Uses: Massage can only be employed to full advantage by fully trained practitioners. A complete list of members of the Chartered Society of Physiotherapy who are qualified to give massage can be obtained on application to the Secretary of the Society, 14 Bedford Row, London, WC1R 4ED (071-242 1941, fax: 071-839 4509). The types of case in which massage is useful are extremely various. Neuralgia, sciatica, and muscular rheumatism are among the painful conditions in which some relief is generally obtained. In muscular wasting, and paralysis due to nerve conditions – such as lead-poisoning, peripheral neuritis, crutch palsy, Bell's paralysis, and poliomyelitis – the muscles affected may be kept in a state of good nutrition till the nerve weakness has disappeared, and so recovery may be materially hastened. In various other nervous conditions, such as hysteria, chorea, loss of sensation, and writer's cramp, massage often proves of great benefit. Several types of joint disease, such as chronic rheumatism and stiffness due to previous slight injuries, such as sprains, are specially amenable to treatment by passive movements combined with deep rubbing, but any such interference with joints which have been recently the seat of tuberculous disease is very dangerous, as by these means the disease may be more widely spread. In several general conditions such as corpulence and constipation associated with a flabby body, massage may be of use.

Massage may be combined with electrical applications. For example, high-frequency and static electricity may be used along with gentle massage to obtain a soothing effect. The interrupted galvanic, sinusoidal, and faradic currents are useful combined with more forcible massage to stimulate muscular contraction in various cases of paralysis. (See also CARDIAC MASSAGE.)

MASSETER: An important muscle of mastication that extends from the zygomatic arch in the cheek to the mandible or jaw bone. It acts by closing the jaw.

MASS HYSTERIA (see HYSTERIA).

MASS MINIATURE RADIOGRAPHY is a method of obtaining X-ray photographs of the chests of large numbers of people at about the rate of two per minute. It has been used on a large scale as a means of screening the population for pulmonary tuberculosis.

MASTALGIA is the term applied to pain in the breast.

MAST CELLS are round or oval cells found predominantly in the loose connective tissues. They contain histamine (q.v.) and heparin (q.v.), and carry immunoglobulin E, the antibody which plays a predominant part in allergic reactions. Although known to play a part in inflammatory reactions, allergy, and hypersensitivity, their precise function in health and disease is still not quite clear.

MASTECTOMY is the operation for removal of a breast. It is an operation that can cause considerable psychological disturbance. Those who find it difficult to adjust to the situation after the operation will obtain helpful advice from the Breast Care and Mastectomy Association of Great Britain, 15–19 Britten Street, London SW3 3TZ (071-867 1103, fax: 071-867 9303).

MASTICATION is the act whereby, as a result of movements of the lower jaw, lips, tongue, and cheek, food is reduced to a condition in which it is ready to be acted on by the gastric juices in the process of digestion. Adequate mastication is an essential part of the digestive process. (See DIGESTION.)

MASTITIS is the term applied to inflammation of the breast. (See BREAST, DISEASES OF.)

MASTOID PROCESS is the large process of the temporal bone of the skull which can be felt immediately behind the ear. It contains numerous cavities, one of which, the mastoid antrum, communicates with the middle ear, and is liable to suppurate when the middle ear is diseased. (See EAR, DISEASES OF.)

MASTURBATION is the production of an orgasm by self-manipulation of the penis or clitoris.

MAT BURN is a combination of a burn and an abrasion which occurs in wrestlers when the skin over the bony points is rubbed against the unyielding canvas mat. It is particularly liable to become infected. Treatment consists of thorough cleansing and the application of a dressing such as gauze and chlorhexidine covered by cotton-wool and firmly fixed by a bandage or elastoplast – depending on the extent of the injury.

MATCH-WORKERS' DISEASE (see PHOS-PHORUS POISONING).

MATERIA MEDICA is that branch of medical study which deals with the sources, preparations, and uses of drugs.

MATERNITY AND CHILD WELFARE: The high rate of infantile mortality which used to prevail in the larger towns drew attention to the great loss of infant life which was produced partly by ignorance on the part of the mothers and partly by poverty. A movement was accordingly begun early in the present century in some of the larger cities to provide trained women as health visitors for giving advice to working-class women on the proper methods of rearing their children. This was at first a voluntary effort conducted by philanthropic agencies, but it was soon taken up by local authorities throughout the country. The necessary information as to the existence of newly born infants was provided by the Notification of Births which was demanded by Acts passed in 1907 and 1915. Women health visitors were appointed to visit the homes of such newly born infants, and shortly afterwards infant consultation centres and clinics were established by various local authorities and voluntary agencies.

At first the movement for child welfare was limited to infants from birth to 1 year of age, but shortly afterwards the necessity for supervising the health of children until they came under school discipline at 5 years was recognized. Still later it became evident that it was desirable to watch over the health of the expectant mother and to provide skilled attendance prior to and during confinement. This led, accordingly, to the establishment of maternity and child welfare centres and clinics by many local authorities. The schemes which have now been devised for combating infantile mortality are very wide. They include better housing, health visitors, consultation centres for mothers, vitamin preparations and iron tablets for expectant and nursing mothers, and hospital accommodation for expectant mothers before and during confinement. The provision of child welfare centres and clinics in general practice to which parents may bring their infants produces valuable results, both by advice to the mothers and by keeping records about the infant. Antenatal clinics, which provide education and assistance for the expectant mother, form an important section of this work.

HEALTH VISITORS have been described as 'truly medico-social workers – playing a full part in both preventive medicine and social action'. Their duties cover maternity and child welfare, school nursing, health education, tuberculosis, venereal disease, infectious diseases, mental illness, welfare of the aged and the handicapped, family welfare services, and co-operation with general practitioners. Their training lasts three years and the courses must be approved by the United Kingdom Central Council for Nursing, Midwifery and Health Visiting.

ANTENATAL CLINICS are considered to be of great value, because the fatality among the unborn from stillbirth, abortion, etc., is higher than the mortality of infants during the first year of life; it is generally believed, further, that by the medical attention provided at such clinics many of these antenatal deaths could be prevented, and the number of infants born prematurely and of weak constitution could be much reduced. Thus, it has been shown that the perinatal mortality rate (q.v.) is nearly five times higher in the children of mothers who are late in attending antenatal clinics than in the children of those who start attending early. Health visitors follow up cases seen at antenatal clinics and ensure that the medical instructions given at the clinic are carried out, and proper steps taken to prepare for the confinement.

Under the National Insurance Acts in Great Britain, a woman receives a maternity grant in respect of each child, and also a home confinement grant if the confinement takes place at home. A woman who ordinarily follows a gainful occupation is also given a maternity allowance for 18 weeks beginning about 11 weeks before her confinement provided that she abstains from work. Under the Employment Protection (Consolidation) Act 1978, a woman has the right to return to work after confinement provided (a) she has been continuously employed for not less than two years and has worked at least 16 hours a week; (b) she was employed until 11 weeks before the expected week of confinement. She is also entitled to maternity pay.

INFANT CONSULTATION CLINICS are conducted usually by local authorities, and, in cases where it is desirable, mothers are urged to bring infants to these clinics regularly. Many of the disabling illnesses of early childhood are thus prevented, and the attendance should continue as required during the first five years of the child's life.

DAY NURSERIES, or crèches, are provided in many places in connection with these clinics, at which children can be left when the mothers are out at work. Many privately run day nurseries are also available.

SPECIAL TREATMENT CLINICS are also provided in many places for the examination and care of teeth, eyes, ears, nose, throat, and skin of children. Also there is at present a movement for the treatment of cases in which children are crippled as the result of early disease. Further, in connection with the clinics, many local authorities possess convalescent homes, or arrange with voluntary agencies for admission to their convalescent homes of children who are in need of special care and open-air regime. Indirectly connected with these clinics in many places there have also been established play centres and kindergartens for young children.

Under the National Health Service Act, 1946, all these services were unified under Local Health Authorities. A statutory duty was imposed upon Local Health Authorities to provide health centres, maternity and child welfare, domiciliary midwifery, health visiting, home nursing, vaccination and immunization, and ambulances. They were also empowered to provide home-help services, and care and aftercare. Maternity and child welfare covers the care of expectant and nursing mothers and of children under 5 years of age who are not attending school. It includes antenatal clinics, postnatal clinics, child-welfare clinics, and a priority dental service for both expectant and nursing mothers and young children. Further reorganization of the National Health Service introduced in 1974, 1982 and 1990 aimed at a closer co-ordination of these services with the hospital service and the family doctor service.

MAXILLA is the name applied to the upper jaw-bones, which bear the teeth.

ME: (see MYALGIC ENCEPHALOMYELITIS).

MEASLES, also known as MORBILLI, is an acute infectious disease occurring mostly in children. The name, measles, comes from the teutonic root, *maes*, meaning a spot. Morbilli is a diminutive of morbus, a disease. It appears to have been known from an early period in the history of medicine, mention being made of it in the writings of Rhazes and others of the Arabian physicians in the tenth century. For long, however, its specific nature was not recognized, and it was held to be a variety of smallpox. Measles and scarlet fever were long confused with each other; and in the account given by Sydenham of epidemics of measles in London in 1670 and 1674, it is evident that even that accurate observer had not as yet clearly perceived their pathological distinction, although it would seem to have been made a century earlier by Ingrassia, a physician of Palermo. The disease known as German measles, or rubella, is a much milder disease than measles. Measles is compulsorily notifiable in Britain.

Causes: Measles is a disease of the earlier years of childhood. Like most other infectious maladies, it is rare in infants under 6 months old on account of the antibodies that they have acquired from their mothers before birth. It is comparatively seldom met in adults because most have undergone an attack in early life, although second attacks can occur. Some countries enjoy long immunity from outbreaks of measles, but in such cases the disease, when introduced, spreads with great rapidity and virulence.

In many countries, such as the United Kingdom and the United States, measles has rarely been absent, especially from large towns, but every two years, especially from December to February, epidemics have arisen and spread among the children who were not protected by a recent attack. In 1990, however, there were only 13,291 cases in England and Wales, a dramatic fall in numbers from 1986 when over 80,000 cases were reported. This is due to the introduction in 1988 of the measles, mumps and rubella vaccine. 1990 was the first year in which no deaths from measles were reported.

There are few diseases so infectious as measles, and its rapid spread in epidemics is no doubt due to the fact that this viral infection is most potent in the earlier stages. Hence the difficulty of timely isolation and the readiness with which the disease is spread, which is mostly by infected droplets from the nose and throat coughed or sneezed into the air. (See INFECTION.)

Symptoms: After the infection has been received into the system, a period of incubation or latency precedes the development of the disease, during which scarcely any disturbance of the health is perceptible. This period appears to vary in duration, but it generally lasts for from ten to fifteen days, when it is followed by the invasion of the symptoms specially characteristic of measles. These consist in the somewhat sudden onset of acute catarrh of the mucous membranes. Sneezing, accompanied with a watery discharge, sometimes bleeding from the nose, redness and watering of the eyes, cough of a short, frequent, and noisy character, with little or no expectoration, hoarseness of the voice, and occasionally sickness and diarrhoea, are the chief symptoms of this stage. The temperature rises to 37·7 to 39 °C (100 to 102 °F), and the pulse is rapid, while headache, thirst, and restlessness are usually present to a greater or less degree. About the fourth day after infection the characteristic eruption appears on the skin, being first noticed on the brow, cheeks, chin, also behind the ears, and on the neck. It consists of small raised spots of a dusky red or crimson colour, that tend to group together into irregular, occasionally crescentic patches. Even before it appears on the skin, the rash is sometimes visible within the mouth, as bluish-white spots on the mucous membrane, known as Koplik spots. By the end of about a week after its first appearance, scarcely any trace of the eruption remains beyond a faint staining of the skin. At the start of the eruptive stage, the constitutional disturbances become aggravated, the temperature often rising to 40·5 °C (105 °F) or more. These symptoms usually decline as soon as the rash has attained its maximum, and often there occurs a sudden and extensive fall of temperature, indicating that the crisis of the disease has been reached.

Treatment: The patient should be isolated, but quarantine of contacts is used much less than it used to be, though it is probably a wise precaution to keep infants away from the infected child. During an epidemic children under the age of 5 years should not be admitted to a nursery school, nursery class or infant school unless they are known to have had the disease or have been immunized against it. Child contacts of measles should be allowed to go to school provided they are sent home on the first suggestion of fever or malaise. The vaccine now available gives substantial protection against the disease. It is usually given during the second year of life, and its use has resulted in a sharp fall in the number of cases.

MEASURES (see WEIGHTS AND MEASURES).

MEAT (see PROTEIN).

MEATUS is a term applied to any passage or opening: e.g. external auditory meatus, the passage from the surface to the drum of the ear.

MECKEL'S DIVERTICULUM is a hollow process sometimes found attached to the small intestine. It is placed on the small intestine about 90 to 120 cm (3 or 4 feet) away from its junction with the large intestine, is several cms long, and ends blindly.

MECONIUM is the brown, semi-fluid material which collects in the bowels of a child prior to birth, and which should be discharged either at the time of birth or shortly afterwards. It consists partly of bile secreted by the liver before birth, partly of debris from the mucous membrane of the intestines.

MEDIA: The middle layer of an organ or tissue, but more usually applied to the wall of an artery or vein, where the media comprises layers of elastic and smooth muscle fibres.

MEDIAL: Near the middle of tissue, organ or body.

MEDIAL TIBIAL SYNDROME is the term applied by athletes to a condition characterized by pain over the inner border of the shin, which occurs in most runners and sometimes in joggers. The syndrome, also known as shin splints, is due to muscular swelling resulting in inadequate blood supply in the muscle: hence the pain. The disorder may be the result of compartment syndrome (build-up of pressure in the muscles), tendinitis, muscle or bone inflammation or damage to the muscle. It usually disappears within a few weeks, responding to rest and physiotherapy, with or without injections. In some cases, however, it becomes chronic and so severe that it occurs even at rest. If the cause is the compartment syndrome, relief is usually obtained by a simple operation to relieve the pressure in the affected muscles.

MEDIASTINUM is the space in the chest which lies between the two lungs. It contains the heart and great vessels, the gullet, the lower part of the windpipe, the thoracic duct, the phrenic nerves, as well as numerous structures of less importance.

MEDICATED: Description of a substance that contains a medicinal drug, commonly applied to items such as sweets and soaps.

MEDULLA: The inside part of an organ or tissue that is distinct from the outer part – for example, the marrow in the centre of a long bone or the inner portion of the kidneys or adrenal glands.

MEDULLA OBLONGATA is the hindmost part of the brain and is continued into the spinal cord. In it are situated several of the nerve-centres which are most essential to life, such as those governing breathing, the action of the heart, swallowing. (See BRAIN.)

MEFENAMIC ACID: is a drug with pain-relieving, anti-inflammatory and antipyretic actions that is proving of value in the treatment of osteoarthritis and rheumatoid arthritis.

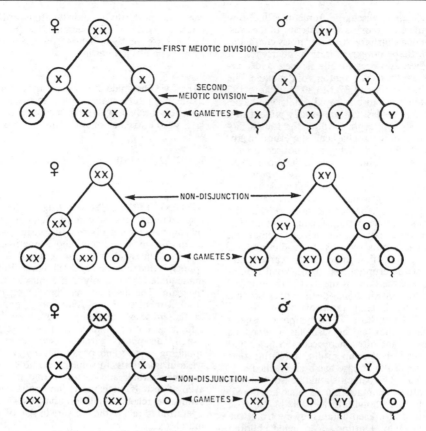

The formation of gametes. Top, normal meiosis. Centre, non-disjunction at first meiotic division. Bottom, non-disjunction at second meiotic division.

MEGA- and MEGALO- are prefixes denoting largeness.

MEGACOLON: A greatly enlarged colon that may be present at birth or develop later. It can occur in all age groups and the condition is typified by severe chronic constipation. Megacolon is caused by obstruction of the colon which may be due to faulty innervation, or to psychological factors. Other causes are Hirschsprung's disease (q.v.) or ulcerative colitis (q.v.). In old people the persistent use of powerful laxative drugs may cause the condition.

MEGALOMANIA is a delusion of grandeur or an insane belief in a person's own extreme greatness, goodness, or power.

MEIBOMIAN GLANDS: Numerous glands within the tarsal plates of the eyelids. Their secretions form part of the tears.

MEIOSIS or REDUCTION DIVISION is the form of cell division that only occurs in the gonads, that is the testis and the ovary, giving rise to the germ cells of the sperms and the ova. Two types of sperm cells are produced. One contains 22 autosomes and a Y sex chromosome and the other contains 22 autosomes and an X sex chromosome. All the ova, however, produced by normal meiosis have 22 autosomes and an X sex chromosome. Two divisions of the nucleus occur and only one division of the chromosomes, so that the number of chromosomes in the ova and sperms is half that of the somatic cells. Each chromosome pair divides so that the gametes receives only one member of each pair. The number of chromosomes is restored to full complement at fertilization so the the zygote has a complete set, each chromosome from the nucleus of the sperm pairing up with its corresponding partner from the ovum.

The first stage of meiosis involves the pairing of homologous chromosomes which join together and synapse lengthwise. The chromosomes then become doubled by splitting along their length and the chromatids so formed are held together by centromeres. As the homologous chromosomes, one of which has come from the mother and the other from the father, are lying together genetic interchange can take place between the chromatids and in this way new combinations of genes arise. All four chromatids are closely interwoven and recombination may take place between any maternal or any paternal chromatids. This process is known as crossing over or recombination.

After this period of interchange homologous chromosomes move apart, one to each pole of the nucleus. The cell then divides and the nucleus of each new cell now contains 23 and not 46 chromosomes. The second meiotic division then occurs, the centromeres divide and the chromatids move apart to opposite poles of the nucleus so there are still 23 chromosomes in each of the daughter nuclei so formed. The cell divides again so that there are four gametes, each containing a half number (haploid) set of chromosomes. However, owing to the recombination or crossing over the genetic material is not identical with either parent or with other spermatozoa.

MELAENA means a condition of the stools in which dark, tarry masses are passed from the bowel. It is due to bleeding from the stomach or from the higher part of the bowel, the blood undergoing chemical changes under the action of the secretions, and being finally converted in large part into sulphide of iron.

MELANCHOLIA is a form of mental illness characterized by great mental and physical depression. (See MENTAL ILLNESS.)

MELANIN is the dark pigment found in the skin and hair, as well as the choroid coat of the eye. It is the amount of melanin which decides the colour of the skin and hair. In white skin it occurs as granules in cells known as melanocytes situated in the stratum basale of the skin (q.v.). On exposure to ultra-violet light these granules are released and pass into the superficial layers of the skin where they produce the brown colour known as sun-tan which protects the skin against the harmful effects of continued exposure to the ultra-violet rays of the sun. Genetic factors play an important role in determining the distribution of melanin in the skin and hence its colour. Thus in those with genetically brown or black skin, as well as sun-tanned white-skinned people, there is a widespread distribution of melanin in the more superficial layers of the skin. This is due more to increased activity of the melanocytes than to an actual increase in their number.

MELANOMA is a tumour arising from the cells that produce melanin (q.v.). A highly malignant form, known as malignant melanoma, arises from the pigmented cells of moles (q.v.) or naevi. Malignant melanoma, which responds well to surgical removal provided this is done at an early enough stage, is much more common in white people living in sunny climes such as Australia, South Africa and parts of the USA, but it can occur in the United Kingdom. The hazards of ultra-violet light in causing malignant melanoma cannot be ignored in the British Isles, particularly in those who holiday abroad. The incidence is steadily rising and, as one expert has pointed out, 'is likely to continue to rise so long as our society remains addicted

to the sun'. He adds: 'Though ultra-violet light is not the sole cause of malignant melanoma, excessive exposure is an important factor . . . particularly in people whose skin has a tendency to go red whether or not it subsequently tans. The prophylactic use of sun-screening agents should be a routine for such people.' (See SUNBURN.)

MELPHALAN is one of the alkylating agents (q.v.) which is proving of value in the treatment of certain forms of malignant disease. (See CYTOTOXIC.)

MEMBRANES (see BRAIN; CROUP; DIPHTHERIA; LABOUR).

MEMORY is the capacity to remember. It is complex and probably occurs in many areas of the brain including the limbic system and the temporal lobes. Despite such poor knowledge of the anatomy of memory, research has revealed much about how the process works. There are three main steps: registration, storage, and recall.

During registration information from the sense organs and the cerebral cortex is put into codes for storage in the short-term memory system. The codes are usually acoustic (based on the sounds and words that would be used to describe the information) but may use any of the five senses. This system can take only a few chunks of information at a time. Research shows, for example, that only about seven longish numbers can be retained and recalled at once – the next new number displaces an earlier one that is then forgotten. And if a subject is asked to describe a person he has just met, he will recall only seven or so facts about that person. This depends on attention span and can be improved by concentration and rehearsal, for example, by reciting the list of things that must be remembered.

Material needing storage for several minutes stays in the short-term memory. More valuable information goes to the long-term memory where it can be kept for any period from a few minutes to a lifetime. Storage is more reliable if the information is in meaningful codes – it is much easier to remember people's names if their faces and personalities are memorable too. Using techniques such as mnemonics takes this into account.

The final stage is retrieval. Recognizing and recalling the required information involves searching the memory. In the short-term memory this takes about 40 thousandths of a second per item, a rate that is surprisingly consistent, even in people with disorders such as schizophrenia.

Most kinds of forgetting or amnesia occur during retrieval. Benign forgetfulness is usually caused by interference from similar items because the required information was not clearly coded and well organized. Retrieval can be improved by recreating the context in which the information was registered. This is why the police reconstruct scenes of crimes, and why revision for exams is more effective if facts are learnt in the form of answers to mock questions.

MENARCHE is the term applied to the beginning of the menstrual function. The average age at which it occurs in British girls is 12½ years. In London girls it is 13·1 years. There is considerable racial and geographical variation.

MENDELISM is the term applied to a law enunciated by G. J. Mendel that the offspring is not intermediate in type between its parents, but that the type of one or other parent is predominant. Characteristics are classed as either dominant or recessive. The offspring of the first generation tend to inherit the dominant characteristics, whilst the recessive characteristics remain latent and appear in some of the offspring of the second generation. If individuals possessing recessive characters unite, recessive characters then become dominant characters in succeeding generations. The law may be expressed by the following formula:

$$n(DD+2DR+RR)$$

in which DD represents dominant offspring, RR recessive offspring, and DR offspring with mixed characters.

MENDELSON SYNDROME: Inhalation of regurgitated stomach contents, usually as a complication of general anaesthesia. It may cause death from anoxia or result in extensive lung damage.

MENIÈRE'S DISEASE, so called after the Frenchman, Prosper Menière, who first described it in 1861, is a disease characterized by tinnitus (q.v.), deafness and intermittent attacks of vertigo. It usually occurs in middle age, and is slightly more common in men than in women. The first manifestation is usually deafness on one side. Then, as a rule many months later, there is a sudden attack, without any warning, of intense vertigo. This often occurs during sleep, waking the patient up. It is soon followed by vomiting and sweating. The acute giddiness usually lasts for two to three hours but, after the attack, some unsteadiness persists for a few days. The time interval between attacks varies from a week to a few months. When they do recur, they tend to occur in clusters. The tinnitus, which tends to be high-pitched, comes on about the same time as the deafness. It is often described as being like rushing water or escaping steam. The deafness becomes gradually worse until it is complete. The condition is due to excessive fluid in the labyrinth of the ears (see EAR). The cause of this accumulation is not known, though it has been suggested that it might be a form of allergy, or might be due to spasm of the small blood-vessels.

Treatment consists of restricting the daily in-

take of fluid to 1·5 litres (2½ pints), and controlling the daily consumption of salt by not adding it to food at the table. A multiplicity of drugs has been recommended, including diuretics such as frusemide (q.v.), drugs to prevent vomiting such as dimenhydrinate (q.v.), and prochlorperazine (q.v.), and vasodilating drugs such as nicotinic acid (q.v.). If these all fail and the condition persists, then destruction of the labyrinth is carried out by operation or by ultrasound. An alternative is to cut the vestibular nerve; this has the advantage of preserving hearing, which the other surgical procedures do not do. (See TINNITUS.)

MENINGES are the membranes surrounding the brain and spinal cord. (See BRAIN.) The membranes include the dura mater, a tough, fibrous membrane closely applied to the inside of the skull; the arachnoid, a more delicate membrane, enveloping the brain but separated from its irregular surface by spaces containing fluid; and the pia mater, a delicate network of fibres containing blood-vessels and uniting the arachnoid to the brain. The two last are sometimes referred to as the pia-arachnoid. These membranes bear the blood-vessels which nourish the surface of the brain and the interior of the skull. Meningeal haemorrhage from these vessels forms one of the chief dangers arising from fracture of the skull.

MENINGISM is a condition with symptoms closely resembling those of meningitis, but due simply to a feverish state.

MENINGITIS is inflammation affecting the membranes of the brain (cerebral meningitis) or

1 arachnoid
2 spinal ganglion
3 ventral nerve root
4 ligamentum denticulatum
5 dura mater, cut and turned backwards
6 dura mater

The membranes of the spinal cord.

spinal cord (spinal meningitis), or both. Either the dura or the pia-arachnoid may be inflamed. In the former case the condition is known as pachymeningitis; in the latter, leptomeningitis. Pachymeningitis is the less common of the two, is often local and secondary to disease of the bone (e.g. tuberculous or syphilitic), and may be cranial or spinal. Leptomeningitis is the more common, is usually extensive in distribution, greatly alters the composition of the cerebrospinal fluid, and may be primary or secondary to infection elsewhere in the body.

Meningitis may be classified according to the infecting organism as viral or bacterial. Viral meningitis is a relatively mild disease but bacterial meningitis is life threatening. Pneumococcal, pyogenic, tuberculous, syphilitic, meningococcal are all bacterial varieties. The all-important evidence is gained by lumbar puncture and examination of the CEREBROSPINAL FLUID (q.v.). In meningitis the pressure of this fluid is increased, changes in its appearance and constituents occur, and the infecting agent can usually be isolated from it. In meningitis the protein and the number of cells increase and the glucose decreases. A decrease in the amount of chlorides of the cerebrospinal fluid is characteristic of tuberculous meningitis. Increase in the number of cells may make the normally clear cerebrospinal fluid opalescent, as in tuberculous meningitis, or turbid, as in pneumococcal and pyogenic meningitis. Clinically, the symptoms are due to irritation of the meninges and rise in the intracranial pressure: headache, vomiting, photophobia, rigidity of the neck, Kernig's sign (q.v.), convulsions, paralyses, coma.

In England, in 1986, there were 2172 cases of acute meningitis, 820 of which were due to the meningococcus. (See MENINGOCOCCAL MENINGITIS.)

PNEUMOCOCCAL MENINGITIS is usually secondary to infection with the pneumococcus elsewhere: for example, empyema or otitis media. This formerly fatal condition is now in many cases successfully treated by penicillin given intravenously.

PYOGENIC MENINGITIS is due to secondary infection with staphylococci, streptococci, *H. influenzae*, gonococci, or anthrax bacilli – especially the first two. The introduction of antibiotics has altered the previously fatal prognosis of these cases. Satisfactory results are obtained from the use of chloramphenicol in the treatment of meningitis due to *H. influenzae*.

TUBERCULOUS MENINGITIS is an inflammation of the membranes caused by the *Mycobacterium tuberculosis*. The disease is most common in children under the age of 10 years, but is by no means confined to that period of life, and may affect adults. The determining factor in the disease is exposure to infection with the bovine or the human *Mycobacterium tuberculosis*. All too often a grandparent with a chronic cough due to pulmonary tuberculosis is the unsuspected source of infection of the grandchild. In numerous cases associated factors are bad hygienic conditions, with insufficient or im-

proper feeding, or some disease of childhood, particularly measles or whooping-cough. When it occurs in adults it is usually secondary to some chronic manifestation of tuberculosis in another part of the body, especially in the lungs.

Treatment: The drugs used in the treatment of tuberculous meningitis are streptomycin, isoniazid, rifampicin and ethambutol. The administration of streptomycin and isoniazid in this condition requires skilled medical and nursing supervision such as is available only in hospital. Every child (or adult) with tuberculous meningitis, or suspected tuberculous meningitis, therefore should be examined as early as possible by an experienced children's (or tuberculosis) specialist, in order that an expert opinion may be obtained.

SYPHILITIC MENINGITIS is usually a chronic inflammation (but sometimes producing acute symptoms) occurring in most cases within the first four years of infection. It may spread from the pia-arachnoid into the brain – a meningoencephalitis – or it may attack the dura mater and the overlying bone. The pressure of the cerebrospinal fluid is raised; the fluid itself is clear and contains an increased number of lymphocytes. Headache is a common symptom. Paralysis of cranial nerves (resulting, for example, in a squint) can occur as a result of strangulation of the nerve in inflamed meninges at the base of the brain. Hydrocephalus may arise suddenly, with headache, vomiting, sleepiness, mental changes, and congestion of the optic discs as symptoms and signs, or syphilitic meningitis may come on acutely. The treatment is as for syphilis.

MENINGOCOCCAL MENINGITIS is the most common form of meningitis. It is a dangerous epidemic condition characterized by painful contractions of the muscles of the neck, retraction of the head, and mental symptoms. It was first distinctly recognized in the year 1837, when it prevailed as an epidemic, chiefly among troops in the south-west of France. In 1846 it appeared in Ireland, especially in the workhouses of Belfast and Dublin. Since that time it has appeared repeatedly both in Europe and America, notably in a severe epidemic in the large towns of Scotland in 1907–09, in a slighter form among the troops during the war of 1914–18, and a fair-sized epidemic in Great Britain in the winter of 1939–40. The disease is notifiable. Epidemics of it sweep across tropical Africa with great regularity.

Causes: When an outbreak takes place, it usually occurs about the months of February, March, and April, and affects a closed community such as a school, garrison, camp, or prison. The direct cause is an organism, the *Neisseria meningitidis* or *meningococcus*, which is found in the exudation round the nervous system, in the blood, and often in the nasal discharge. The organism is of four different types. It is believed that the infection takes place through the nose and that a large number of persons who do not contract the disease harbour the meningococcus in the nasal discharge and form sources of infection to more susceptible people, especially children, by coughing and sneezing – they are known as carriers. Factors favouring infection are a high carrier-rate, the virulence of the organism, a closed community (e.g. a camp), nasopharyngeal catarrh, bad ventilation, insufficient space between beds, introduction of susceptible persons into a closed community, season of the year (winter and spring). Young children are much more susceptible than adults. The incubation period is 2 to 10 days (commonly 2 to 5).

Symptoms: The onset is usually sudden, sometimes startlingly so. As a rule, vomiting, headache, and shivering first appear, followed in a few hours by stiffness of the neck. In children, convulsions are common. In a case of very sudden onset, the patient, while going about as usual, may fall down suddenly in a convulsion, or he may go to bed perfectly well and be found unconscious on the following morning. If the patient is not unconscious, headache and pain with stiffness in the back of the neck continue, squinting is often seen, the tongue is furred and dry, and there is a rise of temperature: 37·8 to 40 °C (100 to 104 °F). The patient is irritable, the body tender to the touch, and the limbs stiff so that bending up of the lower limbs on the abdomen with the knee straight becomes impossible (Kernig's sign). The patient is often sleepless or delirious, and there is a great tendency for the symptoms to go and come. Purpuric spots, from which the disease takes its name of 'spotted fever', appear over the surface of the trunk during the first week of the disease in greater or less numbers in about one-quarter of the cases. Death occurs in a large number of the cases within a week of the onset, taking place very often suddenly from heart failure. After the first week, if life is prolonged, the disease usually abates gradually and in the course of some weeks the rigidity may have disappeared and the temperature may have become normal.

In those patients who die, it is common to find the surface of the brain and the spinal cord covered with thick pus and the blood-vessels markedly congested. If death has occurred at a very early period, nothing more may be visible than very intense congestion of the membranes on the surface of the brain. The interior of the brain shows more than the usual amount of fluid.

The prognosis in this disease has been revolutionized by the introduction of antibiotic drugs. Formerly the mortality rate in epidemics was 70 to 80 per cent, whilst in fulminating cases it might even be 100 per cent. Today, with efficient treatment it has fallen to 7 to 10 per cent. The main factors governing the prognosis are: (1) The age of the patient: the disease is particularly dangerous in infants and old people. (2) The type of onset: a fulminating onset carries a bad prognosis. (3) The stage of the disease at which treatment is begun: the earlier the better.

Treatment: The patient must be isolated and, whenever possible, should be treated in hospi-

tal. Treatment consists essentially of the administration of full doses of penicillin injections intravenously. The patient is confined to bed and given a light nutritious diet. For insomnia sedatives are usually required, whilst the pains in the joints and limbs are usually best relieved by warm baths. The headache usually responds to a combination of aspirin, paracetamol, and codeine but, if particularly severe, lumbar puncture may be necessary.

Quarantine of contacts is useless, but there is some evidence that, in the event of an outbreak in a semi-closed community (e.g. a residential school or a military camp) the administration of sulphadiazine to all contacts may be of value. A vaccine is now available which is proving of value in the control of epidemics in Africa, but the duration of its action is still not certain.

MENINGOCELE is a protusion of the meninges of the brain through a defect in the skull. (See SPINA BIFIDA.)

MENINGOCOCCUS (see NEISSERIA).

MENINGOENCEPHALITIS is the term applied to infection of the membranes, or meninges, of the brain and the underlying brain matter. In practically all cases of meningitis (q.v.) there is some involvement of the underlying brain. It is when this involvement is considerable that the term, meningoencephalitis, is used. One form that has attracted attention in recent years is that caused by amoebae (q.v.), particularly that known as *Naegleria fowleri*, in which the infection is acquired through bathing in contaminated water. Effective chlorination of swimming baths kills this micro-organism.

MENINGOMYELOCELE is a protrusion of the meninges of the spinal cord through a defect in the spine. (See SPINA BIFIDA.)

MENISCUS is the term applied to a crescentic fibro-cartilage in a joint, such as the cartilages in the knee-joint.

MENOPAUSE is the term applied to the cessation of menstruation at the end of reproductive life. Usually it occurs between the ages of 45 and 50, although it may occur before the age of 30 or after the age of 50. It can be a psychologically disturbing experience which is quite often accompanied by physical manifestations. These include hot flushes, tiredness, irritability, lack of concentration, palpitations, aching joints and vaginal irritation. There may also be loss of libido. Most women can and do live happy, active lives through the menopause, the length of which varies considerably. The chauvinists would say that it was a natural event and it is those women that can accept it as such who are least likely to suffer from its manifestations. This is not true. The loss of oestrogen which occurs at the menopause causes atrophy of the genital tract. Vasomotor instability in the form of hot flushes, sweats and palpitations occur and can be very debilitating. The urinary urge, loss of libido and depression are not uncommon manifestations and are remediable with treatment.

One of the major problems of the menopause which does not give rise to symptoms until many years later is the osteoporosis which follows the cessation of menstruation. Osteoporosis is a metabolic bone disease characterized by a reduction in the total amount of bone but without any abnormality in the actual bone present. After the menopause 1 per cent of the bone is lost per annum to the end of life. This accounts for the frequency of fractures of the femur in elderly women as a result of osetoporosis but it can be prevented by hormone-replacement therapy. Oestrogens are more effective than tranquillizers or sedatives in relieving the short-term symptoms such as hot flushes, sweats and vaginal dryness. Atrophic vaginitis and vulvitis also usually respond to treatment with oestrogens. Oestrogen therapy reduces the demineralization of bone which normally occurs after the menopause and, if it is started early and continued for years, it may prevent the development of osteoporosis. Oestrogen is far more effective than calcium supplements and has been shown greatly to reduce fractures affecting the spine, wrists and legs after the age of 50. Cyclical therapy is necessary to avoid abnormal bleeding in women who have reached the menopause. If oestrogens are given alone there is a slightly increased risk of endometrial hyperplasia which may proceed to endometrial cancer. This can be prevented by the administration of oestrogen-progestogen combinations. There is good evidence that a combination of oestrogen and a progestogen – known as hormone replacement therapy (HRT) – avoids the endometrial hyperstimulation produced by the oestrogen alone and relieves most of the symptoms of vasomotor instability of the menopause and prevents the bone loss associated with the menopause. It has been suggested there was a relationship between oestrogen treatment and breast tumours. However a study by the Boston Collaborative Drug Surveillance Program showed that there was no evidence of any association between oestrogen therapy and either benign or malignant breast tumours. There is good evidence that before the age of 50 men are a greater risk of developing myocardial infarction but in the post-menopausal women the risks are the same. It has thus been suggested that the secretion of oestrogens protects against cardiovascular disease in the reproductive years. Nevertheless there is no evidence that the administration of oestrogens in the menopause increases the risk of developing atherosclerotic vascular disease, breast cancer, thrombo-embolic disorders or hypertension.

MENORRHAGIA means an over-abundance of the menstrual discharge.

MENSTRUATION is a periodic change occurring in human beings and the higher apes, and consists chiefly in a flow of blood from the cavity of the womb, and associated with various slight constitutional disturbances. It begins between the ages of 12 and 15, as a rule, although its onset may be delayed till as late as 20, or it may begin as early as 10 or 11. Along with its first appearance the body develops the secondary sex characteristics of the sex: e.g. enlargement of the breasts, characteristic hair distribution. The duration of each menstrual period varies in different persons from two to eight days. It recurs in the great majority of cases with regularity, most commonly at intervals of twenty-eight days or thirty days, less often with intervals of twenty-one or twenty-seven days, ceasing only during pregnancy and lactation, till the age of 45 or 50 arrives, when it stops altogether, as a rule ceasing early if it has begun early, and vice versa. The final stoppage is known as the menopause (q.v.) or the climacteric (q.v.).

Menstruation depends upon a functioning ovary and this upon a healthy pituitary gland. The regular rhythm may depend upon a centre in the hypothalamus, which is in close connection with the pituitary. After menstruation the denuded uterine endometrium is regenerated under the influence of the follicular hormone, oestradiol. The epithelium of the endometrium proliferates, and about a fortnight after the beginning of menstruation great development of the endometrial glands takes place under the influence of progesterone, the hormone secreted by the corpus luteum. These changes are made for the reception of the fertilized ovum. In the absence of fertilization the uterine endometrium breaks down in the subsequent menstrual discharge.

Disorders of menstruation: In the majority of healthy women, menstruation proceeds regularly for thirty years or more, with the exceptions connected with childbirth. In many persons, as the result either of general or local conditions, the process may be absent or excessive, or may be attended with great discomfort or pain. The term *amenorrhoea* is applied to cases in which menstruation is absent, *menorrhagia* and *metrorrhagia* to cases in which it is excessive, the former if the excess occurs at the regular periods, the latter if it is irregular, whilst *dysmenorrhoea* is the name given to cases in which the process is attended by pain.

AMENORRHOEA: If menstruation has never occurred the amenorrhoea is termed *primary*. If it ceases after having once become established it is known as *secondary amenorrhoea*. The only value of these terms is that some patients with either chromosome abnormalities or malformations of the genital tract fall into the primary category. Otherwise the age of onset of symptoms is more important.

The causes of amenorrhoea are numerous and treatment requires dealing with the primary cause. The commonest cause is pregnancy. Hypothalamic disorders such as psychological stress or anorexia nervosa cause amenorrhoea. Poor nutrition or loss of weight by dieting may cause amenorrhoea and any serious underlying disease such as tuberculosis or malaria may also result in the cessation of periods. The excess secretion of prolactin, whether this is the result of a micro-adenoma of the pituitary gland or whether it is drug induced, will cause amenorrhoea and possibly galactorrhoea as well. Malfunction of the pituitary gland will result in a failure to produce the gonadotrophic hormones with consequent amenorrhoea. Excessive production of cortisol, as in Cushing's syndrome, or of androgens, as in the adreno-genital syndrome or the polycystic ovary syndrome, will result in amenorrhoea. Amenorrhoea occasionally follows use of the oral contraceptive pill and may be associated with both hypothyroidism and obesity. It is thus important to take a careful history with emphasis on psychological factors, weight fluctuations and the use of drugs that may stimulate the release of prolactin and it is also important to look for evidence of virilization. A gynaecological examination is necessary in primary amenorrhoea to exclude malformations of the genital tract. Estimations of the gonadotrophic hormone levels will reveal whether the amenorrhoea is primary ovarian failure or secondary to pituitary disease.

In view of the frequent psychosomatic origins of amenorrhoea, reassurance of the patient is of great importance, in particular with reference to marriage and the ability to conceive. When weight loss is the cause of amenorrhoea, restoration of body weight alone can result in spontaneous menstruation. Patients with raised concentration of serum gonadotrophin hormones have primary ovarian failure. It is not amenable to treatment. Cyclical oestrogen/progestogen therapy will usually establish withdrawal bleeding. If the amenorrhoea is due to mild pituitary failure menstruation may return after treatment with clomiphene. Clomiphene is a non-steroidal agent which competes for oestrogen receptors in the hypothalamus. The patients who are most likely to respond to clomiphene are those who have some evidence of endogenous oestrogen and gonadotrophin production.

MENORRHAGIA: Excessive menstruation may be due to the same general conditions which produce amenorrhoea, the same diseases, such as glomerulonephritis or tuberculosis, causing stoppage or excess in different women. Thus, in some people an excessive loss is brought about by these conditions, and the effects of the general disease are much increased by the loss of blood. In heart disease, the womb may share in the general internal congestion, and the menses in consequence are increased. In some people, menstruation at its first appearance is excessive; whilst this is so often the case as to be almost the general rule at the time when the menstrual periods are about to stop, i.e. at the menopause, when they also tend to become irregular. But it is most often a local condition that produces menorrhagia: in this case, as a rule, not only is the periodic loss increased but

there is bleeding at irregular times (metrorrhagia). Polypus, fibroid, and other tumours, displacements of the womb, and some inflammation consequent upon childbirth or miscarriage, are the most common causes of this type. In the treatment, rest and various internal remedies which check haemorrhage, together with careful attention to the general health between the periods, are essential. (See UTERUS, DISEASES OF.)

DYSMENORRHOEA may vary from mere discomfort to agonizing colic, accompanied by prostration and vomiting. Anaemia is sometimes a cause of painful menstruation as well as of stoppage of this function. Chills and exhaustion may produce pain for a single period in women whose periods are usually painless.

Inflammation of various internal organs, e.g. of the womb itself, the ovaries, or the Fallopian tubes, is one of the commonest causes of dysmenorrhoea which comes on for the first time late in life, especially when the trouble follows the birth of a child. In this case the pain exists more or less at all times, but is aggravated at the periods. It is relieved by various local means directed towards checking the inflammation present.

Many cases of dysmenorrhoea appear with the beginning of menstrual life, and accompany every period. It has been estimated that 5 to 10 per cent of girls in their late teens or early twenties are severely incapacitated by dysmenorrhoea for several hours each month. Various causes have been suggested for the pain, one being an excessive production of prostaglandins (q.v.). In not a few – indeed some would say the majority – there is a large psychological factor. This may be the sole cause, or it may be an ancillary cause exacerbating the pain, or discomfort, induced by some physical cause. Whatever the psychological factor – whether due to inadequate sex instruction, fear, mental, domestic, or work disharmony – the sooner it is discovered and dealt with, the more likely is the dysmenorrhoea to come under control. For the temporary relief of dysmenorrhoea, rest in bed, or, at all events, in the recumbent position, a hot water bottle to the lower part of the abdomen, and aspirin orally, are the remedies which prove most useful.

MENTAL HANDICAP is also referred to as intellectual handicap or learning difficulties. Terms such as mental deficiency, mental retardation, mental subnormality, and still more outdated words such as imbecility, feeblemindedness and idiocy, are now regarded as pejorative and offensive to the people they label, as indeed may be the term mental handicap itself.

A person with a mental handicap has been defined as 'an individual who, by reason of developmental intellectual impairment, needs additional services to live a normal life, or as normal a life as possible.' The World Health Organization International Classification of Diseases defines mental retardation as a condition of arrested or incomplete development of mind which is especially characterized by subnormality of intelligence and social functioning. The American Association on mental deficiency defines mental retardation as significantly subaverage intellectual functioning existing concurrently with deficits in adaptive behaviour and manifest during the developmental period. The 1983 Mental Health Act uses the term 'mental impairment' to describe that small minority of mentally handicapped people who also show 'abnormally aggressive or seriously irresponsible conduct'.

The degree of mental handicap is often further subdivided on IQ grounds into profound (under 20), severe (20–35), moderate (35–49), and mild (50–70). The profound, severe and moderate groups are often grouped together as major mental handicap. However it must be emphasized that IQ testing is not a precise science, that due account must be taken of the individual's linguistic, social and cultural background, and that individuals who function normally in society cannot be said to be handicapped.

Occurrence: Estimates vary as to how common mental handicap is, depending on the definitions used and the age of the populations being examined. In general it seems that the incidence (of new cases within a particular period of time) of mental handicap is decreasing in the UK but that, because people with a mental handicap now live longer, the prevalence is increasing. IQ tests are commonly statistically designed to ensure that about 2·5 per cent of the population tested scores below IQ 70. Not all these people will have significant impairment of adaptive function or need special services. For school age children it is generally agreed that major mental handicap occurs in about 0·4 per cent of the population. In countries with a high infant mortality the percentage may well be lower because children with handicaps are more vulnerable.

Causation: All degrees of handicap result from a complex interaction between genetic make-up and past and present and environmental features. The greater the degree of impairment the more likely it is to have an organic basis, i.e. to be caused by maldevelopment of, or damage to the brain. For major mental handicap it is possible to identify a medical cause for the handicap in about three-quarters of those affected. There is less but increasing evidence for an organic component in mild mental handicap.

Forty per cent of major mental handicap is caused by chromosome abnormalities, mainly trisomy 21 (Down's syndrome). Other genetic defects account for a further 15 per cent. Another 10 per cent occur within pregnancy or the perinatal period and 10 per cent of mental handicap occurs after birth as a result of accidents, child abuse, infections and brain tumours. The cause in the remaining quarter is unknown. Prenatal diagnosis is now available for many of the conditions causing major mental handicap.

Medical complications: Since major mental handicap is usually caused by maldevelopment of, or damage to the brain, and sometimes other body systems, it is not surprising that people with such handicaps are also more liable to physical ill health and handicap. Down's syndrome may involve malformation of the heart and intestines, and people with the syndrome are more liable to develop other illnesses subsequently. Some people with major mental handicap are paralysed or have other motor disorders. Sensory handicaps are also more common and must be identified to prevent secondary handicap resulting from them. About one-third of people with major mental handicap have epileptic fits. People with a mental handicap will in the first place use normal primary care services, but may need referral on to specialist medical services.

Psychological and psychiatric needs: The lives many mentally handicapped people lead, their learning difficulties and the presence of brain damage, all predispose to the development of disturbed behaviour. This may require a change of environment or a range of psychiatric and psychological interventions, from behaviour therapy to psychotropic drugs. This may be provided by mental-illness services or specialist mental-handicap services.

Residential needs: It is now recognized that people with a mental handicap neither wish nor need to live in hospitals, though obviously they may need to be admitted when acutely ill. Most live at home, usually with family members but occasionally alone. People with mental handicap may want to leave home or their families may want them to do so. They will need a variety of accommodation: both staffed and unstaffed houses, group homes and hostels with appropriate specialist support.

Education: People who learn slowly obviously have special educational needs. These may be met by special schools or, increasingly, by special provision within mainstream education. The 1981 Education Act requires local authorities to provide for children with special educational needs which are defined in the Warnock Report, including special means of access, equipment or resources, modification of the environment or specialist teaching techniques, the provision of a specialized or modified curriculum, and attention to the social and emotional climate in which education takes place. Each child's special needs must be assessed, and a decision made as to where these can best be met. Parents must be involved in drawing up the statement of special needs under the 1981 Act.

People with a mental handicap are entitled to remain at school until the age of 19 and further education may be available to them. Many can find employment on the open market, but for others specialist help or sheltered employment may be needed.

Parents or other relatives of mentally handicapped children can obtain helpful advice from the Mental Health Foundation, 8 Hallam Street, London W1N 6DH (071-580 0145); The Royal

Society for Mentally Handicapped Children and Adults, 123 Golden Lane, London EC1Y 0RT (071-454 0454); or the Scottish Society for the Mentally Handicapped, 13 Elmbank Street, Glasgow G2 4QA (041-226 4541, Fax: 041-204 4398).

MENTAL ILLNESS: Problems of feeling, thinking and behaving may be regarded as a mental illness if they become excessive for the particular individual in relation to the difficulties experienced.

Mental illness exists in many forms which may overlap with one another. Help and treatment may be sought by the sufferer, or less commonly may be imposed against his or her will. So long as symptoms of mental disorder do not result in behaviour which is markedly opposed to prevailing social custom, society does not interfere with the person in a restrictive way. When people's conduct becomes a risk to their own health and safety, or that of others, they can be compulsorily admitted to a psychiatric unit under the Mental Health Act, 1983 (UK). Approximately 10 per cent of psychiatric admissions in England and Wales are compulsory. A large number of people with socially maladapted personalities may be found in the prison population.

The medical approach, which regards mental disorder as a disease to be treated on the same lines as other diseases, is generally regarded as having begun with the publication of Pinel's *Traité médico-philosophique sur l'aliénation mentale ou la manie* in 1801. A great amount of attention was paid during the next fifty years to the study of mental diseases, and during this period a large number of asylums for the humane treatment of mentally disordered people were founded. The emphasis now, however, is more on care in the community.

The question of legal responsibility may arise in various civil or criminal matters, including the ability to make a valid will. (In order to be 'of sound disposing mind', individuals should know the nature and extent of their property, know the persons having a claim on it as possible beneficiaries and the relative strengths of their claims and be able to express themselves on this question clearly and without ambiguity.) The development of mental illness subject to detention under the Mental Health Act, 1983, does not excuse the patient from the fulfilment of a contract, provided he was not eligible to be detained at the time when the contract was entered into.

When a crime is committed, the question of responsibility is often very difficult to decide. The general principle accepted is that, if the accused person suffers from a delusion, but is not insane in other matters, he is held responsible for his offence, unless he has acted in such a way as would have been permissible if the facts about which his delusion exists had been true. In other words, in order to establish a defence on the ground of insanity, it must be proved that 'at the time of committing the act

the party accused was labouring under such a defect of reason, from disease of the mind, as not to know the nature and quality of the act he was doing or, if he did know it, that he did not know he was doing it, or that he did not know he was doing what was wrong'. The principle is also recognized that, if the mind is so diseased or so defective that there is complete absence of the power of self-control, so that the person acts under an ungovernable impulse, then he is not held responsible. This inability to exercise self-control does not, however, exonerate a person in whom the loss of self-control is due to his own fault, as, for example, when he is intoxicated.

Causes: Mental illness, like normal mental functioning, is complex and a single causal explanation is not often sufficient on its own. Any one causative agent may increase the risk of mental illness but by no means make it inevitable. It may be helpful to think in terms of the predisposing causes and the precipitating causes, and sometimes the perpetuating causes.

PREDISPOSING CAUSES: It is often difficult to distinguish between the roles of genetic inheritance and family upbringing among the more distant predisposing causes. Modern research suggests that, for some illnesses, genetic loading significantly increases the risk but may not be a sufficient cause on its own. Even an identical twin, with exactly the same genetic constitution, has only a substantial risk, rather than a complete certainty, of developing the same illness.

Birth trauma is another physical cause increasing the risk of mental illness, as is the presence of any sort of physical illness.

Socio-cultural factors, such as family size, class or ethnic background may predispose to some illnesses. The individual's psychology and personality, shaped on the basis of inherited features by upbringing, are often relevant in their mental resilience to different types of stresses. Loss of a parent in childhood has been shown in some subjects slightly to increase the risk of depression many years later. Some researchers argue that the characteristic pattern of thinking, or cognitive approach, may make some individuals vulnerable to anxiety or depression.

PRECIPITATING CAUSES: Physical disorders may again be relevant. A depressive episode following influenza is well known, as is emotional disequilibrium following childbirth, even if this more often takes the form of 'the blues', or more rarely a depressive illness. A post-puerperal psychosis is rare. Acute confusional states, especially in the elderly, may have an infective or metabolic origin. Diseases of the *endocrine glands*, particularly myxoedema and thyrotoxicosis but also abnormalities of adrenal function, can cause mental symptoms. Medication related to these, as well as other medication, can be a factor.

Legal but non-therapeutic drugs like alcohol are often implicated, partly because people take them as a way of modifying their response to stress and particularly if there are withdrawal reactions after dependence has occurred. Opiates, such as heroin, cause marked withdrawal reactions which are not regarded as a mental illness. Other drugs, such as amphetamines, cocaine and, rarely, cannabis, can precipitate a psychotic reaction.

There has been much study of social precipitants of mental illness, known technically as life events. Although it is sometimes unclear whether the illness has caused the event (such as loss of job) or vice versa and, although they only increase the risk of illness rather than determine it, the association is well established. Among the most stressful events are bereavement, divorce or separation, moving house and retirement.

PERPETUATING CAUSES may include any of the above factors but the victim may have suffered additional social dislocation as a result of the illness itself, for example, through the loss of job or eviction. Psychologically, patients may experience real or imagined stigma and their self-confidence may have been impaired by the 'breakdown'.

Symptoms of mental disorder: EARLY SYMPTOMS: Mental illness rarely develops suddenly and indications of vulnerability to an approaching mental breakdown may be gathered from some early prodromal symptoms. These are often non-specific symptoms of anxiety or depression including insomnia, mental and physical tension and other bodily symptoms of anxiety such as rapid pulse, sweating and gastrointestinal upset, as well as difficulty concentrating.

GENERAL SYMPTOMS of mental illness may be classed as psychotic and non-psychotic. *Psychotic symptoms*, such as delusions or hallucinations, imply that the patient has lost touch with reality to some degree. A *delusion* is a fixed false belief, held with unshakeable conviction, not in conformity with the information available to the patient or with the social and cultural background of his or her peers. There are many types of delusions. In delusions of reference, for example, patients think people in the street or on the television are referring to them. In paranoid delusions, others, human or supernatural, are intent on harming the person, although there is no basis in reality. Delusions of grandeur or of having remarkable attributes are typically associated with mania. Delusions of guilt, hypochondriacal or 'nihilistic' delusions (that part of the patient's body is being or has been destroyed) are characteristic of the psychotic extremes of depression. Other delusions are religious or jealous. In some delusions people, places or situations may be misidentified or misinterpreted. There may be delusions that feelings, actions, willpower or thoughts are being interfered with or controlled.

Hallucinations are false perceptions of the senses, which occur in the absence of external stimuli. They are not misinterpretations or distortions of actually existing stimuli ('*illusions*'). Patients complain that they hear voices speaking to them when there is no one there. *Pseudo-hallucinations* are experienced within the mind and are not truly psychotic but true.

Auditory hallucinations are heard through the ears. These voices may be well known to them or unknown. They may be persecutory, condemnatory or imperative with direct instructions. They may comment on the patient's actions or several voices may argue. Hallucinations of sight are suggestive of some organic disorder. Hallucinations of smell may imply pathology in the temporal lobe of the brain.

Obsessions are included among the neurotic symptoms. Although an obsessional trait such as over-tidiness is quite common, obsessions are relatively rare. They are the persistent intrusion of unwelcome thoughts, feeling or impulses, despite the fact that the sufferer tries to resist them. They are often repugnant or bizarre, violent, sexual or blasphemous in nature. A 'compulsion' is technically an act which is similarly bizarre but which the individual is compelled to perform, despite resisting. Nevertheless obsessions and compulsions are clearly recognized as part of the subject's own mind and are not delusions.

Phobias are more common than obsessions. The fear is disproportionate to the situation; it cannot be reasoned away or controlled voluntarily. It may cause intense subjective and bodily symptoms of anxiety and the subject characteristically avoids the feared situation. Some fears, of spiders or the dark, are common in childhood. A list of recognized objects of phobia runs well into three figures but is now considered most usefully under three main headings: (a) *agoraphobia*, includes fear of congested places or leaving the house. It does not mean fear of open spaces and psychiatrists do not use the term claustrophobia separately to indicate a fear of closed spaces. Crowded shops, lifts, buses and underground trains are typical feared situations. (b) animal or other *specific phobias*, e.g. of spiders, birds or snakes. (c) *social phobias* of meeting and being exposed to scrutiny by others, going beyond natural shyness, often with feelings of intense anxiety or panic and usually resulting in relative social isolation.

Derealization and depersonalization are rare but normal experiences. Respectively, subjects have a sudden intense feeling that their surroundings are somehow unreal, as if part of a video or stage set, or that they themselves are unreal or even out of their own body. These may be due to a dissociative mechanism in a situation which the subject would otherwise find very stressful and should not be regarded as psychotic phenomena.

Suicide may be the result of profound mental depression but is also more common with schizophrenia. It is associated with men, older years and concurrent painful physical disease. The number of deaths due to suicide in England and Wales is approximately 4,000 a year, but the rate in young men is rising.

Attempted suicide is roughly ten times more common and ranges from a failed serious attempt, to a cry for help or an overdose of tablets to ensure a prolonged sleep. The assessment of someone who has attempted suicide should exclude any serious psychiatric illness and evaluate all the evidence about how determined the attempt was.

MANIA: The term, mania, should strictly be reserved for cases in which there are hallucinations or delusions. Hypomania is less florid and includes all the other symptoms, most typically, elevation of mood. Patients are in a state of over-activity, loquacious, garrulous, often clever in repartee; they flit from one subject to another; the mind never rests and sleeplessness is common. In the more pronounced form there may be pressure leading to incoherence of speech, intense restlessness and distractability. Social, sexual and financial disinhibition may be of concern. Patients may seem to be unaware of fatigue, either of mind or body, and wear themselves out, with very occasionally a fatal result. The illness characteristically occurs in episodes, lasting several weeks or months. When episodes of both depression and hypomania have occurred, the illness is termed manic-depressive disorder.

DEPRESSION is characterized by feelings of misery that are excessive in relation to the circumstances. In milder forms the depression is not very great and may exist only as a symptom on its own, rather than as a cluster of associated symptoms constituting a syndrome or medical illness. Patients may be able to pull themselves together in the presence of strangers and when it is necessary. Sometimes, especially after a severely depressed state has lasted for some time, patients are retarded in their movements, sit staring straight in front of them and are persuaded with difficulty to take food. In severe agitated depression, patients show restlessness and agitation, wringing their hands, swaying their body, weeping, or showing inability for the slightest concentration upon any one subject. Depressive delusions may be present, and patients think they have wronged themselves and their family, that they are responsible for the illness or misfortune of other people, that they are going to be burned, tortured or otherwise maltreated and, in such people, the impulse to suicide may be very strong. Along with the mental symptoms, physical signs are often present, including disordered digestion with constipation. Recovery is usual but a person of depressive personality is liable to subsequent episodes.

PARANOIA is a condition in which there are delusions in the absence of hallucinations, which gradually form into a system that can be complex. Used more loosely, the term applies to abnormal suspiciousness that one is a victim of persecution by others.

SCHIZOPHRENIA is the collective name given to a group of conditions characterized during an acute episode by positive symptoms such as hallucinations (typically taking the form of voices talking to or about the afflicted person), strange experiences (for example, that mental or bodily functions are being interfered with by some outside force such as radio waves or telepathy) and inability to think clearly. Such symptoms may lead to bizarre speech and behaviour. Acute episodes usually respond to treatment with medication, the phenothiazines being the class of drugs most commonly used.

In about 25 per cent of cases the condition clears up completely after one or a few such attacks. Unfortunately, many conditions become chronic and a 'negative' type of syndrome becomes prominent. This is characterized by slowness, lack of energy and social withdrawal. About 25 per cent of those with schizophrenia become severely disabled. The rest, about half, are subject to occasional relapses (particularly if medication is discontinued) and to a moderate degree of disability. About one in a hundred individuals develops schizophrenia at some time during their lives, a proportion that seems to vary by, at most, a factor of 10 between extremes in different parts of the world. The causes are not known but a genetic factor is present in a proportion of cases, indicating a possible biochemical vulnerability.

In recent years there has been an intensive search for a biochemical basis for schizophrenia: a theory apparently supported by the response of the condition to certain potent tranquillizing drugs.

Undue environmental stress can precipitate a relapse. A degree of support may therefore be necessary, although not so great as to discourage the individual from becoming as independent as possible.

Apart from the people who are themselves afflicted by schizophrenia, those chiefly involved are the relatives and close friends. A voluntary organization, the National Schizophrenia Fellowship, has been formed to promote the welfare of sufferers and families. There are branches in most parts of the UK. Enquiries should be addressed to the General Secretary, NSF, London Advisory Centre, 197 Kings Cross Road, London WC1X 9DB (071-837 6436).

ALCOHOLIC PSYCHOSIS: Alcoholism and drug habits are also sometimes regarded as mental disorders and alcohol, in turn, can produce organic changes in the nervous system which lead to chronic mental illness.

CONFUSIONAL STATES: This type of mental disorder usually is due to organic factors, such as infections, metabolic disturbances or poisons such as alcohol. The patient has difficulty in understanding simple questions. Hallucinations are common and patients may see faces in the air or insects crawling on the bedclothes and mistake persons near them for old friends or enemies. Commonly too, patients have no idea where they are. They may also be disorientated with regard to time. Memory is often disordered and restlessness is frequent. Recovery usually depends on the treatment of the underlying condition.

DEMENTIA is a condition of general impairment of most mental faculties. It usually starts gradually with impairment of short-term memory. Approximately 5 per cent of those over 65 in England and Wales have mild and a further 5 per cent severe dementia. The two commonest varieties are due to impairment of blood circulation and Alzheimer's disease. The Alzheimer's Disease Society address is 158/160 Balham High Road, London SW12 9BN, (081-675 6557).

Treatment: *Depression* is the commonest psychiatric disorder encountered both in general practice and in hospital medicine. A relatively mild depression responds to supportive psychotherapy, whilst a psychotic depression with delusions and hallucinations will require admission to hospital and possible electro- convulsive therapy. Depressive illness has a spontaneous remission rate of about 50 per cent within several months and, if anti-depressant drugs are given, the recovery rate increases to over 70 per cent. The advantage of drugs treatment is that recovery is made more rapidly and the patient's suffering is therefore curtailed and the risk of suicide reduced. Tricyclic anti-depressant drugs act, apparently, by promoting the transmission of impulses between nerves by noradrenaline or serotonin. Depressed patients with agitation or anxiety respond best to a sedative tricyclic antidepressant such as amitriptyline or dothiepin. Retarded, apathetic patients are best treated with a less sedative antidepressant, such as imipramine. The side-effects of the tricyclic antidepressants (particularly amitriptyline) are due to atropine-like effects which lead to a dry mouth, constipation, pupillary dilatation and blurring of close vision. The monoamine oxidase inhibitors are best reserved for those neurotic or atypical cases, where the depression is accompanied by a great deal of anxiety and phobic behaviour. The monoamine oxidase inhibitors are associated with severe side-effects if the patient eats cheese or any substance that contains tyramine or catecholamines. Electro-convulsive therapy may also facilitate the transmission of nerve impulses. It is now given under brief general anaesthetic with a muscle relaxant. It is an effective treatment in severe depressive illness and the response is at least as good and probably more rapid than the response to tricyclic antidepressants.

People with *hypomania* require admission to hospital. The most useful drugs are the phenothiazines, such as chlorpromazine and the butyrophenones such as haloperidol, which act by blocking central dopamine receptors. Lithium carbonate has anti-manic properties but as it has little effect for seven to ten days it is generally reserved for prophylaxis of recurrent manic depressive disorder.

In the treatment of anxiety states, patients must be given an opportunity to ventilate their worries and be counselled on stress management and relaxation. Since many patients with anxiety states are often concerned that the commonly associated physical symptoms indicate an underlying organic disorder, they should be reassured (see PSYCHOSOMATIC DISEASES). If an acute stress cannot be managed in this way, long-acting benzodiazepines may be indicated (see BENZODIAZEPINES). Short-acting benzodiazepines are more suitable for elderly patients or patients with renal or hepatic impairment.

These drugs should in general be prescribed only for a few weeks at most, as patients often become tolerant to their effects and dependent on them. In patients who experience a rapid pulse or tremor, beta-blockers (see ADRENERGIC RECEPTORS) are useful and do not cause dependence.

The treatment of *schizophrenia* usually requires admission to a psychiatric unit for clarification of the diagnosis. The treatment is both pharmacological and psycho-social. The drugs most commonly used for the treatment of schizophrenia are neuroleptics including the phenothiazines, such as chlorpromazine, and the butyrophenones, such as haloperidol. The efficacy of neuroleptics in acute schizophrenia is demonstrated by the fact that 75 per cent of patients given phenothiazines are substantially better after four weeks compared to 25 per cent given a placebo. Psycho-social treatment is also important. During the acute phase the schizophrenic patient needs support, reassurance and simple counselling. Schizophrenic individuals are vulnerable to social pressures that most people can take in their stride. Despite the introduction of drug treatment, schizophrenic patients still occupy about one-sixth of all hospital beds in England and Wales. Drug treatment needs to be prolonged as 50 per cent of patients will relapse when drugs are discontinued. As a high proportion of psychiatric outpatients fail to comply with oral medication, long-acting depot-neuroleptics are commonly used, such as fluphenazine and flupenthixol. Patients may experience side-effects with the neuroleptics. These take the form of abnormal muscle movements or rigidity, as well as restlessness in the legs and increased salivation. Some of them can be controlled with other medication and recede with time.

After treatment has been established and florid symptoms are controlled, the patient is encouraged to resume activities by degrees. If living at home is not desirable, a hostel or group home may be indicated.

Like the 1959 Mental Health Act, the 1983 Act continues the principles (1) that as much treatment as possible, both in hospital and outside, should be given on a voluntary and informal basis; (2) that the care of people with mental illness should be shifted as far as possible from the institutions to care within the community. Psychiatric units attached to or in district general hospitals are now regarded as the norm and large separate mental hospitals are being closed.

The 1983 Act strengthened the checks and protected the civil liberties of the 10 per cent of in-patients who are admitted to psychiatric hospitals involuntarily.

Under the Act, mental disorder is defined as mental illness, arrested or incomplete development of mind, psychopathic disorder, or any other disability of mind.

Under Section 2 it provides for the compulsory admission of a patient to hospital for a maximum of 28 days on the grounds: (a) that he is suffering from mental disorder of a nature or degree which warrants his detention for assessment (or for assessment followed by medical treatment); and (b) that he ought to be so detained in the interests of his own health or safety or with a view to the protection of other persons.

Under Section 3 compulsory admission to hospital for treatment is for a maximum of six months, subject to renewal.

Patients detained in hospital must be informed of their rights and may apply to a Mental Health Tribunal to be released. Medical staff and hospital managers also have the power to discharge a patient from the compulsory provisions at any time.

Other sections of the Act permit involuntary detention for shorter periods of time under certain conditions and provide for guardianship in the community, although this last provision has been little used.

Persons coming before the courts who are mentally disordered may be detained in hospital or received into guardianship if the court considers it a suitable course. In certain circumstances higher courts may also make restriction orders, in which case the patient may not be discharged without the consent of the Home Secretary. Persons detained in prison or approved school who are found to be mentally disordered may be transferred to hospital by the Home Secretary.

Institutions, known as Special Hospitals, exist for mentally disordered people who, in the opinion of the minister, require treatment under conditions of special security on account of their dangerous, violent, or criminal tendencies.

The Mental Health Act Commission has been set up to provide special safeguards for detained patients. It gives second opinions in certain matters affecting the treatment of patients, will visit detained patients, investigate complaints, review the use of legal powers and advise staff on good practice. Some treatments are not permitted without the patient's consent and an independent second opinion; some may be given without consent but only if the second opinion agrees, whilst others can be given for up to three months without consent or a second opinion.

The checks on and safeguards of civil liberties of detained patients in the 1983 Act are detailed. Further information can be obtained from the Mental Health Act Commission, Maid Marian House, 56 Houndsgate, Nottingham NG1 6BG (0602-504040, fax: 0602-505998) and from MIND, The National Association for Mental Health, 22 Harley Street, London W1N 2ED (071-637 0741). MIND also acts as a campaigning and advice organization on all aspects of mental health.

MEPACRINE HYDROCHLORIDE is a synthetic acridine product used in the treatment of malaria. It came to the fore during the 1939–45 War, when supplies of quinine were short, and proved of great value both as a prophylactic and in the treatment of malaria. It is also used in the treatment of infestation with tapeworms. (See MALARIA; TAENIASIS.)

MEPROBAMATE is one of the tranquillizer drugs. It is mainly used for the relief of states of tension, mild anxiety states and persistent insomnia.

MEPYRAMINE MALEATE is one of the antihistamine drugs (q.v.).

MERALGIA PARAESTHETICA is a condition characterized by pain and paraesthesia (q.v.) on the front and outer aspect of the thigh. It is more common in men than in women, and the victims are usually middle-aged, overweight and out of condition. It is due to compression of the lateral cutaneous nerve of the thigh. It is exacerbated by an uncomfortable driving position when motoring long distances. Reduction in weight, improvement in general fitness and correction of faulty posture usually bring relief. If these fail, surgical decompression of the nerve may bring relief.

MERCAPTAMINE is a drug that is proving of value in the treatment of paracetamol poisoning.

MERCAPTOPURINE is one of a group of drugs known as antimetabolites which are proving of value in the treatment of certain forms of malignant disease, especially acute leukaemia. It is believed that they act by depriving rapidly dividing malignant cells of factors essential for their metabolism. Hence the generic name for the group of drugs – antimetabolites. It is also proving of value in the treatment of Crohn's disease (q.v.). (See CYTOTOXIC.)

MERCURY, also known as QUICKSILVER or HYDRARGYRUM, is a heavy fluid metal which, with its salts, has been used in medicine for many centuries.
Action: The salts of mercury fall into two groups: the mercuric salts, which are very soluble and powerful in action; and the mercurous salts, which are less soluble and act more slowly and mildly. The mercuric salts are all highly poisonous both to man and to bacterial life, so that they are strongly antiseptic. In strong solutions, several act as caustics, and in weaker solutions they are irritants. Taken internally, the first effect of the mercuric, and to a less degree of the mercurous salts, is by their irritating action to set up copious purging. They are also credited with the power of increasing the flow of bile, and for this reason blue pill, which contains mercury, and mercurous chloride, i.e. calomel, were at one time much used as purgatives.
Uses: Externally the mercuric salts are used as disinfectants and antiseptics. Ammoniated mer-

cury ointment, or white precipitate ointment, is used in the treatment of impetigo. The yellow oxide of mercury ointment is used for an application to the eyelids when a mild antiseptic ointment is required. Internally, mercurial salts were widely used at one time as purges, particularly calomel, the dosage of which is 30 to 200 mg for an adult, and blue pill 250 to 500 mg. They are best taken at night, and followed by a saline draught in the morning. They are seldom used nowadays.

A complex organic salt of mercury (mersalyl) is used as a diuretic in the treatment of oedema but it has largely been replaced by the oral benzothiadiazine and loop diuretics.

MESCALINE is derived from the Mexican peyote cactus, *Anhalonium lewinii*. It is probably the most powerful of all the hallucinogens and has been used for many centuries by Indian tribes in Mexico as an intoxicant to produce ecstatic states for religious celebrations. (See DRUG ADDICTION.)

MESENCEPHALON is the mid-brain connecting the cerebral hemispheres with the pons and cerebellum.

MESENTERY is the double layer of peritoneal membrane which supports the small intestine. It is of a fan shape, and its shorter edge is attached to the back wall of the abdomen for a distance of about 15 cm (6 inches), while the small intestine lies within its longer edge, for a length of over 6 metres (20 feet). The terms mesocolon, mesorectum, etc., are applied to similar folds of peritoneum that support parts of the colon, rectum, etc.

MESMERISM (see HYPNOTISM).

MESOCOLON is the double fold of peritoneum by which the large intestine is suspended from the back wall of the abdomen.

MESOTHELIOMA: A malignant tumour of the pleura, the membrane lining the chest cavity. The condition is commoner in people exposed to asbestos dust. It may be asymptomatic or cause pain, cough, and breathing troubles. Surgery or radiotherapy may be effective but often the disease has spread too far before it is discovered.

MESTEROLONE is a synthetic androgen (q.v.) which is being used in the treatment of hypogonadism (q.v.). (See ANDROGEN.)

METABOLISM means tissue change and includes all the physical and chemical processes by which the living body is maintained, and also those by which the energy is made available for various forms of work. The constructive, chemical and physical, processes by which food materials are adapted for the use of the body are collectively known as anabolism. The destructive processes by which energy is produced with the breaking down of tissues into waste products is known as catabolism. *Basal metabolism* is the term applied to the energy changes necessary for essential processes such as the beating of the heart, respiration, and maintenance of body warmth. This can be estimated, when a person is placed in a state of complete rest, by measuring the amounts of oxygen and carbon dioxide exchanged during breathing under certain standard conditions. (See CALORIE.)

METACARPAL bones are the five long bones which occupy the hand between the carpal bones at the wrist and the phalanges of the fingers. The large rounded 'knuckles' at the root of the fingers are formed by the heads of these bones. (See HAND.)

METAPHYSIS is the extremity of a long bone where it joins the epiphysis (q.v.).

METAPLASIA is the term applied to a change of one kind of tissue into another.

METASTASIS and METASTATIC are terms applied to the process by which malignant disease spreads to distant parts of the body, and also to the secondary tumours resulting from this process. For example, a cancer of the breast may produce metastatic growths in the glands of the armpit, cancer of the stomach may be followed by metastases in the liver.

METATARSAL bones are the five bones in the foot which correspond to the metacarpal bones in the hand, lying between the tarsal bones, at the ankle, and the toes. (See FOOT.)

METATARSALGIA is pain affecting the metatarsal region of the foot. It is common in adolescents associated with flat-foot (q.v.). In adults it may be a manifestation of rheumatoid arthritis. *Morton's metatarsalgia* is a form associated usually with the nerve to the second toe cleft often induced by the compression of tight shoes.

METATARSUS is the group name of the five metatarsal bones in the foot (q.v.). *Metatarsus varus* is the condition characterized by deviation of the forefoot towards the other foot. It is a common condition in new-born babes and almost always corrects itself spontaneously. Only in the rare cases in which it is due to some deformity of the bones or muscles of the foot is any treatment required.

METEORISM means the distension of the abdomen by gas produced in the intestines. (See FLATULENCE.)

METFORMIN is a biguanide (q.v.) which lowers the blood sugar. This it does by increasing cellular uptake of glucose. It is active when taken by mouth and is proving of value in the treatment of certain cases of diabetes mellitus.

METHADONE, or PHYSEPTONE, is an analgesic with morphine-like properties. It has much less hypnotic action than morphine, and is used as a linctus for the alleviation of troublesome cough. It has some of the addiction-forming properties of morphine.

METHAEMOGLOBIN is a derivative of haemoglobin in which the iron has been oxidized from ferrous to ferric form. It does not combine with oxygen and therefore plays no part in oxygen transport. Normal concentration of methaemoglobin in red blood cells is less than one per cent of the total haemoglobin. When a large concentration of the haemoglobin is in the form of methaemoglobin the patient will suffer from hypoxia and will be cyanosed. Most cases of methaemoglobinaemia are due to chemical agents.

METHAEMOGLOBINAEMIA is a condition due to the presence in the blood of methaemoglobin (q.v.). It is characterized by cyanosis (q.v.) which turns the skin and lips a blue colour, shortness of breath, headache, fatigue and sickness. There are two main forms: a *hereditary* form and a *toxic* form. The latter is caused by certain drugs, including acetanilide, phenacetin, the sulphonamides and benzocaine. The treatment of the toxic form is the withdrawal of the causative drug. In the more severe cases the administration of methylene blue or ascorbic acid may also be needed, and these are the drugs used in the hereditary form.

In recent years attention has been drawn to a form known as *infantile methaemoglobinaemia* in bottle-fed babies under the age of 6 months. This is due to the presence of excess nitrate in the drinking water. Nitrate pollution of water has been increasing due to the purification of sewage effluent before its discharge to water-courses, and to changes in agricultural policy leading to better drainage of land and increased use of artificial fertilizers. As a result, especially where rainfall is low and the land low-lying, as in eastern and south-east England, underground supplies of water contain more than 50 mg of nitrate per litre, which is the level recommended by the World Health Organization, and may even exceed the maximum acceptable level of 100 mg per litre. High nitrate concentrations may also occur in surface waters after heavy rain. The cause of the methaemoglobinaemia is nitrite into which the nitrate is converted either in the baby's bottle or in his gut. Few serious cases have been recorded in Britain, and most of those which have occurred have been due to water from private sources.

Arrangements are now in force whereby water authorities inform the appropriate health authority if water with a nitrate content of 50 mg per litre has to be supplied, and alternative low-nitrate water is made available, sometimes in the form of bottled water, by local authorities for infants below the age of 6 months. The EEC has recommended an even more stringent criterion: that water used for baby feeds should not contain more than 25 mg of nitrate per litre.

METHICILLIN (see PENICILLIN, ANTIBIOTIC).

METHOHEXITONE is an ultra-short-acting barbiturate which is proving of value as a short-acting anaesthetic – particularly in dentistry.

METHOTREXATE is an antimetabolite (q.v.) which is proving of value in the treatment of choriocarcinoma (q.v.). (See CYTOTOXIC.)

METHYL is an organic radical whose chemical formula is CH_3, and which forms the centre of a wide group of substances known as the methyl group. For example, methyl alcohol is obtained as a by-product in the manufacture of beet-sugar, or by distillation of wood; methyl salicylate is the active constituent in oil of wintergreen; methyl hydride is better known as marsh gas.

Methyl alcohol, or wood spirit, is distilled from wood and is thus a cheap form of alcohol. It has actions similar to, but much more toxic than, those of ethyl alcohol. It has a specially pronounced action on the nervous system, and in large doses is apt to cause neuritis, especially of the optic nerves, leading to blindness, partial or complete.

METHYLCELLULOSE is a colloid (q.v.) which absorbs water to swell to about 25 times its original volume. It is used in the treatment of constipation and also in the management of obesity. The rationale for its use in obesity is that by swelling up in the stomach it reduces the appetite.

METHYLDOPA is one of the drugs introduced for the treatment of high blood-pressure. It is the drug most commonly used to control high blood-pressure in pregnancy.

METHYLENE BLUE is another name for methylthionin chloride.

METHYLPREDNISOLONE is a preparation with an action comparable to that of prednisolone (q.v.), but effective at a somewhat lower dose.

METHYLTESTOSTERONE is a derivative of the testicular hormone, testosterone (q.v.), which is active when taken by mouth. (See ANDROGEN.)

METHYSERGIDE is a drug that is being used in the prevention of attacks of migraine (q.v.). Its precise value is still not clear, and it has to be used with care because of the toxic effects it sometimes produces, such as nausea, drowsiness and retroperitoneal fibrosis.

METOCLOPRAMIDE is a drug that is proving of value in the treatment of vomiting. It is said to restore normal co-ordination and tone to the upper digestive tract. It is proving of value in the early treatment, and prevention, of migraine (q.v.).

METOLAZONE (see BENZOTHIADIAZINES).

METOPROLOL is a beta-adrenergic receptor blocking agent. (See ADRENERGIC RECEPTORS.)

METRE is the basic unit of length in the modern version of the metric system, known as the International System of Units (SI). (See WEIGHTS AND MEASURES.) It is equivalent to 39·37 inches.

METRITIS means inflammation of the womb.

METRONIDAZOLE is a drug, administered by mouth, which is proving of value in the treatment of various diseases including balantidiasis (q.v.), giardiasis (q.v.), amoebic dysentery (see DYSENTERY) and trichomonal vaginitis. (See TRICHOMONAS VAGINALIS.) It is also active against Gram-negative anaerobic micro-organisms.

METROPATHIA HAEMORRHAGICA, or ESSENTIAL UTERINE HAEMORRHAGE, is a diseased state characterized by haemorrhage from the uterus, cysts in the ovaries, and thickening of the uterine mucosa.

METRORRHAGIA means bleeding from the womb otherwise than at the proper period. It is usually due to a uterine lesion. (See MENSTRUATION.)

METYRAPONE is a drug that is used in the treatment of Cushing's syndrome (q.v.).

MEXENONE is a substance that has the property of absorbing ultra-violet light over a wide range, and is therefore used in the prevention of sunburn. It has the practical advantage of not being readily removed from the skin by washing or sweating, and thereby provides long protection.

MEZLOCILLIN (see ANTIBIOTIC).

MICONAZOLE is a drug that is proving of value in the treatment of the group of diseases known as the mycoses (q.v.).

MICROANGIOPATHY means disease of the capillaries (q.v.).

MICROBE (see BACTERIA).

MICROBIOLOGY is the study of all aspects of micro-organisms (microbes) – that is, organisms which individually are generally too small to be visible other than by microscopy. Few ecological habitats are devoid of micro-organisms – even extreme environments such as salt pans and thermal springs support microbial life – and the range of habitats the microbes can colonize is reflected in their extraordinary diversity in terms of morphology and development; metabolic abilities; and behaviour in response to stimuli in their immediate environment, adverse conditions, and other organisms.

The term micro-organism is applicable to viruses (q.v.); bacteria (q.v.); and microscopic forms of fungi (q.v.), algae, and protozoa. Some micro-organisms have affinities with both plants and animals, and it is preferable to consider micro-organisms as belonging to a separate kingdom, the protista, rather than attempting to categorize them according to the conventional dichotomy of the plant and animal kingdoms.

Among the smallest and simplest micro-organisms are the viruses. First described as filterable agents, and ranging in size from 20–30 nm to 300 nm, they may be directly visualized only by electron microscopy. They consist of a core of deoxyribonucleic or ribonucleic acid (DNA or RNA) (qq.v.) within a protective protein coat, or capsid, whose subunits confer a geometric symmetry. Thus viruses are usually cubical (icosahedral) or helical; the larger viruses (pox-, herpes-, myxo-viruses) may also have an outer envelope. Their minimal structure dictates that viruses are all obligate parasites, relying on living cells to provide essential components for their replication. Apart from animal and plant cells, viruses may infect and replicate in bacteria (bacteriophages) or fungi (mycophages), which are damaged in the process.

Bacteria are larger (0·01–5000μm) and more complex. They are prokaryotes, with a subcellular organization which generally includes DNA and RNA, a cell membrane, organelles such as ribosomes, and a complex and chemically variable cell envelope. Rickettsiae, chlamydia, and mycoplasmas, once thought of as viruses because of their small size and absence of a cell wall (mycoplasma) or major wall component (chlamydia), are now acknowledged as bacteria. Rickettsiae and chlamydia are obligate intracellular parasites of medical importance. Bacteria may also possess additional surface structures, such as capsules and organs of locomotion (flagella) and attachment (fimbriae and stalks). Individual bacterial cells may be spheres (cocci); straight (bacilli), curved (vibrio), or flexuous (spirilla) rods; or oval cells (coccobacilli). On examination by light microscopy bacteria may be visible in characteristic configurations (as pairs of cocci (diplococci), or chains (streptococci), or clusters); actinomycete bacteria grow as filaments with externally produced spores. Bacteria grow essentially by increasing in cell size and dividing by fission, a process which in ideal laboratory conditions some bacteria may achieve about once every 20 minutes. Under natural conditions growth is usually much slower.

As a group bacteria have a wide repertoire of metabolic and physiological capabilities. Some can synthesize their complex organic cellular components and biochemical intermediates if provided with light or chemical energy; others require sources of existing organic molecules from other micro-organisms, plants, or animals.

Eukaryotic micro-organisms comprise fungi, algae, and protozoa. These organisms are larger, and they have in common a well-developed internal compartmentation into subcellular organelles. Algae additionally have chloroplasts, which contain photosynthetic pigments; fungi lack chloroplasts; and protozoa lack both a cell wall and choroplasts but may have a contractile vacuole to regulate water uptake and, in some, structures for capturing and ingesting food. Fungi grow either as discrete cells (yeasts), multiplying by budding, fission, or conjugation, or as thin filaments (hyphae) which bear spores, though some may show both morphological forms during their life cycle. Algae and protozoa generally grow as individual cells or colonies of individuals and multiply by fission.

Micro-organisms of medical importance include representatives of the five major microbial groups that obtain their essential nutrients at the expense of their hosts. Many bacteria and most fungi, however, are saprophytes (q.v.), being major contributors to the natural cycling of carbon in the environment and to biodeterioration; others are of ecological and economic importance because of the diseases they cause in agricultural or horticultural crops or because of their beneficial relationships with higher organisms. Additionally, they may be of industrial or biotechnological importance. Fungal diseases of humans tend to be most important in tropical environments and in immunocompromised subjects.

For the micro-organism to be considered pathogenic and therefore capable of causing disease, it should fulfil a classic set of criteria termed Koch's postulates, which are designed to establish pathogenicity unequivocally. Some pathogens, for example, those that are not cultivable *in vitro* or in an alternative animal host, cannot fulfil all of the criteria and their status as true pathogens may have to rely on indirect methods.

Pathogenic micro-organisms display to a varying extent special characteristics, or virulence factors, that enable them to colonize their hosts and overcome or evade physical, biochemical, and immunological host defences. For bacteria, whose pathogenic properties have been intensively researched, the role of specific virulence factors and their relation to disease is better understood. Thus the presence of capsules, as in the bacteria that cause anthrax (*Bacillus anthracis*), one form of pneumonia (*Streptococcus preumoniae*), scarlet fever (*S. pyogenes*), bacterial meningitis (*Neisseria meningitidis, Haemophilus influenzae*) is directly related to the ability to cause disease because of their antiphagocytic properties. Fimbriae are related to virulence, enabling tissue attachment – for example, in gonorrhoea (*N. gonorrhoeae*) and cholera (*Vibrio cholerae*). Many bacteria excrete extracellular virulence factors; these include enzymes and other agents that impair the host's physiological and immunological functions. Some bacteria produce powerful toxins (excreted exotoxins or endogenous endotoxin), which may cause local tissue destruction and allow colonization by the pathogen or whose specific action may explain the disease mechanism. In *Staphylococcus aureus* exfoliative toxin produces the staphylococcal scalded-skin syndrome, TSS toxin-1 toxic-shock syndrome, and enterotoxin food poisoning. The pertussis exotixin of *Bordetella pertussis*, the cause of whooping cough, blocks immunological defences and mediates attachment to tracheal cells, and the exotoxin produced by *Corynebacterium diphtheriae* causes local damage resulting in a pronounced exudate in the trachea.

Viruses cause disease by cellular destruction arising from their intracellular parasitic existence. Attachment to particular cells is often mediated by specific viral surface proteins; mechanisms for evading immunological defences include latency, change in viral antigenic structure, or incapacitation of the immune system – for example, destruction of CD 4 lymphocytes by the human immunodeficiency virus.

Mechanisms of pathogenicity are generally less well understood for fungi and protozoa; further discussion of these topics is to be found in major textbooks and on medical microbiology.

MICROCEPHALY is abnormal smallness of the head.

MICROCYTE means a small red blood corpuscle.

MICROFILARIA: The mobile embryo of certain parasitic nematode worms which are found in the blood or lymph of patients infected with filarial worms. The microfilariae develop into larva in the body of a blood-sucking insect, for example, a mosquito.

MICROGRAM is the 1/1000th part of a milligram. The abreviation for it is µg.

MICROMETRE, or MICRON, is the 1/1000th part of a millimetre. The abbreviation for it is μm.

MICRO-ORGANISM (see BACTERIA).

MICROPSIA: Condition in which objects appear smaller than normal. It can be due to disease of the macula.

MICROSCOPE: An optical instrument comprising adjustable magnifying lenses that greatly enlarge a small object under study – for example, an insect, blood cells, or bacteria. Some microscopes use electron beams to magnify minute objects such as chromosomes, crystals, or even large molecules. Optical microscopes are also used for microsurgery when the area being operated on is otherwise inaccessible, for example, in eye and inner ear surgery, for the removal of tumours from the brain or spinal cord and for resuturing damaged blood vessels and nerves.

MICROSPORON is the genus of fungi which includes the fungi responsible for ringworm of the scalp. (See RINGWORM.)

MICROSURGERY is surgery performed with the use of an operating microscope. It is used routinely in certain operations on the eye, the ear and the larynx. In recent years it has been used, with increasing success, in attempts to reunite severed legs and arms. Under the operating microscope, surgical sutures invisible to the naked eye are used to reunite blood vessels 0·5 millimetre in diameter. The severed limb will survive for up to eight hours at room temperature, longer if cooled – as by ice in the ambulance taking the patient to hospital. Success depends primarily on restoration of the circulation to the limb. Once this has been achieved, attention is later turned to restoring the continuity of the nerves.

MICROWAVES are non-ionizing electro-magnetic radiations in the frequency range of 30–300,000 megahertz. They are emitted from electronic devices, such as heaters, some domestic ovens, television receivers, radar units and diathermy units. There is no scientific evidence to justify the claims that they are harmful to man or produce any harmful effect in the genes (q.v.). The only known necessary precaution is the protection of the eyes in those using them in industry, as there is some evidence that prolonged exposure to them in this may induce cataract. (See also DIATHERMY.)

MICTURITION means the act of passing water.

MIDDLE EAR: That portion of the ear lying between the tympanic membrane and the inner ear (q.v.). It contains the ossicles, the three small bones that transmit sound. (See EAR.)

MIDGES (see BITES AND STINGS).

MIDWIFE: A member of the profession which provides care and advice during pregnancy, supervises the mother's labour and delivery and looks after her and the baby after birth. Should a pregnancy or labour develop complications, the midwife will seek medical advice. Most midwives are registered general nurses who have also done an 18-month course in midwifery. Trained midwives are registered with the UK Central Council for Midwifery and work in hospitals or a domiciliary setting.

MIDWIFERY (see LABOUR; MIDWIFE).

MIGRAINE, or HEMICRANIA as it is sometimes known from the Greek word for half a skull, is a common condition characterized by recurring intense headaches. It is much commoner in women than men. There are said to be six million victims of it in Britain. It has been defined as 'episodic headache accompanied by visual or gastro-intestinal disturbances, or both, attacks lasting hours with total freedom between episodes'.

It usually begins at puberty and often tends to stop in middle age: e.g. in women attacks often cease after menopause. It often disappears during pregnancy. In susceptible individuals attacks may be provoked by a wide variety of causes including:

Anxiety, emotion, depression, shock, and excitement

Physical and mental fatigue

Prolonged focusing on television or cinema screen

Noise, especially loud and high-pitched sounds

Certain foods: e.g. chocolate, cheese, citrus fruits, pastry

Alcohol

Prolonged lack of food

Irregular meals

Menstruation and the pre-menstrual period

Indeed, it has been said that anything that can provoke a headache in the ordinary individual can precipitate an attack in a migrainous subject. It seems as if there is an inherited predispostion that triggers a mechanism whereby in the migrainous subject the headache and the associated sickness persist for hours, a whole day or even longer.

The precise cause is not known, but the generally accepted view is that in susceptible individuals one or other of these causes produces spasm or constriction of the blood-vessels of the brain. This in turn is followed by dilatation of these blood-vessels which also become more permeable and so allow fluid to pass out into the surrounding tissues. This combination of dilatation and outpouring of fluid is held to be responsible for the headache.

The typical attack is very characteristic. It

consists of an intense headache, usually situated over one or other eye. The headache is usually preceded by a feeling of sickness and blurring of sight. In 15 to 20 per cent of cases this disturbance of sight takes the form of bright lights: the so-called aura of migraine. The majority of attacks are accompanied by vomiting. The duration of the headache varies, but in the more severe cases the victim is usually confined to bed for twenty-four hours.
Treatment consists, in the first place, of trying to avoid any precipitating factor. Patients must find out which drug, or drugs, give them most relief, and they must always carry these about with them wherever they go. This is because it is a not uncommon experience to be aware of an attack coming on and to find that there is a critical quarter of an hour or so during which the tablets are effective. If not taken within this period, they may be ineffective and the unfortunate victim finds himself prostrate with headache and vomiting. In addition he should immediately lie down, and at this stage a few hours' rest may prevent the development of a full attack. When an attack is fully developed, rest in bed in a quiet, darkened room is essential; any loud noise or bright light intensifies the headache or sickness. The less food that is taken during an attack the better, provided the individual drinks as much fluid as he wants. Group therapy, in which groups of around ten migrainous subjects learn how to relax, is often of help in more severe cases, whilst in others the injection of a local anaesthetic into tender spots in the scalp reduces the number of attacks. Drug treatment is not very satisfactory. Perhaps the most effective remedy for the condition is ergotamine tartrate which causes the dilated blood vessels to contract, but this must only be taken under medical supervision. In many cases metoclopramide, followed ten minutes later by three tablets of either aspirin or paracetamol, provides a most effective form of treatment if taken early in an attack. In milder attacks, aspirin, with or without codeine and paracetamol, may be of value.

People with migraine and their relatives can obtain help and guidance from the British Migraine Association, 178A High Road, Byfleet, West Byfleet, Surrey KT14 7ED (0932-352468).

MILIA: These are small keratin cysts appearing as white papules on the cheek and eyelids.

MILIARIA is the name applied to the group of diseases of the skin caused by disturbances of perspiration. The best known is MILIARIA RUBRA, or PRICKLY HEAT (q.v.).

MILIARY is a term, expressing size, applied to various disease products which are about the size of millet seeds: e.g. miliary aneurysms, miliary tuberculosis.

MILIUM is the term applied to a small, whitish nodule in the skin, especially of the face. (See ACNE.)

MILK is the natural food of all animals belonging to the class of mammalia for a considerable period following their birth. It is practically the only form of animal food in which protein, fat, carbohydrate, and salt are all represented in sufficient amount, and it therefore contains all the constituents of a standard diet. Milk is important in human nutrition because it contains first-class animal protein of high biological value, because it is exceptionally rich in calcium, and because it is a good source of vitamin A, thiamine and riboflavine. It also contains a variable amount of ascorbic acid (vitamin C) and of vitamin D, the amount of the latter being higher during the summer months than during the winter months. Raw milk yields 67 Calories per 100 millilitres, in which are present (in grams) 87·6 of water, 3·3 of protein, 3·6 of fat, 4·7 of carbohydrate, and 0·12 of calcium. Heat has no effect on the vitamin A or D content of milk, or on the riboflavine content, but it causes a considerable reduction in the vitamin C and thiamine content.

The ready digestibility of milk, especially when mixed with lime water, or when 125 to 200 mg of citrate of soda have been added for 30 ml of milk in order to soften the curd, makes it a specially suitable food for children, invalids, and people suffering from fever. For a person confined to bed and restricted in the matter of food, 1·5 litres (3 pints) daily afford sufficient nourishment for two or three weeks.
Preparation of milk: Milk may be prepared for food in various ways. *Boiling* destroys the bacteria, especially any *Mycobacteria tuberculosis* which the milk may contain. It also partly destroys vitamin C and thiamine, as does *pasteurization. Curdling* of milk is effected by adding rennet, which carries out the initial stage of digestion and thus renders milk more suitable for people who could not otherwise tolerate it. *Souring* of milk is practised in many countries before milk is considered suitable for food; it is carried out by adding certain organisms such as the lactic acid bacillus, the Bulgarian bacillus, and setting the milk in a warm place for several hours. (See LACTIC ACID BACILLI.) *Sterilization*, which prevents fermentation and decomposition, is usually carried out by raising the milk to boiling temperature (100 °C) for fifteen minutes and then hermetically sealing it. *Condensed, unsweetened milk* – usually known as *evaporated milk* – is concentrated *in vacuo* at low temperature; the milk is then placed in tins, which are sealed, and is sterilized by heat at a temperature of 105 °C. This destroys 60 per cent of the vitamin C and 30 to 50 per cent of the thiamine. *Sweetened condensed milk* is not exposed to such a high temperature. The sugar, which prevents the growth of micro-organisms, is added before the condensing, and finally reaches a concentration

of about 40 per cent. *Dried milk* is prepared by evaporating all the fluid so that the milk is reduced to the form of powder. *Humanized milk* is cow's milk treated to render it closely similar to human milk.

Grades of milk: In the Unted Kingomd the grades of milk that are now officially recognized are: untreated milk and heat-treated milk, which is divided into three categories: pasteurized, sterilized, and ultra heat-treated.

Pasteurized milk is milk that has been treated in one of two ways. One is the 'Holder Process', in which the milk is retained at a temperature of not less than 63 °C and not more than 65·5 °C for at least half an hour and then immediately cooled to a temperature of not more than 10 °C. The other is the 'High Temperature Short Time Process', in which the milk is retained at a temperature of not less than 71·7 °C for at least fifteen seconds and then immediately cooled to a temperature of not more than 10 °C. Pasteurization will not make satisfactory milk that was unsatisfactory in the first instance but, provided satisfactory milk is used in the first instance, it does provide a safe milk of good keeping qualities without affecting its nutritive value to any appreciable extcnt. *Sterilized milk* is milk that has been filtered or clarified, homogenized and then heated to, and maintained at, a temperature of at least 100 °C for such a period as to ensure that it complies with the turbidity test as described in the appropriate regulations. *Ultra heat-treated milk* is milk which has been retained at a temperature of at least 132 °C for not less than one second. It is required to satisfy the bacteriology colony count test as laid down in the appropriate regulations. It keeps much better than pasteurized milk: packed in sterile cartons it will keep for several weeks without refrigeration.

MILK TEETH are the temporary teeth of children. (For the time of their appearance, see TEETH.)

MILLILITRE is the 1000th part of 1 litre. It is practically the equivalent of a cubic centimetre (1 cm^3 = 0·999973 ml); ml is the usual abbreviation.

MINERAL CORTICOID: (see CORTICOSTEROIDS).

MINOCYCLINE is a long-acting tetracycline (q.v.) which is proving of value in the treatment of carriers of meningococci, or *Neisseria meningitidis* (see MENINGITIS), and in some cases of chronic bronchitis.

MIOSIS: Condition of constriction of the pupil.

MISCARRIAGE (see ABORTION).

MITHRAMYCIN (see CYTOTOXIC).

MITHRIDATISM is a term applied to immunity against the effects of poisons produced by administration of gradually increasing doses of the poison itself. The process is named after Mithridates, King of Pontus, who rendered himself immune against poisoning by this means.

MITOCHONDRIA are the rod-like bodies in the cells of the body which contain the enzymes (q.v.) necessary for the activity of the cell. They have been described as the 'power plant of the cell'. (See CELLS.)

MITOSIS is the process of cell division for somatic cells and for the ovum after fertilization. Each chromosome becomes doubled by splitting lengthwise and forming two chromatids which remain held together by the centromere. These chromatids are exact copies of the original chromosomes and contain duplicates of all the genes they bear. When cell division takes place the pull of the spindle splits the centromere and each double chromatid separates, one passing to one pole of the nucleus and the other to the opposite pole. Thc nucleus and the cell itself then also divide, forming two new daughter cells containing precisely the same 23 pairs of chromosomes and carrying exactly the same complement of genes as did the mother cell.

MITRAL INCOMPETENCE: A defect in the mitral valve (q.v.) or the heart (q.v.) allows blood to leak from the left ventricle into the left atrium (qq.v.). It is also known as mitral regurgitation; incompetence may occur along with mitral stenosis (q.v.). The left ventricle has to work harder to compensate for the faulty valve, so it enlarges, but eventually the ventricle cannot cope with the extra load and left-sided heart failure may develop. A common cause of mitral incompetence is rheumatic fever or damage following a heart attack. The condition is treated with drugs to help the heart but in severe cases heart surgery may be required.

MITRAL STENOSIS is the narrowing of the opening between the left atrium and left ventricle of the heart as a result of rigidity of, and adhesion between, the cusps of the mitral valve. It is due, almost invariably, to the infection of rheumatic fever.

MITRAL VALVE, so called from its resemblance to a bishop's mitre, is the valve which guards the opening between the atrium and ventricle on the left side of the heart. (See HEART.)

MMR VACCINE: A combined vaccine that protects a person against measles, mumps, and rubella (German measles). It was introduced in the UK in 1988 for routine immunization and is offered to children in single-dose form in their second year. In the year ending February 1991 89 per cent of children offered MMR were immunized and the figure is rising steadily. Children who have not been immunized as infants should be offered MMR with the pre-school booster doses against diphtheria, tetanus, and polio. The procedure is effective and safe, although minor symptoms such as malaise, fever, and rash may occur 5 to 10 days after immunization. The incidence of the three diseases has dropped markedly since MMR was introduced in the United States and the United Kingdom. (See IMMUNIZATION.)

MOLAR TEETH are the last three teeth on each side of the jaw. (See TEETH.)

MOLE is a term used in two quite different senses. In the first place, a mole on the skin is a darkly pigmented spot, usually raised above the surrounding surface, rough, and covered with hair. These moles are of developmental origin, and malignant growths may spring from some of them late in life. Secondly the term hydatidiform mole is applied to cases in which, following upon conception, a degenerative mass forms in the womb, the embryo dying in the process; whilst the term carneous mole is applied to an ovum that has died in the early months of pregnancy.

MOLLUSCUM CONTAGIOSUM: A disease in which small papules, seldom larger than peas, develop on the surface of the skin. It is due to a virus and is highly contagious, being most commonly conveyed from individual to individual in swimming pools and Turkish baths. They may disappear spontaneously. Treatment is by freezing the nodules with liquid nitrogen. Alternatively, each nodule may be spiked with a sharpened orange stick which has been dipped in pure phenol, or in 10 per cent podophyllin in industrial methylated spirit.

MONGOLIAN BLUE SPOTS are irregularly shaped areas of bluish-black pigmentation found occasionally on the buttocks, lower back or upper arms in new-born infants of African, Chinese and Japanese parentage and sometimes in the babies of black-haired Europeans. They measure from one to several centimetres in diameter, and usually disappear in a few months. They are commonly mistaken for bruises.

MONGOLISM (see DOWN'S SYNDROME).

MONILIASIS is the infection caused by monilia, the genus of fungi now known as *Candida albicans*. The infection may occur in the mouth, where it is known as thrush (q.v.), lungs, intestine, vagina, skin, or nails.

MONKEYPOX is a smallpox-like disease, due to a virus which occurs in monkeys kept in captivity. Since 1970, when first reported, 48 human cases have been recorded. Most of these have been in Zaïre, and all have been in the equatorial rain-forest of West and Central Africa (Zaïre, Liberia, Sierra Leone, Nigeria, Ivory Coast and Cameroon). The case-fatality rate to date has been 17 per cent. It does not appear to be highly infectious and it is not at the moment considered to be a great risk to human beings.

MONOAMINE OXIDASE INHIBITORS are drugs that destroy, or prevent the action of, monoamine oxidase (MAO). Monoamines, which include noradrenaline (q.v.) and tyramine, play an important part in the metabolism of the brain, and there is some evidence that excitement is due to an accumulation of monoamines in the brain. MAO is a naturally occurring enzyme (q.v.) which is concerned in the breakdown of monoamines.

An excessive accumulation of monoamines can induce a dangerous reaction characterized by high blood-pressure, palpitations, sweating and a feeling of suffocation. Hence the care with which MAO inhibitor drugs are administered. What is equally important, however, is that in no circumstances should a patient receiving any MAO inhibitor drug eat cheese, yeast preparations such as Marmite, tinned fish, or high game. The reason for this ban is that all these foodstuffs contain large amounts of tyramine which increases the amount of certain monoamines such as noradrenaline in the body.

There are also certain drugs, such as amphetamine and pethidine, which must not be taken by a patient who is receiving an MAO inhibitor drug.

MONOCLONAL ANTIBODIES: An artificially prepared *antibody* (q.v.) obtained from cell clones – a genetically identical group of cells – and comprising a single type of immunoglobulin. It neutralizes only one specific antigen (q.v.). The antibodies are prepared by linking antibody-forming lymphocytes (q.v.) from the spleen of mice with myeloma cells (q.v.) from mice. Monoclonal antibodies are used in the development of new vaccines and in the study of human cells, hormones, and microorganisms. Research is under way for their use in the treatment of some forms of cancer.

MONOCYTE: A type of white blood cell which has a single kidney-shaped nucleus. Present in the tissues and lymphatic system as well as the circulation, it ingests foreign particles such as tissue debris and bacteria. Monocytes are about 20μm in diameter and 1 mm^3 of blood contains around 7500 of them, many times fewer than the five million erythrocytes (red blood cells).

MONOMANIA is a form of partial insanity, in which the affected person has a delusion upon one subject, though he can converse rationally and is a responsible individual upon other matters.

MONONUCLEOSIS: An acute viral infection in which the patient developes a sore throat, swollen lymph glands and fever. Also known as glandular fever, infectious mononucleosis is caused by members of the Herpes (q.v.) group of viruses – Epstein Barr and cytomegalovirus. The disease is more common among adolescents aged 15 to 17, an age when their immune defence machanisms are not fully developed. In the UK many thousands of teenagers catch the disease every year, and kissing is believed to be the method of transmission among many of them. The blood contains many atypical lymphocytes and the diagnosis is confirmed with the heterophil antibodies test. Patients normally recover within six weeks without treatment, but they may feel tired and depressed for several months afterwards.

MONOPLEGIA means paralysis of a single limb or part. (See PARALYSIS.)

MONOSACCHARIDE is a sugar having six carbon atoms in the molecule, such as glucose, galactose, and laevulose.

MONOZYGOTIC TWINS: Twins who develop from a single ovum fertilized by a single spermatozoa. Also known as identical or uniovular twins (see MULTIPLE BIRTHS).

MORBIDITY: The condition of being diseased. The morbidity rate is the number of cases of disease occurring within a particular number of the population.

MORBILLI is another name for measles.

MORBILLIVIRUSES are the group of viruses which include those responsible for measles, canine distemper and rinderpest.

MORBUS, the Latin word for disease, is used in such terms as morbus cordis (heart disease), morbus coxae (hip-joint disease).

MORIBUND: In a state of dying.

MORON is the term applied to a feeble-minded person whose defect is relatively slight and whose mental age is somewhere between 8 and 12 years.

MORPHINE, or MORPHIA, is the name of the chief alkaloid upon which the action of opium depends. (See OPIUM; DRUG ADDICTION.)

MORPHOEA is a form of circumscribed scleroderma. (See SCLERODERMA.)

MORTALITY (see DEATH, CAUSES OF; DEATH RATE; INFANT MORTALITY).

MORTIFICATION is another name for gangrene. (See GANGRENE.)

MOSAICISM: If non-dysjunction occurs after the formation of a zygote, that is during a mitotic cell division and not a meiotic cell division, some of the cells will have one chromosome constitution and others another. The term mosaicism describes a condition in which a substantial minority of cells differ from the majority in their chromosome content. How substantial this minority is will depend on how early during cleavage the zygote undergoes non-dysjunction.

MOSQUITOES. (See ANOPHELES; BITES AND STINGS.)

MOTILIN is a hormone (q.v.) formed in the duodenum (q.v.) and the jejunum (q.v.) which plays a part in controlling the movements of the stomach and the gut.

MOTION SICKNESS is a characteristic set of symptoms experienced by many people when subjected to the constant changes of position caused, for example, by the pitching and rolling motion of a vessel at sea. Depression, giddiness, nausea and vomiting are the most prominent. **Causes**: Although the vast majority of people appear to be liable to this ailment at sea, they do not all suffer alike. Many endure distress of a most acute and even alarming kind, whilst others are simply conscious of transient feelings of nausea and discomfort. In long voyages, whilst many are affected with sea-sickness for the first few days only, others are affected for the entire period, especially on the occurrence of rough weather. In short voyages, such as across the English Channel, not a few, of those susceptible, escape, while others suffer in an extreme degree, the sickness persisting long after arrival on shore. A smaller proportion of people suffer from air and car sickness.

Many theories have been advanced to account for the connection between the motion of a ship, aeroplane or vehicle and sickness, and there is probably more than one set of causes. In the first place, the movement of the ship or vehicle disturbs that feeling of the relation of the body to surrounding objects upon which our sense of security rests. The nervous system being thus subjected to a succession of shocks or surprises fails to effect the necessary adjustments for equilibrium. Giddiness, nausea and vomiting follow. The changing impressions made upon the vision have been regarded by some as a powerful influence, but attacks of motion sickness occur also in the dark, and in the case of blind persons. Other contributory causes may be mentioned, such as the feeling that sickness is certain to come, which may bring on the attack even before the start of a journey.

Symptoms: The symptoms generally show themselves soon after the journey has started, by the onset of giddiness and discomfort in the head, together with a sense of nausea and sinking at the stomach, which soon develops into intense sickness and vomiting. Along with the sickness there is physical prostration, as shown in the pallor of the skin, cold sweats and feeble pulse, accompanied with mental depression and wretchedness. In almost all instances the attack has a favourable termination, and it is extremely rare that serious results arise, except in the case of persons weakened by other diseases, although occasionally the symptoms are for a time sufficiently alarming.

Treatment: Innumerable preventives and remedies have been proposed, but most of them fall far short of the success claimed for them. No means has yet been discovered which can althogether prevent the occurrence of motion sickness. None of the drugs used possesses infallible properties; a remedy which suits one person will often fail with another. Experience gained during the 1939–45 War has shown that the most satisfactory remedy is hyoscine hydrobromide, 0·6 to 0·3 mg. Other drugs of value in the prevention of sickness include avomine, dramamine, ginger and marzine.

MOTOR NEURON DISEASE (see PARALYSIS).

MOUNTAIN SICKNESS (see ALTITUDE SICKNESS).

MOUTH is the start of the alimentary canal. It is bounded anteriorly by the lips and posteriorly by the fauces which is the narrow passage between the tonsils. Immediately behind the lips are the teeth, embedded in the jaw, and behind the lower teeth is the tongue. The upper part of the mouth is the palate. The anterior or hard palate is firm and immovable as it consists of bone covered by mucosa, while the posterior part is soft and mobile. The soft palate moves during swallowing and speech. The salivary glands discharge their saliva into the mouth through small ducts. Two of these ducts are large and can be easily seen; the parotid duct opens into the cheek opposite the upper second molar tooth and the submandibular gland duct can be seen under the tongue in the midline.

Food in the mouth is prepared for digestion by being broken up by the teeth and mixed with saliva prior to being projected into the stomach via the oesophagus.

MOUTH, DISEASES OF: The mucous membrane of the mouth can indicate the health of the individual and internal organs, e.g. pallor or pigmentation may indicate anaemia, jaundice or Addison's disease. The musculature of the tongue can also act as a guide to the health of other muscles and of the nervous system in generalized disease.

CONDITIONS OF THE TONGUE: At rest the tongue touches all the lower teeth and is slightly arched from side to side. It has a smooth surface with a groove in the middle and an even but definite edge. It is under voluntary control and the tip can be moved in all directions.

Ankyloglossia or tongue-tie is found when the frenum or band connecting the lower surface of the tongue to the floor of the mouth is so short or tight that the tongue cannot be protruded. This is said to interfere with speech but, if it does, it is only to a small degree. The restricted movement makes it difficult to remove food from round the teeth which may encourage decay.

Gross enlargement of the tongue can make speech indistinct or make swallowing and even breathing difficult. This is known as macroglossia and may be such that the tongue is constantly protruded from the mouth. The cause may be congenital as in severe cases of Down's Syndrome or it may occur as a result of acromegaly or be due to abnormal deposits as in amyloid disease.

In general debility the tongue may appear flabby, large and pale with the edge indented by the teeth.

A marked tremor of the tongue when protruded may be seen in various nervous diseases but is common in excessive indulgence in alcohol and cannot be concealed.

After a stroke involving the motor nerve centre the control of one side of the tongue musculature will be lost. This will result in the protruded tongue pointing to the side of the body which is paralysed. The sense of taste on one side of the tongue may also be lost in some diseases of the brain and facial nerve.

The presence of fur on the tongue may be obvious and distressing. This is due to thickening of the superficial layers of the tongue which may appear like hairs which trap food debris and become discoloured. Furring is common in the presence of fever, mouth breathing and smoking. Debility and loss of appetite will prevent the normal cleaning movements of the tongue and result in a build-up of debris between elongated papillae. A prominent brown fur with a yellow edge on a red mucous membrane is commonly seen in typhoid fever. In scarlet fever the description *strawberry tongue* is used when the surface of the tongue is covered with a white fur through which red spots of mucosal papillae project. Constipation and bowel obstruction are associated with a thick white or brownish fissured fur. Gastritis particularly when related to alcohol excess is associated with a thin white fur which wears off as the day progresses. Stomach cancers and ulcers are not particularly associated with furring of the tongue. Inflammatory lesions of the throat such as tonsillitis may accompany a thick moist fur on the tongue.

In some conditions the tongue may appear

dry, red and raw. An inflamed *beefy tongue* is characteristic of pellagra, a disease caused by deficiency of nicotinic acid in the diet. A magenta-coloured tongue may be seen when there is a lack of riboflavin.

THRUSH is characterized by the presence of white patches on the mucous membrane which bleeds if the patch is gently removed. It is caused by the growth of a parasitic mould known as *Candida albicans*. Thrush is frequently found under the upper denture of elderly people who wear their dentures day and night and whose oral hygiene is poor. A more florid form is seen in feeble babies and in adults with a chronic severe illness. A less obvious form may be found in some patients after they have been taking antibiotics. Antifungal agents usually suppress the growth of Candida. Candidal infiltration of the mucosa is often found in cancerous lesions.

LEUKOPLAKIA literally means a white patch. In the mouth it is often due to an area of thickened cells from the horny layer of the epithelium. It appears as a white patch of varying density and is often grooved by dense fissures. There are many causes, most of them of minor importance. If, however, it is associated with spirits, smoking, syphilis, chronic sepsis or trauma from a sharp tooth, then cancer must be excluded.

A bright red bare area of tongue surrounded by a definite whitish yellow margin is known as *geographical tongue*. The areas may change position from week to week and there may be a slight burning sensation. Apart from an association with digestive disorders, it is of no great importance.

Ulcers of the tongue are similar to those elsewhere in the mouth. The most common are aphthous ulcers which are small red and painful and last for about ten days. They are associated with stress, mild trauma, and occasionally with folic acid and vitamin B_{12} deficiency. Ulcers of the tongue are sometimes found in patients with chronic bowel disease.

STOMATITIS (inflammation of the mouth) arises from the same causes as inflammation elsewhere, but among the main causes are the cutting of teeth in children, sharp or broken teeth, excess alcohol, tobacco smoking and general ill-health. The mucous membrane becomes red, swollen and tender and ulcers may appear. The avoidance of spicy foods and other irritants make the patient more comfortable until the condition resolves. Treatment consists mainly of preventing secondary infection supervening before the stomatitis has resolved. Antiseptic mouthwashes are usually sufficient.

Gingivitis (see TEETH, DISEASES OF) is inflammation of the gum where it touches the tooth. It is caused by poor oral hygiene and is often associated with the production of calculus or tartar on the teeth. If it is neglected it will proceed to periodontal disease.

ULCERS OF THE MOUTH: These are usually small and arise from a variety of causes. *Aphthous ulcers* are the most common. They are round with a bright red margin and uncomfortable as they tend to occur near a sharp tooth or on a mobile part of the mucosa where they are easily stretched open or torn. They last about ten days and usually heal without scarring. They may be associated with stress or dyspepsia. There is no ideal treatment.

Herpetic ulcers are similar but usually there are many ulcers and the patient appears feverish and lethargic. It is more common in children and may arise from mothers who have cold sores on their lip.

Undernourished children may develop an ulcer in the cheek which causes pain, an increased flow of saliva and a foetid breath. This rarely progresses to a condition known as cancrum oris in which much of the cheek may be destroyed.

In whooping cough the underside of the tongue may be frequently forced against the lower teeth as it is protruded during the coughing bouts and this will cause an ulcer under the tongue. Larger ulcers may be tuberculous, syphilitic or cancerous in origin.

ALVEOLAR ABSCESS, DENTAL ABSCESS or GUMBOIL: This is an abscess caused by an infected tooth. It may present as a large swelling or cause trismus (inability to open the mouth). Treatment is drainage of the pus, extraction of the tooth or antibiotics.

CALCULUS: (*a*) *Salivary*: A calculus or stone may develop in one of the major salivary gland ducts. This may result in a blockage which will cause the gland to swell and be painful. It usually swells before a meal and then slowly subsides. The stone may be passed but often has to be removed in a minor operation. If the gland behind the calculus becomes infected, then an abscess forms and, if this persists, the removal of the gland may be indicated. (*b*) *Dental*, also called TARTAR: This is a hard substance which adheres to the teeth. Some people produce more than others. It is a mixture of calcified material and bacteria and often starts as the soft debris found on teeth which have not been well cleaned and is called plaque. If not removed, it will gradually destroy the periodontal membrane and result in the loss of the tooth.

RANULA: This is a cystlike swelling found in the floor of the mouth. It is often caused by mild trauma to the salivary glands with the result that saliva collects in the cyst instead of discharging into the mouth. Careful surgical removal is required as cysts can become quite large.

MUCOCOELE or MUCOUS CYST: This is a collection of saliva in the lip following mild trauma. It is similar to a ranula but does not become so large. Treatment is surgical removal.

MUMPS is an acute infective disorder of the major salivary glands. It causes painful enlargement of the glands which lasts for about two weeks.

TUMOURS occur in all parts of the mouth. They may be benign or malignant. Benign tumours are common and may follow mild trauma or are an exaggerated response to irritation. Polyps are found in the cheeks and on the tongue and become a nuisance as they may be bitten frequently. They are easily excised.

A *mucocoele* (q.v.) is found mainly in the lower lip.

An *epulis* is a lump on the gum. One form is seen during pregnancy and may bleed easily but disappears spontaneously at the end of the gestation. Another form is more persistent and may recur after excision and removal of the associated teeth. An *exostosis* or bone outgrowth is often found in the mid-line of the palate and on the inside of the mandible. This only requires removal if it becomes unduly large or pointed and easily ulcerated.

Malignant tumours within the mouth are often large before they are noticed, whereas those on the lips are usually seen early and are more easily treated. The cancer may arise from any of the tissues found in the mouth including epithelium, bone, salivary tissue and tooth-forming tissue remnants. In England and Wales in 1986 there were nearly 3,000 new cases of malignant disease in the mouth and major salivary glands. Nearly 600 of these were in the tongue.

Cancer of the mouth is less common below the age of 40 years and more common in men. It is often associated with chronic irritation from a broken tooth or ill-fitting denture. It is also more common in those who smoke and those who chew betel leaves. Leukoplakia (q.v.) may be a precursor of cancer. Spread of the cancer is by way of the lymph nodes in the neck. Early treatment by surgery or radiotherapy will often give a five-year cure, except for the posterior of the tongue where the prognosis is very poor. Although surgery may be extensive and potentially mutilating, recent advances in repairing defects and grafting tissues from elsewhere have made treatment more acceptable to the patient.

MUCILAGE is prepared from acacia or tragacanth gum, and is used as an ingredient of mixtures containing solid particles in order to keep the latter from settling, and also as a demulcent.

MUCOCOELE is an abnormally dilated cavity in the body due to the accumulation of mucus; such a 'cyst' may therefore form wherever there is mucous membrane.

MUCOCUTANEOUS LYMPH NODE SYNDROME is a disease that has been reported from Japan, Korea, Hawaii, Greece and the USA, but not yet from Britain. The cause is not known. It occurs in young children, usually under the age of 5 years. It is characterized by fever, a generalized rash which becomes bright red on the hands and feet, and enlargement of the glands in the neck. Recovery usually occurs in two to four weeks. Complications sometimes occur in the form of meningitis, arthritis, jaundice, or myocarditis. The

mortality rate is 1 to 2 per cent. There is no specific treatment.

MUCOLYTIC is the term used to describe the property of destroying, or lessening the tenacity of, mucus. It is most commonly used to describe drugs which have this property and are therefore used in the treatment of bronchitis (q.v.). The inhalation of steam, for example, has a mucolytic action.

MUCOMEMBRANOUS COLIC is a disorder in which constipation, abdominal pain, and the passage of mucus or casts of mucus in the stools occur in highly strung or neurotic people, especially women. The spasm of the colon causing these symptoms may be allergic in origin.

MUCOSA: A term for mucous membrane.

MUCOUS MEMBRANE is the general name given to the membrane which lines many of the hollow organs of the body. These membranes vary widely in structure in different sites, but all have the common character of being lubricated by mucus, derived in some cases from isolated cells on the surface of the membrane, but more generally from definite glands placed beneath the membrane, and opening here and there through it by ducts. The air passages, the alimentary canal and the ducts of glands which open into it, and also the urinary passages, are all lined by mucous membrane.

In structure a mucous membrane consists of a basis of fibrous tissue resembling the true skin, though looser and lighter in texture, in which the blood-vessels, nerves, and mucous glands lie. This is covered on its surface by a layer of epithelium resembling the epithelium covering the skin, although the cells are in all cases of a more soft and succulent nature than those on the outer surface of the body.

Ciliated epithelial cells from the air passages.

It is in the character and properties of these cells that the various mucous membranes chiefly differ. In the air passages they are – almost everywhere except over the vocal cords – of a pillar-like shape and provided with thread-like processes, being known as ciliated cells. On the vocal cords the cells, which are exposed to constant friction, resemble those of the skin. In the alimentary system generally they are of a simple pillar-like or columnar type placed side by side, though in the mouth and gullet, where the food causes much friction, the surface, like

1 surface view of the ends of a group of cells
2 columnar cell from the mucous membrane of
   the small intestine
3 side view of a group of cells

Columnar epithelium.

that of the vocal cords, closely resembles the epidermis of the skin.

Lying close beneath the epithelium there is, in most mucous membranes, a thin layer of involuntary muscle fibres, and to this, coupled with the extremely loose attachment of mucous membranes to the organs which they line, is due the great pliability and elasticity of these membranes.

MUCOVISCIDOSIS (see CYSTIC FIBROSIS).

MUCUS is the general name for the slimy secretion derived from mucous membranes. It is mainly composed of a substance called mucin, which varies according to the particular mucous membrane from which it is derived, and it contains other substances, such as cells cast off from the surface of the membrane, ferments, and dust particles. From whatever source derived, mucin has the following characteristics: it is viscid, clear, and tenacious; when dissolved in water it can be precipitated by addition of acetic acid; and when not in solution already, it is dissolved by weak alkalis, such as lime-water.

Under normal conditions the surface of a mucous membrane is lubricated by only a small quantity of mucus; the appearance of large quantities is a sign of inflammation.

MULLERIAN DUCTS: The Mullerian and the Wolffian ducts are separate sets of primordia that transiently co-exist in embryos of both sexes. In female embryos the Mullerian ducts grow and fuse in the midline producing the Fallopian tubes, the uterus and the upper third of the vagina whereas the Wolffian ducts regress. In the male the Wolffian ducts give rise to the vas deferens, the seminal vesicles and the epididymis and the Mullerian ducts disappear. This phase of development requires a functioning testis from which an inducer substance diffuses locally over the primordia to bring about the suppression of the Mullerian duct and the development of the Wolffian duct. In the absence of this substance development proceeds along female lines regardless of the genetic sex.

MULTIGRAVIDA is a pregnant woman who has had more than one pregnancy.

MULTIPARA is a woman who has borne several children.

MULTIPLE BIRTHS: Twins occur about once in eighty pregnancies, triplets once in 6000, quadruplets about once in 500,000. Quintuplets are exceedingly rare. Such is the natural state of affairs. In recent years, however, the position has been altered by the introduction of the so-called fertility drugs, such as clomiphene (q.v.), and human menopausal gonadotrophin which, through the medium of the pituitary gland, stimulate the production of ova. Their wide use in the treatment of infertility has resulted in an increase in the number of multiple births, a recognized hazard of giving too large a dose. So far as fraternal, or binovular, twins are concerned, multiple pregnancy may be an inherited tendency; it certainly occurs more often in certain families, but this may be partly due to chance. A woman who has already given birth to twins is ten times more likely to have another multiple pregnancy than one who has not previously had twins. In 1974, a Swedish mother, who had not had any fertility drugs, gave birth to her third lot of twin girls. Both she and her husband were twins themselves. The statistical chance of a third pair of twins is 1 in 512,000. Identical twins do not run in families.

Twins may be binovular or uniovular. *Binovular*, or *fraternal, twins* are the result of the mother's releasing two ova within a few days of each other and both being fertilized by separate spermatozoa. They both develop separately in the mother's womb and are no more alike than is usual with members of the same family. They are three times as common as *uniovular*, or *identical, twins*, who are developed from a single ovum fertilized by a single spermatozoon, but which has split early in development. This is why they are usually so remarkably alike in looks and mental characteristics. Unlike binovular twins, who may be of the same or different sex, they are always of the same sex.

The relative proportion of twins of each type varies in different races. Identical twins have much the same frequency all over the world: around 3 per 1000 maternities. Fraternal twins are rare in Mongolian races: less than 3 per 1000 maternities. In Whites they occur two or three times as often as identical twins: between 7 (Spain and Portugal) and 10 (Czechoslovakia and Greece) per 1000 maternities. They are more common in Negroes, reaching 30 per 1000 maternities in certain West African populations. (See also SIAMESE TWINS.)

'False twins' are not uncommon, when 'twin' children have been fathered by different men.

Parents of twins can obtain advice and help from the Twins and Multiple Births Association, Hon. Secretary, c/o 59 Sunnyside, Worksop, North Nottinghamshire S81 7LN.

MULTIPLE SCLEROSIS is a disease of the brain and spinal cord, which, though slow in its onset, in time may produce marked symptoms, such as paralysis and tremors, and may ultimately render people suffering from it confirmed invalids. It consists of hardened patches, from the size of a pin-head to that of a pea or larger, scattered here and there irregularly through the brain and cord, each patch being made up of a mass of the connective tissue (neuroglia), which should be present only in sufficient amount to bind the nerve-cells and fibres together. In the earliest stage, the insulating sheaths of the nerve-fibres in the hardened patches break up, are absorbed, and leave the nerve-fibres bare, the connective tissue being later formed between these.

Cause: Although this is one of the most common diseases of the central nervous system in Europe – there are around 50,000 affected individuals in Britain alone – the cause is still not known. The disease comes on in young people (onset being rare after the age of 40), apparently without previous illness. It is more common in first and second children than in those later in birth order, and in small rather than big families. There may be a hereditary factor, but this is by no means proven. If such exists it is of an obscure nature and linked more to a defect in the individual's reaction to infection than to any precise defect in the nervous system. The actual changes in the nervous system appear to be due to the action of some substance which dissolves or breaks up the fatty matter of the nerve-sheaths.

Symptoms: These depend greatly upon the part of the brain and cord affected by the sclerotic patches. Temporary paralysis of a limb, or of an eye muscle, causing double vision, and tremors upon exertion, first in the affected parts, and later in all parts of the body, are early symptoms. Stiffness of the lower limbs causing the toes to catch on small irregularities in the ground and trip the person in walking, is often an annoying symptom and one of the first to be noticed. Great activity is shown in the reflex movements obtained by striking the tendons and by stroking the soles of the feet. The latter reflex shows a characteristic sign (Babinski sign) in which the great toe bends upwards and the other toes spread apart as the sole is stroked, instead of the toes collectively bending downwards as in the normal person. Tremor of the eye movements (nystagmus) is usually found. Trembling handwriting, interference with the functions of the bladder, giddiness, and a peculiar 'staccato' or 'scanning' speech are common symptoms at a later stage. Numbness and tingling in the extremities occur commonly, particularly in the early stages of the disease. As the disease progresses, the paralyses, which were transitory at first, now become confirmed, often with great rigidity in the limbs. Many cases progress very slowly and show little or no tendency to shortening of the duration of life.

People with multiple sclerosis, and their relatives, can obtain help and guidance from the Multiple Sclerosis Society of Great Britain and Northern Ireland, 25 Effie Road, London SW6 1EE (081-736 6267). Another helpful organization is Action and Research for Multiple Sclerosis, 4A Chapel Hill, Stansted, Essex CM24 8AG (0279 815553), which provides a 24-hour telephone counselling service (071-222 3123, 021-476 4229 and 041-945 3939) for those with the disease and their families. Those with sexual or marital problems arising out of the illness can obtain information from SPOD (Association to Aid the Sexual and Personal Relationships of People with a Disability), 286 Camden Road, London N7 0BJ (071-607 8851).

Treatment is unsatisfactory, because the most that can be done is to lead a life as free from strain as possible, to check the progress of the disease. It is important to keep the nerves and muscles functioning, and therefore the patient should remain at work as long as he or she is capable of doing it, and in any case should regularly exercise the lower limbs by walking and the upper limbs by carrying out movements requiring co-ordination, such as knitting or embroidery. Corticosteriods seem to be as effective a means as any of slowing up the progress of the disease, but they can only be used under skilled medical supervision.

MUMPS, also known as EPIDEMIC PAROTITIS, is an infectious disease characterized by inflammatory swelling of the parotid and other salivary glands, often occurring as an epidemic, and affecting mostly young people. Its name comes from the old verb, 'mump', meaning to mope or assume a disconsolate appearance – an apt description of the victim of the disease at its height.

Causes: Mumps is due to infection with a virus and is highly infectious from person to person. It is predominantly a disease of childhood and early adult life, but it can occur at any age. Epidemics usually occur in the winter and spring. It is infectious for two or three days before the swelling of the glands appears. A vaccine is now available that gives a high degree of protection against the disease, the incidence of which is falling sharply.

Symptoms: There is a long incubation period of two to three weeks after infection before the glands begin to swell. The first signs are fatigue, slight feverishness, and sore throat, which may precede the swelling by a day or two. The gland first affected is generally the parotid, situated in front of and below the ear. Along with the swelling there is often some face-ache and considerable rise of temperature to 38·3 or even 40 °C (101 or 104 °F). The swelling usually spreads to the submaxillary and sublingual glands lying beneath the jaw, and to the glands on the side opposite that first affected. There is hardly ever any redness or tendency to suppuration in the swollen parts, although interference with the acts of chewing and swallowing may occasion a good deal of trouble, and the swelling is tender to touch. After continuing four or five days, the swelling abates, the temperature having generally already fallen. In 15 to 30 per cent of males, inflammation of the testicles (orchitis) develops. This usually occurs during the second week of the illness, but may not occur until two or three weeks later. It may result in partial atrophy of the testicles, but practically never in infertility. In a much smaller proportion of females with mumps, inflammation of the ovaries or breasts may occur. Inflammation of the pancreas, accompanied by tenderness in the upper part of the abdomen and digestive disturbances, sometimes occurs. Meningitis is also an occasional complication. The various complications are found much more often when the disease affects adults than when it occurs in childhood.

Treatment: The patient may require bed rest and should be kept in isolation for 14 days from the onset of the disease or 7 days from the subsidence of all swelling. Soft food, and the protection of the inflamed parts by a strip of flannel or by cotton-wool and a handkerchief are all the treatment usually required. If there is much face-ache, it is relieved by warm fomentations or aspirin.

MUNCHAUSEN'S SYNDROME: A condition in which the sufferer complains of pretended or self-induced symptoms. It differs from malingering as it brings no obvious reward for the imagined symptoms. Although the victims of the syndrome are resistant to psychiatric treatment, they should be offered the opportunity to have it as the condition often results in their attending a succession of hospitals or having unnecessary operations. They become skilled in simulating real disease. The cause is not known.

MURMUR is the uneven, rustling sound heard by auscultation over the heart and various blood-vessels in abnormal conditons. For example, murmurs heard when the stethoscope is applied over the heart are highly characteristic of valvular disease of this organ.

MUSCAE VOLITANTES ('FLYING FLIES'): Spots before the eyes due to small opacities in the vitreous humour casting shadows on the retina. In themselves vitreous floaters are harmless but anyone with 'spots before the eyes' of sudden onset should seek specialist advice.

MUSCARINE is the poisonous principle found in some toadstools. (See FUNGUS-POISONING.)

MUSCLE, popularly known as FLESH, is the tissue by which, because of its power of contraction, movements are made in the higher animals. Muscular tissue is divided, according to its function, into two main groups, voluntary muscle and involuntary muscle, of which the former is under control of the will, whilst the latter discharges its functions independently. The term striped muscle is often given to voluntary muscle, because under the microscope all the voluntary muscles show a striped appearance, whilst involuntary muscle is, in the main, unstriped or plain. There are exceptions to the latter statement, for the heart muscle, which is involuntary, is partially striped, while certain muscles of the throat, and two small muscles inside the ear, not controllable by willpower, are also striped.

Structure of muscle: VOLUNTARY MUSCLE is disposed in a regular method over the body, being mainly attached to the skeleton, and hence often called skeletal muscle. There are certain definite muscles, and these vary as to shape only slightly in different persons, although in one person particular muscles may be developed to a much greater bulk than in others. Each muscle is enclosed in a sheath of fibrous tissue, known as fascia or epimysium, and, from this, partitions of fibrous tissue, known as perimysium, run into the substance of the muscle, dividing it up into small bundles. Each of these bundles, if carefully examined, will be found to consist in turn of a collection of fibres, which form the units of the muscle. Each fibre is about 50 micrometres in thickness and ranges in length from a few millimetres to 300 millimetres. If the fibre is cut across and examined under a high-powered microscope, it is seen to be further divided into fibrils. Each fibre is enclosed in an elastic sheath of its own, which allows it to lengthen and shorten, and is known as the sarcolemma. Within the sarcolemma lie numerous nuclei belonging to the muscle fibre, which was originally developed from a simple cell. To the sarcolemma, at either end, is attached a minute bundle of connective-tissue fibres which unites the muscle fibre to its neighbours, or to one of the connective tissue partitions in the muscle, and by means of these connections the fibre produces its effect upon contracting. The sarcolemma is pierced by a nerve fibre, which breaks up upon the surface of the muscle fibre into a complicated endplate, and by this means each muscle fibre is brought under the guidance of the central nervous system, and the discharge of energy which produces muscular contraction is controlled. When the muscle fibre within the sarcolemma is examined by a high magnifying power, it is found to show alternate light and dark transverse stripes, with a fine dotted line, called Dobie's line or Krause's membrane, across the middle of each light stripe. These appearances are due to the fact that the fibre is composed of segments made up partly of fibrous connective material, partly of semifluid contractile tissue, in which visible changes take place as the fibre contracts.

Between the muscle fibres, which have, on account of their relative length and width, a pillar-like shape, run many capillary blood-vessels. They are so placed that the contractions of the muscle fibres empty them at once of blood, and thus the active muscle is ensured a specially good blood supply. None of these vessels, however, pierces the sarcolemma surrounding the fibres, so that the blood does not come into direct contact with the muscular tissue, whose nourishment is carried on by the lymph that exudes from the blood-vessels. The lymph circulation is also automatically varied, as required, by the muscular contractions. Between the muscle fibres, and enveloped in a sheath of connective tissue, lie here and there special structures known as muscle-spindles. Each of these contains thin muscle fibres, numerous nuclei, and the endings of sensory nerves. They appear to be the sensory organs of the muscles. (See TOUCH.)

INVOLUNTARY MUSCLE includes, as already stated, the heart muscle and unstriped muscle. The heart muscle stands in structure between striped and unstriped muscle. Each fibre is short, has a nucleus in its centre, communicates with its neighbours by short branches, shows a faintly striped appearance near its exterior, and is devoid of sarcolemma.

Plain or unstriped muscle is found in the following positions: the inner and middle coats of the stomach and intestines; the ureters and urinary bladder; the windpipe and bronchial tubes; the ducts of glands; the gall-bladder; the uterus and fallopian tubes; the middle coat of the blood- and lymph-vessels; the iris and ciliary muscle of the eye; the dartos muscle of the scrotum; and in association with the various glands and hairs in the skin. The fibres are very much smaller than those of striped muscle, although they vary greatly in size. Each is pointed at the ends, has one or more oval nuclei in the centre, and a delicate sheath of sarcolemma enveloping it. The fibres are grouped in bundles, much as are the striped fibres, but they adhere to one another by cement material, not by the tendon bundles found in voluntary muscle.

Development of muscle: All the muscles of the developing individual arise from the central layer (mesoderm) of the embryo, each fibre taking origin from a single cell. Later on in life, muscles have the power both of increasing in size, as the result of use, for example, in athletes, and also of healing, after parts of them have been destroyed by injury. This takes place partly by the growth and splitting of the original fibres to form new fibres, and partly from reserve cells, known as sarcoplasts, which lie in every muscle between the muscle fibres. An example of the great extent to which unstriped muscle can develop, to meet the demands made upon its power, is given by the womb, whose muscular wall develops so much during pregnancy that the organ increases from the weight of 30 to 40 g (1 to 1½ oz.) to a weight of around 1 kg (2 lb.), decreasing again to its former small size in the course of a month after child-birth.

Physiology of contraction: A muscle is an elaborate chemico-physical system for producing heat and mechanical work. The total energy liberated by a contracting muscle can be exactly measured. From 25 to 30 per cent of the total energy expended is used in mechanical work. The heat of contracting muscle makes an important contribution to the maintenance of the heat of the body. (See also MYOGLOBIN.)

The energy of muscular contraction is derived from a complicated series of chemical reactions. Complex substances are broken down and built up again, supplying each other with energy for this purpose. The first reaction is the breakdown of adenyl-pyrophosphate into phosphoric acid and adenylic acid (derived from nucleic acid); this supplies the immediate energy for contraction. Next phosphocreatine breaks down into creatine and phosphoric acid, giving energy for the resynthesis of adenyl-pyrophosphate. Creatine is a normal nitrogenous constituent of muscle. Then glycogen through the intermediary stage of sugar bound to phosphate breaks down into lactic acid to supply energy for the resynthesis of phosphocreatine. Finally part of the lactic acid is oxidized to supply energy for building up the rest of the lactic acid into glycogen again. If there is not enough oxygen, lactic acid accumulates and fatigue results.

There are some points to be noticed in this version of muscular activity. First, muscle contraction and relaxation take place in the absence of oxygen – the anaerobic phase. Secondly, oxygen comes into the picture in the phase of recovery, and by oxidizing some of the lactic acid winds up the contractile mechanism once more. Thirdly, the energy of contraction does not come directly from the breakdown of glycogen.

All of the chemical changes are mediated by the action of several enzymes.

Involuntary muscle has several peculiarities of contraction. In the heart *rhythmicality* is an important feature, one beat appearing to be, in a sense, the cause of the next beat. *Tonus* is a character of all muscle, but particularly of unstriped muscle in some localities, as in the walls of arteries. Muscles are not held either slack or taut, but in a slightly stretched condition, so that when occasion arises they are ready for instant action, while the arteries owe their elasticity and strength mainly to this fact. The involuntary muscle, forming the middle coat of the bowels, gland-ducts, and other tubes, contracts in the so-called *vermicular movement*, or peristalsis, which means that a ring of contraction passes slowly along the tube, at a rate of about 25 mm (1 inch) per second, the muscle relaxing as the ring of contraction passes on.

Fatigue of muscle comes on when a muscle is made to act for some time. It is due, not to wearing out of the muscle's power, but to the accumulation of waste products, especially sarcolactic acid, produced by the muscle's activity. These substances affect the end plates of the nerve controlling the muscle, and so prevent destructive over-action of the muscle. As they are rapidly swept away by the blood, the muscle, after a rest, particularly if the rest is accompanied by massage or by gentle contractions to quicken the circulation, recovers rapidly from the fatigue. After great muscular activity over the whole body, a more lasting fatigue is produced by the accumulation of these products, and by their action upon the central nervous system, this being recovered from after a prolonged rest, during which the waste substances are excreted by the lungs, kidneys, and other excretory organs.

Another factor that comes into play is the accumulation of fluid in the muscles on unaccustomed exercise. Active tissues swell because of the increased blood flow through them. This results in an increased amount outside the blood-vessels but within the tissues themselves. Normally the body can cope with this state of affairs but on occasion, as when an undertrained individual undertakes excessive exercise, the accumulation of fluid in the muscles may be so great that the body cannot absorb it quickly enough, and the muscles swell and become tense and painful. This is the cause of the muscle stiffness which follows unaccustomed exercise. In those areas of the body where the space available for muscles is restricted, this increase of fluid may cause trouble and produce what is known as the compression syndrome. The classical example of this is the *anterior tibial syndrome*, in which the muscles on the front and outer aspect of the shin, lying within a tight fascial envelope, as they do, become tense and painful, and there may be actual damage to the muscles as a result of interference with their blood supply. (See MUSCLES, DISEASES OF.)

Rigor mortis is a condition which comes on in the muscles after death, and to which the general stiffening of the dead body is due. It consists in a state of permanent, wasteful contraction, beginning in the muscles of the neck and lower jaw at a period which varies from ten minutes to seven hours after death, and spreading gradually over the whole body. It comes on quickest after death from exhaustion, or from some weakening disease; and, occasionally, after violent injuries causing death, it comes on instantaneously, so that the posture of the body is fixed in the attitude in which death occurs. The rigidity lasts usually from sixteen to twenty-four hours, but its duration is extremely variable, being longer, as a rule, when its onset has been slow. (See DEATH, SIGNS OF.)

Muscular system, popularly known as 'the flesh', comprises all the voluntary muscles, and amounts in an average man of 70 kg (154 lb.) to about 35 kg (77 lb.), or half of the whole body weight. The total number of the voluntary muscles, each of which is named, amounts to around 620, including the muscles of both sides. Each muscle constitutes a separate organ, controlled by a special nerve or nerves, which connect it with the spinal cord and brain, where, however, actions and combined movements are represented rather than individual muscles. (See BRAIN.) The fleshy part of the muscle is known as its belly, and there is usually at either end a tendon, by which the muscle is inserted into bone or other structure, upon which it acts. One end is more fixed than the other, as a rule, the rigid end being known as the origin of the muscle, the more mobile end as its insertion.

UPPER LIMB: *Between the trunk and limb* run the following muscles: the trapezius, latissimus dorsi, large and small rhomboids, and levator of the angle of the scapula, behind; and the large and small pectoral, the subclavius, and serratus anterior muscles in front. *In the shoulder region* lie the deltoid, supraspinatus, infraspinatus, large and small teres, and the subscapular muscles. *In the upper arm* the coracobrachialis, biceps, and brachialis occupy the front, while the triceps fills up the back of the arm. *In the forearm* the muscles in front that bend the wrist and fingers, or turn the hand palm downwards, are the pronator teres, the radial flexor of the wrist, the long palmar, the ulnar flexor of the wrist, the superficial and deep flexors of the fingers, the long flexor of the thumb, and the pronator quadratus; while the muscles on the back of the forearm that extend the fingers and bend the wrist backwards, or turn the hand palm upwards, are the supinator, longer and shorter radial extensors of the wrist, extensor of the fingers, extensor of the little finger, ulnar extensor of the wrist, the extensors of the metacarpal bone, of the first joint, and of the second joint of the thumb, and the extensor of the forefinger. *In the palm of the hand* there are four lumbrical muscles, the short palmar muscle, three muscles each for the thumb and little finger, which respectively abduct, oppose, and flex these digits, an adductor of the thumb and, in the spaces between the metacarpal bones, seven interosseous muscles.

LOWER LIMB: *Muscles of the hip* are the iliacus in front, and, behind, the three gluteus muscles forming the prominence of the buttock, with the pyriform, external and internal obturator, two gemelli, and quadratus femoris muscles under cover of the largest gluteal muscle, while to the outer side lies the tensor of the sheath of the thigh. *On the back of the thigh* lie the biceps, semitendinosus, and semimembranosus muscles, whose tendons, standing out prominently behind the knee, are known collectively as the ham-strings. *In front of the thigh* are placed the sartorius, which is the longest, and the quadriceps extensor of the leg, which is the largest muscle of the body. *On the inner side of the thigh* lie the gracilis and pectineus muscles, with the long, the short, and the large adductors. *On the front of the leg* are placed the tibialis anterior, the long extensor of the great toe, the long extensor of the toes, and the peroneus tertius muscles. *On the outer side of the leg* are two muscles, the long and short peroneal muscles, whose tendons pass down behind the outer ankle to the foot. *On the back of the leg* are two groups of muscles. The superficial group of three muscles, consisting of the gastrocnemius, a double-bellied muscle, the soleus, which is flat and projects slightly beneath the gastrocnemius, and the small plantaris muscle, forms the calf of the leg, and ends in the tendo calcaneus, or Achilles tendon, behind the heel. The deep group lies close upon the bones, and consists of the popliteus, long flexor of the toes, long flexor of the great toe, and tibialis posterior muscles, the tendons of the last three passing down behind the inner ankle. *In the foot* there is one muscle, the short extensor of the toes, upon the 'dorsum' or upper surface; while in the sole of

1 frontalis
2 orbicularis oculi
3 masseter
4 orbicularis oris
5 depressor anguli oris
6 sternocleidomastoid
7 pectoralis major
8 latissimus dorsi
9 serratus anterior
10 rectus abdominis
11 external intercostals
12 sheath of rectus abdominis
13 external oblique
14 internal oblique

15 extensor hallucis longus
16 peroneus brevis
17 soleus
18 extensor digitorium longus
19 peroneus longus
20 gastrocnemius
21 anterior tibial
22 vastus medialis
23 vastus lateralis
24 rectus femoris
25 gracilis
26 sartorius
27 adductor longus
28 pectineus

29 tensor fasciae latae
30 iliopsoas
31 iliacus
32 abductor pollicis longus
33 extensor carpi radialis brevis
34 flexor carpi radialis
35 extensor carpi radialis longus
36 brachialis
37 biceps brachii
38 coracobrachialis
39 triceps brachii
40 deltoid
41 sternothyroid
42 sternohyroid

Muscles on the front of the body.

1 temporal
2 sternocleidomastoid
3 splenius capitis
4 trapezius
5 infraspinatus
6 teres minor
7 teres major
8 rhomboid major
9 latissimus dorsi
10 thoracolumbar fascia
11 external abdominal oblique
12 gluteus medius
13 gluteus maximus
14 gracilis
15 flexor digitorum longus
16 peroneus brevis
17 calcaneus tendon (achilles)
18 peroneus longus
19 soleus
20 gastrocnemius
21 plantaris
22 semitendinosus
23 biceps femoris (short head), (long head)

24 semimembranosus
25 adductor magnus
26 vastus externus
27 abductor pollicis
28 flexor carpi ulnaris
29 extensor carpi ulnaris
30 extensor digitorum
31 extensor carpi radialis longus
32 anconeus
33 supinalon brevis
34 brachioradialis
35 triceps brachii lateralis
36 triceps brachii longus
37 deltoid

Muscles on the back of the body.

the foot are four layers of small muscles, comprising the short flexor of the toes, and abductors of the great and little toes; the accessory flexor of the toes, and four lumbrical muscles; the short flexor of the great toe, oblique and transverse adductors of the great toe, and short flexor of the little toe; and in the fourth layer seven interosseous muscles, as in the hand.

FACE AND HEAD: Attached to the auricle of the ear are three weak muscles which raise, draw back, and flatten the auricle. The eyelids, nose, and lips are provided with numerous flattened muscles, which dilate and draw together these openings, and which form the means of varying facial expression.

The movements of the eye-ball are effected by six small muscles. (See EYE.) The movements of the lower jaw in chewing are controlled by four muscles on each side: the masseter muscle, which can be felt on the hinder part of the cheek as the jaws are closed; the temporal muscle, felt in the region of the temple; and the outer and inner pterygoid muscles, attached to the deep surface of the jaw-bone. Within the mouth the tongue consists of certain intrinsic muscle bundles, together with four muscles on each side, which connect it with the lower jaw, hyoid bone, and base of the skull. The floor of the mouth is formed by four muscles, which pass from the hyoid bone in front of the neck up to the lower jaw and base of the skull. The throat or pharynx, which is open in front to the nose, the mouth, and the larynx, one beneath the other, is closed behind by three broad, flat muscles, the superior, middle, and inferior constrictors of the pharynx, and is swung from the base of the skull by the stylopharyngeus muscle on either side. The soft palate, which separates the hinder part of the cavities of nose and mouth from one another, consists of five muscles on each side covered by mucous membrane. The larynx is controlled by eleven small muscles, which open or close its opening, and render the vocal cords more or less tense in the production of the voice.

FRONT OF NECK: The most prominent feature of the neck is the thick sternocleidomastoid muscle, which on each side runs from behind the ear downwards and forwards to the breast-bone and collar-bone. Partly under cover of these and protecting the front of the larynx are four small muscles on each side: the sternohyoid, sternothyroid, thyrohyoid, and omohyoid muscles. Deep in the neck, behind, and to either side of the windpipe, gullet, and large blood-vessels, lie the anterior, middle, and posterior scalene muscles, which pass from the spinal column to the upper two ribs. Lying close upon the spine are three rectus muscles on each side, which bend the head upon the spine, and the long muscle of the neck, which bends the spine in this region.

BACK OF THE NECK AND TRUNK: The muscles in this region form a very complicated system, most arising from the spine or transverse processes of several vertebrae or from a number of ribs, and running upwards to be attached to another series of vertebrae or ribs some distance above, whilst the upper muscles of the set are attached to the hinder portion of the skull. These muscles form a couple of strong columns running the whole length of the back from the loins to the head, with a groove between in which the line of vertebral spines can be felt. The upper and lower serrated muscles of the back are muscles of respiration passing from ribs to spine, and, together with the splenius muscle in the neck, form a superficial layer. Beneath them the erector spinae, the great muscle which supports the back, runs the whole distance from the sacrum to the skull, obtaining at numerous points attachments to the spines and transverse processes of the vertebrae and to the neighbouring portions of the ribs. This muscle, along with those about to be mentioned, is of great power, having, even in moderately strong persons, a lifting power of 90 to 180 kg (200 to 400 lb.). Covered by the erector is the transversospinalis group of muscles, in which all the muscles ascend with an inward inclination; a series of short muscles connecting succeeding vertebrae with one another; and four small muscles passing from the uppermost two vertebrae to the skull. These last-named muscles incline and rotate the trunk and head from side to side.

CHEST: The diaphragm is the chief muscle of this part of the body. (See DIAPHRAGM.) Next in importance come the outer and inner intercostal muscles, which form a double layer of oblique fibres filling up the gaps between the ribs, the fibres of the two muscles running in different directions. There are also levators of the ribs, which pass each from a vertebra to the rib beneath it, and subcostal muscles which are of feeble development. All these muscles share in the act of inspiration.

ABDOMEN: The sides and front of the abdomen, unprotected by any bone beneath the level of the ribs, are enclosed by thick muscular layers strengthened by sheets of fibrous tissue. On the sides of the abdomen are three muscles: the external oblique, consisting of fibres which run downwards and forwards from the lower eight ribs; the internal oblique, under cover of the first, consisting of fibres which run upwards and forwards from the haunch-bone, and fibrous layers in its neighbourhood; and thirdly, the transversalis muscle, the fibres of which run horizontally forward from the lower six ribs, the lumbar vertebrae, and the haunch-bone. The fibres of all three muscles end along a curved line, the semilunar line, which is plainly visible upon the surface of the abdomen, running with a curve from its upper to its lower end, and distant, at the level of the navel, some 10 or 12·5 cm (4 or 5 inches) from the middle line. From the curved line a sheet of dense fibrous tissue runs inwards, those of the two sides meeting down the middle line of the body. Embedded in this fibrous sheet is a strong muscle upon each side, the rectus abdominis, which is 7·5 or 10 cm (3 or 4 inches) broad, almost 25 mm (1 inch) thick in muscular persons, and runs vertically from the front of the pelvis up to the lower part of the chest. It is a muscle of great strength, and is divided into four or five sections, by tendinous intervals, which run across the muscle, and which, in well-developed persons, form distinct transverse depressions on the front of the abdomen. The quadratus lumborum is still another muscle situated, behind, in the gap between the last rib and the haunch-bone. Other small muscles close the lower opening of the pelvis, and are associated with the functions of the bowel and genital organs.

MUSCLE CRAMP is a sudden painful involuntary maximal contraction of a muscle or muscle group. It may last up to 10 minutes and occurs in individuals with no neurological or muscle disease. Cramps usually occur in bed at night when the individual is at rest. Night cramps are especially common in the elderly, during pregnancy and in cases of diabetes or peripheral vascular disease. They can be caused by sodium loss from excessive sweating, vomiting or diarrhoea. It may also be due to hypokalaemia as a result of treatment with diuretics. Drugs such as the beta-adrenergic stimulants may be responsible. Sometimes an attack can be thwarted by actively contracting the opposing muscle. The most common cramp is in the calf or foot, so the foot should be dorsiflexed at the ankle and the leg straightened. When the cramp is in the calf muscles, getting out of bed and standing up will stretch the calf muscles and ease the attack. When attacks of cramp occur frequently at night, treatment with quinine bisulphate is beneficial.

MUSCLE RELAXANTS are drugs which cause relaxation of muscles. The most effective of them, such as tubocurarine (q.v.), gallamine and pancuronium, act by antagonizing the action of acetylcholine (q.v.). Acetylcholine is the natural transmitter of nerve impulses to muscle. When an impulse passes down a motor nerve to voluntary muscle it causes release of acetylcholine at the nerve endings, which in turn causes contraction of the muscle. This it does by action on specific receptors in the muscle. The group of drugs which includes tubocurarine combine with these receptors and so prevent acetylcholine from performing its natural functions. This results in relaxation, or paralysis of the muscle. Other drugs, such as suxamethonium, act principally by reducing the excitability of muscle. Others again, such as some of the tranquillizers (q.v.), act through the brain; these, however, cannot be used as muscle relaxants because of their overpowering sedative action. The main use of muscle relaxants is in anaesthesia to produce adequate relaxation of muscles. They are also used to control convulsions, as in status epilepticus, tetanus, electric convulsion therapy, and poisoning with convulsant drugs such as strychnine.

MUSCLES, DISEASES OF: The muscles are singularly free from liability to diseases which commonly affect other tissues, this being the result, probably, of their activity, good blood supply, and the changes constantly taking place in them. Wasting of muscles sometimes occurs as a symptom of disease in other organs: for example, damage to the nervous system, as in poliomyelitis or in the disease known as progressive muscular atrophy. (See PARALYSIS.)

INFLAMMATION (MYOSITIS) of various types may occur. As the result of injury, an abscess may develop (see ABSCESS), although wounds affecting muscle generally heal well. Tuberculous inflammation in muscles is almost unknown. A growth due to syphilis, known as a gumma, sometimes forms a hard, almost painless swelling in a muscle. Rheumatism is a type of chronic inflammation (see RHEUMATISM) to which muscles are very liable. The most common form of myositis is the result of immunological damage as a result of auto-immune disease. Because it affects many muscles it is called polymyositis.

MYOSITIS OSSIFICANS, or deposition of bone in muscles, may be congenital or acquired. The congenital form, which is rare, first manifests itself as painful swellings in the muscles. These gradually harden and extend until the child is encased in a rigid sheet – the 'stone man' who used to be one of the unfortunate 'freaks' in circus side-shows. There are usually associated congenital abnormalities of the toes and fingers. The condition is fatal sooner or later. There is no effective treatment, though in some cases diphosphonates seem to delay the onset of calcification.

The acquired form arises as a sequel of a direct blow on muscle, most commonly on the front of the thigh. The condition should be suspected whenever there is severe pain and swelling following a direct blow over muscle. The diagnosis is confirmed by hardening of the swelling. Even when the condition is only suspected it is essential to avoid immobilization of the patient, and to avoid massage. Treatment consists of short-wave diathermy (see DIATHERMY) with gentle active movements. Recovery is usually complete, though slow surgical removal of residual calcified areas may be necessary.

RUPTURE of a muscle may occur, without any external wound, as the result of a spasmodic effort. It may tear the muscle right across, as sometimes happens to the feeble plantaris muscle in running and leaping, or part of the muscle may be driven through its fibrous envelope, forming a hernia of the muscle. The severe pain experienced in many cases of lumbago is due to tearing of one of the muscles in the back. These conditions give rise to considerable pain, but are relieved by rest and massage. Partial muscle tears, such as occur in sport, require more energetic treatment. In the early stages this consists of the application of cold (see COLD, USES OF), firm compression, elevation of the affected limb and rest. After forty-eight hours gradual mobilization is started, with active exercises and short-wave diathermy (see DIA-THERMY) or ultrasound (q.v.).

COMPRESSION SYNDROME is the tense painful state of muscles induced by excessive accumulation of interstitial fluid (q.v.) in them, following unusual exercise. It is particularly likely to occur in those parts of the body where the space available for muscles is restricted, as on the front and outer aspect of the shin, where the muscles lie within a tight fascial membrane. Here the syndrome is known as the *anterior tibial syndrome*. Prevention consists of always keeping fit and in training for the amount of exercise to be undertaken. Equally important is what is known in sporting circles as 'warming down': i.e., at the end of training or a game, exercise should be gradually tailed off. Treatment consists of elevation of the affected limb, compression of it by compression bandages, with ample exercise of the limb within the bandage, and massage. In more severe cases diuretics (q.v.) may be given. Occasionally surgical decompression may be necessary.

MYASTHENIA (see MYASTHENIA GRAVIS) is muscle weakness due to a defect of neuro-muscular conduction.

PAIN, quite apart from any inflammation or injury, may be experienced on exertion. This type of pain, known as myalgia, occurs especially in weakly persons, and is then relieved by rest and physiotherapy. It is also one of the common forms of rheumatism. In young children, pains of an aching character are often experienced in the muscles, especially of the legs and back, and are known as growing pains (q.v.). These come on especially after exertion and are relieved by resting.

PARASITES sometimes lodge in the muscles, the most common being *Trichinella spiralis*, producing the disease known as trichinosis (q.v.).

TUMOURS are occasionally met with, the most common being fibroid, fatty, and sarcomatous growths.

MYOPATHY is a term applied to an acquired or developmental defect in certain muscles. (See MYOPATHY.)

MUSCULAR DYSTROPHY (see MYOPATHY).

MUSHROOM POISONING (see FUNGUS-POISONING).

MUSHROOM-WORKER'S LUNG is a form of lung disease that occurs in mushroom workers as a result of their being hypersensitive to mushrooms. (See ALVEOLITIS.)

MUSTINE is the British Pharmacopoeia name for the bis form of nitrogen mustard. The nitrogen mustards have an action comparable to that of ionizing radiation and inhibit cell division. Mustine is used in the treatment of chronic leukaemia and Hodgkin's disease. (See CYTOTOXIC.)

MUTAGEN: A chemical or physical agent that has the property of increasing the rate of mutation (q.v.) among cells. A mutagen does not usually increase the range of mutations. Chemicals, ionizing radiation, and viruses may act as mutagens.

MUTATION: A change occurring in the genetic material (DNA) in the chromosomes of a cell. It is caused by a fault in the replication of a cell's genetic material when it divides to form two daughter cells. Mutations may occur in somatic cells which may result in a local growth of the new type of cells. These may be destroyed by the body's defence mechanism or they may develop into a tumour. If mutation occurs in a germ cell or gamete – the organism's sex cells – the outcome may be a changed inherited characteristic in succeeding generations. Mutations occur rarely but a small steady number are caused by background radiation in the environment. They are also caused by mutagens (q.v.).

MUTISM (see VOICE AND SPEECH).

MYALGIA means pain in a muscle. (See BORNHOLM DISEASE; LUMBAGO; RHEUMATISM.)

MYALGIC ENCEPHALOMYELITIS (ME): A syndrome in which tiredness, muscle pain, lack of concentration, panic attacks, memory loss and depression occur. Its existence and causes have been the subject of controversy reflected in the variety of names given to the syndrome: post-viral fatigue syndrome, Royal Free disease, epidemic neuromyasthenia and Icelandic disease. ME often follows virus infections of the upper respiratory tract or gut. It may occur in epidemics or as individual cases. Physical examination shows no evidence of disease and there is no diagnostic test. The sufferer usually recovers in time, though sometimes recovery may take many months. There is no specific curative treatment, but symptomatic treatment such as resting in the early stages, may help. Sufferers may find it helpful to consult the Myalgic Encephalomyelitis Association, PO Box 8, Stanford-le-Hope, Essex SS17 8EX.

MYASTHENIA GRAVIS is a serious disorder in which the chief symptoms are muscular weakness and a special tendency for fatigue to come on rapidly when efforts are made. The prevalence is around 1 in 30,000. Two-thirds of the patients are women, in whom it develops in early adult life. In men it tends to develop later in life.

It is a classical example of an auto-immune disease (see AUTO-IMMUNITY). The body develops antibodies which interfere with the working of the nerve endings in muscle that are acted on by acetylcholine (q.v.). It is acetylcholine that transmits the nerve impulses to muscles. If this transmission cannot be effected, as in myasthenia gravis, then the muscles are unable to contract. Not only the voluntary muscles, but those connected with the acts of swallowing, breathing, and the like, become progressively weaker, though there is no very marked wasting. Rest and avoidance of undue exertion, so as carefully to husband the strength, are necessary, and regular doses of neostigmine bromide, or pyridostigmine at intervals enable the muscles to be used and in some cases have a curative effect. These drugs act by inhibiting the action of cholinesterase. This is an enzyme (q.v.) produced in the body which destroys any excess of acetylcholine. In this way they increase the amount of available acetylcholine which compensates for the deleterious effect of antibodies on the nerve endings.

The dose of anticholinesterase that gives the maximum therapeutic response must be established. This may not restore muscle strength to normal and patients often have to live with some degree of disability. If the dose of drugs is increased above the maximum response level, in the forlorn hope of improving physical activity, the opposite effect will be produced, with progressive muscle weakness, possibly ending in what is called a cholinergic crisis. Anticholinergic drugs have no affect on the underlying disease, they merely increase the concentration of acetylcholine at receptor level.

The thymus gland plays the major part in the cause of myasthenia gravis, possibly by being the source of the original acetylcholine receptors to which the antibodies are being formed. At all events, thymectomy, or removal of the thymus, is increasingly important in the management of patients with myathenia gravis. The incidence of remission following thymectomy increases with the number of years after the operation. Complete remission or substantial improvement can be expected in 80 per cent of patients.

The other important aspect in the management of patients with myasthenia gravis is immunosuppression. Drugs are now available that suppress antibody production and so reduce the concentration of antibodies to the acetylcholine receptor. The problem is that they not only suppress abnormal antibody production, but also suppress normal antibody production. The main groups of immunosuppressive drugs used in myasthenia gravis are the corticosteroids and azathioprine. Improvement following steroids may take several weeks to become manifest and an initial deterioration is often found during the first week or ten days of treatment. Azathioprine is also effective in producing clinical improvement and reducing the antibodies to acetylcholine receptors. These affects occur more slowly than with steroids and the mean time for an azathioprine remission is nine months.

The Myasthenia Gravis Association has been established to relieve and comfort those who suffer from myasthenia gravis, to bring myasthenics together into a meaningful association where they may be offered help and understanding, and to provide the opportunity where myasthenics also help each other to overcome many of their common problems and disabilities. The association also encourages families and friends to accompany myasthenics in order that they too may learn more about the symptoms and effects of the disorder, and so offer the real help and understanding that is required. The Myasthenia Gravis Association was created and is supported by myasthenics, their families and friends. Its address is Keynes House, 77 Nottingham Road, Derby DE1 3QS (0332- 290219).

MYCOBACTERIUM: A Gram-positive rod-like genus of aerobic bacteria, some species of which are harmful to man and animals. For example, *M. tuberculosis* (Koch's bacillus) and *M. leprae* cause, respectively, tuberculosis and leprosy.

MYCOPLASMA is a genus of micro-organisms which differ from bacteria in that they lack a rigid cell wall. They are responsible for widespread epidemics in cattle and poultry. For a long time the only member of the genus known to cause disease in man was *Mycoplasma pneumoniae* which is responsible for the form of pneumonia known as primary atypical pneumonia (see PNEUMONIA). Another, *Mycoplasma genitalium*, has now been isolated which is responsible for certain cases of non-gonococcal urethritis. (See NON-SPECIFIC GENITAL INFECTION.)

MYCOSIS is the general term applied to diseases due to the growth of fungi in the body. Among some of the simplest and commonest mycoses are ringworm, favus, and thrush. The Madura foot of India, actinomycosis, and occasional cases of pneumonia and suppurative ear disease are also due to the growth of moulds in the bodily tissues. Other forms of mycosis include aspergillosis (q.v.), candidiasis (q.v.), cryptococcosis (q.v.) and histoplasmosis (q.v.).

MYCOSIS FUNGOIDES is a rare neoplastic condition of the reticulo-endothelial system, characterized in its later stages by multiple tumours of the skin. The course is prolonged and almost invariably ends fatally.

MYDRIASIS: Condition of dilatation of the pupil.

MYELIN: A substance made up of protein and phospholipid that forms the sheath surrounding the axons (q.v.) of some neurons (q.v.). These are described as myelinated or medullated nerve fibres (see NERVES), and electric impulses pass along them faster than along non-myelinated nerves. Myelin is produced by Schwann cells which occur at intervals along the nerve fibre.

MYELITIS is inflammation of the spinal cord.

MYELOCYTE is the name given to one of the cells of bone-marrow from which the granular white corpuscles of the blood are produced. They are found in the blood in certain forms of leukaemia.

MYELOGRAPHY is the injection of a radio-opaque substance into the central canal of the spinal cord in order to assist in the diagnosis of diseases of the spinal cord or spine.

MYELOID: An adjective that relates to the granulocyte precursor cell in the bone marrow. For example, myeloid leukaemia, which arises from abnormal growth in the blood-forming tissue of the marrow.

MYELOMA is a tumour made up of bone-marrow cells and generally occurring in the marrow of more than one bone at the same time.

MYELOMATOSIS is a malignant process involving the bone marrow. It runs an invariably fatal course.

MYOCARDIAL INFARCTION (see CORONARY THROMBOSIS).

MYOCARDITIS means inflammation of the muscular wall of the heart.

MYOCARDIUM is the muscular substance of the heart.

MYOCLONUS is a brief, twitching muscular contraction which may involve only a single muscle or many muscles. It may be too slight to cause movement of the affected limb, or so violent as to throw the victim to the floor. The cause is not known, but in some cases may be a form of epilepsy. A single myoclonic jerk in the upper limbs occasionally occurs in petit mal. (See EPILEPSY.) The myoclonic jerks which many people experience in falling asleep are a perfectly normal phenomenon.

MYOGLOBIN is the protein which gives muscle (q.v.) its red colour. It has the property of combining loosely and reversibly with oxygen. This means that it is the vehicle whereby muscle extracts oxygen from the haemoglobin in the blood circulating through it, and then releases the oxygen for use by the muscle.

MYOGLOBINURIA: The occurrence of myoglobin in the urine. This is the oxygen-binding pigment in muscle and mild myoglobinuria may occur during exercise. Severe myoglobinuria will result from severe injuries, particularly crushing injuries, to muscles.

MYOMA is the term applied to a tumour, almost invariably of a simple nature, which consists mainly of muscle fibres. These muscle tumours often occur in the uterus.

MYOMECTOMY: Removal by surgery of FIBROIDS from the muscular wall of the uterus (q.v.).

MYOMETRIUM is the muscular coat of the uterus (q.v.).

MYOPATHY, also known as MUSCULAR DYSTROPHY or IDIOPATHIC MUSCULAR ATROPHY, is a condition in which wasting takes place in certain muscles, with or without previous increase in bulk of these muscles, and apparently without any affection of the nervous system. The cause of the condition is still obscure, although the disease appears to run in families, being transmitted, like some other hereditary diseases, by the mother. Generally the disease appears in early childhood. The changes which are found after death show that a simple wasting away of the muscle fibres takes place, and that these are in some cases to a great extent replaced by fatty and fibrous tissue.
Symptoms: There are three chief types of myopathy. The commonest, known as pseudo-hypertrophic muscular dystrophy, affects particularly the upper part of the lower limbs of children. The muscles of the buttocks, thighs and calves seem excessively well developed, but nevertheless the child is clumsy, weak on his legs, and has difficulty in picking himself up when he falls. In another form of the disease, which begins a little later, as a rule about the age of 14, the muscles of the upper arm are first affected, and those of the spine and lower limbs become weak later on. In a third type, which begins about this age, the muscles of the face, along with certain of the shoulder and upper arm muscles, show the first signs of wasting. All the forms have this in common: that the affected muscles grow weaker till their power to contract is quite lost. In the first form, the patients seldom reach the age of 20, falling victims to some disease which, to ordinary people, would not be serious. In the other forms the wasting, after progressing to a certain extent, often remains stationary for the rest of life. Myopathy may also be acquired when it is the result of disease such as thyrotoxicosis, osteomalacia or Cushing's disease, and the myopathy resolves when the primary disease is treated.
Treatment: The general health must be well maintained. Massage, electricity and exercise short of fatigue are of the utmost importance, and above all, care must be taken that these invalids are not exposed unduly, as they succumb easily to chest affections.

The education and management of these

unfortunate children raise many difficulties. Much help in dealing with these problems can be obtained from the Muscular Dystrophy Group of Great Britain, 35 Macaulay Road, London, SW4 0QP (071-720 8055, fax: 071-498 0670).

MYOPIA (see REFRACTION).

MYOSITIS means inflammation of a muscle. (See MUSCLES, DISEASES OF.)

MYOSITIS OSSIFICANS (see MUSCLE).

MYOTONIA is a condition in which the muscles, though possessed of normal power, contract only very slowly. The stiffness disappears as the muscles are used.

MYRINGOTOMY is the operation of cutting the drum of the ear in cases of acute inflammation of the middle ear.

MYRRH is a gum-resin obtained from *Commiphora molmol*, an Arabian myrtle tree. It stimulates the function of mucous membranes with which it is brought in contact or by which it is excreted. Tincture of myrrh is used for a gargle in sore throat, as a tooth-wash when the gums are inflamed, and as an ingredient of cough mixtures.

MYXOEDEMA is a disease due to underactivity of the thyroid gland. The thyroid gland secretes two hormones – thyroxine and triodothyronine – and these hormones are responsible for the metabolic activity of the body. Hypothyroidism may result from developmental abnormalities of the gland or a deficiency of the enzymes necessary for the synthesis of the hormones. It may be a feature of endemic goitre and cretinism, but the most common cause of hypothyroidism is the auto-immune destruction of the thyroid known as chronic thyroiditis. It may also occur as a result of radio-iodine treatment of thyroid overactivity and is occasionally secondary to pituitary disease in which inadequate TSH production occurs. It is a common disorder, occurring in fourteen per one thousand females and one per one thousand males. Most patients present between the age of thirty and sixty years. The term myxoedema was introduced in 1878 to describe the swelling of the skin and sub-cutaneous tissues that characterized severe forms of hypothyroidism.

Symptoms: As thyroid hormones are responsible for the metabolic rate of the body hypothyroidism usually presents with a general slowing-up. This affects both physical and mental activities. The intellectual functions become slow, the speech deliberate and the formation of ideas and the answers to questions take longer than in healthy people. Physical energy is reduced and patients frequently complain of lethargy and generalized muscle aches and pains. Patients become intolerant of the cold and the skin becomes dry and swollen. The larynx also becomes swollen and gives rise to a hoarseness of the voice. Most patients gain weight and develop constipation. The skin becomes dry and yellow due to the presence of increased carotine. Hair becomes thinned and brittle and even baldness may develop. Swelling of the soft tissues may give rise to a carpal tunnel syndrome and middle-ear deafness. The diagnosis is confirmed by measuring the levels of thyroid hormones in the blood which are low and of the pituitary TSH which is raised in primary hypothyroidism.

Treatment consists of the administration of thyroxine. Although triodothyronine is the metabolically active hormone, thyroxine is converted to triodothyronine by the tissues of the body. Treatment should be started cautiously with a small dose of not more than 0·05 mg of thyroxine and this can be slowly increased to 0·2 mg daily, the equivalent of the maximum output of the thyroid gland. If too large a dose is given initially palpitations and tachycardia are likely to result and in the elderly heart failure may be precipitated.

MYXOMA is a tumour consisting of very imperfect connective tissue, and containing a peculiar mucus-like juice.

MYXOVIRUSES include the influenza viruses A, B and C; the para-influenza viruses, types 1 to 3; and respiratory syncytial virus which is an important cause of respiratory disease in the early years of life.

N

NADOLOL (see ADRENERGIC RECEPTORS).

NAEVUS is the term applied to a mass of dilated blood-vessels. They most commonly occur as birthmarks. These structures may take the form of the large port-wine stain often seen on the face, for which little can be done, or they may occur as swellings of a more restricted nature, usually of a red or bluish colour. Many naevi tend to decrease in size as the child advances in years; if not, the blemish can often be removed by excision of the piece of skin that is involved, or by electrolysis. There is a form known as spider naevi which occur in cirrhosis of the liver. (See LIVER DISEASES.)

NAFCILLIN (see ANTIBIOTIC).

NAIL-BITING is a common practice in schoolchildren, most of whom gradually give it up as they approach adolescence. Too much significance should therefore not be attached to it. In itself it does no harm, and punishment or restraining devices do nothing but harm. It is a manifestation of tension or insecurity, the cause of which should be removed.

NAILS (see SKIN).

NAILS, DISEASES OF: The nails are subject to relatively few diseases. On the other hand, any interference with the natural appearance of the finger-nails is very unsightly, whilst the sensitive matrix of both finger- and toe-nails is extremely tender when diseased.

INFLAMMATION of the nails and of the bed in which they rest occurs in various skin diseases: e.g. psoriasis, eczema, fungus infections (see RINGWORM). The nails then become rough, thickened, irregular, discoloured, and split readily into layers. Most acute febrile diseases are accompanied by irregularities in growth of the nails, producing a transverse furrow in the nail, as it grows onwards, and these furrows on the nails serve to date a severe illness fairly accurately, the furrow gradually approaching the free margin of the nail and disappearing in about six months' time.

Brittle nails tend to be troublesome in the elderly. To reduce this brittleness, nails should be kept trimmed and as short as possible. A hand cream, consisting of equal parts of salicylic acid ointment and glycerin of starch, should be applied all over the finger tips and nails on going to bed every night. In some instances the brittleness may be due to, or associated with, poor local circulation to the finger. This may be ameliorated by taking a small dose (250 mg) of inositol nicotinate daily during the cold weather.

Spoon-shaped or concave nails (KOILONYCHIA) are often associated with iron deficiency, especially in middle-aged women, and become normal when this is treated.

ABSCESS may occur at the root of the nail (see WHITLOW) or underneath it near its edge. As a rule, these abscesses are caused by a minute poisoned wound, such as that due to a splinter of wood. The condition is generally very painful, but is relieved by opening, so as to allow free exit for the pus, the nail being snipped up with a pair of scissors if necessary. The nail in these cases is often cast off.

INJURY to the nail by a blow is often followed by an extravasation of blood beneath it, the nail first turning black, and then often being shed. In all these cases in which the nail is shed, a new nail generally appears quickly, and replaces the old one in six months, unless the matrix has been very seriously diseased or injured. While the new nail is growing, the point of the finger merely requires the protection of a finger-stall.

INGROWING NAIL is a troublesome condition affecting only the nails of the toes. It is due to a variety of causes, chief among which are the pressure of badly fitting shoes, cutting away of the corners in paring the nails, and want of attention to the nails, whereby scarf-skin and dirt collect beneath the nail, and by inflammatory changes causing ulceration of the skin at the sides. The condition commonly occurs in old, bedridden people, mainly for the last-named reason. The treatment is simple, though sometimes tedious. It consists in the wearing of well-made footwear, cutting of the nails square across without paring away the corners and the packing two or three times daily of a shred of boric lint between the corner of the nail and the skin which it is chafing. These measures are generally sufficient after a little time, but sometimes the nail is so much thickened that the edges cannot be raised up to admit the threads of lint. In this case the centre of the nail may be softened by dabbing on caustic potash, and then the nail is easily thinned down by scraping with a sharp knife till it becomes pliable. When the skin at the side of the nail bleeds very readily, this is remedied by touching with bluestone or with nitrate of silver. In severe cases a minor surgical operation may be required. Anyone having trouble with ingrowing toe-nails, especially elderly people, should consult a chiropodist.

NALIDIXIC ACID is a drug, active against Gram-negative micro-organisms, which is proving useful in the treatment of infections of the urinary tract.

NALORPHINE reduces or abolishes most of the actions of morphine and similarly acting narcotics, such as pethidine. It was used as an antidote in the treatment of over-dosage with these drugs but has now been superseded by naloxone (q.v.).

NALOXONE is the most efficient drug in the treatment of morphine poisoning. It blocks the effects of most opiates. Administration by mouth is unreliable but, when given intravenously, it acts within two or three minutes.

NANDROLONE DECANOATE (see ANABOLIC STEROIDS).

NANDROLONE PHENYLPROPIONATE (see ANABOLIC STEROIDS).

NANOMETRE is a millionth of a millimetre. The approved abbreviation is nm.

NAPPY RASH is the eruption which tends to occur on the buttocks of infants, due to too infrequent changing of soiled nappies or inadequate laundering of nappies. There is some evidence that it is more common in bottle-fed, than in breast-fed, babies. It has become much less common since the advent of disposable nappies.

Prevention consists of four main measures. (i) When the baby is bathed, particular attention must be paid to the creases and folds of the skin which must be carefully washed, then equally carefully dried and sprinkled with a bland baby powder. (ii) Nappies must not be washed in strong soaps or detergent solutions. After washing they must be carefully rinsed out in several changes of clean water. (iii) Soiled nappies must be changed frequently. (iv) Waterproof pants should be reserved for special social occasions, and not used every day.

Should the skin become inflamed, washing it with a 1-per-cent solution of sodium sulphate, followed by careful drying and the application of calamine lotion, is often useful. An alternative application which has stood the test of time is zinc and castor oil ointment.

NAPRAPATHY is a system of healing which attributes disease to disorder in the ligaments and connective tissues.

NAPROXEN (see NON-STEROIDAL ANTI-INFLAMMATORY DRUGS).

NARCISSISM is an abnormal mental state characterized by excessive admiration of self.

NARCOLEPSY is a condition in which uncontrollable episodes of sleep occur two or three times a day. It starts at any age and persists for life. The attacks, which usually last for 10 to 15 minutes, come on at times normally conducive to sleep, such as after a meal, or sitting in a bus, but they may occur when walking in the street. In due course, usually after some years, they are associated with cataplectic attacks when for a few seconds there is sudden muscular weakness affecting the whole body. These attacks are commonly brought on by amusement with laughter. In others they may be induced by anger or by a sense of triumph. In the first of these groups the affected individual soon learns to sit down when jokes are going around. The attacks of narcolepsy seem to be reduced in number if the individual takes a 15-minute nap after meals. Affected people should carry 5 mg tablets of dexamphetamine about with them and take one or two to tide them over special occasions when an attack could be embarrassing. Some doctors recommend the regular taking of dexamphetamine, but this is deprecated by others in view of the possible adverse effect of such continued treatment on the mental state. The cataplectic attacks are controlled by imipramine or clomipramine.

Familial narcolepsy is well recognized and recently a near-100-per-cent association between narcolepsy and the histocompatability antigen HLA-DR2 has been discovered. This has given rise to the notion that narcolepsy is an immune-related disease. The Narcolepsy Association (UK) has been founded to help patients with this strange disorder. The address is South Hall, High Street, Farningham, Kent DA4 0DE (0322-863195).

NARCOSIS is a condition of profound insensibility, resembling sleep so far that the unconscious person can still be roused slightly by great efforts, or at all events is not entirely indifferent to sensory stimuli. It is most commonly produced by drugs, such as opium, but may also be due to poisons formed within the body, as in uraemia.

NARCOTICS (see HYPNOTICS).

NARES is the Latin word for the nostrils.

NASOGASTRIC TUBE: A small-bore plastic or rubber tube passed into the stomach through the nose, pharynx and then the oesophagus. It is used either to aspirate gas and liquid from the stomach or to pass food or drugs into it.

NASOPHARYNX is the upper part of the throat, lying behind the nasal cavity. (See NOSE.)

NATAMYCIN is an antibiotic isolated from *Streptomyces natalensis* which is proving of value in the treatment of moniliasis (q.v.).

NATIONAL HEALTH SERVICE (NHS): The United Kingdom's National Health Service came into being on 5 July 1948. Its aim was to provide comprehensive health care to all people, free at the point of delivery. The service was to be funded by a small contribution from National Insurance and from general taxation. (In 1990 Britain spent 6·1 per cent of its gross domestic product on health, 0·9 per cent of this in the private sector.) Various reforms of the system have occurred since, the most recent and far-reaching being the 1990 National Health Service and Community Care Act which came into effect on 1 April 1991. This introduces 'market forces' into the NHS as a way of shaping how health services are provided, with an emphasis on improved management of services and accountability of staff. An NHS policy board, chaired by the Secretary of State for Health, determines the strategy, objectives and funding of the NHS in England and Wales. The NHS management executive is responsible for operational matters. Beneath this are the 14 regional health authorities in England, mainly responsible for setting and monitoring performance criteria. Over 200 district health authorities (boards in Scotland and Northern Ireland) are responsible for the health needs of their populations, with much of the responsibility delegated to individual units. District health authorities are funded on a weighted capitation basis, taking into account the size and needs of their populations. (This is not yet fully implemented.) Districts will be 'purchasers' of services for their population and will shop around among the 'providers' (hospitals and other services) to obtain the best deal. The NHS employs nearly one million people, the largest group being nurses. Hospital staff are salaried employees, but the senior doctors (consultants) are allowed to do private practice as well as their NHS work.

The 1990 Act also allows for the formation of 'NHS hospital trusts' – self-governing hospitals under the control of a board of directors – which will have certain freedoms (e.g. the power to acquire and dispose of assets, decide what services to provide and set their own terms and conditions of service for employees) not available to other units within the NHS.

Most general practitioners have always remained independent practitioners who have contracted with the NHS to provide primary health care for the population. Under the 1990 Act some GPs (depending on their practice size) will become direct fund holders and will be free to negotiate as 'purchasers'. Family health service authorities are responsible for paying general practitioners and monitoring their performance. Payment is by a mixture of capitation fee, salary, item of service fees and bonuses.

Scotland and Northern Ireland have broadly similar arrangements tailored to take account of their national requirements.

The 1990 Act provided for closer co-operation between health and local authorities for the provision of certain social services but implementation of this part of the Act has been delayed.

NATIONAL LISTENING LIBRARY is a charity which produces recorded books for handicapped people who cannot read, with the exception of the blind who have their own separate organization, the Royal National Institute for the Blind. Its address, from which full details can be obtained, is: National Listening Library, 12 Lant Street, London SE1 1QR (071-407 9417). (See also CALIBRE.)

NAUSEA means a feeling that vomiting is about to take place. (See VOMITING.)

NAVEL, or UMBILICUS, is the scar on the abdomen marking the point where the umbilical cord joined the body in embryonic life. (See AFTERBIRTH.)

NEAR SIGHT (see REFRACTION).

NEBULA is the term applied to a slight opacity on the cornea producing a haze in the field of vision, and also to any oily preparation to be sprayed from a nebulizer, an apparatus for splitting up a fluid into fine droplets.

NEBULIZERS: A nebulizer makes an aerosol by blowing air or oxygen through a solution of a drug. Many inhaled drugs such as salbutamol, ipratropium and beclomethasone can be given in this way. It has the advantage over a medihaler in that no special effort is required to co-ordinate breathing and a nebulizer allows a much greater concentration of the drug to be delivered compared with that of a medihaler. The use of higher doses of bronchodilator drugs made possible by the nebulizer means that the risk of unwanted side-effects is also increased.

NECATOR AMERICANUS is a hookworm, closely resembling but smaller than the *Ancylostoma duodenale*. (See ANCYLOSTOMIASIS.)

NECK is that portion of the body which extends from the upper limit of the chest to the base of the skull. Its main function is to support the head. Through its front part run the passages for the air and the food. The great bulk of the neck is composed of seven cervical vertebrae with the muscles attached thereto, in front and behind. (See MUSCLES.) Within the canal formed by the rings of these vertebrae lies the cervical part of the spinal cord, from which proceed the nerves that control the movements of the neck and arms.

In front of the spinal column lies the pharynx, or throat-cavity, extending from the base of the skull above down to the lower edge of the sixth vertebra, where the gullet continues it directly downwards, while the larynx opens out of it in front. The larynx is close to the surface of the front of the neck, and the thyroid cartilage can be readily seen and felt beneath the skin. (See LARYNX.) The larynx is continued downwards by the windpipe, and just beneath the larynx the isthmus of the thyroid gland can be felt crossing the windpipe and connecting the two lobes of the gland which lie one on either side of the larynx. The strong sterno-cleidomastoid muscle is prominent on each side of the neck, running from the mastoid process of the skull down to the breast-bone and inner end of the clavicle; under cover of it lies a fibrous sheath containing the carotid artery, internal jugular vein and vagus nerve. The sternocleidomastoid muscle divides each side of the neck into two triangular areas, in which lie important nerves and branches of these blood-vessels, as well as chains of lymphatic glands. Several large superficial veins run down the neck, and are of importance, because in wounds of the neck they may give rise to much bleeding. The chief of these are the external jugular vein, running straight downwards from the angle of the jaw, and the anterior jugular vein, running downwards from beneath the chin, not far from the middle line. At the root of the neck the apex of each lung projects a short distance from the chest into the neck.

NECROPSY is a post-mortem examination which produces almost no disfigurement. The brain is examined by an opening across the scalp, afterwards hidden by the hair, and the contents of chest and abdomen are inspected through an opening down the middle line in front. If necessary minute pieces of organs are removed for microscopic examination. It is a social duty of the deceased person's relatives to permit or request a post-mortem examination in cases in which the disease was a matter of uncertainty.

NECROSIS means death of a limited portion of tissue, the term being most commonly applied to bones when, as the result of disease or injury, a fragment dies and separates. (See BONE, DISEASES OF.)

NEEDLING is an operation performed by means of a needle, especially in the discission or tearing of a cataract so as to allow the fluid in the anterior chamber of the eye to dissolve it.

NEGATIVISM means a morbid tendency in a person to do the opposite of what he is desired or directed to do. It is specially characteristic of schizophrenia, but is not uncommon in non-psychotic persons.

NEISSERIA is a group, or genus, of rounded bacteria that occur in pairs and are therefore known as diplococci (see MICROBIOLOGY). They are named after Albert Neisser, the German physician who discovered the gonococcus, the causative organism of gonorrhoea (q.v.), which is now known as *Neisseria gonorrhoea*. The group also includes the causative organism of cerebrospinal meningitis (see MENINGITIS): *Neisseria meningitidis*.

NEMATODE is a roundworm. (See ASCARIASIS.)

NEOMYCIN is an antibiotic derived from *Streptomyces fradiae*. It has a wide antibacterial spectrum, being effective against the majority of Gram-negative bacilli. Its use is limited by the fact that it is liable to cause deafness and kidney damage. For this reason it is never given by injections. Its main use is for application to the skin, either in solution or as an ointment, for the treatment of infection of the skin. It is also given by mouth for the treatment of certain forms of enteritis due to *E. coli*.

NEONATAL means pertaining to the first month of life.

NEONATAL MORTALITY is the mortality of infants under one month of age. In England and Wales this has fallen markedly in recent decades: from over 28 per 1000 related live births in 1939 to around 4 in 1990. This improvement can be attributed to various factors: better antenatal supervision of expectant mothers; care to ensure that expectant mothers receive adequate nourishing food; improvements in the management of the complications of pregnancy and of labour. Nearly three-quarters of neonatal deaths occur during the first week of life. For this reason, increasing emphasis is being laid on this initial period of life. Between 1960 and 1990, in England, the number of deaths in the first week fell from 9772 to 2382, representing a fall in the rate per 1000 live births from 13·2 to 3·6. The chief causes of deaths in this period are immaturity of the infant, birth injuries, congenital abnormalities and asphyxia. After the first week the commonest cause is infection.

NEOPLASM, which means literally a 'new formation', is another word for tumour.

NEPHRECTOMY is the operation for removal of the kidney. (See KIDNEYS, DISEASES OF.)

NEPHRITIS means inflammation of the kidneys. (See GLOMERULONEPHRITIS.)

NEPHROLITHIASIS is the term applied to a condition in which calculi are present in the kidney.

NEPHROLOGY: The branch of medicine concerned with the study and management of kidney disease.

NEPHRON: Each kidney comprises over a million of these microscopic units which regulate and control the formation of urine. A tuft of capillaries invaginates the Bowmans capsule which is the blind-ending tube (glomerulus) of each nephron. Plasma is filtered out of blood and through the Bowmans capsule into the renal tubule. As the filtrate passes along the tubule most of the water and electrolytes are reabsorbed. The composition is regulated with the retention or addition of certain molecules (e.g. urea, drugs, etc.). The tubules eventually empty the filtrate, which by now is urine, into the renal pelvis from where it flows down the ureters into the bladder. (See KIDNEYS.)

NEPHROPEXY is the fixation of a floating kidney in its original position.

NEPHROPTOSIS means the condition in which a kidney is movable or 'floating'.

NEPHRORRHAPHY is the operation by which a movable kidney is fastened by stitches in its proper place.

NEPHROSTOMY is the operation of making an opening into the kidney to drain it.

NEPHROTIC SYNDROME is one of proteinuria, hypo-albuminaemia and gross oedema. The primary cause is the leak of albumin through the glomerulus. When this exceeds the liver's ability to synthesise albumin the plasma level falls and oedema results. The nephrotic syndrome is commonly the result of primary renal glomerular disease (see GLOMERULO-NEPHRITIS). It may also be a result of metabolic diseases such as diabetic glomerular sclerosis and amyloidosis. It may be the result of systemic auto-immune diseases such as systemic lupus erythematosis and polyarteritis. It may complicate malignant diseases such as myelomatosis, Hodgkin's disease and lymphocytic leukaemia. It is sometimes caused by nephrotoxins such as gold or mercury and certain drugs, and it may be the result of certain infections such as malaria and Crohn's disease.

NEPHROTOMY means the operation of cutting into the kidney, in search of calculi or for other reasons.

NERVE BLOCK (see ANAESTHESIA, local anaesthetics).

NERVE INJURIES are produced by several causes. Continued or repeated severe pressure may be enough to damage a nerve seriously, as in the case of a badly made crutch pressing into the armpit and causing drop-wrist. Bruising due to a blow which drives a superficially placed nerve against a bone may inflict severe damage upon a nerve such as the radial nerve behind the upper arm. A wound may sever nerves, along with other structures; this accident is specially liable to occur to the ulnar nerve in front of the wrist, owing to falls upon broken glass, and to various nerves in the armpit when the humerus is fractured near its upper end.

Symptoms: When a sensory nerve is injured, sensation is immediately more or less impaired in the part supplied by the nerve. When the nerve in question is a motor one the muscles governed through it are instantly paralysed. In the latter case, the portion of nerve beyond the injury degenerates and the muscles gradually waste, and lose their power of contraction in response to electrical applications. Finally, deformities result and the joints become fixed. This is particularly noticeable when the ulnar nerve is injured, the hand and fingers taking up a claw-like position. The skin may also become cold, glossy and even ulcerate, owing to the loss of its nerve supply.

Treatment: The nerve, if wounded, should be carefully stitched with the ends touching one another, and, if injured by other causes, should be carefully protected from a repetition of the injury. In some cases recovery takes place within a few days, but usually, if the nerve is completely severed or seriously injured, the muscles supplied by it do not regain their power for several weeks at least. The reason for this is that the part cut off from connection with the brain and cord degenerates rapidly, and the new nerve has to grow all the way down the sheath of the old one. (See NERVES.) An operation designed to unite a damaged nerve and relieve paralysis may sometimes be successfully performed even some weeks or months after the wound has closed. When the ends of the damaged nerve are so shortened that they cannot be got to meet, a portion of a sensory nerve or of a nerve from an animal is sometimes inserted and carefully stitched between the divided ends. Nerve anastomosis is also sometimes practised by bringing the ends of the divided nerve up to a neighbouring nerve and carefully stitching them within its sheath. For example, the facial nerve when injured at the side of the face is sometimes anastomosed with the healthy hypoglossal nerve, and the facial paralysis which has resulted is thus relieved. Massage and galvanism of the muscles will keep them from wasting till the nerve is ready to take up its functions again. The power of the

1 Schwann cell   4 myelin
2 node of Ranvier   5 neurilemma
3 axon

Diagram of (left) a healthy nerve, (centre) degenerating nerve cell after two days, (right) and after a week.

to brain

sensory fibres

sense organs

corpuscles

hair

muscle spindle

3

motor fibres

muscle

spinal cord   nerve trunk

Diagram showing nervous connections between the central nervous system
and muscle and skin.

muscles to react again to faradic electricity is a most important sign, as showing that repair of the nerve is taking place.

NERVES: The nervous system consists in part of cells and in part of fibres, each of which is a long process extending from a nerve-cell. The brain and spinal cord are often spoken of together as the central nervous system; the nerves which proceed from them, forty-three on each side, are named the cerebrospinal, or peripheral nerves; whilst the third great division, situated in the neck, thorax and abdomen, and intimately connected with the cerebrospinal nerves (though in its action largely independent of the brain and cord) is known as the autonomic nervous system. The last-named consists of ganglia containing nerve-cells, which are profusely connected by plexuses of nerve-fibres.

The nerve-cells originate, or receive, impulses and impressions of various sorts, which are conveyed from them to muscles, blood-vessels, and elsewhere, by efferent nerves, or received by them through afferent nerves coming from the skin, organs of sense, joints, etc. The autonomic system is concerned mainly with the movements and other functions of the internal organs, secreting glands and blood-vessels, the activities of which proceed independently of the will.

Structure: (1) NERVE-FIBRES: The nerves vary much in size. The sciatic nerve, deeply buried in the muscles on the back of the thigh, is the largest nerve in the body, being as thick as a pencil or more; other nerves reach about the size of goose-quills, and from these there are all gradations, down to the minute single fibres distributed to muscle-fibres or to skin. A nerve, such as the sciatic, possesses a strong, outer fibrous sheath, called the epineurium, within which lie bundles of nerve-fibres, divided from one another by partitions of fibrous tissue, in which run blood-vessels that nourish the nerve. Each of these bundles is surrounded by its own sheath, known as the perineurium, and within the bundle fine partitions of fibrous tissue, known as endoneurium, divide up the bundle into groups of fibres. The blood-vessels and lymphatics of the nerves divide into fine branches, which run in these sheaths and partitions of fibrous tissue. The finest subdivisions of the nerves are the fibres, and these are

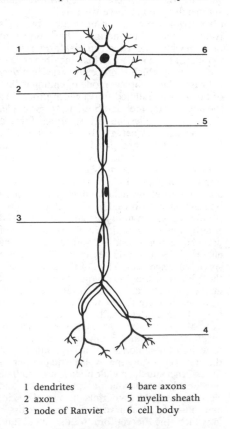

1 dendrites   4 bare axons
2 axon   5 myelin sheath
3 node of Ranvier   6 cell body

Diagram of a nerve.

A nerve cell, showing Nissl's granules.

of two kinds: medullated and non-medullated fibres. The *medullated fibres* vary in thickness from 2 to 15 micrometres, some nerves containing a greater proportion of the small fibres than others. Under the microscope, all have the appearance of tubes, this being due to the fact that each has an outer membranous sheath, the neurilemma, within which is a clear white material, the medullary (or myelin) sheath, in the centre of which runs the axis-cylinder or nerve-fibre proper. The neurilemma is a strong but thin sheath with nuclei at regular intervals on its inner surface. The medullary sheath is composed of fatty material containing lecithin and cholesterin, and to it the white colour of the nerves is mainly due. It is divided at regular intervals by short gaps, situated about 1 mm apart, known as the nodes of Ranvier, but across these gaps the neurilemma and axis-cylinder are continuous. This medullary, or myelin, sheath is regarded as fulfilling a purpose similar to the insulating material upon electric wires and preventing nerve impulses from passing beyond the nerve-fibre by which they are conveyed. The axis-cylinder, or axon, is the conducting part of the nerve, for whilst the neurilemma is absent from the fibre in its course through the brain and spinal cord, and the medullary sheath is absent from non-medullated nerves, the axis-cylinder never fails. It has a striped appearance, seeming to consist of a number of fibrils which, however, cannot be separated from one another. The *non-medullated fibres* are very much thinner than the average of medullated fibres, from which they differ only in the fact of not possessing a medullary sheath, and of being therefore greyish in colour.

(2) NERVE-CELLS, from one of which springs each nerve-fibre, are found in the grey matter of the brain and spinal cord. In the brain alone it is calculated there are some 600,000,000 of these cells. They also exist in the ganglia of the sympathetic system, in connection with some of the nerves of special sense, and on the posterior roots of the spinal nerves. The shape of these nerve-cells varies. The most common appearance is that of a large clear cell, containing an oval nucleus, and running out at various points into long processes, which, as a rule, branch again and again, after the manner of a tree, these dendritic processes, as they are called, meeting with similar processes from neighbouring cells. The ends of the branching processes from one cell meet the ends of similar processes from another cell, the points of apposition being known as *synapses*. The state of closure or openness of these synapses is believed to be of great importance in quickening or blocking nerve impulses. The body of the cell has a mottled appearance, owing to its containing many bodies, known as Nissl's granules, which appear to be of the nature of food material, destined to be used up when the cell is stimulated to work till reduced to a state of fatigue.

In the cerebrum, the cells are distinctly pyramidal in shape, and one of the processes of each cell is much longer than the rest, forming indeed a nerve-fibre, which may run a long distance down the spinal cord. Other cells are bipolar, i.e. they possess just two processes, and others are unipolar, i.e. they possess only one process, which, a short distance from the cell, divides in a T-shaped manner, as, for example, the cells in the ganglia upon the posterior roots of the spinal nerves. Other cells are found in the grey matter of the brain, which are known as neuroglia cells. These are provided with innumerable processes that form a supporting feltwork for the nerve-cells and nerve-fibres, and act merely as connective tissue cells.

(3) NERVE-ENDINGS: Each nerve-fibre proceeds from a nerve-cell to end in a definite organ, to or from which it carries a special form of nerve impulse. The manner in which the fibre ends in the organ to which it proceeds varies in different cases. The simplest mode of ending is that of the non-medullated fibres which proceed to the involuntary muscle-fibres, as, for example, those of the intestine. These fibres form a complex network between the layers of muscle, from which fine fibres pass between the muscle-fibres. In the heart the nerves end in a similar manner. In voluntary muscles the arrangement is more complicated. Each nerve-fibre splits up into numerous branches, which go to neighbouring muscle-fibres. Each branch pierces the membrane surrounding its muscle-fibre, and ends by spreading out into a plate composed of granular material and numerous nuclei. The endings of sensory nerves in the skin have a special arrangement. Most of these end, not in the epidermis, which is devoid of sensation, but in the projections of the corium beneath it, where each nerve-fibre enters a small rounded bulb. Some of these bulbs found beneath the skin of the fingers are known as Pacinian corpuscles: around 2·5 mm long and half that in width. These consist of a large number of thin coats enclosing the swollen end of a nerve-fibre. Other much smaller bodies, around 0·08 mm long, known as touch-corpuscles, are found close beneath the epidermis all over the skin, and consist of a framework of connective tissue in which the nerve-fibre winds round and round. Similar bodies are found on the front of

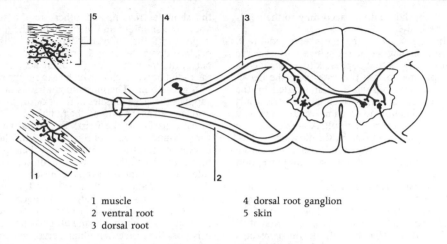

1 muscle   4 dorsal root ganglion
2 ventral root   5 skin
3 dorsal root

Diagram of a reflex arc.

the eye. In other cases the nerves appear to end abruptly in cells in the deepest layer of the epidermis.

Development and repair: The whole nervous system is developed from the ectoderm or outer layer of the embryo, the brain and spinal cord arising from an infolding of the surface along the back to form a tube, and all the nerves being formed directly or indirectly as out-growths from this tube, which increase in length till they reach the muscle, skin or other structure for which they are destined. Each nerve-fibre, as already stated, is the process of a nerve-cell, and, if a nerve is cut, that portion of its fibres which is separated from the cells immediately starts to degenerate, the medullary sheath and axis-cylinder, as a rule, breaking up. Within a few days or weeks, however, a bundle of small new fibres grows out from the cut end of each fibre in that portion which has not been cut off from connection with the nerve-cells, and these grow through the scar and down the sheath of the degenerated portion till they reach the organs to which the nerve originally proceeded. Thus the nerve is restored. This process is quickened when the cut ends have been carefully brought together, and indeed there are reasons for believing that, sometimes when this is done, no degeneration takes place, but the nerve heals and again transmits impulses at once.

Functions of nerves: The greater part of the bodily activity originates in the nerve-cells, food material being used up in the process. As a result of this activity, impulses are sent down the nerves, which act simply as transmitters. The impulse which passes from a nerve-cell along a nerve-fibre to a muscle may be compared to the electric spark which explodes a mine, since the nerve impulse causes sudden chemical changes in the muscles as the latter contract. (See MUSCLES.) Similarly, the impulse which passes from a sensory ending in the skin along a nerve-fibre to affect nerve-cells in the spinal cord and brain, where it is perceived as a sensation, may be compared to the electric

current which passes along a telephone cable to affect the receiver. Nevertheless, it must be understood that the impulse passing along a nerve is a form of motion quite different from electricity: travelling at the slow rate of about 30 metres (100 feet) per second, and probably more nearly resembling the motion of air-particles which produces sound. (See NERVOUS IMPULSE.)

The important fact that the anterior root of each spinal nerve is motor in function was discovered in 1811 by Sir Charles Bell. This was confirmed by Magendie in 1822, and the discovery also made that the posterior roots are sensory in function. They therefore concluded that the anterior roots consist of motor fibres to muscles, the posterior roots of sensory fibres from the skin. The terms, efferent and afferent, are applied to these roots more correctly, because, in addition to motor fibres, fibres through which blood-vessels are contracted and relaxed, and fibres which control secreting glands leave the cord in the anterior roots, while, in addition to sensory fibres, fibres which bring in impulses from muscles, joints and other organs, and inform the sense of locality as well as the sense of feeling, also enter the cord by the posterior roots.

Sensation is popularly supposed to be derived through five senses: smell, sight, hearing, taste and touch. In addition to these, impulses are brought by special nerve-fibres and converted in the brain into sensations which furnish a sense of movement and locality, a sense of pain, and a sense of heat and cold. (See TOUCH.)

The connection between the sensory and motor systems of nerves is important. The simplest form of nerve action is that known as *automatic action*. In this a part of the nervous system, controlling, for example, the lungs, goes on rhythmically, making discharges from its motor cells sufficient to keep the muscles of respiration in regular action, influenced only by occasional sensory impressions and chemical changes from various sources, which increase or diminish its activity according to the needs of the body.

In *reflex action* the parts engaged are a sensory ending, say in the skin; a sensory nerve leading from it to the spinal cord, where it ends by splitting up into processes near the nerve-cells; a nerve-cell which is stimulated by the sensory impulse, and which immediately sends a motor impulse down its nerve; and a muscle which contracts as the result. A simple example of reflex action is given by the drawing away of the hand when it is pricked with a pin, before and independently of the conscious perception of pain.

Voluntary acts are more complicated than reflex ones. The same mechanism is involved, but, in addition, the controlling power of the brain is brought into play. This exerts first of all an inhibitory or blocking effect, which prevents immediate reflex action, and then the impulse, passing up to the cerebral hemispheres, sets up activity in a series of cells there, the complexity of these processes depending upon the intellectual processes involved. Finally, the inhibition is removed and an impulse passes down to motor cells in the spinal cord, and a muscle or set of muscles is brought into play through the motor nerves.

The *trophic function* of nerves is another most important part of their activity, for it appears as if the constant passage of nerve impulses down the nerves of any part were important for its nutrition. Thus, if sensory nerves are diseased or injured, ulceration of the skin, bed sores and other changes are liable to occur, while muscles waste and disappear if their motor nerves are permanently destroyed.

Nervous system: The brain and its twelve pairs of cranial nerves are treated under BRAIN; the spinal cord and the origin of its thirty-one pairs of nerves are treated under SPINAL CORD.

Each of these spinal nerves arises by two roots, the posterior root being larger than the anterior, and being furnished with a ganglion. Just before they emerge from the side of the spinal canal, the two roots unite to form a single nerve, their fibres mix, and then the nerve separates into two divisions.

One division immediately turns backwards to supply the skin and muscles of the back (posterior division), the other runs forwards (anterior division).

These anterior divisions supply the skin on the front and sides of the body and on the limbs, as well as all the muscles of the trunk and limbs, excepting those on the back. They do not run straight to these parts, but form a series of plexuses in which the nerve-fibres from different levels of the cord to the limbs are given off. The upper four cervical nerves unite to produce the *cervical plexus*. From this the muscles and skin of the neck are mainly supplied, and the phrenic nerve, which runs down through the lower part of the neck and the chest to innervate the diaphragm, is given off. The *brachial plexus* is formed by the union of the lower four cervical and first dorsal nerves, and, in addition to nerves which proceed to some of the muscles in

the shoulder region, and others to the skin about the shoulder and inner side of the arm, it gives off the following large nerves that proceed down the arm: the musculocutaneous nerve, the median nerve, the ulnar nerve, and the radial nerve, each of which is about the size of a goose-quill. The musculocutaneous nerve supplies the large muscles in front of the upper arm, as well as the skin on the radial side of the forearm as far as the wrist. The radial nerve winds round the back of the upper arm, where it supplies the triceps muscle, and then gives branches which innervate the skin on the outer side of the arm and forearm, the muscles behind the forearm, and finally the skin on the outer part of the back of the hand and fingers. The median nerve and the ulnar nerve run through the upper arm without giving off branches, and it is possible to feel the ulnar nerve as a cord running between the two marked bony prominences behind the elbow. The median nerve supplies most of the muscles in front of the forearm, a few of the small muscles in the hand and the skin of the palm and front of the thumb, index finger, middle finger and half of the ring finger. The ulnar nerve supplies two muscles in the forearm, most of the small muscles in the hand and the skin down the inner side of the forearm and palm and the skin in front of the little finger and half the ring finger.

The *thoracic* or *dorsal nerves*, with the exception of the first, do not form a plexus, but each runs round the chest along the lower margin of the rib to which it corresponds, whilst the lower six extend on to the abdomen. In this course they supply both the skin and muscle of the trunk.

The *lumbar plexus* is formed by the upper four lumbar nerves, and its branches are distributed to the lower part of the abdomen, and front and inner side of the thigh.

The *sacral plexus* is formed by parts of the fourth and fifth lumbar nerves, and the upper three and part of the fourth sacral nerves. It gives branches directly to the muscles and skin about the hip and fork, and supplies the skin down the back of the thigh, but the main bulk of the plexus is collected into the sciatic nerve. This, the largest nerve in the body, is buried in the muscles on the back of the thigh, which it supplies. It continues down to the back of the knee, and there divides into two branches, the internal popliteal (tibial) nerve and the external (common) popliteal nerve, which between them supply all the muscles below the knee and the greater part of the skin covering the leg and the foot.

The *sympathetic system* is joined by a pair of small branches given off from each spinal nerve, close to the spine. This system consists of two great parts. There is, first, a pair of cords running down on the side and front of the spine, and containing on each side three ganglia in the neck, and beneath this a ganglion opposite each vertebra. From these two ganglionated cords numerous branches are given off, and these unite in the second place to form plexuses connected with various internal organs, and provided with numerous large and irregularly placed ganglia. The chief of these plexuses are the cardiac plexus, the solar or epigastric plexus, the diaphragmatic, suprarenal, renal, spermatic, or ovarian, aortic, hypogastric and pelvic plexuses, the name in each case indicating the organ upon which, or the part of the abdomen within which, the plexus is placed.

NERVOUS DEBILITY (see NEURASTHENIA).

NERVOUS DISEASES: This class of disease is one of the most difficult to diagnose. The brain and spinal cord being enclosed in the skull and spine, beyond the reach of direct examination, and the nerves being almost everywhere deeply buried in the tissues, the nature of nervous diseases must be made out from the disturbances of organs governed by the affected nerves.

The following conditions are discussed under their individual headings: APHASIA; BRAIN, DISEASES AND INJURIES OF; CATALEPSY; CHOREA; CRAMP; EPILEPSY; HYSTERIA; MEMORY; MENTAL HANDICAP; MENTAL ILLNESS; MULTIPLE SCLEROSIS; NERVE INJURIES; NEURALGIA; NEURITIS; PARALYSIS; PSYCHOSOMATIC DISEASES; SPINE AND SPINAL CORD, DISEASES AND INJURIES OF; STROKE; TABES.

NERVOUS IMPULSE: The effects of nervous activity are now believed in all cases to be transmitted chemically, by the formation at nerve-endings of chemical substances. When, for example, a nerve to a muscle is stimulated, there appears at the neuromuscular junction (q.v.) the chemical substance, acetylcholine. Acetylcholine also appears at endings of the parasympathetic nerves and transmits the effect of the parasympathetic impulse. When an impulse passes down a sympathetic nerve, the effect of it is transmitted at the nerve-ending by the chemical liberated there: adrenaline or an adrenaline-like substance.

NETTLE-RASH (see URTICARIA).

NEURALGIA, literally 'nerve pain', is a term which is often employed both technically and popularly in a somewhat loose manner, to describe pains the origin of which is not clearly traceable. In its strict sense it means the existence of pain in some portion of, or throughout the whole of, the distribution of a sensory nerve, without any distinctly recognizable structural change in the nerve or nerve-centres. This strict definition, if adhered to, however, would not be applicable to a large number of cases of nerve pain; for in many instances the pain is connected with pressure on, or inflammation of, the nerve. Hence the word is generally used to indicate pain affecting a particular nerve or its branches, whatever be the cause.

Symptoms: Although the pain is generally localized, it may spread beyond the area where it first occurs. It is usually of paroxysmal charac-

ter, and often periodic: that is to say, it occurs at a certain time of the day or night. It varies in intensity, being often of the most agonizing character, and again less severe and more of a tingling kind. Various forms of perverted nerve function may be found along with or following neuralgia. Thus there may be over-sensitiveness of the skin, loss of feeling, paralysis or alterations of nutrition, such as wasting of muscles, whitening of the hair. Attacks of neuralgia are apt to recur, particularly when the general health is low, and some people unhappily continue to suffer from occasional attacks during the greater part of their lifetime.

Varieties: The nature of the disease is best described under the names of the forms in which it most commonly occurs. These are trigeminal neuralgia (q.v.) or tic douloureux; intercostal neuralgia; and sciatica (q.v.). Other forms, affecting other nerves, are of much less frequent occurrence.

INTERCOSTAL NEURALGIA is pain affecting the nerves which emerge from the spinal cord and run along the spaces between the ribs to the front of the body. This form of neuralgia affects the left side more than the right, is more common in women than in men, and occurs generally in enfeebled states of health. It might be mistaken for pleurisy or some inflammatory affection of the lungs; but the absence of any chest symptoms, its occurrence independently of the acts of respiration, and other considerations establish the distinction. The specially painful points are chiefly where the nerve issues from the spinal canal, and at the extremities towards the front of the body, where it breaks up into filaments which ramify in the skin. This form of neuralgia is occasionally the precursor of an attack of shingles (*herpes zoster*) as well as a result of it. (See HERPES ZOSTER.)

Treatment: With all forms of neuralgia it is of the first importance to ascertain, if possible, whether any constitutional condition is associated with the symptom.

Naturally also one looks for, and as speedily as possible removes, any source of local irritation, such as a decayed tooth, and also any such reflex source as uterine or intestinal disorder.

During the time an acute attack lasts, various local applications give relief, the most useful being, perhaps, hot fomentations applied over the painful part. Bathing with water as hot as can be borne is also beneficial in many cases. Rubbing or painting with anodyne liniment, such as a mixture of the liniments of aconite, belladonna and chloroform (ABC Liniment); or a mixture, in equal parts, of chloral, camphor and menthol, rubbed up together and painted over the part, is soothing, especially perhaps for those cases in which the pain begins as soon as the sufferer gets warm in bed at night. Ointment of aconitine is also recommended by some to be rubbed on the painful spot. Hypodermic injections of morphine, although they give temporary relief, are not to be recommended because of the great danger that their use will become a habit. In the case of purely sensory nerves, like the fifth nerve, injection of pure alcohol into the nerve has a deadening effect and often gives relief for a long time.

Internally, during an acute attack, many remedies are given. Those which are most generally useful, and which may be safely used without any tendency to bring about habitual use, are aspirin, paracetamol and codeine.

Local measures in the chronic state include the application of blisters or counter-irritation by touching the skin with the button-cautery. The blister is made of an oblong shape, with its length corresponding to the line of the nerve, and the spots at which the cautery is applied generally also follow the affected nerve. The use of galvanic electricity is often beneficial in both the acute and the chronic stage. Diathermy is also employed with soothing effect. (See DIATHERMY.) Massage, though it increases the pain in the acute state, may be of great benefit in chronic cases due to some inflammatory process in the nerve.

Some cases resist all forms of medicinal treatment, and for these surgical procedures are sometimes tried, such as division and removal of a portion of the nerve, or injection of absolute alcohol into the nerve.

NEURALGIA TRIGEMINAL: This form of neuralgia affects the sensory nerve which supplies most of the face. Usually two out of the three main branches are involved. It is a severe pain often initiated by light pressure on the skin. It is generally diagnosed after excluding all other likely causes of facial pain. Treatment may be with the long-term use of the analgesic carbamezepine or partial or complete destruction of the appropriate branch of the nerve. The nerve may be destroyed by freezing, coagulating or injection of an alcohol round it. If untreated or suppressed the pain may be present for many months, then disappear, only to recur a year or so later.

NEURASTHENIA means a condition of nervous exhaustion in which, although the patient suffers from no definite disease, he becomes incapable of sustained exertion. It was never a very well-defined entity, and the term has now been largely given up. The condition which it represented is now recognized to be a form of neurosis (q.v.) or psychosomatic disease (q.v.).

NEURECTOMY is an operation in which part of a nerve is excised: for example, for the relief of neuralgia.

NEURILEMMA is the thin membranous covering which surrounds every nerve-fibre. (See NERVES.)

NEURITIS means inflammation affecting a nerve or nerves which may be localized to one part of the body, as, for instance, in sciatica, or which may be general, being then known as multiple neuritis, or polyneuritis. Owing to the fact that the most peripheral parts of the nerves are usually at fault in the latter condition, i.e. the fine subdivisions in the substance of the muscles, it is also known as peripheral neuritis.

Causes: In cases of LOCALIZED NEURITIS the fibrous sheath of the nerve is usually at fault, the actual nerve-fibres being only secondarily affected. This condition may be due to inflammation spreading into the nerve from surrounding tissues, to cold or to long-continued irritation by pressure on the nerve, and the symptoms produced vary according to the function of the nerve, in the case of sensory nerves being usually neuralgic pain (see NEURALGIA), in the case of motor nerves more or less paralysis in the muscles to which the nerves pass.

In POLYNEURITIS, which is always due to some general or constitutional cause, the nerve-fibres themselves in the small nerves degenerate and break down. Hence the very protracted nature of this malady, since, if recovery takes place, it must be brought about by the growth of new nerve-fibres from the healthy part of the nerve, down the sheath of the nerve, to the muscle. The cause of this degeneration may be said, in general terms, to be some poison either taken into or produced in the body, and circulating in the blood. By far the commonest of these poisons is alcohol, and the disease especially affects women who are quiet, steady tipplers. The condition also arises in men, though more rarely, but the abuse of alcohol in this sex tends more to produce delirium tremens, from which women are almost exempt. Next in importance comes lead, wrist-drop and other features of neuritis being among the most prominent symptoms of lead-poisoning. (See LEAD POISONING.) Arsenic is occasionally responsible for neuritis, particularly when the effect of arsenic is combined with over-indulgence in alcohol, as in an epidemic of neuritis, due to beer contaminated with arsenic, in the Midlands of England about the year 1900. Bisulphide of carbon, naphtha and other solvents of rubber are apt to produce the disease when inhaled in large quantity by the workmen in rubber factories. Those who suffer from diabetes mellitus are prone to neuritis, the condition sometimes being the result of deficiency of thiamine in the diet. This deficiency probably also accounts for some cases of alcoholic neuritis. The disease known as beriberi (q.v.) is a form of neuritis which persists in certain localities of the world, in consequence of thiamine deficiency.

Symptoms: The chief symptom of a LOCALIZED NEURITIS, whether pain or paralysis, varies according to the functions of the nerve. In cases following diphtheria, or other infective disease, the neuritis of an outlying nerve often shows, as its most prominent and annoying feature, a paralysis of a group of muscles in the arm or leg, leading to weakness of the part concerned. This may cause inability for some months to grasp objects with the hand, to lift the foot in walking and similar troublesome symptoms. These, however, usually pass off completely in time. The area of skin associated with the affected nerve is, in addition, often much changed, becoming glossy, or developing an ulcer or, especially about the face and trunk, breaking out in shingles. (See HERPES ZOSTER.) A case of neuritis of this type may come on very quickly, developing fully in a few days.

POLYNEURITIS, as a rule, takes longer to show itself. In most cases it begins with vague pains and tingling in the limbs; weakness and wasting of the muscles in the feet and legs, in the hand and arms, or in other parts, following later. Wrist-drop, the peculiar steppage gait in which the person lifts his feet as if he were constantly stepping over small obstacles, squinting, loss of voice, difficulty of breathing, enfeeblement of the heart's action appear according to the muscles whose nerves are affected. The knee-jerks and other deep reflexes are generally lost in all forms of neuritis, if severe in character. A peculiar feature of alcoholic neuritis is the wandering delirium from which the patient often suffers, her imagination conjuring up the most vivid delusions as to journeys she is making, and the mind being quite confused, especially in matters regarding time and place.

The course of the disease is usually very slow, and particularly is this the case when a poison, as in the case of alcohol or lead, has been taken into the system over a long period. Months, or even a year or two, may elapse before health is restored. The ultimate hope of recovery is, however, good. Except in the case of beriberi, which is fatal unless treated, and in those cases of poisoning by alcohol, or of diphtheria, in which the mechanism of the heart or that of respiration becomes affected, the mortality is low.

Treatment: For the treatment of LOCALIZED NEURITIS see under NEURALGIA.

The first essential in the treatment of POLYNEURITIS is to discover and remove the cause by which the nerves are being poisoned. This applies particularly to alcoholism, lead poisoning and neuritis due to manufacture of rubber. In the case of alcoholism there is always the moral difficulty of preventing the patient from obtaining fresh supplies of stimulants, so that treatment must be carried out in a hospital or nursing-home. Rest in bed is the next essential to prevent over-fatigue of the weakened nerves and muscles. In the early stages the muscles are too tender to permit much handling, but, later on, massage helps to prevent wasting of muscles, and the deformities which arise through fixation of the joints in one position. These deformities must be prevented as far as possible during the earlier stages by frequently changing the position of the patient's limbs as he lies in bed. Electrical treatment may also help as recovery advances. Much benefit is sometimes gained from injections of thiamine or administration of foods containing it, such as Bemax or Marmite.

NEURODERMATOSES, sometimes grouped under the name of NEURODERMATITIS, are disorders of the skin in which stress is one of the important factors, if not the most important cause. In some conditions, such as pruritus (see ITCHING) and rosacea (q.v.) this is the principal cause. In others, such as atopic eczema (see ECZEMA) and *Lichen simplex* (see LICHEN), it is a secondary, but none the less often important, factor, any mental or emotional stress or strain bringing on an exacerbation, or flaring up, of the skin condition. In others again, such as *Dermatitis artefacta* the emotional, or mental, instability may be the sole cause, the individual deliberately damaging his or her skin, without divulging the cause. The extreme form of this manifestation of mental illness is parasitophobia, in which the individual has a morbid terror of parasites and is quite convinced that he or she is infested with some parasite which is causing the itching which in turn has been scratched until the skin has broken down.

NEUROFIBROMATOSIS (see VON RECKLING-HAUSEN'S DISEASE).

NEUROGLIA is the name applied to a fine web of tissue and branching cells which supports the nerve fibres and cells of the nervous system. (See NERVES.)

NEUROLEPTICS: Although many of these drugs have sedative properties they should not be regarded as tranquillizers. They are used to quieten disturbed patients, whether this is the result of brain damage, mania, delirium, agitated depression or an acute behavioural disturbance. They relieve the florid psychotic symptoms such as hallucinations and thought disorder in schizophrenia and prevent relapse of this disorder when it is in remission.

Most of these drugs are dopamine antagonists (see DOPAMINE) and act by blocking dopamine receptors. As a result they can give rise to the extra pyramidal effects of Parkinsonism (q.v.) and they may also cause hyperprolactinaemia. The extrapyramidal symptoms are the most troublesome side-effects and they can usually be controlled by anticholinergic drugs. The main anti-psychotic drugs are: (i) chlorpromazine, methotrimeprazine, and promazine. These drugs are characterized by pronounced sedative effects and a moderate anticholinergic and extrapyramidal effect. (ii) pericyazine, pipothiazine and thioridazine. These drugs have moderate sedative effects, marked anticholinergic effects but less extrapyramidal effects than the other groups. (iii) fluphenazine, perphenazine, prochlorperazine, sulpiride and trifluoperazine. These drugs have fewer sedative effects, fewer anticholinergic effects but more pronounced extrapyramidal effects.

NEUROLOGY is the branch of medical practice and science which deals with the nervous system and its diseases.

NEUROMA means a tumour connected with a nerve, such tumours being generally composed of fibrous tissue, and of a painful nature.

NEUROMUSCULAR BLOCKADE: In clinical practice the transmission of impulses at the neuromuscular junction (q.v.) may be competitively blocked in order to paralyse reversibly a patient for a surgical procedure or to assist treatment on the intensive care unit. There are two main types of drug, both of which competitively block the acetylcholine receptors on the motor end plates: (1) Depolarizing neuromuscular blocking agents: these act by first producing stimulation at the receptor and then blocking it. There are characteristic muscle fasciculations before the rapid onset of paralysis which is of short duration (less than five minutes with the commonly used drug, suxamethonium). The drug is removed from the receptor by the enzyme plasma, cholinesterase. (2) Non-depolarizing neuromuscular blocking agents: these drugs occupy the receptor and prevent acetylcholine from becoming attached to it. However, in sufficiently high concentrations acetylcholine will compete with the drug and dislodge it from the receptor and the effect of these drugs is reversed by giving an anticholinesterase, which allows the amount of acetylcholine at the neuromuscular junction to build up. These drugs have varying durations of action but all are slower in onset and of longer duration than the depolarizers.

NEUROMUSCULAR JUNCTION: The specialized area where a motor nerve ends in close proximity to the muscle membrane and is able to initiate muscle contraction. The motor nerve ending is separated from the motor end plate by the synaptic cleft which is only 50–70 nm wide. When a nerve impulse arrives at the motor nerve ending molecules of acetylcholine are released which cross the synaptic cleft and attach to receptors on the motor end plate. This initiates depolarization of the muscle which in turn initiates the process of contraction. Acetylcholinesterase (an enzyme) rapidly breaks down the molecules of acetylcholine, thus ending their action and freeing the receptor in preparation for the next impulse.

NEURON is a single unit of the nervous system, consisting of a nerve cell with its various processes and the nerve fibre or fibres to which it gives origin. As applied to the motor part of the nervous system, two neurons are specially recognized: the *upper neuron*, which includes a cell on the surface of the brain and a fibre extending down into the spinal cord; the *lower neuron*, which consists of a cell in the grey matter of the cord with a nerve fibre extending outwards to end in a fibre of the muscle with which it is connected. The former has a controlling influence over the latter, whilst the latter is more directly concerned with the changes that result in the contraction of the muscle fibre and with nutritional influences over it. (See NERVES.)

NEUROPATHIC BLADDER: A bladder with complete or partial loss of sensation. As there is no sensation of fullness, the individual either develops complete retention of urine or the bladder empties reflexly. The condition predisposes affected individuals to urinary-tract infections and back pressure on the kidneys, leading to renal failure. It may be caused by spinal injury, spina bifida (q.v.) or any disorder which produces neuropathy (q.v.).

NEUROPATHY: A disease affecting nerves. It may affect single nerves (mononeuropathy) or be a generalized disorder affecting many nerves. The symptoms will depend on whether motor, sensory or autonomic nerves are affected.

NEUROSIS is a general term applied to mental or emotional disturbance in which, as opposed to psychosis, there is no serious disturbance in the perception or understanding of external reality. However, the boundaries between neurosis and psychosis are not always clearly defined. Neuroses are usually classified into anxiety neuroses, depressive neuroses, phobias, hysteria and obsessional neuroses.
ANXIETY NEUROSIS, or ANXIETY STATE, constitutes the commonest form of neurosis. Fortunately it is also almost the most responsive to treatment. It is more likely in people of anxious personality. Once the neurosis develops, they are in a state of persistent anxiety and worry, 'tensed up', always feeling fatigue and unable to sleep at night. In addition, there are often physical complaints, e.g. palpitations or headache.
OBSESSIONAL NEUROSES are much less common and constitute only about 5 per cent of all neuroses. Like other neuroses, they usually develop in early adult life. (See MENTAL ILLNESS.)

NEUROSURGERY is surgery performed on some part of the nervous system, whether brain, spinal cord or nerves.

NEUROTIC is a general term of indefinite meaning applied to a person of nervous temperament, whose actions are largely determined by emotions or instincts rather than by reason.

NEUROTRANSMITTER is a substance which transmits the action of a nerve to a cell. It is now recognized that this is how nerves work. If there should be a lack or deficiency of the appropriate neurotransmitter, then the nerve cannot carry out its action. A classical example of this is dopamine (q.v.), lack of which is responsible for the condition known as Parkinsonism (q.v.). Other neurotransmitters include acetylcholine (q.v.) which is the neurotransmitter for the parasympathetic nervous system (q.v.) and noradrenaline which is the neurotransmitter for the sympathetic nervous system.

NEUTRON is one of the particles that enter into the structure of the atomic nucleus. (See ISOTOPES.)

NEUTROPENIA denotes a reduction in the number of neutrophil leucocytes per cubic millimetre of circulating blood to a figure below that found in health. There is still some disagreement over the precise limits of normality, but a count of less than 2500 per mm^3 would be generally accepted as constituting neutropenia. Several infective diseases are characterized by neutropenia, including typhoid fever, influenza and measles. It may also be induced by certain drugs, including chloramphenicol, phenylbutazone, the sulphonamides and chlorpromazine.

NEUTROPHIL: A type of leucocyte (q.v.) or white blood cell (see BLOOD).

NICLOSAMIDE is the drug of choice in the treatment of tapeworm infestation. It is also known as YOMESAN.

NICOTINAMIDE, the amide of nicotinic acid, is sometimes used instead of nicotinic acid (q.v.).

NICOTINE is the active principle in tobacco. (See TOBACCO.)

NICOTINIC ACID, or NIACIN, is a member of the vitamin B complex. It is essential for human nutrition, the normal daily requirement for an adult being about 15 to 20 mg. A deficiency of nicotinic acid is one of the factors in the etiology of pellagra (q.v.), and either nicotine acid or nicotinamide is used in the treatment of this condition. (See HYPERLIPIDAEMIA.)

NIDUS: A site of infection within the body from which it can spread to other tissues.

NIFEDIPINE is a drug that is being used in the treatment of angina pectoris (q.v.). It is said to reduce the requirements of the heart muscle for oxygen. It is also proving of value in the treatment of high blood-pressure. It is one of the calcium antagonists. (See CALCIUM-CHANNEL BLOCKERS.)

NIGHT BLINDNESS (see BLINDNESS).

NIGHTMARE (see SLEEP).

NIGHT SWEATS consist in copious perspiration occurring in bed at night and found in conditions such as tuberculosis, brucellosis and lymphomas.

NIKETHAMIDE is a drug which stimulates the respiratory centre.

NIPPLES, DISEASES OF (see BREASTS, DISEASES OF).

NIRIDAZOLE is a drug which is proving of value in the treatment of schistosomiasis (q.v.) and guinea-worm infections (see DRACUNCULIASIS).

NITRAZEPAM is a tranquillizer introduced as a hypnotic. (See TRANQUILLIZERS, BENZODIAZEPINES.)

NITRIC ACID is one of the strongest of the mineral acids, and is a clear, heavy liquid, becoming brownish with age. It is kept in dark, stoppered bottles, and immediately the stopper is removed from the bottle, irritating white fumes are given off.
Action: In its pure state, nitric acid acts as a powerful caustic upon the tissues of the body, which it turns a bright yellow colour. In weaker solution it is, like all acids, an antiseptic, but is very irritating. Internally, in small doses it has a stimulating action upon the gastric mucous membrane.
Uses: Nitric acid is one of the most effective caustics for warts, and is also used as a powerful antiseptic and caustic for destroying foul ulcers which threaten to spread, leaving clean ulcers in their place. It is applied to warts drop by drop with a glass rod, and its action can be checked by applying similarly a few drops of solution of common salt.

NITRITES are salts which have a powerful effect in paralysing the action of involuntary muscle, and they therefore dilate the blood-vessels, and check spasm of all sorts. The most commonly used nitrites are nitrite of amyl, of ethyl, and of sodium. Erythrol tetranitrate and nitroglycerin have a similar action. (See GLYCERYL TRINITRATE.)

NITROFURANTOIN is a synthetic nitrofuran derivative which has a wide range of antibacterial activity and is effective against many Gram-positive and Gram-negative micro-organisms. It is used mainly in the treatment of infections of the urinary tract.

NITROGEN MUSTARDS are nitrogen analogues of mustard gas. They are among the most important alkylating agents (q.v.) used in the treatment of various forms of malignant disease. They include mustine, trimustine, uramustine, busulphan, chlorambucil and melphalan.

NITROHYDROCHLORIC ACID, or AQUA REGIA, so called because of its power to dissolve gold, is a yellow liquid prepared by adding 1 part of nitric acid to 4 parts of hydrochloric acid. It is a caustic in its pure state, but is only used for internal administration in a diluted form. It is used in the treatment of dyspepsia associated with a low gastric acidity.

NITROUS OXIDE GAS, also known as LAUGHING GAS, is, at ordinary pressures, a gas devoid of odour but of a slightly sweetish taste. Its use in medicine is to produce insensibility to pain, which it does very quickly, and with a great degree of safety, though the effect is of very short duration, not extending beyond two or three minutes. Its use is therefore applicable only for short operations, such as extraction of a tooth, unless it is repeatedly administered in association with oxygen. (See ANAESTHESIA.)

NOCICEPTORS: Nerve endings which detect and respond to painful or unpleasant stimuli.

NOCTURIA denotes excess passing of urine during the night. Among its many causes are glomerulonephritis (q.v.) and enlargement of the prostate. (See also URINE, EXCESS OF.)

NOCTURNAL ENURESIS is the involuntary passing of urine during sleep. It is a condition predominantly of childhood. In a small minority of cases it is due to some organic cause such as infection of the genito-urinary tract, but in the vast majority of cases it is due to inadequate or improper training of the child or psychological ill health. Traditionally it is said to be associated with threadworms, but there is little, if any, evidence to support this tradition.

Before deciding that a child is suffering from nocturnal enuresis, it is necessary to remember that the age at which a child achieves full control of bladder function varies considerably. Such control is usually achieved in the second year, but more commonly in the third year of life, and there are some children who do not normally achieve such control until the fourth, or even fifth, year.

It is a difficult condition to cure in the absence of an organic cause. If there should be an organic cause, treatment consists of its eradication. In the absence of such a cause, treatment consists essentially of reassurance and firm but kindly and understanding training. In quite a number of cases the use of a buzzer alarm which wakens the child should he start passing water is helpful provided that it is backed up by psychological support from the parents and the family doctor.

NODE: The term node is widely used in medicine. For instance, the smaller lymphatic glands are often termed lymph nodes. It is also applied to a collection of nerve cells forming a subsidiary nerve centre found in various places in the sympathetic nervous system, such as the sinuatrial node and the atrio-ventricular node which control the beating of the heart.

NOISE (see DEAFNESS).

NOMA is another name for cancrum oris. (See CANCRUM ORIS.)

NOMIFENSINE (see ANTIDEPRESSANTS).

NON-SPECIFIC GENITAL INFECTION, or NON-SPECIFIC URETHRITIS, is an inflammatory condition of the urethra (q.v.) due to infection with certain types of micro-organism. The most common is *Chlamydia trachomatis* – nearly 27,000 cases were identified by laboratories in England and Wales in 1989. It produces pelvic inflammatory disease in women, which often results in sterility, the risk of ectopic pregnancy (see ECTOPIC), and recurrent pelvic pain. Most cases respond well to tetracycline (q.v.). Abstinence from sexual intercourse should be observed during treatment and until cure is complete. Children born to infected mothers may have their eyes infected during birth, producing the condition known as ophthalmia neonatorum. This is treated by the application to the eye of chlortetracycline eye ointment. The lungs of such a child may also be infected, resulting in pneumonia.

NON-STEROIDAL ANTI-INFLAMMATORY DRUGS act by inhibiting the formation of prostaglandins which are mediators of inflammation. They act both as analgesics to relieve pain and as inhibitors of inflammation. Aspirin is a classic example of such a compound. Newer compounds have been synthesized with the aim of producing fewer and less severe side-effects. They are sometimes preferred to aspirin for the treatment of conditions such as rheumatoid arthritis, osteoarthritis, sprains, strains and sports injuries. Their main side-effects are gastro-intestinal. Gastric ulcers and gastric haemorrhage may result. This is because prostaglandins are necessary for the production of the mucous protective coat in the stomach and, when the production of prostaglandin is inhibited, the protection of the stomach is compromised. They should therefore be used with caution in patients with dyspepsia and gastric ulceration. The various non-steroidal anti-inflammatory drugs differ little from each other in efficacy though there is considerable variation in patient response. Naproxen is one of the first choices in this group of drugs as it combines good efficacy with a low incidence of side-effects and administration is only required twice daily. Other drugs in this series include azapropazone, fenbufen, fenclofenac, fenoprofen, feprazone, flurbiprofen, ibuprofen, indomethacin, indoprofen, ketoprofen, piroxicam, sulindac, tiaprofenic acid and tolmetin.

NORADRENALINE is a precursor of adrenaline (q.v.) in the medulla of the suprarenal glands. It is also present in the brain. Its main function is to mediate the transmission of impulses in the sympathetic nervous system (q.v.). It also has a transmitter function in the brain.

NOREPINEPHRINE (see NORADRENALINE).

NORETHISTERONE is a synthetic preparation that has the action of progesterone (q.v.), but is active when given by mouth.

NORETHYNODREL is a synthetic substance which has a progesterone-like action. (See PROGESTERONE.) Originally, and still, used for the treatment of various menstrual disorders, these progestogens, as they are known, have also the property of inhibiting ovulation. It is this property that led to their use as oral contraceptives. (See CONTRACEPTION.)

NORMAL is a term used in several different senses. Generally speaking, it is applied to anything which agrees with the regular and established type. In chemistry the term is applied to solutions of acids or bases of such strength that each litre contains the number of grams corresponding to the molecular weight of the substance in question. In physiology the term normal is applied to solutions of such strength that, when mixed with a body fluid, they are isotonic and cause no disturbance: e.g. normal saline solution. (See ISOTONIC.)

NORMOBLAST is the term applied to the precursor of a red blood corpuscle which still contains the remnant of a nucleus.

NORMOTENSIVE: Having a blood pressure within the normal range for an individual's age and sex.

NORTRIPTYLINE is an antidepressant drug which is also a sedative. (See ANTIDEPRESSANTS.)

NOSE: The nose has three main functions. It is the natural pathway whereby air enters the body in the course of respiration (q.v.). In the nose the incoming air is warmed, moistened and filtered before passing on into the lungs. It has also a protective function. Irritation of it by dust or the like induces sneezing (q.v.) which expels the irritant from the nose and so prevents it getting into the lungs. It is also the organ of smell (q.v.).

The *external nose* is formed partly of bone and partly of cartilage, covered by skin. In its upper part, the two nasal bones, one on each side, project downwards from the frontal bone for about 25 mm (1 inch) and, supported by a process of the upper jaw-bone, form the hard bridge of the nose between the eyes. The ending of the bony part can be seen or felt on most noses, and, beneath this, two cartilages on each side, the lateral cartilages and the cartilages of the aperture give shape, firmness, and pliability to the lower two-thirds of the nose. The gap between the cartilages of the aperture can be distinctly felt on the point of the nose. The spaces between the cartilages are filled up and the cartilages firmly bound to the bones and to one another by fibrous tissue. When the nose is injured, some of the cartilages are apt to be dislocated, thus altering the shape of this organ. However, most injuries resulting in deformity of the nose are due to injuries to the bones of the nose.

In its *interior*, the nose is completely divided into two narrow cavities, one on each side, by a septum or partition running from front to back. This septum is a thin plate composed partly of bone, partly of cartilage, consisting in about its hinder two-thirds of the central plate of the ethmoid bone and of the vomer bone, and in about its anterior third of a four-sided plate of cartilage, which along one edge touches the nasal bones, the lateral cartilages, and the cartilages of the aperture. On both surfaces this septum is covered by the general mucous membrane that lines the nose.

The cavities on either side of the septum, known as the *nasal fossae*, are extremely narrow, being at their widest point less than 6 mm (¼ inch) in breadth, though in height they correspond to the length of the nose, and run directly backwards about 5 cm (2 inches). At its upper end each cavity is separated from the interior of the skull by a thin plate of bone containing many minute apertures for the passage of the filaments of the olfactory nerve. The front part of each cavity consists of the space enclosed by the cartilages of the nose, is lined by skin, which is furnished with stiff hairs or vibrisae that grow downwards and protect the entrance, and is known as the vestibule. Further back the outer surface of each cavity is rendered very complicated, and the space in the cavity greatly filled up, by three projections known as the nasal conchae or turbinates. These bones form ridges which run from before backwards with an inclination downwards, and, in section, each ridge is curled over so that its edge looks downwards. There are therefore three passages (meatus) running from before backwards, each under cover of a corresponding nasal turbinate. As each of these bones, in common with the whole of the cavity, is covered with very vascular and thick mucous membrane, the air in its passage through the nose is by this arrangement brought in contact with a large surface of mucous membrane, and thus is considerably warmed before it enters the broncial tubes and lungs. In addition, this mucous membrane, which is covered with cilia (q.v.), secretes more that 500 millilitres of sticky mucus every 24 hours. This traps dust particles and the like, which are then moved on by the cilia and usually swallowed unnoticed. It is the excessive production of this mucus, in response to irritations or infection, that is known as nasal catarrh (q.v.). The front portion of the inferior and of the middle nasal concha can be seen as two red projections by looking up the nostril with a bright light, when the nostril is slightly opened by a speculum. The superior meatus beneath the superior nasal concha is a narrow passage, and, upon this bone and passage as well as upon the corresponding part of the septum, the nerves of smell end in the mucous membrane. The wider and longer middle meatus and inferior meatus are the passages through which the air mainly passes out and in during respiration.

Certain *sinuses* lie concealed in the bones of the skull, into which air enters freely by apertures connecting them with the nose. These cavities occupy spaces in the frontal bone over the eyebrow (frontal sinus), in the upper jawbone, filling in the angle between the eye and the nose (maxillary sinus or antrum of Highmore), in the sphenoid bone (sphenoidal sinus), and in the lateral part of the ethmoid bone (ethmoidal sinus). The function of the sinuses is, as yet, unknown. The most capacious is the maxillary sinus, which is a cubical cavity, often over 12 mm (½ inch) in measurement each way. The frontal sinus, maxillary sinus, and ethmoidal sinus open by small apertures about the centre of the middle meatus, the sphenoidal sinus above this. Into the front part of the inferior meatus opens the nasal duct, which carries the tears off from the eye. (See EYE.) The latter fact explains the frequent blowing of the nose which becomes necessary when a person is weeping. On a level with the inferior meatus, but situated in the part of the throat into which the nose opens, is placed the orifice of the Eustachian, or auditory, tube leading to the middle ear. (See EAR.)

NOSE, DISEASES OF: The nose, so far as the skin-covering is concerned, is subject to the same diseases as the skin of other parts. Redness of the skin of this part may, on account of its disfiguring character, be very annoying. It may be due to poor circulation in cold weather, partaking of the nature of a chilblain (see CHILBLAIN); occasionally it is due to acne rosacea. Among the skin diseases, acne (q.v.), lupus (q.v.), and erysipelas (q.v.) are specially prone to affect this site.

ACUTE INFLAMMATION of the nose is generally a viral infection affecting the mucous membrane of the nose and paranasal sinuses and is commonly known as a cold in the head. (See CHILLS AND COLDS.) It may be due, though less commonly, to the inhalation of irritating gases. Boils occasionally develop just within the entrance to the nose, in connection with the hairs there, and in this locality give rise to great pain and considerable danger. (See BOILS.) Diphtheria used to be a form of severe rhinitis but this is now extremely rare. Hay fever is a distressing form of acute rhinitis. (See HAY FEVER.)

MALFORMATIONS OF THE NOSE are of various kinds. The external nose varies much in shape in different races, even in different families, and it is possible for persons who desire for aesthetic reasons to alter the character of their noses to undergo some form of surgery. This is known as rhinoplasty. As to the interior of the nose, the two cavities are practically never of equal size, the septum almost always bulging to one or other side, so that the passage of air is slightly freer on one side than on the other. When this bulging is so marked that the septum touches the nasal conchae on one side, or when, owing to injury or other cause, spurs and crests have developed on the septum, considerable

1 frontal sinus	6 inferior meatus	11 auditory tube
2 atrium of middle meatus	7 maxilla	12 sphenoethmoidal recess
3 middle nasal concha	8 inferior nasal concha	and higher nasal concha
4 middle meatus	9 soft palate	13 superior nasal concha
5 vestibule	10 sphenoidal sinus	14 superior meatus

The lateral wall of the right half of the nasal cavity.

irritation may arise, and this may form the starting-point for chronic inflammation of the nose, hay fever or asthma. These imperfections, though they often exist without the least ill-effect, and are only discovered accidentally, are readily removed by the specialist if necessary, such operations being attended by but little pain. A more common abnormality is that in which the nose becomes obstructed as the result of nasal polyps, adenoids and other causes and in consequence the person breathes through the mouth.

ADENOIDS means an overgrowth of the glandular tissue which is naturally found in small amount on the back of the upper part of the throat, into which the nose opens.

This glandular tissue is similar in structure to the tonsils and lymphatic glands, and in children may be large enough to obstruct the posterior openings of the nose into the nasopharynx. This obstruction therefore leads to nasal obstruction and may also obstruct the Eustachian tubes.

Generally this overgrowth subsides as the child reaches puberty but the continued enlarged state of the adenoids for a prolonged period of time may produce serious problems for the child's health. This constant obstruction often leads to the typical appearance of the child suffering from enlarged adenoids. The mouth is kept constantly open since breathing proceeds through it and, as a result, the child snores at night. The point of the nose is often pinched and the nostrils narrow, and the bridge of the nose is often flattened. The palate is highly arched and the front teeth often prominent. This condition varies in its severity in that there may be minimal symptoms or there may be significant obstruction with excessive mouth breathing, snoring at night and periods in the night where the child actually stops breathing for short spells. This leads to episodes of hypoxia and may have associated cardiovascular implications. Although the parents often think that the child is sleeping well and is in a deep sleep because of the excessive snoring, the sleep pattern is in fact grossly disturbed and the children are often irritable the next day, they may be somnolent, and performance at school may be affected. The association between enlarged adenoids and Eustachian-tube dysfunction remains controversial, but a substantial number of children with enlarged adenoids do have secretory otitis media (glue ear). Children with a problem of enlarged adenoids and some or all of these symptoms should seek specialist opinion.

If symptoms are severe with the complications mentioned above, operation is usually necessary. The operation is called adenoidectomy and may or may not be associated with tonsillectomy if enlarged tonsils are also contributing to the obstruction of the upper airway.

POLYPI: Nasal polyps are growths of soft, jelly-like character, with more or less of a stalk, usually arising from the ethmoid and maxillary sinuses, but they may also grow from the middle nasal turbinate. They arise from chronic inflammation associated with allergic rhinitis, chronic sinusitis, asthma and aspirin abuse. This chronic inflammation leads to oedema or swelling of the mucous membrane of the nose and paranasal sinuses which becomes so extensive as to produce polypi.

When polyps become large they can cause erosion of the nasal bones and should therefore generally be removed.

BLEEDING FROM THE NOSE, or EPISTAXIS (see HAEMORRHAGE).

FOREIGN BODIES At first the foreign body may set up no reaction and produce no symptoms but, in time, there will be obstruction of the affected nostril, with a foul-smelling discharge, which is often bloody from that side. The foreign body may remain in the nose for years until symptoms are noticed, but the presence of a unilateral foul-smelling bloody discharge should always alert one to the possible presence of a foreign body.

Foreign bodies require removal.

LOSS OF SENSE OF SMELL, or ANOSMIA may be temporary or permanent. Temporary anosmia is caused by conditions of the nose which are reversible, whereas permanent anosmia is caused by conditions which destroy the olefactory nerves. Temporary conditions are those such as the common cold, or other inflammatory conditions of the nasal mucosa or the presence of nasal polyps. Permanent anosmia may follow and influenzal neuritis or it may also follow injuries to the brain and fractures of the skull involving the olfactory nerves.

SINUSITIS is of fairly frequent occurrence and most commonly follows an upper-respiratory-tract infection involving the nose and paranasal sinuses. The maxillary sinus is the sinus most commonly prone to sinus infection, followed by the ethmoid sinuses, then the frontal sinuses and, finally, the cells of the sphenoid sinus. Maxillary sinusitis may also arise from dental infection if the roots of the upper teeth penetrate into the floor of that sinus.

When suppuration occurs in the *frontal sinuses*, severe headache is apt to result as well as discharge from the nose. When suppuration takes place in the *sphenoidal sinuses*, there is constant purulent discharge either from the nose or into the throat, and there may be a state of general debility, or inflammatory changes may be set up in the eye or its optic nerve, which lie in close relation to these sinuses.

Sinusitis is generally treated by the administration of antibiotics and decongestants, preferably topical ones. In more severe cases, it may be necessary to drain the sinus through an opening made between the sinus and the nose.

NOSOLOGY is the term applied to scientific classification of diseases.

NOSTALGIA means a form of melancholy or aggravated home-sickness occurring in persons who have left their home.

NOTIFIABLE DISEASES are diseases, usually of an infectious nature, which are required by law to be made known to a health officer or local authority. (See INFECTION.) Certain occupational diseases (q.v.) are also notifiable.

Notifiable Diseases in the U.K. as at 1 October 1991

Acute encephalitis
Acute poliomyelitis
Anthrax
Cholera
Diphtheria
Dysentery (amoebic or bacillary)
Food poisoning
Lassa fever
Leprosy (reported to Chief Medical Officer at the Department of Health)
Leptospirosis
Malaria
Marburg disease
Measles
Meningitis
Meningococcal septicaemia (without meningitis)
Mumps
Ophthalmia neonatorum
Paratyphoid fever
Plague
Rabies
Relapsing fever
Rubella
Scarlet fever
Smallpox
Tetanus
Tuberculosis
Typhoid fever
Typhus
Viral haemorrhagic fever
Viral hepatitis
Whooping cough
Yellow fever

NOVOBIOCIN is an antibiotic derived from cultures of *Streptomyces spheroides* or *Streptomyces niveus*. It is particularly active against staphylococci, and has proved especially useful in the treatment of staphylococcal infections which have not responded to treatment with other antibiotics, or in which the causative micro-organism is resistant to such antibiotics.

NUCHA is the Latin name for the back of the neck.

NUCLEAR MAGNETIC RESONANCE: A non-invasive method of imaging the body and its organs. It may also be used to study tissue metabolism. The body is placed in a magnetic field which causes certain atomic nuclei to align in the direction of the field. Pulses of radio-frequency radiation are then applied and interpretation of the frequencies absorbed and re-emitted allows an image in any body plane to be built up.

NUCLEAR MEDICINE is that branch of medicine that is concerned with the use of radioactive material in the diagnosis, investigation and treatment of disease.

NUCLEIC ACID is a substance constructed out of units known as nucleotides which consist of a purine or pyrimidine base linked to a pentose sugar which in turn is esterified with phosphoric acid. Two types of nucleic acid occur in nature: deoxyribonucleic acid (DNA) and ribonucleic acid (RNA). (See DNA; RNA.)

NUCLEUS means the central body in a cell, which controls the activities of the latter. (See CELLS.)

NUCLEUS PULPOSUS is the inner core of an intervertebral disc. (See SPINAL COLUMN.)

NULLIPARA is the term applied to a woman who has never borne a child.

NUMBNESS (see TOUCH).

NURSING as a profession requires an elaborate training, although people are often called upon to nurse relatives and friends without any previous experience of the subject. Changes are taking place in the organization and training of nurses and full details about openings in nursing, details of training and of training schools can be obtained from the Royal College of Nursing, 20 Cavendish Square, London W1M 0AB (071-409 3333). The Nurses, Midwives and Health Visitors Act 1979 led to the establishment of a United Kingdom Central Council and four National Boards for nursing, midwifery and health visiting. The Central Council, supported by the Boards, has responsibility for registration and the setting and maintaining of standards of education and of conduct of nurses, midwives and health visitors throughout the United Kingdom. Over 380,000 nurses were employed in the NHS in England in 1989.

NUTRITION: The process by which the living organism physiologically absorbs and used food to ensure growth, energy production and repair of tissues. The science of nutrition includes the study of diets and deficiency diseases (see DIET).

NUX VOMICA is the seed of *Strychnos nux-vomica*, an East Indian tree. It has an intensely bitter taste. The medicinal properties of the plant are almost entirely due to two alkaloids, strychnine and brucine, which it contains. (See STRYCHNINE.)

NYSTAGMUS (see EYE, DISEASE AND INJURIES).

NYSTATIN is an antibiotic isolated from *Streptomyces noursei*. It was the first antibiotic to be isolated which was active against fungus diseases, and is proving particularly useful in the treatment of moniliasis (q.v.).

O

OAT CELL: A type of cell found in one highly malignant form of lung cancer. The cell is small and either oval or round. The nucleus stains darkly and the cytoplasm is sparse and difficult to identify. Oat-cell carcinoma of the bronchus is usually caused by smoking and comprises around 30 per cent of all bronchial cancers. It responds to radiotherapy and chemotherapy but, because the growth has usually spread widely by the time it is diagnosed, the prognosis is poor. Results of surgery are unsatisfactory.

OBESITY is a condition in which the energy stores of the body (mainly fat) are too large. It is a prevalent nutritional disorder in prosperous countries. The Quetelet Index or Body Mass Index (BMI), which relates weight in kilograms (W) to height^2 in metres (H^2), is a widely accepted way of classifying obesity in adults according to severity, e.g.

Grade of obseity	BMI (W/H^2)
III	>40
II	30–40
I	25–29·9
not obese	<25

There is no advantage in further classifying obesity according to frame size since this does not improve the accuracy with which levels of body fat are predicted.

Causes: For obesity to occur, energy intake must exceed energy output over a sufficiently long period of time. All aetiological factors must ultimately act by reducing energy output or increasing energy intake or both.

Obesity tends to aggregate in families. This has led to the suggestion that some people inherit a 'thrifty' gene which predisposes them to obesity in later life by lowering their energy output. Indeed patients often attribute their obesity to such a metabolic defect. Total energy output is made up of the resting metabolic rate (RMR), which represents about 70 per cent of the total, the energy cost of physical activity and thermogenesis, i.e. the increase in energy output in response to food intake, cold exposure, some drugs and psychological influences. In general, obese people are consistently found to have a higher RMR and total energy output, per person and also when expressed against fat-free mass, than do their lean counterparts. Most obese people do not appear to have a reduced capacity for thermogenesis. Although a genetic component to obesity remains a possibility, it is unlikely to be great or to prevent weight loss from being possible in most patients by reducing energy intake. Environmental influences are believed to be more important in explaining the familial association in obesity.

An inactive lifestyle is thought to play a minor role in the development of obesity, but it remains unclear if people are obese because they are inactive or are inactive because they are obese.

For the majority of obese people a reduction in energy output does not appear to be the main aetiological factor. It follows then that the explanation must lie in an excessive energy intake. Unfortunately, it is difficult to demonstrate this directly since the methods used to assess habitual energy intake are unreliable. For most obese people it seems likely that the defect lies in their failure to regulate energy intake in response to a variety of cognitive factors (i.e. ease of fitting of clothes) in the long term.

Rarely, obesity has an endocrine basis and is caused by hypothyroidism, hypopituitarism, hypogonadism or Cushing's syndrome (qq.v.)
Symptoms: Obesity has adverse effects on morbidity and mortality which are greatest in young adults and increase with the severity of obesity. It is associated with an increased mortality and/or morbidity from cardiovascular disease, non-insulin-dependent diabetes mellitus, diseases of the gall bladder, osteoarthritis, hernia, gout and possibly certain cancers (i.e. colon, rectum and prostate in men, and breast, ovary, endometrium and cervix in women). Menstrual irregularities and ovulatory failure are often experienced by obese women. Obese people are also at greater risk when they undergo surgery. With the exception of gallstone formation, weight loss will reduce these health risks.
Treatment: Creation of an energy deficit is essential for weight loss to occur. An average deficit of 1000 kcal/day will produce a loss of 1 kg of fat/week and should be aimed for. Theoretically, this can be achieved by increasing energy expenditure or reducing energy intake. In practice, a low-energy diet is the usual form of treatment since attempts to increase energy expenditure, either by physical exercise or a thermogenic drug, are relatively ineffective.

Anorectic drugs, gastric stapling and jaw wiring are sometimes used to treat severe obesity. They are said to aid compliance with a low-energy diet by either reducing hunger (anorectic drugs) or limiting the amount of food the patient can eat. Unfortunately, the long-term effectiveness of gastric stapling is not known and it is debatable if the modest reduction in weight achieved by use of anorectic drugs is worthwhile. For some grossly obese patients jaw wiring can be helpful but a regain of weight once the wires are removed must be prevented. Fitting a waist cord as a means of alerting a person to an increase in weight may help to maintain weight loss.

OBSESSION in medicine means the sudden domination of the mind by an idea or emotion, leading to impulsive acts which are beyond the control of the will, the power of judgment being for a time lost. (See MENTAL ILLNESS.)

OBSTETRICS means the art of midwifery. (See LABOUR.)

OBSTIPATION: Severe constipation.

OBSTRUCTION OF THE BOWELS (see INTESTINE, DISEASES OF).

OCCIPUT is the lower and hinder part of the head where it merges into the neck.

OCCLUSION: The way that the teeth fit together when the jaws close. Also the closing or obstruction of a duct, hollow organ, or blood vessel.

OCCULT: Describing something that is not easily seen. Occult blood in the faeces is present in very small amounts and can be identified only by a chemical test or under the microscope.

OCCUPATIONAL DISEASES: Work has been the cause of human illness and injury for centuries. The earliest accounts concentrated on the rigours of underground mining where, in earliest times, the risks to health were severe enough to relegate such 'occupations' to slaves and criminals. Such activities are inherently dangerous but the advent of industrialization widened and broadened the range of health risks to which employed people could be exposed. Control of workplace exposures in modern industrialized society has limited the toll of disease and injury but cannot abolish it entirely.

In the country such as Britain with 30 million employable people, over 400 are killed and another 150,000 injured each year as a direct result of work. One in 4,500 develops an occupational disease annually. By contrast, the Scandinavian figures for occupational disease are ten time 'worse'. Such differences are more to do with reporting criteria than true differences in occupational health. Whilst compensation for such disease rests with government social-security departments, the control of workplace hazards is in the hands of labour inspectorates. In Britain, this responsibility lies in the Department of Employment with the Health and Safety Commission and its Executive. The Executive includes both inspectorates and a medical division staffed by doctors and nurses who have responsibility for giving advise to employers and employees on workplace risk to health in relation to health and safety legislation. Increasingly the laws governing health and safety at work are moving into a European arena as the European Commission promulgates directives which are binding on member states. Although a new European list of compensatable occupational diseases is currently being drafted, member states have widely differing criteria. What follows are brief notes on the numerically more important compensatable occupational diseases in the United Kingdom.

Inhaled materials: PNEUMOCONIOSIS covers a group of diseases which cause fibrotic lung disease following the inhalation of dust. Around 500 new cases receive benefit each year – mostly due to coal dust with or without silica contamination. Silicosis is the more severe disease. The contraction in the size of the coal-mining industry as well as improved dust suppression in the mines have diminished the importance of this disease, whereas *asbestos-related diseases* now exceed 1,000 per year. Asbestos fibres cause a restrictive lung disease but also are responsible for certain malignant conditions such as pleural and peritoneal mesothelioma and lung cancer. The lung-cancer risk is exacerbated by cigarette smoking.

OCCUPATIONAL ASTHMA is of increasing importance – not only because of the recognition of new allergic agents but also in the number of reported cases. Twenty-two specific agents are listed at present of which the most common offending agents are isocyanates, flour and other grain dusts, soldering flux, epoxy resins and wood dusts. Other notable allergens are platinum salts, proteolytic enzymes, arthropods and crustaceans, antibiotics and reactive dyes. The disease develops after a short symptomless period of exposure and symptoms are temporally related to work exposures and relieved by absences from work. Removal of the worker from exposure does not necessarily lead to complete cessation of symptoms. For many agents, there is no relationship with a previous history of atopy (q.v.). Occupational asthma now accounts for about 10 per cent of all asthma cases.

BYSSINOSIS is considered by many authorities to be a variant of occupational asthma. The condition is, however, broader and more complex than this. In susceptible individuals, exposure to the dusts of cotton, sisal, hemp, or flax can cause acute dyspnoea with cough and reversible airways obstruction. It is first noticed on the first day of the working week and then subsides. Later, with continued exposure, symptoms recur on subsequent days of the week until even weekends and holidays are not free of symptoms.

Other organic dusts can produce extrinsic allergic alveolitis with resultant lowering of respiratory gas transfer in the alveoli. Most of the agents causing this condition are fungal spores and the most common condition in Britain is FARMER'S LUNG (SEE ALVEOLITIS). These diseases frequently start as an influenza-like illness and, if exposure is continued, lead to subacute and chronic pulmonary fibrotic disease.

Dermatitis: The risk of dermatitis caused by an allergic or irritant reaction to substances used or handled at work is present in a wide variety of jobs. This condition is the commonest of all the occupational diseases. Whilst changes in the compensation criteria over the last twenty years have reduced successful claims from 11,000 a year to a few hundred, general-practice-based

Cause	Occupation	Disease
Coal dust	Coal mining	Coal-workers' pneumoconiosis
Silica	Gold mining	Silicosis
	Iron and steel industries (metal casting)	
	Metal grinding	
	Stone dressing	
	Pottery	
Asbestos	Asbestos mining	Asbestosis
	Manufacturer of fireproof and insulating materials	
Iron oxide	Arc welding	Siderosis
Tin dioxide	Tin ore mining	Stannosis
Beryllium	Aircraft and atomic energy industries	Berylliosis
Cotton, flax or hemp dust	Textile industries	Byssinosis
Fungal spores from mouldy hay, straw or grain, bagasse, mushroom compost	Agriculture and related industries	Farmer's lung
		Metalworker's lung
		Bagassosis
		Mushroom worker's lung

Some occupational lung diseases. Davidson and Macleod.

surveys suggest that over 50,000 new cases are diagnosed each year. About three-quarters of these cases are irritant-contact dermatitis due to such agents as acids, alkalis and even soap and water. Allergic contact dermatitis is a more specific response by susceptible individuals to a range of allergens. The main occupational contact allergens include chromates, nickel, epoxy resins, rubber additives, germicidal agents, dyes, topical anaesthetics and antibiotics as well as certain plants and woods.

Musculo-skeletal disorders: Apart from the commonest problems of injured backs from manual handling, there are two groups of disorders caused by repeated injury – the 'beat' conditions and work-related upper-limb disorders. The *beat conditions* such as beat knee and beat elbow are caused by repeated damage to a joint from kneeling or crawling – problems associated with mining and carpet-laying, for example. The *work-related upper-limb disorders* range from clear-cut occupationally induced repetitive movement conditions such as tendinitis, tenosynovitis (q.v.), carpal tunnel syndrome (q.v.) and epicondylitis to less well-defined disorders of prolonged or repetitive posture disturbances which may lead to shoulder or cervical spine discomfort. These disorders are common in the general population and their occupational attribution is frequently controversial. Particular high-risk occupations include poultry processors, packers, electronic assembly workers, data processors, supermarket check-out operators and telephonists. These jobs often contain a number of the relevant exposures of dynamic load, static load, a full or excessive range of movements and awkward postures.

Physical agents: A number of physical agents cause occupational ill health of which most important is *occupational deafness*. Workplace noise exposures in excess of 85 decibels for a working day are likely to cause damage to hearing which is initially restricted to the vital frequencies associated with speech – around 3–4 KHz. Protection from such noise is imperative as hearing aids do nothing to ameliorate the neural damage once it has occurred.

Hand–arm vibration syndrome is a disorder of the vascular and/or neural endings in the hands leading to episodic blanching and numbness which is exacerbated by low temperature. The condition, which is caused by vibrating tools such as chain saws and pneumatic hammers, is akin to Raynaud's disease (q.v.) and can be disabling.

Decompression sickness is caused by a rapid change in ambient pressure and is a disease associated with deep-sea divers, tunnel workers and high-flying aviators. Apart from the direct effects of pressure change such as ruptured tympanic membrane or sinus pain, the more serious damage is indirectly due to nitrogen bubbles appearing in the blood and blocking small vessels. Central and peripheral nervous-system damage and bone necrosis are the most dangerous sequelae.

Radiation: *Non-ionizing radiation* from lasers or microwaves can cause severe localized heating leading to tissue damage of which cataracts are a particular variety. *Ionizing radiation* from radioactive sources can cause similar acute tissue damage to the eyes as well as cell damage to rapidly dividing cells in the gut and bone marrow. Longer-term effects include genetic damage and various malignant disorders of which leukaemia and aplastic anaemia are notable. Particular radioactive isotopes may destroy or induce malignant change in target organs, for example, I^{131} (thyroid), Sr^{90} (bone).

Other occupational cancers: Occupation is directly responsible for about 5 per cent of all cancers and contributes to a further 5 per cent. Apart from the cancers caused by asbestos and ionising radiation, a number of other occupational exposures can cause human cancer. The International Agency for Research on Cancer lists 50 agents or processes of which occupational agents or processes account for 31. The more important of these are polynuclear aromatic hydrocarbons such as mineral oils, soots, tars (skin and lung cancer), the aromatic amines in dyestuffs (bladder cancer), certain hexavalent chromates, arsenic and nickel refining (lung cancer), wood and leather dust (nasal sinus cancer), benzene (leukaemia) and vinyl chloride monomer (angiosarcoma of the liver). Elimination of all known occupational carcinogens, if possible, would lead to an annual saving of 5,000 premature deaths in Britain.

Infections: Two broad categories of job carry an occupational risk. These are workers in contact with animals (farmers, veterinary surgeons and slaughtermen) and those in contact with human sources of infection (health care staff and sewage workers). Estimates of current annual incidences of work related cases are leptospirosis (q.v.) (40 cases), tuberculosis (q.v.) (30 cases), hepatitis B (q.v.) (25 cases), chlamydiosis (see CHLAMYDIA) (16 cases), Q fever (q.v.) (12 cases), brucellosis (q.v.) (10 cases). The less severe orf (q.v.) accounts for at least 50 cases but this is even more of an underestimate than the figures for the other diseases. Other compensatable infections are anthrax, glanders, ancylostomiasis (qq.v.), streptococcus suis, and hydatidosis.

Poisonings: In earlier decades, chemical poisonings by lead, phosphorus, arsenic, mercury, cadmium and a number of organic solvents were much more common. Today, around 2,000 poisonings are reported annually with 20–30 fatalities. The commonest agents are now solvents, gases, acids, alkalis and irritant vapours. The lead regulations specify that persons with blood lead levels above 69μg/100 ml (above 39 for females of reproductive age) should be suspended from working with lead. In 1989–90, of 22,000 male lead workers, there were 534 suspensions. The success in diminishing morbidity is largely one of prevention.

Prevention: There are certain principles of prevention which, if followed, can significantly diminish the risk of occupationally induced diseases. Indeed as these diseases cannot be eliminated from the world – in comparison with smallpox – prevention is the utmost importance. This is a hierachy of control measures. The ideal solution is elimination of the offending substance or process. Failing this, substitution by a less hazardous material or process could be undertaken and/or more effective enclosure or exhaust ventilation, thereby diminishing exposure of the worker. The least satisfactory method is personal protection for the worker.

OCCUPATIONAL THERAPY is the treatment of physical and psychiatric conditions through specific selected activities in order to help people reach their maximum level of function and independence in all aspects of daily life.

Occupational therapists work from hospital and community bases. They do much more than keep patients occupied with diverting hobbies. The arts and crafts still have a place in modern therapy techniques but these now also include household chores, industrial work, communication techniques, social activities, sports and educational programmes. An Occupational Therapy Department may have facilities for woodwork, metalwork, printing, gardening, cooking, art and drama. Occupational thera-

pists will use any combination of activities to strengthen muscles, increase movement and restore co-ordination and balance. With mentally ill people similar activies are used. They help provide order, comfort and support and aim to build up self-confidence. Occupational therapists plan courses of treatment which are individually tailored to the needs of the patient. The aim is to help the patient practise all the activites involved in daily life. The therapists are part of a team including doctors, nurses, social workers, home helps, housing officers, physiotherapists, speech therapists and psychologists. Occupational therapists are mainly employed by the National Health Service and by Local Authority Social Services and they work in hospitals, special centres and in the handicapped person's own home. State Registration is essential for employment as an occupational therapists. There are 15 occupational therapy schools in the United Kingdom where the course leading to the diploma of the College of Occupational Therapists can be followed. The course lasts three academic years. (See REHABILITATION; REMPLOY.)

OCHRONOSIS is a rare condition in which the ligaments and cartilages of the body, and sometimes the conjunctiva, become stained by dark brown or black pigment. This may occur in chronic carbolic poisoning, or in a congenital disorder of metabolism in which the individual is unable to break down completely the tyrosine of the protein molecule, the intermediate product, homogentisic acid, appearing in the urine – this being known as alkaptonuria.

OEDEMA means an abnormal accumulation offluid beneath the skin, or in one or more of the cavities of the body.

Causes: Oedema is not a disease, although this is a popular idea, supported by the fact that at one time many deaths were recorded as due to 'dropsy' without a further statement of the cause. Oedema may be due to one of three conditions: (1) weakening of the walls of the capillary vessels, by injury of the part in which oedema occurs, by ill-health of the body generally, by poverty of the blood circulating through and nourishing the vessels, or by poisonous materials in the blood; (2) obstruction to the blood-flow through the veins; (3) a watery condition of the blood allowing fluid to escape through the capillary walls. Oedema may also result from obstruction to the flow of lymph in the lymph channels.

Heart disease, which produces increased pressure in the veins, and also an impaired circulation of the blood, in consequence of the defective pumping action of the heart, and *glomerulonephritis* in which the kidneys fail in their functions of excreting poisonous substances and a certain amount of water from the blood, are the main causes of general oedema. In heart disease the oedema is more marked after exertion; in kidney disease it is found chiefly after resting. Thus one of the chief characters of oedema due to glomerulonephritis is that it appears in the morning, affects loose tissues like the skin beneath the eyes, and passes off as the day advances. Oedema due to heart disease, on the other hand, tends to appear towards evening, affects dependent parts like the feet, and diminishes during the night.

In *hunger oedema* due to diminution of the amount of protein in the blood as a result of starvation, the oedema is generalized, but in the earlier stages is most marked in the feet and legs, especially after exertion. The swelling which sometimes follows snake bites, bee-stings or the eating of poisonous shell-fish, and constitutes an extreme and rapidly ensuing form of *nettle-rash*, is a special variety of oedema. *White-leg*, which may appear after some acute disease like typhoid fever or pneumonia, or after the birth of a child, due to a thrombosis or plugging of the main vein in the affected limb, is one of the localized forms of oedema. A similar condition may be caused by a *tumour* pressing upon a large vein of the arm or leg. Oedema in the legs may be due to varicose veins. *Cirrhosis*, tumours, and other diseases of the liver may, by interference with the circulation through it, cause oedema, first of the abdomen and later of the lower limbs.

Treatment: There is no general treatment which will meet every case. The particular cause has, in each case, to be removed. Oedema due to heart or kidney disease yields as the disease producing it is alleviated. In cases of localized oedema, elevation of the oedematous part is of great importance, and the person should adopt the recumbent position. In the case of heart disease, digitalis, which improves the action of the heart, and benzothiadiazine diuretics form the chief means employed. In acute kidney disease the treatment of the oedema consists in the routine treatment of glomerulonephritis. In oedema due to liver conditions, occasional purges with blue-pill or calomel may help the condition. When the oedema will not yield to drugs, some of the fluid may have to be drawn off (see ASPIRATION); when this is done partially, the kidneys are sometimes enabled to cope with the remainder of the fluid.

OEDEMA OF THE LUNGS results when the left ventricular myocardium is unable to handle the blood delivered to it. There is an abrupt increase in the venous and capillary pressure in the pulmonary vessels followed by flooding of fluid into the interstitial spaces and alveoli. The commonest cause of acute pulmonary oedema is myocardial infarction which reduces the ability of the left ventricular myocardial muscle to handle the blood delivered to it. Pulmonary oedema may result from other causes of left ventricular failure such as hypertension or valvular disease of the mitral and aortic valves. The initial symptoms are cough with breathlessness and occasionally with wheezing. The patient becomes extremely short of breath with a sensation of imminent death. In a severe attack the patient is pale, sweating and cyanosed and obviously gasping for breath. Frequently frothy sputum is produced which may be blood stained.

OEDIPUS COMPLEX: A description used by psychoanalysts of the subconscious attraction of a child for its parent of the opposite sex. This is accompanied by a wish to get rid of the parent of the same sex. The origin of the phrase lies in the Greek story in which Oedipus kills his father without realizing who he is and then marries his mother.

OESOPHAGOSCOPE is an instrument constructed on the principle of the telescope, which is passed down the oesophagus and enables the observer to see the state of the oesophagus. (See ENDOSCOPE.)

OESOPHAGUS, or GULLET, is the tube which conveys the food and drink from the throat down to the stomach. It begins above at the level of the sixth cervical vertebra, and, lying close against the left side and front of the spinal column, passes downward through the neck and chest to pierce the diaphragm, and then opens into the stomach. It consists of three coats: a strong outer coat of muscle fibres in two layers, the outer running lengthwise, the inner being circular; inside this a loose connective tissue coat containing blood-vessels, glands, and nerves; and finally a strong mucous membrane lined by epithelium, which closely resembles that of the mouth and skin.

OESOPHAGUS, DISEASES OF: The oesophagus, or gullet, may be the seat of catarrhal or inflammatory conditions causing discomfort in swallowing, but the more important ailments are those which arise from local injuries, such as the swallowing of scalding or corrosive substances. This may cause ulceration followed by the formation of a scar which narrows the passage and produces the symptoms of *stricture* of the oesophagus: namely, pain and difficulty in swallowing, with regurgitation of the food. In all cases of organic stricture the food does not necessarily return at once, but seems as if it has passed into the stomach. In reality, however, it has passed into the dilated or pouched portion of the gullet, which is almost always present immediately above the seat of stricture, where it remains until, from its amount, it regurgitates back into the mouth, when it can be seen, by the absence of any evidence of digestion, that it has never been in the stomach. The severity of the case will necessarily depend upon the amount of narrowing and consequent mechanical obstruction, but in some instances this has occurred to such an extent as practically to close the canal. Cases of oesophageal stricture of this kind may sometimes be dilated by the use of suitable instruments.

A still more serious and frequent cause of oesophageal stricture is that due to *cancer*, which may occur at any part, but is most common at the lower end, in the vicinity of the entrance into the stomach. The chief symptoms of this condition are increasing difficulty in the passage downwards of the food, steady decline in strength, together with enlargement of the glands in the neck. The diagnosis is rendered the more certain by the absence of any cause, such as local injury, for the formation of a stricture, and by the age (as a rule at or beyond middle life). Traditionally it is said to be much more common in men than women, but of the 3572 fatal cases in England in 1980, 1518 were in women, compared with 2054 in men. In many cases treatment can only be palliative, but recent advances in surgery are producing promising results. In some cases treatment with irradiation produces relief, if not cure. In those in whom neither operation nor radiation can be performed life may be prolonged and freedom from pain obtained by fluid food which is either swallowed or passed down a tube. The operation of gastrostomy, by which an opening is made through the front of the abdomen, allows food to be directly introduced into the stomach.

Strictures of the oesophagus may also be produced by the pressure of tumours or aneurysms within the cavity of the chest but external to the gullet.

An important cause of difficulty in swallowing is the condition known as *cardiospasm* or *achalasia of the cardia*. The latter is the more accurate description as the condition is due to failure of the cardiac sphincter (the sphincter at the lower end of the oesophagus) to relax when food is swallowed. The cause is not known. The condition occurs usually in young adults, who complain of food sticking behind the chestbone. This results in vomiting and, of course, loss of weight. Treatment consists of passing special bougies down the oesophagus to dilate the sphincter. As this may need to be done before every meal for several months, the patient learns to pass the bougie himself. Such treatment, though prolonged, is usually successful.

Finally, difficulty in swallowing sometimes occurs in certain serious nervous diseases from paralysis affecting the nerves supplying the muscular coats of the pharynx, which thus loses its propulsive power (*bulbar paralysis*). When such complications occur, they usually denote an advanced stage of the brain disease with which they are connected, and a speedily fatal termination.

Foreign bodies which lodge in the respiratory part of the throat, i.e. at the entrance to, or in the cavity of, the larynx, set up immediate symptoms of choking. (See CHOKING.) Those which lodge in the gullet, on the contrary, do not usually set up any immediately serious symptoms, although their presence causes considerable discomfort. Such bodies are divided, for practical purposes, into two classes. One class includes smooth bodies like coins or fruit stones, which may be pushed down into the stomach or pulled up into the mouth by means of a bougie or a special instrument known as a coin-catcher, or, better still, by forceps passed down under the direct guidance of the oesophagoscope. The other, and more dangerous, class comprises bodies which are too large to be pushed down into the stomach and safely passed by the bowels, or too rough to be pulled back into the mouth, such as large pieces of bone, or large plates of artificial teeth. In cases in which it is impossible to dislodge a foreign body up or down, it becomes necessary to perform an operation in order to remove the body from the gullet directly through the side of the neck.

OESTRADIOL is the name given to the oestrogenic hormone secreted by the ovarian follicle. Oestradiol is responsible for the development of the female sexual characteristics, of the breasts, and of part of the changes that take place in the uterus before menstruation.

OESTRADIOL VALERATE (see OESTROGEN).

OESTRIOL (see OESTROGEN).

OESTROGEN is the term applied to any substance that will induce oestrus or 'heat'. In human medicine it is applied to the substances, natural or synthetic, that induce the changes in the uterus that precede ovulation. They are also responsible for the development of the secondary sex characteristics in women: that is the physical changes that take place in a girl at puberty, such as enlargement of the breasts, appearance of pubic and axillary hair and the deposition of fat on the thighs and hips. They are used in the management of disturbances of the menopause, and also in the treatment of cancer of the prostate and certain cases of cancer of the breast.

The oestrogenic hormones of the ovary are oestradiol and oestrone and they are interconvertible. The natural oestrogens, like the hormones of the testis and the adrenal cortex, are steroids. They are rapidly metabolized in the body and excreted in the urine as inactive conjugates. The rapid degradation of natural oestrogens limits their use as therapeutic agents. Chemical substitution of the steroid molecule, as in ethinyl oestradiol, or the use of a non-steroidal synthetic oestrogen such as stilboestrol, greatly reduces the rate of degradation and enhances the therapeutic action. A further development has been the use of compounds which are not actually oestrogenic themselves, but which are slowly metabolized to oestrogenic substances, or substances such as chlorotrianisene, which are taken up in the body fat and then slowly released into the circulation. There is in fact little to choose between the various synthetic oestrogens. Preparations such as equine oestrogens or chlorotrianisene have little therapeutic advantage and are considerably more expensive. Ethinyl oestradiol is the most potent oral oestrogen, being twenty times more active than stilboestrol.

The following oestrogens are in therapeutic use: chlorotrianisene, cyclofenil, cyproterone, dinoestrol, equine oestrogens, ethinyl oestradiol, hexoestrol, methallenoestril, oestradiol valerate, oestriol, oestrone, piperazine oestrone sulphate, quinestradol, stilboestrol, stilboestrol diphosphate, quinestrol.

OESTRONE (see OESTROGEN).

OFFICE OF POPULATION CENSUSES AND SURVEYS: A central government department in the United Kingdom that compiles and publishes statistics of local and national populations as well as the demography of births, marriages, and deaths. It also records the medical cause of deaths. Every ten years the OPCS conducts a national survey of the population on a particular night. The figures it provides are used by other government departments and local authorities for planning services for the public.

OINTMENTS are semi-solid mixtures of medicinal substances with lard, benzoated lard, paraffin or yellow soft paraffin, and wool- fat (lanolin), intended for external application. They are used for three main purposes: (i) as emollients, that is to soften the skin; (ii) as a protective preparation to be applied to the skin; (iii) as a means for the local application of medicaments to be absorbed through the skin.

Other substances occasionally used to form the body of an ointment are almond oil, beeswax, camphor, glycerin, oleic acid, spermaceti, and prepared suet.

Among the most useful ointments are the following: *Simple Ointment* BP, which contains 5 per cent each of wool fat, hard paraffin, and cetostearyl acid in white or yellow soft paraffin, and is used for application to chafed surfaces. *Cold Cream*, made of beeswax, spermaceti, almond oil, rose water, and attar of rose, is used for a similar purpose. *Zinc and Castor Oil Ointment* BP, which contains 7·5 per cent zinc oxide and 50 per cent w/w castor oil has a well-earned reputation for the prevention and treatment of napkin rash. *Mercuric Oxide Eye Ointment* BPC, or yellow oxide of mercury eye ointment as it is sometimes known, is used for treating inflammation about the eye.

OLD AGE (see AGE, NATURAL CHANGES IN).

OLEANDOMYCIN is an antibiotic derived from *Streptomyces antibioticus*. It is active against many Gram-positive micro-organisms and some Gram-negative micro-organisms.

OLEIC ACID is the commonest of naturally occurring fatty acids, being present in most fats and oils in the form of triglyceride. It is used in the preparation of ointments, but not eye ointments.

OLFACTORY NERVE, the nerve of smell, is the first cranial nerve.

OLIGAEMIA means a diminution of the quantity of blood in the circulation.

OLIGOMENORRHOEA is infrequent menstruation.

OLIGURIA means an abnormally low excretion of urine, such as occurs in acute nephritis.

OLIVE OIL is the oil obtained by pressure from the fruit of *Olea europaea*. It is practically a pure fat.

OMENTUM is a long fold of peritoneal membrane, generally loaded with more or less fat, which hangs down within the abdominal cavity in front of the bowels. It is formed by the layers of peritoneum that cover the front and back surfaces of the stomach in their passage from the lower margin of this organ to cover the back and front surfaces of the large intestine. Instead of passing straight from one organ to the other, these layers dip down and form a sort of fourfold apron. It is to the increasing deposit of fat in this structure that the prominence of the abdomen is largely due in people of middle age who are large eaters. This omentum is known as the greater omentum, to distinguish it from two smaller peritoneal folds, one of which passes between the liver and stomach (the hepatogastric omentum), and the other between the liver and duodenum (the hepatoduodenal omentum). Together they are known as the lesser omentum.

OMPHALOCELE is another name for exomphalos – a hernia of abdominal organs through the umbilicus.

ONCHOCERCIASIS is infestation with the filarial worm, *Onchocerca volvulus*. It is found in many parts of tropical Africa south of the Sahara, in Central and South America, and in the Yemen and Saudi Arabia. It is estimated that there are more than 20 million victims of it. It is transmitted by gnats of the genus *Simulium*. After a period of nine to eighteen months, the young filarial worms, injected into the body by the bite of an infected *Simulium*, mature, mate and start producing young microfilariae. The females live for up to fifteen years and during this period each may produce several thousand microfilariae a day. It is these microfilariae, which have a life-span of up to two years, that produce the characteristic features of the disease: an itching rash of the skin and the appearance of nodules in different parts of the body. There may also be involvement of the eyes and the worm may invade the optic nerve and so cause blindness; hence the name of African river blindness. Treatment consists of diethylcarbamazine and suramin. An international campaign is now under way in an attempt to destroy *Simulium* in the affected zones. Meanwhile the only means of prevention is to avoid so far as possible being bitten by the gnat. One means of achieving this is by wearing long trousers, shoes and socks.

ONCOGENE is a specific segment of DNA (q.v.) which confers the property of malignancy.

ONCOLOGY is that part of medical science which is concerned with the management of malignant disease such as cancer.

ONYCHIA means an inflammation affecting the nails. (See NAILS, DISEASES OF.)

ONYCHOGRYPHOSIS is a distortion of the nail in which it is much thickened, overgrown and twisted on itself. This usually affects a toenail and is the result of chronic irritation and inflammation.

ONYCHOLYSIS means separation of the nail from the nail-bed.

OÖCYTE: An immature ovum (q.v.). When the cell undergoes meiosis in the ovary it becomes an ovum and is ready for fertilization by the spermatozoa. Only a small number of the many oöcytes produced survive until puberty (q.v.), and not all of them will become ova and be ejected into the fallopian tubes (q.v.).

OÖPHORECTOMY is a term applied to removal, by operation, of an ovary. When the ovary is removed for the presence of a cyst, the term ovariotomy is usually employed.

OÖPHORITIS is another name for ovaritis or inflammation of an ovary.

OÖPHORON is another name for the ovary.

OPHTHALMOLOGY: The study of the structure and function of the eye and the diagnosis and treatment of the diseases that affect it.

OPHTHALMOPLEGIA means paralysis of the muscles of the eye. Internal ophthalmoplegia refers to paralysis of the iris and ciliary body, external ophthalmoplegia refers to paralysis of one or all of the muscles that move the eyes.

OPHTHALMOSCOPE: An instrument for examining the interior of the eye. There are different types of ophthalmoscope, all have a light source to illuminate the inside of the eye and a magnifying lens to make examination easier.

OPIATE is a preparation of opium (q.v.).

OPIOID: A substance with a pharmacological action that is like that of opium or its derivatives.

OPIPRAMOL is a drug with antidepressant properties.

OPISTHOTONOS is the name given to a position assumed by the body during one of the convulsive seizures of tetanus. The muscles of the back, by their spasmodic contraction, arch the body in such a way that the person for a time may rest upon the bed only by his heels and head.

OPIUM is the dried juice of the unripe seed-capsules of the white Indian poppy, *Papaver somniferum*. It is cultivated mainly in India, but it is also produced in Iran, China, and the Asiatic provinces of Turkey. Opium possesses its medicinal properties only when produced

optic disc
optic cup
fovea centralis
retinal artery
retinal vein

View through an ophthalmoscope of the fundus of the right eye.

under favourable conditions of soil and climate, and the juice of other species of poppies grown in temperate climates is almost useless. The juice is obtained by scarifying the seed-capsules of the poppies before they are ripe, and next day collecting the gummy sap which has exuded from the cuts. This is dried with great care, kneaded, and carefully tested. Good opium should contain about 10 per cent of morphine, to which its action is chiefly due. It is a brown, resinous-looking substance, or brown powder, with characteristic smell and bitter taste. The action of opium depends upon the twenty to twenty-five alkaloids it contains. Of these, the chief is morphine, the amount of which varies from around 9 to 17 per cent. Other alkaloids include codeine, narcotine, thebaine, papaverine, and naceine, and as the action of these differs considerably, the effect of the opium naturally varies according to the proportion of each that it contains. Turkish opium, which is purest in morphine, is generally regarded as the best, the use of Indian opium, which contains a large proportion of narcotine, being more apt to cause sickness. Opium, which is exported from the country of its production in balls or cakes, is often adulterated with sugar, vegetable extracts, gum, molasses, and even stones concealed in the middle of the cakes, and it is therefore very carefully tested before sale.

The importation into Britain of opium is very carefully regulated under the *Dangerous Drugs Acts*. Similar regulations govern the sale and distribution of any preparation of morphine or diamorphine (heroin) stronger than 1 part in 500.

The alkaloids, morphine and codeine, are administered in various forms. Morphine hydrochloride and morphine sulphate are given in doses from 7·5 to 20 mg; codeine phosphate in doses from 10 to 60 mg. Morphine hydrochloride solution (containing 1 per cent of morphine) is used in doses from 0·5 to 2 ml.
Action: The action of opium varies considerably, according to the source of the drug and the preparation used; it varies even more according to the age, race, and temperament of the individual. Children are profoundly affected by even the smallest doses, so that the drug is unsuited for use, except with great care, during childhood.

In small doses, opium produces a state of gentle excitement, the person finding his imagination more vivid, his thoughts more brilliant, and his power of expression greater than usual. This stage lasts for some hours, and is succeeded by languor. In larger, i.e. medicinal, doses this stage of excitement is short and is followed by deep sleep, from which the person can still be aroused as from natural sleep. When very large, i.e. poisonous, doses are taken, sleep comes on quickly, and passes into coma and death. The habitual use of opium produces great tolerance, so that opium users require to take large quantities daily before experiencing its pleasurable effects. The need for opium also confers tolerance, so that people suffering great pain may take, with apparently little effect

beyond dulling the pain, quantities which at another time would be dangerous.

It checks all secretions, except the sweat, and slows the processes of tissue change, this action being sometimes useful, sometimes a hindrance to its employment. (See DRUG ADDICTION.)

OPIUM POISONING: Perhaps there is no drug in which the amount that can produce serious consequences varies so much as in the case of opium.
Symptoms: When a poisonous dose of any of the preparations of the drug has been taken, sleep rapidly comes on, becomes deeper and deeper, and passes gradually into a state of complete insensibility, usually within half-an-hour, although the effect may be postponed for several hours, particularly when the drug is taken along with alcoholic liquor. Convulsions sometimes occur, especially in children, and vomiting may take place before sleep becomes deep, or as the person is recovering. The breathing is slow, quiet, and shallow; and these characteristics become more and more marked as death approaches, the person dying, indeed, as the result of paralysis of the respiratory centre in the brain. The lips and face become livid and covered with cold sweat, and the pupils are much contracted. As a rule, death occurs in from seven to eighteen hours after the dose has been taken.
Treatment: An emetic should be given as soon as possible (see EMETICS), and after this has acted, a cup of strong coffee should be swallowed. Even after an emetic has acted, and certainly if it fails to act, the stomach should be washed out with water containing potassium permanganate, which destroys the alkaloids of the opium. As an antidote, full doses of naloxone, levallorphan or nalorphine should be given. Should none of these be immediately available, injections of caffeine sodium benzoate or nikethamide may be given.

It is important to keep the patient awake. Strong coffee, and other stimulants may be given internally. If, in spite of all these measures, he becomes unconscious and the breathing begins to fail, artificial respiration must be performed. Generally speaking, by twelve hours after taking the poison the patient is either dead or is showing signs of recovery.

OPPORTUNISTIC: A description usually applied to infection resulting from an organism that does not normally cause disease in a healthy individual. It is also used to describe widespread infection by an organism that usually causes local infection. The body's defence mechanism can usually combat these organisms but if it is impaired – as happens in AIDS – opportunistic infection, such as pneumonia, may develop. Some viral and fungal infections behave in this way. Antimicrobial treatment is often effective, even though the weakness in the body's defence mechanism cannot be rectified.

OPSONINS are substances present in the serum of the blood which act upon bacteria, so as to prepare them for destruction by the white corpuscles of the blood.

OPTIC ATROPHY: A deterioration in the fibres of the optic nerve resulting in partial or complete loss of vision. It may be caused by damage to the nerve from inflammation or injury, or the atrophy may be secondary to disease in the eye.

OPTIC CHIASMA: This is formed by a crossing over of the two optic nerves which run from the back of the eyeballs to meet in the midline beneath the brain. Nerve fibres from the nasal part of the retina cross to link up with fibres from the outer part of the retina of the opposite eye. The linked nerves form two separate optic tracts which travel back to the occipital lobes of the brain.

OPTIC DISC: Otherwise known as the blind spot of the eye, the disc is the beginning of the optic nerve, the point where nerve fibres from the retina's rods and cones – the light- and colour-sensitive cells – leave the eyeball.

OPTICIAN: Someone who fits and sells glasses or contact lenses. An ophthalmic optician is trained to perform eye examinations to test for long and short sightedness but they do not treat disorders of the eye.

OPTIC NERVE (see EYE).

ORAL: An adjective referring to the mouth or to substances taken by mouth.

ORAL CONTRACEPTIVES: A contraceptive taken by mouth. It comprises one or more synthetic female hormones. (See CONTRACEPTION.)

ORANGE is an excellent source of vitamin C: 100 millilitres of orange juice contain 50 mg of ascorbic acid (ie. vitamin C). It is also used as a flavouring agent in the form of infusion, tincture and syrup of the peel. Fresh orange is also employed, often mixed with glucose, in feverish conditions for the action of the citric acid it contains. (See CITRIC ACID.)

ORBIT (see EYE).

ORCHIDECTOMY is the operation for the removal of the testicles (one or both).

ORCHIDOPEXY: When testes do not descend into the scrotum normally in young children (cryptorchidism) an operation is necessary to bring the testes in to the scrotum. This is called surgical orchidopexy.

ORCHITIS means inflammation of the testicle. (See TESTICLE, DISEASES OF.)

ORF is a widespread viral infection of sheep and goats which is sometimes transmitted to man, in whom it manifests itself as a skin eruption, usually on the hands, fingers, forearms and face.

ORGAN: A collection of different tissues that form a distinct structure in the body with a particular function or functions. The liver, for example, comprises a collection of different metabolic cells bound together with connective tissue and liberally supplied with blood vessels that performs vital functions in the breakdown of substances absorbed from the gastrointestinal tract. Other examples of organs are the kidneys, brain and heart.

ORGANIC DISEASE is a term used in contradistinction to the word functional, to indicate that some structural change is responsible for the faulty action of an organ or other part of the body.

ORGANIC SUBSTANCES are those which are obtained from animal or vegetable bodies, or which resemble in chemical composition those derived from this source. Organic chemistry has come to mean the chemistry of the carbon compounds.

ORGANO-PHOSPHORUS INSECTICIDES are a group of insecticides which act by inhibiting the action of cholinesterase. (See ACETYLCHOLINE.) For this reason they are also toxic to man and must therefore be handled with great care. The most widely used are parathion (q.v.) and malathion (q.v.).
Some of them are of value in agriculture because, when applied to plants, they are absorbed, and distributed to all parts of the plant, where they may kill sucking insects such as aphids.

ORGASM: The climax of sexual intercourse. In men this coincides with ejaculation of the semen when the muscles of the pelvis force the seminal fluid from the prostate into the urethra and out through the urethral orifice. In women orgasm is typified by irregular contractions of the muscular walls of the vagina followed by relaxation. The sensation is more diffuse in women than men and tends to last longer with successive orgasms sometimes occurring.

ORIENTAL SORE, also known as DELHI BOIL and as ALEPPO EVIL, is a disease of tropical climates in which an ulcer begins in a small pimple, spreads, and then heals very slowly; leaving an unsightly scar. (See LEISHMANIASIS.)

ORNITHOSIS is an infection of birds with the micro-organism known as *Chlamydia psittaci*, which is transmissible to man.

ORPHENADRINE is a drug used in the treatment of Parkinsonism (q.v.).

ORTHODONTICS is the branch of dentistry concerned with the prevention and treatment of dental irregularities and malocclusion.

ORTHOPAEDICS: Originally the general measures, surgical and mechanical, which can be used for the correction or prevention of deformities in children. Now, that branch of medical science dealing with skeletal deformity, congenital or acquired.

ORTHOPNOEA is a form of difficulty in breathing so severe that the patient cannot bear to lie down, but must sit or stand up. As a rule, it occurs only in serious affections of the heart or lungs.

ORTHOPTIC TREATMENT involves the examination and treatment by exercises of squints and their sequelae.

OSGOOD-SCHLATTER'S DISEASE is the form of osteochondrosis (q.v.) involving the tibial tubercle – the growing point of the tibia (q.v.). It occurs around puberty, mainly in boys, and first manifests itself by a painful swelling over the tibial tubercle at the upper end of the tibia. The pain is worst during and after exercise. A limp with increasing limitation of movement of the knee joint develops. Treatment consists of immobilization of the knee joint in plaster of Paris for six to eight weeks, with gradual return to activity over the next few months. Thereafter progressive return to sport may be allowed, but intense activity must be banned for many months.

OSMOLARITY: The osmotic pressure of a particular concentration of an osmotic solute dissolved in water. It is defined by the number of active particles in a set volume.

OSMOSIS means the passage of fluids through a membrane, which separates them, so as to become mixed with one another. Osmotic pressure is a term applied to the strength of the tendency which a fluid shows to do this, and depends largely upon the amount of solid which it holds in solution.

OSSICLE: A small bone, the term is usually applied to the three small bones of the middle ear – malleus, incus, and stapes – that conduct sound from the eardrum to the inner ear (q.v.). (See EAR.)

OSSIFICATION means the formation of bone. In early life, centres appear in the bones previously represented by cartilage or fibrous tissue, and from these the formation of true bone and deposit of lime salts proceed. When a fracture occurs, the bone mends by ossification of the clot which forms between the fragments. (See FRACTURES.) In old age an unnatural process of ossification often takes place in parts which should remain cartilaginous, e.g. in the cartilages of the larynx and of the ribs, making these parts unusually brittle.

OSTEITIS means inflammation in the substance of a bone. *Traumatic osteitis* is a condition particularly common in footballers, in which the victim complains of pain in the groin following exercise, particularly if this has involved much hip rotation. Examination reveals difficulty in spreading the legs and marked tenderness over the symphysis pubis. It responds well to rest and the administration of anti-inflammatory drugs such as indomethacin.

OSTEITIS DEFORMANS (see PAGET'S DISEASE OF BONE).

OSTEITIS FIBROSA CYSTICA is a pathological rather than a clinical entity. The term refers to the replacement of bone by a highly cellular and vascular connective tissue. It is the result of osteoclastic and osteoblastic activity and is due to excessive parathyroid activity. It is thus seen in a proportion of patients with primary hyperparathyroidism and in patients with uraemic osteodystrophy; that is, the secondary hyperparathyroidism that occurs in patients with chronic renal disease.

OSTEOARTHRITIS is a term used for joint problems where the primary problem is seen as a change in structure of cartilage and bone, rather than an inflammatory synovitis. Osteoarthritis usually implies a loss of the central load-bearing area of articular hyaline cartilage by a process of fibrillation, fissuring and fragmentation. This is usually associated with outgrowth of cartilage at the articular margin with subsequent ossification to form bony outgrowths known as osteophytes. Unfortunately there is confusion because the term is also used to cover joint pain that appears to have a mechanical basis in the absence of clinical or radiographic evidence of cartilage loss. Osteophytes form with increasing age, whether or not there is significant cartilage loss, and in the elderly osteophytes may lead to local frictional symptoms, and in the spine nerve compression. Despite major efforts, it has proved impossible to produce a single clear definition of osteoarthritis and this probably reflects the muddled nature of a concept which will need replacing.

The important problem of loss of central load-bearing articular cartilage occurs increasingly with age but is by no means inevitable. It has a wide range of causes, of which some, like dysplasia and trauma, are known and others have yet to be identified. The main clinical problems occur in the hip and knee. The cartilage loss in the hip usually occurs in the sixth or seventh decade. It may affect both hips in fairly rapid succession, or only one hip and such patients often have no problems in other joints. Cartilage loss in the knee occurs from the fifth decade onwards and is often associated with cartilage loss in small joints in the hand and elsewhere. Cartilage loss in the distal interphalangeal joints of the hand is associated with the formation of bony swellings known as Heberden's nodes.

Treatment: Management is largely directed at maintaining activity, with physical and social support as necessary. Analgesics may be of some value, particularly in the management of night pain. Non-steroidal anti-inflammatory agents may help patients with early morning stiffness and may also reduce pain on movement and night pain. Their benefit, however, tends to be less marked than in rheumatoid arthritis and their long-term usage has considerable toxicity problems. Advanced cartilage loss is best treated by joint replacement.

People with arthritis and their relatives can obtain help and advice from Arthritis Care, 18-20 Stephenson Way, London NW1 2HD (071-916 1500).

OSTEOCHONDRITIS is inflammation of both bone and cartilage. It is a not uncommon cause of backache in young people, particularly gymnasts.

OSTEOCHONDROSIS includes a group of diseases involving degeneration of the centre of ossification (see BONE) in the growing bones of children and adolescents. They include Kohler's disease, Osgood-Schlatter's disease (q.v.), and Perthes' disease (q.v.).

OSTEOCYTE: A bone cell formed from an osteoblast or bone-forming cell that has stopped its activity. The cell is embedded in the matrix of the bone.

OSTEOGENESIS IMPERFECTA is a hereditary disease due to an inherited abnormality of collagen (q.v.). It is characterized by extreme fragility of the skeleton, resulting in fractures and deformities. It may be accompanied by blue sclera (the outermost, normally white coat of the eyeball), transparent teeth, hypermobility (excessive range of movement) of the joints, deafness, and dwarfism (shortness of stature). The cause is not known, though there is some evidence that it may be associated with collagen formation (see COLLAGEN). Parents of affected children can obtain help and advice from the Brittle Bone Society, 112 City Road, Dundee DD2 3QT (0382-817771).

OSTEOMALACIA is the adult form of rickets. It is due to inadequate mineralization of osteoid tissue caused by a deficiency of vitamin D. This deficiency may arise because of inadequate intake or it may be due to impaired absorption such as occurs in intestinal malabsorption. It may also be due to renal disease as the kidney is responsible for the hydroxylation of cholecalciferol, which has virtually no metabolic action, to dihydroxy-cholecalciferol, the metabolically active form of the vitamin. (See VITAMIN D.)

OSTEOMYELITIS means inflammation in the marrow of a bone. (See BONE, DISEASES OF.)

OSTEOPATHY is the name applied to a system of healing in which diseases are treated by manipulating bones and other parts with the idea of thereby restoring functions in the bodily mechanism that have become deranged. Properly qualified osteopaths are included on the General Council and Register of Osteopaths, 56 London Road, Reading, Berkshire RG1 4SQ (0734-576585).

OSTEOPHYTES are bony spurs or projections. They occur most commonly at the margins of points involved in osteoarthritis (q.v.).

OSTEOPOROSIS is a reduced mass of normal bone. It is due to excessive resorption of bone rather than decreased bone synthesis. The quality of the bone that is present is normal, it is just the quantity that is deficient. It is a feature of ageing so that osteoporosis is common in the elderly. After the menopause women lose one per cent of their bone each year so that post-menopausal osteoporosis is a common disorder unless hormone-replacement therapy is given. Osteoporosis is also a feature of Cushing's syndrome and of patients who have been on long-term treatment with corticosteroids. Information and advice about the disease can be obtained from the National Osteoporosis Society, PO Box 10, Radstock, Bath BA3 3YB (0761-432472).

OSTEOSARCOMA is the most common, and most malignant, tumour of bone. It occurs predominantly in older children and young adults. The commonest site for it is at the ends of the long bones of the body: i.e. the femur, tibia and humerus. Treatment is by amputation of the limb followed by radiotherapy and chemotherapy. The 5-year survival rate is only 20 per cent.

OSTEOTOMY is the operation of cutting of a bone.

OS TRIGONUM is a small accessory bone behind the ankle joint which is present in about 7 per cent of the population. It may be damaged by energetic springing from the toes in ballet, jumping or fast bowling.

OTITIS means inflammation of the ear. (See EAR, DISEASES OF.)

OTOLOGY is that branch of medical science which is concerned with disorders and diseases of the organ of hearing, one practising this branch being called an OTOLOGIST.

OTORRHOEA means discharge from the ear. (See EAR, DISEASES OF.)

OTOSCLEROSIS is a condition in which abnormal bone is deposited around the foot-plate of the stapes resulting in fixation of that bone and causing a progressive conductive hearing loss due to immobility of the ossicular chain. There is an hereditary pattern to the disease and its onset is usually in the third decade. It tends to be slightly commoner in women and is often accelerated in pregnancy. Treatment involves supplying a hearing aid or performing an operation known as stapedectomy. Rarely the deposition of abnormal bone may affect the inner ear as well.

OTOSCOPE: (see AURISCOPE).

OUABAIN, or Strophanthin-G, is a glycoside first obtained from the African tree, *Acokanthera ouabaio*: it was used as an arrow poison in West Africa. It is now obtained from the African tree *Strophanthus gratus*. It is a cardiac stimulant, having a similar action to that of digitalis.

OUTPATIENT: A patient attending hospital on a day basis. He or she is not admitted to a bed. Most patients attend an outpatients' department after referral for a specialist opinion by their general practitioner. An increasing number of investigations and treatments, including surgery, are being done on an outpatient basis.

OVARIES are the glands in which are produced, in the female sex, the ova, capable, if fertilized, of developing into new individuals. They are situated, one on each side, in the cavity of the pelvis, corresponding on the surface of the body approximately to the centre of the groin. Each is shaped something like an almond, is about 3 cm long, 1·5 cm wide, and 1 cm in thickness, and is whitish in colour. It is attached to the broad ligament running from the womb to the side of the pelvis, by one edge along which blood-vessels and nerves enter. One end is connected to the expanded end of the Fallopian tube, as well as by a ligament to the side of the pelvis, and the other end to a ligament to the side of the womb. The ovary therefore lies to a considerable extent free in the pelvis.

The chief bulk of the ovary is made up of connective tissue, which differs from ordinary fibrous tissue in being composed of spindle-shaped cells. On the surface is a layer of columnar cells, and beneath this a dense connective tissue layer, the tunica albuginea. Beneath the tunica albuginea the structure appears to the naked eye to be of a granular character, this appearance being due to the presence of a layer of follicles, estimated at around 2,000,000 in number in each ovary at birth. By puberty they are reduced to around 40,000 in each ovary, a mere 400 of which will be shed at ovulation during the child-bearing period. Each follicle contains one (seldom more) ovum, each of these ova being capable of developing into a new individual. Every follicle consists essentially of a hollow ball of cells, embedded in which is a single large cell, the ovum. Each ovary contains follicles in all stages of maturity, from the rudimentary ones described above to several which are greatly increased in size to 35 micrometres in diameter through multiplication of the cells surrounding the ovum and the formation among them of a cavity distended with fluid. One at least of these follicles comes to maturity, when it is known as a Graafian follicle, about half-way between two menstrual periods, distends till it reaches the surface of the ovary, and finally bursts allowing the escape of the contained ovum, measuring 110 micrometres in diameter, which finds its way down the corresponding Fallopian tube into the womb. This process is know as ovulation. (See MENSTRUATION.)

For ovarian secretions, see Ovaries under ENDOCRINE GLANDS, and also OESTRADIOL; OESTROGEN; PROGESTERONE.

OVARIES, DISEASES OF: When diseased, the ovaries can be responsible for much ill-health.

INFLAMMATION OF THE OVARY (OVARITIS) seldom, if ever, occurs alone and is usually associated with inflammation of the Fallopian tubes (i.e. salpingitis) and of the pelvic peritoneum. It may be acute or chronic. The acute form is due to gonorrhoea, infection during the puerperium or following abortion, or infection from the alimentary tract: e.g. the appendix. If the acute form is not successfully overcome, it is liable to become chronic with exacerbations. In the chronic stage adhesions form which bind down and displace the ovaries, the Fallopian tubes, and the uterus. Bladder function is also liable to be interfered with. In all cases of infection of the ovaries and Fallopian tubes the possibility of this being due to tuberculosis must be considered, particularly in young patients.

Symptoms: In the acute form these may be mild or severe, consisting of pain in the lower part of the abdomen, usually during or just after menstruation, prolongation of menstruation, and fever. There may also be pain on passing water, sickness and vomiting. In severe cases with high temperature there may be rigors. In chronic cases there may be backache, usually worse after a day's work, fatigue, excessive or painful menstruation, pain on passing water, sterility and debility. In more severe cases there may be a discharge from the vagina (ie. leucorrhoea) and anaemia. Sometimes an abscess develops in the ovary or in the Fallopian tubes, and in these cases the general health is more likely to suffer because of toxic absorption.

Treatment: In the acute cases this consists of rest in bed and the administration of an antibiotic. Hot fomentations are useful to relieve pain. Hot douches to the vagina are not used as much as they were at one time, as they are sometimes liable to increase the pain. The diet should be light and nourishing. Care is necessary to ensure regular emptying of the bowels, but violent purgatives must not be used for this purpose. The majority of cases respond to such treatment. Operation is only indicated when there are signs of general peritonitis, or when there is no evidence of the condition responding to medical treatment in two to three weeks. The treatment of chronic cases is similar, but here hot douches to the vagina twice daily are also of value. Operation is required for chronic cases if the general health is affected, if there are acute exacerbations, or if there is much persistent local pain and menorrhagia.

OVARIAN TUMOURS may be of several kinds. Solid tumours, either simple or malignant, are relatively rare, though cancer of the ovary causes the death of more than 3000 women in Britain every year. Far commoner are the cystic forms, which often reach a huge size. The largest ever reported weighed 148 kg (328 pounds). These cysts are of several types, sometimes consisting of a distended condition of the Graafian follicles, at other times being simple cysts filled with a complex papillary growth, again being dermoid tumours and containing fat, hair, teeth, and other structures associated with the skin, and yet again arising from the distension of some part of the parovarium, a rudimentary structure attached to the ovary.

The fluid in these cysts is sometimes of a greenish-grey or brown colour and viscid, ropy consistence, at other times clearer and thinner, and, in the case of dermoid tumours, usually of a greasy nature.

Symptoms: These cystic tumours generally remain painless till the weight and distension caused by their increasing size give trouble. They arise often in young women without any apparent cause. If they are not removed, some, which stand on the verge of being malignant tumours, increase rapidly in size, and all lead to great discomfort and loss of health, and finally shorten life.

Treatment: The one method of treatment adopted now consists in *oöphorectomy* i.e. removal of the affected ovary. This operation should be performed early in the course of the disease, because, as the tumour grows, it contracts adhesions to surrounding organs, and these are the source both of most distressing symptoms and of the chief difficulty and danger in a later operation. Most cases operated upon at an early stage recover well, the operation being one of the safest major operations in surgery.

OVARIOTOMY or oöphorectomy is the operation of removal of an ovary or an ovarian tumour.

OVULATION: The development and release of an ovum (q.v.) (egg) from the ovary into the fallopian tube. Ovulation is initiated by the secretion of luteinizing hormone by the anterior pituitary gland and occurs half way through the menstrual cycle. If the ovum is not fertilized, it is lost during menstruation.

OVUM is the single cell derived from the female, out of which a future individual arises, after its union with the spermatozoon derived from the male. It is about 35 micrometres in diameter. (See FETUS; OVARIES.)

OXALIC ACID is not used in medicine, but it is of importance because it is an irritant poison, and has a domestic use for cleaning purposes: e.g. removing ink stains and iron mould, and cleaning leather. Oxalic acid, or binoxalate of potassium (salt of sorrel), is occasionally taken by mistake for Epsom salts or for cream of tartar. This substance is also important, because oxalate of lime is found in urinary sediment, and sometimes composes urinary calculi. (See BLADDER, DISEASES OF.) Oxalate of lime in the urine is derived partly from articles of food, like rhubarb, that contain it, and is partly produced within the body as the result of tissue change.

When poisoning is the result of taking oxalic acid or binoxalate of potassium, chalk or whiting well diluted with water should be given, and, if vomiting is not already present, an emetic; afterwards the irritation resulting in the stomach and bowels is to be soothed by demulcents. The antidote to oxalic acid is Calcium Gluconate Injection BP.

OXIMETRY: The measurement by an oximeter of the proportion of oxygenated haemoglobin (q.v.) in the blood.

OXPRENOLOL (see ADRENERGIC RECEPTORS).

OXYCEPHALY, or STEEPLE HEAD, describes a deformity of the skull in which the forehead is high and the top of the head pointed. There is also poor vision and the eyes bulge.

OXYGEN is a colourless gas, devoid of smell, slightly heavier than common air. It was discovered by Joseph Priestley in 1772. It forms rather more than one-fifth by volume of the atmosphere. It may be obtained by the fractional distillation of liquid air, or by the electrolysis of water. It is stored at high pressure (up to 120 atmospheres) in steel cylinders, from which it is obtained at any desired rate by turning a stop-cock.

Action: Oxygen is necessary to life, and the process of respiration (see RESPIRATION) has, as one of its main objects, the supply of oxygen to the blood (see also HAEMOGLOBIN). Applied to the unbroken skin, oxygen has little effect, but when brought in contact with a wound or ulcer, it increases the circulation and acts as a stimulant.

The condition of oxygen want, or anoxia, may be produced by various conditions, such as damage to the lung by tumours, or defects of the circulation, e.g. valvular disease of the heart, in which the circulation is so slow that the tissues do not receive their proper amount of oxygen, and in cases of anaemia and poisoning where the blood is not capable of carrying its normal amount of oxygen. In these states, and above all in cases of anaemia and valvular disease, when the pulse is quick and feeble, when the patient's lips and ears are blue, and when the breathing is rapid and shallow, the administration of oxygen gives great relief.

Uses: In severe cases of anoxia the rate at which oxygen may require to be delivered to the patient is between 4 and 6 litres per minute. A tube is attached to the head of the cylinder, which passes through the tubes of a wash-bottle and is continued to either a mask, which fits over the patient's nose and mouth, or to a catheter which is passed into one of the nostrils and fixed in position at the side of the face by a strip of sticking plaster. The use of the latter is unaccompanied by any sense of oppression to the patient.

Great advances have been made in recent years in the development of both oxygen masks and tents. The advantage of the latter is that the patient is breathing all the time in an atmosphere saturated with oxygen.

A recent development in oxygen therapy is what is known as *hyperbaric oxygen*. This is the use of oxygen at high pressures, such as 3 atmospheres. Originally introduced as an adjunct to radiotherapy in the treatment of cancer, it is now being used in the treatment of carbon monoxide poisoning, *Clostridium welchii* infections (q.v.) and coronary thrombosis. The most convenient method of administering hyperbaric oxygen is in a special pressure chamber.

Substances which contain oxygen and are capable of giving it off, such as permanganate of potassium, and peroxide of hydrogen, have a powerful effect as disinfectants either by destroying organisms or oxidizing noxious products of their growth. Such substances are therefore used in the treatment of ulcers and various skin diseases and as antiseptics.

OXYGEN DEFICIT: A normal physiological state that occurs in living cells when there is a temporary oxygen shortage. The body needs extra energy when it is undergoing exertion. After the available oxygen has been used the cells break down glucose. The resultant products are acidic and cause muscle cramps. The oxygen needed to dispose of the breakdown products – the oxygen deficit – must be made available when the effort stops.

OXYGEN TOXICITY: The damaging effect of oxygen on the lung was first described at the turn of the century. If too strong a concentration of oxygen – over 50 per cent – is breathed for too long, more than 24 hours, the cells in the lung are damaged. This may occur when patients are treated with oxygen or when deep-sea divers inhale oxygen for prolonged periods.

OXYMETHOLONE (see ANABOLIC STEROIDS).

OXYPERTINE is an anti-psychotic drug related to the phenothiazines.

OXYTETRACYCLINE is an antibiotic derived from a soil organism, Streptomyces rimosus. Its range of antibacterial activity is comparable to that of tetracycline (q.v.).

OXYTOCIC means hastening parturition or stimulating uterine contraction, or a drug or procedure that has this effect.

OXYTOCIN is the extract isolated from the pituitary posterior lobe which stimulates the uterine muscle to contract. It can also be synthesized. (See PITUITARY BODY.)

OXYURIS is another name for the threadworm.

OZAENA is a chronic disease of the nose of an inflammatory nature, combined with atrophy of the mucous membrane and the formation of extremely foul-smelling crusts in the interior of the nose. (See NOSE, DISEASES OF.)

OZONE is a specially active and poisonous form of oxygen in which three volumes of the gas are condensed into the space ordinarily occupied by two. It has a characteristic smell and is a strong oxidizing agent. Formed when an electrical charge is passed through oxygen or air, it is found at high altitudes in the atmosphere where it screens out much of the sun's ultraviolet radiation. The ozone layer, as it is called, is being damaged by pollutant gases from earth and, unless this damage is reversed, lethal quantities of ultraviolet radiation could penetrate to the earth's surface.

P

PACEMAKER (see cardiac pacemaker).

PACHYDERMIA means hypertrophy or thickening of the skin. PACHYDERMIA LARYNGIS is a name applied to thickening of the vocal cords due to chronic inflammation or irritation.

PACHYMENINGITIS means inflammation of the dura mater of the brain and spinal cord. (See MENINGITIS.)

PACINIAN CORPUSCLES, or lamellated corpuscles, are minute bulbs at the ends of the nerves scattered through the skin and subcutaneous tissue, and forming one of the end-organs for sensation.

PACKED CELL VOLUME: That fraction of the blood's total volume made up of red cells. The packed cell volume is established by centrifuging blood in a tube and measuring the depth of the column of red cells as a fraction of the whole column of blood.

PACKS (see WET PACK).

PAEDIATRICS means the branch of medicine dealing with diseases of children.

PAGET'S DISEASE OF BONE, or OSTEITIS DEFORMANS, is a chronic disease in which the bones – especially those of the skull, limbs, and spine – gradually become thick and also soft, causing them to bend. It is said to be the commonest bone disease in the world, and it is estimated that some 600,000 people in England may suffer from it. It seldom occurs under the age of 40. Pain is its most unpleasant manifestation. The cause is not known, and there is no known cure, but satisfactory results are being obtained from the use of calcitonin (q.v.) and a group of drugs known as diphosphonates (eg. etidronate). Those with the disease can obtain help and advice from the National Association for the Relief of Paget's Disease, University of Manchester Department of Medicine, Hope Hospital, Salford M6 8HD (061-787 4949).

PAIN is a necessary part of conscious existence, all our sensations being accompanied by more or less feeling of pleasure or pain. In the former case we seek the repetition of the sensations; in the latter case we instinctively avoid them, unless, by an act of will, we avoid the sense of pleasure or bear that of pain for some ulterior motive. The ability to perceive pain constitutes a special sense which the body has evolved, or with which it has been furnished, in order that it may preserve itself, by avoiding conditions that produce damage.

Pain is of various types. The most important is that caused by injury of the skin, as by a prick, burn, or pinch. This sense is quite distinct from that of touch. There are special nerve-fibres for the conduction of painful impressions, running up the spinal cord near its central canal, while the fibres conveying the impressions for touch run up in the posterior part of the cord. This is proved by the destruction of the sense of pain in the disease known as syringomyelia (which affects the central part of the cord), notwithstanding the fact that the slightest touch can still be felt in the parts of the body incapable of feeling pain. It is probable that these nerves of pain have special endings in the skin, since pain does not appear to be felt uniformly, but, like the other senses, at special spots thickly scattered over the surface. And it is also likely that there is a special centre in the brain for the reception of painful impressions.

Internal parts are much less sensitive than the skin, and diseases in them usually give rise to quite a different sensation. Indeed these parts, not being liable to damage by external objects, are not endowed with the power of feeling pain due to sudden injury, so that the bowel, when brought out through the skin, may be cut with scissors or knife, though the individual, unless he sees it, is quite unaware of what is taking place; tendon, muscle, and bone are also very insensitive, so that the two former may be cut or scraped without more than a slightly sickening sensation, or the ends of a broken bone rubbed together without causing severe pain.

Nevertheless inflammatory changes in these deep-seated structures, and disturbances in their functions, are capable of influencing the brain so as to produce the severest type of pain. This inflammation, particularly when seated in dense structures which cannot expand so as to prevent the congested blood-vessels of the part from pressing upon its nerves, is accompanied by throbbing pain, and, in bone particularly, this is apt to be of a boring, excruciating character. The gnawing pain of a tumour invading surrounding tissues is of a similar nature, and any source of irritation on the course of a nerve is apt to produce the severe pain of neuralgia. Over-action of a weak part or muscle leads to continued pain of an aching character, due probably to an irritating deposit of the chemical products of muscular activity, or may produce spasm, as in the stitch of the side caused by unwontedly violent exercise. Of a similar nature is the colic or griping pain, caused by irritation of the bowels, bile-ducts, and ureters, which in its severest forms may properly be designated agony. (See COLIC.) The burning pain of certain forms of dyspepsia is due to the action of an excessively acid gastric juice, and, like burns of the skin, is apparently due to irritation of the sensitive nerve-endings at points where the surface of the mucous membrane has become eroded.

Ordinary sensations of all sorts become painful when they are excessive, and thus liable to damage the organ in question: e.g. bright light, loud sound.

Painful sensations depend much also upon the state of the nervous system, varying according to the power of the nerves to conduct, and of the brain to receive, impressions. Some people are notoriously better at bearing pain than others, and the healthy and strong are less affected by trivial injuries than those whose nervous system is in a state of ready irritability through chronic ill-health. People with strong will-power can undoubtedly inhibit painful impressions, like those from a surgical operation, just as they can control irregular movements. Thus by a mental effort not only do such people bear pain better, but they actually feel less pain. Similarly the mind that is dominated by an idea unconsciously inhibits painful impressions, so that they gain no entrance for the time, as in the case of soldiers wounded in the heat of battle.

On the other hand, pain may be of a purely functional character, and a person may suffer pain without any external cause, the mind misinterpreting or exaggerating sensations. (See HYSTERIA.)

These facts are well known to those faith-healers and others who attempt to cure by a direct mental impression.

Pain in a certain part is not necessarily due to disease in the same part. In the case of injury to the skin covering the body, the mind, as the result of experience, very accurately refers the painful impressions down the nerves which bring them, to the parts from which they come. But when impressions come to the central nervous system from organs or parts of the body not usually liable to injury or disease, the mind is apt to refer the pain to some other part which is more commonly the seat of pain, and whose nerve-fibres enter the same part of the brain or spinal cord as do those coming from the part which is really affected. For example, in the early stages of hip-joint disease, the pain is more often felt down the inner side of the thigh and knee than in the deep-seated hip-joint, since branches from the same nerves (obturator and femoral) supply the hip-joint and the skin of this particular area. For the same reason, the pain of spinal disease, due to pressure upon the large nerve roots close to the point where they enter the cord, is often referred, not to this unfamiliar seat of pain, but to the sides and front of the body where these nerves end in the skin. Pain felt equally on both sides of the body is almost always due to some affection of the central nervous system.

In the case of the internal organs whose nervous control is derived from the sympathetic nervous system (in the case of the heart, lungs, stomach, and bowels partly also from the tenth cranial, or vagus, nerve), through which they often obtain complicated and very distant connections with the brain and cord, pain is often referred, in what seems at first sight to be a bizarre manner, to distant points. *Referred pain* is often, in the case of the heart, stomach, liver, and bowels, felt on the surface situated over these organs, and the skin may be so tender that gentle pressure or even the slightest touch cannot be borne. Heart conditions are liable also to cause pain running down the inner side of the left, and in some cases of the right, arm to the elbow. In dyspepsia, due to irritation of the stomach, the pain is often referred to the pit of the stomach or middle of the back. In conditions affecting the liver there may be pain in the region of the right shoulder. Affections of the lower end of the bowel commonly cause pain down the back of the thighs, especially of the left thigh, to the knee. Pain due to disorders of the womb is felt internally much less often than in the lowest part of the back and the thighs; and, when the ovaries or fallopian tubes also are affected, the pain may have a wide distribution, including the small of the back, the groin, and the front of the thigh, or it is occasionally referred to the hip or knee-joint, so that the case may for a time be mistaken for disease in one of these joints.

Treatment of pain: There are three general principles by which the relief of pain may be attempted. (1) The most natural way is to remove the cause of pain, such as a decayed tooth, ulcer, abscess, or inflammatory condition of some internal organ, or to soothe the nerves of the affected part by warmth or some other means. (2) The nerves which convey impressions from the affected region may be treated so that their conducting power is lessened or stopped, as, for example, by administration of sedatives, use of electricity, local anaesthetics, or by chordotomy (see NEURALGIA). (3) The part of the brain which receives the impressions of pain may be dulled by drugs, or the influence of these impressions may be inhibited by powerful mental impressions, as, for example in hypnotism, faith-healing. Patients with severe persistent pain are now commonly treated in pain clinics staffed by doctors who specialize in the alleviation of pain. (See also ANAESTHESIA; ANALGESICS; ANODYNES; TRANSCUTANEOUS ELECTRICAL NERVE STIMULATION; and under the headings of the various diseases that give rise to pain.)

PAINS (see LABOUR).

PAINTER'S COLIC (see COLIC; LEAD POISONING).

PALATE is the partition between the cavity of the mouth, below, and that of the nose, above. It consists of the *hard palate* towards the front, which is composed of a bony plate covered below by the mucous membrane of the mouth, above by that of the nose; and of the *soft palate* further back, in which a muscular layer, composed of nine small muscles, is similarly covered. The hard palate extends a little further back than the wisdom teeth, and is formed by the maxillary and palate bones. The soft palate is concave towards the mouth and convex towards the nose, and it ends behind in a free border, at the centre of which is the prolongation known as the uvula. When food or air is passing through the mouth, as in the acts of swallowing, coughing, or vomiting, the soft palate is drawn upwards so as to touch the back wall of the throat and shut off the cavity of the nose. Movements of the soft palate, by changing the shape of the mouth and nose cavities, are important in the production of speech.

PALATE, MALFORMATIONS OF: The palate is subject to certain alterations, as the result of defective development. The hard palate may be much more arched than usual: this is sometimes due to the failure to breathe through the nose, caused by the presence of adenoid vegetations in the throat. (See NOSE, DISEASES OF.)

In early embryonic life (see FETUS) there are certain clefts in the region of the throat and face, the nose being formed by the junction of one process which grows down from between the eyes (fronto-nasal process) and two which grow in, one from either side (maxillary processes). The fronto-nasal process produces the external nose, the septum of the nose, the central part of the upper lip, and that part of the upper jaw which carries the two front teeth. The maxillary processes form the remainder of the upper jaw and the palate on each side. These three should unite completely prior to birth, but if they fail to do so, a Y-shaped gap is left. This gap runs from the back of the palate forward to a point a little distance behind the front teeth, from which point a limb of the gap runs forwards to each nostril and through the upper lip. A complete state of *cleft palate* may occur; or there may be only a partial gap in the soft palate, the parts having closed in front; or again, there may be closure behind and only a notch be left in the lip or a single cleft in the edge of the upper jaw. The notch of the lip is known as *hare-lip*, from a fanciful resemblance to the hare, which has a notch in the centre of its lip.

The incidence of cleft lip (hare-lip) and cleft palate seems to be increasing and one child in approximately 700 normal births has some degree of cleft lip and palate. The increase is probably due to more of these babies surviving, as a result of improved surgical techniques, and getting married and having children. As a rough guide, it can be said that if a child is born with a cleft, and there is no family history as far back as the parents' grandparents, the chances of another malformed child is about the same as in the general population. When one parent is affected, the risk is around 1 in 80 but, when a mother with a cleft palate produces a daughter with a cleft palate, the risk to a second daughter is as high as 1 in 7.

Cleft-palate and hare-lip should, if possible, be rectified by operation, because both are a serious drawback to feeding in early life, while later, hare-lip is a great disfigurement, and cleft-palate gives to the voice a peculiar twang. When there is merely a slight degree of hare-lip, it is usual to operate a few weeks or even some days after birth, although, when the notch is very large, it may be necessary to wait till the child is several months old. The closure of a large cleft in the palate, which is a more formidable operation, is usually deferred till the child has gained some strength, and the most suitable time is generally held to be between eighteen months and two and a half years of age, because the fault must be remedied before the child has learned to speak. The operations performed vary greatly in details, but all consist in paring the edges of the gap and drawing the soft parts together across it.

Until a hare-lip has been remedied, it is often necessary to feed the child with a spoon, as he cannot suck. When a cleft palate is too wide for operation, its effects can be diminished in later life by wearing an artificial palate.

Parents of such children can obtain help and advice from the Cleft Lip and Palate Association, 1 Eastwood Gardens, Kenton, Newcastle-upon-Tyne NE3 3DQ (091–2859396), or the Dental and Maxillofacial Department, Hospital for Sick Children, Great Ormond Street, London WC1N 3JH.

PALINDROMIC RHEUMATISM is a form of rheumatism in adults characterized by multiple, afebrile attacks of acute arthritis, and inflammation of the surrounding tissues, with pain, swelling, redness, and disability of one or more small or large joints, the attacks coming on suddenly, lasting a few hours to a few days then disappearing completely, to recur at irregular intervals.

PALLIATIVE is a term applied to the treatment of incurable diseases, in which the aim is to mitigate the sufferings of the patient, not to effect a cure.

PALLOR: Unusual paleness of the skin caused by a reduced flow of blood or a deficiency in normal pigments. Pallor may be a sign of shock, anaemia, or other diseases.

PALPATION means the method of examining the surface of the body and the size, shape, and movements of the internal organs, by laying the flat of the hand upon the skin.

PALPEBRAL: Relating to the eyelid.

PALPITATION is a condition in which the heart beats forcibly or irregularly, and the person becomes conscious of its action.
Causes: As a rule we are quite unconscious of the beating of the heart, but when the nervous system is unduly excited its action may become unpleasantly palpable. A disorder of the rhythm of the heart (arrhythmia) may cause the heart to beat rapidly and give rise to palpitations. Sudden emotions, such as fright, and occasionally dyspepsia, may bring it on. A common cause consists in over-use of tobacco, tea, coffee, or alcohol. Sometimes it may appear in cases of organic heart disease.

Symptoms: There may simply be a fluttering of the heart and a feeling of weakness, which is often expressively described as 'gone-ness', or the heart may be felt pounding and the arteries throbbing, causing great distress to the affected person. In some cases the subject of palpitation is conscious of the heart missing beats.

Treatment: Mental quietness is the great requisite to still the overaction, and all sources of excitement must be avoided. The person should understand that, however unpleasant the condition may be, there is no danger from it, and that serious disease is not usually the cause. Moderate exercise is a good thing. If the person is a heavy smoker, this is probably the cause, and tobacco should be given up. Similarly tea, coffee, and alcohol should be partaken of sparingly, and any food likely to cause flatulent dyspepsia should be avoided. In the cases due to organic disease, the condition causing palpitation must be treated. The beta adrenoreceptor antagonists are the most useful drugs in controlling the palpitations of anxiety and those due to some cardiac arrhythmias.

PALSY is another name for paralysis. (See PARALYSIS.)

PALUDRINE (see PROGUANIL HYDROCHLORIDE).

PAN- is a prefix meaning all or completely.

PANACEA is a term applied to a remedy for all diseases, or more usually to a remedy which benefits many different diseases.

PANCARDITIS means inflammation of the pericardium, myocardium, and endocardium at the same time.

PANCREAS, or SWEETBREAD, is a long secreting gland situated in the back of the abdomen, at the level of the first and second lumbar vertebrae. It lies behind the lower part of the stomach, an expanded portion, called the head of the pancreas, occupying the bend formed by the duodenum or first part of the small intestine, whilst a long portion known as the body extends to the left, ending in the tail, which rests against the spleen. A duct runs through the whole gland from left to right, joined by many small branches in its course, and, leaving the head of the gland, unites with the bile duct from the liver to open into the side of the small intestine about 7·5 to 10 cm (3 or 4 inches) below the outlet of the stomach.

Minute structure: The gland resembles one of the salivary glands, being composed of tubes of columnar cells bound together by loose connective tissue. These cells are arranged with one end abutting on a central lumen into which the secretion of the cells passes, and each group of tubes ends in a small duct, which unites with other small ducts to join the main pancreatic duct running to the intestine. The cells present an outer, clear zone, and an inner zone filled with granules of the materials secreted by the activity of the cell. Blood-vessels and nerves in large numbers run in the connective tissue of the gland.

Scattered through the pancreas are collections of cells known as the islets of Langerhans, of which there are around a million in a normal individual. These do not communicate with the duct of the gland, and the internal secretion of the pancreas – insulin – is formed by these cells and absorbed directly into the blood.

Functions: The most obvious function of the pancreas is the formation of the pancreatic juice, which is poured into the small intestine after the partially digested food has left the stomach. This is the most important of the digestive juices, is alkaline in reaction, and contains, in addition to various salts, four enzymes. These enzymes are: trypsin and chymotrypsin, which digest proteins; amylase, which converts starchy foods into the disaccharide maltose; lipase, which breaks up fats. For the action of these see DIGESTION.

Inadequate production of insulin by the islets of Langerhans leads to the condition known as diabetes mellitus (q.v.). In addition to insulin, another hormone is produced by the pancreas. This is glucagon which has the opposite effect to insulin and raises the blood sugar by promoting the breakdown of liver glycogen.

PANCREAS, DISEASES OF: Abscesses, cysts, calculi, and tumours may occur in the pancreas as in other organs, but are not very common. The most important disease of the pancreas, though again, fortunately, not very common, is acute pancreatitis. This is sudden in onset, accompanied by acute pain, and causes severe shock and collapse. It carries a mortality rate of around 20 per cent, even when treated adequately and early. Chronic pancreatitis is a much more indeterminate disease, commonly associated with disease of the gall-bladder, particularly gall-stones, and chronic alcoholism. Pancreatitis may occur as a complication of mumps. Cancer of the pancreas is on the increase and around 7,000 cases are now diagnosed every year in the UK. There is an established association with heavy cigarette smoking, and it is twice as common in patients with diabetes mellitus as compared with the general population. Reference has already been made to the association between the islets of Langerhans (q.v.) and diabetes mellitus (q.v.).

PANCREATIN contains three ferments: trypsin, lipase, and amylase. Thereby it hydrolyses fats to glyceryl and fatty acids, changes protein to proteoses and derived substances, and converts starch into dextrins and sugars (see DIGESTION). It is given by mouth for the relief of pancreatic deficiency in conditions such as pancreatitis (see PANCREAS, DISEASES OF) and fibrocystic disease of the pancreas (see CYSTIC FIBROSIS). It is also used for the preparation of predigested, or so-called peptonized, foods. For peptonizing milk, pancreatin is added to tepid water to which milk previously heated to 38 °C is added. The mixture is stirred and maintained at 38 °C for 15 minutes, and then raised to boiling point. It is then transferred to a cool place. It should be used within 24 hours. Various farinaceous foods may be similarly predigested.

PANCYTOPENIA: A fall in the number of red and white blood cells as well as of platelets. The condition is found in aplastic anaemia, bone-marrow tumours, enlarged spleen, and other disorders.

PANDEMIC is an epidemic which affects a vast area, such as a country or a continent.

PANHYSTERECTOMY is an operation by which the uterus is completely removed.

PANNICULITIS means inflammation of the subcutaneous fat, and may occur anywhere on the body surface.

PANNUS: Blood vessels growing into the cornea beneath its epithelium. Seen in trachoma and to a lesser extent in patients who are long-term soft-contact-lens wearers.

PANTOTHENIC ACID, which has now been prepared synthetically, is part of the vitamin B complex. It is known as the chick anti-dermatitis factor because if it is absent from the chick's diet the bird develops dermatitis, and degeneration of nerve-fibres in the spinal cord also occurs. In rats lack of pantothenic acid produces greying of the hair, but there is no evidence that in man greying is due to lack of this vitamin. Indeed, little is known about the significance of pantothenic acid in man, except that it is one of the essential constituents of the diet. The daily requirement is probably around 10 milligrams. It is widely distributed in foodstuffs, both animal and vegetable. Yeast, liver, and egg-yolk are particularly rich sources.

PAPAIN, PAPYAOTIN, and PAPOID are names given to a ferment, or mixture of ferments, obtained from the juice of the pawpaw, the unripe fruit of *Carica papaya*, which has an action similar to that of the ferments of the gastric and pancreatic juices. It is accordingly sometimes used to peptonize foods for invalids, as it does not give them the same bitter taste that pepsin gives. It is widely used as a meat tenderizer.

PAPANICOLAOU TEST: (see CERVICAL SMEAR).

PAPAVERETUM consists of the hydro-chlorides of alkaloids of opium (q.v.). It has the pain-relieving and narcotic effects of morphine (q.v.), but fewer side-effects. It is largely used in association with anaesthesia.

PAPILLA means a small projection, such as those with which the corium of the skin is covered, and which project into the epidermis and make its union with the corium more intimate; or those covering the tongue and projecting from its surface.

PAPILLITIS is the term applied to inflammation of any papilla, but especially of the prominence formed by the end of the optic nerve in the retina, also known as optic neuritis.

PAPILLOEDEMA: Swelling of the optic disc specifically due to raised intra-cranial pressure.

PAPILLOMA means a tumour composed of papillae growing from the surface of skin or mucous membrane. These tumours may be either simple or malignant in nature. Such a tumour is found occasionally in the bladder, and the chief symptom of its presence is the painless presence of blood in the urine.

PAPOVAVIRUS is a group of viruses, one of which is responsible for warts (q.v.).

PAPULE means a pimple.

PARA- is a prefix meaning near, aside from, or beyond.

PARA-AMINO SALICYLIC ACID was one of the early antituberculous antibiotics. It tended to cause a lot of dyspepsia and has been replaced by newer antituberculous drugs with fewer side-effects. The first-line drugs for tuberculosis are now rifampicin, isoniazid, and ethambutol.

PARACENTESIS is the puncture by hollow needle or trocar and cannula of any body cavity (e.g. abdominal, pleural, pericardial), for tapping or aspirating fluid pathologically accumulated. (See ASPIRATION.)

PARACETAMOL has antipyretic and analgesic actions similar to those of aspirin. The dose is 500 to 1000 milligrams.

PARACETAMOL POISONING: Paracetamol is one of the safest of drugs when taken in correct dosage. When an overdose is taken, however, it is a very dangerous one because of the toxic effect on the liver. This is why cases of poisoning with it must be taken to hospital as quickly as possible. In the early stages there is only sickness and vomiting without any loss of consciousness. Once in hospital, treatment consists of washing out the stomach, and the administration of drugs, such as cysteamine and acetylcysteine, to protect the liver.

PARACUSIS means any perversion of the sense of hearing.

PARAESTHESIA is a term applied to unusual feelings, apart from mere increase, or loss, of sensation, experienced by a patient without any external cause: for example, hot flushes, numbness, tingling, itching. Various paraesthesiae form a common symptom in some nervous diseases.

PARAFFIN is the general name used to designate a series of saturated hydrocarbon bodies, discovered by Reichenbach in 1830 and first produced as a commercial product by Young in 1850. The higher members of the series, paraffin-waxes, are solid at ordinary temperatures, some being hard, others soft. Lower in the scale comes petroleum, which is liquid at ordinary temperatures. Naphtha, petroleum spirit, and hydramyl are lower members of the series which are very volatile, and lowest comes methane, better known as marsh-gas, which is a gaseous body.
Uses: In the form of the *British Pharmacopoeia* preparation, liquid paraffin, it is used in the treatment of constipation.

Externally, the hard and soft paraffins are used in various consistencies, being very useful as ointments and lubricants as they are apparently harmless.

PARAFORMALDEHYDE is used as a source of formaldehyde. For disinfecting rooms it is prepared in the form of tablets which are vaporized on an electric hotplate. It is also used as lozenges. These should be allowed to dissolve slowly in the mouth. To keep catheters and other surgical instruments aseptic, it is enclosed with them in airtight containers.

PARAGANGLIOMA is the term used to describe two types of tumour. One known as a CHROMAFFINOMA or PHAEOCHROMOCYTOMA, is a tumour containing chromaffin cells (q.v.), most often found in the medulla of the suprarenal gland, where chromaffin cells are normal constituents. An important sign of these tumours is paroxysmal high blood-pressure. The other, also known as a CHEMODECTOMA, occurs in the carotid body (q.v.) and the comparable aortic body. It is usually quite small and is more common in women than men.

PARAGONIMIASIS is the condition caused by *paragonimus*, a genus of trematode or fluke, the most common being *Paragonimus westermani*, which is most often found in the Far East, but is also found in India, South America and parts of Africa. The disease is also known as endemic haemoptysis, as the presenting feature is haemoptysis, or the coughing up of blood, due to the worm settling in the lungs. The infection is acquired by eating inadequately cooked crayfish or crab. Bithionol is the drug most commonly used in treatment. Chloroquine is also used.

PARAGRAPHIA is misplacement of words, or of letters in words, or wrong spelling, or use of wrong words in writing as a result of a lesion in the speech region of the brain.

PARAINFLUENZA VIRUSES are divided into four types, all of which cause infection of the respiratory system. Infection with type 3 begins in May, reaches a maximum in July or August and returns to baseline level in October. Types 1 and 2 are predominantly winter viruses. In 1981, 455 cases of parainfluenza type 3 infection were reported. Children aged 1 to 11 months were the most commonly affected age-group. The manifestations include croup (q.v.), fever, a rash, and occasionally convulsions. It is of interest that the virus was isolated from the upper respiratory tract of three children, aged 7 weeks, 2 months and 4 months, with a diagnosis of cot death (see SUDDEN INFANT DEATH SYNDROME).

PARALDEHYDE is a clear, colourless liquid with a penetrating ethereal odour, and a burning taste followed by a cool sensation in the mouth. Although in small quantities it may cause excitement, in larger doses it is a soporific, with little depressing effect, and productive of quiet, refreshing sleep.
Uses: It is given when a powerful hypnotic action is required, and is particularly useful in inducing sleep in mentally unstable patients. Its unpleasant taste restricts its use, but has the compensatory advantage that it usually prevents the patient receiving paraldehyde from becoming an addict. It is sometimes given per rectum as a general anaesthetic.

PARALYSIS, or PALSY, means loss of muscular power due to interference with the nervous system. When muscular power is weakened as the result of some affection of the nervous system, but not entirely lost in the parts concerned, the term *paresis* is often used instead of paralysis. Various terms are used to designate paralysis distributed in different ways. Thus *hemiplegia* is the term applied to paralysis affecting one side of the face, with the corresponding arm and leg, as the result of disease on one side of the brain; *diplegia* means a condition of more or less total paralysis, in which both sides are affected in this manner; *monoplegia* is the term applied to paralysis of a single limb; and *paraplegia* signifies paralysis of both sides of the body below a given level, usually from about the level of the waist; *quadriplegia* is paralysis of all four limbs.

Paralysis should be regarded rather as a symptom than as a disease by itself, and it is generally connected with well-marked disorder of some portion of the nervous system. According to the locality and extent of the nervous system affected, so will be the form and completeness of the paralysis.

Reference can here be made only to the more common types of paralysis, and that merely in general terms.

(1) PARALYSIS DUE TO BRAIN DISEASE: Of this, by far the most common form is palsy affecting one side of the body, or *Hemiplegia*. It usually arises from disease of the hemisphere of the brain opposite to the side of the body affected, such disease being in the form of haemorrhage into the brain substance (*cerebral haemorrhage*), or the plugging up of blood-vessels by a locally formed clot (*cerebral thrombosis*) or by a clot dislodged from some other part of the

Brain and spinal cord, showing motor paths and positions of injuries causing various forms of paralysis. 1 position of haemorrhage causing paralysis of left arm; 2 face; 3 position of haemorrhage causing complete paralysis of left side; 4 position of haemorrhage followed by paralysis of left arm and leg with right side of face (crossed paralysis); 5 cerebellum; 6 spinal cord; 7 position of disorder causing paralysis of both lower limbs (paraplegia); 8 position of the disease responsible for poliomyelitis in the left leg; 9 to leg; 10 to arm; 11 medulla oblongata; 12 seventh nerve (facial); 13 pons; 14 lentiform nucleus; 15 thalamus; 16 cerebral hemisphere; 17 leg; 18 arm.

body (*cerebral embolism*), and consequent arrest of blood supply to an area of the brain; or again, it may result from an injury, or be due to a tumour in the tissues of the brain. The character of the seizure and the amount of paralysis vary according to the situation of the disease or injury, its extent, and its sudden or gradual occurrence. The attack may come on as a stroke (see STROKE), in which the patient becomes suddenly unconscious, and loses completely the power of motion of one side of the body, or a like result may arise more gradually and without loss of consciousness. In either type of complete hemiplegia, the paralysis affects on one side the muscles of the face, tongue, body, and limbs. Speech is indistinct and thick, and the tongue, when protruded, points towards the paralysed side owing to the unopposed action of its muscles on the unaffected side. The muscles of the face implicated are chiefly those about the mouth. The paralysed side hangs loose, and the corner of the mouth is depressed, but the muscles closing the eye are, as a rule, unimpaired, because movements like that of shutting the eyes, which are performed usually on both sides together, are controlled from either side of the brain. As a result the eye on the paralysed side can be shut, unlike what occurs in another form of facial paralysis (Bell's palsy), in which the fault lies in the nerve. The muscles of respiration on the affected side are seldom more than slightly weakened for deep breathing, but those of the arm and leg are completely powerless. Sensation may at first be impaired (anaesthesia), but as a rule returns soon, unless the portion of the brain affected is connected with this function. Rigidity of the paralysed members is usually present as a later symptom. In many cases of even complete hemiplegia, improvement takes place after the lapse of weeks or months, and is in general indicated by a return of motor power, first in the face, next in the leg, while that of the arm follows after a longer or shorter interval, and is rarely complete. Such recovery of movement is, however, only partial in a large proportion of cases and the side remains weakened. In such instances the gait of the patient is characteristic. In walking, he leans to the sound side and swings round the affected limb from the hip, the foot scraping the ground as it is raised and advanced. The paralysed parts retain their contractility when stimulated by electric currents, but they are apt to suffer in their nutrition from disuse and to assume an attitude of rigidity unless treatment is carefully carried out.

Besides hemiplegia, various other forms of paralysis may arise from cerebral disease. Thus occasionally there is CROSSED PARALYSIS, one side of the face and the opposite side of the body being affected simultaneously. Or again, as is often observed in the case of tumours of the brain, the paralysis may be limited to the distribution of one or more of the cranial nerves, and may produce a combination of symptoms (such as squinting, drooping of the eyelid, and impairment or loss of vision) which may enable the seat of the disease to be accurately localized. The condition of DIPLEGIA, in which both sides are affected, sometimes occurs in infants, and is due generally to some inflammation of the brain occurring soon after birth.

TREMBLING PALSY, PARALYSIS AGITANS; PARKINSONISM or SHAKING PARALYSIS (see PARKINSONISM). CEREBRAL PALSY (q.v.).

FUNCTIONAL PARALYSIS includes other forms of paralysis which, being of cerebral origin, should be mentioned here, although they are not connected with any discoverable disease of the brain. These forms of paralysis are amenable to psychological treatment, the cause of the paralysis often being traceable to some deepseated mental conflict having its origin in childhood. (See HYSTERIA.)

(2) PARALYSIS DUE TO DISEASE OF THE SPINAL CORD: Of paralysis from this cause, there are numerous varieties, depending on the nature, the site, and the extent of the disease. Frequently defects in muscular action, due to disease in the spinal cord, are not of a paralytic nature, and these must be carefully distinguished.

PARAPLEGIA, paralysis of both lower extremities, including usually the lower portion of the trunk, and occasionally also the upper portion – indeed, all the parts below the seat of the disease in the spinal cord – is a form of paralysis which is a common result of injuries or disease of the vertebral column; also of inflammation

affecting the spinal cord (myelitis), as well as of haemorrhage or tumours involving its substance. When it is due to disease, this is generally situated in the lower portion of the cord. The symptoms necessarily vary in relation to the locality and the extent of the disease in the cord. Thus, if in the affected area the posterior part of the cord, including the posterior nerve roots, suffer, the function of sensation in the parts below is impaired because the cord is unable to transmit the sensory impressions from the surface of the body to the brain, and the condition of ataxia affects the power of motion. If, on the other hand, the anterior portion of the cord and the anterior nerve roots be affected, the motor impulses from the brain cannot be conveyed to the muscles below the seat of the injury or disease, and consequently their power of movement is abolished. Whilst, if the lateral portions of the cord be affected, a condition of spastic paralysis is set up. In many forms of this complaint, particularly in the case of injuries, the whole thickness of the cord is involved (transverse myelitis), and both sensory and motor functions are lost below the level at which the cord is affected. Further, the functions of the bladder and bowels are apt to suffer, and either spasm, or more often paralysis, of these organs is the result. The nutrition of the paralysed parts tends to become affected, and bed sores and wasting of the muscles are common. Occasionally, more especially in cases of injury, recovery takes place, but in general

right side   left side

1 conscious muscle sense, direct touch
2 unconscious muscle sense
3 voluntary control of striated muscle
4 involuntary control of striated muscle
5 pain, heat and cold
6 crossed touch
7 ventral corticospinal tract (pyramidal)

8 ventral spinothalmic tract
9 ventral spinocerebellar tract
10 lateral spinothalmic tract
11 rubrospinal tract (extrapyramidal
12 lateral corticospinal tract (pyramidal)
13 dorsal spinocerebellar tract
14 posterior columns

Diagram of a cross-section of spinal cord. Nerve
tracts are shown on the right and their function
on the left.

this is incomplete, the power of walking being more or less impaired. When the paralysis is due to pressure caused by a diseased or injured spine, an operation often designed to relieve this pressure is often completely successful, and entire power is restored, even after the paralysis has lasted for several months. Advances in recent years, however, have gone a long way towards ameliorating the lot of the paraplegic patient and allowing him or her to lead a reasonably active life at home and in the community. Patients and their relatives can obtain help and advice from the Spinal Injuries Association, Newpoint House, 76 St James's Lane, Muswell Hill, London N10 3DF (081-444 2121) and the Scottish Spinal Cord Injury Association, Unit 22, 100 Elderpark Street, Glasgow G51 3TR (041-440 0960).

INFANTILE PARALYSIS (see POLIOMYELITIS).

MOTOR NEURON DISEASE is a disease usually occurring in middle life. Pathologically it is characterized by degeneration: (*a*) of the anterior horn cells of the grey matter of the spinal cord, with corresponding degeneration of the peripheral motor nerves and wasting of the muscles innervated by them; (*b*) of the nerve cells in the bulb of the brain from which the motor cranial nerves arise: hypoglossal, facial, trigeminal, oculomotor, accessory, glossopharyngeal, vagus; (*c*) in some cases the large motor neurons of the cerebral cortex that give rise to the cortico-spinal tract. There is diffuse atrophy of the white matter of the spinal cord, excepting the posterior, sensory columns. The cause of the degeneration is not known. Approximately one person in 50,000 develops it each year, and it is estimated that there are around 5000 victims of it in the United Kingdom.

BULBAR PARALYSIS may occur as a form of motor neuron disease, or as a complication of other diseases, including rabies, diphtheria, and polyneuritis. The muscles of facial expression, of mastication, of articulation, and of swallowing suffer progressive loss of power.

Treatment: All forms of motor neuron disease run an inexorable course to a fatal termination. There is no treatment in the strict sense of the term, but much can be done to make the lot of the victim more comfortable.

Much help can be obtained from the Motor Neurone Disease Association, PO Box 246, Northampton NN1 2PR (0604-25050 or 22269, fax: 0604-24726).

PROGRESSIVE MUSCULAR DYSTROPHY, MYOPATHY, or PSEUDOHYPERTROPHIC MUSCULAR DYSTROPHY, is one of the muscular dystrophies. (See MYOPATHY.)

(3) PERIPHERAL PARALYSIS, or local paralysis of individual nerves, is of frequent occurrrence. Only the most common and important examples of this condition will be briefly referred to.

FACIAL PARALYSIS and BELL'S PALSY are the terms applied to paralysis involving the muscles of expression supplied by the seventh cranial nerve. It is unilateral. The cause is not known, but it sometimes follows exposure of one side of the head to a draught of cold air, which sets up inflammation of the nerve. It may also be due to injury or disease either affecting the nerve near the surface or deeper in the bony canals through which it passes, or in the brain itself, involving the nerve at its origin. The paralysis is manifested by a marked change in the expression of the face, the patient being unable to move the muscles of one side in such acts as laughing, and whistling, or to close the eye on that side. Recovery usually takes place in about six weeks, the improvement being first shown in the power of closing the eye, which is soon followed by the disappearance of the other signs. Recovery may be speeded up by the administration of prednisolone (q.v.), especially if this is given at an early stage of the disease. It is more effective in younger patients (under the age of 45) than older ones. When the paralysis proceeds from damage to the nerve, disease of the temporal bone, or from tumours in the brain, it is more apt to be permanent.

A form of peripheral paralysis often results from chronic alcoholism. Other poisons also act similarly, as, for example, lead and arsenic. (See NEURITIS.) Injury to a nerve may cause paralysis in the muscles which it should supply, and this may follow on wounds, severe bruises, or even long-continued pressure, as in crutch-palsy. (See DROP-WRIST; NERVE INJURIES.)

Treatment: Generally speaking, the treatment consists of measures which aim at supporting the patient's strength and maintaining his health while the nervous system is slowly restoring itself.

An important point in the treatment is that, since paralysed muscles tend to undergo degenerative changes, their action should be maintained as long as possible. With the view of improving the circulation in the muscles, and also in order to prevent stiffening of the joints, massage is very useful.

In the case of paraplegia there is a necessity for highly skilled nursing, since not only the patient's comfort but his life depends upon careful management, directed towards preventing bed sores (see BED SORES), and inflammation of the bladder (see CATHETERS) in cases in which the act of urination is interfered with.

PARAMEDICAL: A description applied to those professions closely linked to and working with the medical profession. Paramedical workers have expert knowledge or skill in their particular area of health but they do not have a medical degree. Examples are nurses, physiotherapists, occupational therapists, radiographers, and dietitians.

PARAMETER: A measurement of a certain factor – for example, pulse rate, blood pressure, or haemoglobin concentration – that is relevant to a disorder under investigation.

PARAMNESIA is a derangement of the memory in which words are used without a comprehension of their meaning; it is also applied to illusions of memory in which a person in good faith imagines and describes experiencès which never occurred to him.

PARANOIA is a form of mental illness characterized by fixed delusions, usually of persecution. Many sufferers are able to go about freely and carry out activities with which their delusions do not interfere. In loose English usage, 'paranoia' means 'subject to any sorts of feelings of persecution'. (See MENTAL ILLNESS).

PARAPHASIA is misplacement of words, or use of wrong words, in speech as a result of a lesion in the speech region of the brain.

PARAPHIMOSIS: The constriction of the penis behind the glans by an abnormally tight foreskin that has been retracted. The condition causes swelling and severe pain. Sometimes the foreskin can be returned by manual manipulation after an ice pack has been applied to the glans. Sometimes an operation to cut the foreskin is required to release it.

PARAPHRENIA is a form of paranoia (q.v.). (See also MENTAL ILLNESS.)

PARAPLEGIA means paralysis of the lower limbs, accompanied generally by paralysis of bladder and rectum. (See PARALYSIS.)

PARAQUAT is a contact herbicide widely used in agriculture and horticulture. A mouthful is enough to kill. Its major misuse has resulted from its being decanted from the professional pack into soft-drink bottles and kept in the domestic kitchen. The resultant potential for accidental and probably fatal ingestion is obvious. It is involved in around 40 cases of suicide every year. The eyes and skin must be carefully protected so as not to come into contact with it. So widespread is its use that nineteen medical centres have been set up throughout the country to provide treatment in cases of poisoning with it. Details of these can be obtained from the National Poisons Information Service centres in London (071-407 7600), Edinburgh (031-229 2477) and Cardiff (0222-711711).

PARASITE: An organism which lives in or on another organism, known as the host. A parasite derives all its nourishment from the host but provides no benefits in return. It may damage the host's bodily functions and in extreme cases cause the death of the host. Human parasites include worms, fungi, bacteria and viruses.

PARASITICIDE is a general term applied to agents or substances destructive to parasites.

PARASUICIDE is non-fatal self-poisoning or self-injury, or attempted suicide. It is most common in the 12–15 age-group. The intention is not as a rule to commit suicide, but a cry for help to resolve an acute domestic upset.

PARASYMPATHETIC NERVOUS SYSTEM is that part of the autonomic nervous system which is connected with the brain and spinal cord through certain nerve centres in the midbrain, medulla, and lower end of the cord. The nerves from these centres are carried in the 3rd, 7th, 9th, and 10th cranial nerves and the 2nd, 3rd, and 4th sacral nerves. The action of the parasympathetic system is usually antagonistic to that of the sympathetic system. Thus it inhibits the action of the heart and augments the action of the intestine, whereas the sympathetic augments the action of the heart and inhibits that of the intestine.

PARATHION is one of the organo-phosphorus insecticides (q.v.). It is highly toxic to man and must therefore be handled with the utmost care.

PARATHYROID is the name applied to four small glands, about 5 mm in diameter, which lie to the side of and behind the thyroid gland. These glands regulate the metabolism of calcium and of phosphorus. If for any reason there is a deficiency of the secretion of the parathyroid glands, the amount of calcium in the blood falls too low and the amount of phosphorus increases. The result is the condition known as tetany (q.v.), in which there is great restlessness and spasm of muscles. The condition is checked by the injection of calcium gluconate – which causes an increase in the amount of calcium in the blood. The commonest cause of this condition, or hypoparathyroidism as it is known, is accidental injury to or removal of the glands during the operation of thyroidectomy for the treatment of Graves' disease (q.v.). This is one of the hazards of thyroidectomy in view of the very close relationship of the parathyroid glands to the thyroid gland. If there is over-production of the parathyroids there will be an increase of calcium in the blood. This extra calcium is drawn from the bones, in which, as a consequence, thin cysts form and greatly weaken the bones, these breaking easily as a result. This cystic disease of bone is known as OSTEITIS FIBROSA CYSTICA (q.v.). Tumours of the parathyroid glands result in this overactivity of the parathyroid hormone, and the resulting increase in the amount of calcium in the blood leads to the formation of stones in the kidneys. The only available treatment is surgical removal of the tumour. This state of increased activity of the parathyroid glands, or hyperparathyroidism, is always considered as a possible cause in dealing with a case of stones in the kidneys. (See KIDNEYS, DISEASES OF.)

PARATYPHOID FEVER (see ENTERIC FEVERS).

PAREGORIC, or CAMPHORATED OPIUM TINCTURE, is a preparation of opium much used for cough mixtures. It contains 5 per cent of tincture of opium, together with oil of anise, benzoic acid and camphor. The dose is 2 to 10 ml. Scotch paregoric, or ammoniated opium tincture, contains 10 per cent of tincture of opium, together with dilute ammonia solution, oil of anise and benzoic acid. The dose is 2 to 4 ml.

PARENCHYMA is a term meaning originally all the soft tissues of internal organs except the muscular flesh, though now reserved for the secreting cells of the glandular organs.

PARENTERAL is the word applied to the administration of drugs by any route other than by the mouth or by the bowel.

PARENTERAL NUTRITION: In severely ill patients, especially those who have had major surgery or with sepsis, burns, acute pancreatitis and renal failure, the body's reserves of protein become exhausted. This results in weight loss, reduction of muscle mass, a fall in the serum albumin and lymphocyte count and an impairment of cellular immunity. Severely ill patients are unable to take adequate food by mouth to repair the body protein loss so that enteral or parenteral nutrition is required. Enteral feeding is through the gastro-intestinal tract with the aid of a naso-gastric tube. Parenteral nutrition involves the provision of carbohydrate, fat and proteins by intravenous administration. Intitally the carbohydrate glucose was the sole energy substrate used, but it soon became appreciated that regimes supplying an equal proportion of carbohydrate and fat were preferable in the vast majority of cases. Over the last decade a multitude of nitrogen solutions have been developed for the purpose of intravenous nutrition. As with enteral nutrition there are few indications for the administrations of pure amino acids. All patients requiring intravenous nutrition will require, in addition, a supply of vitamins and essential minerals.

Methods of vascular access have improved remarkably over recent years. The preferred route for the infusion of hyperosmolar solutions is via a central venous catheter. If parenteral nutrition is required for more than two weeks it is advisable to use a long-term type catheter such as the Broviac, Hickman or extra corporeal type, which is made of silastic material and is inserted via a long subcutaneous tunnel, which not only helps to fix the catheter but minimizes the risk of ascending infection.

Dextrose is considered the best source of carbohydrate and may be used as a 20-per-cent or 50-per-cent solution. Amino acids should be in the laevo form and should contain the correct proportion of essential and non-essential amino acids. Preparations such as Vamin glucose 9, Synthamin 9 (low nitrogen solution), Synthamin 14 and 17 (high nitrogen solutions) are available with or without electrolytes. Intralipid is the safest fat emulsion and is used either as 10 per cent or 20 per cent solution.

The main hazards of intravenous feeding are blood-borne infections made possible by continued direct access to the circulation, and biochemical abnormalities related to the composition of the solutions infused. The continuous use of hypertonic solutions of glucose can cause hyperglycaemia and glycosuria and the resultant polyuria may lead to dehydration. Treatment with insulin is needed when hyperosmolality occurs, and in addition the water and sodium deficits will require to be corrected.

PARESIS means a state of partial paralysis. (See PARALYSIS.)

PARIETAL is the term applied to anything pertaining to the wall of a cavity: e.g. parietal pleura, the part of the pleural membrane which lines the wall of the chest.

PARIETAL LOBE: A major section of each cerebral hemisphere (see BRAIN). The two lobes lie under the parietal bones and contain the sensory cortex.

PARKINSONISM, or PARKINSON'S DISEASE, so called after the London general practitioner who first described the condition in 1817, is also known as PARALYSIS AGITANS. It is a progressive disease of insidious onset which comes on in the second half of life, and is due to degenerative changes in the ganglia at the base of the cerebrum. This results in a deficiency of a neurotransmitter known as dopamine (q.v.), and it is this deficiency of dopamine which is responsible for most cases. In some, however, deficiency of neurotransmitters other than dopamine may be the cause. It is much commoner in men than in women. In some cases the disease is a sequel to encephalitis lethargica. The disease first manifests itself by increasing rigidity of the muscles. In the face this results in a loss of the natural play of expression and produces a mask-like expression. The voice is also affected by the rigidity of the muscles of the larynx, tongue and lips, loses its tone and inflexion and develops into a monotone. Later the limbs become rigid, and this is typified by the peculiar running gait. The patient always seems to be tottering and taking short steps as if running after himself. Later a coarse tremor develops in the muscles, best typified in the rolling movements of the fingers as if a cigarette were always being rolled. The tremor is exaggerated by excitement and self-consciousness and ceases during sleep. In the hands and arms it may interfere grossly with eating and dressing.

Treatment: There is now an increasing number

of drugs that keep the condition under control. None is curative, and the effort to find the most suitable one for any given individual is usually a matter of trial and error, the successful outcome of which depends largely upon understanding co-operation between family doctor and patient. The most promising one at the moment is levodopa which is a precursor of dopamine. Its introduction has revolutionized the outlook in this disease. Unfortunately it has considerable side-effects, which means that it must only be administered under skilled medical supervision. Current opinion is that it produces spectacular improvement in one-fifth of patients, moderate improvement in two-fifths, modest improvement in one-fifth, and no improvement in one-fifth. A recently introduced drug proving of value in supplementing the benefit of levodopa is selegiline.

Patients with the disease and their relatives, seeking advice and help, are recommended to get in touch with the Parkinson's Disease Society of the UK, 22 Upper Woburn Place, London WC1H 0RA (071-383 3513, fax: 071-383 5754).

PARONYCHIA is the term applied to inflammation near the nail. In the *acute* form it is usually due to infection with *Staphylococcus aureus*, and is most often seen in nurses and others handling septic material. It usually starts at one corner of the nail-fold and then spreads to the other side and deeply under the base of the nail. There is local pain and tenderness, with swelling of the nail-fold. Treatment in mild cases consists of applying an adhesive dressing and giving penicillin. In more severe cases the swelling has to be opened. A new nail grows in two or three months, displacing the old one in front of it. *Chronic paronychia* occurs usually in women who have their hands much in water. In men it occurs in fishmongers and chefs. It may affect one or more fingers. Treatment consists of keeping the finger dry and giving a suitable antibiotic. (See WHITLOW.)

PAROSMIA means a perverted sense of smell; everything usually smells unpleasant to the affected individual. The most common cause is some septic condition of the nasal passages, but it may occasionally be due to a lesion in the brain involving the centre responsible for the sense of smell.

PAROTID GLAND is one of the salivary glands (q.v.). It is situated just in front of the ear, and its duct runs forwards across the cheek to open into the interior of the mouth on a little projection opposite the second last tooth of the upper row. The parotid gland is generally the first of the salivary glands to become enlarged in mumps.

PAROTITIS means inflammation of the parotid gland. Epidemic parotitis is another name for mumps (q.v.).

PAROXYSM: A sudden temporary attack that may take the form of a convulsion or spasm. It may also occur when a patient with a disease suddenly deteriorates.

PARTHENOGENESIS is non-sexual reproduction. In other words, development of the ovum into an individual without fertilization by a spermatozoon. It has been produced in animals experimentally. There is, however, no certain record of the birth of a parthenogenetic animal. The most that has been achieved is that parthogenetic mice and rabbit embryos have developed normally to about halfway through pregnancy but have then died and been aborted.

PARTOGRAM is a method of recording the degree of dilatation, or opening, of the cervix (or neck) of the uterus in labour, which is of value in assessing how labour is progressing.

PARTURITION (see LABOUR).

PARVOVIRUSES (from *parvus*, Latin for small) is a group of viruses responsible for outbreaks of winter vomiting disease (q.v.).

P.A.S. is a commonly used abbreviation for para-aminosalicylic acid (q.v.).

PASSIVE MOVEMENT: A movement induced by someone other than the patient. Physiotherapists manipulate joints by passive movement in order to retain and encourage function of a nerve or muscle that is not working normally because of injury or disease.

PASTEURELLA is a group of bacilli. They are essentially animal parasites that under certain conditions are transmitted to man. They include the micro-organism responsible for plague and tularaemia.

PASTEURIZATION is a method of sterilizing milk. In many parts of the world pasteurization has done away with milk-borne infections, of which the most serious is bovine tuberculosis, affecting the glands, bones, and joints of children. Other infections conveyed by milk are scarlet fever, diphtheria, enteric fever (typhoid and paratyphoid), undulant fever (brucellosis), and food poisoning (eg. from salmonellae or the toxins of the staphylococcus). The case therefore is very clear for the compulsory pasteurization of all milk. Yet 10 per cent of all milk retailed in Scotland is neither pasteurized nor heat treated in any way. The comparable figure for England and Wales is 3 per cent. HIGH-TEMPERATURE SHORT-TIME (HTST) PASTEURIZATION consists in heating the milk at a temperature not less than 71·7 °C (161 °F) for at least fifteen seconds, followed by immediate cooling to a temperature of not more than 10 °C (50 °F).

LOW-TEMPERATURE PASTEURIZATION, or 'HOLDER' PROCESS, consists in maintaining the milk for at least half-an-hour at a temperature between 63 to 65 °C (145 °F and 150 °F), followed by immediate cooling to a temperature of not more that 10 °C (50 °F). This has the effect of considerably reducing the number of bacteria contained in the milk and of preventing the diseases conveyed by milk referred to above. This procedure is sufficient for the sale of milk as 'pasteurized milk' in England. (See MILK.)

PATCH TEST: This is used to identify possible substances that may be causing a patient's allergy. Small amounts of different substances are placed on the skin, usually the back or arm. If the patient is allergic a red flare and swelling will appear, usually within about 15 minutes. Sometimes the reaction may take longer – up to three days – to develop.

PATELLA, also known as the knee-pan or knee-cap, is a flat bone shaped somewhat like an oyster-shell, lying in the tendon of the extensor muscle of the thigh, and protecting the knee-joint in front. (See BONE; KNEE; FRACTURES.)

PATELLAR REFLEX (see REFLEX ACTION).

PATENT DUCTUS ARTERIOSUS (see DUCTUS ARTERIOSUS).

PATHOGENIC means disease-producing, and is a term, for example, applied to bacteria, capable of causing disease.

PATHOGNOMONIC is a term applied to signs or symptoms which are specially characteristic of certain diseases, and on the presence or absence of which the diagnosis depends. Thus the discovery of the *Mycobacterium tuberculosis* in the expectoration is said to be pathognomonic of pulmonary tuberculosis.

PATHOLOGY is the science which deals with the causes of, and changes produced in the body by, disease.

PATIENT-CONTROLLED ANALGESIA: A technique whereby a patient can deliver an analgesic substance in amounts related to the extent of the pain he is suffering. For example, to combat postoperative pain some hospitals use devices which allow patients to give themselves small intravenous amounts of opiates when they are needed. Pain is more effectively controlled if it is not allowed to reach a high level, a situation which tends to happen when patients receive analgesics only on ward drug rounds or when they ask the nursing staff for them.

PAUL-BUNNELL TEST is a test for mononucleosis (q.v.) which is based upon the fact that patients with this disease develop antibodies which agglutinate sheep red blood cells.

PECTIN is a polysaccharide substance allied to starch, contained in fruits and plants, and forming the basis of vegetable jelly. It has been used as a transfusion fluid in place of blood in cases of haemorrhage and shock.

PECTORAL means anything pertaining to the chest, or a remedy used in treating chest troubles.

PECTORILOQUY means the resonance of the voice, when spoken or whispered words can be clearly heard through the stethoscope. It is a sign of consolidation, or of a cavity, in the lung.

PEDICLE: A narrow tube of tissue formed by folded skin which links a piece of tissue used for surgical grafting to its site of origin. A pedicle graft is used by the surgeon when the site under repair is unsuitable for an independent graft, usually because the blood supply at the recipient site is inadequate.

A pedicle is also found occurring between a tumour and its tissue of origin, and the term is used in anatomy to refer to any slim tubular process.

PEDICULOSIS is infestation with lice.
PEDICULI, or lice, are of three species, which vary in shape and size as well as in the area of the body they infest.
PEDICULUS HUMANUS var. CAPITIS (*Pediculus capitis*), or the head louse, is similar in practically all respects to the body louse, except that it occurs in the head and not on the trunk of the body. It is more common in girls and women than boys and men. The eggs, commonly known as nits and visible as little white specks, are usually laid in the hairs of the back of the head; behind the ears is also a favourite site. On infested heads the hairs are often matted together by the exudate which results from irritation and scratching. The glands behind the ears and in the back of the neck are often enlarged.
PEDICULUS HUMANUS var. CORPORIS (*Pediculus vestimenti*), or the body louse, is found on the underclothing on the trunk and upper arms, rather than on the skin. The female louse, which has a life of almost a month, lays seven to ten eggs a day. The eggs hatch out in 7 to 10 days and become mature in another week. Without food the adult dies in nine days and the newly hatched louse in two days. The eggs are viable for much longer (up to a month) and are usually found in the more inaccessible parts of the clothing: e.g. the seams.
PEDICULUS PUBIS, popularly known as the crab louse, is broader and shorter. It is found predominantly on the short hairs of the pubic

region, to which it adheres very tenaciously. It may also infest the eye-lashes, beard, and leg and under-arm hairs. It causes intense itching. So far as is known, it does not carry any disease. It is most commonly transmitted from one person to another by sexual contact. Live lice have been found on lavatory seats, and the eggs may be spread from a lousy person by attachment of their infected hairs to towels and clothing.

(For further details, see INSECTS IN RELATION TO DISEASE.)

PEDUNCLE: A stalk-like structure that usually acts as a support.

PELLAGRA is a nutritional disorder, showing a number of nervous, digestive, and skin symptoms.

Causes: It occurs in those parts of the world where the inhabitants live on a diet of maize without adequate first-class protein in the form of milk and meat. It is due to deficiency of the nicotinic acid component of the vitamin B complex, in association with deficiency of protein. For long the puzzling feature was that it occurred predominantly in maize-eating areas of the world, yet maize has as much nicotinic acid as wheat but the disease did not occur in wheat-eating areas. The explanation is that the nicotinic acid in maize is in a bound form that the consumer cannot utilize. Further, maize is deficient in the amino-acid, tryptophan, from which the human body can make nicotinic acid.

Symptoms: Pellagra is known as the disease of the three D's: dermatitis, diarrhoea and dementia. The course of pellagra lasts many years, with digestive disturbances including loss of appetite and diarrhoea or constipation, headache, and irritability of temper. The skin manifestations consist at first of redness resembling severe sunburn on the parts of the body exposed to the sun, such as the hands, forearms, chest, neck, and face. The irritation usually lasts about a fortnight, is followed by desquamation, and the skin remains rough, thickened, and permanently brownish in colour. This brownish and roughened appearance on the hands is the most prominent feature of the disease, and from this the disease takes its name. Tremors, sleepiness, and weakness of the legs also appear. For several years the disease may recur in this manner every spring, the attacks gradually becoming more severe, the patient slowly growing emaciated and in some cases completely paralytic or demented.

Treatment: The disease is prevented or cured by adding to the diet foods such as fresh meat, eggs, milk, liver, and yeast extracts, and nicotinic acid, as well as by improvement of the general conditions of life.

PELVIC INFLAMMATORY DISEASE: Acute or chronic infection of the ovaries, fallopian tube, or uterus. The condition is usually caused by infection spreading from the vagina or from a nearby infected organ – for example, the appendix. Blood-borne infection may also be the cause. Lower abdominal pain, sometimes severe, is characteristic of the condition. Treatment may be by antibiotics or sometimes surgery.

PELVIMETRY: Measurement of the internal dimensions of the pelvis. The four diameters measured are: transverse, anterioposterior, and left and right oblique. These measurements help to establish whether a fetus can be delivered normally. If the outlet is abnormally small, the mother will have to be delivered by Caesarian section.

PELVIS is that divison of the skeleton which is made up of the haunch-bones, one on each side, and the sacrum and coccyx behind. It connects the lower limbs with the spine. Each haunch-bone is composed of three originally separate bones, in the adult pelvis firmly fused together: the ilium; the ischium, with a rounded part below, the tuberosity, upon which the body rests in sitting; and the pubis in front. The expanded parts of the iliac bones incompletely surround the lower part of the abdomen, known as the false pelvis, and are separated by a distinct line, known as the brim or inlet, from the true pelvis beneath. The true pelvis, as its name implies, is basin-shaped; though in the dried state it has a wide outlet beneath, yet in the living body this is well closed and rounded off by ligaments and muscles so as to leave small openings only for the urinary and genital passages and for the rectum. This soft floor of the pelvis is composed mainly of two muscles, the levators of the anus, whilst the deep notch, between the haunch-bone and sacrum behind, is closed in by a pair of strong sacro-sciatic ligaments.

The pelvis varies considerably in the two sexes. In the female it is shallower and the ilia are more widely separated, giving great breadth to the hips of the woman; the inlet is more circular and the outlet larger; whilst the angle beneath the pubic bones (subpubic angle), which is an acute angle in the male, is obtuse in the female. All these points are of importance in connection with child-bearing.

The contents of the pelvis are the urinary bladder and rectum in both sexes; in addition the male has the seminal vesicles and the prostate gland surrounding the neck of the bladder, whilst the female has the womb, ovaries, and their appendages.

In addition to these sex differences, there are differences in the pelvis of different races, those of certain races, such as the Negro race, being, generally speaking, longer from before back and from above down than those of Caucasians: the so-called anthropoid pelvis.

PEMPHIGOID (see PEMPHIGUS).

PEMPHIGUS is an autoimmune skin condition characterized by the appearance of large blebs. *Pemphigus neonatorum* is really a form of impetigo in which bullae (or large blisters) occur. (The term pemphigus neonatorum is misleading and should be abandoned.) It is liable to occur in nurseries and maternity hospitals and is highly infectious. Strict isolation of cases is essential and the prognosis is satisfactory provided active treatment is started at an early stage. In addition to the local treatment recommended for impetigo in older children and adults, an antibiotic or sulphonamide should be given provided the staphylococcus responsible or the condition is sensitive to it. Unfortunately *Staphylococcus aureus*, especially that which occurs in hospital, is so often resistant to penicillin that this antibiotic is of no avail, and some other has to be used. *Pemphigus vulgaris*, which occurs in the middle-aged, particularly Jews, is a comparatively rare condition. The skin eruption is accompanied by marked constitutional disturbances and, until the introduction of the corticosteroids (q.v.) it was almost invariably fatal, though it still carries a mortality rate of 30–50 per cent. With large doses of corticosteroids, however, the condition can usually be kept under control. The local application of zinc cream or calamine lotion is soothing. *Pemphigus foliaceus*, in which practically the whole of the skin may be involved, is not marked by such constitutional disturbances. Treatment is as for pemphigus vulgaris. *Pemphigoid* is the form of the disease as it occurs in old age. It responds well to corticosteroids. It may occur as a complication of penicillamine or gold therapy and usually clears on withdrawal of the offending drug.

PENICILLAMINE is a metabolite of penicillin which is a chelating agent (q.v.). It is sometimes used in rheumatoid arthritis that has not responded to the first-line remedies and it is particularly useful when the disease is complicated by vasculitis. Penicillamine is also used as an antidote to poisoning by heavy metals, particularly copper and lead, as it is able to bind these metals and so remove their toxic effects. Because of its ability to bind copper it is also used in Wilson's disease where there is a deficiency in the copper-binding protein so that copper is able to become deposited in he brain and liver, damaging these tissues.

PENICILLIN is the name given by Sir Alexander Fleming, in 1929, to an antibacterial substance produced by the mould *Penicillium notatum*. This mould was first described in 1911 in Scandinavia, where it was discovered in decaying hyssop. The story of penicillin is one of the most dramatic in the history of medicine, and its introduction into medicine initiated a new era in therapeutics comparable only to the introduction of anaesthesia by Morton and Simpson and of antiseptics by Pasteur and Lister. The two names that will always be primarily associated with penicillin are those of

Sir Alexander Fleming, of St Mary's Hospital, London, who discovered its anti-bacterial action, and Lord Florey, of Oxford, who did so much to develop its practical use during the 1939–45 War. The two great advantages of penicillin are that it is active against a large range of bacteria and that, even in large doses, it is non-toxic. Among the organisms against which it is active are: staphylococcus, streptococcus, pneumococcus, meningococcus, gonococcus, and the organisms responsible for syphilis, and for gas gangrene.

Penicillin has been synthesized in the laboratory, but it is such a complex and unstable substance that there is no reason to believe that it will be possible to synthesize it on a commercial scale – at least not for a long time to come. This means that the main method of obtaining penicillin is by the laborious technique of cultivating the penicillin mould, *Penicillium chrysogenum*. Partial synthesis of penicillin, however, has been achieved by the isolation of the penicillin nucleus – 6-aminopenicillanic acid. This can still only be obtained by culture of the penicillin mould but, now that the nucleus can be isolated, it has proved possible to add side-chains to it and so produce a large number of different – semi-synthetic as they are known – penicillins.

Various forms of penicillin are now available. *Benzylpenicillin* is available as the sodium or potassium salt. It is given intramuscularly, and is the form that is used when a rapid action is required. It can also be given by mouth but, as the proportion absorbed varies greatly, it is unreliable in action when given in this way. *Procaine penicillin* is a relatively insoluble form of penicillin. A single daily intramuscular injection of 600,000 units will maintain a bacteriostatic level in the blood for twenty-four hours. *Benzathine penicillin* is a relatively insoluble derivative of penicillin which is often given by mouth. When given intramuscularly it gives low but very prolonged blood levels of penicillin. *Phenoxymethylpenicillin* is given by mouth but is absorbed inconstantly.

Phenethicillin was the first of the penicillins obtained by adding a side chain to the penicillin nucleus. It is effective when taken by mouth and produces a blood concentration of penicillin which is twice as great as that following a comparable dose of phenoxymethylpenicillin. *Ampicillin* is another of the penicillins derived by semi-synthesis from the penicillin nucleus. It, too, is active when taken by mouth, but its special feature is that it is active against Gram-negative micro-organisms such as *E. coli* and the salmonellae. *Cloxacillin* is yet another of the semi-synthesized penicillins. It has a relatively weak antibacterial action, but has the advantage of being active against penicillin-resistant staphylococci. *Propicillin* is alpha-phenoxypropyl penicillin, which is active when taken by mouth, and against penicillin-resistant staphylococci. *Phenbenicillin* is potassium phenoxybenzylpenicillin and is active when taken by mouth.

Methicillin is another penicillin derived from

the penicillin nucleus. It is active against peni-cillin-resistant staphylococci but has to be given by injection as it is destroyed by the acid secretion of the stomach. *Carbenicillin*, a semi-synthetic penicillin, must be given by injection, which may be painful. Its main use is in dealing with infections due to *Pseudomonas pyocanea*. It is the only penicillin active against this micro-organism. *Carfecillin* is another semi-synthetic penicillin. It is given by mouth and in the body is converted into carbenicillin, to which it owes its antibiotic properties. It is proving of particu-lar value in the treatment of infection of the urinary tract such as cystitis and pyelonephritis. *Flucloxacillin*, also a semi-synthetic penicillin, is active against penicillin-resistant staphylococci and has the practical advantage of being active when taken by mouth. *Amoxycillin* and *talampicillin* are orally administered semi-syn-thetic penicillins with the same range of action as ampicillin but less likely to cause side-effects. *Mezlocillin*, another semi-synthetic penicillin, is comparable to ampicillin in its range of action, but is particularly active against *H. influenzae*, gonococci, and *Proteus* micro-or-ganisms. *Mecillinam* is yet another in this series, though of slightly different chemical origin. It is of value in the treatment of infections with salmonellae (see FOOD POISONING), including typhoid fever, and with *E. coli* (see ESCHERICHIA). It is given by injection. There is a derivative, *Pivmecillinam*, which can be taken by mouth.

PENIS is the organ down which, in the male, passes the urethra, the tube by which the contents of the urinary bladder and those of the seminal vesicles escape (see EJACULATION).

PENTAMIDINE is a drug that is used in the prevention and treatment of African trypan-somiasis, and in the treatment of leishmaniasis.

PENTAZOCINE is a pain-relieving drug with similar actions and uses to those of morphine, but much less likely to lead to addiction. It is given, usually by injection, for the relief of moderate to severe pain, especially postopera-tive pain, and to relieve the pain of myocardial infarction, or coronary thrombosis.

PEPPERMINT is the leaves and tops of *Mentha piperita*. It has an aromatic odour, due to the presence of an oil from which is obtained menthol, a camphor-like substance. Pepper-mint water is a useful remedy for flatulence and colic in infants. Oil of peppermint is used like the other volatile oils.

PEPSIN is the name given to a ferment found in the gastric juice which digests proteins by converting them into peptides and amino-acids. Pepsin is used in medicine in cases of weak digestion either to digest food before it is taken or more frequently to administer after meals. It is a light yellowish-brown or white

powder prepared from the fresh mucous mem-brane of the stomach of pigs, sheep, or calves. (For the predigestion of food, see PEPTONIZED FOODS.)

PEPTIC ULCER is the term commonly ap-plied to ulcers in the stomach and duodenum. (See DUODENAL ULCER; STOMACH, DISEASES OF.)

PEPTIDE is a compound formed by the union of two or more amino-acids.

PEPTONIZED FOODS are foods which have been predigested by pancreatin (q.v.) and thereby rendered more digestible.

PERCUSSION is an aid to diagnosis practised by striking the body with the fingers, in such a way as to make it give out a note. It was introduced in 1761 by Leopold Auenbrugger (1722–1809) of Vienna, the son of an innkeeper, who derived the idea from the habit of his father tapping casks of wine to ascertain how much wine they contained. According to the degree of dullness or resonance of the note, an opinion can be formed as to the state of consolidation of air-containing organs, the presence of abnormal cavities in organs, and the dimensions of solid and air-containing organs, which happen to lie next to one an-other. Still more valuable evidence is given by auscultation (q.v.).

PERCUTANEOUS is a term applied to any method of administering remedies by passing them through the skin, as by rubbing in an ointment or carrying in drugs on the galvanic current.

PERFORATION is one of the serious dangers attaching to any ulcerated condition of the stomach or bowels. When a perforation from one of these hollow organs takes place into the peritoneal cavity, many bacteria, are poured into this cavity and there set up peritonitis. (See PERITONITIS.) The immediate signs that a perfo-ration has taken place are usually a state of collapse, and increase of pain over the abdo-men, together with, in some cases, the evidence of free fluid and gas in the peritoneal cavity.

PERFUSION: The transfer of fluid through a tissue. For example, when blood passes through the lung tissue, dissolved oxygen perfuses from the moist air in the alveoli to the blood. Fluid may also be deliberately introduced into a tissue by injecting it into the blood vessels supplying the tissue.

PERI- is a prefix meaning around.

PERIARTERITIS NODOSA (see POLY-ARTERITIS NODOSA).

PERICARDITIS means inflammation of the pericardium. (See HEART DISEASES.)

PERICARDIUM is the smooth membrane that surrounds the heart. (See HEART.)

PERICHONDRITIS: Inflammation of cartilage (q.v.) and the tissue surrounding it, usually as a result of chronic infection.

PERICYAZINE (see NEUROLEPTICS).

PERIMETRITIS means a localized inflammation of the peritoneum surrounding the womb.

PERINATAL MORTALITY consists of deaths of the fetus after the 28th week of pregnancy and deaths of the new-born child during the first week of life. Today, more individuals die within a few hours of birth than during the following forty years. It is therefore not surprising that the perinatal mortality rate, which is the number of such deaths per 1000 total births, has come to be looked upon as a valuable indicator of the quality of care provided for the mother and her new-born baby. In 1990, the perinatal mortality rate was 8·1 in England, compared with 32·5 in 1960.

The causes of perinatal mortality include intrapartum anoxia (that is, difficulty in the birth of the baby, resulting in lack of oxygen), congenital abnormalities of the baby, antepartum anoxia (that is, conditions in the terminal stages of pregnancy preventing the fetus getting sufficient oxygen), and injuries to the brain of the baby during birth.

In 1990 perinatal deaths in England numbered 5,450 (which number includes still births). The deaths during the first weeks of life numbered 2,382. The commonest cause of perinatal death was some complication of placenta, cord or membranes. The next most common was congenital abnormality. Intra-uterine hypoxia and birth asphyxia comprised the third most common cause.

PERINEUM, or FORK, or CROTCH, is the region situated between the opening of the bowel behind and of the genital organs in front. In women it is apt to be lacerated in the act of childbirth.

PERIOD (see MENSTRUATION).

PERIODIC PARALYSIS is a condition characterized by the onset of weakness of the voluntary muscles. It usually occurs in young adults. As a rule the onset is in the morning on awakening. The weakness usually lasts for several hours. Attacks may also be brought on by a heavy meal or severe cold. It is a familial condition of obscure origin. There is one form, probably the most common, which is apparently due to a low level of potassium in the blood and is relieved by the taking of potassium chloride – 10 grams in water. There are other forms, however, in which the blood potassium may be raised or normal.

PERIODONTAL: An adjective that relates to the tissues around the teeth.

PERIODONTAL MEMBRANE (see TEETH).

PERIOSTEUM is the membrane surrounding a bone. The periosteum carries blood-vessels and nerves for the nutrition and development of the bone. When it is irritated, an increased deposit of bone takes place beneath it; if it is destroyed, the bone may cease to grow and a portion may die and separate as a sequestrum. (See BONE.)

PERIOSTITIS means inflammation on the surface of a bone affecting the periosteum. (See BONE, DISEASES OF.)

PERIPHERAL NEURITIS means inflammation of the nerves in the outlying parts of the body. (See NEURITIS.)

PERISTALSIS is the worm-like movement by which the stomach and bowels propel their contents. It consists of alternate waves of relaxation and contraction in successive parts of the tube. When any obstruction to the movement of the contents exists, these contractions become more forcible and are liable to be accompanied by the severe form of pain known as colic.

PERITONEOSCOPY is viewing of the peritoneal cavity through a tube fitted with mirrors and light. The instrument (see ENDOSCOPE) is entered just below the umbilicus. The peritoneal cavity is then inflated with air. This simple operation may obviate a more drastic one: for example, if peritoneoscopy shows deposits of cancer in the peritoneum or the liver. Colour photographs of the liver have been taken through the peritoneoscope.

PERITONEUM is the membrane lining the abdominal cavity, and forming a covering for the organs contained in it. That part lining the walls of the abdomen is called the parietal peritoneum, and that part covering the viscera is known as the visceral peritoneum. The two are continuous with one another at the back of the abdomen, and form a closed sac. One may understand its relation to the organs by conceiving them to have been pressed against the outside of this sac from behind, and each to have become wrapped up in the hinder part of the sac without being forced through to its interior, while the front wall of the sac remains quite smooth. The folds of peritoneum passing from one organ to another are thus very complicated, and receive special names in various parts. (See MESENTERY; OMENTUM.)

Although the peritoneum is said to form a closed sac, there is an exception in the female, the Fallopian tube on each side having an opening into the cavity at its end large enough to admit a bristle. There is, however, no large outlet for drainage of fluid, so that a small amount is always present to lubricate the membrane, while a large amount collects in conditions that are associated with dropsy. From this arises one great reason for the danger of inflammation affecting this membrane, since there is no escape from it for the pus and other products of inflammation, which accumulate and increase the state of irritation.

In structure the peritoneum consists of a dense, though thin and elastic, fibrous membrane covered, on its inner side, by a smooth glistening layer of plate-like epithelial cells. Here and there between the cells are minute openings (stomas), each of which communicates with a lymphatic vessel, so that the fluid in the cavity is constantly draining off into the general lymphatic circulation.

PERITONITIS means inflammation of the peritoneum or membrane investing the abdominal and pelvic cavities and their contained viscera. It may exist in an acute or a chronic form, and may be either localized in one part or generally diffused. Inflammation of this membrane varies much as regards its causes, severity, and danger, according as it is acute or chronic.

ACUTE PERITONITIS: **Causes**: As a rule it arises in consequence of the entrance of micro-organisms into the peritoneal cavity, which gain entrance through wounds from the exterior or pass out of some of the abdominal organs. The great danger which follows upon stabs and other penetrating wounds of the abdomen originates from the risk of peritonitis. On the other hand, the danger may come from within, and all conditions which lead to perforation of the stomach, bowels, bile-ducts, bladder, and other hollow organs may produce it. Thus gastric ulcer, typhoid fever, gall-stones, rupture of the bladder, strangulated hernia, and obstructions of the bowels may end in peritonitis. Again, abscesses and cysts developed in connection with various organs may burst and so produce it, appendicitis, abscesses of the ovary and Fallopian tubes being specially dangerous. Peritonitis may also arise within a few days after delivery.

The changes which take place in the peritoneum are similar to those undergone by other serous membranes when inflamed: (1) congestion; (2) exudation of fibrin in greater or less abundance, at first greyish in colour and soft, thereafter yellow and becoming tough in consistence, causing the folds of intestine to adhere together, and so tending to limit the spread of the inflammation; (3) effusion of fluid, either clear, turbid, bloody, or purulent; (4) absorption, more or less complete, of the fluid and

fibrin, or, in cases which proceed to a serious issue, the formation of grey or greenish-grey pus. Occasionally shreds or bands of unabsorbed fibrin remain, and become converted into fibrous tissue, thus producing adhesions which constitute a subsequent danger of strangulation of the bowel, although this risk follows more often upon recovery from the chronic form.

In some cases the peritonitis becomes *localized* by adhesions between neighbouring organs due to the deposit of fibrin upon their surface. This process takes place with great rapidity, and it makes a great deal of difference to the result of the disease whether it be thus shut in to one part of the abdomen or whether it spreads so rapidly, or is of so virulent a type, as quickly to become *general*.

The bacteria causing peritonitis are numerous, but among the most common are the *Escherichia coli*, which is always present in the intestine; streptococci, which produce the most virulent form of inflammation; and the gonococcus.

Symptoms: The symptoms usually begin by a rigor, together with vomiting and pain in the abdomen of a peculiarly severe and sickening character, accompanied with extreme tenderness, so that the slightest pressure causes intense aggravation of the pain. The patient lies on the back with the knees drawn up, and the hands often rest upon the head, and it will be noticed that the breathing is rapid and shallow and performed by movements of the chest only, the abdominal muscles remaining rigid, unlike what takes place in healthy respiration. The abdomen becomes swollen by flatulent distension of the intestines, which increases the patient's distress. There is usually constipation. The skin is hot, and the temperature rises to 40 to 40·5 °C (104 or 105 °F), although there may be no perspiration; the pulse is small in volume; the urine is scanty and high coloured, and passed with pain. The patient's aspect is one of anxiety and suffering. These symptoms and signs may subside in a day or two, but if they do not, the case is apt to go on rapidly to a fatal termination. In such an event, the pain and tenderness subside, the abdomen becomes more distended, hiccup and vomiting of brown or blood-coloured matter occurs, the temperature falls, the face becomes pinched, cold, and clammy, the pulse exceedingly rapid and feeble, and death takes place from collapse, the patient's mental faculties generally remaining clear till the close. When the peritonitis is due to perforation, as may happen in the case of a gastric ulcer, or the ulcers of typhoid fever, the above-mentioned manifestations and the fatal collapse may all take place in from twelve to twenty-four hours. But usually the disease lasts four or five days, and the patient sometimes survives as long as a week. The puerperal form of this disease, which comes on within a day or two after parturition, is always very serious.

Treatment: The patient should lie recumbent on the back, with a pillow beneath the knees, so as to bend up the thighs, and a cage over the abdomen to support the weight of the bed-clothes. Externally, either an ice-bag or hot laudanum fomentations give relief, though sooner or later morphine or pethidine is necessary to give relief from the pain. The patient must be given ample fluid, but this must not be given by mouth or in the form of enemas. It must be given parenterally – preferably intravenously but, if facilities for this are not available, it can be given subcutaneously. The fluid may be normal saline (see ISOTONIC) or one-fifth normal saline with 4·2 per cent dextrose. If it is to be given intravenously, plasma or blood is given. Once vomiting occurs, it is usual in hospital to pass a tube through the nose into the stomach (a naso-gastric tube) and keep the stomach clear by aspirating the stomach contents through this tube.

The introduction of antibiotics greatly improved the outlook for this serious condition.

The question of operation arises in every case of peritonitis. In cases due to perforation of the stomach or intestine which are discovered early, operation is always advisable, because there is a good prospect of freeing the abdomen from the septic material which has entered it, and, if no operation is performed, the patient will almost certainly die. In cases in which peritonitis has become localized the question of when to operate is often a difficult one and can only be answered by an experienced doctor or surgeon. The operation consists in making an opening into the abdomen, carefully cleansing the outer surface of the bowels, and attending to the original cause of the peritonitis, whether it be a perforation, obstruction, abscess, or appendicitis, after which it is usual to insert drainage tubes.

CHRONIC PERITONITIS: In the great majority of cases this is tuberculous in origin and secondary to tuberculous disease of bones, joints, glands, or bowels. There is also a localized form of chronic peritonitis, which is non-tuberculous.

PERITONSILLAR ABSCESS is the term applied to a collection of pus or an abscess which occurs complicating an attack of tonsillitis. The collection of pus forms between the tonsil and the superior constrictor muscle of the pharynx. This condition is also known as quinsy. The treatment of this condition involves drainage of the abscess and the administration of appropriate antibiotics.

PERNICIOUS ANAEMIA is an auto-immune disease in which the sensitized lymphocytes destroy the parietal cells of the stomach. These cells normally produce intrinsic factor which is the carrier protein for vitamin B_{12} that permits its absorption in the terminal ileum. Without intrinsic factor, vitamin B_{12} can not be absorbed and this gives rise to a macrocytic anaemia. The skin and mucosa become pale and the tongue smooth and atrophic. A peripheral neuropathy is often present and this is commonly manifest by paraesthesiae and numbness, and even ataxia. The more severe neurological complication of

sub-acute combined degeneration of the cord is fortunately more rare. The anaemia gets its name from the fact that before the discovery of vitamin B_{12} it was uniformly fatal. Now a monthly injection of vitamin B_{12} is all that is required to keep the patient healthy.

PERONEAL is the name given to structures, such as the muscles, and nerves, on the outer or fibular side of the leg.

PERPHENAZINE (see NEUROLEPTICS).

PERSEVERATION is the senseless repetition of words or deeds by a person with a disordered mind.

PERSONALITY DISORDER: Condition in which the sufferers fail to learn from experience or to adapt to changes. The outcome is impaired social functioning and personal distress. There are three broad overlapping groups. One group is characterized by eccentric behaviour with paranoid or schizoid overtones. The second group shows dramatic and emotional behaviour with self-centredness and antisocial behaviour as typical components of the disorder. In the third group anxiety and fear are the main characteristics, which are accompanied by dependency and compulsive behaviour. These disorders are not classed as illnesses but psychotherapy and behavioural therapy may help. The individuals affected are notoriously resistant to any help that is offered, tending to blame other people, circumstances or bad luck for their persistent difficulties.

PERSPIRATION, or SWEAT, is an excretion from the skin, produced by microscopic sweat-glands, of which there are around 2·5 million, scattered over the surface. There are two different types of sweat-glands, known as eccrine and apocrine. Perspiration takes place constantly by evaporation from the openings of the sweat-glands, and this insensible perspiration amounts in twenty-four hours to considerably over a litre. Under certain circumstances, as when the skin is heated or the person exerts himself, drops of sensible perspiration appear on the skin; to these the term sweat is generally confined, and the amount of sweat secreted may become very large: up to 3 litres an hour for short periods of time.

Eccrine sweat is a faintly acid, watery fluid containing less than 2 per cent of solids, made up mainly of salts and to a slight extent of fatty material, and including 0·3 per cent of urea (about the same concentration as in the blood), the substance which the kidneys excrete in large amount. When the action of the kidneys is defective, for example in glomerulonephritis, urea and other substances, which the kidneys normally excrete, pass out in increased amounts through the skin. This action of the skin is so marked that in a case of uraemia crystals of urea may be deposited on the surface as the sweat evaporates.

The *eccrine sweat-glands* in man are situated in greatest numbers on the soles of the feet and palms of the hands, and with a magnifying glass their minute openings or pores can be seen in rows occupying the summit of each ridge in the skin. Perspiration is most abundant in these regions, though it also occurs all over the body.

The chief object of perspiration is to regulate the amount of heat lost from the surface of the body and so maintain an even body temperature. Accordingly muscular activity, which sets free a great deal of heat, is the chief cause of sweating, and external heat is another. The process is regulated by nerves, some of which are the nerves controlling the size of the blood-vessels (vasomotor), and therefore the amount of blood in a part, whilst other nerves proceed to the sweat-glands (secretory) and directly influence secretion. These belong to the sympathetic nervous system (q.v.).

The *apocrine sweat-glands* are found in the armpits, the eyelids, around the anus in association with the external genitalia and in the areola and nipple of the breast. (The glands that produce wax in the ear are modified apocrine glands.) They are developed in close association with hairs and their ducts often open into hair follicles. They do not start functioning until puberty. The flow of apocrine sweat is evoked by emotional stimuli such as fear, anger, or sexual excitement. It is the decomposition of apocrine sweat in the armpits by the bacteria of the skin that produces the characteristic smell of armpit sweat.

Abnormalities of perspiration: LESSENED sweating under certain conditions may occur, as in the early stages of fever, in diabetes, and in some forms of glomerulonephritis. Certain persons are peculiar in the fact of being unable to sweat copiously after muscular exertion, or when exposed to heat, and such persons are often seriously affected by exposure to a hot sun or to the heat of an engine-room. (See HEAT-STROKE.)

EXCESSIVE sweating or HYPERIDROSIS, may take place in any feverish condition, tending to be particularly marked in rheumatic fever, and, above all, in advanced pulmonary tuberculosis, where the night sweats are often copious enough to drench the patient's night-clothes and bedding. Such copious night-sweats also occur in certain cases of undulant fever. In a slighter degree, weak people of feeble muscular power are apt to perspire very freely on exertion or when exposed to heat. It may also be due to hyperthyroidism, obesity, diabetes mellitus, or an anxiety state. There is also a form of hyperidrosis, which may be localized or generalized, due to some disturbance of the nervous control of the sweat-glands. The troublesome form of excessive sweating in the armpits tends to run in families. Rare in children and the aged, it is usually induced or exacerbated by emotional stress.

OFFENSIVE perspiration, or BROMIDROSIS, is not uncommon. But it is sweating of the feet or armpits that is most offensive of all, this condition being often due to decomposition of the skin secretions by bacteria.

Treatment: LESSENED perspiration is treated when necessary by various drugs known as diaphoretics, and by hot-air baths.

EXCESSIVE sweating occurring in febrile diseases, e.g. pulmonary tuberculosis, is diminished by treatment of the condition responsible for the fever. In conditions such as pulmonary tuberculosis, in which the sweating is liable to be prolonged and is particularly irritating to the patient, sponging the skin with vinegar in water may be helpful. In other cases the administration of extract of belladonna by mouth may help.

Hyperidrosis, in which the perspiration is often offensive, is best treated by frequent baths. Regular shaving of the axillary, or armpit, hair is also helpful. The feet, armpits, and other sources of perspiration should be washed daily with hexachlorophane, coal-tar, or other mildly antiseptic soap, carefully dried, and thereafter dusted with talcum powder or bathed with hydrogen peroxide. Socks must be frequently changed. Shoes should be worn in preference to boots, so as to allow freer access of air to the feet, and for the same reason it is a good plan not to wear rubber soles. Sandals should be worn in hot weather. Sweating may also be considerably checked, if it is very copious, by rubbing the feet and armpits with liniment of belladonna or with spirit. Another useful plan in the case of excessive sweating of the feet is to soak the soles (not the entire foot) in 3 per cent formalin solution for five to ten minutes every night. There is also available a wide range of antiperspirant preparations, the active ingredient of which is often an aluminium salt. One of the most effective of these aluminium salts, is 25 per cent aluminium chloride hexahydrate in absolute alcohol, but this must only be used under medical supervision. A deodorant in powder form which has stood the test of time consists of: zinc peroxide 20 per cent; zinc stearate 10 per cent; boric acid 10 per cent; talc 60 per cent. In severe cases of localized excessive sweating, treatment by X-rays may be necessary and may give satisfactory results. Alternatively, in cases of excessive sweating in the armpits, which fails to respond to any other form of treatment, removal, by surgery or cryosurgery (q.v.), of a small area of skin (4 × 2·5 cm) at the dome of the armpit, where 70 to 80 per cent of the sweat-glands are present, may bring the condition under control.

PERTHES' DISEASE is an affection of the hip in children, due to fragmentation of the epiphysis (or spongy extremity) of the head of the femur. It occurs in the age-group, 4 to 10 years, with a peak between 6 and 8. It is ten times more common in boys than girls, and is bilateral in 10 per cent of cases. The initial manifestation is a lurching gait with a limp, accompanied by pain. Treatment consists of bed rest and traction of the affected limb so long as there is pain and spasm. The child is then allowed up and about with a walking calliper splint (q.v.) until the condition has healed. Spontaneous recovery occurs in about two years.

PERTUSSIS is another name for whooping-cough. (See WHOOPING-COUGH.)

PES CAVUS is the technical name for claw-foot (q.v.).

PES PLANUS is the technical name for flat-foot (q.v.).

PESSARIES are either instruments designed to support a displaced womb, or solid bodies suitably shaped for insertion into the vagina, which are made of oil of theobromine or a glycerin basis and are used for applying local treatment to the vagina.

PESTICIDES may be defined as any substance or mixture of substances intended for preventing or controlling any unwanted species of plants and animals, and includes any substances intended for use as plant growth regulators, defoliants or dessicants. The main groups of pesticides are: *herbicides* to control weeds; *insecticides* to control insects; *fungicides* to control or prevent fungal disease.

PETECHIAE are small spots on the skin, of red or purple colour, resembling flea-bites. They are small haemorrhages in the skin, as in purpura.

PETHIDINE HYDROCHLORIDE is a synthetic analgesic and antispasmodic drug, which is used in the treatment of painful and spasmodic conditions in place of morphine and atropine. It was at first thought that the drug would have an advantage over morphine in not encouraging addiction, but this has not proved to be the case.

PETIT MAL means the lesser type of epileptic seizure. (See EPILEPSY.)

PETRI DISHES are shallow, circular glass dishes, usually 10 cm in diameter, which are used in bacteriology laboratories for the growth of micro-organisms.

PEYER'S PATCHES are conglomerations of lymphoid nodules in the ileum, or lower part of the small intestine. They play an important part in the defence of the body against bacterial invasion, as in typhoid fever.

PEYRONIES DISEASE: Painful and deformed erection of the penis caused by the formation of fibrous tissue. The cause is unknown but it may be associated with Dupuytren's contracture (q.v.). The condition may be improved by surgery.

pH: A measurement of the concentration of hydrogen ions in a solution that is calculated as a negative logarithm. A neutral solution has a pH of 7·0 and this figure falls for a solution with increasing acidity and rises if the alkalinity increases.

PHAEOCHROMOCYTOMA: A disorder in which a vascular tumour of the adrenal medulla develops. The tumour may also affect the structurally similar tissues associated with the chain of sympathetic nerves. There is uncontrolled and irregular secretion of adrenaline and noradrenaline (qq.v.) with the result that the patient suffers from episodes of high blood pressure, raised heart rate, and headache. Surgery to remove the tumour may be possible; if not, drug treatment may help.

PHAGOCYTE: Cells, including white blood cells and macrophages, that envelop and digest bacteria, cells, cell debris, and other small particles. These cells are a vital part of the body's defence system.

PHAGOCYTOSIS is a process by which the attacks of bacteria upon the living body are repelled and the bacteria destroyed through the activity of the white corpuscles of the blood.

The first observations upon this point were made by Metchnikoff in the case of the Daphnia or water-flea. This little animal, which exists in large numbers in pools of stagnant water, may often be observed to devour the large spores of a species of fungus. Metchnikoff observed that these spores, perforating the intestine of the Daphnia, found their way into its body cavity and there multiplied. They were, however, attacked at once by the white corpuscles circulating in the creature's vessels, which surrounded and took into their substance these spores, apparently in time digesting them, so that they broke down and disappeared. In some cases, however, he found that the spores developed quickly, the white corpuscles appeared to be sluggish in attacking them, and the creature died.

Similar observations have been made in the case of other bacteria in higher animals. The processes which precede phagocytosis – the slowing of the blood-stream in the part, collection of the white corpuscles on the walls of the vessels, their passage out of the vessels into the tissues (diapedesis), and their approach to the bacteria – are described under ABSCESS and INFLAMMATION. When bacteria are very virulent they seem to repel the white corpuscles instead of attracting them, and no phagocytosis takes place, but the bacteria develop unimpeded. (See OPSONINS.)

PHALANX is the name given to any one of the small bones of the fingers and toes. The phalanges are fourteen in number in each hand and foot, the thumb and great toe possessing only two each, whilst each of the other fingers and toes has three.

PHALLUS: An alternative name for the penis (q.v.), this word may also be used to describe a penis-like object. In embryology the phallus is the rudimentary penis before the urethral duct has completely developed.

PHANTASY, or FANTASY, is the term applied to an imaginary appearance or day dream.

PHANTOM LIMB: Following the amputation of a limb it is usual for the patient to experience sensations as if the limb were still present. This condition is referred to as a phantom limb. In the vast majority of cases the sensation passes off in time.

PHARMACOKINETICS: The way in which the body deals with a drug. This includes the drug's absorption, distribution in the tissues, metabolism, and excretion.

PHARMACOLOGY is the part of medical science dealing with knowledge of the action of drugs.

PHARMACOPOEIA is an official publication dealing with the recognized drugs and giving their doses, preparations, sources, and tests. Most countries have a pharmacopoeia of their own. That for Great Britain and Ireland is prepared by the British Pharmacopoeia Commission under the direction of the Medicines Commission. Many hospitals and medical schools have a small pharmacopoeia of their own, giving the prescriptions most commonly dispensed in that particular hospital or school. The *British National Formulary* (q.v.) is a useful pocket book for those concerned with the prescribing or dispensing of medicines.

PHARMACY is the term applied to the art of preparing and compounding medicines, or to a place where this is carried out.

PHARYNGITIS is an inflammatory condition affecting the wall of the pharynx or throat proper. It is most commonly due to a viral upper respiratory tract infection. It may be confined to the pharynx or may also involve the rest of the upper respiratory tract, i.e. the nose and the larynx. On examination the mucous membrane is red and glazed with enlarged lymph-follicles scattered over it. It produces considerable irritation, tickling in the throat and discomfort which may last longer if not treated. If a viral cause is suspected, then only symptomatic treatment is instituted, consisting of analgesia and various gargles. This may include the sucking of medicated pastilles or lozenges. If a bacterial cause is suspected, an antibiotic should be prescribed and in both conditions irritants, such as smoking and highly spiced foods should be avoided.

PHARYNX is another name for the throat. The term throat is popularly applied to the region about the front of the neck generally, but in its strict sense it means the irregular cavity into which the nose and mouth open above, from which the larynx and gullet open below, and in which the channel for the air and that for the food cross one another. It extends from the base of the skull down to the 6th cervical vertebra, separated from the upper six vertebrae only by some loose fibrous tissue, and is about 12·5 cm (5 inches) long.

It is completely closed behind by a layer of muscles, and by mucous membrane, but in front it opens into the nose, mouth, and larynx in succession from above down. In its upper part, the Eustachian tubes open one on either side, and between them on the back wall grows a mass of glandular tissue known as the third tonsil, which, if enlarged, produces the condition known as adenoids. (See NOSE, DISEASES OF.) The muscles which close in the sides and back of the pharynx are three in number on each side, and spring, one from the jawbone, the second from the hyoid bone, the third from the side of the larynx, each of these constrictors spreading out like a fan on the back of the pharynx. Two other small muscles run downwards on each side.

PHENACETIN is a white crystalline coal-tar product, at one time much used in fevers, influenza, headaches, and neuralgias of all kinds, on account of its power of reducing temperature and of deadening pain. As its regular use is not without danger, particularly to the kidneys, it is gradually being discarded, and in Britain is only now available on a doctor's prescription.

PHENAZOCINE is a powerful pain-reliever, or analgesic, which is said to be more potent, but less habit-forming, than morphine.

PHENAZONE is an antipyretic and analgesic.

PHENCYCLIDINE (see DRUG ADDICTION).

PHENELZINE is one of the widely used antidepressant drugs which are classified as monoamine oxidase inhibitors (q.v.). (See ANTIDEPRESSANTS.)

PHENETHICILLIN (see PENICILLIN, ANTIBIOTIC).

PHENINDIONE is a synthetic anticoagulant (q.v.) which is effective by mouth, and is used for the same purpose as heparin. It is slower in action than heparin, the full anticoagulant effect not being obtained until 36 to 48 hours after the initial dose.

PHENOBARBITONE is the *British Pharmacopoeia* name for one of the most widely used of all the barbiturate group of drugs. It is given in doses of 30 to 125 mg to control epilepsy. Phenobarbitone Sodium is a soluble preparation which can be given by injection.

PHENOL is another name for carbolic acid (q.v.).

PHENOLPHTHALEIN is a substance much used as an indicator of reaction in urine, and gastric juice, for example, being colourless in acid media, brilliant red with alkalis, and varying in tint according to the acid concentration. It is also given internally in 60 to 300 mg doses as an aperient.

PHENOTHIAZINES are the group of major tranquillizers which are proving of value in the treatment of the psychoses (q.v.). They include chlorpromazine, prochlorperazine and thioridazine.

PHENOTYPE: An individual's characteristics as determined by the interaction between his genotype – his quota of genes – and the environment.

PHENOXYBENZAMINE is an alpha-adrenoceptor blocking drug (see ADRENERGIC RECEPTORS) that is proving of value in the treatment of some cases of enlargement of the prostate. (See PROSTATE GLAND.)

PHENOXYMETHYLPENICILLIN (see PENICILLIN).

PHENYLKETONURIA is one of the less common, but very severe, forms of mental deficiency. The incidence in populations of European origin is around 1 in 15,000 births. It is due to the inability of the baby to metabolize the amino-acid, phenylalamine. Its outstanding interest lies in the fact that, if it is diagnosed soon after birth – and this can be done by a simple urine test or by a test carried out on a drop of blood – and the infant is then given a diet low in phenylalamine, the chances are that the infant will grow up mentally normal. Parents of children with phenylketonuria can obtain help and information from the National Society for Phenylketonuria and Allied Disorders (NSPKU), Worth Cottage, Lower Scholes, Pickels Hill, Keighley, West Yorkshire BD22 0RR (0535 44865).

PHENYTOIN SODIUM is one of the most effective drugs for the treatment of epilepsy. One of its advantages is that it does not make the patient feel particularly sleepy. Its use is not without risk and it must therefore be used only under medical supervision.

PHEROMONES are chemicals produced and emitted by an individual which produce changes in the social or sexual behaviour when perceived by other individuals of the same species. The precise role of these odours, for it is by their smell that they are recognized, in man is still not clear, but there is growing evidence of the part they play in the animal kingdom. Thus if a strange male rat is put into a group of female rats, this may cause death of the fetus in any pregnant rats, and this is attributed to the pheromones emitted by the male rat.

PHIMOSIS is a condition of great narrowing at the edge of the foreskin, for which the operation of circumcision (q.v.) may be necessary.

PHLEBITIS means inflammation of a vein. (See VEINS, DISEASES OF.)

PHLEBOGRAPHY is the study of the veins, particularly by means of X-rays after the veins have been injected with a radio-opaque substance.

PHLEBOLITH is the term applied to a small stone formed in a vein as a result of calcification of a thrombus.

PHLEBOTOMY is an old name for the operation of blood-letting by opening a vein. (See VENESECTION.)

PHLEGM is a popular name for mucus, particularly that secreted in the air passages. (See BRONCHITIS; EXPECTORANTS; MUCUS.)

PHLEGMASIA DOLENS is another name for white leg (q.v.).

PHLYCTENULE: A hypersensitivity reaction of the conjunctiva. At the turn of the century the commonest cause was tuberculosis. Nowadays it is most commonly due to hypersensitivity to *staphylococci*.

PHOBIA is an irrational fear of particular objects or situations. A well-known American medical dictionary lists 206 'examples' of phobias, ranging, alphabetically, from air to writing. Included in the list are phobophobia (fear of phobias) and triskaidekaphobia (fear of thirteen at table). It is a form of obsession, and not uncommonly one of the features of the anxiety. (See MENTAL ILLNESS.) Those who suffer from what can be a most distressing condition can obtain help and advice from the Phobics Society, 4 Cheltenham Road, Chorlton-cum-Hardy, Manchester M21 1QN (061–881 1937).

PHOCOMELIA: This is a great reduction in the size of the proximal parts of the limbs. In extreme cases the hands and feet may spring directly from the trunk.

PHOLCODINE is the 3-(2-morpholinoethyl) ester of morphine. As it resembles codeine in suppressing cough, it is used for the relief of unproductive coughs.

PHONOCARDIOGRAPH is an instrument for the graphic recording of heart sounds and murmurs.

PHOSPHATES are salts of phosphoric acid, and, as this substance is contained in many articles of food as well as in bone, the nuclei of cells, and the nervous system, phosphates are constantly excreted in the urine. The continued use of an excess of food containing alkalis, such as green vegetables, and still more the presence in the urine of bacteria which lead to its decomposition, produce the necessary change from the natural mild acidity to alkalinity, and lead to the deposit of phosphates and to their collection into stones.

PHOSPHATURIA means the presence in the urine of a large amount of phosphates.

PHOSPHORIC ACID, either as the dilute acid or in the form of phosphates, forms a constituent of many so-called 'tonics'. Phosphate of lime is used in cases of debility and especially of bone disease. Sodium phosphate and effervescent sodium phosphate are much used as mild aperients, and acid sodium phosphate is used in cases of cystitis.

PHOSPHORUS BURNS: If particles of phosphorus settle on or become embedded in the skin, the resulting burn should be treated with a 2 per cent sodium bicarbonate solution, followed by application of a 1 per cent solution of copper sulphate. Fats and oils should not be employed.

PHOSPHORUS POISONING is now rare, and is produced only by the yellow, soluble form of phosphorus. Red phosphorus, from which safety matches are made, is harmless or nearly so. The main cause of acute phosphorus poisoning at the present moment is the swallowing of a rat poison containing phosphorus. When taken internally phosphorus acts first as an irritant poison, and, being thereafter absorbed, produces profound degenerative changes in the liver and other abdominal organs. There is also a chronic form of phosphorus poisoning, usually due to exposure to phosphorus fumes in chemical works. This consists of profound debility, and the occurrence of disease in the lower jaw-bone (phossy jaw), which necroses and comes away in large fragments, over a period of months or years. It is now believed by some authorities that this disease in the bone is due partly to infection occurring in the jaw as a result of toxic effects produced by the phosphorus.

Symptoms: When a child, for example, has taken a large dose he speedily suffers from pain, vomiting, colic, diarrhoea, and perhaps convulsions, and may die in a few hours. There is often a smell of garlic in the breath. Or partial recovery may take place, and the sufferer survive for several days, later developing jaundice and blood-stained urine.

Treatment: As phosphorus is absorbed slowly, washing out the stomach may succeed in removing the poison up to two hours after it has been swallowed. Copper sulphate, a 1 in 1000 solution, in water, may be given every ten minutes until vomiting occurs. Gastric lavage with a 1 in 5000 solution of potassium permanganate or with hydrogen peroxide solution may be tried instead. After emesis and gastric lavage 56 or 112 ml of liquid paraffin and a big dose of a saline purge should be given. No oils, fats, or milk should be taken so long as any phosphorus remains in the gastro-intestinal tract, for phosphorus is soluble in fats. If damage to the liver is threatened then treatment with sodium bicarbonate, glucose and insulin is indicated.

Chronic poisoning is prevented in chemical works dealing with phosphorus, by free ventilation, cleanliness, and periodic examination of the teeth of the match-workers.

PHOTOCOAGULATION: Coagulation of the tissues of the retina by laser for treatment of diseases of the retina such as diabetic retinopathy (see RETINA, DISORDERS OF).

PHOTODERMATOSIS, or PHOTODERMATITIS, is the term applied to an eruption on areas of the skin exposed to sunlight, caused by sensitivity to sunlight. (See POLYMORPHIC LIGHT ERUPTION.) In some cases the sensitivity is caused by certain drugs, cosmetics or chemicals.

PHOTOPHOBIA: Sensitivity to light. It can occur in disorders of the eye, or in meningitis.

PHOTOPSIA: This is a description of the flashing lights which are a not uncommon aura preceding an attack of migraine.

PHOTOSENSITIVITY: Abnormal reaction to sunlight. The condition usually occurs as a skin rash appearing in response to light falling on the skin, and it may be caused by substances that have been eaten or applied to the skin.

These are called photosensitizers and may be dyes, chemicals in soaps, or drugs. Sometimes plants act as photosensitizers – for example, buttercups and mustard. The condition may occur in some illnesses such as lupus erythematosus (q.v.).

PHOTOTHERAPY is treatment by means of light rays, the source of which is usually fluorescent light strips. Its main use is in the treatment of jaundice in the newborn infant. It is the blue section of the visual spectrum that is most effective in this respect. (See JAUNDICE.)

PHRENIC NERVE is the nerve which chiefly supplies the diaphragm. It springs from the 3rd, 4th, and 5th cervical spinal nerves, and has a long course down the neck, and through the chest to the diaphragm.

PHRENOLOGY is an old term applied to the study of the mind and character of individuals from the shape of the head. As the shape of the head has been shown to depend chiefly upon accidental characteristics, such as the size of the air spaces in the bones, and not upon development of special areas in the contained brain, this branch of science is now generally discredited.

PHTHISIS means wasting, and is the general term applied to that progressive enfeeblement and loss of weight that arise from tuberculous disease of all kinds, but especially from the disease as it affects the lungs.

PHYSIOLOGY is the branch of medical science that deals with the healthy functions of different organs, and the changes that the whole body undergoes in the course of its activities.

PHYSIOTHERAPY is the form of treatment involving the use of physical measures, such as exercise, heat and massage in the treatment of disease. An alternative name is PHYSICAL MEDICINE.

PHYSOSTIGMINE, or ESERINE, is an alkaloid obtained from Calabar bean, the seed of *Physostigma venenosum*, a climbing plant of West Africa. Calabar bean is known also as the ordeal bean, because preparations derived from it were at one time used by the natives of West Africa to decide the guilt or innocence of accused persons, the guilty being supposed to succumb to its action, while the innocent escaped. Its action depends on the presence of two alkaloids, the one known as physostigmine or eserine, the other as calabarine, the former of these being much the more important.
Action: Physostigmine produces the same effect as stimulation of the parasympathetic nervous system (q.v.): i.e. it constricts the pupil, stimu-

lates the gut, increases the secretion of saliva, stimulates the bladder, and increases the irritability of voluntary muscle. In poisonous doses it brings on a general paralysis.
Uses: It is used in medicine in the form of physostigmine salicylate. Its main use is to contract the pupil and thereby reduce the pressure inside the eyeball. For this purpose it is used as eye-drops or as lamellae. It is also given by subcutaneous injection to stimulate the gut when this is paralysed or atonic. It is the specific antidote (q.v.) to atropine and is therefore used in the treatment of atropine poisoning (q.v.).

PHYTOMENADIONE is the *British Pharmacopoeia* name for vitamin K. (See VITAMIN.)

PIA MATER is the membrane closely investing the brain and spinal cord, in which run blood-vessels for the nourishment of these organs. (See BRAIN; SPINAL CORD.)

PICA (Latin for magpie) is a term which means an abnormal craving for unusual foods. It is not uncommon in pregnancy. Among the unusual substances for which pregnant women have developed a craving are soap, clay pipes, bed linen, charcoal, ashes – and almost every imaginable foodstuff taken in excess. In primitive races it is taken to mean that it indicates the growing fetus requires such food. It is also not uncommon in children. (See APPETITE; LEAD POISONING.)

PICORNAVIRUSES derive their name from pico (small) and RNA (because they contain ribonuleic acid). They are a group of viruses which includes the enteroviruses (q.v.) and the rhinoviruses (q.v.).

PICRIC ACID, or TRINITROPHENOL, is used for preparing explosives, and so is employed in medicine only in solution. As it coagulates albumin, it produces a soothing pellicle over any raw surface with which it is brought into contact. It has antiseptic properties, but is rapidly going out of use because of its toxic effects.

PIGEON BREAST (see CHEST, DEFORMITIES OF).

PIGMENT is the term applied to the colouring matter of various secretions, blood, etc.; also to any medicinal preparation of thick consistence intended for painting on the skin or mucous membranes.

PILES, or HAEMORRHOIDS, consist of a varicose and often inflamed condition of the veins about the lower end of the bowel, known as the haemorrhoidal veins.
Varieties: It is usual to divide haemorrhoids

into external piles, internal piles, and mixed piles. To understand this division, it is important to remember that at the margin of the anus the skin joins the mucous membrane of the bowel in a sharp line, and that the bowel is kept closed by two circular muscles, the external sphincter and internal sphincter. The external sphincter is a weak muscle situated immediately beneath the skin, while the internal sphincter is a stronger circular band, extending up the bowel for about 25 mm. External piles are found outside the bowel, and are covered by skin, being brown or dusky purple in colour; internal piles are within the opening, covered by mucous membrane, and are bright red or cherry-coloured. Mixed piles are those situated just on the margin, and covered half by skin, half by mucous membrane. Even internal piles do not extend past the position of the internal sphincter muscle.

Causes: There is always a tendency for the veins in this situation to become distended, partly because they are unprovided with valves, partly because they form the lowest part of the portal system and are very apt to become overfilled when there is the least interference with the circulation through the portal vein, and partly because the muscular arrangements for keeping the rectum closed interfere with the circulation through the haemorrhoidal veins. Probably most people of middle life are troubled by this condition to some extent, especially men of sedentary habits who indulge in over-eating and are troubled by constipation, as well as women who have borne many children. Habitual constipation is perhaps the principal cause of the presence of piles, and sitting on a cold stone or damp seat, or even a general chill, may suffice from time to time to irritate them and bring on what is popularly known as an 'attack of piles'.

It must be remembered, however, that in a certain number of cases piles are merely a symptom of disease higher up on the portal system, causing interference with the circulation. They often come on during pregnancy, passing off when this condition has terminated. They are common in heart disease, liver complaints, such as cirrhosis or congestion, and any disease affecting the bowels.

Symptoms: EXTERNAL PILES may be present for years and give no trouble whatever, beyond occasioning pain of a cutting or burning character now and then when a very costive motion is passed. When, in consequence of a chill or other cause, they become inflamed, they are very painful and tender from chafing against the thighs and clothing in walking, and from pressure upon the chair on which the person sits. The pile, or piles, in these circumstances become enlarged and red, and give off a thin blood-stained discharge. They may become so badly inflamed as to suppurate, and this sometimes results in a natural cure, or they may cure by filling with blood-clot and shrivelling up into hard little knots. Such an 'attack of piles' lasts generally a week or two, and then subsides.

INTERNAL PILES may be slight, and may give no sign of their presence beyond occasional bleeding, which may vary from a mere streak, when the bowels are opened, to a discharge of several ounces of dark blood. They are apt to produce a constant discharge of mucus tinged with blood which soils the linen, but unless very severe are not, as a rule, painful. These discharges of blood may, when copious and frequent, cause anaemia and become a serious menace to the health, though they are never fatal. When internal piles are large they may come down with the movement of the bowels, and may then become inflamed and painful from time to time, just like external piles.

Treatment: Constipation must, in the first place, be corrected. While the use of violent and irritating purgatives should be avoided, care must be taken, by regulation of the diet and other means, to secure soft motions. (See CONSTIPATION.) The diet should include plenty of fruit and vegetables, and should in all cases be of a simple nature. Alcoholic beverages tend to produce and perpetuate piles, and should therefore in bad cases be entirely abandoned. Regular exercise is necessary in order to carry off the blood to the limbs and so relieve the portal circulation.

Locally, great care must be taken not to irritate the piles, and when they are inflamed they should be washed with water and cotton-wool every time the bowels move. Bleeding and the tendency to inflammation may be controlled by applying a sponge full of very hot water, or by smearing on cocaine or adrenaline ointment after the motion. In the case of internal piles which come down at stool it is very important that they should be returned within the bowel each time by gentle steady pressure with the fingers. If they are down and inflamed, a hot bath followed by a cocaine and morphine suppository gives relief.

Often these means suffice to keep the piles from causing trouble or to cure them completely, but occasionally surgical treatment is necessary. The external piles are simply removed. Internal piles require, according to their size and position, to be ligatured, destroyed by clamp and cautery, or, when they extend all round the bowel, to be removed *en masse* along with the last inch of mucous membrane lining the bowel. In many cases, however, the most satisfactory treatment of internal piles consists of injecting them with a 5-per-cent solution of phenol in arachis oil, to which 0·5 per cent of menthol has been added, or some other comparable solution. Alternative non- surgical methods of treatment that are now being advocated are ligation of the piles with rubber bands, cryosurgery (q.v.), and manual dilatation of the anus.

PILLS are small round masses containing active drugs held together by syrup, gum, glycerin, or adhesive vegetable extracts. They are sometimes without coating, being merely rolled in French chalk, but often they are covered with sugar, gelatin, or gilt. Some pills, designed to act upon the bowels only, are coated with keratin, salol or other substances which are insoluble in the gastric juice.

PILOCARPINE is an alkaloid derived from the leaves of *Pilocarpus microphyllus* (jaborandi). It produces the same effects as stimulation of the parasympathetic nervous system: i.e. it has exactly the opposite effect to atropine (q.v.), but cannot be used in the treatment of atropine poisoning as it does not antagonize the action of poisonous doses of atropine on the brain. Its main use today is in the form of eye-drops to decrease the pressure inside the eyeball in glaucoma (q.v.).

PILONOIDAL SINUS: A sinus (q.v.) that contains hairs, usually occurring in the cleft between the buttocks. It may get infected and cause considerable pain. Treatment is by antibiotics and, if necessary, surgical removal.

PIMPLES, technically known as papules, are small, raised, and inflamed areas on the skin. On the face the most common cause is acne (q.v.). Boils (q.v.) start as hard pimples. The eruption of smallpox and that of chicken-pox begin also with pimples. (See also SKIN DISEASES.)

PINEAL BODY is a small reddish structure, 10 mm in length and shaped somewhat like a pine cone (hence its name), situated on the upper part of the mid-brain. Many theories have been expounded as to its function, but there is increasing evidence that, in some animals at least, it is affected by light and plays a part in hibernation and in controlling sexual activity and the colour of the skin. This it seems to do by means of a substance it produces known as melatonin. There is also growing evidence that it may play a part in controlling the circadian rhythms of the body – the natural variations in physiological activities throughout the 24-hour day.

PINNA: The part of the ear, formed of cartilage and skin, that is external to the head. In animals it is an important element in detecting the direction of sound.

PINS AND NEEDLES is a form of paraesthesia (q.v.), or disturbed sensation, such as may occur, for example, in neuritis (q.v.) or poly-neuritis (q.v.).

PINT is a measure of quantity containing 16 fluid ounces (wine measure) or 20 fluid ounces (Imperial measure). The metric equivalent is 568 millilitres. (See WEIGHTS AND MEASURES.)

PINWORM (see ENTEROBIASIS).

PIPERACILLIN (see ANTIBIOTIC).

PIPERAZINE is a drug used for the treatment of threadworms and ascariasis. (See ASCARIASIS; ENTEROBIASIS.)

PIPOTHIAZINE (see NEUROLEPTICS).

PIROXICAM (see NON-STEROIDAL ANTI-INFLAMMATORY DRUGS).

PITHIATISM is a group of disorders in which the patient is subject to cure by persuasion or suggestion, the term being used as an equivalent for hysteria. (See HYSTERIA.)

PITUITARY BODY, also known as the PITUITARY GLAND and the HYPOPHYSIS, is an ovoid structure, weighing around 0·5 gram in the adult, attached to the base of the brain, and lying in the depression in the base of the skull known as the sella turcica on account of its resemblance to a Turkish saddle. It consists of an anterior and a posterior section divided by a clear line of cleavage. For long these two parts were known, respectively, as the anterior and the posterior lobes of the pituitary body, and the part of the gland that connected it to the brain was known as the stalk or infundibulum. This, however, was too simple a classification to be accurate, as was realized once information concerning the multifarious functions of the gland began to accumulate. It was therefore decided to divide it up according to its origin. The reason for this is that the pituitary has a double origin. The anterior part is derived in the embryo from the ectoderm (see FETUS) of the primitive mouth, and this part of the gland is now known as the adenohypophysis. The posterior part is derived from the brain and is now known as the neurohypophysis. The gland is connected to the hypothalamus (q.v.) of the brain by a stalk known as the hypophyseal or pituitary stalk. The confusing thing about this new 'classification' of the pituitary is that it involves a certain amount of overlapping with the old classification. Thus, the adenohypophysis is made up of the anterior lobe which, in turn, is subdivided into a pars distalis and a pars tuberalis, and the pars intermedia of the posterior lobe. The neurohypophysis is also made up of three parts: the infundibular process (or neural lobe) of the posterior lobe, the nervous part of the stalk known as the infundibular or neural stalk, and the median eminence of the tuber cinereum.

The pars distalis, which accounts for the greater part of the gland, is composed of masses of cells which fall into three main groups: (1) chromophobe cells which do not stain and constitute about 50 per cent of the total; (2) acidophil cells which stain with acid dyes and constitute about 35 per cent of the total; and (3) basophil cells which stain with basic stains and constitute about 15 per cent of the total. The pars intermedia consists only of a few cells, whilst the pars tuberalis contains non-granular cells. The neurohypophysis is composed of nerve fibres and brown granular cells known as pituicytes.

The pituitary gland is the most important ductless, or endocrine, gland in the body. (See ENDOCRINE GLANDS.) It has been described as the master gland of the endocrine system, or the conductor of the endocrine orchestra. This over-all control it exerts through the media of a series of hormones which it produces. The adenohypophysis is the major producer of these, and those it produces will be dealt with first. Those which function through the media of other endocrine glands are known as trophic hormones and have therefore been given names ending with 'trophic' or 'trophin'. The thyro-trophic hormone, or thyroid-stimulating hor-mone (abbreviated to TSH) as it is also known, exerts a powerful influence over the activity of the thyroid gland. The adrenocorticotrophic hormone, also known as corticotrophin (ACTH), stimulates the cortex of the adrenal glands. The growth, or somatotrophic, hor-mone, also known as somatotrophin (SMH), controls the growth of the body. There are also two gonadotrophic hormones which play a vital part in the control of the gonads: these are the follicle-stimulating hormone (FSH), and the luteinizing hormone (LH) which is also known as the interstitial-cell-stimulating hor-mone (ICSH). (See GONADOTROPHINS.) The lactogenic hormone, also known as prolactin, mammotrophin and luteotrophin, induces lac-tation. The neurohypophysis produces two hormones. One is oxytocin which is widely used because of its stimulating effect on contraction of the uterus. The other is vasopressin, or the antidiuretic hormone (ADH), which acts on the renal tubules and the collecting tubules (see KIDNEYS) to increase the amount of water that they normally absorb.

Gigantism is the result of the over-activity of, or tumour formation of, the acidophil cells in the adenohypophysis which produce the growth hormone. If this over-activity occurs after growth has ceased a condition known as acromegaly (q.v.) arises, in which there is gross over-growth of the ears, nose, jaws, and hands and feet. Dwarfism may be due to lack of the growth hormone. Diabetes insipidus (q.v.), a condition characterized by the passing of a large volume of urine every day, is due to lack of the antidiuretic hormone. Enhanced pro-duction of ACTH by the basophil cells of the pituitary leads to Cushing's syndrome (q.v.). Excessive production of prolactin by micro or macro adenomas leads to hyperprolactinaemia and consequent amenorrhoea and galactorrhoea. Some chromophobe adenomas do not produce any hormone but cause effects by damaging the pituitary cells and inhibiting their hormone production. The most sensitive cells to extrinsic pressure are the gonadotrophin-producing cells and the growth-hormone producing cells, so that if the tumour occurs in childhood growth-hormone will be suppressed and growth will cease. Gonadotrophin hormone suppression will prevent the development of puberty and if the tumour occurs after puberty will result in amenorrhoea in the female and lack of libido in both sexes. The thyroid-stimulating hormone cells are the next to suffer and the pressure effects on these cells will result in hypo-thyroidism. Fortunately the ACTH-producing cells are the most resistant to extrinsic pressure and this is teleologically sound as ACTH is the one pituitary hormone that is essential to life. However, these cells do suffer damage from intracellular tumours, and adrenocortical in-sufficiency is not uncommon.

PITYRIASIS ALBA is a form of chronic eczema which occurs mainly in children. It is characterized by rounded, scaly, white patches, usually on the face, but also sometimes on the upper arms and back. It is a self-limiting condition, but may drag on for several years. A bland cream controls the scaling if this is troublesome.

PITYRIASIS ROSEA is a skin eruption of unknown origin that occurs in young people. It starts characteristically with an oval, slightly red and scaly area – known as the herald patch – between the shoulder blades or on the lower abdomen. Three or four days later the eruption spreads all over the trunk. It consists of pink papules (q.v.) and oval brownish macules (q.v.), which tend to itch considerably. It usually lasts about six weeks, and does not usually recur. No specific treatment is called for. Hot baths should be avoided as they tend to accentuate the itching. If this itching is unpleasant, it can be relieved with calamine lotion or antihista-mine tablets.

PIVAMPICILLIN (see ANTIBIOTIC).

PIVMECILLINAM is a derivative of the anti-biotic, mecillinam. It differs from the latter in being active when taken by mouth. (See PENI-CILLIN, ANTIBIOTIC.)

PLACEBO: No treatments of specific value are found in all the pages of Hippocrates. Never-theless the placebo response occurred with sufficient frequency to enable the physician to command respect. The therapeutic opportuni-ties are now very different. However, man himself has not changed. He still wants and expects to take medicine when he is ill and is still just as subject to persuasion and suggestion. Despite the scientific advances of this century the physician is still the most important thera-peutic agent.

Placebo is the Latin for 'I will please'. Traditionally, placebos were used to pacify without actually benefiting the patient. They were inactive substances formerly given to please or gratify the patient but now only used in controlled studies to determine the efficacy of drugs. We now realise that pharmacologically inert compounds can relieve symptoms and we call this the placebo effect. The reassurance that is associated with placebo administration is accompanied by measurable changes in body function which are affected through autonomic pathways and humoral mechanisms. Alterations in blood pressure and pulse frequency are especially common. Placebos have the ability to relieve a variety of symptoms in a consistent proportion of the population. On average, one third of patients with symptoms such as pain or cough will respond to placebo medications and an even higher proportion of patients with psychological symptoms such as anxiety or insomnia is relieved. Current scientific jargon defines the placebo as any therapy or component of therapy that is deliberately or unknowingly used for its non-specific psychological or psycho-biological effect and that is without specific activity for the condition being treated.

PLACENTA is the technical name for the afterbirth. (See AFTERBIRTH.)

PLACENTA PRAEVIA: Implantation of the placenta in the bottom part of the uterus adjacent to or over the cervix. The condition may cause few problems during pregnancy or labour; it may, however, cause vaginal bleeding late in pregnancy and this requires medical attention.

PLACENTOGRAPHY is the procedure of rendering the placenta, or afterbirth (q.v.), visible by means of X-rays. This can be done either by using what is known as soft-tissue radiography, or by injecting a radio-opaque substance into the blood-stream or into the amniotic cavity. (See AMNION.) The procedure is not without danger to both mother and fetus, and must therefore only be carried out under expert supervision but it is sometimes of value in assessing the cause of antepartum haemorrhage. The placenta and fetus can now be visualized by the non-invasive and safe method of ultrasound (q.v.).

PLAGUE, or BUBONIC PLAGUE, is an infectious epidemic disease common to man and many of the lower animals. Its main characters are fever, swelling of the lymphatic glands, a rapid course, and a very high mortality, which has made it a much dreaded scourge. In the Middle Ages it was known as the BLACK DEATH, which again and again ravaged Europe, though for the past century it has been almost confined to warm climates. The ancients referred to a disease which they called 'pestis', a term which possibly included several severe epidemic maladies; but, according to Hirsch, there is a recognizable description of an epidemic of what we know as plague infesting Libya, Egypt, and Syria between the second and third centuries BC. The first occurrence of the disease in Europe was the plague of Justinian, which swept through the

Roman Empire in AD 542, devastating cities and country as it spread. Subsequently it periodically invaded Europe from the east, and spread westward, though with lessening severity in successive epidemics. The last occasion on which England was seriously invaded was at the time of the Great Plague in 1664–65, when 70,000 people died in London out of the total population of 460,000. In Glasgow a small outbreak occurred in 1900, which was quickly supressed. The disease had not invaded America till 1899–1900, when it broke out in Brazil, the Argentine Republic, San Francisco, and Mexico. At the present day 1000 to 6000 cases occur annually, with 100 to 200 deaths.

Causes: The disease is probably always present (endemic) in certain localities, such as in the south-west of China, among the hill people of India, and in East Africa. From these areas it spreads outwards at intervals, sometimes creeping from village to village, at other times being disseminated widely along trade-routes.

The bacillus (*Yersinia pestis*) which is the immediate cause was discovered independently by Kitasato and Yersin in 1894. (See MICROBIOLOGY.) It is found in the enlarged lymphatic glands, and the sputum in pneumonic cases, as well as in the blood of septicaemic cases.

Plague occurs first as an epizoötic (q.v.) in rats: especially in the black rat, *Rattus rattus*. The infection is then conveyed to man by the rat flea, especially *Xenopsylla cheopis*. The plague bacilli multiply in the gastro-intestinal tract of the flea, which may remain infectious for as long as six weeks. In pneumonic plague the bacillus may pass from man to man as a droplet infection.

The rat is not the only rodent which serves as a reservoir for *Yersinia pestis*. In the Caucasus, Siberia, and Manchuria the marmot is an important reservoir, whilst in Argentina it has been found in wild guinea-pigs. In the USA between the Rocky Mountains and the west coast plague is widespread among ground squirrels, wood rats, and prairie dogs. Between 1900 and 1951 rodent plague had spread through fifteen of the western states of the USA. This carries with it the risk of starting plague in any city with a large rat population. In South Africa, too, plague is prevalent in rodents, and human cases have cropped up from time to time. In England the last outbreak was in Suffolk in 1910.

Symptoms: After infection, an incubation period, varying from two to six days for bubonic plague, and three to four days for pneumonic plague, elapses, and then the disease sets in suddenly with fever, headache, great lassitude, and aching of the limbs. The temperature soon rises to 39·5 °C (103 °F) or more, the skin is hot and dry, the tongue furred, while thirst, prostration, and a feeling of utter weakness assail the sufferer. His features become drawn, his eyes sunken, and he sinks into a state of stupor or passes sometimes into wild delirium. There is often also sickness and vomiting.

In over two-thirds of all cases there are

swollen glands, known as buboes, from which the malady has received the name of *bubonic plague*. These are situated most commonly in the groins, less often in the armpits, and give sometimes the first sign that the person has contracted the plague. There are also haemorrhages under the skin in many cases, which sometimes produce black gangrenous patches that lead to large ulcers, and hence the old name of black death. In favourable cases the fever abates at about the end of a week, the strength gradually returns, and the buboes soften, burst, and discharge foul-smelling pus.

There is a rapidly fatal form, associated with great weakness, in which the bacteria enter the blood, and the person dies on the second or third day, sometimes even in a few hours, before the buboes have time to form (*septicaemic plague*).

In other cases the lungs especially become affected, and pneumonia comes on, with death on the fourth or fifth day. This is said to be both the most infectious and the most fatal form of the disease (*pneumonic plague*).

In all epidemics, especially at the beginning and end of the epidemic, mild cases occur, in which the persons continue to go about, the buboes being almost the only sign of the malady. The matter from the buboes of such slight cases is, nevertheless, infectious, and these cases are therefore specially dangerous to other people.

The death-rate in untreated cases varies in different epidemics from 25 to 50 per cent. Untreated septicaemic plague and pneumonic plague are usually fatal, but modern treatment has reduced the fatality considerably, even in pneumonic plague.

Treatment: Preventive treatment is all-important in this disease. Plague is one of the six internationally quarantineable diseases, the others being cholera, louse-borne relapsing fever, smallpox, louse-borne typhus, and yellow fever. Contacts of plague are quarantined for six days. The strictest quarantine is apt to be ineffective, and measures directed against the spread of plague are essential. This includes the disinfestation of all contacts with insecticide powder, such as 5 to 10 per cent DDT powder. Clothes, skins, any soft merchandise which have been in contact with the plague-stricken preserve the bacilli, and consequently their infectiousness, for several months. Such articles must therefore be either destroyed or disinfected with DDT. Houses or huts in which plague has occurrred should either be carefully disinfected with DDT or, if valueless, burned to the ground. The inhabitants of a plague-infected village or district are not allowed to migrate, carrying infection with them, to other localities, but all who have been in contact with a plague-stricken person should be isolated as contacts or suspects in special houses or camps and dusted with DDT.

In time of plague, or when plague is approaching, a war of extermination should be waged against rats and other rodents which are responsible for spreading the disease, and the bodies should also be carefully examined. Various devices are adopted against the rats on ships. Thus the ships are generally moored a little way distant from the quay, the hawsers are rendered 'rat-proof' by slipping hollow metal cones round them, and sulphurous acid gas or hydrocyanic acid is pumped into the holds under closed hatches to kill vermin which may be among the merchandise.

Personal protection is gained by good feeding, and by living in bright, well-ventilated rooms or out of doors. The wearing of high boots and special clothing impervious to fleas is important for those who go into the neighbourhood of plague cases. The use of antiseptics for the hands and of disinfectant mouth-washes is important for those nursing the plague-stricken, and special precautions must be taken to seal up any small wounds on the hands, and so guard against inoculation.

Vaccination affords partial protection for six months, and is used in the control of local outbreaks of plague. The administration of the sulphonamides, sulphadiazine, sulphamerizine, or sulphadiamine, is recommended for the protection of those who have been exposed, particularly to pneumonic plague.

In the treatment of the disease the best results are obtained from streptomycin or one of the broad-spectrum antibiotics.

PLANTAR: Describing anything related to the sole of the foot.

PLANTAR DERMATOSIS is a condition usually affecting children, characterized by cracks, or fissures, in the skin of the soles of the feet. The skin also assumes a glazed appearance. It is usually relieved by the regular rubbing in of paraffin ointment BPC, or one of its proprietary equivalents.

PLANTAR FASCIITIS (See FASCIITIS.)

PLAQUE is a coating of the teeth which forms as a result of neglect. It consists of food debris and bacteria and later calcium salts will be deposited in it to form calculus. It is therefore associated with both caries and periodontal disease.

PLASMA is the name applied to the fluid portion of the blood composed of serum and fibrinogen, the material which produces clotting. When the plasma is clotted, the thinner fluid separating from the clot is the serum.

PLASMA EXCHANGE involves the removal of the circulating plasma (q.v.) from the patient. It is done by removing blood from a patient and returning the red cells with a plasma expander. The plasma exchange is carried out through an in-dwelling cannula in the femoral vein and the red cells and plasma are separated by a hemonetics separator.

Usually a sequence of three or four sessions is undertaken, at each of which two to three litres of plasma are removed. The lost plasma can either be replaced by human serum albumin or a plasma expander.

In auto-immune disorders the disease is due to damage wrought by circulating antibodies or sensitized lymphocytes. If the disease is due to circulating humoral antibodies, removal of these antibodies from the body should theoretically relieve the disorder. This is the principle on which plasma exchange was used in the management of auto-immune diseases due to circulating antibodies. Such disorders include Goodpasture's syndrome, systemic lupus erythematosis and myasthenis gravis. One of the problems in the use of plasma exchange in the treatment of such diseases is that the body responds to the removal of antibody from the circulation by enhanced production of that antibody by the immune system. It is therefore necessary to suppress this homeostatic response with cytotoxic drugs such as azathioprine. Nevertheless remissions can be achieved in auto-immune diseases due to circulating antibodies by the process of plasma exchange.

PLASMAPHERISIS: A way of removing plasma (q.v.) from the blood. Blood is taken from a donor and allowed to settle in a vessel after which the separated plasma is extracted. The blood cells are transfused back into a vein. The process may be repeated and is used to treat some auto diseases caused by antibodies circulating in the patient's plasma. (See AUTO-IMMUNITY.)

PLASMA TRANSFUSION is sometimes used instead of blood transfusion. Plasma, the fluid part of blood from which the cells have been separated, may be dried and in powder form kept almost indefinitely; when wanted it is reconstituted by adding sterile distilled water. In powder form it can be transported easily and over long distances. Transfusion of plasma is especially useful in the treatment of shock. One advantage of plasma transfusion is that it is not necessary to carry out testing of blood groups before using it. (See TRANSFUSION OF BLOOD.)

PLASMINOGEN: A precursor of plasmin, an enzyme that digests the protein fibrin, the main constituent of blood clots. When tissue is damaged, activators are released which provoke the conversion of plasminogen into plasmin.

PLASMODIUM is the general term applied to minute protoplasmic cells, and particularly to those which cause malaria and allied diseases. (See MALARIA.)

PLASTER OF PARIS is a form of calcium sulphate, which, after soaking in water, sets firmly. For this reason it is widely used as a form of splinting in the treatment of fractures. It is used for this purpose in the form of bandages which consist of bleached cotton cloth impregnated with the plaster and suitably adhesive. Its great advantage, compared with an ordinary splint, is that it can be moulded to the shape of the limb. This technique was originally introduced by a Dutchman in 1852. A predecessor of it, which seemed to serve its purpose well, was a bandage stiffened by soaking in egg white and flour – a method still in use in parts of Africa.

PLASTIC SURGERY is that branch of surgery which is concerned with the reformation and restoration of parts of the body which are damaged, lost, or deformed.

PLATELETS: Blood platelets, or thrombocytes, are small spherical bodies in the blood, which play an important part in the process of blood coagulation. Normally, there are around 300,000 per cubic millimetre of blood.

PLATING is a term used in connection with bacteriological investigation to mean the cultivation of bacteria on flat plates containing nutrient material. The term is also applied in surgery to the method of securing union of fractured bones by screwing to the sides of the fragments narrow metal plates, which hold them firmly together while union is taking place.

PLETHORA means a condition of fullness of the blood-vessels in a particular part or in the whole body. The term is applied to a condition in which the volume of the blood is increased above normal; there may or may not be an increase in the total number of red blood corpuscles.

PLETHYSMOGRAPH is an apparatus for estimating changes in the size of any part placed in the apparatus; in this way changes in the volume of blood in a part can be measured.

PLEURA, or PLEURAL MEMBRANE, is the name of the membrane which, on either side of the chest, forms a covering for one lung. The two pleurae are distinct, though they touch one another for a short distance behind the breastbone. (See LUNGS.)

PLEURAL CAVITY: The normally restricted space between the parietal and visceral pleura (q.v.), which slide over one another as the individual breathes in and out. If gas or fluid are introduced as a result of injury or infection, the pleural surfaces are separated and the pleural space increases in volume. This usually causes breathing difficulties.

PLEURISY, or PLEURITIS, means inflammation of the pleura or serous membrane investing the lung and lining the inner surface of the ribs. It is a common condition, and may be either acute or chronic, the latter being usually tuberculous in origin.

The changes which take place are as follows. (1) Inflammatory congestion and infiltration of the pleura, which may spread to the tissues of the lung on the one hand, and to those of the chest wall on the other. (2) Exudation of fibrin on the pleural surfaces. This exudation consists mainly of coagulated fibrin along with epithelial cells and red and white blood corpuscles. Its presence causes roughening of the two pleural surfaces by material which may later break up or may become organized by the development of new blood-vessels and formation of fibrous tissue. This, by forming permanent adhesions, may obliterate the pleural sac throughout a greater or less space, and interfere with the free play of the lungs. (3) Effusion of fluid into the pleural cavity. This fluid may vary in its characters. Most commonly it is clear or slightly turbid, of yellowish-green colour, sero- fibrinous, and containing flocculi of fibrin. The amount may vary from an almost inappreciable quantity to 4–6 litres. When large in quantity, it may fill the pleural sac to distension, bulge out the thoracic wall externally, and compress completely the lung, which may in such cases have all its air displaced and be reduced to a mere fraction of its natural bulk lying squeezed up upon its own root. Other organs, such as the heart and liver, may in consequence of the presence of the fluid be shifted away from their normal position. In favourable cases the fluid is absorbed more or less completely and the pleural surfaces may unite by adhesions; or, all traces of inflammatory products having disappeared, the pleura may be restored to its normal condition. When the fluid is not speedily absorbed, it may remain long in the cavity and compress the lung to such a degree as to render it incapable of re-expansion as the effusion passes slowly away. The consequence is that the chest wall falls in, the ribs become approximated, the shoulder is lowered, the spine becomes curved and internal organs permanently displaced, while the affected side scarcely moves in respiration. Sometimes the unabsorbed fluid becomes purulent, and an *empyema* is the result. In such a case the pus may point as an abscess upon the chest or abdominal wall, or, on the other hand, burst into the lung and be discharged by the mouth, if it is not evacuated by surgical means.

Many cases of pleurisy are associated with only a little effusion, the inflammation consisting chiefly in exudation of fibrin. To this form the term *dry pleurisy* is applied. Further, pleurisy may be limited to a very small area, or, on the contrary, may affect, throughout a greater or less extent, the pleural surfaces of both lungs.

Causes: Pleurisy is often associated with other forms of inflammatory disease within the chest, more particularly pneumonia, bronchiectasis, and tuberculosis, and also occasionally accompanies pericarditis. It may also be due to carcinoma of the lung, or be secondary to abdominal infections such as subphrenic abscess. Further, wounds or injuries of the thoracic walls are apt to set up pleurisy. The connection of pleurisy with tuberculosis is important. Sometimes it happens that an attack of pleurisy, which apparently has passed off, returns and is eventually followed by tuberculosis, it may be after several years.

Symptoms: The symptoms of pleurisy vary, being generally well marked, but sometimes obscure.

DRY PLEURISY: In the case of dry pleurisy, which is, on the whole, the milder form, the chief symptom is a sharp pain in the side, felt especially on breathing. Fever may or may not be present. There is a slight, dry cough, which the individual does his best to suppress because of the pain which it causes. The breathing is quicker than normal and shallow. Should a deep breath be taken, it ends with a characteristic catch, due to the pain which it causes. If much pain is present, the body leans somewhat to the affected side, to relax the tension on the intercostal muscles and their covering, which are even tender to touch. On listening to the chest with the stethoscope the physician recognizes sooner or later friction, a superficial rough rubbing sound, occurring only with respiration and ceasing when the breath is held. It is due to the coming together during respiration of the two pleural surfaces which are roughened by the exuded fibrin. The patient may himself be aware of this rubbing sensation, and its vibration or fremitus may be felt by the hand laid upon the thoracic wall during breathing. This form of pleurisy may be limited or may extend over the greater part of one or both sides. It is a frequent complication of pulmonary tuberculosis. In general it disappears in a short time, and complete recovery takes place; or, on the other hand, extensive adhesions may form between the surfaces of the pleura covering the ribs and the lung, preventing uniform expansion of the lung in respiration, and leading to emphysema. Although not of itself attended with danger, dry pleurisy must always be treated as a serious condition, as it may be accompanied by disease in the underlying lung.

PLEURISY WITH EFFUSION is usually more severe than dry pleurisy, and, although it may in some cases develop insidiously, it is in general ushered in sharply by shivering and fever, like other acute inflammatory diseases. Pain is felt in the side or breast, of a severe cutting or stabbing character. The pain is greatest at the outset, and tends to abate as the effusion takes place. A dry cough is almost always present, which is particularly distressing, owing to the increased pain the effort excites. The breathing is painful and difficult, tending to become shorter and shallower as the disease advances, and the lung on the affected side becomes compressed. The patient at first lies most easily on the sound side, but as the effusion increases he finds his most comfortable position on his back or on the affected side.

In most instances the termination is favourable, the acute symptoms subsiding, and the fluid (if not drawn off) gradually or rapidly becoming absorbed, sometimes after re-accumulation. On the other hand, it may remain long without undergoing much change, and thus a condition of *chronic pleurisy* becomes established. Such cases are to be viewed with suspicion, particularly in those who are predisposed to tuberculosis, of which it is sometimes the precursor.

In some cases the pleurisy is on the undersurface of the lung. This condition, known as *diaphragmatic pleurisy*, gives few signs on examination and is liable, when the symptoms are severe, to be mistaken for some acute inflammation of the abdomen.

The chief dangers in pleurisy are the occurrence of a large and rapid effusion, particularly if both sides be affected, causing much embarrassment to the breathing, and tendency to collapse; the formation of an *empyema* (often marked by recurring fever); severe collateral congestion of the other lung; imperfect recovery, and the supervention of tuberculosis.

Acute pleurisy is often merely an accompaniment of the severer condition of lobar pneumonia.

Treatment: The treatment varies greatly with the form and severity of the attack. If it is tuberculous in origin, a full course of chemotherapy is given as for pulmonary tuberculosis. (See TUBERCULOSIS.) Should it be associated with an underlying infection of the lung, such as pneumonia, the appropriate antibiotics are given.

So far as the treatment of the pleurisy itself is concerned, in the early inflammatory stage, one of the chief symptoms calling for treatment is the pain, which may be soothed by opiates in the form of morphine, along with the application to the chest of heat in the form of hot poultices, fomentations or a hot water bottle. Instead of these, an ice-bag may be applied to the side, and this has the effect of almost immediately soothing the acute pain.

In the case of pleurisy with effusion, in addition to these measures, aspiration of the fluid may be required. (See ASPIRATION.) The operation is all the more necessary if the accumulated fluid is interfering with the function of other organs, such as the heart, or is attended with marked embarrassment of the breathing. The chest is punctured in the lateral or posterior regions, and most physicians prefer to draw off not more than 850 ml or thereabout at one time and to repeat the operation if necessary. In general, the operation is unattended with danger, although not entirely exempt from such risks as sudden fainting. In many instances, not only is the removal of distressing symptoms speedy and complete, but the lung is relieved from pressure in time to enable it to resume its normal expansion. When there is any evidence that the fluid is purulent, the operation should be performed early. In such cases it is sometimes necessary to establish for a time a drainage of the pleural cavity by introducing a drainage tube through an opening in the lower part of the side, a portion of a rib being usually removed to admit the tube. The pleural cavity is then irrigated through the opening at regular intervals, and treated exactly as any other large abscess cavity. (See EMPYEMA.)

The convalescence from pleurisy requires care, and the expansion of the lung may be assisted by suitable breathing exercises.

After an attack of pleurisy, and particularly after a second attack, the person should submit himself from time to time to medical examination, in order to make sure that tuberculosis does not develop in the lung. He will thus be enabled, if this serious disease should show itself, to start its treatment at an early stage, when a cure may be expected.

PLEURODYNIA means a painful condition of the chest-wall. It may be due to rheumatism of the intercostal muscles or to neuralgia of the intercostal nerves, or, when of the sharp nature popularly known as a 'stitch in the side', to cramp.

PLEXUS is a network of nerves or vessels: e.g. the brachial and sacral plexuses of nerves and the choroid plexus of veins within the brain.

PLUMBISM is another name for lead poisoning. (See LEAD POISONING.)

PLUMMER-VINSON SYNDROME is a syndrome associated with certain cases of hypochromic anaemia. It consists of hyochromic anaemia, and difficulty in swallowing due to an oesophageal web. It is found practically only in women. (See ANAEMIA.)

PNEUMOCONIOSIS is the general name applied to a chronic form of inflammation of the lungs which is liable to affect workmen who constantly inhale irritating particles at work. It has been defined by the Industrial Injuries Advisory Council as: 'Permanent alteration of lung structure due to the inhalation of mineral dust and the tissue reactions of the lung to its presence but does not include bronchitis and emphysema'. Some of the trades liable to suffer are those of stone-masons, potters, steel-grinders, ganister workers, colour-grinders, coal-miners, millers, and workers in cotton, flax, or wool mills. Annually about 400 workers are diagnosed as having coalminer's pneumoconiosis; 120 other workers have asbestosis and under 100 silicosis. (See OCCUPATIONAL DISEASES; TUBERCULOSIS.)

PNEUMONECTOMY is the operation of removing an entire lung in such diseases as bronchiectasis, tuberculosis, and cancer of the lung.

PNEUMONIA: Inflammation of the lung may be caused by allergic reactions, when the term *alveolitis* is used, or by chemical or physical agents, when the term *pneumonitis* is used. The classical division of pneumonia into lobar and bronchial pneumonia is no longer relevant. The aetiology and management of pneumonia depends on whether it occurs in a healthy person or in a person who has some underlying chronic disease that has lowered his local bronchial defences or his general resistance to infection. In the latter case a multitude of organisms may be responsible, many of which have no special affinity for the lungs. Conditions predisposing to the lowering of local or general resistance are chronic bronchitis, diabetes mellitus, malnutrition, alcoholism, and in those patients in whom the immune mechanism is suppressed either by a disease such as leukaemia or by the treatment with immunosuppressive drugs which is always necessary after an organ transplant.

When pneumonia arises in a previously healthy person the three most common organisms are the streptococcus pneumoniae, a virus or mycoplasma pneumoniae. Staphlylococcus aureus is an important cause of pneumonia following an attack of influenza. Rarer causes of pneumonia in a previously healthy person include psittacosis, which is caused by a chlamydia, Q fever caused by a rickettsia, and legionnaire's disease which is caused by a bacterium. Organisms responsible for pneumonia in patients with pre-existing disease include Strep. pneumoniae, Staphlylococcus aureus, Haemophilus influenziae, Stre. pyogenes, Klebsiella and Gram Negative bacilli such as Pseudomomas aeruginosa, Escherichia coli and Proteus.

Immunosuppressive drugs predispose to what are called opportunist infections of the lung, which are infections by organisms that rarely cause pneumonia in ordinary circumstances. These include bacteria such as nocardia, cytomegalovirus, fungi and protozoa (Pneumocystic carinii).

Symptoms: The common symptoms with which pneumonia presents are cough, fever, especially when accompanied by rigors, pleuritic pain, dyspnoea or cyanosis. The elderly or infirm may have no fever. The sputum is usually purulent in patients with chronic bronchitis and watery and rusty in those with an overwhelming infection. In other cases sputum may be difficult to obtain during the early stages of the disease and this is partly because coughing is suppressed by pleuritic pain. It is however important to obtain a specimen of sputum so that the nature of the pneumonia can be ascertained by culturing the organism responsible.

Certain physical signs are usually present. Diminished movement of the affected side is noticeable, the healthy side of the chest performing most of the respiratory function. On percussion over the affected area a dull note is obtained which becomes particularly marked if fluid has collected in the pleural cavity. On auscultation over the affected area the breathing is usually harsh and high-pitched (bronchial breathing) but it sometimes shows no deviation from normal, especially in cases in which the deeper parts of the lung only are affected. Accompanying the breathing in the early stages of the disease crackling sounds may be heard.

It is advisable to obtain a specimen of sputum and to do a blood culture before antibiotics are given.

Treatment: The treatment of pneumonia requires eradication of the infection, correcting hypoxia, relieving cough and pleuritic pain, and dealing with any complications that may arise. If the patient is drowsy, cyanosed or confused, hospital admission is indicated. Treatment of the infection with antibiotics should start at the earliest possible moment. The choice of antibiotic is based on the clinical judgement of the type of pneumonia with any microbiological support that is available. Microscopic examination of the sputum with the relevant stains will provide a clue to the nature of the prevailing organism but the results of culture may take 24 to 48 hours. Pus cells in the sputum and a leucocytosis suggest that the infection is bacterial rather than viral in origin. Pneumonia in a previously healthy person, particularly if there are rigors and herpes labialis and if there are pus cells and diplococci in the sputum, means that pneumonia is almost certainly due to Strep. pneumoniae and the antibiotic of choice is benzylpenicillin. If the clinical symptoms and signs suggest that the pneumonia is due to a virus, mycoplasma or other non-bacterial infection, then a broad spectrum antibiotic such as erythromycin or tetracycline or ampicillin is indicated. Pneumonia complicating chronic bronchitis should be treated with a broad spectrum antibiotic such as ampicillin or co-trimoxazole. Acute fulminating pneumonia accompanied by signs of respiratory or circulatory failure is probably staphylococcal in origin and this requires urgent intravenous treatment with flucloxacillin and either gentamicin or tobramicin. The optimum duration of antibiotic treatment depends on the response of the patient and the nature of the infection. Good nursing is also important. Pain and difficulty in breathing may be relieved by the application of hot-water bottles and by the administration of analgesics. Cough may be relieved by expectorants. Excessive fever may be controlled by sponging with tepid water. As regards feeding, the digestive powers are much reduced in such an acute infection and the patient should be fed with milk, soups and other light forms of nourishment. Oxygen is important for the hypoxic patient. However if the patient has chronic obstructive airways disease oxygen is the drive to respiration and if oxygen is given in too great a concentration respiration will be suppressed and the patient will die of hypercapnia and acidosis. Oxygen is therefore administered in a concentration of 28 per cent usually through a Venturi mask.

PNEUMONITIS is an inflammation of the lung due to chemical or physical agents. When the inflammation of the lung is due to infections it is called pneumonia and when it is caused by allergic reactions it is known as alveolitis.

PNEUMOPERITONEUM means a collection of air in the peritoneal cavity. Air introduced into the peritoneal cavity collects under the diaphragm which is thus raised and collapses the lungs. This procedure was sometimes carried out in the treatment of pulmonary tuberculosis in the pre-antibiotic days as an alternative to artificial pneumothorax.

PNEUMOTHORAX means a collection of air in the pleural cavity, into which it has gained entrance by a lesion in the lung or a wound in the chest wall. When air enters the chest the lung immediately collapses towards the centre of the chest, but, air being absorbed from the pleural cavity, the lung expands again in a short time. (See LUNGS, DISEASES OF.)

Artificial pneumothorax was an operation often performed in the pre-antibiotic days by which in a case of pulmonary tuberculosis air was run into the pleural cavity to cause collapse of one lung, which rests it and allows cavities in it to heal.

PODAGRA is another name for gout affecting the foot. (See GOUT.)

PODOPHYLLIN is a resin derived from the root of *Podophyllum peltatum*, a plant of the United States and Canada, or from *Podophyllum emodi*, a plant which grows in the Himalayas. It has a purgative action but is seldom used for this purpose now. It is also used as a local application in the treatment of venereal warts.

POIKILOCYTOSIS: This is a term used to describe the variation seen in the shape of red blood cells in some bone marrow disorders.

POISONS: 'Poison' is a common word, often used without regard for the definition. By law, in the United Kingdom, it is singled out under the Offences Against the Person Act, 1861, as 'any destructing or noxious thing'. But this, in itself, is too generalized, for a gun could be so described. Rather is a *poison* a substance that proves inimical to living matter, whether that be a micro-organism or a more complex structure. In so doing, it acts chemically more than physically, although strong acids, caustics and corrosives owe their adverse effects almost entirely to their physical properties.

Synonymously, a *toxin*, or *toxic substance* is a poison, these terms deriving their meaning etymologically from the ancient practice of tipping arrow heads with noxious material to intensify their primary wounding effects. Thus, the study of poisoning is nowadays designated as *toxicology*.

Pertinent to all poisons and poisoning is the concept of dose-response, for there is no clear separation between those substances which are toxic and those which are not. Morphine is an admirable analgesic, but in excess it can kill. Selenium is an element essential for metabolism, whereas in excess it can be destructive. So, Paracelsus's dictum of more than four centuries ago still holds true: 'All substances are poisons; there is none which is not a poison. The right dose differentiates a poison and a remedy.' Too often, nowadays, the force of this principle is overlooked, with the mere presence of a substance's being assumed to exert a toxic effect.

Aetiology: In human toxicology, poisoning can arise in various ways: (i) deliberately – murder, or suicide; (ii) accidentally, including therapeutic misadventures; (iii) occupationally; (iv) environmentally.

The traditional association of poisoning only with homicide is out of date. Moreover, the toxic phenomenon may be acute, when a relatively brief exposure leads to prompt manifestations, or chronic, when prolonged or repetitive exposure is eventually followed by adverse reactions.

Statistics: Accurate statistics of the incidence of poisoning overall are lacking in the United Kingdom, for this is not a notifiable disease. Diagnostic validation, except where death ensues, so often proves elusive. So, whereas the mortality figures are substantially reliable, those for morbidity are generally too vague.

Even so some guide can be gained from hospital records. In England and Wales, some 120,000 cases are admitted annually and, of these, about 20,000 apply to children under 5 years of age. But deaths number only around 5,000, of which 200 are children, with 150 or so of these succumbing to carbon monoxide.

Most of the deaths take place before the patient reaches medical care and it has been estimated that, of all the poisoned patients reaching hospital alive, fewer that 1 per cent fail to recover.

Closer analysis shows that most poisonings, at least in the developed countries, are due to overdoses of drugs, chiefly pain killers and other psychotropic agents. Some of these are undoubtedly accidental. Most, however, are intentional, not wilfully suicidal, but rather gestures of unhappy people wishing to draw attention to their plight.

Murder by poisoning is rare, possibly because it must be premeditated, but more so, perhaps, because the chances of detection are high.

Occupationally, compared with other causes of injury and death, poisoning is not a major hazard. Unease, nevertheless, persists because of the possibility, proved demonstrably in several instances, that continuing and relatively low exposure can be attended eventually by diseases such as asbestosis (q.v.), haemangioma of the liver from vinyl acetate monomer, bone marrow disease from benzene, etc.

Environmentally the extent of poisoning is largely speculative, with public anxiety and media sensationalism clouding the picture. What is needed is disciplined epidemiology to establish accurate information.

Diagnosis: There are no distinctive symptoms or signs by which poisoning can surely be recognized. Indeed, reliable causation can be difficult to establish.

Diagnosis rests upon: (i) the presence, location and amount of the toxin; (ii) the extent to which it gains access to the body, i.e. exposure (association and availability are not sufficient to establish a diagnosis); (iii) the eliciting of symptoms and signs characteristic of the known effects of the particular toxin, or toxins, coupled sometimes with the results of specific tests and investigations.

In default of these conditions, no more than *suspected poisoning* should be assumed.

Treatment: Despite popular belief to the contrary, the indications for specific antidotes are few. Examples of toxic substances for which there are specific antidotes include morphine and other opioid overdose, poisoning from carbon monoxide, paracetamol, digoxin, organophosphorus pesticides, mercurials, lead, iron salts and thallium. Otherwise and additionally, prudent management depends upon general resuscitative measures – ensuring a free airway, maintaining respiration, supporting the cardiovascular system, paying heed to the victim's fluid and electrolyte balance, along with kidney function, and, above all, expert nursing care (see APPENDIX: BASIC FIRST AID).

Especially with occupational and environmental poisoning, the victim should be withdrawn, at once, from any ongoing exposure, with treatment being practised as above.

Prevention: Increasing efforts are being devoted to poisoning prevention. Suicidally inclined patients are being denied access to dangerous stocks of tablets, capsules and the like. To protect children, child-resistant containers have been widely adopted. As a curb on would-be malefactors, the sale and supply of dangerous substances are statutorily regulated.

Occupationally, more emphasis is being placed on work-place hygiene, backed increasingly by official controls, such as the Control of Substances Hazardous to Health in the United Kingdom. Environmentally, too, the policies for overcoming pollution and contamination are being progressively strengthened.

A National Poisons Information Service has been set up to give advice, preferably to doctors, on the diagnosis and treatment of cases of poisoning. It has centres in London (071-407 7600), Edinburgh (031-229 2477) and Cardiff (0222-711711). (See also SELF-POISONING.)

POLIOMYELITIS, or INFANTILE PARALYSIS, is an infectious disease involving the spinal cord and the brain.

Cause: The first epidemic of poliomyelitis to be recorded occurred in Sweden in 1881. The disease then became of increasing importance, particularly in Scandinavia, USA and Australia, but with the successful introduction of poliomyelitis vaccination it rapidly became a relatively rare disease. In Great Britain the disease has been notifiable since 1912. Although sporadic cases may occur at any time, there is a definite seasonal incidence, epidemics tending to occur in the late summer and early autumn in the northern hemisphere and in March and April in the southern hemisphere. In the tropics infection continues throughout the year. The annual number of cases of poliomyelitis in the UK is in single figures, and in some years there are no cases reported.

The infecting organism is a virus, of which there are three types. Infection occurs from ingestion of the virus by mouth. The virus then passes to the lower alimentary tract and is excreted in the stools. It has been shown that the viruses are excreted by 90 per cent of paralytic cases, particularly children, and they are also excreted in the stools by healthy contacts of cases. It is in this way that the disease is spread: through contamination of the hands and then contamination of the mouth from such contaminated hands. Children are the most susceptible members of families, but during recent years there has been a definite tendency to severe paralytic cases' occurring among young adults. One attack usually produces permanent immunity; second attacks are rare.

Pathology: The sites of selection for the virus are the motor cells in the anterior horn of the spinal cord, and there is a tendency for this to be more marked in the lumbar part of the cord. The cranial nerves and certain nuclei in the brain are also involved in some cases.

Symptoms: The incubation period is 3 to 21 days, commonly 7 to 12 days. The onset may be either sudden or gradual. In the case of the latter the child may merely be 'off colour' for a day or two and complain of aches or pains in the limbs; there may be only a slight rise in temperature. This may gradually pass into the stage of weakness, and then paralysis, of the limbs. In other cases, after a few days' vague illness, the paralysis of the limbs may come on quite suddenly, usually with a sharp rise in temperature. In cases of sudden onset, the victim complains of headache and aches and pains, and the temperature rises to 39·5 °C (103 °F) or higher. In other cases, particularly in children, the limbs may be found to be paralysed when the child wakens in the morning, although he was apparently quite well when he went to bed the previous evening.

The site and the distribution of the paralysis depend upon the extent to which the spinal cord and brain are involved. The most serious cases are those in which the diaphragm and the muscles of respiration (the intercostal muscles) are involved, as this prevents the patient breathing, and he may die in a very short space of time unless he is placed on a respirator. When the cranial nerves and brain are involved, there may be nystagmus (q.v.), hoarseness, and difficulty in swallowing. Convulsions may occur in young children. The cerebrospinal fluid contains an excess of cells in the first and second weeks and an increased amount of protein in the third week.

Prophylaxis: A high degree of protection is given by poliomyelitis vaccine. This is now given by mouth, and its use has practically banished the disease. Of the 6 cases in England in 1979, none had been immunized. The vaccine is given in childhood, but a booster dose should be given to adults, particularly young adults, when they are going to a country of high poliomyelitis incidence, which in practice means any country outside Europe and North America. It is also recommended that unvaccinated parents of a child being given oral vaccine should be given the vaccine at the same time.

In the presence of an epidemic the following measures should be taken. Children should not be allowed to go into crowded buildings such as cinemas. Public swimming baths should be avoided. Children, especially younger ones, should not be allowed to get overtired, particularly in hot weather. Particular care should be taken to protect food from flies and to ensure that the highest standards of cleanliness are observed in the handling of food. No operations for the removal of tonsils or adenoids should be performed. Immunization against diphtheria and whooping-cough and measles vaccination should, if at all possible, be postponed until the epidemic is over.

Treatment: The patient must be put to bed on the first sign of the disease, and the affected limbs completely rested. This is the one definite practical fact that has resulted from all the careful investigation of the disease during recent years: that the earlier the disease is detected, and therefore the earlier the patient is put to bed and the affected parts rested, the better the ultimate result. Splints may be necessary at this stage to give adequate rest to the affected muscles. Later, careful physiotherapy is necessary. If the breathing is affected, it may be necessary to put the patient on a respirator. To ensure the best possible results, after-treatment may need to be continued for two or three years. In cases in which severe paralysis and wasting of limbs persist, surgical treatment may be necessary to reduce the resulting disability to a minimum.

POLIOSIS means premature greying of the hair. It is also the term applied to whitening of the hair in segments, such as a forelock.

POLLEN consists of microspores formed in flowering plants and conifers. Between 4 and 7 million tons of it are said to be shed annually throughout the world. From ancient days it has had the reputation of being a specific against old age, and recent reports from Russia claim that bee-keepers live longer because they eat pollen. It contains protein, vitamins A, B, C, D and K, small amounts of minerals including calcium, copper, iron, magnesium, manganese, phosphorus, potassium, and sulphur, as well as several enzymes. It has a bitter taste, which is traditionally disguised by honey – the ambrosia of the Bible, the Koran and the Talmud. Sufferers from hay fever should not eat it during the hay-fever season as it may induce allergic reactions.

POLLEX is a Latin term for thumb.

POLYARTERITIS NODOSA, or PERIARTERITIS NODOSA as it is sometimes known, is a disease of unknown origin, in which prolonged fever and obscure symptoms referable to any system of the body are associated with local areas of inflammation along the arteries, giving rise to nodules in their walls. Recovery occurs in about 50 per cent of cases.

POLYCHROMASIA and POLYCHRO-MATOPHILIA are terms applied to an abnormal reaction of the red blood corpuscles in severe anaemia, whereby they have a bluish tinge instead of the normal red colour in a blood film stained by the usual method. It is a sign that the cell is not fully developed.

POLYCYSTIC DISEASE OF KIDNEY: An inherited disease in which the kidneys contain many cysts. These grow in size until normal kidney tissue is largely destroyed. Cysts may also occur in other organs such as the liver. In adults the disease will cause hypertension and kidney failure. There is also a juvenile form. There is no effective treatment, though symptoms can be alleviated by dialysis and sometimes kidney transplant.

POLYCYSTIC OVARY SYNDROME: In 1935 Stein and Leventhan described seven hirsute and infertile women with amenorrhoea or oligomenorrhoea in whom bilateral cystic ovarian enlargement was found at laparotomy and thereby gave their names to a polycystic ovarian disorder. Since then, however, the protean manner of clinical presentation and the variability of biochemical changes in patients with this condition have lead some people to doubt the existence of a disease entity. Enlarged cystic ovaries may occur in the absence of the classical clinical characteristics originally described. Polycystic ovaries may be found in those who have conceived and are not hirsute, and they may be seen in infertile women who menstruate regularly and even in some patients with menorrhagia. On the other hand, the clinical features of oligomenorrhoea, hirsutism and infertility may occur in the absence of bilateral ovarian enlargement and cystic change may be found in normal sized or small ovaries.

Polycystic ovaries may have several causes. Whether large or small ovaries result may be determined by the duration and severity of the particular cause. Sclerocystic ovarian change would therefore be a better description, but the term polycystic is now firmly established by common usage. The choice of treatment is determined by the clinical presentation and the main complaint. If hirsutism is the main problem and there is evidence of androgen suppression after dexamethasone, then corticosteroid treatment should be tried. The anti-androgen, cyproterone acetate, has recently been introduced and is probably more effective. If, however, fertility is the prime consideration then clomiphene should be given and wedge ressection of the ovaries considered if pregnancy does not result after three courses of the drug.

POLYCYTHAEMIA is an excess in the number of red corpuscles in the blood.

POLYCYTHEMIA RUBRA VERA: A disorder in which the red blood cells increase in number along with an increase in the number of white blood cells and platelets. The cause is unknown. Severe cases may require treatment with cytotoxic drugs or radiotherapy.

POLYDACTYLY means the presence of extra, or supernumerary, fingers or toes.

POLYDIPSIA means excessive thirst, which is a symptom of diabetes mellitus and some other diseases.

POLYMER FUME FEVER occurs in people who work with polytetrafluoroethylene (PTFE, Teflon). The fever is caused by degradation products, including hydrofluoric acid, which are produced at temperatures of 170 °C and upwards. The likeliest source of these injurious products is cigarette smoking. Even the tiniest particles of PTFE on a burning cigarette will yield sufficient of these degradation products to cause fume fever.

The illness consists of an influenza-like illness, which lasts for a few hours.

POLYMORPH is a name applied to certain white corpuscles of the blood which have a nucleus of irregular and varied shape. These form between 70 and 75 per cent of all the white corpuscles. (See BLOOD.)

POLYMORPHIC LIGHT ERUPTION is a photodermatosis (q.v.) which occurs predominantly in females, appearing first as a rule in adolescence or early adult life. The eruption, which consists of a mixture of erythema (q.v.), papules (q.v.) and vesicles (q.v.), occurs on those parts of the body exposed to the sun, mainly the back of the hands, the forearms, the front of the neck, the cheeks and the nose. There are usually several attacks a year, depending on the amount of sunlight. The attacks start in the spring and continue until the winter. Apart from the fact that the rash is provoked by sunlight, the precise cause is not known. Treatment consists of avoiding sunlight, wearing protective clothing, and using sunscreening preparations. (See SUNBURN.)

POLYMYALGIA RHEUMATICA is a form of rheumatism characterized by gross early morning stiffness, which tends to ease off during the day, and pain in the shoulders and sometimes round the hips. It affects women more than men, and is rare under the age of 60. The cause is still obscure. It responds well to prednisolone, but treatment may need to be long continued. On the other hand the condition is not progressive and does not lead to crippling.

POLYMYOSITIS: A disease of the muscles throughout the body. The disorder may be acute or chronic but it usually affects the muscles of the shoulders or hip areas. The muscles weaken and are tender to the touch. Diffuse inflammatory changes occur and symptomatic relief may be obtained with corticosteroid drugs (q.v.).

POLYMYXIN is the name applied to the group of antibiotics derived from various species of *Bacillus polymyxa*. Polymyxin B is the one available commercially, and is the antibiotic of choice in the treatment of infections due to *Ps. pyocyanea*.

POLYNEURITIS means an inflammatory condition of nerves in various parts of the body. (See NEURITIS.)

POLYPEPTIDE: A molecule in which several amino-acids (q.v.) are joined together by peptide bonds. Protein (q.v.) molecules are polypeptides.

POLYPHARMACY is a term applied to the administration of too many drugs to one person. Sometimes combinations of drugs are an effective means of treatment, reducing the risk of drug resistance. Polypharmacy, however, worsens the risk of drug interactions and of adverse effects, especially in the elderly.

POLYPOSIS means the presence of a crop, or large number, of polypi. The most important form of polyposis is that known as *familial polyposis coli*. This is a hereditary disease characterized by the presence of large numbers of polypoid tumours in the large bowel. Every child born to an affected parent stands a fifty-fifty chance of developing the disease. Its importance is that sooner or later one or more of these tumours undergoes cancerous change. If the affected gut is removed surgically before this occurs, and preferably before the age of 20, the results are excellent.

POLYPUS or POLYP is a general name applied to tumours which are attached by a stalk to the surface from which they spring. The term refers only to the shape of the growth and has nothing to do with its structure or nature. Most polypi are of a simple nature, though malignant polypi are also found. The usual structure of a polypus is that of a fine fibrous core covered with epithelium resembling that of the surrounding surface. The sites in which polypi are most usually found are the interior of the nose, the outer meatus of the ear, and the interior of the womb, bladder, or bowels (see POLYPOSIS).

Their removal is generally easy, as they are simply twisted off, or cut off, by some form of snare or ligature. Those which are situated in the interior of the bladder or bowels, and whose presence is usually recognized by the presence of blood in the urine or stools, require a more serious operation to reach the organ into which they project.

POLYSACCHARIDE: A carbohydrate comprising several monosaccharides linked in long chains. Polysaccharides store energy – as starch in plants and glycogen in animals – and they also form the structural parts of plants (as cellulose) and animals (as mucopolysaccharides).

POLYTHELIA is the condition in which extra or supernumerary nipples appear along a line between the armpit and the groin.

POLYTHIAZIDE (see BENZOTHIADIAZINES).

POLYURIA means the passage of an amount of urine considerably in excess of the 1500 ml or thereabout which is the usual daily quantity. It is a symptom of diabetes mellitus, diabetes insipidus, chronic renal failure and psychogenic polydipsia.

POMPHOLYX is a form of eczema characterized by the appearance of deeply set vesicles (q.v.) on the palms and soles, fingers and toes. When it occurs on the fingers and hands it is known as CHEIROPOMPHOLYX. On the toes and feet it is known as PODOPOMPHOLYX.

PONS VAROLII is the bridge of the brain, mainly composed of strands of white nerve-fibres which unite various parts of the brain. (See BRAIN.)

POPLITEAL SPACE, or HAM, is the name given to the region behind the knee. The muscles attached to the bones immediately above and below the knee bound a diamond-shaped space through which pass the main artery and vein of the limb (known in this part of their course as the popliteal artery and vein), the tibial and common peroneal nerves (which continue the sciatic nerve from the thigh down to the leg), the external saphenous vein, as well as several small nerves and lymphatic vessels. The muscles, which bound the upper angle of the space and which are attached to the leg bones by strong prominent tendons, are known as the hamstrings. The lower angle of the space lies between the two heads of the gastrocnemius

muscle, which makes up the main bulk of the calf of the leg.

POPPY as used in medicine is of two species: *Papaver somniferum*, the white opium-poppy (see OPIUM), and *Papaver rhoeas*, the red corn-poppy. The corn-poppy is chiefly used as a colouring agent, the syrup made from it having a brilliant crimson colour.

PORE: A small opening. The word is usually used to describe an opening in the skin that releases sweat or sebum, a waxy material secreted by the sebaceous glands in the skin.

PORPHYRIA is a condition, or rather a series of conditions, characterized by an excessive production and excretion of porphyrins. Porphyrins are constituents of various blood and respiratory pigments found throughout the animal kingdom, including human beings. They are also found in plants and micro-organisms.

In porphyria there is some disturbance of their metabolism and this results in a variegated picture which includes discoloration of the urine due to excessive excretion of porphyrins, skin rashes due to sensitization of the skin to light, various forms of indigestion and mental disturbances.

PORPHYRINS: Complex organic compounds which are sensitive to light and form the basis of respiratory pigments, for example, haemoglobin and myoglobin. Porphyrins are crucial to many metabolic oxidation/reduction reactions in animals, plants, and micro-organisms.

PORT-A-CATH: The Port-a-cath system consists of a silicon catheter connected to a stainless steel chamber in which there is a silicon injection port. The catheter is inserted into a central vein and connected by a sub-cutaneous tunnel to the portal which is implanted subcutaneously on the chest wall. Its purpose is to provide a central venous access while avoiding repeated cannulation with its inevitable risk of sepsis.

PORTAL HYPERTENSION: Raised blood pressure in the portal vein. This results in increased pressure in the veins of the oesophagus and upper stomach and these grow in size to form varices – dilated tortuous veins. Sometimes these varices rupture causing bleeding into the oesophagus. The raised pressure also causes fluid to collect in the abdomen and form ascites. The commonest reason for portal hypertension is cirrhosis (see LIVER DISEASES) (fibrosis) of the liver. Thrombosis in the portal vein may also be a cause. Treatment requires the cause to be tackled, but bleeding from ruptured vessels may be stopped by injecting a sclerosant or hardening solution into and around the veins. Sometimes a surgical shunt may be done to divert blood from the portal vein to another blood vessel.

PORTAL SYSTEM: A vein or collection of veins which finish at both ends in a bed of capillary blood vessels. An important example is the hepatic portal system, comprising the portal vein and its tributaries. Blood from the stomach, pancreas, spleen and intestines drains into the veins that join up to comprise the portal vein into the liver, where it branches into sinusoids.

PORTAL VEIN is the vein which carries to the liver blood that has been circulating in many of the abdominal organs. It is peculiar among the veins of the body in that it ends by breaking up into a capillary network instead of carrying the blood directly to the heart, a peculiarity which it shares only with certain small vessels in the kidneys. The portal system begins below in the haemorrhoidal plexus of veins round the lower end of the rectum, and from this point, along the whole length of the intestines, the blood is collected into an inferior mesenteric vein upon the left, and a superior mesenteric vein upon the right side. The inferior mesenteric vein empties into the splenic vein, and the latter, uniting with the superior mesenteric vein immediately above the pancreas, forms the portal vein. The portal vein is joined by veins from the stomach and gall-bladder, and finally divides into two branches which sink into the right and left lobes of the liver. (For their further course, see LIVER.)

The organs from which the portal vein collects the blood are the large and small intestines, the stomach, spleen, pancreas, and gall-bladder.

POSITRON-EMISSION TOMOGRAPHY: A method for assessing the metabolic activity of tissues in the brain. The operator measures emissions of radiation from specially radiated deoxyglucose. The brain cells accept this substance in the same way as they do glucose. Metabolic activity is slowed down in injured brain tissues, which can therefore be identified. This type of tomography is used to diagnose and treat patients with cerebral palsy and similar brain damage.

POSSETTING is the technical term used to describe the quite common habit of healthy babies to regurgitate, or bring up, small amounts of the meal they have just taken.

POST- is a prefix signifying after or behind.

POST-COITAL CONTRACEPTION: Action taken to prevent conception after intercourse (see CONTRACEPTION).

POST-COITAL TEST: A test for infertility. A specimen of cervical mucus, taken up to 24

hours after coitus (during the post-ovulatory phase of the menstrual cycle), is examined microscopically to assess the motility of the sperms. If motility is above a certain level then sperms and mucus are not interacting abnormally, thus eliminating one cause of sterility.

POST-MORTEM EXAMINATION (see NECROPSY).

POST-OPERATIVE: Relating to the period after an operation, to the patient's condition after operation or to any investigations or treatment during this time.

POST-PARTUM is the term applied to anything happening immediately after child-birth: for example, post-partum haemorrhage.

POST-VIRAL FATIGUE SYNDROME (see MYALGIC ENCEPHALOMYELITIS).

POSTURAL DRAINAGE is the process whereby the drainage of secretions from dilated bronchi of the lungs is facilitated. The patient lies on an inclined plane head downwards and is encouraged to cough up as much secretion from the lungs as possible. The precise position depends on which part of the lungs is affected. It may need to be carried out for up to three hours daily in divided periods. It is of particular value in bronchiectasis (q.v.) and lung abscess.

POTASH, or POTASSA, is the popular name for potassium carbonate. Hydrated oxide of potassium is usually known as caustic potash, and its solution as potash solution.

POTASSIUM is a metal which, on account of its great affinity for other substances, is not found in a pure state in nature. Its salts are used to a great extent in medicine but, as their action depends in general not on their metallic radicle but upon the acid with which it is combined, their uses vary greatly and are described elsewhere. All salts of potassium have a depressing effect on the heart's action by virtue of the potassium ion.

POTASSIUM ASCORBATE EYE-DROPS were originally introduced for the treatment of glaucoma. They are now largely used in helping to prevent ulceration and perforation of the cornea (SEE EYE, DISEASE AND INJURIES) following acid and alkali burns of the eye.

POTASSIUM CHLORATE, in addition to the general actions exerted by potassium salts, has a soothing action upon inflamed mucous membranes, and is used for a gargle in sore throat of every description.

POTT'S DISEASE is a name often applied to the angular curvature of the spine which results from tuberculous disease. (See SPINE AND SPINAL CORD, DISEASES AND INJURIES OF.) The disease is named after Percivall Pott, an English surgeon (1714–88), who first described the condition.

POTT'S FRACTURE is a term applied to a variety of fractures around the ankle, accompanied by a varying degree of dislocation of the ankle. In all cases the fibula is fractured. Named after Percivall Pott, who suffered from this fracture and was the first to describe it (see FRACTURES), it is often mistaken for a simple sprain of the ankle.

POULTICES (see also FOMENTATION) are soft moist applications to the surface of the body, generally used hot. They soften the parts with which they come in contact, soothe irritated nerve-endings, relax spasmodically contracted muscle-fibres, and, after being applied for some time, dilate the vessels of the part they cover and increase the circulation through it. These applications are consequently used in all stages of inflammation to soothe pain and promote resolution, or in the late stages, when pus is forming, to aid the rapid formation of an abscess. (See ABSCESS.)

POUPART'S LIGAMENT, also known as the inguinal ligament, is the strong ligament lying in the boundary between the anterior abdominal wall and the front of the thigh.

POWDERS form a method in which drugs are prescribed, powerful drugs being made up with inert substances like sugar, gum, or ginger in order to give them sufficient bulk. The best known powders were Dover's powder (ipecacuanha and opium powder), containing opium; Gregory's powder (compound rhubarb powder); and Seidlitz powder (compound effervescent powder). Powders have largely been replaced by tablets.

PRAZEPAM (see BENZODIAZEPINES).

PRAZIQUANTEL is a drug that is proving of value in the treatment of schistosomiasis (q.v.).

PRE- is a prefix meaning before.

PRECIPITIN: An antibody that combines with an antigen and forms the immune complex as a precipitate. The reaction is used in some diagnostic serological tests to indentify antigens in the serum.

PRECORDIAL REGION is the area on the centre and towards the left side of the chest, lying in front of the heart.

PREDNISOLONE is a derivative of cortisone, which is five or six times as active as cortisone and has less of the salt- and water-retaining properties of cortisone. It is given by mouth.

PREDNISONE is the official name for deltadehydrocortisone, and has the same action as prednisolone.

PRE-ECLAMPSIA is a complication of pregnancy characterized by oedema, high blood-pressure and the presence of albumin in the urine. It is so called because, unless adequately treated in time, it may be a prelude to the onset of eclampsia (q.v.).

PREGNANCY: This state is a natural one, although it sets up great changes, not only in the womb, but throughout the whole body. Most of these changes subside quickly after delivery is accomplished, and though a few minor alterations persist throughout life, the mother returns to her normal state within about one month after the child is born.
Duration of pregnancy: It is generally accepted that pregnancy lasts about 280 days from the first day of the last menstrual period. In exceptional cases there may be considerable variation, but it is generally agreed that the shortest duration of a normal pregnancy is 240 days and the longest duration 313 days. The cause of these variations is not understood. For the purpose of calculating the probable date of confinement, it is usual to take the first day of the last period that occurred, to allow seven days for the duration of this and then to add 273 days for the duration of gestation, making in all 280 days from the beginning of the last menstruation.
Signs of pregnancy: (a) The stoppage of the menstrual flow is the first sign. This symptom may, however, be due to many other causes (see MENSTRUATION), but if it occurs quite suddenly it may usually be counted upon as an important sign. It is a popular mistake to suppose that pregnancy cannot occur in a woman while she is suckling a previous child, for this does occur even while the menses are in abeyance. (b) Swelling of the breasts is another important sign, appearing even in the second or third month of pregnancy. A thin fluid, known as colostrum, can, even at this early stage, be pressed from the nipples. At the same time the veins on the breasts become enlarged and visible, and the pigmented ring round the nipple (areola) becomes much darker than before, as well as showing small nodules (Montgomery's tubercles) round its edge. (c) Sickness in the morning immediately on rising is also a common sign, occurring in about two-thirds of all women. When the sickness is marked, however, it is a valuable sign, because it appears early in the course of pregnancy, during the second month, and lasts usually about a couple of months. (d) Quickening, or the fluttering sensation felt by the mother in consequence of the

child's rapid movements, is a very important sign, though it does not usually occur till some time during the fifth month of pregnancy or even later. It is the first sign of life felt by the mother, though it is a popular error to suppose that the child only then begins to live. (*e*) Enlargement of the abdomen is a pronounced sign, though for the first three months the enlargement is not apparent. It must not be forgotten, however, that enlargement may be due to other causes, such as tumours or increasing development of fat. It is not an uncommmon mistake for an elderly childless woman to delude herself with the hope that she is about to bear a child, when the abdomen is enlarging simply for the last-named reason. This condition is known as pseudocyesis or false pregnancy. (*f*) One certain sign of pregnancy is the beating of the fetal heart which can be heard by auscultation over the lower part of the abdomen. The heart-sounds are rapid, much resembling the ticking of a watch, and are heard, in general, from the middle of the fifth month onwards. (*g*) There are various minor signs which are sometimes present, sometimes absent, such are the occurrence of varicose veins, mucous discharge from the vagina, changes in the neck of the womb.

Hygiene of pregnancy: It is unnecessary for a healthy woman to make any great change in her ordinary mode of life during pregnancy. Her diet must be good, but should be simple and moderate. Alcoholic drinking and smoking should be stopped during pregnancy. Because of the possible risk to the unborn child, no drugs should be taken during early pregnancy except on medical advice. A pregnant woman should drink at least half a litre (one pint) of milk a day, on account, amongst other things, of the calcium it contains. Cheese should also be taken for its calcium. (The fetus in the uterus needs calcium for its bones.) Iron- containing foods are also important for the development of the fetus's red blood corpuscles. Iron is present in such foods as eggs, green leafy vegetables, and in liver and meat. Vitamins are also of great importance to the pregnant woman, and these are present in such foods as eggs, milk, cheese, butter, wholemeal bread, brown bread, fresh vegetables, and fruit (especially oranges, lemons, currants, potatoes, and tomatoes), and fat fish, such as herring and salmon; in the winter months compound vitamin tablets may well be taken in addition. Constipation should be avoided by a suitable diet containing vegetables, fruit, and the like, or by mild aperients. The skin should be kept in good condition by regular bathing. Moderate exercise should be taken every day and late hours avoided. The dress should be loose and comfortable. It is inadvisable for sexual intercourse to take place during the last month of pregnancy. During pregnancy a healthy woman gains an average of 12·5 kg (28 pounds), but this varies considerably.

Special ailments: Digestive disturbances are common. Thus the natural morning sickness may become very troublesome, or even dangerous, and require special treatment. Constipation or diarrhoea may be troublesome, but either of them is treated much as under ordinary circumstances. Varicose veins in the legs, piles, swelling of the feet, and cramps in the legs are all liable to be caused in the later months by pressure of the increasing womb upon the large vessels and nerves within the pelvis. These, however, are not serious signs, and they quickly improve after delivery. Varicose veins, if very severe, should be supported by elastic stockings or by bandaging the legs, and cramps may be relieved by the usual means. (See CRAMP.) Irritability of the bladder, showing itself by frequency of making water, is also a temporary inconvenience, similarly due to pressure.

More serious symptoms occasionally arise, such as those of kidney disease, various nervous disorders, and especially hypertension and the condition known as eclampsia, in which convulsions occur. A sudden gain in weight in late pregnancy may indicate the onset of pre-eclampsia (q.v.).

It is because of the possibility of such ailments, whether mild or serious, occurring during pregnancy that every pregnant mother should be seen by her doctor, or attend an antenatal clinic, at regular intervals throughout pregnancy.

PREGNANCY TESTS: There are several tests for pregnancy in its early stages, and these can be done on blood or urine; some of the urine tests may be carried out at home.

The Hogben test: This test is based upon the observation that the injection of pregnancy urine promotes ovulation in the female South African clawed toad (*Xenopus laevis*). It gives a result within twenty-four hours.

The Haemagglutination Inhibition test: This, and the subsequent tests to be mentioned, are known as immunological tests, as opposed to that already mentioned which is known as a biological test. They are based upon the effect of the urine from a pregnant woman upon the interaction of red-blood cells, which have been sensitized to human gonadotrophin (q.v.), and anti-gonadotrophin serum. They have the great practical advantage of being performed in a test-tube or even on a slide, and therefore not requiring animals. Because of their ease and speed of performance (a result can be obtained in two hours), these tests are being used on an increased scale. The *Latex test* and the *Gravindex test* are modifications of the haemagglutination test.

PREGNANDIOL is the excretion product of the hormone, PROGESTERONE (q.v.), manufactured by the corpus luteum of the ovary. Pregnandiol is excreted in the urine during the second half of the menstrual period, and its excretion rises steadily throughout pregnancy.

PREMATURE BEAT (see ECTOPIC BEAT).

PREMATURE BIRTH (see ABORTION; FETUS) is one that takes place before the end of the normal period of gestation, usually before 37 weeks. In practice, however, it is defined as a birth that takes place when the baby weighs less than 2·5 kilograms (5½ pounds). Between 5 and 10 per cent of babies are born prematurely and in around 40 per cent of premature births the cause is unknown. Pre-eclampsia is the commonest known cause; others include hypertension, chronic kidney disease, heart disease and diabetes mellitus. Multiple pregnancy is another cause. In the vast majority of cases the aim of management is to prolong the pregnancy and so improve the outlook for the unborn child. This consists essentially of rest in bed and sedation, but there are now several drugs, such as ritodrine (q.v.), that may be used to suppress the activity of the uterus and so help to delay premature labour. Prematurity was once a prime cause of infant mortality but modern medical care has greatly improved survival rates in development countries.

PREMATURE EJACULATION: A disorder in which ejaculation occurs before or immediately after the penis penetrates the vagina. The commonest sexual problem in men, persistent premature ejaculation, may have psychological causes, although many adolescents and some adults experience it occasionally. Sexual counselling may help to alleviate the condition.

PREMEDICATION: A drug or drugs given to a patient to produce sedation before an operation. A narcotic analgesic drug is usually used as this relieves pain as well as anxiety. An antisecretory drug is often added to reduce the secretions in the airways and thus lessen the risk of general anaesthesia. Premedication reduces the amount of anaesthetic needed to make the patient unconscious.

PREMENSTRUAL SYNDROME has been defined as 'any combination of emotional or physical features which occur cyclically in a woman before menstruation and which regress or disappear during menstruation'. It is characterized by mood changes, discomfort, swelling and tenderness in the breasts, swelling of the legs, a bloated feeling in the abdomen, headache, fatigue and constipation. The mood changes range from irritability and mild depression to outbursts of violence. It may last for three up to 14 days. How common it is is not known, as only the more severe cases are seen by doctors, but it has been estimated that 1 in 10 of all menstruating women suffer from it severely enough to require treatment. The cause is not known, but it is probably due to some upset of the hormonal balance of the body. In view of the multiplicity of causes that have been put forward, it is not surprising that there is an equal multiplicity of treatments. Among these one of the most widely used is progesterone (q.v.). Others include pyridoxine

(q.v.), danazol (q.v.), and gamma linolenic acid available in the form of oil of evening primrose. Whatever drug may be prescribed, psychological treatment is equally essential and, in many cases, is all that is required.

PREMOLAR: The two teeth on each side of the jaw positioned between the canines and the molars in the adult. The teeth are used with the molars for holding and grinding food.

PRENATAL DIAGNOSIS: AMNIOCENTESIS: This method of antenatal diagnosis involves examining fetal cells from the amniotic fluid, which surrounds the fetus. Guided by ultrasound (q.v.) a fine needle is inserted through the mother's abdomen into the amniotic cavity, and a sample of amniotic fluid is withdrawn.

The fetal cells are then cultured and the genetic make-up of the fetus determined. This allows testing for chromosonal abnormalities such as Down's syndrome (q.v.) and other birth defects. The fluid may be checked for its alpha fetoprotein content, which is helpful in the diagnosis of spina bifida (q.v.).

The test is usually offered to pregnant women who have had a previously affected child, a family history of genetic abnormalities or are over the age of 35. (The risk of genetic abnormalities increases with age; at the age of 40 the risk of having a baby with Down's syndrome is 1 in 100).

Traditionally amniocentesis is carried out between 15 and 16 weeks of pregnancy but may in future be available as early as 10 weeks. As it takes about 4 weeks to obtain results of the cell culture this would be a significant advance. Counselling is important and allows the parents to make an informed choice, which may not necessarily involve terminating the pregnancy if an abnormality is found. Currently termination of an abnormal fetus is performed around 19–20 weeks.

The risk of miscarriage following the procedure is about 0·5–1 per cent.

CHORIONIC VILLUS SAMPLING (CVS): In this method of antenatal diagnosis a small sample of placental tissue (afterbirth) is removed between the 9th and the 11th week of pregnancy and tested for genetic abnormalities. Under ultrasound guidance a needle is introduced into the placenta, either through the vagina and the neck of the womb or through the abdomen.

The advantages of the technique are that the results are available within a week. This allows termination relatively early in pregnancy before other people have become aware of the pregnancy.

The procedure has a miscarriage rate of 3–4 per cent and results can sometimes be difficult to interpret, in which case amniocentesis will still be required later in the pregnancy.

CORDOCENTESIS: In this method of antenatal diagnosis a sample of the blood from the fetus is taken from the umbilical cord (q.v.) which connects the fetus to the placenta by inserting a needle through the mother's abdomen under ultrasound guidance. It may be performed after 18 weeks of pregnancy and offers an accurate diagnosis of genetic abnormalities within three days. Blood disorders and infections in the baby, such as German measles (q.v.) or toxoplasmosis may also be detected by the test.

In skilled hands the risk of fetal death after cordocentesis is 0·5–1 per cent.

Ultrasound scanning (q.v.) is widely used to assess the progress of a pregnancy.

PREPUCE is the free fold of skin that overlaps the glans penis and retracts when the penis becomes erect.

PRESBYACUSIS is the deafness that comes on with increasing years. It is caused by increasing loss of elasticity in the hearing mechanism, combined with the slowing down of the mental processes that accompanies old age. It is characterized by particular difficulty in hearing high notes such as the telephone and the voices of women and children. Hearing in a background of noise, is also early affected. Modern, miniaturized, transistor 'within-the-ear' hearing aids are now available that are proving helpful in making life more bearable for the elderly in this respect. (See also DEAFNESS; HEARING AIDS.)

PRESBYOPIA (see ACCOMMODATION; REFRACTION).

PRESCRIPTION means the written direction given by the doctor to the chemist for the compounding of medicine suitable to a patient's case.

Prescriptions are written in terms of milligrams and grams and in the *British Pharmacopoeia* and *British National Formulary* dosages are given in terms of the metric system only. (See also DOSAGE; DRUGS.)

Restrictions on prescribing and dispensing at public expense came into effect in the United Kingdom on 1 April 1985. The restrictions have helped to reduce the expenditure on pharmaceutical remedies in the National Health Service. The aim was to exclude more expensive proprietary preparations when equivalent non-proprietary remedies were available at much less expense. The following groups of drugs were involved:

Antacids.

Laxatives.

Analgesics – used for mild or moderate pain.

Cough and cold remedies.

Bitters and tonics, vitamins.

Benzodiazepine tranquillisers and sedatives.

Medicines should be prescribed only when they are essential. This is particularly important in patients who are pregnant, where the risk to both patient and fetus must be considered – there are many drugs for which there is not sufficient evidence to be quite certain that they are harmless to the fetus. The most

dangerous time is the first trimester of pregnancy.

Non-proprietary titles should normally be prescribed as this will enable the pharmacist to dispense any of the proprietary equivalents that he has in stock and thus avoid delay to the patient and expense to the Health Service. The pharmacist is not allowed to dispense a controlled drug unless the specific requirements of the 'Misuse of Drugs Regulations' of 1973 are met. The *British National Formulary* gives classified notes on drugs and preparations used in the treatment of diseases and their recommended doses. It is intended for the guidance of medical practitioners, pharmacists, nurses and other health workers. The councils of the British Medical Association and the Pharmaceutical Society have agreed that the name of the preparation should appear on the label of the bottle unless the prescriber indicates otherwise.

PRESENILE: Describing the condition of premature ageing. The mental and physical faculties are adversely affected in presenility to an extent that does not usually occur until old age (see DEMENTIA).

PRESENTATION means the appearance in labour of some particular part of the child's body at the mouth of the womb. This is a head presentation in 96 per cent of cases, but in a certain number the breech (or buttocks) may present, or the face, or foot, or even a part of the trunk in cases of cross-birth.

PRESSOR is the term applied to anything that increases the activity of a function: for example, a pressor nerve or pressor drug.

PRESSURE SORES (see BED SORES).

PREVALENCE: An epidemiological term describing the proportion of a defined group in the population having a condition at one point in time. It is an appropriate measure only in relatively stable conditions for example, chronic bronchitis – and is not suitable for measuring acute illnesses.

PREVENTIVE MEDICINE: The branch of medicine concerned with the prevention of disease. Prevention is achieved by public health measures such as health education, health-screening programmes, immunization procedures against infectious diseases, the provision of clean water and the maintenance of a clean environment (see PUBLIC HEALTH).

PRIAPISM: A persisting painful erection of the penis (q.v.) occurring without sexual stimulation. It is a rare but acute condition that requires immediate treatment. The cause is the failure of blood to drain from the spongy corpus caversonum tissues of the penis, thus maintaining an erection. This may happen because of infection, damage to the nerves controlling the blood vessels, or a clotting defect in the blood.

PRICKLY HEAT, or MILIARA RUBRA, is a troublesome skin condition affecting Europeans in tropical climates. It consists in the appearance of numbers of minute vesicles, produced by blocking of the outlet of the sweat or sebaceous glands in the skin, and accompanied by intolerable itching.

Causes: Nearly every European suffers from prickly heat during the early years of residence in the tropics, when the hot season comes round. It is due probably to the cells on the surface of the skin becoming sodden by the constant perspiration, and so swelling and blocking the outlets of the minute gland-ducts. Anything that leads to perspiration, such as hot drinks, hot soup, close rooms, or warm clothing, aggravates the condition.

Symptoms: The surface is covered by minute vesicles which cause extreme itching and pricking. The scratching which this entails often leads to the formation of boils and pustules, but the condition is not in itself a dangerous one. The extreme discomfort, and the loss of sleep arising from it, may, however, be a serious matter for invalids.

Treatment: The most important point is to avoid, so far as possible, all causes of excessive perspiration, such as warm drinks and rough underclothing. Curtailing the intake of salt and maintaining an adequate intake of fluid are also said to be helpful. Common soap should not be used in the bath, and each time after bathing, the skin should be dusted with an astringent and antiseptic dusting powder, such as one composed of boric acid, zinc oxide, and starch in equal parts. Equally effective is the use of an emollient cream or bath oil. If nothing else is immediately available, the application of olive oil is often helpful.

As a preventive, rubbing the body over after the bath with the juice of a lemon has been recommended. Calamine lotion (either alone or incorporating some menthol crystals) or carbolic acid lotion relieves the itching temporarily.

PRIMIDONE is a drug used for the treatment of epilepsy.

PRIMIGRAVIDA: A woman who is undergoing her first pregnancy.

PRIMIPARA is the term applied to a woman who has given birth, or is giving birth, to her first child.

PRO- is a prefix meaning forwards.

PROBE is a slender, flexible instrument usually made of metal designed for introduction into a wound or cavity either to explore its depth and direction, to discover the presence of foreign bodies, or to introduce medicinal substances.

PROBENECID is a benzoic acid derivative. It interferes with the excretion by the kidney of certain compounds, including penicillin and para-aminosalicylic acid, and was originally introduced into medicine for this reason, as a means of increasing and maintaining the concentration of penicillin in the body. It has also proved of value in the treatment of chronic gout.

PROBUCOL (see HYPERLIPIDAEMIA).

PROCAINAMIDE is a derivative of procaine, which has been introduced for the treatment of certain cardiac arrythmias.

PROCAINE, or PROCAINE HYDROCHLORIDE, is a synthetic substance having a similar action to the natural alkaloid, cocaine. It is a powerful local anaesthetic with transitory effect. Procaine possesses the anaesthetic properties of cocaine, but has an advantage over the latter in being very much less poisonous, so that it can be administered in larger doses, and also in producing no tendency to contract a habit for its use.

PROCAINE PENICILLIN (see PENICILLIN).

PROCARBAZINE is a drug that is proving useful in the treatment of various forms of tumour, especially Hodgkin's disease (q.v.). It acts by interfering with the process of mitosis (q.v.), whereby the cells of the body, or tumours, reproduce themselves.

PROCHLORPERAZINE is an anti-psychotic drug. It is also an effective drug for the prevention or treatment of vomiting, and has therefore been used in the treatment of Menière's disease (q.v.). (See NEUROLEPTICS.)

PROCIDENTIA is another term for prolapse (q.v.).

PROCTALGIA is neuralgic pain in the anus or rectum. The term is usually reserved for rectal pain without local disease in the rectum to account for it.

Proctalgia fugax is a condition characterized by cramp-like pains in the rectum which may be excruciatingly painful. They are more common in men than women. They occur during the night, last up to fifteen minutes and may be accompanied by a feeling of faintness. The cause is not known. The taking of food or drink may bring relief, as may pressure on the perineum (eg. by sitting astride the edge of the bath). A finger in the rectum may also bring relief. The sucking of a 1 mg tablet of glyceryl trinitrate is said by some to bring prompt relief. The attacks are said to cease after the age of 50.

PROCTITIS means inflammation situated about the rectum or anus.

PRODROMATA is a term applied to the earliest symptoms of a disease, or those which give warning of its presence.

PROFLAVINE is a valuable antiseptic. It is an acridine derivative. Like all the acridine derivatives it is effective against both Gram-positive and Gram-negative bacteria and is not inactivated by body fluids or pus. It is also non-toxic and non-irritating.

PROGERIA is premature old age.

PROGESTERONE is the hormone of the corpus luteum (q.v.). After the escape of the ovum from the ruptured follicle, the corpus luteum secretes progesterone, which stimulates the growth and secretion of the endometrial glands of the uterus during the fourteen days before menstruation. In the event of pregnancy, the secretion of progesterone continues until parturition. (See also ETHISTERONE; NORE-THISTERONE; NORETHYNODREL; PREGNANDIOL; CONTRACEPTION; MENSTRUATION.)

PROGESTOGEN is a preparation with an action like that of progesterone (q.v.).

PROGLOTTIS is a segment of a tapeworm.

PROGNATHISM: Abnormal protusion of the lower jaw or sometimes of both jaws. The condition may make biting and chewing difficult, in which case corrective surgery is necessary.

PROGNOSIS is the term applied to a forecast as to the probable result of an illness or disease, particularly with regard to the prospect of recovery.

PROGRESSIVE MUSCULAR ATROPHY (see PARALYSIS).

PROGUANIL HYDROCHLORIDE is a synthetic antimalarial drug which has proved of value both in the treatment and the prevention of malaria, particularly the form known as malignant tertian malaria.

PROLACTIN is the pituitary hormone which initiates lactation. The development of the breasts during pregnancy is ascribed to the action of oestrogens (q.v.). Prolactin starts them secreting. If lactation does not occur or fails, it may be started by injection of prolactin.

The secretion of prolactin is normally kept under tonic inhibition by the secretion of a prolactin inhibitory hormone. This is formed in the hypothalamus and secreted into the portal capillaries of the pituitary stalk to reach the anterior pituitary cells. The prolactin inhibitory hormone has now been identified as the catecholamine dopamine. Drugs that deplete the brain stores of dopamine or antagonize dopamine at receptor level will cause hyperprolactinaemia and hence the secretion of milk from the breast and amenorrhoea. Methyldopa and reserpine deplete brain stores of dopamine and the phenothiazines act as dopamine antagonists at receptor level. Other causes of excess secretion of prolactin are pituitary tumours, which may be minute and are then called microadenomas, or may actually enlarge the pituitary fossa and are then called macroadenomas. The commonest cause of hyperprolactinaemia is a pituitary tumour. The patient may present with infertility, because patients with hyperprolactinaemia do not ovulate, or the patient may present with amenorrhea and even galactorrhoea.

Bromocriptine is a dopamine agonist. Treatment with bromocriptine will therefore control hyperprolactinaemia and restore normal menstruation and ovulation and suppress galactorrhoea. If the cause of hyperprolactinaemia is a macroadenoma, surgical treatment should be considered.

PROLAPSE means slipping down of some organ or structure. The term is applied chiefly to downward displacements of the rectum and womb. When the lower end of the bowel prolapses each time the bowels move – as may occur in children – it should be carefully sponged with cold water, replaced, and, if necessary, retained in place by a soft pad and bandage attached to a waist- belt, or by strapping the buttocks together with plaster. The condition tends to pass off as the child grows older. Prolapse which affects the womb may, in the earlier stages, cause protrusion of a fold of the bowel or bladder through the vagina, and in the later stages the womb itself may protrude to the exterior. The condition, which affects elderly women, is mainly due to injuries caused by childbirth. It may often be remedied by wearing a suitably shaped pessary, or by an operation designed to unite the torn parts.

PROLAPSED INTERVERTEBRAL DISC: The spinal column (q.v.) is built up of a series of bones, known as vertebrae, placed one upon the other. Between these vertebrae lies a series of thick discs of fibro-cartilage known as intervertebral discs. Each disc consists of an outer portion known as the annulus fibrosus, and an inner core known as the nucleus pulposus. The function of these discs is to give flexibility and resiliency to the spinal column and to act as buffers against undue jarring. In other words, they are most efficient shock absorbers. They may, however, prolapse, or protrude, between the two adjacent vertebrae. If this should happen they press on the neighbouring spinal nerve and cause pain. As the most common sites of protrusion, or prolapse, are between the last two lumbar vertebrae and between the last lumbar vertebra and the sacrum, this means that the pain occurs in the back, causing lumbago (q.v.) or down the course of the sciatic nerve causing sciatica (q.v.). The prolapse is most likely to occur in middle age, which suggests that it may be associated with degeneration of the disc involved, but it can occur in early adult life as well. It usually occurs when the individual is performing some form of exercise which involves bending, as in gardening. The onset of pain may be acute and sudden, or gradual and more chronic in intensity.

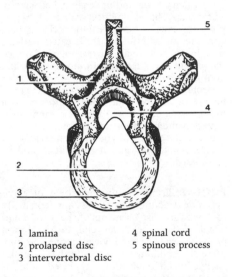

1 lamina   4 spinal cord
2 prolapsed disc   5 spinous process
3 intervertebral disc

Diagram of prolapsed intervertebral disc.

Treatment varies, depending, amongst other things, on the severity of the condition. In the acute phase rest in bed is essential. Later, exercise and physiotherapy are helpful, and in some cases manipulation of the spine brings relief by allowing the herniated, or prolapsed, disc to slip back into position. The injection of a local anaesthetic into the spine (epidural anaesthesia) is yet another measure that often helps the more chronic cases. The ultimate form of treatment is an operation to remove the prolapsed disc, but this is a procedure that is not now performed nearly as often as it once was. An alternative form of treatment is the injection into the disc of chymopapain, an enzyme (q.v.) obtained from the paw-paw, which dissolves the disc.

PROMAZINE (see NEUROLEPTICS).

PROMETHAZINE HYDROCHLORIDE is a widely used antihistamine drug with a prolonged action and a pronounced sedative effect. (See ANTIHISTAMINE DRUGS.)

PROMETHAZINE THEOCLATE, or AVO-MINE, is a drug that is widely used in the alleviation or prevention of sea-sickness.

PRONATION is the movement whereby the bones of the forearm are crossed and the palm of the hand faces downwards.

PRONE: Lying with the face down, or positioning the arm and hand so that the palm faces downwards.

PROPANTHELINE, or PROPANTHELINE BRO-MIDE, is a substance with an anti-cholinergic, or atropine-like action, which is used in the treatment of conditions such as duodenal ulcer and spastic colon.

PROPHYLAXIS means treatment or action adopted with the view of warding off disease.

PROPRANOLOL is a drug that is used in the treatment of angina pectoris, myocardial infarction, certain abnormal rhythms of the heart, and high blood-pressure. It is also proving of value in preventing attacks of migraine, and in certain anxiety states, particularly those associated with unpleasant bodily sensations, such as palpitations. It is a beta-adrenoceptor-blocking drug. (See ADRENERGIC RECEPTORS.)

PROPRIETARY NAME: The trade name of a drug registered by the pharmaceutical company which has developed and patented it. This protects the name, ingredients and manufacturing technique for a set period of time. Doctors may prescribe a drug by its trade name or by its official, approved name, though the NHS encourages the latter.

PROPRIOCEPTORS: Sensory nerve endings in the muscles, tendons and joints which signal to the brain their position relative to the outside world and the state of contraction of the muscle. During movement of a regular flow of information to the brain from the proprioceptors, the eyes and ears ensure that actions are co-ordinated and the body's balance maintained.

PROPTOSIS: A condition in which the eye protrudes from the orbit. Some causes include thyroid disorders, tumours within the orbit, inflammation or infection of the orbit. Proptosis due to endocrine abnormality, e.g. thyroid problems, is known as *exophthalmos*.

PROSTACYCLIN is a prostaglandin (q.v.) produced by the endothelial lining of the blood vessels. It inhibits the aggregation of platelets (q.v.), and thereby reduces the likelihood of the blood clotting. It is also a strong vasodilator.

PROSTAGLANDINS, so called because they were first discovered in the semen and thought to arise in the prostate gland, are a group of recently discovered substances with a wide range of activity. The richest known source is semen, but they are also present in many other parts of the body. Their precise mode of action is not yet clear, but they are potent stimulators of muscle contraction and they are also potent vasodilators (q.v.). They cause contraction of the womb and have been used to induce labour. They are also being used as a means of inducing therapeutic abortions. They play an important part in the production of pain, and it is now known that aspirin relieves pain by virtue of the fact that it prevents, or antagonizes, the formation of certain prostaglandins. In addition, they play some, though as yet incompletely defined, part in producing inflammatory changes. (See INFLAMMATION, NON-STEROIDAL ANTI-INFLAMMATORY DRUGS.)

Thus prostaglandins have potent biological effects but their instability and rapid metabolism make them short acting. They are produced but not stored by most living cells and act locally. The two most important prostaglandins are prostacycline and thromboxane. Prostacycline is a vaso-dilator and an inhibitor of platelet aggregation and may cause relaxation of the myometrium. Thromboxanes have the opposite effects and cause vaso-constriction and platelet aggregation. The non-steroidal anti-inflammatory drugs act by blocking an enzyme called cyclo-oxygenase which converts arachidonic acid to the precursors of the various prostaglandins. Despite their potent pharmacological properties, the role of prostaglandins in current therapeutics is limited and controversial. They have been used most successfully as an inhibitor of platelet aggregation in extra-corporeal haemoperfusion systems. The problems with the prostacyclines is that they have to be given intravenously as they are inactive by mouth, and continuous infusion is required because the drug is rapidly eliminated with a half-life of minutes. Side-effects tend to be severe because the drug is usually given at the highest dose the patient can tolerate. The hope for the future lies in the exploitation of the novel compound to generate stable orally active prostacycline analogues which will inhibit platelet aggregation and hence thrombotic events, and yet have minimal effects on the heart and blood vessels.

PROSTATE GLAND is a structure which lies at the neck of the bladder in men and surrounds that part of the urethra lying within the pelvis. This gland is of importance, especially because in late life it is apt to increase in size and change in shape in such a way as to obstruct the exit of urine from the bladder. Accordingly, great difficulty occurs in urinating. In some cases relief can be obtained, for a time at least, by the administration of phenoxybenzamine. In the large majority of cases, however, in which enlargement of the prostate produces such obstruction, removal by means of operation is now recommended. This operation, if performed by experienced surgeons, carries a relatively low mortality rate – 0·75 to 1 per cent – even though it is often carried out on old men who are far from fit. It has been estimated that one in every ten men will undergo this operation. The prostate is also one of the common sites of cancer in men, for which treatment takes various forms, including removal of the gland by operation, orchidectomy (q.v.), radiotherapy (q.v.), and administration of stilboestrol (q.v.).

PROSTATISM is the condition induced by benign enlargement of the prostate gland (q.v.).

PROSTHESES: A prosthesis is an artificial replacement, such as an artificial limb or eye, or a denture. It is often necessary, for aesthetic or practical reasons, to replace part of the body, lost by injury or disease, with copies of the original, or PROSTHESES as they are now known. From ancient times this has been the case: Herodotus speaks of a man with a wooden foot; the Romans carried the manufacture of limbs to a high degree of efficiency, as witnesssed by a leg, the oldest known artificial limb in existence, neatly formed of thin bronze plates, leather and iron, found in a tomb at Capua and dating from around 300 BC; the Etruscans fashioned gold teeth five centuries before the Christian era; Goetz von Berlichingen (1480–1562), to supply his lost right hand, had one made of iron and thus became known as Goetz of the Iron Hand; and Ambroise Paré, who wrote on surgery in the sixteenth century, has a chapter upon artificial limbs. From then there was little advance until 1800 when James Potts, of London, patented an artificial leg made of two hollow wooden cones with a steel knee joint and a wooden ankle joint. It became known as the Anglesey leg after its owner, the Marquis of Anglesey and, with few modifications, remained the basis of British designs until the 1914–18 War. Since the 1939–45 War there have been striking advances, particularly in artificial hands, as the result of the introduction of electronics and myoelectric means of control.

Arms: Owing to the very delicate movements which the upper limb has to carry out, it is never amputated if there is any possibility of its being of any use. When amputation is decided upon, as little as possible of the arm is removed. Great strides have been made in the provision of artificial arms and hands, and it is now found that 50 per cent efficiency can be obtained when the amputation has been above the elbow, and 75 per cent efficiency when it is below the elbow. Appliances are now available which allow an individual who has lost an arm to engage, for example, in carpentry, many branches of engineering, and the electrical trades. Such an individual can also write, shoot, play golf and cricket, and even fly-fish.

Legs: An artificial substitute can come much nearer to the usefulness of the original in the lower than in the upper limb. As result of experience gained in the two World Wars artificial lower limbs are now so efficient that the individual often suffers little disability. This applies particularly to amputations below the knee, but even in the case of amputations high in the thigh many individuals can often resume their old occupations. In addition, they can often ride a bicycle or a horse, or drive a car, whilst tennis and golf are quite normal pastimes. One of the great secrets of success in the fitting of artificial limbs is to restore the patient's morale and to stimulate his sense of independence. A considerable time must elapse after amputation, to allow for shrinkage of the stump, before a permanent prosthesis can be fitted. To overcome the practical disadvantages of this delay, a pneumatic post-amputation mobility aid is now available. This fits over the bandaged stump, and is inflated to 40 mm Hg to support a rigid frame. It can be fitted by nurses and paramendical staff without any special training in prosthetics. Using this device patients can now start learning to walk again within a week of their amputation. It is suitable for amputation below, above and through the knee.

Eyes: Artificial eyes are worn both for appearance and to protect the socket from dust, though, of course, vision is impossible. They are made of glass or plastic, and are thin shells of a boat-shape. representing the front half of the eye which has been removed. The stump which is left has still the eye-muscles in it, and so the artificial eye still has the power of moving with the other, though to a less extent, and it is often difficult for this reason to tell at a short distance that a person has a false eye. A glass eye has to be replaced by a new one every year. Plastic eyes have the advantage of being more comfortable to wear, and more durable and of being unbreakable.

Dental prosthesis is any artificial replacement of a tooth. There are three main types, a crown, a bridge and a denture. A crown is the replacement of the part of a tooth which sticks through the gum. It is fixed to the remaining part of the tooth and may be made of metal, porcelain, plastic or a combination of these. A bridge is the replacement of two or three missing teeth and is usually fixed in place. The replacement teeth are held in position by being joined to one or more crowns on the adjacent teeth. A denture is a removable prosthesis used to replace some or all the teeth. The teeth are made of plastic or porcelain and the base may be of plastic or metal. All these prostheses are individually made by skilled technicians and are matched to the patient's own teeth for size, shape and colour. Removable teeth may be held more firmly by means of implants.

Nose: The making of a new nose is the oldest known operation in plastic surgery, Hindu records of such operations dating back to 1000 BC. Loss of a nose may be due to eroding disease, war wounds, gun-shot wounds or dog bites. In essence the operation is the same as that practised a thousand years before Christ: namely the use of a skin graft, brought down from the forehead. Alternative sources of the skin graft today are skin from the arm, chest or abdomen. As a means of support the new nose is built round a graft of bone or of cartilage from the ear.

PROTEIN is the term applied to members of a group of non- crystallizable nitrogenous substances widely distributed in the animal and vegetable kingdoms and forming the characteristic materials of their tissues and fluids. They are essentially combinations of amino-acids. They mostly dissolve in water and are coagulated by heat and various chemical substances. Typical examples of protein substances are white of egg and gelatin.

Proteins constitute an essential part of the diet as a source of energy and for the replacement of protein lost in the wear and tear of daily life. Their essential constituent from this point of view is the nitrogen they contain. To be absorbed, or digested, proteins have to be broken down into their constituent amino-acids. The adult human body can maintain nitrogenous equilibrium on a mixture of eight amino-acids, which are therefore known as the essential amino-acids. They are isoleucine, leucine, lysine, methionine, phenylalanine, threonine, tryptophan and valine. In addition, infants require histidine. It is because some of these essential amino-acids, particularly lysine, are lacking in cereals and pulses that these cannot alone constitute an adequate diet. Generally speaking, the major source of protein is animal food, although some vegetables, notably the pulses, contain protein. The use of a certain amount of nitrogenous food is necessary to the system, as from this source alone can the body derive all the building material it requires to repair daily waste. Even carbohydrate foods contain a certain amount of protein, but if all the necessary protein were to be obtained from these it would incur the waste of much starch, or its formation into fat in the bodily tissues. Hence the main value of a mixed diet.

Meat, in structure, consists of long cylinders of semi-fluid, protein material enclosed in thin, fibrous tubes, and known as muscle fibres. (See MUSCLE.) These are bound together by fibrous tissue, enclosing more or less fat in its meshes. The protein material consists mainly of myosin, which clots when the muscle dies, and contains also albumin and haemoglobin. In addition, there are several chemical substances which can be extracted by steeping the meat in hot water, and which are therefore known as extractives. To these the flavour of meat is due, and the varying taste of different meats is to be explained by slight chemical differences in the extractives present. The feeding and habits of animals have much to do with these differences, and explain the variety in taste between the flesh of wild and tame rabbits, and of grouse and poultry. The shape of the muscle fibres has much to do with the digestibility of meat, short or fine fibres, as in poultry, being the most quickly dissolved. The fatness of meat, or rather the extent to which the fat is interspersed between the meat fibres, is of more importance in connection with digestibility and explains why pork, duck, and goose have a reputation for being indigestible. Sweetbreads and tripe, being held together by loose connective tissue, are, on the other hand, quickly digested, and therefore suitable for invalids. Liver and kidney, which contain much nuclein, a substance closely allied to uric acid, are bad for gout.

Jellies contain little but gelatin, obtained from the fibrous tissue of meat and sinews, and when made with a large quantity of water, i.e. weak in gelatin, they are easily digested. Gelatin is of little or no use as building material, and the main value of jellies is to add bulk and variety to the invalid diet.

Soup consists of a small quantity of gelatin, fat, salts and extractives in hot water. To make soup or beef-tea from meat does not remove the nutritious materials, although it extracts all the flavour and hardens the meat. Clear soup contains practically no nourishment, although it is stimulating to the digestion by reason of the extractives it contains. Thick soup is nutritious only by reason of the vegetables and gelatin added to it. The same is true of the extract of meat introduced by Baron Liebig in 1865, and of its many more recent imitations. Each pint of beef-tea made from this extract represents the salts and extractives in about half a pound of lean meat, although it contains little or none of the nutritive materials. Its use is valuable, because it appears to play a part in helping on the processes of nutrition. It is useful therefore in fevers and in feeble conditions, when little food is needed, or when the digestive powers are weak. Beef-juice, obtained by chopping meat up finely, mixing with a little water and squeezing out cold, is quite another article, and contains a larger proportion of the nutritive materials as well as extractives.

Fish is an excellent source of protein, and, in the case of fatty fish, such as herring and mackerel, has the additional advantage of containing vitamins A and D. Haddock and whiting are among the most digestible fish, some of which, like cod, have a coarse fibre, and others, like salmon, are very fat. Herring is one of the most palatable forms of nitrogenous food, and two herrings contain as much animal protein as need enter into the daily dietary of an ordinary working man.

Milk is practically the only form of animal food in which protein, fat, carbohydrate and salt are all represented in sufficient amount. It contains 2 to 3 per cent of casein, from which cheese, an almost purely protein and fatty food, is made; a small quantity of milk-albumin; 4 per cent of fat in the form of a fine emulsion, which gradually rises to the surface as cream; and 4 to 5 per cent of milk-sugar, to the decomposition of which souring of milk is due. (See INFANT FEEDING; MILK.)

Eggs, each of which contains the material necessary to form a chicken, present the building material for the formation of bone and muscle in an easily convertible form, and are therefore an excellent food for convalescents, and for children. They do not contain any carbohydrate material, and therefore, to form a good article of general diet, should be mixed with rice, flour or other cereals, as is done in the shape of puddings. The digestibility is increased when an egg is beaten up with milk or water, and still more when the eggs are lightly boiled. One egg corresponds in nutritive value to about half a tumblerful of good milk, or to about 30 grams of meat.

Pulses, of which the chief are peas, beans and lentils, have been called the poor man's beef. This, however, is misleading because, though they are cheap, they are not so digestible, contain little first-class protein, and are far from being so completely absorbed as meat unless carefully cooked, while in some people the gases formed by their decomposition in the bowels give rise to great flatulence. Nevertheless, the pulses form a valuable form of food.

PROTEINURIA means a condition in which proteins, principally albumin, are present in the urine. It is of immense importance because it is often a symptom of serious heart or kidney disease.

Causes (1) *Kidney disease* is the most important cause of proteinuria, and in some cases the discovery of proteinuria may be the first evidence of such disease. This is why an examination of the urine for the presence of albumin constitutes an essential part of every medical examination. Almost any form of kidney disease will cause proteinuria, but the most frequent form to do this is glomerulonephritis. In the subacute (or nephrotic) stage of glomerulonephritis the most marked proteinuria of all may be found. Proteinuria is also found in infections of the kidney (pyelitis) as well as in infections of the bladder (cystitis) and of the urethra (urethritis). The development of proteinuria in pregnancy is always an indication for the individual to receive careful medical treatment, as it may be the first sign of one of the most dangerous complications of pregnancy: toxaemia of pregnancy, glomerulonephritis, or eclampsia (q.v.).

(2) *Heart failure* is always accompanied by proteinuria, particularly when the right side of the heart is failing. In severe cases of failure, accompanied by oedema, the proteinuria may be marked. It is due to congestion of the kidneys.

(3) *Fever* is practically always accompanied by proteinuria, even though there is not actual kidney disease. The proteinuria disappears soon after the temperature becomes normal.

(4) *Drugs and poisons*: These include arsenic, lead, mercury, gold, copaiba, salicylic acid and quinine.

(5) *Anaemia*: A trace of albumin may be found in the urine in severe cases of anaemia.

(6) *Functional or orthostatic albuminuria*: Almost any normal person may have a transitory proteinuria after severe muscular exertion or after a cold bath, and it may occasionally appear after eating a large amount of protein: e.g. raw eggs. The form commonly known as *orthostatic* or postural proteinuria is much more common and is of importance because, if the true cause is not recognized, it may be taken as a sign of kidney disease. In the 1914–18 War it was found in 4 per cent of healthy British soldiers, and in an American investigation it was found in 5 per cent of healthy university freshmen. The cause is still doubtful, but it is probably due to temporary congestion of the kidneys caused by adoption of the upright position in individuals with some slight disturbance of the circulation of the blood in the kidneys. At one time it was thought that individuals with this type of proteinuria were more prone to develop glomerulonephritis later in life than individuals in whom it was not present, but this has now been definitely disproved. The features of this type of proteinuria are that it usually occurs in young people, usually between the ages of 8 and 18 years, and that it is not present while the patient is at rest. Thus, the specimen of urine obtained the first thing in the morning, before the individual getss up, contains no albumin, while a specimen obtained later in the day, after the individual has been up and about, will contain albumin.

Proteinuria and life assurance: Most companies will not issue a life policy to anyone with permanent proteinuria in case this is due to glomerulonephritis. Even cases in which no serious disease manifests itself have, if the proteinuria persists, a shorter expectation of life than other people, and so require a higher premium. In cases of doubt, tests to measure the function of the kidney may be carried out. If the tests show normal function, then the proteinuria takes on a much less serious aspect.

Treatment: The treatment is that of the underlying disease. (See GLOMERULONEPHRITIS, etc.) In the case of functional proteinuria due to excessive exercise, cold baths, or excessive ingestion of protein, treatment consists of removal of the cause. Individuals who have orthostatic or postural proteinuria are usually adolescents or young adults who are not in good training, and the treatment consists of getting them into good condition.

PROTHROMBIN: An inactive substance in the blood plasma that is the precursor of the enzyme thrombin, which clots the blood. The conversion occurs when a blood vessel is damaged and the process of blood coagulation occurs (see COAGULATION).

PROTOPLASM is the viscid, translucent, glue-like material containing fine granules and composed mainly of proteins, which makes up the essential material of plant and animal cells and has the properties of life.

PROTOZOA: A simple, primitive animal comprising a single cell. Protozoa are microscopic in size but are much larger than bacteria. Most protozoa live freely but around 30 are parasitic in humans causing disease such as amoebiasis and giardiasis (intestinal infections), malaria, kala-azar and sleeping sickness. Some protozoa are able to excrete, respire, and absorb food particles and they may move around like a mobile jelly or by means of flagellae.

PROTRIPTYLINE is an antidepressant drug. (See ANTIDEPRESSANTS.)

PROXIMAL is a term of comparison applied to structures which are nearer the centre of the body or the median line as opposed to more distal, or distant, structures.

PRURIGO is the name of a chronic skin disease in which small papules (q.v.) develop in the skin, accompanied by intense itching. The condition may either be permanent or may come and go.

PRURITUS is another name for itching (q.v.).

PRUSSIC ACID POISONING (see CYANIDE POISONING).

PSEUDOCYESIS means spurious or false pregnancy, a condition characterized by enlargement of the abdomen, and even enlargement of the breasts and early morning sickness, the unfortunate woman being quite convinced that she is pregnant.

PSEUDOHYPERTROPHIC MUSCULAR DYSTROPHY, or PSEUDOHYPERTROPHIC PARALYSIS, is a condition in which certain muscles enlarge owing to a fatty and fibrous degeneration, giving a false appearance of increased strength. (See MUSCLES, DISEASES OF.)

PSEUDOXANTHOMA ELASTICUM: This is a hereditary disorder of elastic tissue. Degenerating elastic tissue in the skin produces lesions in the skin which look like soft yellow papules. Elastic tissue in the eye and blood vessels is also involved, giving rise to visual impairment, raised blood pressure and haemorrhages.

PSITTACOSIS is a contagious infection of parrots sometimes communicated to man and caused by a micro-organism known as *Chlamydia psittaci*. In 1979 five cases were reported in England attributable to an ill parrot in a consignment of parrots from Brazil which spent a few days in transit in an animal quarantine station at an airport before being shipped abroad. Four out of six persons in contact with the parrots in the quarantine station developed the disease, as did a man who had taken part in unloading the birds and driving them to the quarantine station. In 1980, there were 43 cases in which the source of infection were 'psittacine and other exotic birds'. The number of laboratory reports received at the Communicable Disease Surveillance Centre at Colingdale for Chlamydia B were 362 in 1983 and 410 in 1984.

PSOAS is a powerful muscle which arises from the front of the vertebral column in the lumbar region, and passes down, round the pelvis and through the groin, to be attached to the inner side of the thigh-bone not far from its upper end. The act of sitting up from a recumbent posture, or that of bending the thigh on the abdomen, is mainly accomplished by the contraction of this muscle. Disease of the spine in the lumbar region is apt to produce an abscess which lies within the sheath of this muscle and makes its way down to the front of the thigh, where it threatens to burst. Such an abscess is known as a psoas abscess. (See ABSCESS, CHRONIC.)

PSORIASIS is a disease of the skin in which raised, rough, reddened areas appear, covered with fine silvery scales. This eruption consists of a chronic inflammatory process in the corium, the papillae of which become considerably lengthened and more vascular than usual, together with changes in the epidermis which cause a defect in the horny formation that naturally takes place on the surface and results in an increased production of epidermal cells. The nails are also involved in about 50 per cent of cases. (See SKIN.)
Causes: The condition generally appears for the first time around adolescence or early adult life and, it has been estimated, affects around 2 per cent of the population in Britain. It is often a family disease. A child with one affected parent has a 25-per-cent chance of developing the disease. The risk rises to 60 per cent if both parents are affected. If parents without the disease have a child with psoriasis the risk for a subsequent child is 17 per cent. It may be associated with arthritis and rarely gout. In some persons, psoriasis appears repeatedly at a particular season of the year, especially in the spring and autumn, but it is not infectious. Depressing influences seem to have something to do with its appearance, and people who are liable to it are troubled by its reappearance at any time when the general health is below par.
Symptoms: The eruption almost always appears first round the back of the elbows and front of the knees. It begins as small pimples, each covered with a white cap of scales, which enlarge in breadth till they form patches 5 to 7·5 cm (2 or 3 inches) wide. At the same time, patches appear on other parts of the body, trunk, back, limbs, scalp and in the more extensive disease the face is also affected. The disease is divided into several varieties according to the size, shape, and distribution of these patches.
Treatment: It is essential first of all to attend to the general health. A sympathetic approach to the patient is very important and an adequate explanation of the nature of the condition, the treatments available and what can be expected of these often helps to alleviate many an anxiety. It is important also for the individual to be well motivated, as the success of therapy depends to a great extent on his or her willingness to apply what are often messy creams several times a day for long periods. There is no cure for the condition and the best that can be hoped for is that it can be kept under control. Tar and dithranol are among the chief and most successful external applications. Satisfying results can also be obtained from the use of creams or ointments containing one or other of the corticosteroid preparations. Natural sunlight, or ultra-violet light, alone or in combination with tar preparations, produces a marked improvement in many cases. The latest form of treatment is that known as PUVA (q.v.). More recently, synthetic vitamin A is being used to treat one type of psoriasis, while cyclosporin (a drug used to prevent rejection in patients who have received a kidney transplant) is used in severe resistant cases. Patients with psoriasis can obtain help and advice by contacting the Psoriasis Association, 7 Milton Street, Northampton NN2 7JG (0604-711129).

PSYCHEDELIC DRUGS are drugs, such as lysergic acid diethylamide (LSD), that expand consciousness and perception. (See DRUG ADDICTION.)

PSYCHIATRY is that branch of medical science which treats mental disorder and disease.

PSYCHO-ANALYSIS is the term applied to the theories and practice of the school of psychology originating with Freud. It depends upon the theory that states of disordered mental health have been produced by a repression of painful memories or of conflicting instincts. By such repression these hurtful memories or instincts are kept constantly in a subconscious condition. As a result, the individual's mental power is needlessly occupied and diverted from the proper objects with which it should be concerned and he finds difficulty in concentrating his attention upon and adapting himself to the practical realities of everyday life.
Psycho-analysis aims at discovering these repressed memories which are responsible for the diversion of mental power and of which the affected person usually is only dimly aware or quite unaware. The fundamental method of psycho-analytical treatment is the free expression of thoughts, ideas and fantasies on the part of the patient. To facilitate this, in classical

analysis, he or she lies on a couch to relax mind and body, and the analyst may sit so as to observe the patient but not to be observed by him. The analyst's task is to adopt a neutral attitude to the patient, to encourage the free association of ideas and to explain where explanation is necessary for the continuance of free association. The analyst will receive by way of transference good and bad fantasies of the patient and represent for him or her from time to time objects of love and hate, especially members of the patient's family. In the course of analysis the patient will re-explore his early emotional attitudes and tensions.

There is much that is speculative in the theories of psycho-analysis by the standards of orthodox experimental science but, at the same time, its fundamental conceptions have been widely adopted and developed by other schools of psychology to their enrichment. The new approaches to the study of the mind in health and disease opened up by the concepts of Freud have changed the attitude of the lay and the medical public to the problems of the neurotic, the morbidly anxious, the fearful and to the mental and emotional development of the child.

PSYCHOLOGY is the branch of science that deals with the mind and its methods of working.

PSYCHONEUROSIS is a general term applied to various functional disorders of the nervous system. (See NEUROSIS.)

PSYCHOPATHIC: Psychopathic disorder is defined by the Mental Health Act 1983 as a persistent disorder or disability of mind (whether or not including significant impairment of intelligence) which results in abnormally aggressive or seriously irresponsible conduct. The cardinal features are as follows: (1) Absence of normal feelings for other people such as love, affection, sympathy and condolence. (2) A tendency to anti-social impulsive acts with no forethought of the consequences. (3) A failure to learn by experience and to be deterred from crime by punishment. (4) Absence of any other form of mental disorder that would explain the unusual behaviour. The corresponding American terminology is 'anti-social personality disorder'.

PSYCHOSIS is a term applied to serious disorder of the mind, amounting to insanity.

PSYCHOSOMATIC DISEASES are illnesses resulting from the effects of excessive or repressed emotions upon bodily function or structure. They affect vast numbers of patients who are not out of their minds and yet do not have any organic disease to account for their illness. Functional symptoms must not be regarded as invented or imagined or as a mysterious state affecting an inferior personality. In psychosomatic disease the will may be strong and the mind normal, yet the emotions require treatment. Disorders precipitated by emotional factors may be psychotic, psychoneurotic or psychosomatic. In psychotic and psychoneurotic illnesses the symptoms are predoninantly psychological, whilst in psychosomatic disorders the symptoms may be entirely somatic. The concept of emotional disturbances contributing to bodily disease is not new. It was over 2400 years ago that Socrates stressed that 'as you ought not to attempt to cure the eyes without the head, or the head without the body, so you should not treat body without mind'. The rapid advances of scientific medicine have encouraged a preoccupation with the measurable and a neglect of the intangible. It has been estimated that one third of medical outpatients have psychiatric illness. In another third symptoms are largely dependent on an emotional factor even though organic disease is present. In gynaecological clinics emotional tensions are even more commonly encountered and exceed physical disease as a cause of illness. Over one quarter of all absence from work due to sickness is a result of an illness having an emotional basis.

The three major problems that lead to psychosomatic disorder are marital relationships; occupation, which includes the frustrations, disappointments and feelings of unfulfilment provoked by the patient's work; and finally, social relationships – the feelings which prevail between friends, neighbours and relations.

The many somatic symptoms due to anxiety result from enhanced activity of the sympathetic nervous system. Pain may be a manifestation of psychosomatic disease. Psychogenic factors may produce muscle tension and and cause a pain that is organic. The tension headache is due to the increased tone of the muscles of the neck and scalp.

The visceral reactions of emotional stimuli are of two types:

(1) *Sympathetic*. This is the part of the autonomic nervous system concerned with emergency situations in the external environment, the so-called preparation for fight or flight. The sympathetic nervous system which adjusts the body to such stresses inhibits the metabolic processes of the body and increases the heart rate and blood pressure, and mobilizes carbohydrate reserves. Its effects are mediated through the hormones adrenaline and noradrenaline.

(2) *Parasympathetic*. This is concerned with the conservation and anabolic processes of the body. Hence there is stimulation of gastrointestinal and bronchial secretions, a storing of sugar in the liver, and protective reflexes such as contraction of the pupil and spasm of the bronchiolar muscles as a protection against irritant substances. Parasympathetic effects are mediated through the secretion of acetylcholine. As a result of excess acetylcholine there is a feeling of warmth and flushing due to vasodilatation, and sweating due to cholinergic stimulation of the sweat glands. This is associ-

ated with nausea, vomiting and abdominal colic due to increased peristalsis and contraction of the intestines and the stomach. Thus, when emotional impulses are repressed, two possibilities arise. The patient may be in a constant state of preparedness for action and if this is never executed the sympathetic overactivity persists with a chronic increase in muscle tension, tachycardia and raised blood pressure, and these may give rise to symptoms. An alternative reaction is emotional withdrawal from action into a dependent state of para-sympathetic overactivity. This would include diarrhoea, gastric acid hypersecretion, oesophageal spasm and other parasympathetic effects on the gastro-intestinal tract. Since the autonomic nervous system innovates practically every portion of the body, a somatic manifestation of emotional tension may be related to any area.

Autonomic nervous overactivity may be manifest in the various systems as follows:

(1) *Central nervous system.* Headache. Often described as a pressure on the head. Dizziness, feelings of faintness, nervousness, tremors, sleeplessness and physical exhaustion.

(2) *Cardiovascular system* Tachycardia, arrhythmia and precordial pains.

(3) *Respiratory symptoms.* Sighing respirations and a feeling of an inability to breathe deeply. Vasomotor rhinitis, chronic sore throat and asthma.

(4) *Gastro-intestinal system.* Anorexia, nausea, vomiting, indigestion, wind, heartburn, diarrhoea, constipation and sensations of a lump in the throat.

(5) *Skin.* Itching, sweating, parasthesiae and neuro-dermatitis.

Direct observations on the human colon through fistulae and colostomy openings and on the gastric mucosa through gastrostomy have shown that fear, anxiety and pain can cause an increase in peristalsis with reddening and swelling of the mucous membrane, whilst depression causes reduced motility and pallor of the mucosa. Psychosomatic symptoms may be the result of disorders of secretory functions, such as salivation, dry mouth, hyperchlorhydria, functional hyperinsulinism and mucous colitis, or alternatively they may be due to disorders of motor function such as oesophageal spasm, gastric hypermotility, spastic colon, constipation and diarrhoea. The skin plays an important part in the regulation of body temperature by sweating and its functions are controlled by the autonomic nervous system.

Vasoconstriction, vasodilatation, pilomotor activity and sweating are the four common physiological processes of the skin and are all largely controlled by the autonomic nervous system. Emotional sweating is most evident on the palms and soles and in the axilla. The influence of emotion on respiratory function is well recognized by the everyday expression, 'it took my breath away'. The autonomic innervation of the respiratory tract, which includes the nasal mucosa, consists of sympathetic and para-sympathetic nerves. Para-sympathetic

nerves exert a constrictor effect on the smooth muscle of the respiratory tract and the sympathetic nerves have a relaxing influence. If parasympathetic stimulation is excessive, mucous cells oversecrete and vasodilatation of blood vessels occurs. This produces swelling of the bronchial mucosa and congestion of airways.

Functional illness has its own characteristics and the diagnosis is not established by the mere exclusion of organic disease. It is suggested by the existence of emotional disturbance as a precipitating factor, by the presence of certain characteristic symptoms, by a family history of a similar disorder and by a phasic course characterized by remissions and relapses. It must always be remembered that organic disease may cause anxiety and may provide the stressful factor needed to precipitate psychosomatic disease.

PSYCHOSURGERY was introduced in 1936 by Egas Moniz, Professor of Medicine in Lisbon University, for the surgical treatment of certain psychoses. For his work in this field he shared the Nobel prize in 1949. The original operation, known as leucotomy, consisted of cutting white fibres in the frontal lobe of the brain. It was accompanied by certain hazards such as persistent epilepsy and undesirable changes in personality. Pre-frontal leucotomy is now regarded as obsolete. Modern stereotactic surgery may be indicated in certain intractable psychiatric illnesses in which the patient is chronically incapacitated, especially where there is a high suicide risk. Patients are only considered for psychosurgery when they have failed to respond to routine therapies. One contra-indication is marked histrionic or anti-social personality. The conditions in which a favourable response has been obtained are intractable and chronic obsessional neuroses, anxiety states and severe chronic depression.

Psychosurgery is now rare in Britain. The Mental Health Act 1983 requires not only consent by the patient, confirmed by an independent doctor, and two other representatives of the Mental Health Act Commission, but that the Commission's appointed medical representative must also advise on the likelihood of the treatment's alleviating or preventing a deterioration in the patient's condition.

PSYCHOTHERAPY is the term applied to any form of treatment which operates through the mind. Almost every type of disease or injury has a mental aspect, even if this relates only to the pain or discomfort that it causes. In some diseases and with some temperaments, the mental factor is much more pronounced than in others; for such cases psychotherapy is particularly important. The chief methods employed are the following:

Suggestion is a commonly employed method, used in almost every department of medicine. It may consist, in its simplest form, merely of emphasizing that the patient's health is better, so that this idea becomes fixed in the patient's mind. A suggestion of efficacy may be conveyed by the physical properties of a medicine or by the appearance of some apparatus used in treatment. Again, suggestion may be conveyed emotionally, as in religious healing. In occasional cases a therapeutic suggestion may be made to the patient in a hypnotic state.

Persuasion is a method of treatment in which appeal is made to a patient's reasoning faculties.

Analysis consists in the elucidation of the half-conscious or subconscious repressed memories or instincts that are responsible for some cases of mental disorder or personal conflicts.

Group therapy is a method whereby patients are treated in small groups and encouraged to participate actively in the discussion which ensues amongst themselves and the participating therapists. A modification of group therapy is *drama* therapy. Large group therapy also exists.

Education and employment may be important factors in rehabilitative psychotherapy.

Supportive therapy consists of sympathetically reviewing the patient's situation with him or her and encouraging the patient to identify and solve problems.

Short-term supportive psychotherapy is aimed at stabilizing and strengthening the psychological defence mechanisms of those patients who are confronted by a crisis which threatens to overwhelm their ability to cope, or who are struggling with the aftermath of major life events.

Long-term supportive psychotherapy is needed for patients with personality disorders or recurrent psychotic states, where the aim of treatment is to prevent deterioration and help the patient to achieve an optimal adaptation, making the most of his psychological assets. Such patients may find more profound and unstructured forms of therapy distressing.

Behavioural therapy and *cognitive therapy*, often carried out by psychologists, attempt to clarify with the patient specific features of behaviour or mental outlook respectively and identify step-by-step methods the patient can use for controlling the disorder. Behaviour therapy is commonly used for agoraphobia and other phobias, and cognitive therapy has been used for depression and anxiety.

PSYCHOTROPIC: Affecting the mind. Psychotropic drugs include hallucinogens (q.v.), sleeping drugs, sedatives, tranquillisers (q.v.) and neuroleptic (q.v.) drugs.

PTERYGIUM: A degenerative disorder of the conjunctiva which grows over the cornea medially and laterally. The overgrowths look like wings. They are commonly seen in people who live in areas of bright sunlight, particularly when reflected from deserts or snowfields. Treatment involves excision of the overgrowth.

PTOSIS (see EYE, DISEASE AND INJURIES).

PTYALIN is the name of the enzyme contained in the saliva, by which starchy materials are changed into sugar, and so prepared for absorption. It is identical with the amylase of pancreatic juice. (See DIGESTION; PANCREAS.)

PUBERTY means the change that takes place when childhood passes into manhood or womanhood. This change is generally a very definite one, taking place at about the age of fourteen years, although it is modified by race, climate, and bodily health, so that it may appear a year or two earlier or several years later. At this time the sexual functions attain their full development, the contour of the body changes from a childish to a more rounded womanly, or sturdy manly form, and great changes take place in the mode of thought and feeling. In girls it is marked by the onset of menstruation and development of the breasts. Development of the breasts is usually the first sign of puberty to appear, and may occur from 9 years onwards. Most girls show signs of breast development by the age of 13. The time from the beginning of breast development to the onset of menstruation is usually around two years but may range from six months to five years. The first sign of puberty in boys is an increase in testicular size between the age of 10 and 14. The larynx enlarges in boys, so that the voice after going through a period of 'breaking', finally assumes the deep manly pitch. Hair appears on the pubis and later in the armpits in both boys and girls, whilst in the former it also begins to grow on the upper lip, and skin eruptions are not uncommon on the face. (See ACNE.)

The period is one of transition from a physical and mental point of view. Puberty is not to be regarded as a physiological 'coming of age', for full development is not attained till between twenty and thirty years of age. (See also MENARCHE; MENSTRUATION.)

PUBIS is the bone that forms the front part of the pelvis. The pubic bones of opposite sides meet in the symphysis and protect the bladder from the front.

PUBLIC HEALTH: Disease and health status can be studied and altered in populations as well as individuals. This understanding is central to the concept of public health. The term refers to a broad spectrum of activity organized at all levels of society. This activity, either directly or indirectly, aims to improve the health of the population by preventing disease, prolonging life or promoting health. The determinants of the health of the population are numerous. They range from personal habits such as smoking to environmental conditions such as housing and social factors such as unemployment. Public-health activity can thus include the work of diverse professions: civil engineers improving sewer systems, veterinary scientists controlling animal-feed practices, government ministers changing alcohol taxation and health workers planning community services.

The term 'public health' can be used more specifically to refer to a public-health system. This is a publicly funded service, the primary aim of which is to improve health by the use of population-based measures. The structure of these systems varies from country to country, reflecting differing social composition and political priorities. There are, however, some general elements that can be extracted.

(1) Surveillance: the collection, collation and analysis of data to produce useful information about the distribution and determinants of health and disease in populations. These activities form the basis of epidemiology, which is often considered the backbone of public-health practice.

(2) Intervention: the design and implementation of policies to improve health. This may be through the provision of preventive medical care, environmental measures, influencing the behaviour of individuals or the provision of appropriate services to limit disability and handicap.

(3) Evaluation: assessment of the first two steps in order to determine their impact. This enables further action to be taken as required.

The practice of public health: The situation in the United Kingdom will be described as, even though public-health systems vary, it will give the reader a general impression of the type of work that is covered.

HISTORY: Initially public-health practice related to the environment and the control of infectious disease. Early examples include quarantine for plague and leprosy during the Middle Ages and the development of vaccination in the 18th century. However it was during the 19th century, in response to the health problems of rapid urban growth, that the foundations of a public-health system were created. The concept of the 'sanitary idea' was fundamental to these developments. This suggested that overcrowding in insanitary conditions was the root of disease epidemics. Consequently sanitation measures such as improved sewerage systems and water supplies would prevent disease outbreaks. Although not based on the later, more accurate, knowledge relating the causes of disease to bacteriology, this idea led to the public-health legislation of the 1870s. This gave local authorities the responsibility for sanitation and created the post of medical officer of health. These were the first official public-health doctors.

The role of the medical officer of health increased in importance in the first half of this century. It eventually encompassed not only sanitation but also food hygiene, maternal and child health, clinics for tuberculosis and sexually transmitted diseases and hospital administration. The medical officer of health was employed by local authorities but, in the reorganization of local government and the NHS in the 1970s, the post was abolished and the medical specialty of community medicine was formed and moved across to the health service.

This drew together the existing medical officers of health and the academic discipline of social medicine. These changes altered the nature of the work the new public-health doctors carried out. The organization of the discipline has been further changed as part of the management reforms that took place in the NHS during the 1980s.

CURRENT PRACTICE: There are a number of key personnel and structures that make up today's public-health system.

Public-health doctors: The medical specialty of community medicine changed its name to public-health medicine in 1990. These doctors are usually attached to local public-health departments within the health service, but can be employed in national units within government or in research establishments.

Public-health departments employ public-health doctors, statisticians, social scientists, health economists and other relevant information and research specialists. One of the primary roles of these departments is to assess the health needs of the population and to plan and evaluate services designed to meet those needs. For instance, they may advise health authorities how many hip replacements they need to provide. This would involve assessing the criteria for hip replacement and estimating how many of a given population fit these criteria. In addition the cost of providing the service may be calculated and competing priorities considered.

Disease prevention and health promotion are addressed through advice, co-ordination or evaluation of activities such as cancer-screening programmes, immunization schemes and health-education campaigns.

The spread of HIV infection and AIDS and the increased incidence of food and waterborne disease has emphasized the continued importance of the role of public-health workers in infectious-disease control. Certain public-health doctors have a statutory responsibility for this control.

National Departments such as the Department of Health, the Office of Population Censuses and Surveys (OPCS) and the Communicable Disease Surveillance Centre (CDSC) have a variety of roles. The one they share in common is surveillance and the co-ordinated production of statistics for the public-health system.

Environmental-health officers are based in local authorities. These authorities have a statutory role in enforcing many aspects of public-health legislation. These laws relate primarily to sanitation and environmental aspects of public health. These officers thus deal with food hygiene, pollution and environmental nuisance such as insanitary housing, pest and noise control. They also help with investigating outbreaks of infectious disease, for example food poisoning and legionnaire's disease.

PUERPERAL FEVER, or CHILD-BED FEVER, used to be the great dread of those attending women in child-birth but it is now rare in developed countries.

Causes: This fever is of various types and grades of severity. After the birth of a child, the mother is specially liable, for several reasons, to contract any infectious disease to which she may be exposed. In the first place, she is weakened by the strain through which she has passed, and often by the loss of a considerable quantity of blood. In the second place, the injuries incidental to child-birth produce raw surfaces in the genital tract, from which absorption occurs with great facility. The organism most commonly involved is the *Streptococcus haemolyticus* (q.v.).

Symptoms: The symptoms vary according to the form that the infection takes, and most commonly appear on the second or third day after labour, the first three days being regarded as the critical period in recovery. Thus the organisms may, in the mildest form, develop on the raw or wounded surface, to which they gain access without entering the system. In such a case, there are general discomfort and feverishness, rise of temperature, and quickening of the pulse.

When the organisms gain access to the surrounding lymphatic vessels and veins, inflammation in the cellular tissue of the pelvis results, and may be followed by abscesses, peritonitis, either localized or general (see PERITONITIS), or, later on, by the condition known as white leg, caused by blocking of the veins in one lower limb. In these conditions, which are less common, the symptoms are more severe. There are considerable fever, shivering, prostration, and quickening of the pulse as early signs, together with pain in the lower part of the abdomen, followed later on by the symptoms belonging to peritonitis, white leg, or other condition set up by the inflammation. The condition may be recovered from in a week or two, or long-continued ill-health may result, or the patient may speedily succumb.

If the organisms gain access to the general circulation, the serious condition known as septicaemia results (see BLOOD-POISONING), and is accompanied by high fever, great prostration, delirium, and increasing feebleness of the heart's action.

Treatment: The prevention of the condition is of the greatest importance. For this reason, care in the choice of a lying-in room, great care to shield the patient from every risk of infection, and above all, scrupulous cleanliness on the part of all the attendants, are necessary. (See also LABOUR.)

Treatment resolves itself into careful nursing, blood transfusion if haemoglobin falls below 6 g/dl, and administration of penicillin or the appropriate antibiotic.

PUERPERIUM is the period which elapses after the birth of a child until the mother is again restored to her ordinary health. It is generally regarded as lasting for a month. One of the main changes that occur is the enormous decrease in size that takes place in the muscular wall of the womb. (See MUSCLE.) There are often afterpains during the first day in women who have borne several children, less often after a first child. (See AFTERPAINS.) The discharge is blood-stained for the first two or three days, then clearer till the end of the first week, after which it becomes thicker and less in quantity, finally disappearing altogether, if the case goes well, at the end of two or three weeks. The breasts, which have already enlarged before the birth of the child, secrete milk more copiously, and there should be a plentiful supply on the third day of the puerperium.

Management: It is now realized that prolonged rest in bed is not necessary for the mother after a normal birth. Indeed, it may be harmful. The mother should start practising exercises to help to ensure that the stretched abdominal muscles regain their normal tone. There is no need for any restriction of diet, but care must be taken to ensure an adequate intake of fluid, including at least 580 ml (a pint) of milk a day. The bowels are generally sluggish and it is usual to take an aperient on the second or third day.

Milk, as already stated, appears copiously on the third day, but this is preceded by a secretion from the breast, known as colostrum, which is of value to the new-born child. The child should therefore be put to the breasts within six to eight hours of being born, in order to obtain the small amount of fluid they are secreting, and also because suckling stimulates both the breasts and the natural changes taking place during this period. Suckling is beneficial for both child and mother.

PULMONARY DISEASES (see LUNGS, DISEASES OF).

PULMONARY EMBOLISM is the condition in which an embolus (see EMBOLISM), or clot, is lodged in the lungs. The source of the clot is usually the veins of the lower abdomen or legs in which clot formation has occurred as a result of the occurrence of thrombophlebitis. (See VEINS, DISEASES OF.) Thrombophlebitis, with or without pulmonary embolism, is a not uncommon complication of surgical operations, especially in older patients. This is one reason why nowadays such patients are got up out of bed as quickly as possible, or, alternatively, are encouraged to move and exercise their legs regularly in bed. The severity of a pulmonary embolism, which is characterized by the sudden onset of pain in the chest, with or without the coughing up of blood, and a varying degree of shock, depends upon the size of the clot. If large enough it may prove immediately fatal. In other cases immediate operation may be needed to remove the clot, whilst in less severe cases anticoagulant treatment, in the form of heparin (q.v.), is given to prevent extension of the clot.

PULMONARY HYPERTENSION: In this condition increased resistance to the blood flow through the lungs occurs. This is usually the result of lung disease and the consequence is an increase in pulmonary artery pressure and in the pressure in the right side of the heart and in the veins bringing blood to the heart. Chronic bronchitis or emphysema (qq.v.) commonly constrict the small arteries in the lungs, thus causing pulmonary hypertension.

PULMONARY OEDEMA is a type of water-logging in the lungs caused by left ventricular failure or mitral stenosis (q.v.).

PULMONARY STENOSIS: A disorder of the heart in which obstruction of the outflow of blood from the right ventricle (see HEART) occurs. Narrowing of the pulmonary valve at the exit of the right ventricle and narrowing of the pulmonary artery may cause obstruction. The condition is usually congenital though it may be caused by rheumatic fever. In the congenital condition pulmonary stenosis may occur with other heart defects and is then known as Fallot's tetralogy. Breathlessness and enlargement of the heart and eventual heart failure may be the consequence of pulmonary stenosis. Surgery is usually necessary to remove the obstruction.

PULP (see TEETH).

PULSATION, or throbbing, is an appearance seen or felt naturally below the fourth and fifth ribs on the left side, where the heart lies, and also at every point where an artery lies close beneath the surface. In other situations, it may be a sign of aneurysm. In nervous people, particularly if thin, great pulsation can often be seen and felt in the upper part of the abdomen, due to the throbbing of the normal abdominal aorta.

PULSE: If the tip of one finger is laid gently on the front of the forearm, about 2·5 cm (one inch) above the furrows that mark the wrist, and about 1 cm (half an inch) from the outer edge, the pulsations of the radial artery can be felt. This is known as *the pulse*, but a pulse can be felt wherever an artery of large or medium size lies near the surface.

The cause of the pulsation lies in the fact that, at each heart-beat, 80 to 90 millilitres of blood are driven into the aorta, and a fluid wave, distending the vessels as it passes, is in consequence transmitted along the arteries all over the body. This pulsation gets less and less marked as the arteries grow smaller, and is finally lost in the minute capillaries, where a steady pressure is maintained. For this reason, the blood in the veins flows steadily on without any pulsation. Immediately after the wave has passed, the artery, by virtue of its great elasticity, regains its former size. In this wave the physician has a valuable means of studying both the state of the artery as regards elasticity and the heart's action.

The pulse rate is usually about 70 per minute, but it may vary in health from 50 to 100, and is quicker in childhood and slower in old age than in middle life; it increases in all feverish states.

Further, the character of the vessel wall is of great importance. In childhood and youth the vessel wall is so thin that, when sufficient pressure is made to expel the blood from it, the artery can no longer be felt. In old age, however, and in some degenerative diseases, the vessel wall becomes so thick that it may be felt like a piece of whipcord rolling beneath the finger. The extent to which this change has taken place gives the physician valuable infor-mation as to the state of the arteries.

Different types of heart disease have special features of the pulse associated with them. In atrial fibrillation the great character is irregu-larity. In cases in which the aortic valve is incompetent, the pulse has the peculiarity of rising very quickly and collapsing suddenly.

An instrument known as the sphygmograph has been devised, whereby the artery is made to register these waves. Another instrument known as the polygraph enables tracings to be taken from the pulse at the wrist and from the veins in the neck and simultaneous events in the two compared.

The pressure of the blood in various arteries is estimated by an instrument known as the sphygmomanometer. (See BLOOD-PRESSURE.)

PULSES are the seeds of the *Leguminosa* family. They include peas, beans and lentils and constitute a valuable source of food. Most contain around 20 grams of protein per 100 grams of dry weight but the biological value of this protein requires supplementation to ensure an adequate intake of first class, or essential, amino- acids (q.v.). They have been described as 'the poor man's protein', and a combination of pulse and cereal proteins may have a nutri-tive value comparable to that of animal protein. They are a good source of the B group of vitamins with the exception of riboflavine. (See also DIET.)

PUNCTATE BASOPHILIA (see BASOPHILIA.)

PUNCTUM (see EYE).

PUPIL (see EYE).

PURGATIVES are drugs or other measures which produce evacuation of the bowels.
Varieties and action: Purgatives are divided into several groups, according to the manner and degree of violence with which they act.
LAXATIVES are those which gently stimulate the bowels and render the motions slightly more frequent and softer without causing any grip-ing. Most articles of food that leave a large

indigestible residue upon which the intestine can contract, such as cabbage, brown bread, and oatmeal porridge, act in this way. Those fruits which contain rough seeds, sugar, and vegetable acids act similarly. Among the laxatives are honey, tamarinds, figs, raspberries, strawberries, prunes, stewed apples, senna and magnesia. Liquid paraffin also produces this effect.

SIMPLE PURGATIVES, or APERIENTS, produce one or more copious and slightly liquid movements, often accompanied or preceded by griping pains. Examples of this class are aloes, rhubarb, cascara sagrada, senna, castor oil.

SALINE PURGATIVES are salts of the alkaline metals and alkaline earths. Such are sulphate of potassium, sulphate of sodium (Glauber's salt), sulphate of magnesium (Epsom salts), phosphate of sodium, bitartrate of potassium (cream of tartar), tartrate of potassium and sodium (Seidlitz powder), and citrate of magnesium. Taken in large doses, many of these salines also act as hydragogues, removing water from the system.

Purgatives produce their effects either by stimulating the mucous membrane so that the amount of fluid in the intestine becomes larger, or by stimulating the muscular coat so that peristaltic contractions become more vigorous. Most purgatives have the double action, though one or other preponderates.

Uses: The most common use of purgatives is to remove the contents of the bowels when their action is sluggish. (See CONSTIPATION.) In many cases of diarrhoea, due to the presence of irritating material in the intestine, a single dose of purgative medicine, such as castor oil, is given with the object of getting rid of the offending material, after which the diarrhoea ceases. In cases of inflammation affecting the bowels, saline purgatives are often given with the view of diminishing the congestion in the bowel-wall.

PURPURA is a disease characterized by the occurrence of purple spots upon the surface of the body, due to extravasations of blood in the skin, associated occasionally with haemorrhages from mucous membranes.

Causes: The condition is due either to an increased permeability of the smallest blood-vessels (ie. the capillaries) which allows blood to pass through their walls, or to a shortage of blood platelets which normally play an important part in sealing off any damage which may occur to the walls of the capillaries. The damage to the capillary wall may arise as a result of an infection, e.g. septicaemia; a toxic factor, e.g. certain drugs; or in scurvy.

A common cause of a lack of platelets is their auto-immune destruction in idiopathic thrombocytopenic purpura. Capillary damage is commonly due to anaphylactoid purpura which is an allergic condition, the increased permeability of the capillary wall being due to the individual's coming in contact with, inhaling, or ingesting, some substance to which he is sensitized. Two special forms of anaphylactoid purpura are recognized. One is *Henoch's purpura*, in which the purpuric haemorrhages occur in the wall of the intestine, causing symptoms resembling an acute abdominal emergency. This form occurs in children and young adults. The other is *Schönlein's purpura*, in which the purpura occurs around the joints causing them to be painful and tender. This form principally affects young adults.

Symptoms: The complaint is usually ushered in by lassitude and feverishness. This is soon followed by the appearance on the surface of the body of the characteristic spots in the form of small red points scattered over the skin of the limbs and trunk. Their colour soon becomes deep purple or nearly black; but after a few days they undergo the changes which are observed in the case of an ordinary bruise, passing to a green and yellow hue and finally disappearing. When of minute size they are termed petechiae, when in patches of considerable size ecchymoses. They may come out in fresh crops over a lengthened period.

Treatment: The treatment of *secondary purpura* consists of that of the underlying cause: e.g. scurvy. The treatment of *primary thrombocytopenic purpura* consists of the administration of one of the cortisone-like drugs: e.g. prednisolone. In cases which do not respond to such therapy, removal of the spleen is often helpful, especially in children. In severe cases, with heavy loss of blood, blood transfusion may be necessary. The treatment of *anaphylactoid purpura* consists of the administration of antihistamine drugs. If these fail, then it is worth trying the effect of prednisolone. If, as is often the case, there is any anaemia, this must be treated by the administration of full doses of iron: e.g. ferrous sulphate.

PUS, or MATTER, is a thick, white, yellow, or greenish fluid, which is found in abscesses, on ulcers, and on inflamed and discharging surfaces generally. Its colour and consistency are due to the presence, in great numbers, of pus corpuscles. These are derived mostly from the white corpuscles of the blood, and consist also of the superficial cells of granulation tissue or of a mucous membrane which die and are shed off in consequence of the inflammatory process. (See ABSCESS; PHAGOCYTOSIS.)

PUSTULE means a small collection of pus. (See ABSCESS.) Malignant pustule is one of the forms taken by woolsorters' disease. (See ANTHRAX.)

PUTREFACTION is the change that takes place in the bodies of plants and animals after death, whereby they are ultimately reduced to carbonic acid gas, ammonia, and other simple substances. The change is almost entirely due to the action of bacteria, and, in the course of the process, various offensive and poisonous intermediate substances are formed. In the case of the human body, putrescine, cadaverine, and other alkaloids are among these intermediate products.

The first sign of putrefaction is the appearance of a greenish tinge over the lower part of the abdomen, visible on the second or third day after death. This is not to be confused with the lividity seen on the back, due to the blood running down into the dependent parts, which is visible within eight or twelve hours. In from two to three weeks the body is greenish-brown throughout, the skin beginning to give way, and the features almost unrecognizable. By the end of one year, none of the organs is recognizable. After the lapse of four to seven years, bodies buried in gravel or sandy soil have lost all trace of the soft parts, the bones alone remaining.

When bodies decompose in water, particularly that drained from peaty soil, the skin becomes white and sodden and the changes take place more slowly. Sometimes, in these circumstances, instead of going through the usual changes, the body undergoes a process of saponification, and the tissues are converted into a mixture of soaps, fatty acids, and volatile substances known as *adipocere*. This does not readily undergo further changes, and so bodies lying in ponds or damp graves may become changed in the course of some months or years into this wax-like substance, after which they may be preserved with the smallest details of feature for many years.

Mummification may prevent putrefaction in the dry air of deserts, and even in the case of a body lying in a strong draught of air these changes may be indefinitely postponed by gradual drying. A similar result has been known to occur in the bodies of people who have taken antimony for a long period prior to death, the antimony deposited all through the body acting as an antiseptic.

PUTRID FEVER is an old name for typhus fever.

PUVA is a method of treating severe cases of psoriasis (q.v.) which do not respond to other forms of treatment. This consists of giving the patient a tablet of a psoralen preparation which sensitizes the skin cells to sunlight and then exposing him in a special cubicle to high-intensity long-wave ultraviolet radiation (UVA). Hence the name PUVA: a combination of P for psoralen and UVA. Initially this treatment is given twice a week. Although not curative, it has proved highly effective, but can only be carried out in specially equipped hospital departments.

PYAEMIA means a form of blood-poisoning in which abscesses appear in various parts of the body. (See BLOOD-POISONING.)

PYELITIS means inflammation of that part of the kidney known as the pelvis, which is connected with the ureter. It is now realized,

however, that the infection is seldom restricted to the pelvis, but involves the kidney tissue as well. In other words the correct diagnosis is pyelonephritis.

The inflammation may spread upwards from the bladder or may follow on febrile diseases in which bacteria leave the body by the urine. One of the commonest organisms productive of this condition is the *Escherichia coli*, which produces a highly acid state of the urine accompanied by the presence of pus. Pyelitis sometimes occurs as a complication of pregnancy. There are generally symptoms of feverishness, general malaise, loss of weight, discomfort in the region of the loins, and frequency in passing water. Examination reveals the presence of the infecting organism and of pus in the urine.

Treatment: In some cases the administration of alkalis and the drinking of ample bland fluids are all that is required. As a rule, however, more active treatment is necessary and this consists of the administration of an antibiotic. As pyelitis may be due to some other condition of the kidney, such as a stone, a full investigation is necessary, as such cases will not clear up unless the underlying cause is removed.

PYELOGRAPHY is the term applied to the process whereby the kidneys are rendered radio-opaque, and therefore visible on an X-ray film. It constitutes a most important part of the examination of a patient with kidney disease. (See SODIUM DIATRIZOATE.)

PYELONEPHRITIS (see PYELITIS).

PYLEPHLEBITIS means inflammation of the portal vein. It usually results from disease in the intestine and is part of a general blood-poisoning.

PYLORIC STENOSIS: Narrowing of the pylorus (q.v.), the muscular exit from the stomach. It is usually the result of a pyloric ulcer or cancer near the exit of the stomach. The result is that food is delayed when passing from the stomach to the duodenum and vomiting occurs. The stomach may become distended and peristalsis (muscular movement) may be seen through the abdominal wall. Unless surgically treated the patient will steadily deteriorate, losing weight, becoming dehydrated and developing alkalosis. Congenital pyloric stenosis occurs in babies (commonly boys) about 3 to 5 weeks old, and surgery produces a complete cure.

PYLOROSPASM means spasm of the pyloric portion of the stomach. This interferes with the passage of food in a normal, gentle fashion into the intestine and causes the pain that comes on from half an hour to three hours after meals and is associated with severe disorders of digestion. It is often produced by an ulcer of the stomach or duodenum.

PYLORUS is the lower opening of the stomach, through which the softened and partially digested food passes into the small intestine.

PYO- is a prefix attached to the name of various diseases to indicate cases in which pus is formed, such as pyonephrosis.

PYODERMIA GANGRENOSUM: This is a disorder in which large ulcerating lesions appear suddenly and dramatically in the skin. It is the result of underlying vasculitis. It is usually the result of inflammatory bowel disease such as ulcerative colitis or Crohn's disease but can be associated with rheumatoid arthritis.

PYOGENIC is a term applied to those bacteria which cause the formation of pus and so lead to the formation of abscesses. Although many bacteria have this property, the most common cause of abscess is one of the rounded forms of bacterium (e.g. streptococcus).

PYORRHOEA is the name given to any copious discharge of pus. For *Pyorrhoea alveolaris* see under TEETH, DISEASES OF.

PYREXIA means fever. (See FEVER.)

PYRIDOXINE, or vitamin B$_6$, plays an important part in the metabolism of a number of amino-acids. Deficiency leads to atrophy of the epidermis, the hair follicles, and the sebaceous glands, and peripheral neuritis may also occur. Young infants are more susceptible to pyridoxine deficiency than adults: they begin to lose weight and develop a hypochromic anaemia; irritability and convulsions may also occur. Liver, yeast, and cereals are relatively rich sources of it. Fish is a moderately rich source, but vegetables and milk contain little. The minimal daily requirement in the diet is probably about 2 mg.

PYRIMETHAMINE is an antimalarial drug which is particularly valuable as a prophylactic.

PYROSIS (see WATERBRASH).

PYURIA means the presence of pus in the urine, in consequence of inflammation situated in the kidney, bladder, or other part of the urinary tract. (See URINE.)

Q

Q FEVER is a disease of worldwide distribution due to the organism *Coxiella burneti*. It is characterized by fever, severe headache and often pneumonia. It was first described in 1937 amongst abattoir workers in Brisbane. The disease was given the name 'Q' fever, the Q (?) referring to the unknown cause of the disease. The aetiology of the infection was later established by Burnet who cultured a micro-organism from the blood of an infected patient. This rickettsia-like organism was originally called *Rickettsia burneti* but was later renamed *Coxiella burneti* when Cox found that it had certain features which differentiated it from the true rickettsia.

The principal reservoir of human infection in Britain is probably cattle and sheep in which the infection is usually sub-clinical. The diagnosis is confirmed by the detection of serum antibodies to *Coxiella burneti*. The organism is sensitive to tetracycline.

QUADRANTANOPIA: Inability to see in one quarter of the visual field. Homonymous quadrantanopia is loss of vision in the same quarter of the field in each eye.

QUADRICEPS is the large four-headed muscle occupying the front and sides of the thigh, which straightens the leg at the knee-joint and maintains the body in an upright position.

QUADRIPLEGIA means paralysis of the four limbs of the body.

QUADRUPLETS (see MULTIPLE BIRTHS).

QUARANTINE is the principle of preventing the spread of infectious disease by which people, baggage, merchandise, and so forth likely to be infected or coming from an infected locality are isolated at frontiers or ports till their harmlessness has been proved to the satisfaction of the authorities. (See INFECTION.)

Originally quarantine, as its name implies, involved detention for forty days; but, as this proved intolerable for people engaged in business, the time of detention is now calculated so as simply to cover the incubation period of the disease, the presence of which is suspected.

Numerous international conferences upon the subject have been held with the view of arriving at a uniform practice as regards quarantine in different countries. The diseases to which quarantine applies are cholera, yellow fever, plague, smallpox, typhus and relapsing fever.

The general practice with regard to quarantine is that when a serious disease breaks out in any country, the government of that country notifies surrounding governments as to the ports and other places that have become centres of infection. Any people travelling from these centres and attempting to enter another country, are subject to measures prescribed in the appropriate Regulations. These measures vary with the disease involved; as often as not, today they merely involve keeping under the surveillance of the local medical officer through the incubation period of the disease in question.

Disease	Patients	Contacts
Chickenpox	6 days from the date of the appearance of the rash.	None.
Diphtheria	Until 3 consecutive throat and nose swabs are negative.	Until nose and throat swabs are bacteriologically clear.
German measles	5 days from the appearance of the rash.	None.
Measles	7 days after the appearance of the rash if the child appears well.	Infants who have not had the disease should be excluded for 14 days from the date of appearance of the rash in the last case in the house. Other contacts can attend school. Any contact suffering from a cold, chill or red eyes should be immediately excluded.
Mumps	9 days from the onset of the disease or 7 days from the subsidence of all swelling.	None.
Whooping-cough	21 days from the beginning of the characteristic cough.	Infants who have not had the disease should be excluded for 21 days from the date of onset of the disease in the last case in the house.

Quarantine periods for the commoner infectious diseases.

QUARTAN FEVER: Description of intermittent fever with paroxysms developing every fourth day. Usually applied to malaria (q.v.).

QUASSIA is the wood of *Picrasma excelsa*, a large West Indian tree. Its virtues depend upon the presence of an active principle, quassin, which is excessively bitter and also irritating. The various preparations of the wood are mainly used as a bitter tonic. Quassia cups were for long to be found in many households. Made of quassia wood, they were filled with hot water. This resulted in a bitter water which was drunk as a 'bitter' to stimulate the appetite. These quassia cups could be used over and over again for several years, retaining their ability to produce a bitter extract. (See BITTERS.)

QUICKENING (see PREGNANCY).

QUINIDINE is an alkaloid obtained from cinchona bark and closely related in chemical composition and in action to quinine. It is commonly used in the form of quinidine sulphate in doses of 200 to 600 mg. It is used in the treatment of the cardiac irregularity known as atrial fibrillation, being particularly useful in cases of recent onset.

QUININE is an alkaloid obtained from the bark of various species of cinchona trees. This bark is mainly derived from Peru and neighbouring parts of South America and the East Indies. For the story of its introduction see MALARIA. Other alkaloids and acid substances are also derived from cinchona bark, such as quinidine and cinchonine.

Quinine is generally used in the form of one of its salts, such as the sulphate of quinine, or dihydrochloride of quinine. All are sparingly soluble in water, much more so when taken along with an acid.

Action: Quinine lessens the activity of simple forms of life. It is therefore a powerful antiseptic. Its best-known action is in checking the recurrence of attacks of malaria, and this action it exerts by virtue of its destructive power against the malarial parasite in the blood. In fevers it acts as an antipyretic (q.v.).

In small doses it has a stimulating effect upon the stomach, although larger doses are capable of acting upon an irritable stomach to produce nausea and vomiting. Small doses have also a stimulating action upon the nervous system and a general tonic effect, whilst large doses cause decided depression of the respiration and the heart's action.

Among the other unpleasant effects, due to large doses, are ringing in the ears, temporary impairment of vision, and sometimes irritation of the kidneys: all these pass off when the drug is discontinued.

Uses: The most important use of quinine is its original one in malaria, attacks of which it quickly cuts short or prevents altogether, but it has largely been replaced by the more effective and less toxic anti-malarial drugs now available. (See MALARIA.) For intravenous injection, when this is necessary in cases of malaria, a soluble form of quinine, the dihydrochloride, is used in doses of 300 to 600 mg. Ammoniated solution of quinine given in teaspoonful doses in water is a favourite household remedy in feverish colds and other mild febrile attacks. Quinine and urea hydrochloride is employed as a local anaesthetic with a prolonged effect. Quinine hydrochloride has been used with urethane as a sclerosing agent in the treatment of varicose veins (q.v.).

QUINSY is a corruption of *cynanche*, and is an old name for a peritonsillar abscess (q.v.).

QUINTUPLETS (see MULTIPLE BIRTHS).

R

RABIES is an acute and fatal disease which affects animals, particularly carnivora, and may be communicated from them to man. Infection from man to man is very rare, but those in attendance on a case should take precautions to avoid being bitten or allowing themselves to be contaminated by the patient's saliva as this contains the causative virus.

Cause: The disease is in existence constantly among dogs and wolves in some countries, and from these it spreads widely now and then in epidemics. It also occurs in foxes, coyotes and skunks, as well as vampire bats. Thanks to quarantine measures, it has been practically stamped out in Great Britain since 1897. The last case of human infection contracted in Britain was in 1911. Since 1946, several cases have been diagnosed in Britain, in all of which the infection was acquired overseas. Recent cases of rabies in dogs in this country demonstrate that continuing, indeed increasing, vigilance is necessary if the United Kingdom is to be protected from the ravages of this dread disease. Such vigilance is necessary because the disease in animals is now spreading across Europe. In the whole of Western Europe, only Denmark and Britain are now free of rabies. The most worrying feature from the British point of view is that the current European epidemic of animal rabies, which started in Poland in 1939, is advancing at an annual rate of 30–60 kilometres and is now approaching the English Channel coast line. Restrictions have accordingly been tightened up and under The Rabies Act 1974, which came into force in February 1975, all mammals, except farm livestock, brought into the country must come through designated ports (Dover [Eastern Docks], Harwich [Navy Yard Wharf], Hull, Liverpool, Southampton, and International Hoverport at Ramsgate) and airports (Birmingham, Edinburgh, Glasgow, Leeds, London [Gatwick and Heathrow], Manchester and Prestwick), have an import licence and undergo a compulsory six months' quarantine. Any animals brought in illegally may be destroyed on the spot, and the offender fined an unlimited amount, sentenced up to a year's imprisonment, or both. It also empowers the Government, in the event of the disease being confirmed in Britain again, to destroy foxes, control movement of domestic pets, ban hunts and dog and cat shows, and destroy stray animals.

It is highly infectious from the bite of an animal already affected, but the chance of infection from different animals varies. Thus only about one person in every four bitten by rabid dogs contracts rabies, whilst the bites of rabid wolves and cats almost invariably produce the disease. The disease is due to a virus which has a special affinity for attacking the nervous system.

Symptoms: In animals there are two types of the disease: mad rabies and dumb rabies. In the former, the dog runs about, snapping at objects and other animals, unable to rest; in the latter, which is also the final stage of the mad type, the limbs become paralysed, and the dog crawls about or lies still.

In man the incubation period is usually six to eight weeks, but may be as short as ten days or as long as two years. The disease begins by mental symptoms, the person becoming irritable, restless, and melancholy. At the same time, feverishness and difficulty of swallowing gradually come on. After a couple of days or so, the irritability passes into a state of wildness or terror, and there is great difficulty in swallowing either food or drink. Even the mere sight of fluid may induce spasm of the muscles of the mouth and throat: hence the common name for the disease: hydrophobia (fear of water). Breathing, too, becomes difficult, because of spasm of the respiratory muscles. The flow of saliva is great, and therefore the patient is constantly spitting, and has a dry, short cough. About four days after the onset of the disease, the patient dies of exhaustion.

Treatment: The best treatment is, of course, preventive. The current regulations in the United Kingdom are a quarantine period of six months, and that the animal be given a dose of an inactivated rabies vaccine on entry into quarantine and another dose 28 days later. If a person has been bitten by a dog supposed to be rabid, the dog should not be killed at once, but should be carefully isolated for ten days; if, after this period it is still alive, it was non-infective at the time of biting.

Local treatment consists of immediate, thorough, and careful cleansing of the wound surfaces and surrounding skin with 20 per cent soap solution or any other detergent followed by flushing out with some antiseptic such as benzalkonium or cetrimide. Special attention should be paid to any deep fang punctures, which should be carefully probed with a swabstick dipped in strong nitric acid. Immediate suture of lacerations should not be carried out.

This is followed by a course of rabies vaccine therapy. Only people bitten or in certain circumstances licked, either by a rabid animal or by one thought to be infected with rabies need treatment with rabies vaccine and antiserum and immunoglobulin (q.v.). A person previously vaccinated against rabies who is subsequently bitten by a rabid animal should be given three to four doses of the vaccine. The vaccine is also used to give protection to those liable to infection, such as kennel workers and veterinary surgeons.

RADIAL ARTERY: This artery arises from the brachial artery at the level of the neck of the radius. It passes down the forearm to the wrist where it is easily palpated laterally. It then winds around the wrist to the palm of the hand to supply the fingers.

RADIAL NERVE: This nerve arises from the brachial plexus in the axilla. At first descending posteriorly and then anteriorly it ends just above the elbow by dividing into the superficial radial and interosseous nerves. It supplies motor function to the muscles which extend the arm, wrist, and some fingers and supplies sensation to parts of the posterior and lateral aspects of the arm, forearm, and hand.

RADIATION: Energy in the form of waves or particles. It includes, among others, X-rays, gamma rays, infra-red, ultraviolet, and the visible spectrum.

RADIATION SICKNESS is the term applied to the nausea, vomiting, and loss of appetite which may follow the use of radiotherapy in the treatment of cancer and other diseases. The phenothiazine group of tranquillizers, such as chlorpromazine (q.v.), as well as the antihistamine drugs (q.v.), are of value in its prevention and treatment. Radiotherapy may also be accompanied by irritation and itching of the skin. To prevent this, or at least to reduce its incidence, the skin should be protected from all unnecessary irritation by avoiding, for example, tight collars, hot baths, brisk towelling, wet shaving and cosmetics. Should itching occur, this may be relieved by a weak solution of sodium bicarbonate (1 teaspoonful in a cup of warm water) applied to the skin and dabbed dry with cotton-wool. The application of a bland dusting powder, such as a baby powder, also helps.

RADIOACTIVE ISOTOPES (see ISOTOPES).

RADIOGRAPHY (see X-RAYS).

RADIO-IMMUNO ASSAY is a technique introduced in 1960 which enables the minute quantities of circulating hormones to be measured. A radio-immuno assay depends on the ability of an unlabelled hormone to inhibit, by simple competition, the binding of isotopically labelled hormone by specific antibodies. The requirements for a radio-immuno assay include adequate amounts of the hormone; a method for labelling the hormone with a radio active isotope; the production of satisfactory antibodies; and a technique for separating antibody-bound from free hormone. Radio-immuno assay is more sensitive than the best bio-assay for a given hormone and most sensitive radio-immuno assays permit the detection of picogram ($pg = 10^{-12}g$) and femtogram ($fg = 10^{-15}g$) amounts of material.

RADIOLOGY (see X-RAYS).

RADIONUCLIDE is another word for a radioactive isotope. (See ISOTOPES.)

RADIO-OPAQUE: Substances which absorb X-rays, rather than transmitting them, appear white on X-rays and are known as radio-opaque. This is true of bones, teeth, certain types of gallstones, renal stones and contrast media used to enhance the accuracy of radiographic imaging. (See X-RAYS.)

RADIOTHERAPY is treatment by radium or other radioactive matter, including X-rays. For long, radium and X-rays were the only sources available. Developments in our knowledge of atomic energy, however, have changed the picture entirely, and we have now at our disposal radioactive isotopes (see ISOTOPES) and X-ray machines which have largely replaced radium, except in the case of certain tumours.

Supervoltage X-ray machines are now available capable of producing X-rays generated at up to 22 million electron volts (22 MeV). These include linear accelerators which produce X-rays at four or more million electron volts, and betatrons which produce X-rays at 22 million electron volts. The advantage of these supervoltage machines is that it is predominantly gamma-rays they produce, which are penetrating rays and can therefore be used to treat deep-seated tumours.

Almost equally high concentrations of gamma-rays can now be obtained from the use of certain radioactive isotopes, particularly cobalt and caesium. Thus a telecobalt machine is now in use which contains 2000 curies or more of radioactive cobalt (Co^{60}), an amount equivalent to 3000 grams of radium (an unheard-of amount in the pre-1939 days when the ordinary radium beam units contained only 10 grams of radium). Not only does this machine give a high concentration of gamma-rays (equivalent to that from a 3 million-volt X-ray machine), it is absolutely safe for both patient and operators, and allows the beam to be directed accurately on the tumour.

Other forms of radiant energy are now coming into use in radiotherapy. One of these is electron-beam therapy. The usual source of electrons, one of the particles in the atomic nucleus, is the betatron, which can produce either electrons or X-rays at energies ranging from 18 to 42 MeV. Whilst the effect of electrons in the tissues of the body is the same as that of X-rays, their great practical advantage is that their effect can be concentrated on the part being treated, without any adverse effect on the surrounding normal tissue. The other form of radiant energy now being used is neutron therapy. Neutrons of 6 MeV energy are obtained from a cyclotron. One of the advantages of neutron therapy is that even if a cell is only partially damaged by neutrons it never recovers, but inevitably dies.

RADIUM: The radiations of radium consist of: (1) alpha-rays, which are positively charged helium nuclei; (2) beta-rays, negatively charged electrons; (3) gamma-rays, similar to X-rays but of shorter wave-length.

At the present day the use of radium is largely restricted to the treatment of carcinoma of the neck of the womb, the tongue, and the lips.

Neither X-rays nor radium supersede active surgical measures when these are available for the complete removal of a tumour.

RADIUS is the outer of the two bones in the forearm. (See BONE.)

RÂLE (see CREPITATIONS).

RANITIDINE is a drug used in the treatment of duodenal ulcer (q.v.) by reducing the hyperacidity of the gastric juice. It is a histamine antagonist to the type-2 receptor.

RANULA is a swelling which occasionally appears beneath the tongue, caused by a collection of saliva in the distended duct of a salivary gland. (See MOUTH, DISEASES OF.)

RAPHE means a ridge or furrow between the halves of an organ.

RAREFACTION is the term applied to the diminution in the density of a bone as a result of withdrawal of calcium salts from it.

RASH (see ERUPTION).

RAT-BITE FEVER is an infectious disease following the bite of a rat. There are two causative organisms – *Spirillum minus* and *Actinobacillus muris* – and the incubation period depends upon which is involved. In the case of the former it is 5 to 30 days; in the case of the latter it is 2 to 10 days. The disease is characterized by fever, a characteristic skin rash and often muscular or joint pains. It responds well to penicillin.

RAUWOLFIA is a drug used in the treatment of high blood-pressure, and as a tranquillizer. It is derived from the root of *Rauwolfia serpentina*, a plant which grows widely in India, Ceylon, Burma, and Malaya. The active medicinal properties, which reside mainly in the root of the plant, have been recognized for centuries in India, where extracts of the root were used for the treatment of fevers, insomnia, and nervousness.

It is mainly used in the form of reserpine, which is an alkaloid obtained from the root of the plant. (See ESSENTIAL HYPERTENSION; TRANQUILLIZER.)

RAYNAUD'S DISEASE, so called after Maurice Raynaud (1834–81), the Paris physician who published a thesis on the subject in 1862, is a condition in which the circulation becomes suddenly obstructed in outlying parts of the body. It is supposed to be due to spasm of the smaller arteries in the affected part, as the result of nervous influences, and its effects are increased both by cold and by various diseases involving the blood-vessels. It is predominantly a disease of women, the majority of cases occurring before the age of 40.

Symptoms: The condition is most commonly confined to the occurrence of dead fingers, the fingers or the toes, ears, or nose becoming white, numb, and waxy looking. This condition may last for some minutes, or may not pass off for several hours, or even for a day or two.

Treatment: People who are subject to these attacks should be careful in winter to protect the feet and hands from cold, and should always use warm water when washing the hands. In addition, the whole body should be kept warm, as spasm of the arterioles in the feet and hands may be induced by chilling of the body. Victims of this disease should be advised to give up smoking. Vasodilator drugs are helpful, especially the calcium antagonists (q.v.). In all cases which do not respond to such medical treatment, surgery should be considered in the form of sympathectomy: i.e. cutting of the sympathetic nerves to the affected part. This results in dilatation of the arterioles and hence an improved blood supply. This operation is more successful in the case of the feet than in the case of the hands.

REACTIVE ARTHRITIS is an aseptic arthritis secondary to an episode of infection elsewhere in the body. It often occurs in association with enteritis caused by Salmonella and certain Shigella strains and in both yersinea and campylobacter enteritis. Non-gonococcal urethritis, usually due to clamydia, is another cause of reactive arthritis and Reiter's syndrome is a particularly florid form with mucocutaneous and ocular lesions. The synovitis usually starts acutely and is frequently asymmetrical with the knees and ankles most commonly affected. Often there are inflammatory lesions of tendon sheaths and entheses such as plantar faschitis. The severity and duration of the acute episode are extremely variable. Individuals with the histocompactibility antigen HLA-B27 are particularly prone to severe attacks.

RECEPTOR: (1) Organs, which may consist of one cell or a small group of cells, which respond to different forms of external or internal stimuli by conveying impulses down nerves to the central nervous system, alerting it to changes in the internal or external environment.

(2) A small, discrete area on the cell membrane or within the cell with which molecules or molecular complexes (e.g. hormones, drugs, and other chemical messengers) interact. When this interaction takes place it initiates a change in the working of the cell.

RECESSIVE: Tending to recede. In genetic terms a recessive gene is one whose expression remains dormant if paired with an unlike allele.

The trait will only be manifest in an individual homozygous for the recessive gene. (See GENES.)

RECOMBINANT DNA: DNA (q.v.) or deoxyribonucleic acid containing genes from various sources that have been combined by genetic engineering.

RECRUDESCENCE: The reappearance of a disease after a period without signs or symptoms of its presence.

RECTUM is the last part of the large intestine. It pursues a more or less straight course downwards through the cavity of the pelvis, lying against the sacrum at the back of this cavity. This section of the intestine is about 23 cm (9 inches) long. Its first part is freely movable and corresponds to the upper three pieces of the sacrum, the second part corresponds to the lower two pieces of the sacrum and the coccyx, whilst the third part, known also as the anal canal, is about 25 mm (1 inch) long, runs downwards and backwards, and is kept tightly closed by the internal and external sphincter muscles which surround it. The opening to the exterior is known as the anus. The structure of the rectum is similar to that of the rest of the intestine. (See INTESTINE.)

RECTUM, DISEASES OF: Owing to the fact that this part of the intestine is more exposed to external influences than the rest of the bowels, and that it forms the place of lodgment of the stools prior to the evacuation of the bowels, and is therefore often subject to considerable irritation, the rectum is specially liable to various diseases.

Peculiarities of the motions are treated under STOOLS, while PILES and FISTULA are described under these headings. DIARRHOEA and CONSTIPATION are also treated separately.

IMPERFORATE ANUS, or absence of the anus, may occur in newly born children, and, unless the condition is relieved by operation within a few days, the child dies.

ITCHING at the anal opening, or PRURITUS ANI, is often very troublesome. It may be due to slight abrasions, piles, the presence of threadworms, and anal sex. The anal area should be bathed once or twice a day. Clothing should be loose and smooth – preferably cotton or linen next to the skin. Calamine lotion, containing 1 per cent phenol, or 0·1 to 0·5 per cent camphor, is soothing – applied as a compress on gauze at night and dabbed on during the day. The local application of Eurax or hydrocortisone ointment is often effective.

PAIN of an acute cutting character, at stool, is often due to the presence of a small ulcer or 'fissure'. Pain of an aching nature is not uncommonly caused by the presence of piles. (See also PROCTALGIA.)

ABSCESS in the cellular tissue at the side of the rectum, known from its position as an ischio-

rectal abscess, is fairly common and may produce a fistula. (See FISTULA.)

PROLAPSE or protrusion of the rectum is sometimes found in children, usually between the ages of 6 months and 2 years. In slight cases, where a ring of bright red mucous membrane 12 or 25 mm (½ or 1 inch) in width protrudes as the result of straining at stool, the condition is generally easily curable. Any irritable condition of the bowels due to diarrhoea, constipation or worms, must be removed and the evacuations regulated by diet and laxatives, so as to avoid all straining. Each time the bowels move, the protruded portion must be returned by steady pressure with a cloth or sponge wrung out of cold water. When the protruded part is very large and the condition does not yield to simple treatment it can be remedied by operation but this is not usually necessary, as the prolapse ceases to occur as the child grows older.

TUMOURS of small size situated on the skin near the opening of the bowel, and consisting of nodules, tags of skin, or cauliflower-like excrescences, are common, and may give rise to pain, itching, and watery discharges. These are easily removed if necessary. Polypi occasionally develop within the rectum, and may give rise to no pain, though they may cause frequent discharges of blood. Like polypi elsewhere, they may often be removed by a minor operation. (See POLYPOSIS.)

CANCER of the rectum is fairly common. In 1989, in England and Wales there were 9,327 registrations of new cases of cancer of the rectum and anus (5,168 in men), and in 1990 5,696 people (3,198 men) died of anorectal cancer. It is a disease of later life, seldom affecting young people, and its appearance is generally insidious. The tumour begins commonly in the mucous membrane, its structure resembling that of the glands with which the membrane is furnished, and it quickly infiltrates the other coats of the intestine and then invades neighbouring organs. Secondary growths in most cases occur soon in the lymphatic glands within the abdomen and in the liver. The symptoms appear gradually and consist of diarrhoea, alternating with attacks of constipation, and, later on, discharges of blood or of thin blood-stained fluid from the bowels, together with increasing loss of weight and weakness, and pains about the lower part of the back and down the thighs. Upon examination, the tumour can be felt projecting from one side or in a ring-form into the interior of the bowel. These cases are usually far advanced before they give rise to much disturbance, but a lot can now be done to help them by surgical operation. In the majority of cases this consists of removal of the whole of the rectum and the distal two-thirds of the sigmoid colon, and the establishment of a colostomy (q.v.). Approximately 50 per cent of the patients who have this operation are alive and well after five years. In some cases in which the growth occurs in the upper part of the rectum it is now possible to remove the growth and preserve the anus so that the patient is saved the discomfort of having a colostomy.

RECURRENT LARYNGEAL NERVE is a branch of the vagus nerve which leaves the latter low down in its course, and, hooking round the right subclavian artery on the right side and round the arch of the aorta on the left, runs up again into the neck, where it enters the larynx and supplies branches to the muscles which control the vocal cords. The importance of this nerve is the fact that it is apt in its long course either to be injured by surgical procedures to the neck, by trauma to the neck, or to be pressed upon by enlarged lymph glands in the neck, by aneurysms of the aorta or right subclavian artery, resulting in defects of vocalization. These defects may therefore arise within the larynx itself or may arise from disease in the chest, which affects the left recurrent laryngeal nerve. If both recurrent laryngeal nerves are involved in the disease process or are injured, the vocal cords come to lie in the midline, causing embarrassment of the airway and this may necessitate some form of airway intervention, usually in the form of a tracheostomy.

RED BLOOD CELL (see ERYTHROCYTE and BLOOD).

REDUCTION: The manipulation of part of the body from an abnormal position to the correct one (e.g. fractures, dislocations or hernias).

REFERRED PAIN: Pain felt in one part of the body which is actually arising from a distant site (e.g. pain from the diaphragm is felt at the shoulder tip). This occurs because both sites develop from similar embryological tissue and therefore have common pain pathways in the central nervous system.

REFLEX ACTION is one of the simplest forms of activity of the nervous system. (For the mechanism upon which it depends, see NERVES.) Reflex acts are divided usually into three classes. *Superficial reflexes* comprise the sudden movements which result when the skin is brushed or pricked, such as the movement of the toes that results from stroking the sole of the foot. *Deep reflexes* depend upon the state of mild contraction in which muscles are constantly maintained when at rest, and are obtained, as in the case of the knee-jerks, by sharply tapping the tendon of the muscle in question. *Visceral reflexes* are those connected with various organs, such as the narrowing of the pupil when a bright light is directed upon the eye, and the contraction of the bladder when distended by urine.

Faults in these reflexes, both in the direction of excess and of diminution, give valuable evidence as to the presence of nervous diseases and the part of the nervous system in which such disease is situated. Thus, absence of the knee-jerk, when the patellar tendon is tapped, means some interference with the sensory nerve, nerve-cells, or motor nerve upon which the act depends, as, for example, in poliomyelitis, or peripheral neuritis; whilst an excessive jerk implies that the controlling influence exerted by the brain upon this reflex mechanism has been cut off, as, for example, by a tumour high up in the spinal cord, or in the disease known as multiple sclerosis (q.v.).

The condition of the plantar reflex (obtained by stroking the skin of the sole of the foot) is an important point in diagnosing organic disease of the nervous system. The normal reflex consists in bending downwards of the toes towards the sole. In organic disease of the higher parts of the nervous system the great toe tends to bend upwards with spreading out of the other toes (extensor plantar response).

The reflex of the pupil to light is also of great diagnostic importance. The pupil quickly contracts when light falls upon the eye or when the eyes are directed suddenly to a near object. In certain serious diseases of the nervous system, especially in general paralysis and tabes dorsalis the contraction on looking at a near object remains, while the effect of light is lost (Argyll-Robertson pupil).

REFLUX: Fluid flowing in the opposite direction to normal (e.g. backflow). Often refers to regurgitation of stomach contents into the oesophagus.

REFRACTION: The deviation of rays of light on passing from one transparent medium into another of different density. The refractive surfaces of the eye are the anterior surface of the cornea (which accounts for approximately two-thirds of the focusing or refractive power of the eye) and the lens (one-third of the focusing power of the eye). The refractive power of the lens can change, whereas that of the cornea is fixed. *Errors of refraction* (Ametropia) will occur when the focusing power of the lens and cornea do not match the length of the eye, so that rays of light parallel to the visual axis are not focused at the fovea centralis (see EYE). There are three types of refractive error: (i) *Hypermetropia* or long sightedness: the refractive power of the eye is too weak, or the eye is too short so that rays of light are brought to a focus at a point behind the retina. Long-sighted people can see well in the distance but generally require glasses with convex lenses for reading. Uncorrected long sight can lead to headaches and intermittent blurring of vision following prolonged close work, i.e. *eye strain*. As a result of ageing the eye becomes gradually long sighted, resulting in many people's needing reading glasses in later life. This normal process is known as *presbyopia*. A particular form of long sightedness occurs after cataract extraction. (ii) *Myopia* (short sight or near sight): rays of light are brought to a focus in front of the retina because the refractive power of the eye is too great or the eye is too short. Short-sighted people can see close to but need spectacles with concave lenses in order to see in the distance. (iii) *Astigmatism*: the refractive power of the eye is not the same in each meridian. Some rays of light may be focused in front of the retina while others are focused on or behind the retina. Astigmatism can accompany hypermetropia or myopia. It may be corrected by cylindrical lenses (these consist of a slice from the side of a cylinder, i.e. curved in one meridian and flat in the meridian at right angles to it).

REFRACTORY: Unresponsive or resistant to treatment.

REGIMEN: A course of treatment, possibly combining drugs, exercise, diet, etc., designed to bring about an improvement in health.

REGIONAL ANAESTHESIA (see ANAESTHESIA, Local).

REGIONAL HEALTH AUTHORITY (see NATIONAL HEALTH SERVICE).

REGIONAL ILEITIS (see under ILEITIS).

REGISTRAR: (1) A grade of British junior hospital doctor between senior house officer and senior registrar. Under recent government recommendations registrar numbers should be regulated to ensure a balance with the National Health Service's need for consultants, the senior grade for career doctors in hospitals. (2) A public official responsible for registering births, deaths, and marriages.

REGURGITATION is a term used in various connections in medicine. For instance, in diseases of the heart it is used to indicate a condition in which, as the result of valvular disease, the blood does not entirely pass on from the atria of the heart to the ventricles, or from the ventricles into the arteries. The defective valve is said to be incompetent, and a certain amount of blood leaks past it, or regurgitates back, into the cavity from which it has been driven. (See HEART DISEASES.)

The term is also applied to the return to the mouth of food already swallowed and present in the gullet or stomach.

REHABILITATION is the restoration to health and working capacity of a person incapacitated by disease, mental or physical, or by injury. It is a word that came into prominent use during the 1939–45 War, reflecting the growing awareness of the medical profession that the treatment of a sick or injured person does not end at the moment of recovery from the immediate effects of illness or injury. For example, a man with a fractured limb or spine has to recover full use not only of the injured part but of his whole body; and he has to recover confidence in his ability to work and enjoy life. (See DISABLED PERSONS; REMPLOY.)

REITER'S SYNDROME: For some 40 years the concurrence of polyarthritis, non-gonococcal urethritis and ocular inflammation has been called Reiter's Syndrome. The syndrome has over the years been associated with promiscuous sexual contact because urethritis is a common feature. The evidence for this is, however, circumstantial. It is now well recognized that urethritis can occur unrelated to sexual contact as a result of gastro-intestinal infection with *Yersinia enterocolitica*. Possession of the HLA antigen B27 affects the severity of the disease and the prognosis, but the syndrome is not confined to patients with this antigen. (See REACTIVE ARTHRITIS.)

REJECTION: A term used in transplant medicine to describe the body's immunological response to foreign tissue. Various drugs, such as cyclosporin A, can be used to dampen the host's response to a graft and reduce the risk of rejection.

RELAPSE means the return of a disease during the period of convalescence.

RELAPSING FEVER, so-called because of the characteristic temperature chart showing recurring bouts of fever, is an infectious disease caused by spirochaetes. There are two main forms of the disease.

LOUSE-BORNE RELAPSING FEVER is an epidemic disease, usually associated with wars and famines, which has occurred in practically every country in the world. For long confused with typhus and typhoid, it was not until the 1870's that the causal organism was described by Obermeier. It is now known as the *Borrelia recurrentis*, a motile spiral organism 10 to 20 micrometres in length. The organism is transmitted from man to man by the louse, *Pediculus humanus*.

Symptoms: The incubation period is up to 12 days, usually 7 days. The onset is sudden, with high temperature, generalized aches and pains, and nose-bleeding. In about half the cases a rash appears at an early stage, beginning in the neck and spreading down over the trunk and arms. Jaundice may occur; and both the liver and the spleen are enlarged. The temperature subsides after five or six days, to rise again in about a week. There may be up to four such relapses (see the introductory paragraph above). **Treatment**: Preventive measures are the same as those for typhus (q.v.). Rest in bed is essential, as are good nursing and a light, nourishing diet. There is usually a quick response to penicillin. The tetracyclines and chloramphenicol are also effective. Following such treatment the incidence of relapse is about 15 per cent. The mortality rate is low, except in a starved population.

TICK-BORNE RELAPSING FEVER is an endemic disease which occurs in most tropical and subtropical countries. The causative organism is *Borrelia duttoni*, which is transmitted by a tick, *Ornithodorus moubata*. David Livingstone suggested that it was a tick-borne disease, but it was not until 1905 that Dutton and Todd produced the definite evidence.

Symptoms: The main differences from the louse-borne disease are: (*a*) the incubation period is usually shorter, 3 to 6 days, but may be as short as 2 days or as long as 12; (*b*) the febrile period is usually shorter and the afebrile periods are more variable in duration, sometimes only lasting for a day or two; (*c*) relapses are much more numerous.

Treatment: Preventive measures are more difficult to carry out than in the case of the louse-borne infection. Protective clothing should always be worn in 'tick country'. Old, heavily infected houses should be destroyed. Curative treatment is the same as for the louse-borne infection.

RELATE MARRIAGE GUIDANCE: The idea of a marriage guidance council came from a group of doctors, clergy and social workers who were concerned for the welfare of marriage. It is based upon two major concepts: that marriage provides the best possible way for a man and woman to live and love together and rear their children, and that the counsellors share a basic respect for the unique personality of the individual and his (or her) right to make his (or her) own decisions. The organization consists of between 120 and 130 Marriage Guidance Councils throughout the country, comprising about 1250 counsellors. These Councils are affiliated to Relate National Marriage Guidance, which is responsible for the selection, training and continued supervision of all counsellors. Anyone seeking help can telephone or write for an appointment. No fees are charged, but those receiving help are encouraged to donate what they can. The address of Relate Marriage Guidance is Herbert Gray College, Little Church Street, Rugby, Warwickshire CV21 3AP (0788-573241, fax: 0788-535007).

REMITTENT FEVER is the term applied to the form of fever in which, during remissions, the temperature falls, but not to normal.

REMPLOY is Britain's largest employer of severely disabled people, set up under the provisions of the 1944 Disabled Persons (Employment) Act.

The company currently has about 9,000 severely disabled employees in 94 production units in Scotland, England and Wales, manufacturing over 100 different products and services. Full details may be obtained from Remploy Ltd, 415 Edgware Road, London NW2 6LR (081-452 8020).

REMISSION: A period when a disease has responded to treatment and there are no signs or symptoms present.

REM SLEEP: Rapid-eye-movement sleep – a stage during sleep in which the eyes are seen to move rapidly beneath the lids and during which dreaming occurs. It occurs for several minutes at a time approximately every 100 minutes.

RENAL Related to the kidney.

RENAL DISEASES (see KIDNEYS, DISEASES OF).

RENIN is a protein-like substance extracted from the kidney which, when injected into animals, causes a rise of blood-pressure. This it does, apparently, by reacting with a substance normally present in the blood plasma to produce angiotensin. Angiotensin has been obtained in crystalline form, and it is angiotensin which causes the rise in blood-pressure. This work may have an important bearing on the problem of high blood-pressure in man.

RENNET is a substance prepared from the stomach of the calf, in order to curdle and partially digest milk. Its activity depends upon a ferment known as rennin. Rennet is used for the preparation of junket and in the making of cheese.

REPAIR of tissues after injury is described generally under WOUNDS, and the repair of special tissues which present various peculiarities is described under BONE; MUSCLE; NERVES, etc.

REPETITIVE STRAIN INJURY (see TENDINITIS).

REPRODUCTIVE SYSTEM: A collective term for all the organs involved in sexual reproduction. In the female these are the ovaries, fallopian tubes, uterus, vagina and vulva. In the male these are the testes, vasa deferentia, prostate, seminal vesicles, urethra and penis.

RESECTION is the name given to an operation in which a part of some organ is removed, as, for example, the resection of a fragment of dead bone.

RESERPINE is an alkaloid obtained from the root of Rauwolfia (q.v.), and is used as an antihypertensive and a tranquillizing agent.

RESINS are solid or semi-solid exudations from plants, which are insoluble in water, mostly soluble in alcohol or ether, soften or melt at moderate temperatures, and burn with a smoky flame. They are transparent when pure, but opaque when they contain water. They are non-conductors of electricity. Some of them are acids and combine with alkalis to form soaps. A *natural resin* is one that occurs as an exudation, such as mastic. A *prepared resin* is made from a drug, such as podophyllin, or from a natural oleoresin such as rosin which is obtained from various species of *Pinus*. *Oleoresins* may be either natural oleoresins, which are mixtures of volatile oils and resins generally obtained by incising trunks of trees, such as turpentine and copaiba; or prepared oleoresins which are concentrated liquid preparations made from drugs containing both volatile oil and resin, such as capsicum. *Gum resins* are natural mixtures of gums and resins, usually obtained as exudations from plants, such as myrrh and asafoetida. (See also ION EXCHANGE RESINS.)

RESOLUTION is a term applied to infective processes, to indicate a natural subsidence of the inflammation without the formation of pus. Thus a pneumonic lung is said to resolve when the material exuded into it is absorbed into the blood and lymph, so that recovery takes place naturally; an inflamed area is said to resolve when the inflammation fades away and no abscess forms; a glandular enlargement is said to resolve when it decreases in size without suppuration. Resolvents was an old term applied to procedures capable of assisting this process. (See BLISTERS; INFLAMMATION.)

RESONANCE means the lengthening and intensification of sound produced by striking the body over an air-containing structure. Decrease of resonance is called dullness and increase of resonance is called hyper-resonance. The process of striking the chest or other part of the body to discover its degree of resonance is called percussion, and according to the note obtained, an opinion can be formed as to the state of consolidation of air-containing organs, the presence of abnormal cavities, and the dimensions and relations of solid and air-containing organs lying together. (See also AUSCULTATION.)

RESORCIN, or RESORCINOL, is a white, crystalline, antiseptic substance soluble in water, alcohol, and oils. It is mainly used in skin diseases which require a stimulating and antiseptic application.

RESPIRATION is the process in which air passes into and out of the lungs with the object of allowing the blood to absorb oxygen and to give off carbon dioxide and water. This occurs 18 times a minute in a healthy adult at rest, this being known as the respiratory rate. In other words we inspire more than 25,000 times a day and during this time inhale around 16 kg of air.

Mechanism of respiration: For the structure of the respiratory apparatus see AIR PASSAGES; CHEST; LUNGS. The air passes rhythmically into and out of the air passages, and mixes with the air already in the lungs, these two movements being known as inspiration and expiration.

INSPIRATION is due to a muscular effort which enlarges the chest in all three dimensions, so that the lungs have to expand in order to fill up the vacuum that would otherwise be left, and the air accordingly enters these organs by the air passages. There is no direct pull upon the lungs, each of which is simply suspended within the corresponding pleural cavity by its root, and made to fill this cavity in all conditions of the chest by the pressure of the outer air exerted through the nose, mouth, and air passages. The increase of the chest in size from above downwards is mainly due to the diaphragm, the muscular fibres of which, by their contraction, reduce its domed shape and cause it to descend, pushing down the abdominal organs beneath it. The increase from before back is mainly due to a tilting forwards of the lower end of the breast-bone, and of the lower rib cartilages. The increase from side to side can best be understood by examining a skeleton, noting the very oblique position of the lower ribs, and observing how greatly the capacity of the chest is increased when each is raised, in the manner of a bucket-handle, taking its fixed points at the spine and breast-bone. (See RIBS.)

The muscles which chiefly bring about these changes in ordinary quiet inspiration are the diaphragm, intercostal muscles, and levators of the ribs, whilst in forced or extraordinary inspiration, when a specially deep breath is taken, the sternocleidomastoid, serratus magnus, trapezius, and pectoral muscles are also brought powerfully into play. Many other muscles take part to a slight extent, steadying the spine and the upper and lower ribs, while even the muscles of the face and of the larynx are thrown rhythmically into activity, dilating the nostrils and the entrance to the larynx at each breath.

EXPIRATION is in ordinary circumstances simply an elastic recoil, the diaphragm rising and the ribs sinking into the position that they naturally occupy, when muscular contraction is finished. Expiration occupies a slightly longer period than inspiration. In forced expiration many powerful muscles of the abdomen and thorax are brought into play, and the act may be made a very forcible one, as, for example, in coughing.

Nervous control: Respiration is usually either an automatic or a reflex act, each expiration sending up afferent, sensory impulses to the central nervous system, from which efferent impulses are sent down various other nerves to the muscles that produce inspiration. It appears that there are several centres which govern the rate and force of the breathing, although all are presided over by a chief respiratory centre in the medulla oblongata, which is sometimes spoken of as the vital knot (*noeud vital*).

Although this centre appears to be absolutely essential to life, it in turn is under the control of the higher centres in the cerebral hemispheres, through which the will acts, so that breathing can be voluntarily stopped, quickened, or otherwise changed at will. It would be impossible, however, to cause death by voluntarily holding the breath, because, as the blood becomes more venous, the vital centre in the medulla again assumes control and breathing starts again. Apart from changes due to willpower, the respirations follow one another rhythmically at the rate of about 18 per minute, being in general one for every four heart-beats. **Quantity of air**: The lungs do not by any means completely empty themselves at each expiration and refill at each inspiration. An amount equivalent, in quiet respiration, to less than one-tenth of the total air in the lungs passes out and is replaced by the same quantity of fresh air, which mixes with the stale air in the lungs. This renewal, which in quiet breathing amounts to about 500 millilitres, is known as the *tidal air*. By a special inspiratory effort, one can, however, draw in about 3000 millilitres, this amount being known as *complemental air*. By a special expiratory effort, too, after an ordinary breath one can expel much more than the tidal air from the lungs, this extra amount being known as the *supplemental* or *reserve air*, and amounting to about 1300 millilitres. If one takes as deep an inspiration as possible and then makes a forced expiration, one breathes out the sum of these three, which is known as the *vital capacity*, and amounts to about 4000 millilitres in a healthy adult male of average size. These figures all apply to a man of average height. Figures for women are about 25 per cent lower. The vital capacity varies with size, sex, age and ethnic origin. The following formulae, incorporating age, height and sex, give an approximate guide to the vital capacity:

Men:
vital capacity (*in millilitres*)
$$= [27\cdot63 - (0\cdot112 \times \text{age})] \times \text{height}$$
(*in centimetres*)

Women:
vital capacity (*in millilitres*)
$$= [21\cdot78 - (0\cdot101 \times \text{age})] \times \text{height}$$
(*in centimetres*)

Over and above the vital capacity, the lungs contain air which cannot be expelled by the strongest possible expiration. This *residual air*, as it is known, which remains in the lungs even after death, amounts to another 1500 millilitres.

Tests of respiratory efficiency are being increasingly used to assess lung function in health and disease. The most widely used one is based on an analysis of a single forced expiration after a maximal inspiration. The volume expelled in the first second of expiration (known as FEV_1) correlates well with the respiratory efficiency. Normal values for FEV_1 vary with age, sex and, to a lesser extent, with the size of the body but, by and large, healthy persons can breathe out 15 per cent or more of vital capacity within the first second.

Abnormal forms of respiration: Apart from mere changes in rate and force, respiration is modified in several important ways, either involuntarily or voluntarily. *Sighing* is a long-drawn inspiration following a pause when breathing has been checked by mental preoccupation. This form of breathing also characterizes some conditions of extreme weakness of the nervous system, such as shock and diabetic coma. *Sobbing* is a series of convulsive inspirations, at each of which the larynx is partially closed; it follows grief or great exertion. *Snoring* (q.v.), or stertorous breathing, is due to a flaccid state of the soft palate causing it to vibrate as the air passes into the throat, or simply to sleeping with the mouth open, which has a similar effect. *Coughing* (q.v.) is a series of violent expirations, at each of which the larynx is suddenly opened after the pressure of air in the lungs has risen considerably; its object is to expel some irritating substance from the air passages. *Sneezing* (q.v.) is a single sudden expiration, which differs from coughing in that the sudden rush of air is directed by the soft palate up into the nose in order to expel some source of irritation from this narrow passage. *Cheyne-Stokes breathing* (q.v.) is a type of breathing found in persons suffering from apoplexy, heart disease, and some other conditions, in which death is impending; it consists in an alternate dying away and gradual strengthening of the inspirations. Other disorders of breathing are found in CROUP and in ASTHMA (qq.v.).

RESPIRATORY DISTRESS SYNDROME

may occur in adults as adult respiratory distress syndrome or in new-born children, when it is also known as hyaline membrane disease (q.v.). The adult syndrome consists of pulmonary oedema of non-cardiac origin. It is a complication of shock, systemic sepsis and viral respiratory infections. It was first described in 1967 and despite advances with assisted ventilation it remains a serious disease with a mortality of more than 50 per cent. The maintenance of adequate circulating blood volume, peripheral perfusion, acid base balance and arterial oxygenation is important and assisted ventilation should be instituted early. The aetiology is not understood though the process begins when tissue damage stimulates the autonomic nervous system, releases vaso-active substances precipitates complement activation and produces abnormalities of the clotting cascade – the serial process that leads to clotting of the blood. The activation of complement causes white cells to lodge in the pulmonary capillaries where they release substances which damage the pulmonary endothelium.

RESPIRATORY SYNCYTIAL VIRUS, or RS

VIRUS as it is usually known, is one of the myxoviruses (q.v.). It is the major cause of bronchiolitis and pneumonia in infants under the age of 6 months.

RESTLESS LEGS SYNDROME: A condition in which the patient experiences unpleasant sensations, and occasionally involuntary movements, in the legs when at rest, especially at night. No pathological changes have been identified. It is sometimes indicative of iron-deficiency anaemia, but in many cases the cause remains a mystery and the variety of cures offered are a testimony to this. Some anti-epileptic drugs are said to help.

RESUSCITATION (see APPENDIX: BASIC FIRST AID).

RETARDATION: Slowing down; developmental delay.

RETCHING is an ineffectual form of vomiting. (See VOMITING.)

RETENTION OF URINE (see URINE, RETENTION OF).

RETICULOCYTES are newly formed red blood corpuscles, in which a fine network can be demonstrated by special staining methods.

RETICULO-ENDOTHELIAL SYSTEM consists of highly specialized cells scattered throughout the body, but found mainly in the spleen, bone marrow, liver, and lymph glands. Their main function is the ingestion of red blood cells and the conversion of haemoglobin to bilirubin. They are also able to ingest bacteria and foreign colloidal particles.

RETICULOSES is the term used to describe a group of conditions characterized by progressive widespread proliferation of the cells of the reticulo-endothelial system. The two most important members of this group are Hodgkin's disease (q.v.) and lymphosarcoma (q.v.).

RETINA (see EYE).

RETINA, DISORDERS OF: The retina can be damaged by disease that affects the retina alone, or by diseases affecting the whole body. *Retinopathy* is a term used to denote an abnormality of the retina without specifying a cause. Some retinal disorders are discussed below.

DIABETIC RETINOPATHY: Retinal disease occurring in patients with diabetes mellitus. It is the commonest cause of blind registration in Great Britain of people between 20 and 65 years of age. Diabetic retinopathy can be divided into several types. The two main causes of blindness are those that follow, first, development of new blood vessels from the retina, with resultant complications and, second, those following 'water logging' (oedema) of the macula. Treatment is by maintaining rigid control of blood-sugar levels combined with laser treatment for certain forms of the disease – in particular to get rid of new blood vessels.

HYPERTENSIVE RETINOPATHY: Retinal disease secondary to the development of high blood pressure. Treatment involves control of the blood pressure.

SICKLE CELL RETINOPATHY: People with sickle cell disease can develop a number of retinal problems including new blood vessels from the retina.

RETROLENTAL FIBROPLASIA: A disorder affecting low-birth-weight premature babies exposed to high oxygen pressures. Essentially new blood vessels develop which cause extensive traction on the retina with resultant retinal detachment and poor vision.

RETINAL ARTERY OCCLUSION, RETINAL VEIN OCCLUSION: These result in damage to those areas of retina supplied by the affected blood vessel. The blood vessels become blocked. If the peripheral retina is damaged the patient may be completely symptom free, although areas of blindness may be detected on examination of field of vision. If the macula is involved, visual loss may be sudden, profound and permanent. There is no effective treatment once visual loss has occurred.

SENILE MACULAR DEGENERATION ('senile' indicates age of onset and has no bearing on mental state) is the leading cause of blindness in the elderly in the western world. The average age of onset is 65 years. Patients initially notice a disturbance of their vision which gradually progresses over months or years. They lose the ability to recognize fine detail, e.g. they cannot read fine print, cannot sew or recognize people's faces. They always retain the ability to recognize large objects such as doors and chairs. They are therefore able to get around and about reasonably well. There is no effective treatment in the majority of cases.

RETINITIS PIGMENTOSA: A group of rare, inherited diseases characterized by the development of night blindness and tunnel vision. Symptoms start in childhood and are progressive. Many patients retain good visual acuity, although their peripheral vision is limited. One of the characteristic findings on examination is collections of pigment in the retina which have a characteristic shape and are therefore known as 'bone spicules'. There is no effective treatment.

RETINAL DETACHMENT usually occurs because of development of a hole in the retina. Holes can occur because of degeneration of the retina, because of traction on the retina by the vitreous, or due to injury. Fluid from the vitreous passes through the hole causing a split within the retina. The inner part of the retina becomes detached from the outer part, the latter remains in contact with the choroid. Detached retina loses its ability to detect light with consequent impairment of vision. Retinal detachments are more common in the short sighted, in the elderly or following cataract extraction. Symptoms include spots before the eyes (*floaters*), flashing lights and a shadow over the eye with progressive loss of vision. Treatment by laser is very effective if caught early, at the stage when a hole has developed in the retina but the retina has not become detached. The edges of the hole can be 'spot welded' to the underlying choroid. Once a detachment has occurred, laser therapy cannot be used, the retina has to be repositioned. This is usually done by indenting the wall of the eye from the outside to meet the retina, then making the retina stick to the wall of the eye by inducing inflammation in the wall. This is done by freezing the wall. The outcome of surgery depends largely on the extent of the detachment and its duration. Complicated forms of detachment can occur due to diabetic eye disease, injury or tumour. Each requires a specialized form of treatment.

RETINOIC ACID is a synthetic vitamin A derivative. (See VITAMIN.)

RETINOL is the official chemical name of vitamin A. (See VITAMIN.)

RETINOPATHY (see RETINA, DISEASES OF).

RETRACTOR: An instrument for pulling apart the edges of an incision to allow better surgical access to the organs and tissues being operated on.

RETRO- is a prefix signifying behind or turned backward.

RETROBULBAR NEURITIS: Inflammation of the optic nerve behind (rather than within) the eye. It usually occurs in young adults and presents with a rapid deterioration in vision over a few hours. Colour vision is also impaired. Usually vision recovers over a few weeks, but colour vision may be permanently lost. It can be associated with certain viral illnesses and with multiple sclerosis.

RETROFLEXION means bending of an organ so that its top is thrust backwards. Retroversion is a similar displacement in which the whole organ is turned backwards. These terms are particularly applied to the uterus.

RETROGRADE: Movement in a contrary or backward direction from normal (e.g. a retrograde pyelogram introduces dye into the pelvis of the kidney by passing it up the ureters).

RETROPHARYNGEAL ABSCESS is an abscess occurring in the cellular tissue behind the throat. It is the result in general of disease in the upper part of the spinal column.

RETROVERSION: An abnormal position of the uterus, occurring in about 20 per cent of women, in which its long axis is pivoted backwards in relation to the cervix and vagina instead of forwards.

REYE'S SYNDROME is a condition which occurs predominantly in young children following a virus infection of the upper respiratory tract or a viral infection such as chickenpox or influenza. The cause is not known, but there is some evidence that aspirin may play a part in its causation. It is of worldwide distribution, but relatively rare in Western Europe. The initial feature is severe, persistent vomiting and fever. This is followed by outbursts of wild behaviour, delirium and convulsions terminating in coma and death. The mortality rate is around 23 per cent, and 50 per cent of the survivors may have persistent mental or neurological disturbances. The younger the patient the higher the death rate and the more common the permanent residual effects.

RHABDOVIRUSES is a group of viruses which includes the rabies virus.

RHATANY, or KRAMERIA, is the root of *Krameria triandra*, a South American plant, which contains an astringent principle. It is mainly used in diarrhoea in the form of a tincture or extract, and to make lozenges for use in cases of relaxed throat.

RHESUS FACTOR (see BLOOD GROUPS).

RHEUMATIC FEVER describes an acute febrile illness, usually seen in children which may include arthralgia, arthritis, chorea (qq.v.), carditis and rash. The illness has been shown to follow a streptococcal infection and a streptococcal cause is now implicit in the term.

Rheumatic fever has become extremely uncommon in developed countries, but remains common in developing areas. It is rare before the age of 3, occurring most commonly in midchildhood and adolescence. If chorea is excluded (commoner in girls), the disease is equally common in the two sexes. Recurrences of the acute illness may occur over a period of years. Long-term consequences include damage to heart valves and less commonly a non-erosive deforming arthritis or persistent neurological problems.

The streptococci responsible are the beta haemolytic type. Their presence may be confirmed by a positive throat swab or a rising antistreptolysin antibody titre in serum.

Clinical features: Fever is marked with attacks of shivering or rigor. Joint pain and swelling affect the knee, ankle, wrist or shoulder and may migrate from one joint to another. Tachycardia may be out of proportion to other constitutional features and indicate cardiac involvement. Subcutaneous nodules may occur, particularly over the back of the wrist or over the elbow or knee. Erythema marginatum is a red rash characteristic of the condition.

Cardiac involvement includes pericarditis, endocarditis, and myocarditis (qq.v.). The main long-term complication is damage to the mitral and aortic valves (qq.v.).

The chief neurological problem is chorea (St Vitus's dance) which may develop after the acute symptoms have subsided.

Treatment: Eradication of streptococcal infection is essential. Other features are treated symptomatically. Paracetamol may be preferred to aspirin as an antipyretic in young children. A non-steroidal anti-inflammatory drug (q.v.) may benefit the joint symptoms. Corticosteroids (q.v.) may be indicated for more serious complications.

Patients who have developed cardiac valve abnormalities require antibiotic prophylaxis during dental treatment and other procedures where bacteria may enter the bloodstream. Secondary cardiac problems may occur several decades later and require replacement of affected heart valves.

RHEUMATISM: is an obsolete medical term which no longer has a defined meaning. It remains a lay term covering any painful condition of the arms, legs or spine.

RHEUMATOID ARTHRITIS: is the term used to describe a chronic inflammation of the synovial lining of several joints, tendon sheaths or bursae which is not due to sepsis or a reaction to crystals. Most cases show a typical symmetrical pattern, suggesting a single aetiology. However, several atypical patterns occur. It is likely that the problem is of multifactorial origin, and that there is some variation in the genetic and environmental factors involved in individual cases. Rheumatoid arthritis is distinguished from other patterns of inflammatory arthritis by the symmetrical involvement of a large number of peripheral joints, by the common association with serum rheumatoid factor antibody, by the presence of bony erosions around joints and, in a minority, the presence of subcutaneous nodules with necrobiotic (decaying) centres.

Causes: There is a major immunogenetic predisposition to rheumatoid arthritis in people carrying the HLA-DR4 antigen. Other minor immunogenetic factors have also been implicated. In addition, there is a degree of familial clustering which suggests other unidentified genetic factors. Genetic factors cannot alone explain aetiology, and environmental and chance factors must be important, but these have yet to be identified. Rheumatoid arthritis appears to be more common in developed countries and in rural populations that have moved to an urban lifestyle. No convincing effect of diet has been demonstrated.

Epidemiology: Rheumatoid arthritis most commonly occurs in women from the age of 30 onwards, the sex ratio being approximately 4 to 1. Typical rheumatoid arthritis may occur in adolescence, but in childhood chronic synovitis (q.v.) usually take one of a number of different patterns, classified under juvenile chronic arthritis.

Pathology: The primary lesion is an inflammation of the synovial lining, with an accumulation of macrophages on the lining surface and an infiltration of the deeper tissue with lymphocytes, plasma cells, macrophages, and small numbers of neutrophil polymorphs. The synovial fluid becomes diluted with inflammatory exudate, containing a mixture of leukocytes. If inflammation persists for several months, there is often progressive destruction of articular cartilage and bone. Cartilage is replaced by inflammatory tissue known as pannus. A similar tissue invades bone to form erosions. Synovitis also affects tendon sheaths, and may lead to adhesion fibrosis or attrition and rupture of tendons. Subcutaneous and other bursae may be involved. Necrobiotic nodules also occur at sites outside synovium, including the subcutaneous tissues, the lungs, the pericardium and the pleura.

Clinical features: Rheumatoid arthritis varies from the very mild to the severely disabling. Many mild cases probably go undiagnosed. At least 50 per cent of known cases continue to lead a reasonably normal life, about 25 per cent are significantly disabled in terms of work and leisure activities and a minority become markedly disabled and are limited in their independ-

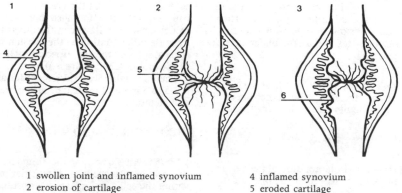

1 swollen joint and inflamed synovium   4 inflamed synovium
2 erosion of cartilage   5 eroded cartilage
3 loss of cartilage and erosion of bone   6 erosion of bone

Changes in a joint caused by rheumatoid arthritis.

ence. There is often an early acute phase, followed by substantial remission, but in other patients gradual stepwise deterioration may occur, with progressive involvement of an increasing number of joints.

The diagnosis of rheumatoid arthritis is largely based on clinical symptoms and signs. Approximately 70 per cent of patients have rheumatoid factor antibodies in the serum but, because of the large number of false positives and false negatives, this test cannot be considered diagnostic and has very little value in clinical practice. It may be a useful pointer to a worse prognosis in early cases if the titre is high. The erythrocyte sedimentation rate (see ESR) and plasma viscosity (stickiness) are usually raised during periods when the patient has clinical symptoms. They may remain abnormal during periods of clinical remission. Their value in long-term management is arguable. Joint radiographs will show progressive loss of the cartilage joint space and the development of body erosions in many cases. Radiographs may assist in diagnosis in early cases and are particularly helpful when considering surgery or possible complications such as pathological fracture. Patients commonly develop anaemia, which may be partly due to gastrointestinal blood loss from anti-inflammatory drug treatment. Treatment involves physical, pharmacological, and surgical measures, together with psychological and social support tailored to the individual patient's needs. Regular activity should be maintained. Resting of certain joints such as the wrist with splints may be helpful at night or to assist prolonged manual activities. Sound footwear is important. Drug treatment includes simple analgesics, non-steroidal anti-inflammatory agents and slow-acting antirheumatics including gold, penicillamine, sulphasalazine and azathioprine. The non-steroidal agents are largely effective in reducing pain, and early morning stiffness, and have no effect on the chronic inflammatory process. The slow-acting drugs take approximately three months to act but have a more global effect on chronic inflammation with a greater reduction in swelling and an associated fall in erythrocyte sedimentation rate and rise in the level of haemoglobin. Local corticosteroids are useful, given into individual joints. Systemic corticosteroids carry serious problems if continued long term, but may be useful under special circumstances.

RHEUMATOLOGY: The medical speciality concerned with the study and management of diseases of the joints and connective tissues.

RH FACTOR (see BLOOD GROUPS).

RHINITIS means inflammation of the mucous membrane of the nose. (See NOSE, DISEASES OF.)

RHINOPHYMA is the condition characterized by enlargement of the nose due to enormous enlargement of the sebaceous glands which may develop in the later stages of rosacea (q.v.).

RHINOPLASTY means the repair of the nose or modification of its shape by operation. This operation is performed by plastic and ENT surgeons alike. It may involve alteration of the bony skeleton of the nose and/or alteration of the septum (septorhinoplasty). It is mostly performed for cosmetic reasons. However, any disease process or injury which has caused defect in the nose may be repaired as well. The latter problem would usually involve the utilization of some form of skin flap, whereas this would not be required for cosmetic surgical purposes.

RHINOVIRUSES are a large group of viruses; to date around 80 distinct rhinoviruses have been identified. Their practical importance is that some of them are responsible for around one- quarter of the cases of the common cold.

RHIZOTOMY is the surgical operation of cutting a nerve root, as, for example, to relieve the pain of trigeminal neuralgia.

RHONCHI denotes the harsh cooing, hissing, or whistling sounds (wheezing) heard by auscultation over the bronchial tubes when they are the seat of infection. (See BRONCHITIS.)

RHYTHM METHOD: A method of contraception which attempts to prevent conception by avoiding intercourse during the fertile part of the menstrual cycle. (See CONTRACEPTION; SAFE PERIOD.)

RIBOFLAVINE is the *British Pharmacopoeia* name for what used to be known as vitamin B_2. Riboflavine belongs to a group of animal and plant pigments which give a greenish fluorescence on exposure to ultra-violet rays. It is present especially in milk, and is not destroyed during pasteurization. Other rich sources are eggs, liver, yeast and the green leaves of broccoli and spinach. It is also present in beer. Deficiency of riboflavine in the diet is thought to cause inflammation of the substance of the cornea, sores on the lips, especially at the angles of the mouth (cheilosis (q.v.)), and dermatitis.

The minimal daily requirement for an adult is 1·5 to 3 mg, but is greater during pregnancy and lactation.

RIBONUCLEIC ACID (see RNA).

RIBOSOME: Granules either found free within the cell or attached to a reticular network within the cell's endoplasm. Consisting of approximately 65 per cent RNA and 35 per cent protein, they are the sites where protein is made.

RIBS are the bones, twelve on each side, which enclose the cavity of the chest. The upper seven are joined to the breast-bone by their costal cartilages and are therefore known as true ribs. The lower five do not reach the breast-bone, and are therefore known as false ribs. Of the latter, the 8th, 9th and 10th are joined by their costal cartilages, each one to the rib immediately above it, while the 11th and 12th are free from any such connection, and are therefore known as floating ribs. Each rib has a head, by which it is joined to the upper part of the body of the vertebra with which it corresponds, as well as to the vertebra immediately above. Next comes a narrow part known as the neck, and then a tubercle, by which the rib is joined to the transverse process of the corresponding vertebra. Finally, the greater part of the bone is made up of the shaft, which runs at first outwards and at the angle turns sharply forwards. On the lower margin of the shaft is a groove, which lodges the corresponding intercostal artery and nerve.

RICE-WATER is a useful diluent drink for invalids, similar to barley-water.

RICKETS is a disease of childhood characterized chiefly by a softened condition of the bones, and by other evidence of perverted nutrition.

Causes: This disease is the result of deficiency of vitamin D in the diet. Healthy bones cannot be built up without calcium (or lime) salts, and the body cannot utilize these salts in the absence of vitamin D. Want of sunlight and fresh air in the dwellings where the children are reared is also of importance. Once a common condition in industrial areas, it had almost disappeared in Great Britain, but there has been a recurrence of it in recent years that is giving rise to concern.

The changes that take place in the bones are due to an irregular process of bone formation. The periosteum, the membrane enveloping the bones, becomes inflamed, and in consequence the bone formed beneath it is defective in lime salts and very soft. At the growing ends of the bones there is an even more striking change. The epiphyseal plate of cartilage, from which growth takes place, is much thickened, the cellular elements in it much increased in number, and the bone which it produces markedly deficient in lime salts. The new bone shows a deficiency of lime amounting to 25 or 35 per cent, and this, too, notwithstanding the fact that there is abundance of lime in the body, as shown by its excessive excretion in the urine. The disease rarely occurs under the age of 6 months, from which it may be assumed that exposure to unsuitable conditions for several months is necessary before rickets ensues. It is most common between 1 and 2 years of age and is increasingly rare after the age of 3.

Symptoms: The symptoms of rickets most commonly attract attention about the end of the first year, and the disease rarely appears for the first time after the age of 5. The symptoms, which precede the outward manifestations of the disease, are marked disorders of the digestive and alimentary functions. The child's appetite is diminished; there is frequent vomiting and diarrhoea; or irregularity of the bowels appears, the evacuations being clay-coloured and unhealthy. In infants, convulsions are sometimes a symptom of rickets and disappear under the treatment appropriate to this disease. At the same time there is tenderness of the bones as shown by crying when the child is moved or handled. A little later it is noticed that there is delay in learning to sit up and walk, so that the child who has begun to walk loses this power.

Gradually changes in the shape of the bones becomes visible, first chiefly noticed at the ends of the long bones, as in those of the arm, causing enlargement at the wrists, or in the ribs, producing a row of knobs at the junction of their ends with the rib cartilages (rickety rosary). Because of their softened condition the bones also tend to become distorted and bent both by the action of the muscles and by the weight of the body resting upon them. Those of the legs are bent outwards and forwards and the child becomes bow-legged or knock-kneed, often to an extreme degree. The trunk of the body likewise shows various alterations and deformities owing to curvatures of the spine, flattening of the lateral curves of the ribs, and the projection forward of the breast-bone. (See CHEST, DEFORMITIES OF.) The cavity of the chest may thus be contracted and interference produced with the development of the thoracic organs, whose functions thus become embarrassed. The liver is pushed outwards and the abdomen becomes protuberant (pot belly). The pelvis undergoes distortion which may reduce its capacity to such a degree that in females serious difficulties may arise later in life in the course of labour. The head of the rickety child is square with high 'intellectual' forehead; the individual bones of the cranium remain long ununited, while the soft fontanelle remains unclosed long after the end of the second year, the time by which it should have disappeared; the face is small and ill-developed; and the teeth appear late and fall out or decay early.

The disease usually terminates in recovery with more or less of deformity and dwarfing, the bones, although altered in shape, becoming ultimately firmly ossified. On the other hand, during the progress of the disease, various intercurrent ailments are apt to arise which may cause death, such as bronchitis and other chest complaints, meningitis, convulsions, laryngismus.

Treatment: The treatment of rickets is more hygienic and dietetic than medicinal. The specific remedy is vitamin D, given as a rule in the form of calciferol (vitamin D_2). A full diet is of course essential, with emphasis upon a sufficient supply of milk. Rickets practically does not occur in breast-fed children but it is a wise precaution to give breast-fed babies supplementary vitamin D. After the child is weaned, the provision of suitable food is of the greatest importance, supplemented by the administration of some source of vitamin D.

Deficiency of vitamin D in adults results in osteomalacia (q.v.).

RICKETTSIA is the general term given to a group of micro-organisms, which are intermediate between bacteria and viruses. They are the causal agents of typhus and a number of typhus-like diseases, such as Rocky Mountain spotted fever, Japanese River fever, and scrub typhus. These micro-organisms are usually conveyed to man by lice, fleas, ticks, and mites. VISCERAL RICKETTSIA is a disease transmitted by mites from an infected house mouse, which occurs in the USA, South Africa, Korea and USSR. The causal organism is *Rickettsia akari*. The incubation period is 7 to 14 days. The characteristic features are fever, headache, and a non-irritating rash on the face, trunk and extremities. The disease is non-fatal and responds rapidly to tetracyclines.

RIFAMPICIN is an antibiotic derived from *Streptomyces mediterranei*, which is proving of value in the treatment of tuberculosis and leprosy. It contains a dye which is excreted in the urine and gives it a red colour.

RIFT VALLEY FEVER is a virus disease, transmitted by mosquitoes, at one time confined to Sub-Saharan Africa and predominantly found in domestic animals, such as cattle, sheep and goats. The only human beings affected were veterinary surgeons, butchers and others exposed to heavy infection by direct contact with infected animals. These usually recovered. Thus in 1975, only four people died of it. In 1977, it suddenly flared up as a human infection in Egypt, involving 200,000 people and killing 600 of these. It recurred as a human disease in 1978 and 1979, and is now threatening to spread throughout the Middle East, and possibly further afield. This human outbreak is attributed to a new virulent strain of virus. The illness in man is characterized by fever, haemorrhages, encephalitis (q.v.) and involvement of the eye. There is an efficient vaccine which protects both animals and human beings against the disease.

RIGIDITY: Stiffness, resistance to movement. The term is often used in neurology, e.g. limb rigidity is a sign of Parkinson's disease (q.v.). Smooth rigidity is described as being 'plastic' and jerky rigidity as 'cogwheel'.

RIGOR means shivering. If prolonged, it is generally accompanied by raised temperature, and may be a sign of the onset of some acute febrile disease, such as influenza, pneumonia, or some internal inflammation. *Rigor mortis* is the name given to the stiffness that ensues soon after death. (See DEATH, SIGNS OF; MUSCLE.)

RINGWORM, or TINEA, is the name given to inflammatory affections of the skin produced by a fungus. The main forms of ringworm in man are: (i) *Tinea capitis*, or ringworm of the scalp; (ii) *Tinea barbae*, or ringworm of the beard; (iii) *Tinea cruris*, or ringworm of the groin, and also known as dhobie itch; (iv) *Tinea pedis*, or ringworm of the feet; (v) *Tinea corporis*, or ringworm of the body; (vi) *Tinea unguium*, or ringworm of the nails; (vii) *Tinea favosa*, favus, or honeycomb ringworm, affecting scalp; (viii) *Tinea versicolor*.

RINGWORM OF THE SCALP, a disease of childhood, is usually due to a human species of fungus, *Microsporum audouini*; some 5 per cent of cases are due to infection by microspora acquired from cats and dogs. Boys are more infected than girls, and in both it disappears spontaneously at adolescence, being excessively rare in adults. It is most contagious. The incidence of the disease fell rapidly in the 1920–30s, and by 1939 was a rare condition in many parts of the country. The typical appearance is that of circular patches of lustreless, greyish, broken hairs scattered over the scalp. The scalp itself is covered with fine greyish-white scabs. Under Wood's light (the rays of a mercury vapour lamp screened through a special glass) the infected hairs have a bright green colour, which is diagnostic.

Treatment: As in all other forms of ringworm, the outlook has been radically changed by the introduction of the antibiotic, griseofulvin (q.v.). When used under medical supervision, this is the most effective method of treatment yet discovered, curing the condition in a high proportion of cases. Treatment should be continued for four weeks or until there is complete cure. In order to prevent reinfection, the infected hairs should be removed either manually, or by clipping and shaving, after three weeks' treatment with griseofulvin. A daily application of an anti-fungal preparation is not essential but is of value in preventing the spread of infection to other parts of the scalp or to other children. The child should be excluded from school until cured.

RINGWORM OF THE BEARD is one of the forms of barber's rash. There is a form occurring in grooms and cattlemen, in which the infection is acquired from animals.

Treatment: This consists of the administration of griseofulvin (q.v.). If suppuration is also present, hot fomentations of 2-per-cent sodium thiosulphate should be applied.

RINGWORM OF THE GROIN, or DHOBIE ITCH, is caused by a fungus of the same group as is responsible for ringworm of the foot: *Epidermophyton*. It occurs at any age, but is most common in young adult males. The eruption is a sharply defined, slightly raised reddish area, which begins in the inner aspect of the upper third of the thigh and tends to spread over the perineum. It is accompanied by considerable irritation at times.

Treatment: This consists of the administration of topical antifungal creams until the condition clears. Since a warm moist atmosphere encourages fungal growth, the groin should be kept dry and loose fitting underpants should be worn.

RINGWORM OF THE FOOT, or athlete's foot as it is often known, is one of the most common forms of ringworm at the present day. It is due to an *Epidermophyton*. Most common among adolescent and young adult males, the infection is usually acquired by walking with bare feet on infected floors: e.g. hotel and school bathrooms, public swimming baths, and pithead baths. The eruption begins between the toes as a rule, but may also be found on the soles of the feet. There are two main forms of eruption: (*a*) the *vesicular*, in which the affected area is covered with small blisters – this form begins on the sole; (*b*) the *intertriginous*, in which the skin between the toes becomes white and sodden, and peels off, leaving a raw red area. Before beginning to treat this type of ringworm it is particularly important to demonstrate the fungus in material removed from the affected area, as a superficially similar appearance may be produced by other infecting organisms or even by excessive sweating alone.

Treatment: Careful hygiene of the feet, particularly for those who tend to perspire freely in the feet, is essential: (*a*) to prevent infection; (*b*) to aid in curing the condition once acquired; (*c*) to prevent relapses. Such hygiene consists of washing the feet every night in warm water, drying them thoroughly but carefully. A fresh pair of socks should be worn every day and rubber footwear is best avoided. Once the infection is acquired, the treatment depends upon the local condition. Treatment is with antifungal creams, such as clotrimazole, miconazole, or econazole. More severe inflammatory conditions may require creams which combine an antifungal agent and a corticosteroid. Dusting powders have no place in treatment except for cosmetic purposes, perhaps, and indeed some powders can cause skin irritation. More resistant cases may require oral griseofulvin.

RINGWORM OF THE BODY, which may occur with ringworm of the scalp, may be due to either a microsporum or a tricophyton. The eruption consists of circular discs, usually red in colour at first, but later tending to become pale in the centre, and blisters may appear in the surrounding ring. There is considerable itching.

Treatment is as for other forms of ringworm of the skin.

RINGWORM OF THE NAILS is not common but is most resistant to treatment. Several nails are usually affected, and they turn a greenish-grey colour, and become brittle, separated from the nail-bed, and thickened and, as a result, difficult to manicure.

Treatment consists of the administration of griseofulvin, but treatment may need to be continued for long periods: for up to six months or longer. Toe-nails are particularly resistant to griseofulvin.

FAVUS is due to a fungus of the genus, *Tricophyton*. It occurs on the scalp, skin, and nails, and consists of thick yellow cups of crust. It is rare in Great Britain. It responds to griseofulvin.

TINEA VERSICOLOR, due to *Malassazia furfur*, is characterized by thin, faint yellowish patches on the chest and abdomen. Treatment consists of the local daily application of lotion of selenium sulphide (q.v.). Ketoconazole orally is usually effective. It usually recurs despite treatment.

KERION, or TINEA KERION, is a complication of ringworm of the scalp. It takes the form of a boggy mass involving several hair follicles. Small beads of pus may be seen on the surface. Treatment consists of oral griseofulvin and, in very severe inflammation, oral corticosteroids.

RINNES TEST: A hearing test in which a vibrating tuning fork is placed on the mastoid process (see EAR). When the subject can no longer hear the ringing, it is placed beside the ear. Normal subjects can then hear the noise once more, but in people with conductive deafness air conduction does not persist after bone conduction has ceased. It can help to distinguish between nerve and conduction deafness.

RIPPLE BEDS are a modern development of the conventional air-bed (q.v.). Their essential feature is a mattress which is alternately pressurized by a compressor to create a gentle rippling effect along the entire length of the mattress. This provides a continuous massaging motion which stimulates the circulation and helps to maintain the nutrition of the skin, thereby reducing the risk of bed sores (q.v.).

RISK FACTOR: An environmental or genetic factor which makes the occurrence of a disease in an individual more likely.

RISUS SARDONICUS is the term used for describing the facial appearance when the muscles of the forehead and the face go into spasm in tetanus, giving the effect of a sardonic grin.

RITODRINE is a drug that is used in the management of premature labour. It acts by suppressing the activity of the uterus. (See PREMATURE BIRTH.)

RNA is the abbreviation for ribonucleic acid, one of the two types of nucleic acid (q.v.) that exist in nature. It is present in both the cytoplasm and nucleus of the cells of the body, but principally in the former. With DNA (q.v.) it is an essential component of the genetic code. It exists in three categories known, respectively, as ribosomal (r), transfer (t), and messenger (m) RNA. Genetic information resides in the linear sequence of nucleotides (see NUCLEIC ACID) in DNA and is transcribed into messenger RNA before protein is synthesized. In the language of the computer, the genetic code consists of 64 three-letter code-words, or codons. The code in DNA is comparable to a tape which contains information written linearly in the form of these codons, each of which is the code for one of the 20 amino-acids (q.v.) from which proteins are made. The genetic information encoded in DNA is used to programme the manufacture of proteins in two stages.

In the first the information is transcribed from DNA on to a molecule of mRNA. In the second the messenger RNA-intermediary transports the information to the protein-manufacturing centres of the cell where the information is translated from the linear sequence of codons in the RNA into a linear sequence of amino-acids which are concurrently converted into protein.

ROCKY MOUNTAIN SPOTTED FEVER is a fever of the typhus group. It received its name from the fact that it was first reported in the Rocky Mountain States of USA. These are still the most heavily infected States, but it is now found in all parts of the United States. The causative organism is *Rickettsia rickettsi*, which is transmitted to man by tics. (See also TYPHUS FEVER.)

RODENT ULCER is a chronic form of ulcer, which is found chiefly about the nose and face of elderly people, and which gradually increases in size. It stands between a simple chronic ulcer and a cancer, being much slower in its growth than the latter. Treatment consists in cutting out the ulcer with the healthy skin for a little distance all round. It is also very amenable to treatment by X-rays, radium, and other forms of radiant energy.

ROMBERGISM is a term applied to marked unsteadiness in standing with the eyes shut. It is found as a symptom in some nervous diseases, such as peripheral neuropathy and tabes dorsalis.

ROOT FILLING or root-canal therapy is the treatment given when the nerve of a tooth has been exposed while the tooth is being prepared for a filling, or if it has died or become infected. The nerve debris is removed with thin files and, when the chamber is clear of infection, an inert radio-opaque material is inserted to seal off the root. This is generally effective.

RORSCHACH TEST is a method of investigating personality and disorders of personality. It was devised by a Swiss psychiatrist, Hermann Rorschach (1884–1922), who determined individuals' reactions to a series of symmetrical ink-blots, ten in number and standardized by him. The person investigated is shown the ink-blots in a defined order and is asked to describe what he sees. His descriptions and ideas about the blots are noted and an elaborate system of scoring is said to afford indications of the kind of personality and psychological make-up of the person investigated. Much work has been done on the test and it is thought highly of by experienced psychiatrists.

ROSACEA, or ACNE ROSACEA as it is sometimes known, is a condition in which there is chronic congestion of the flush areas of the face and forehead, leading to the formation of red papules. In the earlier stages the erythema, or redness of the skin, tends to wax and wane, being more marked after a meal or excessive drinking of alcohol or exposure to sunlight. Ultimately, however, the erythema becomes permanent, and may be accompanied by gross enlargement of the sebaceous glands (see SKIN), leading to the gross enlargement of the nose known as rhinophyma (q.v.) or grog blossoms. **Symptoms**: In the milder forms there is simple redness, burning, and tingling of the nose, the redness lasting at first only for a few hours every day, but later tending to become permanent, and also to appear upon the cheeks, forehead and chin. In the severer form the nose becomes very red and the skin thick and lumpy, while the openings of the sebaceous glands are seen as quite wide pits. In exceptional cases, more commonly in men than in women, there may be enormous enlargement of the sebaceous glands of the nose, the condition known as rhinophyma.
Treatment: Tetracycline is the treatment of choice and most patients respond to 250 mg twice daily for a period of 3 to 6 months.

ROSEOLA is a term applied to any rose-coloured rash.

ROSE-WAALER TEST is a blood test which is proving of value in the diagnosis of rheumatoid arthritis. It is positive in over 70 per cent of patients with this disease, compared with only 4 per cent of people not suffering from rheumatoid arthritis.

ROSE-WATER is prepared by soaking rose-petals in water and distilling over part of the fluid. It is used as an ingredient of cold-cream, etc. Rose oil, or attar of rose, is prepared by distilling the fresh flowers of *Rosa damascena*. It is largely used in perfumery, and in lozenges, dentifrices and ointments.

ROTAVIRUSES are a group of viruses (so-called from their wheel-like structure: *rota* is Latin for wheel) which are a common cause of gastroenteritis in infants (see DIARRHOEA). They are rarely found in children over 6 years of age. They cause from 25 to 80 per cent of childhood diarrhoea in different parts of the world. In the United Kingdom they are responsible for 60 to

65 per cent of cases. They infect only the cells lining the small intestine. In the United Kingdom death from rotavirus is rare.

ROUGHAGE, or dietary fibre, has long been known to affect bowel function. How it does this is still not quite clear but the probability is that it achieves this through its capacity to hold water in a gel-like form. But fibre is not an inert substance as was long thought to be the case. It is digested and metabolized in the colon by the micro-organisms there. This digestive process alters the properties of dietary fibre, including an increase in the amount of bile acids in the stools. The full significance of these changes is not yet known. Many claims are being made for the value of dietary fibre in maintaining health and preventing disease. What does seem to be clear is that it plays a role in the prevention of constipation, diverticular disease (see DIVERTICULOSIS) and the irritable bowel syndrome (q.v.). There is also some evidence that it may reduce the incidence of cancer of the colon. Though bran is not the panacea it is made out to be by some, there seems little doubt that modern western diets do not contain as much roughage, such as wholemeal flour, as they should.

ROULEAUX is the term applied to the heaps into which red blood corpuscles collect as seen under the microscope.

ROUNDWORMS (see ASCARIASIS).

ROUS SARCOMA is a malignant tumour of fowls which is caused by a virus. This tumour has been the subject of much experimental work bearing upon the nature of cancer.

RUBBING (see MASSAGE; LINIMENTS).

RUBEFACIENTS (see BLISTERS AND COUNTERIRRITANTS).

RUBELLA is another name for GERMAN MEASLES (q.v.).

RUPTURE is a popular name for hernia. (See HERNIA.)

RYLE'S TUBE (see NASOGASTRIC TUBE).

S

SABIN VACCINE: An oral vaccine used against poliomyelitis. The virus is cultured and with special treatment its strength is attenuated so that it may be safely injected but is still capable of stimulating the body's defence mechanism to produce appropriate antibodies and hence confer immunity. The oral vaccine is used for immunization in the United Kingdom (see SALK VACCINE).

SACCHARIN is a soluble coal-tar product of white crystalline appearance. It has an extremely sweet taste, being prepared in various strengths so as to equal in sweetness from 300 to 500 times its own weight of cane-sugar. It escapes from the body unchanged, having practically no effect upon the tissues beyond its influence upon the sensation of taste. Accordingly it is used by diabetics, fat people and others to whom sugar is harmful. It tends to give a bitter flavour to drinks to which it is added.

SACCHAROMYCES is another name for yeast.

SACRAL NERVES: The five pairs of spinal nerves that leave the spinal column in the sacral area. They carry motor and sensory fibres from the anal and genital regions and from both legs.

SACRAL VERTEBRAE: The five fused vertebrae that link the thoracic spine and the coccyx and form the sacrum.

SACROILEITIS: Inflammation of one or both of the sacroiliac joints, which lie between the sacrum and the iliac bones. The condition may be the result of rheumatoid arthritis, ankylosing spondylitis, Reiter's syndrome (qq.v.), or the arthritis that occurs with psoriasis (q.v.) or infection. Sacroileitis causes pain in the lower back, buttocks, thighs, and groin. Stiffness may occur with ankylosing spondylitis. Non-steroidal anti-inflammatory drugs relieve the symptoms and if the cause is infection antibiotics should be used.

SACRUM is the portion of the spinal column near its lower end. The sacrum consists of five vertebrae fused together to form a broad triangular bone which lies between the two haunch-bones and forms the back wall of the pelvis.

SADISM (Marquis de Sade) is the term applied to a form of sexual perversion, in which satisfaction is derived from the infliction of cruelty upon another person.

SAFE PERIOD is that period during the menstrual cycle when fertilization of the ovum is unlikely to occur. Ovulation usually occurs about 15 days before the onset of the menstrual period. A woman is commonly believed to be fertile for about 11 days in each menstrual cycle: i.e. on the day of ovulation and for 5 days before and 5 days after this. This would be the eighth to the eighteenth day of the usual 28-day menstrual cycle. Outside this fertile period is the SAFE PERIOD: the first week and the last ten days of the menstrual cycle. On the other hand, there is increasing evidence that the safest period is the last few days before menstruation. In the case of irregular menstruation it is not possible to calculate the safe period. In any event the safety is not absolute.

SAFETY OF DRUGS: The Medicines Act of 1968, which came into force in 1971, is a comprehensive measure replacing most of the previous legislation on the control of medicines for human and veterinary use. It is administered by the Health and Agriculture Ministers of the United Kingdom. It decreed the setting up of a Medicines Commission by the Ministers to give them advice generally relating to the execution of the provisions of the Act. On the advice of the Medicines Commission a series of expert advisory committees was set up. These are Standing Committees of independent experts, and consist of the Committee on Safety of Medicines, the Committee on the Review of Medicines, the Committee on Dental and Surgical Materials, the British Pharmacopoeia Commission which is responsible for the production of the *British Pharmacopoeia*, and the Veterinary Products Committee.

The Committee on Safety of Medicines (CSM) has the function of scrutinizing the efficacy, quality and safety of new drugs before clinical trial and before marketing, as well as the surveillance of each drug after marketing so that adverse reactions are monitored and documented, and warnings issued as required. Early clinical trial for a drug can only be carried out after a clinical trial certificate has been issued by the licensing authority: i.e. all Ministers specified in the Act. In the case of human medicines the Minister acts through the Medicines Division of the Department of Health.

The major defect in this carefully worked out system is the difficulty in obtaining reports of adverse reaction. The present evidence suggests that at most about 10 per cent of such reactions are reported. One method of trying to obtain this information is the yellow card system. It is so called because it is based on the distribution of yellow cards to all doctors and dentists, on which they are asked to report any adverse reaction they may encounter to a drug even though initially the evidence may not be 100 per cent certain. Alternatively the CSM has a Freephone line for practitioners to use. Even though the annual number of adverse reactions reported in this way has risen from aound 5,000 in 1975 to over 17,000 in 1990, there is ample evidence that this represents only a fraction of the adverse reactions that actually occur.

Two further committees in this safety screen are the Joint Committee on Vaccination and Immunization and the Adverse Reactions to Vaccines and Immunological Substances Committee. The function of the Committee on Review of Medicines is to review all medicinal products on the British market.

SAGITTAL is the term applied to a structure or section running from front to back in the body.

ST VITUS'S DANCE is an out moded name for CHOREA (q.v.).

SALBUTAMOL is a drug that is proving of value, and safe, for the relief of spasm of the bronchi in asthma.

SALICYLIC ACID is a white substance in fine crystals, of sweetish taste, and sparingly soluble in water.
Action: Salicylic acid is an antiseptic. Externally it is used in ointments to check various skin affections due to bacteria, and, since it has in addition a softening action on the surface of the skin, salicylic acid plasters are used to remove corns and various other superficial overgrowths.

SALINES are purgatives belonging to the class of salts which produce watery evacuations. (See PURGATIVES.) For normal or isotonic saline solution see ISOTONIC.

SALIVA is the fluid which is always present to some extent in the mouth, and is secreted in specially copious amount during a meal, or when the salivary glands are stimulated, as for example by an acid substance placed in the mouth. Saliva contains much mucus and a ferment known as ptyalin, which changes starch into dextrose and maltose (see DIGESTION); also many cells of different types. About 750 millilitres are produced daily.

The principal function of saliva is to aid in the initial processes of digestion. When food is taken into the mouth, an increased output of saliva is evoked. This saliva is essential for the process of mastication (q.v.), whereby food is reduced to a homogeneous mass before being swallowed. In addition, the ptyalin in the saliva initiates the digestion of starch in the food.

An excessive flow of saliva known as *salivation* occurs as the result of taking certain drugs over a considerable period. Salivation also occurs as the result of irritation in the mouth, as for instance, in the teething child, and from dyspepsia. Dribbling of saliva is a common symptom of bulbar paralysis. The converse state of lack, or deficiency, of saliva is known as xerostomia (q.v.).

SALIVARY GLANDS are the glands situated near, and opening into, the cavity of the mouth, by which the saliva is manufactured. They include the *parotid gland*, placed in the deep space that lies between the ear and the angle of the jaw; the *submandibular gland*, lying beneath the horizontal part of the jaw-bone; and the *sublingual gland*, which lies beneath the tongue.

Each gland is made up of branching tubes closely packed together, and supported by strong connective tissue. These tubes are lined by large cells that secrete the saliva, and from their interior lead ducts that unite with one another to form ultimately the large main ducts that open into the mouth. The appearance and character of the secreting cells vary in different glands. In the parotid gland they secrete a clear fluid containing the ferment, ptyalin; in the sublingual gland they mainly produce mucus, whilst the submandibular gland contains cells of both types.

SALK VACCINE: Treating the poliomyelitis virus with formalin stops it causing the disease but still allows the virus to stimulate the production of antibodies. Salk vaccine is given by injection and protects the recipient against the disease. The orally given Sabin vaccine is used in the United Kingdom.

SALMONELLA INFECTIONS, or SALMO-NELLOSIS (see FOOD POISONING).

SALMON PATCHES are small pink patches found in some new-born infants – on the eyelids, on the forehead between the eyes, and on the nape of the neck. Those on the first two of these three sites have usually faded by the baby's first birthday, but those on the nape of the neck may be more persistent. (See also BIRTH-MARKS.)

SALPINGITIS is inflammation situated in the Fallopian tubes.

SALPINGO- is a prefix indicating a connection with either the Fallopian (or uterine) tubes or the Eustachian (or auditory) tubes.

SALT is the substance produced by the replacement of the acidic hydrogen of an acid by a metal or basic radical. It is also a synonym for common salt or sodium chloride.

SALTPETRE (see NITRE).

SAL VOLATILE is another name for aromatic solution of ammonia, a liquid of burning taste and great stimulating powers. Its action depends upon various volatile oils, ammonia, and bicarbonate of ammonia which it contains. It is used as a stimulating expectorant in cough mixtures, and is valuable as a stimulant in faints. The dose is from half to one teaspoonful (1 to 5 millilitres) in a wineglassful of water. (See AMMONIA.)

SANDFLY FEVER, also known as PHLEBO-TOMUS FEVER, THREE-DAY FEVER, and PAPATACI FEVER, is a short, sharp fever occurring in many parts of the tropics and subtropics, including most of the Mediterranean littoral, due to a virus conveyed by the bite of a small hairy midge or sandfly (*Phlebotomus papatasi*). The incubation period is three to seven days.
Symptoms: There are headache, feverishness, general sensations like those of influenza, flushed face and bloodshot eyes, but no signs of catarrh. The fever passes off in three days, but the patient may take some time to convalesce.
Treatment: As there is no specific remedy, prophylaxis is important. This consists of the spraying of rooms with an insecticide such as Gammexane; the application of insect repellents such as dimethyl phthalate to the exposed parts of the body (e.g. ankles, wrists and face), particularly at sunset; and the use of sandfly nets at night. Once the infection is acquired, treatment consists of rest in bed, light diet and aspirin and codeine.

SANGUINEOUS means containing blood.

SAPHENOUS is the name given to the two large superficial veins of the leg. The small saphenous vein which runs up the outside and back of the leg joins the deep veins at the bend of the knee; the great saphenous vein, the longest vein in the body, which has a long course from the inner ankle to the groin, is specially subject, with its branches, to become the site of varicose veins.

SAPO is the Latin name for soap.

SAPROPHYTE is the term applied to organisms which live usually upon decaying and dead matter and produce its decomposition.

SARCO- is a prefix signifying flesh or fleshy.

SARCOIDOSIS is a chronic disease of unknown origin. It involves the skin, lymph nodes, eyes, salivary glands, lungs, heart and bones of the hands and feet. The Kveim Test is used to confirm the diagnosis. The disease is usually self limiting but occasionally treatment with corticosteroids is required.

SARCOMA (see CANCER).

SARCOPTES SCABIEI is the mite which causes scabies (q.v.).

SAUNA is a hot-air, steam or smoke bath, combined with ice-cold water bathing or douching. An old Finnish practice, practically every house or block of flats there has its sauna. Originally, these log cabins were heated by wood-burning stoves made of rough stones, but the modern sauna has an electric oven surrounded by stones. The sauna cabin has a tightly fitting door and narrow vents in the walls, but no windows. The bathers sit or lie naked, according to their preferences, on wooden benches. Before entering the sauna, with its temperature of 110 °F (43.3 °C), a cold shower is taken. Periodically the bathers come out and plunge into a nearby ice-cold lake or have another cold shower. At some stage of the sauna massage is given, or alternatively the bathers beat each other with birch twigs. After this a further session is spent in the heat, and the course ends with a cold bath. The bather should rest for twenty minutes or until he has ceased to sweat before beginning to dress. The precise therapeutic value of saunas may not be clear, though the Finns claim that they are a well-proven means of maintaining health. There is some evidence that they may be good for the skin, the upper air passages, weight reduction, and for the relief of rheumatic pains.

SCAB is the crust which forms on superficial injured areas. It is composed of fibrin, which is exuded from the raw surface, together with blood corpuscles and epithelial cells entangled in its meshes. Healing takes place naturally under this protection, and the scab dries up and falls off when healing is complete. Scabs appearing on the face without any previous abrasion are often of infectious nature. (See IMPETIGO.)

SCABIES is a skin disease caused by the *Sarcoptes scabiei* which resembles the cheese mite in appearance. It is a minute oval-shaped mite possessing four pairs of legs. It is just visible to the naked eye, the female measuring about 250 to 350 micrometres in length; the male is smaller. The female burrows in the skin, particularly that on the front of the wrist, the web and sides of the fingers, the buttocks, the genitals, and the feet, forming small tunnels in which she lays her eggs (25 to 30). The sides and legs may also be affected in the same way, though rarely the upper parts of the body. The eggs hatch in the burrows in four to five days, and it is the movement of the larvae which causes the intense itching which gives scabies its popular name of itch. The scratching caused by this itching is responsible for much of the eruption of scabies. The larvae ultimately leave the burrows and develop in the skin, a female becoming mature in about two weeks.

Scabies is rife among the population of Great Britain. Personal contact is the most important factor in keeping this infestation going. This is why it is so important that all members of a household in which a case occurs should be carefully examined, and treated if found to be infected. Less stress is now laid on dissemination of the mite by infested clothes and blankets.

Symptoms: The person complains of great itchiness and heat, felt particularly soon after he goes to bed, and preventing sleep in the early part of the night. The spaces between the fingers, the backs of the hands, and the front of the wrists are red and scabbed as the result of scratching, or the surface in these localities may even be much inflamed.

Treatment: The patient is scrubbed with soft soap in a hot bath, to open up the burrows. Immediately after drying, the official *British Pharmacopoeia* 25 per cent preparation of benzyl benzoate, known as Benzyl Benzoate Application BP, is applied to the whole surface of the body below the chin. A second and a third application is made at twelve-hourly intervals. The patient then has a bath, puts on clean underclothes, and has his bed clothes changed. In infants and young children, in whom benzyl benzoate may cause unpleasant stinging, monosulfiram or 1 per cent gamma benzene hexachloride may be used as an alternative.

SCALDS (see BURNS AND SCALDS).

SCALP is the soft covering of the skull on the top of the head. It consists of five layers, which from the surface inwards are as follows: the skin, thickly furnished with hair; next a subcutaneous layer of fat, rendered tough and stringy by many bands of fibrous tissue passing through it to bind the skin and the third layer together; thirdly, a tough membrane composed of fibrous tissue, known as the epicranium; fourthly, a loose layer of connective tissue attaching the epicranium to the deepest layer, and permitting the free movements of which the scalp is capable; and, finally, another fibrous layer clinging closely to the skull, and known as the pericranium.

SCANNING SPEECH: A speech disorder in which articulated syllables are wrongly spaced and each is given the same vocal emphasis. The condition occurs as a result of disease in the cerebellum or its connecting nerves.

SCALPEL is a small, straight, surgical knife.

SCAPHOID BONE: The outside bone on the thumb side of the hand in the row of carpal (wrist) bones nearest to forearm. Fracture of the scaphoid is a common wrist injury that usually occurs when someone falls on to their outstretched hand. The fracture may be missed in which case pain in and permanent damage to the wrist can occur.

SCAPULA is the technical name for the shoulder-blade. (See SHOULDER-BLADE.)

SCAR is the name applied to a healed wound, ulcer or breach of tissue. A scar consists essentially of fibrous tissue, covered by an imperfect formation of epidermis in the case of scars on the surface of the skin. The fibrous tissue is produced by the connective tissue corpuscles that wander into the wound in the course of its repair (see WOUNDS), and is at first delicate in texture and richly provided with blood-vessels. Accordingly a scar at first is soft and has a redder tint than the surrounding skin

Gradually this fibrous tissue contracts, becomes more dense, and loses its blood-vessels, so that an old scar is hard and white.

The more specialized textures are not repaired when a scar forms: thus on the skin-surface the scar does not reproduce hairs and sweat-glands, only the general epithelium growing over the wounded surface. Similarly in the case of internal organs, such as the stomach, no glands form in the scar. When muscles or nerves are wounded, however, new muscle- or nerve-fibres grow into the scar. Bone is repaired by a formation of fibrous tissue, which is produced just as in the soft parts, and later lime salts are deposited in the scars. (See BONE.)

The contraction that takes place in a scar has already been mentioned. The more quickly the surfaces of a wound are brought into contact with one another, the less fibrous tissue is produced for the union. Consequently a wound whose edges are accurately brought together and in which healing is rapid shows far less contraction afterwards, and leaves a fainter scar, than one in which the wound is allowed to gape, and in which healing is slow. Burns are therefore followed by very marked scars and great contraction, which often produces marked deformity of the part concerned. Similarly, when inflammation takes place, as when an operation wound becomes infected, or when such a disease as lupus is present, causing great irritation of the wound, a wide, unsightly scar results and causes much puckering of the surrounding skin as it contracts. Such scars are also of low vitality, stretch easily, so as to become still more evident, and if irritated, as, for example, by the pressure of a boot or badly fitting artificial limb, readily give way and produce an ulcer which is slow to heal. Unsightly scars, on the face for example, can often be removed by the plastic surgeon.

Scars are sometimes extremely painful, especially those which are left after the amputation of part of a limb. This is caused in general by the involvement of a sensory nerve in the hard contracting tissue of the scar. (See also KELOID.)

SCARLET FEVER is caused by the erythrogenic toxin of the streptococcus. The symptoms of pyrexia, headache, vomiting and a punctate erythematous rash follow a streptococcal infection of the throat or even a wound. The rash is symmetrical and does not itch. The skin subsequently peels. In the latter half of the 19th century it was the commonest cause of death in children over the age of one year. The mortality was already decreasing by the year 1900 and had virtually ceased by 1965.

Symptoms: The period of incubation (i.e. the time elapsing between the reception of infection and the development of symptoms) varies somewhat. In most cases it lasts only two to three days, but in occasional cases the patient may take a week to develop his first symptoms. The invasion of fever is usually short and sharp, with rapid rise of temperature to 40 °C (104 °F) or thereabouts in the first few hours. There also

occur shivering, vomiting, headache, sore throat and marked increase in the rate of the pulse. In young children convulsions or delirium may also usher in the fever. The rash usually appears within 24 hours of the onset of fever. Sometimes the redness is accompanied by small vesicles containing fluid. The rash is at its height in about two days and then begins to fade, being gone at the end of a week from its first appearance.

Complications: The most common and serious of these is *inflammation of the kidneys*, or *glomerulonephritis*, which may arise during any period in the course of the fever, but is specially apt to appear in convalescence, while desquamation is in progress. Occasionally this condition does not wholly pass off, and consequently lays the foundation for chronic glomerulonephritis. (See GLOMERULONEPHRITIS.) Another complication is *suppuration of the ears*, due to the extension of the inflamatory process from the throat along the Eustachian tube into the middle ear. (See EAR, DISEASES OF.) Other disorders affecting the heart and lungs occasionally arise in connection with scarlet fever, the chief of these being *endocarditis*, which may lay the foundation of valvular disease of the heart later in life. Arthritis or *scarlatinal rheumatism* is another complication of the disease, producing swelling and pain in the smaller rather than in the larger joints. This complication usually occurs in the second week of illness.

Treatment: In view of the mild type of scarlet fever at present prevailing there is a tendency in Great Britain not to admit such cases to hospital unless they are particularly severe, the home conditions are unsatisfactory, or there is some risk to the public: e.g. a member of the household works in a dairy and may therefore be responsible for infecting milk. Children who have been in contact with cases of scarlet fever are allowed to go to school provided they are sent home at the first suggestion of fever or malaise.

As scarlet fever is predominantly a streptococcal infection, penicillin should be given.

SCHISTOSOMIASIS, also known as BILHARZIASIS, is one of the most important diseases in the tropics. The estimated global incidence is 200 million cases. The responsible parasites, *schistosomes* or blood flukes, which are responsible for the disease, occur in Egypt, the Middle East, many parts of tropical Africa, the Far East, and South America. The male is about 12 millimetres long. The female, which is about 24 millimetres in length, lies partly enclosed in a groove down the body of the male. The ova, or eggs, are provided with a sharp spike which is terminal in *S. haematobium* and lateral in *S. mansoni*. The schistosomes live in the portal vein and its branches. The ova ultimately reach either the bladder (*S. haematobium*) or the rectum (*S. mansoni* and *S. japonicum*), whence they are voided in the urine or faeces. The next stage of development takes place in certain snails. Human infection occurs by wading or bathing in infected water, the infection occurring through the skin, whence the immature schistosome ultimately reaches the portal vein.

SCHISTOSOMA HAEMATOBIUM is widely distributed throughout North Africa, including Egypt, East Africa, and South Africa. It is also found in the Middle East, Portugal and Cyprus. As the ova are excreted through the bladder, the main symptoms are cystitis and haematuria (i.e. the passage of blood in the urine). In chronic cases there may be formation of stones in the bladder, and sometimes cancer develops in the bladder.

SCHISTOSOMA MANSONI is found predominantly in the Nile valley, East Africa, and West Africa. It is also found in Israel, Yemen, Central and South America and the Caribbean Islands. As the ova are mainly excreted through the rectum, the first manifestation of the disease is usually diarrhoea, with the passage of much blood in the stools. As with *S. haematobium* infections, there is often irritation of the skin or dermatitis, and there is always some anaemia, which may become severe. The spleen usually becomes enlarged, sometimes to a very considerable extent.

SCHISTOSOMA JAPONICUM is confined to the Far East, particularly the Yangtse valley, and South East Asia, particularly Indonesia. Here again the ova are found in the rectum, and the main manifestations of the infection are chronic dysentery, enlargement of the liver and the spleen, and anaemia.

Treatment: While prevention is the ideal way of coping with the disease, this is often difficult in practice. Drugs used in treating the disease include various preparations, such as metriphonate for *S. haematobium* infections, oxamniquine for *S. mansoni* infections, and praziquantel which is active against all three varieties.

SCHIZO- is a prefix signifying splitting.

SCHIZOPHRENIA (See MENTAL ILLNESS.)

SCHWANN CELL: The cells that produce the myelin (q.v.) sheath of the axon (q.v.) of a medullated nerve. They are wrapped around a segment of the axon, forming concentric layers.

SCIATICA means pain in the distribution of the sciatic nerve. It is often accompanied by pain in the back, or lumbago. It may be due to a number of causes, such as a tumour in the spine or spinal column, tuberculosis of the spine, ankylosing spondylitis (see SPINE AND SPINAL CORD, DISEASES AND INJURIES OF) or a tumour in one of the organs in the pelvis such as the uterus. In the majority of cases, however, it is due to a prolapsed intervertebral disc (q.v.) pressing on one or more of the nerve roots issuing from the lower part of the spinal cord that make up the sciatic nerve. The precise distribution of the pain will thus depend on which of the nerve roots are affected. As a rule, the pain is felt in the buttock, the back of the thigh and the outside and front of the leg, sometimes extending on to the top of the foot. In other cases the pain is felt in the buttock, the back of the thigh and the calf, and then along the outer border of the foot towards the little toe. What probably happens is that degenerative changes take place in the annulus fibrosus. (See SPINAL COLUMN.) Ultimately this ruptures, either as a result of some special strain such as is induced by heavy lifting, or spontaneously. The cushioning disc between the two neighbouring vertebral bodies slips through the rent in the annulus fibrosus, and presses on the neighbouring roots, thus causing the pain.

The condition usually occurs in adults under the age of 60. The pain may come on suddenly when the person concerned is undertaking some unusual effort, such as heavy lifting, and may be so severe that the victim faints and, when he comes to, he may be locked in one position. More commonly it comes on gradually and keeps on recurring over long periods of time. In these cases the amount of pain varies tremendously: from little more than a recurrent nuisance to a pain of almost unbearable intensity.

Treatment consists essentially of rest in bed in the early stages until the acute phase is over. Boards should be placed underneath the mattress to ensure adequate support for the back. Alternatively, the mattress may be put on the floor for the patient to sleep on. Anodynes, such as aspirin and codeine, are given to relieve the pain. A few days' rest in bed at the beginning of the trouble probably reduces the risk of further trouble. Expert opinion varies as to the desirability of wearing a plaster of Paris jacket or a specially made corset. Some contend that such support is advisable. Others contend that it is seldom necessary. Certainly a corset of this type is uncomfortable to wear, and there is a tendency for some victims of the disease to become too dependent on it. Equally, opinion differs as to the desirability of manipulation of the spine and operation. By and large the tendency in recent years has been for a reduction in the number of operations performed for prolapsed intervertebral disc.

SCIRRHUS is a hard form of cancer in which much fibrous tissue develops.

SCLERA (see EYE).

SCLERITIS (see EYE, DISEASE AND INJURIES).

SCLERODERMA is a condition in which the skin becomes hard – like leather – causing stiffening of the joints, and leading to gradual wasting of the muscles.

SCLEROSIS means literally hardening, and is a term applied to conditions in which portions of organs become hard and useless as the result of an excessive production of connective tissue. The term is especially applied to a change of this type taking place in the nervous system. (See MULTIPLE SCLEROSIS.) When a change of this nature takes place in other organs it is generally known as cirrhosis or fibrosis. (See CIRRHOSIS.) These conditions are generally attributed to some form of chronic inflammation.

SCLEROTHERAPY: A treatment that involves injecting varicose veins (see VEINS, DISEASES OF) with a sclerosing fluid. This causes fibrosis of the lining of the vein and its eventual obliteration. Sclerotherapy is also used to treat varicose veins in the legs, anus (haemorrhoids) and at the junction of the oesophagus (q.v.) with the stomach.

SCOLIOSIS is the name applied to curvature of the spine consisting partly of a bend to one side, partly of a rotary twist. It may result from disease of the spine, but in weakly children it may arise from so slight a cause as a bad habit in standing or in leaning one arm on the table at lessons. It also arises from disease affecting one side of the chest, such as chronic pleurisy or tuberculosis. (See SPINE AND SPINAL CORD, DISEASES OF.)

SCOTOMA: An area of blindness in the field of vision.

SCREENING TEST: The screening of apparently healthy people to identify those who may have treatable diseases. Cervical smears are done when screening women to detect if they have cancer or precancer of the neck of the womb (cervix). Factors to be assessed when planning screening procedures include the severity, frequency, and distribution of the disease and the availability and effectiveness of treatment. Convenience, safety, sensitivity and cost should also be assessed.

SCRIVENER'S PALSY is another name for writer's cramp. (See CRAMP.)

SCROFULA, or STRUMA, is tuberculosis of the glands in the neck. It was formerly known in England as 'king's evil', from the belief that the touch of the sovereign could effect a cure. This superstition can be traced back to the time of Edward the Confessor in England, and to a much earlier period in France. Samuel Johnson was touched by Queen Anne in 1712, and the same supposed prerogative of royalty was exercised by Prince Charles Edward in 1745. The disease, which is treated with antituberculous drugs, is now rare and usually affects young children.

SCROMBOTOXIN POISONING occurs from eating poorly preserved scromboid fish such as tuna, mackerel and other members of the mackerel family. In such fish, a toxic histamine-like substance is produced by the action of bacteria or histidine, a normal component of fish flesh. This toxin produces nausea, vomiting, headache, upper abdominal pain, difficulty in swallowing, thirst, itching (q.v.) and sometimes urticaria (q.v.). The condition settles as a rule in 12 hours. Antihistamine drugs (q.v.) are sometimes of value in ameliorating the condition.

SCROTUM is the pouch of integument within which the testicles are suspended. It consists of a purse-like fold of skin, within which each testicle has a separate investment of muscle fibres, several layers of fibrous tissue, and a serous membrane known as the tunica vaginalis.

SCRUM-POX, or PROP-POX, is a popular name for a contagious affection of the face affecting Rugby football players. It is most likely to occur in forwards as a result of face-to-face contact with cases in the opposing side of the scrum. In one recent investigation, 47 of 48 cases were forwards. Other possible sources of infection are changing rooms and communal baths. The condition may take the form of impetigo (q.v.) or herpes simplex (q.v.).

SCURF, or DANDRUFF, is a popular name for the scaly condition that is often found on the scalp, and often precedes baldness. (See SEBORRHOEA.)

SCURVY, or SCORBUTUS, is a deficiency disease characterized by the occurrence of extravasations of blood in the tissues of the body, and due to an insufficiency of vitamin C, or ascorbic acid, in the diet.
Causes: In former times this disease was extremely common among sailors, and was responsible for a high mortality rate. It is now of rare occurrence at sea, its cause being well understood and its prevention readily secured by simple measures. Scurvy has also frequently broken out among soldiers on campaign, in beleaguered cities, as well as among communities in times of scarcity, and in prisons, workhouses and other public institutions. In all such instances it has been found to depend closely upon the character and amount of the food, the occurrence of serious illness, and a diet too limited, either in amount or variety. These conditions predispose to scurvy, but the essential cause lies in deprivation of fresh food and especially of fresh vegetables for a period of four to six months. The want of vitamin C, which is soluble in water and is found chiefly in citrus fruits, potatoes, green vegetables and black currants, is the essential deficient factor. Besides this essential defect, a diminution in the total amount of food, the large use of salted meat or fish, and all causes of a depressing kind, such as exposure, anxiety, bad hygiene, will contribute to the development of the disease.

Infants, too, may suffer from scurvy as the result of insufficiency of vitamin C in the diet.

Symptoms: The symptoms of scurvy come on gradually, and its onset is not marked by any special indications beyond a certain failure of strength, most manifest on making efforts. Breathlessness and exhaustion are thus easily induced, and there exists a corresponding mental depression. The countenance acquires a sallow or dusky hue; the gums are tender and the breath offensive almost from the first. These preliminary symptoms may continue for weeks, and in isolated cases may readily escape notice, but can scarcely fail to attract attention where they affect large numbers of men. Later the gums are livid, spongy, ulcerating and bleeding; the teeth are loosened and drop out; and the breath is excessively foetid. Extravasations of blood now take place in the skin and elsewhere. These may be small, like the petechial spots of purpura (q.v.), but are often large, and cause swellings of the muscles in which they occur, having the appearance of extensive bruises, and tending to become hard and brawny. These extravasations are most common in the muscles of the lower limbs; but they may be formed anywhere, and may easily be produced by very slight pressure upon the skin or by injuries to it. Bleeding into joints is a troublesome symptom because it produces stiffness later. In addition, there are bleedings from mucous membranes, such as those of the nose, eyes and alimentary or respiratory tracts, whilst effusions of fluid take place into the pleural, pericardial or peritoneal cavity. Painful, extensive, and destructive ulcers are apt to break out on the limbs. There is also a considerable amount of anaemia. The further progress of the malady is marked by profound exhaustion, with a tendency to fainting, and with various complications, such as diarrhoea and lung or kidney troubles, any of which may bring about a fatal result. On the other hand, even in desperate cases, recovery may be hopefully anticipated when the appropriate remedy can be obtained.

Treatment: No disease is more amenable to treatment, both as regards prevention and cure, than scurvy. This consists of the administration of vitamin C in adequate amounts, either in the form of tablets of ascorbic acid or foodstuffs rich in this vitamin. Potatoes, cabbages, tomatoes, swede turnips, many fresh fruits, especially black currants, oranges, grapefruit and lemons, are of great service for this purpose. Orange-juice or lemon-juice is often employed, either fresh or canned. The use, in a fresh state, of lime-juice in the British Navy, which has been practised since 1795, had the effect of virtually extinguishing scurvy in the Service, whilst similar regulations introduced by the British Board of Trade in 1865 had a like beneficial result in the mercantile marine. It is only when these regulations have not been fully carried out, or when the supply of lime-juice has become exhausted, that scurvy among sailors has been noticed in recent times. The anaemia and debility are best overcome by the continued administration of iron, aided by fresh air and other measures calculated to promote the general health.

SEA-SICKNESS (see MOTION SICKNESS).

SEBACEOUS CYST is the term applied to a cyst in the skin formed as a result of blockage of the duct of a sebaceous gland.

SEBACEOUS GLANDS are the minute glands situated alongside of hairs and opening into the follicles of the latter a short distance below the point at which the hairs emerge on the surface . These glands secrete an oily material, and are especially large upon the nose, where their openings form pits that are easily visible. Some varieties of eczema, as well as acne, result from disorders of these glands. (See SKIN.)

SEBORRHOEA is a group of diseases of the skin in which the sebaceous or oil-forming glands are at fault. It manifests itself either by accumulation of dry scurf, or by the formation of an excessive oily deposit on an otherwise healthy skin.

Seborrhoeic dermatitis (or **eczema**), which is also known as SEBORRHOEA CAPITIS, is the form of seborrhoea which involves the scalp. In its mildest form it is little more than an exaggeration of the normal casting off of the superficial layers of the skin of the scalp (see SKIN), which manifests itself as the white scales popularly known as dandruff or scurf. In the more severe cases the amount of scaling is increased and is accompanied by redness of the scalp. This in turn may progress to such a stage that it is accompanied by a profuse discharge, sufficient to soak the victim's pillow at night. In these more severe cases the condition may spread to the forehead, eyebrows and back of the neck. There may indeed be involvement of these sites with minimal scalp disease.

Treatment in the milder cases consists of washing the hair twice weekly with spirit soap or a soapless shampoo. Shampoos containing tar extracts, for example Polytar, may be useful and they are also used to treat psoriasis of the scalp. Selenium sulphide shampoos are also of benefit, though no more so than others. In more severe cases, lotions containing combinations of corticosteroids and salicylic or salicylic acid and sulphur are effective.

SEBUM is the secretion of the sebaceous glands (q.v.). It acts as a natural lubricant of the hair and skin and protects the skin from the effects of moisture or excessive dryness. It may also have antibacterial action.

SECONDARY PREVENTION: The early detection of disease that reduces or prevents its serious outcome. Routine regular examination of particular age groups – for example, children or the elderly – and screening tests are examples of secondary prevention.

SECONDARY SEXUAL CHARACTERISTICS: The physical characteristics that develop during puberty as the body matures sexually. Girl's breasts and genitals increase in size and like boys they grow pubic hair. Boys also grow facial hair, their voice breaks and their genitals grow to adult size.

SECRETIN is a hormone secreted by the mucous membrane of the duodenum, the first part of the small intestine, when food comes in contact with it. On being carried by the blood to the pancreas, it stimulates the secretion of pancreatic juice.

SECRETION is the term applied to the material formed by a gland as the result of its activity. For example, saliva is the secretion of the salivary glands, gastric juice that of the glands in the stomach wall, bile that of the liver. (See GLANDS.) Some secretions consist apparently of waste material which is of no further use in the chemistry of the body. These secretions are often spoken of as excretions: for example, the urine and the sweat. (For further details, see SALIVA; URINE; ENDOCRINE GLANDS, and also under the headings of the various organs.)

SECTION: (1) A thin slice of a tissue specimen taken for examination under a microscope. (2) The act of cutting in surgery; for example, an abdominal section is done to explore the abdomen. (3) The issuing of an order under the United Kingdom's Mental Health Act to admit someone compulsorily to a psychiatric hospital.

SECUNDINES is another name for the afterbirth, consisting of the placenta and membranes expelled in the final stage of labour.

SECUNDUM ARTEM is a Latin expression meaning in a skilful professional manner.

SEDATIVES are drugs and other measures which soothe over-excitement of the nervous system, whether the effect of this excitement is pain, sleeplessness, delirium or muscular spasm. Those sedatives that soothe pain are generally spoken of as anodynes; sedatives in sleeplessness or delirium are known as hypnotics; sedatives of spasm are called antispasmodics. (See ANODYNES; COLIC; HEADACHE; HYPNOTICS; NEURALGIA; PAIN.)

SEDIMENTATION RATE (see ESR).

SELENIUM SULPHIDE is used as a shampoo in the treatment of dandruff (see SEBORRHOEA)

and seborrhoeic eczema (or dermatitis) of the scalp. In view of its potential toxicity it should only be used under medical supervision. It must never be applied to inflamed areas of the scalp, and it must not be allowed to get into the eyes, as it may cause conjunctivitis or keratitis. It is also used in the treatment of tinea versicolor. (See RINGWORM.)

SELF-POISONING has increased dramatically over the past 30 years and is now one of the commonest causes of acute admission to hospital. Drugs are usually taken in overdosage on impulse because of a crisis in coping with social or personal difficulties and most patients have previously been prescribed psychotrophic drugs. It is predominently a disease of young people, the mean age being in the 30s with a peak incidence in the 20s. There is a higher incidence of female patients. Fortunately about 98 per cent of patients admitted with drug overdosage will recover. Even so, there were around 300 deaths from suicide by overdose among young people in 1989 in England and Wales. There have been changes in the types of drugs used in deliberate self-poisoning. In 1962 barbiturates were used in 55 per cent of episodes whereas the benzodiazapines are now the most common drug used. The incidence of salicylate poisoning has declined but overdosage with paracetamol has become more common. Admission to hospital for self-poisoning reached its peak in 1977 and the figures have been falling steadily almost every year since then. This is also true of the number of fatal suicidal poisonings. There may be more than one explanation for this decrease but the most likely cause is that since 1976 the annual number of prescriptions for hypnotics and tranquillizers has also fallen steadily. The tranquillizers which are so popular for overdoses are prescribed for the very patients who are most likely to wish to poison themselves. There was, in fact, a parallel decrease in the rate of carbon monoxide poisoning when carbon monoxide was removed from domestic gas.

Treatment: Emptying the stomach by gastric lavage is sometimes necessary but the risks of this procedure must be balanced against the toxicity of the ingested poison. The danger of gastric aspiration is the inhalation of stomach contents and it should not be attempted in drowsy patients unless there is good cough reflex or unless the airway can be protected by a cuffed tube. A tube should not be passed after corrosive poisoning. Emptying the stomach by gastric lavage is of doubtful value more than four hours after ingestion of a poison. There are, however, two exceptions, namely salicylates and tricyclic antidepressants. Salicylates may be recovered up to 24 hours and tricyclic antidepressants up to 8 hours after ingestion. Gastric lavage is seldom practical or desirable before the patient reaches hospital.

The more common poisons seen today include the amphetamine-related drugs, aspirin and other salicylates, tranquillizers, iron salts,

lithium salts, morphine, paracetamol, phenothiazines, tricyclic antidepressants, carbon
monoxide, paraquat and organophosphorus
insecticides.

SELLA TURCICA is the deep hollow on the
upper surface of the sphenoid bone in which the
pituitary gland (q.v.) is enclosed.

SEMEN is the richly albuminous fluid in which
spermatozoa are suspended.

SEMILUNAR CARTILAGES are two crescentic layers of fibro- cartilage on the outer
and inner edges of the knee-joint, which form
hollows on the upper surface of the tibia in
which the condyles at the lower end of the
femur rest. The inner cartilage is especially
liable to be displaced by a sudden and violent
movement at the knee. (See KNEE.)

SEMINAL VESICLE is one of the small paired
sacs lying on either side of the male urethra
(q.v.), which collect and store spermatozoa.
(See TESTICLE.)

SENILE DEMENTIA: Dementia has traditionally been divided into presenile and senile
types. This is increasingly recognized as an
arbitrary division of a condition in which there
is a general and often slow decline in mental
capabilities. Around 10 per cent of people over
65 years of age and 20 per cent over 75 are
affected by dementing illness, but people under
65 may also be affected. Treatable causes such
as brain tumour, head injury, encephalitis and
alcoholism are commoner in younger people.
Other causes such as cerebrovascular disease,
which is a major factor, especially among older
people, or Alzheimer's disease are not readily
treatable, although antihypertensive treatment
for the former disorder may help and symptomatic treatment for both is possible. Individuals with dementia suffer a gradual deterioration
of memory and of the ability to grasp what is
happening around them. They often cover up
their early failings and the condition may first
become apparent as a result of emotional
outbursts or uncharacteristic behaviour in public. Eventually personal habits and speech
deteriorate and they become thoroughly confused and difficult to look after. Treatment is
primarily a matter of ameliorating the symptoms, coupled with a sympathetic handling of
the sufferer and the relatives. Admission to
hospital or nursing home may be necessary if
relatives are unable to look after the patient at
home.

SENILITY (see AGE, NATURAL CHANGES IN).

SENNA is the leaves of various species of
Cassia senna, being known as Tinnerelly senna
and Alexandrian senna, according to its source.

It is one of the most active of the simple laxative
drugs, producing considerable griping if used
alone. Senna is excreted in the urine, giving it
a dark red or yellow colour. In the case of
nursing mothers, some of the drug is excreted
in the milk and may have a purgative effect
upon the nursling. A standardized preparation
of senna, Senokot, is now available which has
none of the disadvantages of senna itself and is
widely used for the management of constipation in old people.

SENSATION (see PAIN; TOUCH).

SENSITIVITY: The extent to which a screening test (q.v.) detects the proportion of true
cases of the disease being screened.

SENSITIZATION (see ALLERGY; ANAPHYLAXIS).

SEPSIS means poisoning by the products of
the growth of micro- organisms in the body,
and the general symptoms which accompany it
are those of inflammation. (See INFLAMMA-
TION.) It is prevented by the various procedures
mentioned under ASEPSIS, and is neutralized,
when it has occurred, by various substances
(See ANTISEPTICS.)

SEPTAL DEFECT: A congenital abnormality
of the heart affecting about 260 babies in every
100,000 in which there is a hole in the septum
– the dividing wall – between the left and right
sides of the heart. The effects of the defect
depend on its size and position. A defect in the
wall between the atria (upper chambers of the
heart) is called an atrial septal defect and that
between the ventricles a ventricular septal defect, the commonest form (25 per cent of all
defects). Both defects allow blood to circulate
from the left side of the heart, where pressures
are highest, to the right. This abnormal flow of
blood is described as a shunt and the result is
that too much blood flows into the lungs
Pulmonary hypertension occurs and, if the
shunt is large, heart failure may develop. A
small septal defect may not need treatment but
a large one will need to be repaired surgically

SEPTICAEMIA is a serious form of blood
poisoning due to the multiplication in the blood
of bacteria – in fact, it is an infection of the
blood. (See BLOOD-POISONING.)

SEPTIC SHOCK: A dangerous disorder char
acterized by a severe fall in blood pressure and
damage to the body tissues as a result of
septicaemia (q.v.). The toxins from the septi
caemia cause widespread damage to tissue
provoke clotting in small blood vessels and
seriously disturb the circulation. The kidneys
lungs, and heart are particularly affected. The
condition occurs most commonly in people
who already have a chronic disease such a

cancer, cirrhosis of the liver or diabetes mellitus. Septic shock may also develop in patients with immunodeficiency illnesses such as AIDS. The symptoms are those of septicaemia, coupled with those of shock, cold, cyanotic limbs, fast thready pulse and a lowered blood pressure. Septic shock requires urgent treatment with antibiotics, intravenous fluids, and oxygen.

SEPTUM: A dividing wall within a structure in the body. Examples are the divisions between the chambers of the heart and the layer of bone and cartilage that separates the two nostrils of the nose.

SEQUELAE is the term applied to symptoms or effects which are liable to follow certain diseases. For example, bronchitis and other chest complaints may be sequelae of measles; heart disease is often a sequel of rheumatic fever; paralysis may follow diphtheria.

SEQUESTRUM is the name given to a fragment of dead bone cast off from the living bone in the process of necrosis. (See BONE, DISEASES OF.) A sequestrum often remains in contact with, and partly enveloped by, newly formed bone, so that a sinus is produced, and a constant discharge goes on, till the dead bone is removed.

SEROCONVERSION: The production of specific antibodies to antigens present in the body. This may happen as a result of infection by a virus or immunization with a vaccine.

SEROTONIN: A substance widely distributed in the body tissue, but especially in the platelets in the blood, the lining of the gastrointestinal tract and the brain. Serotonin is believed to have a similar function to that of histamine in inflammation. In the gut it inhibits gastric secretion and stimulates smooth (involuntary) muscle in the walls of the intestine. Serotonin participates in the transmission of nerve impulses and may have a function in controlling mood and states of consciousness.

SEROTYPE: A classification of a substance according to its serological activity. This is done in the context of the antigens (q.v.) it contains or the antibodies (q.v.) it may provoke. Micro-organisms of the same species may be classified according to the different antigens that they produce.

SEROUS: Relating to, containing or resembling serum.

SEROUS MEMBRANES are smooth, transparent membranes that line certain large cavities of the body. The chief serous membranes are the peritoneum, lining the cavity of the abdomen; the pleurae, one of which lines each

side of the chest, surrounding the corresponding lung; the pericardium, in which the heart lies; and the tunica vaginalis on each side, enclosing a testicle. The name of these membranes is derived from the fact that the surface is moistened by thin fluid derived from the serum of blood or lymph. Every serous membrane consists of a visceral portion, which closely envelops the organs concerned, and a parietal portion, which adheres to the wall of the cavity. These two portions are continuous with one another so as to form a closed sac, and the opposing surfaces are close together, separated only by a little fluid. This arrangement enables the organs in question to move freely within the cavities containing them. For further details see under PERITONEUM.

SERPIGINOUS is a term used in connection with ulcers or eruptions that spread in a creeping manner.

SERUM is the fluid which separates from blood, lymph and other fluids of the body when clotting takes place in them. (See HAEMORRHAGE.) Blood plasma is the name given to the fluid of the blood circulating in the vessels, by which the corpuscles are carried along. As clotting takes place, fine threads of fibrin form from the fibrinogen contained in the plasma. These threads produce a network of increasing density in which the corpuscles are entangled, and, as a result, the fluid (serum) which is left outside this clot is clear, unmixed with corpuscles, and of a pale yellow colour.

The relation of these substances is shown below:

$$Blood = \begin{cases} Plasma = \begin{cases} Serum \\ Fibrin \end{cases} \\ Corpuscles \end{cases} = Clot$$

Serum is a clear, yellowish fluid and contains, in addition to water, about 7 per cent of albumin and globulin, with smaller quantities of salts, fat, sugar, urea, uric acid and other extractives, as well as minute amounts of other albuminous bodies, which are of great importance in the prevention of disease. (See IMMUNITY.) The chief salt in the serum is common salt.

Serum is derived from the lymph also, and the fluid which is found in effusions into the pleura and other cavities of the body is similar in composition.

The serum used for the administration of antitoxins in cases of diphtheria, tetanus, and other diseases, is generally derived from the blood drawn from horses which have been subjected to a long course of treatment. (See IMMUNITY; IMMUNOLOGY.)

SERUM SICKNESS is a hypersensitivity reaction due to circulating antigen antibody complexes. It got its name because it was a not uncommon reaction to the administration of foreign serum which used to be given as a form of passive immunity before the days of antibiotics. By definition it is a manifestation of sensitivity to serum but the same clinical and pathological picture can occur one to three weeks after the administration of drugs such as penicillin, streptomycin and sulphonamides. It is characterized by fever, arthralgia and lymphadenopathy and is usually self-limiting as it resolves when the supply of antigen is used up.

SERUM THERAPY (see IMMONOLOGY).

SESAMOID BONES are rounded nodules of bone usually embedded in tendon. They are usually a few millimetres in diameter, but some are larger, such as the patella (q.v.), or kneecap.

SESSILE: A growth or tumour that has no stalk.

SEX CHROMOSOMES: In the human being there are 23 pairs of chromosomes. Male and female differ in respect of one pair. In the nucleus of the female somatic cell the two members of the pair are identical and are called X-chromosomes. In the male nucleus there is one X-chromosome and another, unequal, dissimilar chromosome called the Y-chromosome. In the sex cells, after reduction division, all cells in the female will contain X-chromosomes. In the male, half will contain X-chromosomes and half Y-chromosomes. If, then, a sperm with an X-chromosome fertilizes an ovum (with, of course, an X-chromosome) the offspring will be female. If a sperm with a Y-chromosome fertilizes the ovum the offspring will be male. It is the sex chromosomes which determine the sex of an individual.

Sometimes during cell division chromosomes may be lost or duplicated, or abnormalities in the structure of individual chromosomes may occur. The surprising fact is the infrequency of such errors. About one in two hundred live-born babies has an abnormality of development caused by a chromosome and two-thirds of these involve the sex chromosomes. There is little doubt that the frequency of these abnormalities in the early embryo is much higher but because of the serious nature of the defect early spontaneous abortion occurs.

Chromosome studies on such early abortions show that half have chromosome abnormalities with errors of autosomes being three times as common as sex chromosome anomalies. Two of the most common abnormalities in such fetuses are triploidy with 69 chromosomes and trisomy of chromosome 16. These two anomalies almost always cause spontaneous abortion. Abnormalities of chromosome structure may arise because of:

(1) *Deletion*: where a segment of a chromosome is lost.

(2) *Inversion*: where a segment of a chromosome becomes detached and re-attached the other way around. Genes will then appear in the wrong order and thus will not correspond with their opposite numbers on homologous chromosomes.

(3) *Duplication*: where a segment of a chromosome is included twice over. One chromosome will have too little nuclear material and one too much. The individual inheriting too little may be non-viable and the one with too much may be abnormal.

(4) *Translocation*: where chromosomes of different pairs exchange segments.

(5) *Errors in division of centromere*: sometimes the centromere divides transversely instead of longitudinally. If the centromere is not central, one of the daughter chromosomes will arise from the two short arms of the parent chromosome and the other from the two long arms. These abnormal daughter chromosomes are called isochromosomes.

These changes have important bearings on heredity as the effect of a gene depends not only on its nature but on its position on the chromosome with reference to other genes. Genes do not act in isolation but against the background of other genes. Each gene normally has its own position on the chromosome and this corresponds precisely with the positon of its allene on the homologous chromosome of the pair. Each member of a pair of chromosomes will normally carry precisely the same number of genes in exactly the same order. Characteristic clinical syndromes, due to abnormalities of chromosome structure, are less constant than those due to loss or gain of a complete chromosome. This is because the degree of deletion, inversion and duplication is inconstant. However, translocation between chromosomes 15 and 21 of the parent is associated with a familial form of mongolism in the offspring and deletion of part of an X chromosome may result in Turner's syndrome.

NON-DISJUNCTION: Whilst alterations in the structure of chromosomes arise as a result of deletion or translocation, alterations in the number of chromosomes usually arise as a result of non-disjunction occurring during maturation of the parental gametes. The two chromosomes of each pair (homologous chromosomes) may fail to come together at the beginning of meiosis and continue to lie free. If one chromosome then passes to each pole of the spindle, normal gametes may result but if both chromosomes pass to one pole and neither to the other, two kinds of abnormal gametes will be produced. One kind of gamete will contain both chromosomes of the pair and the other gamete will contain neither. Whilst this results in serious disease when the autosomes are involved, the loss or gain of sex chromosomes seems to be well tolerated. The loss of an autosome is incompatible with life and the malformation produced by a gain of an autosome is proportional to the size of the extra chromosome carried.

Only a few instances of a gain of an autosome

are known. An additional chromosome 21 (one of the smallest autosomes) results in mongolism and trisomy of chromosome 13 and 18 are associated with severe mental, skeletal and congenital cardiac defects. Diseases resulting from a gain of a sex chromosome are not as severe. A normal ovum contains 22 autosomes and an X sex chromosome. A normal sperm contains 22 autosomes and either an X or a Y sex chromosome. Thus as a result of non-disjunction of the X chromosome at the first meiotic division during the formation of female gametes the ovum may contain two X chromosomes or none at all, whilst in the male the sperm may contain both X and Y chromosomes (XY) or none at all. (See aso CHROMOSOMES, GENES.)

SEX HORMONES: These hormones control the development of primary and secondary sexual characteristics. They also regulate sex-related functions – for example, menstruation and the production of sperm and eggs. The three main types of sex hormone are androgens, or male sex hormones; oestrogens, or female sex hormones; and progesterones, which are involved in pregnancy.

SEX-LINKED INHERITANCE: The way in which a characteristic or an illness determined by the sex chromosomes in an individual's cells is passed on to the succeeding generation. Men have one X and one Y sex chromosome and women have two X chromosomes. Disorders that result from an abnormal number of sex chromosomes include Klinefelter's syndrome, which affects only men, and Turner's syndrome, which affects only women (qq.v.). Recessive genes on the X chromosome cause most other sex-linked characteristics and in women these may well be masked because one of their two X chromosomes carries a normal (dominant) gene. In men, who have but one X chromosome, no such masking occurs, so more men than women are affected by X-linked characteristics or diseases.

SEXUAL ABUSE: (see CHILD ABUSE).

SEXUAL DYSFUNCTION: Inadequate sexual response may be due to a lack of sexual desire or to an inadequate performance, or it may be that there is a lack of satisfaction or orgasm. The lack of sexual desire may be due to any generalized illness or endocrine disorder or to the taking of drugs that antagonize endocrine function. Disorders of performance in men can occur during arousal, penetration and ejaculation. In the female dyspareunia and vaginismus are the main disorders of performance. Diabetes mellitus (q.v.) can cause a neuropathy which results in loss of erection. Impotence can follow nerve damage from operations on the prostate and lower bowel and can be the result of neurological diseases affecting the autonomic system. Disorders of satisfaction include, in

men, emission without forceful ejaculation and pleasureless ejaculation. In women such disorders range from the absence of the congestive genital response to absence of orgasm.

Sexual dysfunction may be due to physical or psychiatric disease, or it may be the result of the administration of drugs. The main group of drugs likely to cause sexual problems are the anti-convulsants, psychotrophic drugs, the anti-hypertensive drugs and drugs such as metoclopramide that induce hyperprolactinaemia. The benzodiazepine tranquillizers can reduce libido and cause failure of erection. Tricyclic antidepressives may cause failure of erection and clomipramine may delay or abolish ejaculation by blockade of alpha-adrenergic receptors. The mono-amine oxidase inhibitors often inhibit ejaculation. The phenothiazides reduce sexual desire and arousal and may cause difficulty in maintaining an erection. Methyldopa causes impotence in over 20 per cent of patients on large doses. The beta-blockers and the diuretics can also cause impotence. The main psychiatric causes of sexual dysfunction include stress, depression and guilt.

SEXUALLY TRANSMITTED DISEASES (see VENEREAL DISEASES).

SHAKING PALSY is another name for Parkinsonism (q.v.).

SHELLFISH POISONING in the United Kingdom occurs in two main forms. Shellfish may be the cause of typhoid fever (see ENTERIC FEVERS) as a result of their contamination by sewage containing the causative organism. They may also be responsible for what is known as paralytic shellfish poisoning. This is caused by a toxin, or poison, known as saxotoxin, which is present in certain planktons which, under unusual conditions, multiply rapidly, giving rise to what are known as 'red tides'. In these circumstances this toxin accumulates in mussels, cockles and scallops which feed by filtering plankton. The manifestations of such poisoning are loss of feeling in the hands, tingling of the tongue, weakness of the arms and legs, and difficulty in breathing. There is also growing evidence that shellfish poisoning may be due to a virus infection. (See FOOD POISONING.)

SHELL-SHOCK was a form of war neurosis which presented one of the major medical problems in the 1914–18 War.

SHELTERED HOUSING: Accommodation that has been adapted to cater for the special requirements of those elderly people who can largely look after themselves but benefit from some discreet supervision. The accommodation is usually a small flat and a warden will supervise a group of flats. Meals and other services may be provided, and the payment system varies depending on whether the accommodation is privately owned or run by a local social-services department.

SHIGELLA is the name given to a group of rod-shaped, Gram-negative bacteria that are the cause of bacillary dysentery. (See DYSENTERY.)

SHINGLES is a popular name for herpes zoster, which forms more or less of a belt round the body. (See HERPES ZOSTER.)

SHIN SPLINTS (see MEDICAL TIBIAL SYNDROME).

SHOCK is a state of acute circulatory failure in which the cardiac output is inadequate to provide normal perfusion of the major organs. It represents a failure of blood flow rather than a failure of blood pressure. While shock is accompanied by a fall in arterial blood pressure, a fall in blood pressure is not necessarily indicative of shock. Shock can arise from a variety of causes and produce variable clinical signs according to the state of deterioration of the underlying disease. Direct bedside measurements of blood flow are not available so that physicians must usually rely on indirect evidence of inadequate perfusion. Shock is therefore a clinical syndrome and is characterized by systemic arterial hypotension (arterial blood pressure less than 80 mm of mercury) sweating and signs of vasoconstriction. These signs include pallor, cyanosis, a cold clammy skin and a low-volume pulse. These may be associated with clinical evidence of poor tissue perfusion, such as mental apathy, confusion or restlessness and oliguria. In haemodynamic terms shock is a state of circulatory failure associated with a low cardiac output and high peripheral resistance.

Shock results from many situations which give rise to inadequate perfusion of tissues and organs. It may occur because of increased resistance to blood flow, pooling or loss of blood or because of cardiac insufficiency, but the end result of impaired tissue perfusion is the same. As perfusion depends on blood flow and not blood pressure the sphygmomanometer reading is a poor indicator of circulatory failure.

The blood volume is approximately 5 litres. The heart puts out this volume each minute, a stroke volume of 70 ml being ejected 70 times per minute in the resting subject. Only 15 per cent of the blood volume lies in the arterial bed so that variations in arterial calibre have little effect on the vascular capacity. The arterioles are extremely muscular vessels and the tone of the arteriolar muscle varies the blood flow enormously. Because the greatest decline in pressure occurs at this level the arterioles are called resistance vessels. Over two-thirds of the circulating blood volume lies on the venous side of the circulation, particularly in the venules. Hence the venous system is called the capacitance system. The veins are less muscular than

the arterioles but are also under autonomic nervous control. The pressure in veins is only about 7 mm of mercury. They have a relatively large diameter and correspondingly low resistance. The tension of venous musculature, although not great, has a critical influence on venous return and on venous pressure. Passive assumption of the erect posture will reduce the cardiac output by 25 per cent. Nervous adjustment through the sympathetic nervous system is intended to prevent pooling in the capacitance system. Failure of venous tone with pooling of blood in venules and capillaries is associated with a large fall in cardiac output and failure of the peripheral circulation. Failure of arteriolar tone, on the other hand, with consequent arteriolar dilatation is associated with hypotension but blood flow remains normal and there is only a transient decrease in the venous return to the heart. The normal regulatory mechanisms for the circulation, that is the Baro receptors and the autonomic innervation of the arterioles and venules, are geared to cope with the adjustments necessary in postural alterations, physical exercise and acute trauma. The adrenergic system regulates blood pressure, the distribution of blood, the capacity of the venous system and the force and rate of cardiac contraction. The autonomic nervous system can adequately compensate for 10 per cent alterations in blood volume, moderate systemic infections and a good deal of myocardial damage, by shunting away blood from visceral organs into cerebral, coronary and skeletal muscle beds. The haemodynamic response to shock inevitably produces inadequate perfusion of viscera in order to preserve circulation to the brain and coronary vessels. If this is prolonged the effects are disastrous. The ischaemic intestine permits the transfer of toxic bacterial products and proteins across its wall into the blood. Renal ischaemia prevents the maintenance of a normal electrolyte and acid base balance.

Shock may result from loss of blood or plasma volume. This may occur as a result of haemorrhage or severe diarrhoea and vomiting. It may also result because of peripheral pooling of blood due to such causes as toxaemia or anaphylaxis. The toxaemia is commonly the result of a septicaemia. Another form of shock is called cardogenic shock which is due to failure of the heart as a pump. It is most commonly seen as a result of myocardial infarction. The treatment of shock is dependent on its cause. If it is the result of haemorrhage or diarrhoea or vomiting, replacement of blood and lost electrolytes is of prime importance. If it is due to septicaemia the treatment of the infection is of paramount importance and in addition intravenous fluids and vasopressor drugs will be required.

SHOCK LUNG (see ADULT RESPIRATORY DISTRESS SYNDROME).

SHORT-SIGHT is a condition in which objects near at hand are seen clearly, while objects at a distance are blurred. The condition is technically known as myopia. (See REFRACTION; SPECTACLES; VISION.)

SHOULDER is the joint formed by the upper end of the humerus and the shoulder-blade or scapula. The acromion process of the scapula and the outer end of the collar-bone form a protective bony arch above the joint, and from this arch the wide and thick deltoid muscle passes downwards, protecting the outer surface of the joint, and giving to the shoulder its rounded character. The joint itself is of the ball-and-socket variety, the rounded head of the humerus being received into the hollow glenoid cavity of the scapula, which is further deepened by a rim of cartilage. One tendon of the biceps muscle passes through the joint, grooving the humerus deeply, and being attached to the upper edge of the glenoid cavity. The joint is surrounded by a loose fibrous capsule, strengthened at certain places by ligamentous bands. The main strength of the joint comes from the powerful muscles that unite the upper arm with the scapula, clavicle and ribs.

SHOULDER-BLADE, or SCAPULA, is a flat bone, about as large as the flat hand and fingers, placed on the upper and back part of the thorax. Many of the large muscles that move the arm are attached to it. It is not in contact with the ribs, and its only attachment to the trunk of the body is through a joint between its acromion process and the clavicle on the tip of the shoulder and by the powerful muscles which suspend it from the backbone and ribs. With the arm hanging by the side the scapula extends from the second to the seventh rib, but, as the arm is raised and lowered, it slides freely over the back of the chest. From the hinder surface of the bone springs a strong process, the spine of the scapula, which arches upwards and forwards into the acromion process. The latter forms the bony prominence on the top of the shoulder, where it unites in a joint with the outer end of the clavicle.

SHUNT: Passage of blood through a channel that is not its normal one. This may occur as a result of a congenital deformity (see SEPTAL DEFECT) or of surgery – for example, a portocaval shunt in which the main portal vein is joined up to the inferior vena cava.

SIALAGOGUES are substances which produce a copious flow of saliva.

SIAMESE TWINS, or CONJOINED TWINS, is the term applied to twins who are united bodily but are possessed of separate personalities. Their frequency is not known, but it has been estimated that throughout the world six or more conjoined twins are born every year who are capable of separation. The earliest case on record is that of the 'Biddendon Maids' who were born in England in 1100. The 'Scottish Brothers' lived for 28 years at the court of James III of Scotland. Perhaps the most famous, however, were Chang and Eng, who were born of Chinese parents in Siam in 1811. It was they who were responsible for the introduction of the term, 'Siamese twins', which still remains the popular name for 'conjoined twins'. They were joined together at the lower end of the chest bone, and achieved fame by being shown in Barnum's circus in the United States. They subsequently married English sisters and settled as farmers in North Carolina. They died in 1874.

The earliest attempt at surgical separation is said to have been made by Dr Farius of Basle in 1689. The first successful separation in Great Britain was in 1912. Both twins survived the operation and one survived well into adult life. This is said to be the first occasion in which both twins survived the operation. The success of the operation is largely dependent upon the degree of union between the twins. Thus, if this is only skin, subcutaneous tissue and cartilage, the prospects of survival for both twins are good, but if some vital organ such as the liver is shared the operation is much more hazardous.

SIBLING is a brother or sister.

SICKLE-CELL ANAEMIA is a form of anaemia in black people, so-called because of the sickle shape of the red blood cells. The fundamental abnormality is the presence of an abnormal form of haemoglobin. This leads to the sickle shape of the red blood cell. Such a cell is more fragile than the normal red blood cell, and it is this fragility of the cell which is responsible for the anaemia. Advice can be obtained from the Sickle Cell Society, Green Lodge, 54 Station Road, London NW10 4UA (081-961 7795/ 4006, fax: 081-961 8346).

SICKNESS (see VOMITING; MOTION-SICKNESS).

SIDE-EFFECT: A consequence of or reaction to treatment that is extra to the effect the doctor wants. The term is usually applied to harmful or unwanted consequences and generally refers to drug treatment. A side-effect may also be a stronger action of the drug than expected or it may be quite unrelated to the intention of the treatment – for example, the drowsiness that occurs from antihistamine drugs given to combat an allergy. Sometimes the side-effects may be potentially lethal as happens when a person develops anaphylactic shock after the administration of, say, antitetanus vaccine. Doctors are expected to report side-effects of drugs to the manufacturers and the committee on safety of medicines (see SAFETY OF DRUGS).

SIDEROSIS is the name given to chronic fibrosis (q.v.) of the lungs occurring in iron-workers and due to the inhalation of fine iron particles. The term is also applied to the condition in which there is an excessive deposit of iron in the tissues of the body.

SIDS (see SUDDEN INFANT DEATH SYNDROME).

SIGHT (see VISION).

SIGMOIDOSCOPY: Examination of the rectum and sigmoid colon with a viewing device called a sigmoidoscope. The procedure is done to investigate rectal bleeding or presistent diarrhoea with the aim of detecting or excluding cancer of the rectum and colitis. Sigmoidoscopy, which nowadays is performed with a flexible instrument, can usually be performed in the outpatients department. (See ENDOSCOPE.)

SILICA is a major constituent of the earth's crust. Its main danger to health arises from free silica, present mainly as quartz and flint and as an important constituent of granite, sandstone and slate. (See SILICOSIS.)

SILICONES are organic compounds of silicon, with a structure of alternate atoms of silicon and oxygen with organic groups, such as methyl and phenyl attached to the silicone atoms. As they produce a flexible and stable water-repellent film on the skin, they are used as barrier creams (q.v.).

SILICOSIS constitutes the most important industrial hazard in those industries in which silica is encountered: i.e. the pottery industry, the sandstone industry, sand-blasting, metal grinding, the tin-mining industry, anthracite coal mines. It is a specific form of pneumoconiosis (q.v.) caused by the inhalation of free silica. Among pottery workers the condition has for long been known as potter's asthma, whilst in the cutlery industry it was known as grinder's rot. For the production of silicosis the particles of silica must measure 0·5 to 5 micrometres in diameter and they must be inhaled into the alveoli of the lungs, where they produce fibrosis. This diminishes the efficiency of the lungs, which manifests itself by slowly progressive shortness of breath. The main danger of silicosis, however, is that it is liable to be complicated by tuberculosis. The incidence of silicosis is steadily being reduced by various measures which diminish the risk of inhaling silica dust. These include adequate ventilation to draw off the dust; the suppression of dust by the use of water; the wearing of respirators where the risk is particularly great and it is not possible to reduce the amount of dust: e.g. in sand-blasting; periodic medical examination of workpeople exposed to risk. In 1976, there were 171 notified cases.

SIMMONDS' DISEASE, or PITUITARY CACHEXIA, is a rare condition in which wasting of the skin and the bones, impotence, and loss of hair occur as a result of destruction of the pituitary gland.

SINGER'S NODULE is a small excrescence on the vocal cords which causes hoarseness. This tends to develop in people who abuse their voices, e.g. singers, people who shout excessively.

SINOATRIAL NODE: This is the natural pacemaker of the heart and comprises a collection of specialized muscle cells in the wall of the upper chamber (atrium) of the heart. The cells initiate electrical impulses at a rate of up to 100 a minute. These impulses stimulate the muscles of the heart to contract. The rate is altered by the effects of certain hormones and various impulses from the nervous system. Damage or disease of the node affects the regular beating of the heart.

SINUS is a term applied to narrow cavities of various kinds, occurring naturally in the body, or resulting from disease. Thus it is applied to the air-containing cavities which are found in the frontal, ethmoidal, sphenoidal and maxillary bones, and which communicate with the nose. The function of these paranasal sinuses, as they are known, is doubtful, but they do lighten the skull and add resonance to the voice. They enlarge considerably around puberty and in this way are a factor in the alteration of the size and shape of the face. The term is also used in connection with the wide spaces through which the blood circulates in the membranes of the brain. Cavities which are produced when an abscess has burst but remain unhealed, are also known as sinuses. (See ABSCESS; FISTULA.)

SINUSITIS is inflammation of a sinus. It is usually applied to inflammation of the sinuses in the face. (See NOSE, DISEASES OF.)

SINUSOID: A small blood vessel like an enlarged capillary occurring, for example, in the liver, which contains a large number of them. The sinusoids in the liver are drained by the hepatic veins.

SI UNITS: The international system of measurement units used throughout the sciences. SI Units, which derive from metres, kilograms, and seconds, comprise seven basic units and two supplementary ones. Among the other base units are ampere (electric current) and mole (amount of a substance). Derived SI units include joule (energy), pascal (pressure), becquerel (activity), and newton (force). (See WEIGHTS AND MEASURES).

SJOGREN'S SYNDROME: Sjogren described the association of dryness of the mouth (xerostomia) and dryness of the eye (kerato conjunctivitis sieca) with rheumatoid arthritis. It occurs in approximately 10 per cent of patients with rheumatoid arthritis but it can occur, and frequently does so, independently of rheumatoid disease. The lack of tears gives rise to symptoms of dryness and grittiness of the eyes. The dry mouth can occasionally be so severe as to cause a dysphagia. The disease is due to the auto-immune destruction of the salivary glands and the lacrimal glands. The disorder is usually associated with specific HLA antigen. The treatment is unsatisfactory and is limited to oral and ocular hygiene as well as the provision of artificial tears in the form of cellulose eye drops.

SKELETAL MUSCLE: Muscle under a person's voluntary control. (See MUSCLE and VOLUNTARY MUSCLE).

SKELETON is the comprehensive term applied to the hard structures that support or protect the softer tissues of the body. Many animals are possessed of an exoskeleton, consisting of superficial plates of bone, horn, or the like; but in man the skeleton is entirely an endoskeleton, covered everywhere by soft parts, and consisting mainly of bones, but in places also of cartilage. The chief positions in which cartilage is found in place of bone are the larynx and the front of the chest. (For the details of the skeleton, see BONE.)

SKIN is the membrane which envelops the outer surface of the body, meeting, at the various orifices of the body, with the mucous membrane which lines the internal cavities. The skin consists of two distinct layers which differ entirely in structure and in origin. These are (a) *the epidermis*, also known as *scarf-skin*, *cuticle*, or *epithelium*, which is a cellular covering formed from the outer layer of the embryo; and (b) *the corium*, also known as the *cutis vera*, *true skin*, or *dermis*, which is a fibrous covering developed from the middle embryonic layer.
(a) **The epidermis** is the cellular layer which covers the outer surface of the body, varying in thickness from 1 mm on the palms and soles to 0·1 mm on the face. It is composed of four layers, which, from the surface inwards, are as follows:
(1) THE HORNY LAYER, or STRATUM CORNEUM, made up of several thicknesses of flat cells, forming an impervious covering pierced only by the openings of the sweat-glands and by the hairs. The flat cells are rubbed off the surface constantly as minute white scales, being replaced by growth from below.
(2) THE CLEAR LAYER, or STRATUM LUCIDUM, in which the cells are firmly fixed together into a kind of membrane.
(3) THE GRANULAR LAYER, or STRATUM GRANULOSUM, in which the cells are undergoing

a change in form and substance from those of the fourth layer to those of the two on the surface.
(4) THE MALPIGHIAN LAYER, or GERMINATIVE ZONE, as it is sometimes known, which is made up of the STRATUM SPINOSUM (or PRICKLY CELL LAYER) and the STRATUM BASALE, in which the cells are soft, tender and living. These cells live in several rows, the deepest (the stratum basale) being set directly upon the uneven surface of the true skin, which is richly supplied with blood-vessels that nourish the cells. These cells divide continually and as they multiply they are pushed upwards to supply the constant wear and tear on the surface of the horny layer. There are no blood-vessels in the epidermis, but fine sensory nerves terminate between the cells of the Malpighian layer. These cells are joined together by cement substance and by minute processes that are continued from each cell into its neighbours. The cells in the stratum basale include the melanocytes which are responsible for the production of melanin, the pigment responsible for suntan. (See MELANIN; SUNBURN.)
NAILS are analogous to the horny layer, but the cells of which they are composed are harder and more adherent. Beneath the nail is the nail bed, which is made up of the germinative zone together with the corium. Underneath the greater part of the nail the corium has a very liberal blood supply, which gives the nail its pink colour. Towards the root of the nail, however, the nail becomes denser and the corium has a less liberal blood supply. As a result the nail is whiter. This is the part known as the lunule, which is most evident in the thumb, and gradually becomes covered by the nail fold towards the little finger where the lunule is usually hidden completely. The stratum corneum of the nail fold is prolonged over the nail as a thin fold known as the eponychium. All growth of the nail occurs at its root. Finger nails grow at an average rate of 0·5 mm a week. There is a gradual slowing of the rate with age, and a slight variation from finger to finger, the longer the finger the faster the rate of growth. Growth is quicker in summer than in winter. Toe nails grow more slowly than finger nails – at about a fourth of the rate of the latter.
A *blister* is a collection of fluid separating the Malpighian layer from the superficial ones.
(b) **The corium** is the fibrous layer which forms the chief part of the bodily covering. It varies greatly in thickness from about 0·5 to 3 mm, being coarser on the back than on the front of the body, and thicker in men than in women. It contains many nerves, which play an important part in affording sensations of touch, pain and temperature, and blood-vessels which, in addition to nourishing the skin, are largely concerned in regulating the temperature of the body. The corium bears also the hairs which pierce the epidermis, and the sweat-glands, whose ducts also penetrate the epidermis to reach the surface. Beneath the corium lies a loose fibrous layer of subcutaneous tissue which joins the skin to deeper parts and contains more

1 horny zone	5 stratum basale	8 stratum spinosum
2 germinative zone	6 vascular papilla of corium	9 stratum granulosum
3 blood vessels	7 oval corpuscle in corium (tactile)	10 stratum lucidum
4 nerves		11 stratum corneum

Vertical section of epidermis and corium

or less fat, according to the stoutness of the person.

The fibrous tissue of the corium is composed of interlacing bundles of white fibrous tissue that form a dense feltwork. Here and there, elastic fibres are mixed with the others, and these serve to give the skin pliability, and at the same time to keep it always stretched. On the surface the network is very fine and close, and the skin is raised up into projections, known as papillae, which fit into corresponding depressions on the under-surface of the epidermis, and thus render the two inseparable. The corium is crossed everywhere by numerous folds, which are specially plentiful over joints and on the palms of the hands, and which are followed closely by the epidermis. There is a special arrangement on the palms and soles, where the papillae are so placed as to form continuous ridges with intervening grooves. These ridges remain permanent throughout life, and, as the formation by them of whorls and loops upon the finger-tips is distinctive and unchanging in each individual, an impression, or fingerprint, of these in ink is a most effective and reliable means of identifying a person. Hence their world-wide adoption as a means of identifying criminals. On the summit of each ridge, with the help of a magnifying glass,

the orifices of the sweat-glands can be seen arranged in a row.

The endings of the sensory nerves in the skin are described under NERVES.

HAIRS spring from the true skin, each having a root and a stem or shaft. The stem is generally rounded, and varies greatly in thickness, while in the case of curly hair it is oval or flattened in section. The surface is covered by scales, imbricated like the tiles on a roof, and it is in consequence of their projecting edges that felted or matted hair is so difficult to separate. The chief part of the stem is of a fibrous character, the fibres being composed also of elongated cells. Running up the centre, some hairs have a pith composed of soft cells with air-spaces between them. The varying tint of hair is due to pigment scattered in varying amount throughout the hair, while a white hair is produced by the formation of very numerous air-spaces throughout the cells composing it. The root of the hair ends in a knob, and is set upon a fibrous papilla, from which the hair appears to derive its principal nutriment. This root is set deep in the corium, and is the growing part of the hair which pushes the older part of the hair out through the epidermis. In the scalp each hair grows steadily and continuously for three to five years at a rate of a little over 0·3 mm daily. Growth then ceases and after three to four months the hair is shed. In the latter half of this resting period the follicle forms a new hair which replaces the old one. The average daily moult varies from 50 to 100 hairs. The tube which contains the part of the hair embedded in the skin is known as the hair follicle and is lined by a fibrous coat derived from the true skin and a cellular coat developed from the cuticle, each of which consists of three layers. When a hair is roughly pulled out, the clear membrane that is often found surrounding it is part of the cellular root sheath. The follicle does not run straight down into the skin, but has a considerable obliquity, so that the part of the hair above the surface has a natural slope to one side. Attached to the underside of each sloping hair-follicle, near its deep end, is a small muscle, whose other end is attached to the surface of the true skin a little distance off. These muscles have the action of raising the hair, and also of producing goose-flesh, when

stimulated to contract by the influence of cold or of fear.

GLANDS are found in immense numbers in the skin, and are of two kinds: *sebaceous glands*, which secrete a fatty substance, and *sweat glands*, which secrete a clear, watery fluid.

The *sebaceous glands* lie in the true skin, and open into the follicles of the hairs a little way from the surface. Each consists of a bunch of small sacs, within which fatty material is produced. The secretion reaches the surface by the hair-follicle, and serves to lubricate the hair and give pliability to the surface of the skin.

Sweat glands, or sudoriparous glands, are very numerous (there are around 3 million of them), are found all over the surface of the body at a slightly deeper level than the sebaceous glands, and have no connection with the hairs. Each consists of a long tube, coiled up into a ball, from which a duct leads in a zigzag manner up towards the surface. The outlets of these ducts can just be seen with the naked eye as

1 stratum corneum	6 bulb of hair	11 sebaceous gland
2 stratum lucidum	7 dermic coat, outer root-sheath	12 vessel
3 stratum spinosum	8 dermic coat, inner root-sheath	13 stratum basale
4 corium	9 medulla of hair	14 stratum granulosum
5 papilla of hair	10 arrector pili muscle	15 cortex of hair

Section through the skin showing the epidermis and corium, a hair in its follicle, the arrector pili muscle which raises the hair, and sebaceous glands opening into the hair follicle.

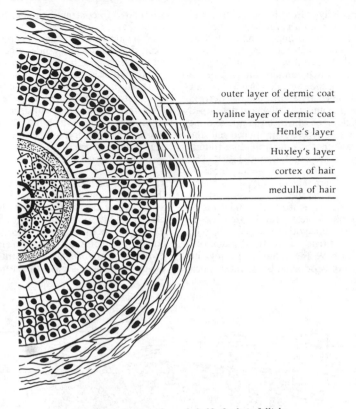

outer layer of dermic coat
hyaline layer of dermic coat
Henle's layer
Huxley's layer
cortex of hair
medulla of hair

Transverse section through half of a hair follicle.

minute openings (pores), though with a magnifying glass they are readily visible. The number is said to vary from 400 in a square inch, on the lower limbs and back, to 2800 in the same area on the palm of the hand. The structure of these glands is simple. Each is a coiled-up tube, which is lined by a layer of cells surrounded by muscle fibres, and these again by a thin membrane. In the fibrous tissue between the coils of the glands run many small blood-vessels, and from the blood in these the materials that form the sweat are extracted.

Functions of the skin: The main use of the skin is a *protective* one. It covers the underlying muscles, both protecting them from injury and, especially by virtue of the layer of fat immediately beneath the skin, warding off extremes of temperature. The epidermis forms a highly impenetrable surface, its horny character and elasticity being well calculated to resist wounds; whilst the sebaceous matter with which it is provided renders it almost waterproof. Thus poisons, drugs, and the like are not absorbed in any appreciable amount through the unbroken skin, unless combined with some fatty material, as in ointments, and diligently rubbed in, or alternatively by molecular diffusion. This latter method is known as the Transdermal Therapeutic System.

Secretion is an important function of the skin, the two secretions being sebaceous material and perspiration. Of these, the former is a lubricant for the hair and skin, the latter is treated of under PERSPIRATION.

Heat regulation is one of the most important functions of the skin. Man is a warm-blooded animal, that is to say, his temperature remains constant in health between 36·7 and 37·2 °C (98 and 99 °F), no matter what the temperature of the surrounding medium may be. In order to maintain this constancy, it is evident that he must be provided with some means of quickly developing heat which will come into action when the body is cooled down by exposure to cold, and also some mechanism which can quickly get rid of heat when necessary. The main source of heat in the body lies in the muscular tissue, which develops heat every time a contraction takes place. The skin also plays a prominent part in this connection. When cold air or water come into contact with the surface, the skin blanches, the numerous blood-vessels of the true skin contracting and thus preventing much blood from circulating through the skin, and being thereby unduly cooled. On the other hand, when the surface is exposed to a temperature approaching that of the body, say one of 26·7 or 32·2 °C (80 or 90 °F), or when an excessive amount of heat is produced by great muscular efforts, the blood-vessels of the surface dilate, the skin reddens as much blood comes to the surface, and there is a copious secretion of perspiration, which produces great cooling as it evaporates from the surface. These actions of narrowing and dilatation of vessels, and of sweat secretion, are brought about through reflex nerve influence. When the temperature rises so high that these processes are unable to take place, very serious results ensue. (See HEAT-STROKE.) It can be readily understood why the body tolerates high temperatures at a dry heat much better than continued moist heat, since evaporation of the perspiration takes place more readily the drier the surrounding air, and thus produces more rapid cooling.

Respiration is a function of the skin which in man is not of so great importance as in the lower animals. In the frog, the lungs and skin are of equal importance as breathing organs, although in man the amount of carbon dioxide given off by the skin is only about $1/150$ or $1/200$ of the amount given off by the lungs. It is probable however, that much of the organic matter which gives to impure air its disagreeable smell and contributes to its poisonous properties is given off by the skin.

Social function: The skin, it has been said, also provides a major pathway for social communication, by virtue of its vascular responses associated with signalling of emotional states, muscular responses of expression, creating a complex sign language, and by the equally subtle possibilities of tactile communication. In primates, it has been noted, the skin forms a signalling system related to complicated instinctive behaviour patterns, but 'how far the signals mediated in man by facial expression and other factors causing alterations in skin appearance are linked to instinctive behaviour patterns rather than to conditioned behaviour is debatable in adults, although studies in children indicate the fusion of these two elements in a complex fashion'.

SKIN DISEASES: These form a large and important class. They are very extensive, owing to the varied forms of change which the skin texture may undergo, and to the different structures in the skin which may be specially affected. Skin diseases are of great importance, not only from the fact that they have an influence on the general health, but also because these diseases are often the expression of constitutional conditions, inherited or acquired, the recognition of which is essential to their effectual treatment.

CANCER of the skin occurs in various forms. *Rodent ulcer* (q.v.), or basal cell epithelioma responds well to treatment. Cure is obtained in 98 per cent of cases if treated early. Anyone over the age of 50 with a persistent superficial

1 epidermis	5 papilla of hair	9 sebaceous gland
2 corium	6 hair follicle	10 papilla of corium
3 subcutaneous fatty tissue	7 body of sweat gland	11 hair
4 oblique section through a lamellated corpuscle	8 arrector pili muscle	12 duct of sweat gland

Schematic vertical section of skin.

crusted ulcer on the cheek or the side of the nose which has not healed over a period of months should seek medical advice in case it is a rodent ulcer. *Squamous cell carcinoma* which usually starts as a hard nodule, is usually the result of long excessive exposure to sunlight. *Malignant melanoma* (see MELANOMA) develops in a pigmented spot. Cancer of the skin may also be induced by exposure to tar, pitch, bitumen, the mineral oils, and X-rays.

(See also ACNE; BOILS; BROMIDROSIS; DERMATITIS; ECTHYMA; ECZEMA; ERYSIPELAS; ERYTHEMA; ERYTHRASMA; HERPES SIMPLEX; HERPES ZOSTER; HYPERIDROSIS; ICHTHYOSIS; IMPETIGO; ITCHING; KERATOSIS; LEUCODERMA; LICHEN; LUPUS; MOLLUSCUM CONTAGIOSUM; NAPPY RASH; NEURODERMATOSES; PEMPHIGUS; PITYRIASIS ROSEA; POMPHOLYX; PRURIGO; PRURITUS; PSORIASIS; RING-WORM; ROSACEA; SEBORRHOEA; URTICARIA.)

SKIN-GRAFTING is an operation in which large breaches of surface due to wounding or ulceration are closed by transplantation of skin from other parts. There are three methods by which this is done. Most frequently the epidermis only is transplanted, according to a method introduced by Reverdin and by Thiersch, and known by their names. For this purpose, a broad strip of epidermis is shaved off the thigh or upper arm, after the part has been carefully purified, and is transferred bodily to the raw or ulcerated surface, or is cut into smaller strips and laid upon it. By a second method, small pieces of the skin in its whole thickness are removed from the arm and thigh, or even from other people, and are implanted and bound upon the raw surface. This method has the disadvantage that the true skin must contract at the spot from which the graft is taken, leaving an unsightly scar. When very large areas require to be covered, a third method is sometimes adopted, as follows. A large flap of skin, amply sufficient to cover the gap, is raised from a neighbouring or distant part of the body, in such a way that it remains attached along one margin, so that blood-vessels can still enter and nourish it. It is then turned so as to cover the gap; or, if it be situated on a distant part, the two parts are brought together and fixed in this position till the flap grows firmly to its new bed. The old connection of the flap is then severed, leaving it growing in its new place.

SKULL is the collection of 22 flat and irregularly shaped bones which protect the brain and form the face. The names of the individual bones composing the skull are given under BONE.

Arrangement of the bones: In early life the brain and organs of special sense are enclosed in a case which is formed partly of cartilage, partly of fibrous membrane. At various parts of this investment, ossification begins early in life, and the bone gradually spreads outwards from each of these centres. Certain of the bones so formed fuse together in early childhood, thus constituting the twenty-two bones of the adult skull,

which maintain their independence throughout the greater part of life. In old age, however, the bones fuse so completely that the cranium comes to be a solid bony case. Even before this happens, the bones are fastened to one another by sutures so tightly that their separation without breaking is very difficult. The sutures are joints in which each edge is locked with the edges of neighbouring bones by exactly fitting projections and depressions, resembling a complicated mortise-work. Occasionally small bones develop in the sutures between the ordinary, named ones, these extra bones being known as sutural bones.

The growth of the bones spreads outwards, as already stated, from certain centres, and at the time of birth the growth of several bones has not been quite completed, so that an infant's head presents six soft spots or fontanelles where the brain is covered only by skin and membranes, and at some of which the pulsations of its blood-vessels can be seen. One of these spots, the anterior fontanelle, situated on the top of the head, does not completely close till the child is 2½ years old. Another change takes place as age advances, consisting in the development of an outer and inner hard table in each of the cranial bones, the tables being separated by a layer of cancellous bone (*diplöe*), and in some positions by spaces containing air, which communicate with the respiratory passages. (See SINUS.) This change begins at the age of 10 years, and leads to great thickening and increased strength in the skull.

Parts of the skull: The skull consists of two distinct parts: the cranium, which encloses the brain and consists of eight bones; and the face, which forms a bony framework for the eyes, nose, and mouth, and is composed of fourteen bones. These two parts can be detached from one another. The lower jaw is connected with the base of the cranium by a movable joint on each side, and when the bones are bare of soft parts there is no union between them. The ear, which lies just behind and above this joint, is enclosed in the substance of the temporal bone, lying beneath the brain and separated from it in places only by a very thin shell of bone. The interior of the cranium is moulded so as to form a support for the brain. Its base is divided by bony ridges into three fossae, which from before back support the frontal lobes, the temporosphenoidal lobes, and the cerebellum. Further, the inner surface of the bone shows grooves and hollows corresponding to the convolutions and blood-vessels of the brain. The bones, especially on the base of the skull, are pierced by many small canals (*foramina*) which transmit nerves, blood-vessels and the like. Of these, the largest is the foramen magnum, through which the medulla oblongata and the spinal cord are continuous with one another.

Shape of the skull: In the lower animals, the cranium is placed in the back part of the head, and the face looks upwards to a great extent as well as forwards. In man, as a consequence of the great development of the cerebral hemispheres of the brain, in connection with his mental activity, the cranium extends above, as well as behind, the face, which therefore looks straight forwards. One method of classification is obtained by taking what is known as the cephalic index: i.e. the percentage that the skull's breadth forms of its length. Long-headed peoples, like the Australian aborigines, are known as *dolichocephalic*; peoples with rounded heads, like most European races, are called *mesocephalic*; while races with broad heads, like some American Indians, are said to be *brachycephalic*.

Age makes considerable changes in the skull. The persistence of soft spots in the skull during the first two years of life, as well as the gradual obliteration of the sutures in later life, have been already mentioned. In children the size of the cranium is large compared with that of the face, which measures only one-eighth of the whole head, but increases till in adult life cranium and face are of almost equal propor-tions. In old age the face once more decreases, owing largely to loss of the teeth and conse-quent absorption of their bony sockets, which allows the cheeks to sink inwards and gives the appearance known as nut-cracker jaws. A similar result is produced earlier in life by premature extraction of the teeth. The child's head is gently rounded, and does not show the prominences above the eyebrows and behind the ears, due to the presence of air-cells at these localities in the full-grown skull. Further, the skull is thinner in childhood, does not show the heavy ridges for attachment of muscles dis-played in later life, and is more vertical on the front and sides.

Sex also makes some differences, so that, as a rule, though not invariably, the skull of a woman can be told from that of a man. In the woman the characters resemble those of the child, the skull being lighter, smoother, and having less marked prominences. The woman's skull has on an average nine-tenths the capacity of the male skull.

Deformities result from various causes. The head is rarely symmetrical, one side almost always bulging more than the other. Premature closure of one of the sutures leads to increased growth at other sutures. Thus if the suture running from before backwards on the vertex of the head (sagittal suture) close too early, the result is a very long boat-shaped head. Some races, as, for example, the flat-head Indians of North America, show striking deformities of the head produced by applying boards and bandages in infant life.

SLAPPED CHEEK DISEASE (see ERYTHEMA).

SLEEP is a periodic resting condition of the body, and especially of the nervous system. It is more than rest. It is a phase that ensures that the whole body, including the nervous system, can recuperate. It has been shown in animals that the formation of protein is more active during sleep, and the same presumably holds in man. It is the brain that controls sleep, and the benefit of sleep is most obvious for the brain. The highest rate of synthesis, or formation, of brain protein takes place during sleep.

CAUSES OF SLEEP: There is a natural rotation of sleeping and waking every twenty-four hours, and sleep comes on commonly during the night when little work can be done. Sleep is not, however, a necessary consequence of darkness, as is proved by those people who have to work in the night and sleep by day, and who speedily adapt themselves to this condition. Many peo-ple, too, such as sailors, gain the power of sleeping as soon as they turn in, and for them short four-hourly periods of sleep and work become natural.

Many theories have been advanced as to the cause of sleep. One theory is that sleep is due to cerebral anaemia, or a poor blood supply to the brain. Against this is the fact that it has been shown that the total blood flow through the brain is not altered during sleep. On the other hand, this does not exclude the possibility that there may be local alterations in certain parts of the brain, such as the midbrain which is known to be concerned with the process of sleeping.

Another theory is the chemical one that sleep is due to want of oxygen in the nerve centres. It has been shown that, of the oxygen taken in during the twenty-four hours, 67 per cent is taken in during the twelve hours of day and 33 per cent during the twelve hours of night, while of the carbon dioxide given off, 58 per cent is the amount by day and 42 per cent by night. It is also well known that vitiated air containing an excess of carbon dioxide is capable, like many other substances, of causing drowsiness followed by unconsciousness. But these facts – while making it plain that want of oxygen or the presence of carbon dioxide and other products of activity in the tissues may cause sleep – do not explain why sleep comes on regularly in people who are not exhausted by their day's work, nor why many people are able to com-pose themselves and fall asleep at any time they find convenient.

A third theory raises the question as to whether the mind remains active during the period of sleep. This theory brings forward the fact that all sensations, volitions, and other acts of consciousness are accompanied by chemical disturbances in the brain-cells that stimulate the mind to activity. When external impressions are cut off by closing the eyes and otherwise composing oneself for sleep, the mind ceases to be stimulated, and tranquil sleep ensues. What might be described as a slightly less fanciful variation of this theory is that during waking hours there is an accumulation in the brain of a sleep-inducing substance, and that after a period of time this ultimately induces sleep. None of these theories explains the direct cause of sleep, although each probably accounts for the main cause in different circumstances.

Sleep is not one steady process of gradually deepening sleep, as was at one time thought. It consists of several cycles of alternation between two stages: NREM (*Non-Rapid-Eye Movement*) or orthodox sleep, and REM or paradoxical sleep. On falling asleep we pass straight into the orthodox phase which lasts for about an hour or so. This is followed by the REM, so called because it is accompanied by *Rapid Eye Movement* (hence the abbreviation, REM) which lasts for two or fifteen minutes. This is the stage during which dreaming occurs. When it is over we pass back into the orthodox stage and so we alternate during the night, the orthodox stages tending to last longer in the earlier stages of sleep. By and large, however, orthodox sleep occupies about three-quarters of the sleep period in adults. In infants, however, it occupies only about half of the sleep period.

When sleep comes on, the eyes are closed as a rule, though in man, even when they are left open, the sense of sight is quickly lost as the sleep deepens. The pupils contract, also, during sleep, and dilate widely as the person awakes. Hearing is lost more slowly, and a person can be wakened even from deep sleep by a loud noise. In natural sleep, touch remains the least affected of the senses, and even the lightest touch will awaken many people from deep sleep. This does not hold good for sleep caused by drugs, many of which have a special effect in dulling general sensation, though much less effect upon the sense of hearing. With regard to the onset of sleep as it affects the mind, willpower is the first faculty to go and the last to appear in wakening. The association of ideas and power of reasoning next disappear, and people are often worried in light sleep by some simple idea which they cannot explain or understand. Memory and imagination remain longest, and, in dreams, the mind is presented with a series of bright, unconnected pictures, all jumbled together, which it does not attempt to explain. The part of the brain which regulates the power of movement is late in falling asleep, sleeps only lightly – since people may turn and make various other movements without waking – and usually wakens before the intellectual faculties and the special senses.

Other parts of the body, as well as the brain, rest during sleep. Thus the kidneys secrete less urine, the stomach secretes less gastric juice, the liver secretes less bile, the heart beats less strongly, the blood-pressure falls, and the respirations are slower and shallower than in the waking state. The skin becomes flushed with blood, so that it is specially necessary to keep the surface well covered during sleep in order to avoid chills. Some parts of the body never have a continued rest throughout life. Thus the heart, during the course of the two to three thousand million beats which it makes throughout an average life, never ceases longer than the fraction of a second that intervenes between each pair of beats, and, in each of these brief intervals, it recuperates itself for its next effort. Similarly the vital centres in the brain may be said never to sleep.

The amount of sleep suitable at different ages varies considerably as it also does from individual to individual. Some people keep going quite happily with five hours a night; others need eight hours or even more. Young people sleep easily but with increasing age sleep becomes more difficult. It becomes more broken and also less deep. At the same time there is a tendency for the elderly to require less sleep.

DREAMS: The mind, like the vital centres, is probably never completely inactive during sleep, but is constantly receiving slight impressions which produce only a faint and quickly forgotten sensation. This is borne out by the fact that a sleeper may be awakened, not only by a loud sound or light touch, but by the ceasing of a continuous sound, as when machinery stops. A sleeper is also especially easily awakened by some sound or other sensation that he expects, and, in further proof of this constant wakefulness of the mind, may be mentioned the fact that many people have the power of wakening after having slept for a period which they have previously determined. It has been already stated that the different parts of the brain and the different faculties of the mind go to sleep usually in a certain order. When the higher intellectual faculties of will and reason have become dulled, but deeper sleep does not at once come on, memory and imagination become increasingly vivid, so that brilliant pictures are presented to the mind. Often these are mingled with misinterpreted sensations from the surface of the body or from disordered internal organs, which serve to give them an unpleasant tinge. For example, dyspepsia may give rise to sensations of falling over precipices, of vague depression, or of other unpleasant experiences which are in part memories of past events. Again, a wakeful memory and imagination may be associated with wakefulness of the motor portion of the brain, as when the person dreams that he is making desperate efforts to achieve some object or to escape pursuit, and his limbs go through movements associated with the ideas presented in his dream. Any sensation received from the surface of the body or from a disordered organ may suffice to produce the condition of partial sleep in which dreams occur, or it may become sufficiently strong to awaken the sleeper altogether. Again, the impression of the dream may produce so great an effect upon consciousness that the dream is remembered on waking, or it may fade so completely that only a sense of something forgotten is present, and a feeling that the slumber has been unrefreshing to the weary mind. Much attention has been paid to dreams with the object of finding out repressed memories responsible for mental unrest in the person concerned. These often become more evident during sleep than in the waking hours, and, if the dreams are remembered, they give a guide to the identity of the disturbing memories. Appearances seen and things felt or heard in dreams often have a symbolic meaning; and the interpretation of this by those who practise psychotherapy often plays an important part in treatment. Dreams are usually in black and white, but occasionally in colour.

NIGHT TERRORS occur in nervous children and are allied to dreaming. The child goes to sleep after a day of unusual excitement or fatigue, or perhaps after eating an indigestible meal, and in a short time, when sleep should be sound and dreamless, he awakens with a start and in a state of terror. Frequently the child screams with fear, cannot be pacified, and for several minutes does not seem to recognize those near him. When quieted, he can often give no reason for his fear, or he may attribute his behaviour to a dream. Children who suffer in this way should be guarded from excitement and fatigue, and, should the night terrors, or nightmares, persist, help should be sought from a child-guidance clinic or child psychologist.

SOMNAMBULISM, or habitual sleep-walking, is an imperfect form of sleep, in which the muscular apparatus, and the portion of brain controlling it, remain awake though the intellectual faculties are buried in slumber. In children it is not uncommon as an isolated phenomenon and is seldom of any significance, especially if it is ignored. Occasionally it may be associated with something that is worrying the child, either at home or at school. This is usually revealed by discreet enquiry, and relatively easily settled. In adults it may be a manifestation of a hysterical personality (see HYSTERIA) precipitated by some mental stress or strain, though this may be difficult to ascertain in the hysteric. While the somnambulistic state persists the individual is unaware of his actions, though he may see and avoid objects in his path, or may hear and answer questions, though seldom with coherence. It is almost unknown for somnambulists to injure themselves. On awakening they remember nothing of the episode.

PARALYSED WAKEFULNESS is a condition of which people sometimes complain. This is the converse of somnambulism, the person waking from sleep to full consciousness and finding himself unable to make any movement for several seconds or minutes. In this condition the motor part of the brain seems to lag behind the intellectual and sensory part in waking up, but the condition is a transitory and unimportant one, though it can be quite terrifying for the victim.

INSOMNIA, or sleeplessness, is a condition that often causes annoyance, and by depriving the person of natural rest produces interference with the full activity during the day-time. When it becomes a habit, it may be damaging to health.

It may be due to a variety of causes, and these may act so effectively as to keep the person awake altogether, or they may serve, when present in a lesser degree, to produce one of the forms of dreaming and unrefreshing slumber already mentioned. In temporary cases of sleeplessness or dreaming, in which the affected person suffers from a disturbed night now and then, the cause is usually to be sought in some external source of irritation. A slight degree of pain, coldness, or even the presence of cold feet may prevent the brain from attaining the necessary degree of repose. Indigestion, due to eating a heavy meal shortly before retiring to rest, or some other internal disorder may act in a similar manner, even although there be no severe pain. In cases of habitual sleeplessness, a voluntary limitation of the hours of sleep, combined with overstudy, worry, or grief, is often instrumental in forming a bad habit which it is exceedingly hard to break. The brain in these cases remains fully active, despite attempts by the sleepless person to go to sleep. A similar effect may result from poisonous materials circulating in the blood, as in fevers, malaria, gout, intemperance, and over-indulgence in tobacco. Another cause of sleeplessness or dreaming is found in persons suffering from depression who are often affected in such a way that they fall asleep on retiring to rest, enjoy only a light and partial slumber for an hour or two, and then lie wide awake till morning.

TREATMENT OF DISORDERED SLEEP: This varies greatly, depending the cause. A greater amount of exercise during the day, and care with regard to the diet may be sufficient in some of the slighter cases to remedy insomnia. In other cases a hot drink, e.g. milk, just before retiring is an excellent sedative. In old people a hot whisky is often a most effective nightcap. As cold feet is a not uncommon cause of insomnia in old people, the wearing of bed-socks may ensure a good night's sleep. A comfortable warm bed can be better than any hypnotic. Where any known cause of pain or irritation exists, this must of course be remedied. Headache is not uncommonly a cause of sleeplessness, and the relief of this condition is often sufficient to restore natural sleep. (See HEADACHE.) When a mental cause is at the root of the condition, the habit of overstudy, business worry, and the like which was originally responsible for the want of sleep, must be abandoned. Some change of occupation in the later part of the evening, such as reading some simple book or engaging in conversation, often helps to quiet the overworked brain. Cases which resist these simple means often yield to hypnotics. (See HYPNOTICS.) Finally, any bad habits, like intemperance and excessive smoking, require appropriate treatment.

COMA is the name applied to a state of deep sleep from which the person cannot be roused. (See COMA.) The condition may be due to stroke, compression or concussion of the brain, poisoning by excess of alcohol or by narcotic poisons such as opium. (See OPIUM.)

APPARENT DEATH is a condition deeper than coma, in which persons are to all appearance dead. Cases have occurred of supposed death in which the person has been in a deep sleep or trance, from which some sudden shock has awakened him after several hours or even days. In all such cases, however, careful examination would reveal signs of life. (See CATALEPSY; DEATH, SIGNS OF.)

SLEEPING SICKNESS, or AFRICAN TRYPANOSOMIASIS is a disease occurring in West, East, Central and South Africa, between 14° N and 25° S latitude, and characterized by increasing weakness, lethargy, and a constant tendency to sleep, with gradual emaciation and finally death. It is one of the group of diseases caused by the presence in the blood of minute parasites known as *trypanosomes*. The discovery of these parasites in the blood in cases of sleeping sickness was first made in 1902. Later it was shown that this parasite is transmitted by various forms of the tsetse fly. The disease also occurs in cattle, when it is known as nagana. The most important species of trypanosomes are *Trypanosoma gambiense*, which only affects man, and *Trypanosoma rhodesiense*, which affects mainly man. *Trypanosoma brucei, Trypanosoma vivax*, and *Trypanosoma congolense* are all found in wild animals and are fatal to cattle and other domestic animals, but harmless to man. The tsetse flies responsible for the transmission of the disease are *Glossina morsitans* in the case of *Trypanosoma rhodesiense*, and *Glossina morsitans, Glossina swynnertoni*, and *Glossina palpalis* in the case of *Trypanosoma gambiense*.

Other forms of the disease transmitted by other insects are also known, such as a disease occurring in Central and South America called *American trypanosomiasis*, or Chagas' disease (q.v.).

The parasite, when introduced into the blood, produces its effects by developing in the small blood-vessels and in the lymphatic glands, around which its presence causes inflammation.

Symptoms: A few days after the person has been bitten by the fly, fever accompanied by a slight rash develops. This fever subsides but recurs at irregular intervals of a few days or weeks. Gradually the fever becomes more pronounced, and in time the patient becomes weakened and anaemic. The glands of the neck and other parts of the body become enlarged and tender, and this state may last for months or even for years. Some cases appear to recover at this stage even after an illness of many months, and the parasite may disappear altogether from the blood. In most cases, however, the stage known as sleeping sickness gradually appears, although the lethargy may not set in for as long as seven years after the original infection. The patient now becomes disinclined for exertion, is slow mentally and weak physically, often complains of headache, and has an increasing tendency to sleep, although at first he is able to engage in conversation and to take his food. As time goes on, the weakness increases and the patient becomes more and more emaciated, bed sores form, and death finally takes place from weakness or from some intercurrent disease. The later symptoms appear to be due to the development of the parasites in the minute blood-vessels of the brain, around which, in consequence, inflammatory changes occur, with disorganization of the nervous tissues.

Treatment: For the prevention of sleeping sickness the chief essential is the avoidance of the flies which carry the disease. Fortunately, the occurrence of the flies is very definitely localized to certain regions, and, when such regions have to be traversed, the journey is made during the night-time when the flies do not feed. Those who live in fly-infested regions should have their houses and persons carefully protected against the fly. The wearing of long trousers and long-sleeved shirts gives some protection, as does the use of insect repellents such as dimethyl phthalate (q.v.). As the flies are mostly found close to streams, much has been done in certain localities by clearing the neighbourhood of streams in infested districts of all vegetation which would shelter the flies. The use of insecticides is proving more difficult than in the case of certain other insect-borne diseases, but promising results are being obtained from the hand-spraying of belts of vegetation bordering roads and tracks, and from aerial spraying of larger areas.

Suramin is the drug of choice in the treatment of *Trypanosoma rhodesiense* infections, and pentamidine in the treatment of *Trypanosoma gambiense* infections. Melarsoprol, a trivalent melaminyl arsenical, has replaced tryparsamide in the treatment of advanced cases of the disease, but it is a drug which must be administered with great care on account of its toxicity.

SLING means a hanging bandage for the support of injured or diseased parts. Slings are generally applied for support of the upper limb, in which case the limb is suspended from the neck. The lower limb may also be supported in a sling from an iron cage placed upon the bed on which the patient lies, the object usually being to aid the circulation, and so quicken the healing of ulcers on the leg.

SLIPPED DISC is the popular name for a prolapsed intervertebral disc (q.v.). (See SPINAL COLUMN.)

SLOUGH means a dead part separated by natural processes from the living body. The term is applied to hard external parts which the lower animals cast off naturally in the course of growth, like the skin of snakes or the shell of crabs. In man, however, the process is generally associated with disease, and is then known as gangrene. (See GANGRENE.) Sloughs may be of very small size, as in the case of the core of a boil, or they may include a whole limb, but in general a slough involves a limited area of skin or of the underlying tissues. The process of separation of a slough is described under gangrene.

SLOW VIRUSES: A group of viruses whose effects take a long time to show after their initial infection of the nervous system. The diseases may take years to develop during which time gradual but widespread damage of the nerve tissue occurs. The outcome is a loss of brain function and eventually death. Slow-virus disease was many years ago recognized as causing scrapie in sheep, and more recently bovine spongiform encephalopathy (BSE) has been identified in cows, the disease being spread through feedstuffs contaminated with nervous tissue from sheep and cattle. In humans the Creutzfeldt-Jakob syndrome (a type of dementia) (q.v.), kuru (laughing sickness) (q.v.) and a type of meningitis are among several diseases thought to be caused by a slow virus.

SMALLPOX, so called to distinguish it from syphilis, the great pox (pox being the plural of pock, the Old English term for a pustule (q.v.)), is also known as VARIOLA (from *varus*, the Latin for pimple). It is an acute, highly infectious disease due to a virus.

Until recent times it was one of the major killing diseases. In the 1960s the World Health Organization undertook an eradication scheme by means of mass vaccination. As a result, the last naturally occurring case was recorded in October 1977, and on 8 May 1980, the World Health Assembly solemnly agreed a Resolution confirming that smallpox has finally been eradicated from the world. This was indeed a historic occasion; the first occasion on which man has attempted to eradicate a disease and has succeeded in so doing. The public lack of interest in it is explained by the fact that so few of those living today have had any experience of it – even doctors.

Since 1960, there have been only 141 reported cases, with 28 deaths, in England and Wales, and not a single naturally occurring case since 1973. (See VACCINATION.)

SMEGMA is a thick, cheesy secretion formed by the sebaceous glands of the glans penis. A bacillus, closely resembling the tubercle bacillus morphologically, develops readily in this secretion.

SMELL: The sense of smell is picked up in what is known as the olfactory areas of the nose. Each of these is about 3 square centimetres in area and contains 50 million olfactory, or smelling, cells. They lie, one on either side, at the highest part of each nasal cavity. This is why we have to sniff if we want to smell anything carefully, as in ordinary quiet breathing only a few eddies of the air we breathe in reaches an olfactory area. From these olfactory cells the olfactory nerves (one on each side) run up to the olfactory bulbs underneath the frontal lobe of the brain (q.v.), and here the impulse is translated into what we describe as smell.

SMELLING SALTS (see AMMONIA).

SMOKE INHALATION: Smoke is made up of small particles of carbon in hot air and gases. The particles are covered with organic chemicals and smoke may also contain carbon monoxide and acids. When smoke is inhaled the effects on breathing may be immediate or delayed depending on the density of smoke and its composition. Laryngeal stridor (obstruction of the larynx), lack of oxygen and pulmonary oedema are life-threatening symptoms that require urgent treatment. Immediate removal of the victim from the smoke is imperative, as is the administration of oxygen. The victim may require admission to an intensive-care unit.

SMOKING (see TOBACCO).

SMOOTH MUSCLE: Muscle that is under the 'involuntary' control of the central nervous system (see MUSCLE).

SNAKE-BITE (see BITES AND STINGS).

SNEEZING means a sudden expulsion of air through the nose, designed to expel irritating materials from the upper air passages. In sneezing, a powerful expiratory effort is made, the vocal cords are kept shut till the pressure in the chest has risen high, and air is then suddenly allowed to escape upward, being directed into the back of the nose by the soft palate. One sneeze projects 10,000 to 100,000 droplets a distance of up to 10 metres at a rate of over 60 kilometres an hour. As such droplets may contain micro-organisms, it is clear what an important part sneezing plays in transmitting infections such as the common cold. Though usually transitory, sneezing may persist for days on end – up to 204 days have been recorded.

Sneezing may be caused by the presence of irritating particles in the nose, such as snuff, the pollen of grasses and flowers. It is also an early symptom of colds, influenza, measles, and hayfever, being then accompanied or followed by running at the nose.

SNELLEN CHART: The most commonly used chart for testing the acuity of distant vision. The chart comprises rows of capital letters with the letters in each row being smaller than the one above. The top line of large letters can be seen by a normally sighted person standing 60 metres away. The subject under test sits six metres from the screen and, if he can read the six metre line of letters, his visual acuity is normal at 6/6 (see VISION).

SNORING is usually attributed to vibrations of the soft palate, but there is evidence that the main fault lies in the edge of the posterior pillars of the fauces (q.v.) which vibrate noisily. Mouth breathing is necessary for snoring, but not all mouth-breathers snore. The principal cause is blockage of the nose, such as occurs during the course of the common cold or chronic nasal catarrh. Such blockage also occurs in some cases of deviation of the nasal septum or nasal polypi. (See NOSE, DISEASES OF.) In children, mouth-breathing, with resulting snoring, is often due to enlarged tonsils and adenoids. A further cause of snoring is loss of tone in the soft palate and surrounding tissues due to smoking, overwork, fatigue, obesity, and general poor health. One in eight people are said to snore regularly. The intensity, or loudness, of snoring is in the range, 40 to 69 decibels. (Pneumatic drills register between 70 and 90 decibels.)

Treatment therefore consists of the removal of any of these causes of mouth-breathing that may be present. Should these not succeed in preventing snoring, then measures should be taken to prevent the victim from sleeping lying on his back, as this is a habit which strongly conduces to snoring. Simple measures include sleeping with several pillows so that the head is raised quite considerably when asleep. Alternatively, a small pillow may be put under the nape of the neck. If all these measures fail, there is much to be said for the old traditional method of sewing a hair-brush, or some other hard object such as a stone, into the back of the snorer's pyjamas. This means that if he does turn on to his back while asleep, he is quickly awakened and therefore able to turn on his side again. (See also STERTOR.)

SNOW BLINDNESS results from exposure to ultraviolet light reflected from snowfields. It causes pain, photophobia and watering of the eyes. Examining the eye shows that there are hundreds of punctate areas of corneal epithelial damage. The symptoms and appearance are exactly the same as in *Arc Eye*, acquired by using an arc welder without adequate eye protection. (See EYE, DISEASE AND INJURIES, *radiant energy injuries*). Treatment is to keep the eye covered with a pad for twenty-four hours.

SNUFFLES is the name applied to noisy breathing in children due to the constant presence of nasal discharge. (For treatment, see NOSE, DISEASES OF.)

SOAP is a substance made by boiling a fat or oil with an alkali. The most commonly used oil is olive oil, and the most frequent alkali is caustic soda. In the process of manufacture the fatty acids of the oil unite with the alkali, glycerin separating out. In soft soap or green soap, caustic potash is used in place of soda; marine soap is made with coconut oil; curd soap has tallow for its fat: while many toilet soaps have palm oil or almond oil. Barilla soap is made from soda got by burning plants; in superfatted soaps care is taken that the fatty part is in excess, so that no crude alkali is left to irritate the skin; whilst glycerin soaps have a specially emollient action. Medicated soaps of various kinds are prepared, the chief drugs added to soap being of an antiseptic nature, such as carbolic acid, coal-tar, formalin, hexachlorophane, terebene.

Uses: The chief use of soap is, mixed with water, as a cleansing agent. Internally, hard soap is often used to make up the bulk of pills contain-ing very active ingredients. As a purgative enema, soap is used made up into a strong solution in warm water. Soap liniment, better known as 'opodeldoc', is used as a popular remedy for stiffness or sprains.

SOCIAL CLASSES: As factors such as the cause of death and the incidence of diseases vary in different social strata, the Registrar-General evolved the following social classification, which has now been in official use for many years:

Class I Professional occupations, such as lawyers, clergymen, and commissioned officers in the Armed Forces.

Class II Intermediate occupations, such as teachers, managers and nurses.

Class III N Non-manual – for example, clerical workers.

Class III M Skilled manual occupations such as miners and bricklayers.

Class IV Partly skilled occupations, such as agricultural workers.

Class V Unskilled occupations, such as building and dock labourers.

SODIUM is a metal, the salts of which are white, crystalline, and very soluble. The fluids of the body contain naturally a considerable quantity of sodium chloride.

SODIUM CARBONATE, commonly known as SODA or WASHING SODA, has a powerful softening action upon the tissues.

SODIUM BICARBONATE, or BAKING SODA, is used as an antacid in relieving indigestion associated with increased acidity of the gastric secretion. It is taken in doses of 600 or 1,200 mg, as a rule. The citrate and the acetate of sodium are used as diuretics and in the treatment of inflammatory conditions of the kidneys and bladder, though the corresponding potassium salts are more often used.

SODIUM CHLORIDE is the chemical name for common salt.

SODIUM CROMOGLYCATE is the main drug used in the prophylaxis of asthma. It is administered by inhalation and can reduce the incidence of asthmatic attacks but is of no value in the treatment of an acute attack. It acts by preventing the release of pharmacological mediators of bronchospasm, particularly histamine, by stabilizing mastcell membranes. It is thus of particular use in patients whose asthma has an allergic basis. The dose frequency is adjusted to the patient's response but is usually administered by inhalation four times daily.

SODIUM DIATRIZOATE is an organic iodine salt that is radio-opaque and is therefore used as a contrast medium to outline various organs in the body in X-ray films. It is given intravenously. Its main use is in pyelography (q.v.), that is in rendering the kidneys radio-opaque, but it is also used to outline the blood-vessels (angiography) and the gall-bladder and bile ducts (cholangiography).

SODIUM HYPOCHLORITE is a disinfectant by virtue of the fact that it gives off chlorine. For domestic use, as, for example, for sterilizing baby feeding bottles, it is available in a variety of proprietary preparations. (See also CHLORINATED LIME.)

SODIUM VALPROATE is a drug that is proving of value in the treatment of some cases of epilepsy which will not respond to any of the other drugs used for the treatment of this condition. It must be used with care as it may cause liver damage.

SODOMY: Sexual intercourse in which the penis penetrates the anus and rectum. Sodomy may occur between men, between a man and a woman or between a man and an animal (bestiality).

SOLARIUM is a room enclosed by glass in which sun baths are taken while protection is afforded from the weather.

SOLAR PLEXUS: A large network of sympathetic nerves and ganglia situated in the abdomen behind the stomach, where it surrounds the coeliac artery. Branches of the vagus nerve, the most important part of the parasympathetic system, lead into the solar plexus, which in turn distributes branches to the stomach, intestines and several other abdominal organs. A severe blow in the solar plexus may cause temporary unconsciousness.

SOLUTION or LIQUOR as it used to be known, is a liquid preparation containing one or more soluble drugs, usually dissolved in water.

SOLVENT ABUSE: Also known as volatile-substance abuse, this is the deliberate inhalation of intoxicating fumes given off by some volatile liquids. Glue sniffing was the most common type of solvent abuse, but inhalation of fuel gases such as butane, especially in the form of lighter refills, is now the major problem in the United Kingdom. The problem has become common among children, particularly teenagers. Solvents or volatile substances are applied to a piece of cloth or put into a plastic bag and inhaled, sometimes until the person loses consciousness. He or she may become acutely intoxicated; chronic abusers may suffer from ulcers and rashes over the face as well as damage to peripheral nerves. Death can occur, probably as a result of an abnormal rhythm of the heart. Tolerance to the volatile substances may develop over months, but acute intoxication may lead to aggressive and impulsive behaviour. Treatment of addiction is difficult and requires professional counselling. Victims with acute symptoms require urgent medical attention. In 1990 about 130 deaths in the United Kingdom were associated with volatile substance abuse, mostly in young people under 20 years of age; 80 per cent of the deaths were in males. This compares with 82 deaths in 1983.

SOMATIC means relating to the body, as opposed to the mind.

SOMNAMBULISM means sleep-walking. (See SLEEP.)

SOPORIFICS are measures which induce sleep. (See HYPNOTICS.)

SORE is a popular term for ulcer (q.v.).

SOTALOL (see ADRENERGIC RECEPTORS).

SOUND is a rod with a curve at one end used mainly for passing into the bladder to determine whether a stone is present or not. (See BLADDER, DISEASES OF.)

SOUTHEY'S TUBES are long, fine tubes for drawing off fluid slowly from cases of oedema. (See ASPIRATION.)

SOYA BEAN is the bean of *Glycine soja*, a leguminous plant related to peas and beans. The outstanding characteristic of the soya bean is its high protein and fat content. There is an almost complete absence of starch, but a large amount of mineral matter. Soya flour contains 40 per cent of protein and 20 per cent of fat. It yields 470 Calories per 100 grams as compared with 370 Calories for white wheat flour. Soya flour contains 0·2 per cent of calcium (about ten times as much as in white flour). It also contains a variable but large amount of iron: 6·7 to 30 mg per 100 grams of soya flour compared with 1 mg in white flour and 3 mg in 100 grams of wholemeal flour. It is a good source of thiamine and riboflavine, and of vitamin A in the form of carotene. (See BEANS.)

SPANISH FLY is a popular term for cantharides, which is used as a blistering agent. (See CANTHARIDES.)

SPASM means an involuntary, and, in severe cases, painful contraction of a muscle or of a hollow organ with a muscular wall. Spasm may be due to affections in the muscle where the spasm takes place, or it may originate in some disturbance of that part of the nervous system which controls the spasmodically acting muscles. Spasms of a general nature are usually spoken of as convulsions; spasms of a painful nature are known as cramp when they affect the muscles of the limbs, and as colic when they are situated in the stomach, bowels, or other organs of the abdomen. Spasm of the heart receives the name of breast-pang or angina pectoris, and is both a serious and an agonizing condition. When the spasm is a prolonged firm contraction, it is spoken of as tonic spasm; when it consists of a series of twitches or quick alternate contractions and relaxations, it is known as clonic spasm. Spasm is a symptom of many diseases.

SPASMODIC TORTICOLLIS is the term applied to a chronic condition in which the neck is rotated or deviated laterally, forwards, or backwards, often with additional jerking or tremor. It is a form of focal dystonia, and should not be confused with the far commoner transient condition of acute painful wry-neck. (See DYSTONIA.)

SPASMOLYTICS are remedies which diminish spasm. They may achieve this in one of three ways: (a) by interfering with the transmission of the nerve impulses that are causing the spasm; (b) by a direct action on the affected muscle; (c) by depressing the central nervous system.
Varieties: In the past many of the favourites in this field, such as oil of cinnamon, oil of cloves, oil of peppermint, and valerian, achieved their reputation by virtue of their depressing effect on the sensitivity of the nerve endings. Others, such as lobelia and stramonium, often in the form of cigarettes to be inhaled, achieved a wide reputation as asthma cures.

Today, a more scientific approach is maintained, though there is still much to be said for the use of preparations, such as oil of cinnamon or of peppermint for the relief of mild spasm of the gut, and not a few asthmatics have implicit faith in the relieving power of lobelia or stramonium. The most widely used spasmolytics today are atropine and its derivatives, or its many synthetic substitutes. These act by paralysing the action of the parasympathetic nerve fibres that induce contraction of smooth muscle. They are most widely used in relieving spasm in the alimentary and renal tracts. For the relief of the spasm of asthma adrenaline and ephedrine are still great standbys, though isoprenaline and other similarly acting drugs are being used to an increasing extent. All these act through the sympathetic nervous system.

Of the spasmolytics acting directly on muscle, the best known group is the nitrites – amyl nitrite and glyceryl trinitrate – which are the great standby for the relief of the spasm that induces angina pectoris. Other drugs that act in this way are theophylline and aminophylline. If the spasm is really severe, and therefore painful enough, general depression of the brain may be necessary by means of general anaesthetics. In less severe cases, the lesser degrees of depression of the brain induced by hypnotics may have a spasmolytic action, and, though it should seldom be used for this purpose because of its habit-forming propensities, even alcohol could rank as a spasmolytic.

SPASTIC is a term applied to any condition showing increased muscle tone: e.g. spastic gait. This is specially associated with some disease affecting the upper part of the nervous system connected with movement (upper neuron), so that its controlling influence is lost and the muscles are in a state of over-excitability.

SPASTIC COLON (see IRRITABLE BOWEL SYNDROME).

SPATULA is a flat, knife-like instrument used for spreading plasters and ointments, and also for depressing the tongue when the throat is being examined.

SPECIAL HEALTH AUTHORITY (see NATIONAL HEALTH SERVICE).

SPECIFICITY: An epidemiological term describing the extent to which a screening test (q.v.) throws up false positives. A specific test has few false positives.

SPECTACLES can be worn for a variety of reasons including correction of a refractive error, correction of a squint, for protection (from foreign bodies or, with tinted lenses, from bright light), or occasionally to hold a prosthesis.

SPECULUM is an instrument designed to aid the examination of the various openings on the surface of the body. Many specula are provided with small electric lamps so placed as to light up the cavity brilliantly.

SPEECH DISORDERS: Speech is the ability to express oneself orally, using exclamations, words and sentences. A child needs to know how to do this and difficulties may occur either through problems during pregnancy, at birth, childhood illnesses or delayed development. For example, a child with severe cleft lip and palate may need to undergo surgery before being able to produce speech which is intelligible to his family. This may discourage talking, and language development may fall behind. In another instance, a child with recurrent ear infections may find it less easy to listen to others and therefore his experience of spoken language is limited. In rare cases a child may develop normally except for the sole area of language development. The result is *childhood dysphasia* and he may need specialist education if he is to develop his full potential.

Adults may lose the ability to talk having acquired it in early childhood in the usual way. This is usually due to a stroke (see DYSPHASIA, STROKE), or to a head injury. They may also have difficulty in articulating words as the result of illness (see DYSARTHRIA). Stammering may persist into adulthood (see STAMMERING).

Children and more often adults, particularly those who use their voices during working hours to a great extent (e.g. teachers) may be prone to hoarse voice.

A very small minority of adults will undergo an operation for removal of the larynx and may need help in using other methods to communicate (see LARYNGECTOMY).

Increasing recognition is being given to those children and adults who are intellectually handicapped and of the impairment of articulation and language which often occurs. Social skills and communication in general are often impaired with those who are severely psychiatrically disturbed. (See also VOICE AND SPEECH.)

DUMBNESS means an inability to pronounce the elementary sounds which make up words.

Varieties: The important classification of cases of deficient power of speech is into (a) those associated with deafness and (b) those in which hearing is good. In a case associated with deafness, the person may be dumb merely because he has been born deaf, and, having no knowledge of sound, cannot understand or make intelligible sounds, although provided with good voice mechanism; or a person who has lost his hearing by some disease in childhood may be unable to speak otherwise than as a child for the same reason. It is estimated that 1 per 1000 deaf children are so deaf that natural speech is impossible. When hearing is good, on the other hand, dumbness is due generally to some mental defect or sometimes to some failure in the organs of voice production.

Causes: Deafness is the most important cause, because the one most capable of treatment. Of those due to some congenital brain-deficiency, some arise in children of parents who were themselves deaf-mutes. Another class of cases, in which there is also mental deficiency, arises from brain disease, such as that due to syphilis. Those children who are mentally bright and whose hearing is good have occasionally some structural defect, such as tongue-tie or enlarged tonsils and adenoids in the throat, which allow of attempts at speaking but prevent proper formation of words. Dumbness is sometimes a hysterical manifestation. Lisping and lalling speech are slight forms of dumbness due to inefficient control of the voice mechanism, but can generally be cured by careful training. (See STAMMERING; VOICE AND SPEECH.)

Treatment: A dumb child is cut off from other people and so cannot develop normally, unless adequately treated; a careful examination should be made of any child who does not speak by two years of age. Deafness is easily discovered by finding that the child pays no attention to noises made behind its back. Mental ability can be measured by special tests. Physical obstructions, like tongue-tie or large tonsils, should be removed if present.

Deaf-mutes may be trained to read the lips and throat movements of others by sight, and to use their powers of voice through a complicated process, which should begin about the age of six or seven. It is hard for adults to pick this up, and people who are to be instructed in this method should not learn the finger language first.

The training required for this 'oral' method is long, and, if the deaf person is to gain a modulated voice and a fair command of language, the constant attention of an expert tutor is necessary all through childhood and youth. In England and Wales a local education authority can compel a parent of any child of two years of age or over to submit the child for medical examination. If this shows that special educational treatment is required, the authority must provide such treatment. In the case of deaf-mutes, attendance is compulsory between the ages of 5 and 16.

Training in lip-reading should be started as soon as possible, and special educational methods should be begun as soon as possible after the age of two years.

SPEECH THERAPY is a small independent graduate profession. Speech therapists assist, diagnose and treat the whole spectrum of acquired or developmental communication disorders. They work in medical and education establishments often in an advisory or consultative capacity. The medical conditions in which speech therapy is employed include: dysgraphia, dyslexia, dysathria, dysphasia, dysphonia, dyspraxia, autism, Bell's palsy, cerebral palsy, deafness, disordered language, delayed speech, disordered speech, Down's syndrome, laryngectomy, macroglossia, mental subnormality, motor neurone disease, malformations of the palate, Parkinsonism, psychiatric disorders, stammering, stroke and disorders of voice production.

It is a caring profession; most speech therapists work for the National Health Service in community clinics and hospitals. They may also work in schools or in units for the handicapped, paediatric assessment centres, language units attached to primary schools, adult training centres and day centres for the elderly.

A speech therapist undergoes a four-year degree course which covers the study of disorders of communication in children and adults, phonetics and linguistics, anatomy and physiology, psychology and many other related subjects. Further information on training can be obtained from the College of Speech Therapists, 6 Lechmere Road, London NW2 5BU (081-459 8521).

If the parents of a child are concerned about their child's speech, they may approach a speech therapist for assessment and guidance. Their general practitioner will be able to give them local addresses or they should contact the district speech therapist. Adults are usually referred by hospital consultants.

The College of Speech Therapists keeps a register of all those who have passed a recognized degree or equivalent qualification in speech therapy. It will be able to direct you to your nearest NHS or private speech therapist.

SPERMATIC is the name applied to the blood-vessels and other structures associated with the testicle.

SPERMATORRHOEA is the passage of semen without erection of the penis or orgasm.

SPERMATOZOON (plural: SPERMATOZOA) is the male sex or germ cell which unites with the ovum to form the embryo or fetus. It is a highly mobile cell approximately 4 micrometres in length, much smaller than an ovum, which is about 35 micrometres in diameter. Each millilitre of semen (q.v.) contains on average about 100 million spermatozoa, and the average volume of semen discharged during ejaculation in sexual intercourse is between 2 and 4 ml. Once ejaculated during intercourse it travels at a rate of 1·5 to 3 millimetres a minute and remains mobile for several days after insemination, but quickly loses its potency for fertilization. As it takes only about 70 minutes to reach the ovarian end of the uterine tube, it is assumed that there must be factors other than its own mobility, such as contraction of the muscle of the womb and uterine tube, that speed it on its way. (See also FETUS.)

SPHAGNUM MOSS, or peat or bog moss, has been used as a wound dressing from time immemorial. A skeleton from the Bronze Age in Scotland showed a large pad of sphagnum moss applied to what had been a chest wound. It was used on a large scale as a wound dressing in the 1914–18 War. It is widely distributed in Scotland, Ireland and Western England. Its main value lies in its great absorptive powers: it can absorb up to seven times its weight of water. It is deodorizing and does not allow discharges from wounds to pass through it as does cotton wool.

SPERMICIDE: Contraceptive preparations that kill sperm. They may be in the form of gels, pessaries, cream, or foam and should be used with a barrier contraceptive such as a diaphragm or a condom.

SPHENOID is a bone lying in the centre of the base of the skull, and supporting the others like a wedge or keystone. (See SKULL.)

SPHINCTER means a circular muscle which surrounds the opening from an organ, and, by maintaining a constant state of moderate contraction, prevents the escape of the contents of the organ. Sphincters close the outlet from the bladder and rectum, and in certain nervous diseases their action is interfered with, so that the power to relax or to keep moderately contracted is lost, and retention or incontinence of the evacuation results.

SPHYGMOGRAPH is an instrument for recording the pulse. (See PULSE.)

SPHYGMOMANOMETER is the name of an instrument for measuring blood-pressure in the arteries. It usually consists of a pneumatic armlet, the interior of which communicates by a rubber tube with an air-pressure pump and a gauge. The armlet is bound about the upper arm and pumped up sufficiently to obliterate the pulse as felt at the wrist or as heard in the artery at the bend of the elbow. The pressure registered on the gauge at this point is regarded as the pressure of the blood at each heart-beat (systolic pressure). The pressure at which the sound heard in the artery suddenly changes its character marks the diastolic pressure.

SPINA BIFIDA is one of the commonest of the congenital malformations. There are marked regional variations. It takes two main forms. SPINA BIFIDA OCCULTA is much the commoner of the two and consists of a defect in the posterior wall of the spinal wall, usually in the lumbar region. As a rule it has no deleterious effects unless the underlying spinal cord is affected. It has been said that one in every ten individuals has such a defect.

SPINA BIFIDA CYSTICA, the other form, is a much more serious condition. Here the defect in the spinal canal is accompanied by protrusion of the spinal cord which, in turn, may take one of two forms. One is a *meningocele*, in which the meninges (q.v.), containing cerebrospinal fluid, protrude through the defect. The other is a *meningomyelocele*, in which the protruding sac contains spinal cord and nerves. This is much the more serious condition of the two and, unfortunately, much the commoner, accounting for 90 per cent of all cases.

The overall incidence of spina bifida varies from one part of the country to another, but in the United Kingdom the incidence is about 40 per 100,000 births, a figure that has fallen in recent years for reasons that are unclear. The cause is not known but there is a strong genetic factor. Thus, a couple who have had one baby affected with spina bifida have a 5 to 8 per cent chance that any subsequent babies they have will have a major malformation of the central nervous system. If they have already had two or more affected infants, the risk of any further having a similar condition is about 1 in 4 to 1 in 8. Tests are now available, whereby severe cases of spina bifida (and anencephaly) can be recognized in the unborn child during pregnancy.

The usual site of the defect is in the lumbo-sacral, or lower, part of the spine. When the baby is born the protruding sac is quite soft, but if it is a meningomyelocele, as it usually is, the baby's condition rapidly deteriorates, with the development of paralysis and incontinence, and a high risk of meningitis. This is why it is now recommended that the baby should be operated on as soon as possible – preferably in a special centre. Many of these babies also have hydrocephalus (q.v.). So successful are the results of operation on carefully selected cases in special centres that it is now claimed that 'the majority of adequately treated children with spina bifida associated with hydrocephalus will grow up with a normal intelligence, although the average intelligence of the whole group falls below the 100 IQ figure which applies to the general population'. The emphasis here, however, is on 'carefully selected cases', and 'adequately treated' and 'special centre'. Indeed, the decision as to how to deal with a severe case of spina bifida can be especially difficult.

There is a growing volume of evidence of the value of vitamin supplements preceding and during pregnancy in reducing the incidence of this pathetic congenital abnormality.

Parents of children with spina bifida or hydrocephalus are recommended to join the Association for Spina Bifida and Hydrocephalus, ASBAH House, 42 Park Road, Peterborough PE1 2UQ (0733-555988, fax: 0733-555985) which has branches in all parts of the country, or The Scottish Spina Bifida Association, 190 Queensferry Road, Edinburgh EH4 2BW (031–332 0743). In this way they will receive continuing help, advice and encouragement.

SPINAL ANAESTHESIA: A method of anaesthesia that involves injecting an anaesthetic drug into the cerebrospinal fluid, which surrounds the spinal cord. This suppresses sensation in a part of the body, the area affected being dependent on the level at which the anaesthetic is injected and the strength of drug used. Two types are used for surgery. In one, epidural, the anaesthetic is injected into the outer lining of the cord. In the other, subarachnoid, the drug is injected into the lumbar region of the vertebral column, the needle being inserted between the vertebrae.

The technique is valuable in patients who cannot take a general anaesthetic because, for example, they have heart or chest disease. Spinal anaesthesia is also useful in obstetrics or in circumstances in which a skilled general anaesthestist is unavailable. It is more often used in the United States and Scandinavia than in the United Kingdom.

Spinal anaesthesia also describes the loss of sensation in an area of the body as a result of disease or injury to the spinal cord, the extent of anaesthesia depending on the location of the disease or injury. (See ANAESTHESIA.)

SPINAL COLUMN, also known as the SPINE, CHINE, BACKBONE, and VERTEBRAL COLUMN, forms an important part of the skeleton, acting both as the rigid pillar which supports the upper parts of the body and as a protection to the spinal cord and nerves arising from it. The spinal column is built up of a number of bones placed one upon another, which, in consequence of having a slight degree of turning-movement, are known as the vertebrae. The possession of a spinal cord supported by a vertebral column distinguishes the higher animals from the lower types, and gains for them the general name of vertebrates. Of the vertebrates, man alone stands absolutely erect, and this erect carriage of the body gives to the skull and vertebral column certain distinctive characters.

The human backbone is about 70 cm (28 inches) in length, and varies little in full-grown people; differences in height depend mainly upon the length of the lower limbs. The number of vertebrae is 33 in children, although in adult life 5 of these fuse together to form the sacrum, and the lowest 4 unite in the coccyx, so that the number of separate bones is reduced to 26. Of these there are 7 in the neck, known therefore as *cervical vertebrae*; 12 with ribs attached, in the region of the thorax, and known as *thoracic* or *dorsal vertebrae*; 5 in the loins, called *lumbar vertebrae*; 5 fused to form the *sacrum*; and 4 joined in the *coccyx*. These numbers are expressed in a formula thus: C7, D12, L5, S5, Coc4 = 33. Although the vertebrae in each of these regions have distinguishing features, all the vertebrae are constructed on the same general plan. Each has a thick, rounded, bony part in front, known as the body, and these bodies form the main thickness of the column. Behind the body of each is a ring of bone, the neural ring, these rings placed one above another forming the bony canal which lodges the spinal cord. From each side of the ring a short process of bone known as the transverse process stands out, and from the back of the ring a larger process, the spinous process, projects. These processes give attachment to the strong ligaments and muscles which unite, support, and bend the column. The spines can be seen or felt beneath the skin of the back lying in the centre of a groove between the muscular masses of the two sides, and they give to the column its name of the spinal column. One of these spines, that of the 7th cervical vertebra, is especially large and forms a distinct bony prominence, where the neck joins the back. Between the bodies of the vertebrae lies a series of thick discs of fibro-cartilage known as intervertebral discs. Each disc consists of an outer portion, known as the annulus fibrosus, and an inner core, known as the nucleus pulposus. To these 23 discs the upper part of the spine owes much of its pliability, as well as a great deal of its resiliency and power of diminishing the effect of jars and blows communicated through the feet or head. There is also a small joint at each side upon the ring of the vertebra so that each vertebra comes in contact with the one above and the one beneath in three places.

The first and second cervical vertebrae are modified in a very special manner. The first vertebra, known as the atlas, is devoid of a body, but has a specially large and strong ring with two hollows upon which the skull rests, thus permitting of nodding movements. The second vertebra, known as the axis, has a pivot upon its body which fits into the first vertebra and thus permits of free rotation of the head from side to side.

An important feature of the spinal column, and one especially marked in human beings, is the presence of four curves from behind forwards. Thus the cervical vertebrae are arranged with a curve whose hollow looks backwards, the dorsal vertebrae have a marked curve with the hollow forwards; in the lumbar region the hollow is directed backwards, while the sacrum and coccyx form a marked hollow to the front. The effect of the dorsal and sacral curves is greatly to increase the size of the cavities of chest and pelvis, while the compensating curves of the neck and loins serve to keep the general axis of the spinal column in a vertical line. The curves have also an action very similar to that of the springs of a vehicle, in minimizing jolting and jarring of the internal organs. There is usually a very slight curve to one side in the upper dorsal region, resulting from the greater development and use of one arm.

The neural rings placed one above another form a canal, which is wide in the neck, smaller and almost round in the dorsal region, and wide again in the lumbar vertebrae. This canal lodges the spinal cord, and the nerves that issue from the cord pass out from the canal by openings between the vertebrae which are produced by notches on the upper and lower margins of each ring. The intervertebral foramina formed by these notches are so large in comparison with the nerves passing through them that there is no chance of pressure upon the latter, except in very serious injuries which dislocate and fracture the spine.

SPINAL CORD is the lower portion of the central nervous system which is situated within the spinal column. Above, it forms the direct continuation of the medulla oblongata, this part of the brain changing its name to spinal cord at the *foramen magnum*, the large opening in the base of the skull through which it passes into the spinal canal. Below, the spinal cord extends to about the upper border of the second lumbar vertebra, where it tapers off into a fine thread, known as the filum terminale, that is attached to the coccyx at the lower end of the spine. The spinal cord is thus considerably shorter than the spinal column, being only 37 to 45 cm (15 to 18 inches) in length, and weighing around 30 grams. In its course from the base of the skull to the lumbar region the cord gives off thirty-one nerves on each side, each of which arises by an anterior and a posterior root that join before the nerve emerges from the spinal canal. The openings for the nerves formed by notches on the ring of each vertebra have been mentioned under SPINAL COLUMN. To reach these openings the upper nerves pass almost directly outwards, whilst lower in the series their obliquity increases, until below the point where the cord terminates there is a sheaf of nerves, known as the cauda equina, running downwards to leave the spinal canal at their appropriate openings. In shape the cord is a cylinder, about the thickness of the little finger, and slightly flattened from before

1 second lumbar vertebrae
2 second sacral vertebrae
3 spinal medulla or cord
4 filum terminale
5 subarachnoid space, containing cerebo-spinal fluid

Diagram of the lower end of the spinal cord.

backwards. It has two slightly enlarged portions, one in the lower part of the neck, the other at the last dorsal vertebra, and from these thickenings arise the nerves that pass to the upper and lower limbs. (See NERVES.) The spinal cord, like the brain, is surrounded by three membranes, the dura mater, arachnoid mater, and pia mater, from without inwards. The arrangement of the dura and arachnoid is much looser in the case of the cord than their application to the brain. The dura especially forms a wide tube which is separated from the cord by fluid and from the vertebral canal by blood-vessels and fat, this arrangement protecting the cord from pressure in any ordinary movements of the spine.

IN SECTION, the spinal cord consists partly of grey, but mainly of white, matter. It differs from the upper parts of the brain in that the white matter in the cord is arranged on the surface, surrounding a mass of grey matter, while in the brain the grey matter is superficial. The arrangement of grey matter, as seen in a section across the cord, resembles the letter H, each half of the cord possessing an anterior and a posterior horn, and the masses of the two sides being joined by a wide posterior grey commissure. In the middle of this commissure lies the central canal of the cord, a small tube which is the continuation of the ventricles in the brain. The horns of grey matter reach almost to the surface of the cord, and from their ends arise the roots of the nerves that leave the cord, but elsewhere the grey matter is completely surrounded by white matter. The white matter is divided almost completely into two halves by a posterior septum and anterior fissure that project inwards from the back and front surfaces, the posterior septum reaching down to the grey commissure, but the anterior fissure being separated from it by a small anterior white commissure that joins the white matter of the two sides together. The white matter is further divided into three columns, on each side, by the horns of grey matter and the nerve roots passing from them to the surface; these are known as the anterior, lateral, and posterior columns.

Functions: The cord is, in part, a receiver and originator of nerve impulses, and in part merely a conductor of such impulses along fibres which pass through it to and from the brain. The presence of centres in the cord, capable of receiving sensory impressions and originating motor impulses, is proved by several facts. Thus, it has been calculated that the number of nerve-fibres entering or leaving the cord by the spinal nerves is twice as great as the number of fibres contained in the upper end of the cord, where it is continued into the brain. Again, if the cord is severed in the dorsal region, as by a fracture of the spine, the centres which govern the evacuation of the bladder and bowel do not lose their power of controlling these organs immediately upon being severed from the brain. Many of these centres are known to exist in the cord, such as centres for regulating the size of the blood-vessels, for altering the size of the pupil of the eye, for sweating, for breathing. Over most, if not all, of these centres, however, the brain exerts a controlling influence, and before any incoming sensation can produce an effect upon consciousness, it is in all probability necessary that it should obtain a clear passage up to the brain.

Many of these centres act in a rhythmical or *automatic* way. Other cells of the cord are capable of originating movements in response to impulses brought direct to them through sensory nerves, such activity being known as *reflex* action. (For a fuller description of the activities of the spinal cord, see NERVES.)

By observing the process of degeneration that takes place when nerve-fibres are cut off by disease or injury from the cells to which they belong, and by observing also the manner in which the fibres in different portions of the cord develop, it has been found possible to divide the three white columns of the cord into tracts, in each of which the fibres have a special function. Thus the posterior column consists of the *fasciculus gracilis* and the *fasciculus cuneatus* both conveying sensory impressions upwards. The lateral column contains the ventral and the dorsal spino-cerebellar tracts passing to the cerebellum, the crossed pyramidal tract of motor fibres carrying outgoing impulses downwards together with the rubro-spinal, the spino-thalamic, the spino-tectal, and the postero-lateral tracts. And, finally, the anterior column contains the direct pyramidal tract of motor fibres and an anterior mixed zone. The pyramidal tracts have the best-known course. Starting from cells near the central sulcus on the brain (see BRAIN), the motor nerve-fibres run down through the internal capsule, pons, and medulla, in the lower part of which many of those coming from the right side of the brain cross to the left side of the spinal cord, and vice versa. Thence the fibres run down in the crossed pyramidal tract to end beside nerve-cells in the anterior horn of the cord. From these nerve-cells other fibres pass outwards to form the nerves that go direct to the muscles. Thus the motor nerve path from brain to muscle is divided into two sections of neurons, of which the upper exerts a controlling influence upon the lower, while the lower is concerned in

1 posterior white column	6 anterior horn
2 lateral white column	7 lateral horn
3 central canal	8 thoracic nucleus
4 anterior white column	9 posterior horn
5 anterior median tissue	10 posterior median septum

Transverse section through the spinal cord in the thoracic region. Magnified eight times.

maintaining the muscle in a state of health and good nutrition, and in directly calling it into action.

SPINE AND SPINAL CORD, DISEASES AND INJURIES OF

SPINE AND SPINAL CORD, DISEASES AND INJURIES OF: SCOLIOSIS is a condition where the spine is curved to one side. The spine is normally straight when seen from behind. The deformity may be mobile and reversible or fixed. If fixed, it is accompanied by vertebral rotation and does not disappear with changes in posture. Fixed scoliosis is idiopathic (q.v.) in 65–80 per cent of cases. There are three main types. The infantile type occurs in boys under three and in 90 per cent of cases resolves spontaneously. The juvenile type affects 4-to-9-year-olds and tends to be progressive. The commonest is adolescent idiopathic scoliosis. Girls are affected in 90 per cent of cases and the incidence is 4 per cent. Treatment may be conservative with a Milwaukee or Boston brace, or surgical fusion may be needed if the curve is greater than 45 degrees. Scoliosis can occur as a congenital condition and in nuromuscular diseases where there is muscle imbalance such as Friedreich's ataxia.

KYPHOSIS is a backward curvature of the spine causing a hump back. It may be postural and reversible in obese people and tall adolescent girls who stoop but it may be fixed. Scheuermann's disease is the term applied to adolescent kyphosis. It is more common in girls. Senile kyphosis occurs in elderly people who probably have osteoporosis (bone weakening) (q.v.) and vertebral collapse.

DISC DEGENERATION is a normal consequence of ageing. The disc loses its resiliance and becomes unable to withstand pressure. Rupture (prolapse) of the disc may occur with physical stress. The disc between the fourth and fifth lumbar vertebrae is most commonly involved. The jelly-like central nucleus pulposus is usually pushed out backwards, forcing the annulus fibrosus to put pressure on the nerves as they leave the spinal canal.

Pain is felt in the back and in the distribution of the compressed nerve. If the disc prolapses forwards into the centre of the spinal canal, it may compress the cauda equina.

Treatment is bed rest with traction and pain relief. Rarely removal of the disc is needed. Compression of the cauda equina is a surgical emergency.

ANKYLOSING SPONDYLITIS is a rheumatic disease of young adults, mostly men. It is a familial condition which starts with lumbar pain and stiffness which progresses to involve the whole spine. The discs and ligaments are replaced by fibrous tissue making the spine rigid. Treatment is physiotherapy and anti-inflammatory drugs to try to keep the spine supple for as long as possible.

A National Association for Ankylosing Spondylitis has been formed which is open to those with the disease, their families, friends and doctors. Those interested should apply to the Secretary, 5 Grosvenor Crescent, London SW1X 7ER (071-235 9585).

SPONDYLOSIS is a term which covers disc degeneration and joint degeneration in the back. Osteoarthritis is usually implicated. Pain is commonly felt in the neck and lumbar regions and in these areas the joints may become unstable. This may put pressure on the nerves leaving the spinal canal and in the lumbar region pain is generally felt in the distribution of the sciatic nerve – down the back of the leg. In the neck the pain may be felt down the arm. Treatment is physiotherapy; often a neck collar or lumbar support helps. Rarely surgery is needed to remove the pressure from the nerves.

SPONDYLOLISTHESIS means that the spine is shifted forward. This is nearly always in the lower lumbar region and may be familial, or due to degeneration in the joints. Pressure may be put on the cauda equina. The usual complaint is of pain after exercise. Treatment is bed rest in a bad attack with surgery indicated only if there are worrying signs of cord compression.

SPINAL STENOSIS is due to a narrowing of the spinal canal which means that the nerves become squashed together. This causes numbness with pins and needles (paraesthia) in the legs. Computed tomography and nuclear magnetic resonance imaging scans can show the amount of cord compression. If improving posture does not help, surgical decompression may be needed.

WHIPLASH INJURIES occur to the neck usually as the result of a car accident when the head and neck are thrown backwards and then forwards rapidly. This causes pain and stiffness in the neck and the arm and shoulder may feel numb. Often a support collar relieves the pain but recovery commonly takes between 18 months to three years.

TRANSECTION OF THE CORD occurs usually as a result of trauma when the vertebral column protecting the spinal cord is fractured and becomes unstable. The cord may be concussed or it may have become sheared by the trauma and not recover (transected). Spinal concussion usually recovers after 12 hours. If the cord is transected the patient remains paralysed.

SPINNER'S FINGER is a cricket injury. Bowlers are liable to develop callosities (q.v.) of the fingers of the bowling hand. These tend to crack, and this is the condition known as spinner's finger.

SPIRAMYCIN is an antibiotic isolated from *Streptomyces ambofaciens*, which is useful in the treatment of certain cases of staphylococcal infection.

SPIRILLUM is a form of micro-organism of wavy or spiral shape. (See MICROBIOLOGY.)

SPIRIT is a strong solution of alcohol in water. (See ALCOHOL.) Proof spirit is one containing 57 per cent of alcohol by volume or 49 per cent by weight, and is so named because it can stand the proof of just catching fire. Rectified spirit contains 90 per cent of alcohol by volume or over 85 per cent by weight. Proof spirit is generally used in the preparation of tinctures. Spirits of various drugs contain a solution of any given drug in rectified spirit, examples include aromatic spirit of ammonia (sal volatile), and spirit of ether. Methylated spirit (also known as wood naphtha or wood spirit) is distilled from wood. When taken internally, it is a dangerous poison producing neuritis, especially neuritis of the optic nerves which may result in blindness. Methylated spirit is used to harden the skin for the prevention of bed sores and foot soreness.

SPIRITS consist of medicinal substances or flavouring agents dissolved in alcohol.

SPIROCHAETE is an order of bacteria which has a spiral form.

SPIROMETER: A test of how the lung is working used to assess the effects of lung disease or the progress of treatment. The spirometer records the total volume of air breathed out – the forced vital capacity. The machine also records the volume of air breathed out in one second – the forced expiratory volume. In diseases such as asthma, in which the airways are obstructed, the ratio of the forced expiratory volume to the forced vital capacity is reduced.

SPIRONOLACTONE belongs to the group of substances known as spirolactones. These are steroids similar to aldosterone (q.v.) in structure which competitively act as inhibitors of it. They can thus antagonize the action of aldosterone in the renal tubules. As there is evidence that there is an increased output of aldosterone in oedematous conditions, such as congestive heart failure, which accentuates the oedema, spironolactone is used, along with other diuretics, in resistant cases of oedema – to antagonize the fluid-retaining action of aldosterone. (See DIURETICS.)

SPLANCHNIC means anything belonging to the internal organs of the body as distinguished from its framework.

SPLEEN is an organ deeply placed in the abdomen.
Position and size: The spleen lies behind the stomach, high up on the left side of the abdomen, and corresponds to the position of the 9th, 10th, and 11th ribs, from which it is separated by the diaphragm. It is a soft, highly vascular, plum-coloured organ, and has a smooth surface, being almost completely covered by peritoneum. There are two wide peritoneal ligaments that support the spleen, the one attaching it to the stomach, the other to the kidney. Through the latter ligament the

1 capsule
2 venous sinuses
3 arterial capillaries ending in sinuses
4 small arteries
5 Malphigi capsules
6 artery
7 vein
8 central artery of Malphigi corpuscle
9 trabecula of capsule

Diagram of spleen.

large vessels that supply the spleen with blood make their way. The size of the spleen varies widely. It is usually about 12·5 to 15 cm (5 to 6 inches) in length, and weighs about 170 grams or more, but these dimensions depend upon the amount of blood contained in it, for it contracts from time to time, and after meals is much smaller than at other times. In diseased conditions the organ may reach a weight of 8 to 9 kg.
Structure: The spleen is enveloped by peritoneal membrane like the stomach and intestines, and this smooth coat greatly facilitates its movements. Beneath the peritoneum is a strong elastic tunic, composed partly of fibrous tissue containing many elastic fibres, and partly of unstriped muscle. This elastic coat allows of the free expansion and contraction of the organ according to the varying amount of blood present in it. From the inner surface of the membrane fibrous partitions known as trabeculae run down into the substance and form a network in which the dark spleen pulp is contained. If the spleen is cut open and the pulp washed away, these trabeculae stand out as shaggy projections on the cut surface. The pulp consists of delicate connective tissue fibres passing between the various trabeculae and of white and red blood corpuscles lying in this meshwork. Round the smaller arteries there are condensed areas of this pulp formed of developing white blood corpuscles, and known as Malpighian bodies or corpuscles.
BLOOD-VESSELS pass to the spleen, and are so large compared with the size which would be

necessary in order simply to carry nutritive material to the spleen as to render it clear that the organ has some important action connected with the maintenance of the blood. The arteries which enter the spleen at the hilum become smaller and smaller till they end in capillaries, which open freely into the pulp. The blood thus escapes readily into the substance of the spleen, and, after passing through its meshwork, is collected by veins that unite into larger trunks till they form the splenic vein, which leaves the organ and joins the portal vein. There are also numerous lymphatics in the organ, which run in the trabeculae or surround the veins.

Functions: The organ produces lymphocytes and acts as a reservoir of red blood cells for use in emergencies. It is also one of the sites for the manufacture of red blood cells in the fetus, but not after birth. Useless or worn-out red and white blood corpuscles and blood platelets are broken up by this organ. This results in the production of bilirubin (q.v.), which is conveyed to the liver, and of iron, which is used in the bone marrow for the production of new red blood cells. Nevertheless the spleen does not appear to be absolutely essential to life, since its removal is followed by increase in size of the lymphatic glands all over the body, and does not necessarily interfere with health.

SPLEEN, DISEASES OF: In certain diseases associated with marked changes in the blood, such as leukaemia, and malaria, the spleen becomes chronically enlarged. In some of the acute infectious diseases, it becomes congested and acutely enlarged: for example, in typhoid fever, anthrax, and infectious mononucleosis. Rupture of the spleen may occur, like rupture of other internal organs, in consequence of extreme violence, but in malarious countries, where many people have the spleen greatly enlarged and softened as the result of malaria, rupture of this organ occurs now and then as the result of some quite trivial blow upon the left side. The spleen, in consequence of its structure, bleeds excessively when torn, so that this accident is generally followed by collapse, signs of internal haemorrhage – and death if not dealt with promptly by operation.

SPLENECTOMY means removal of the spleen. This operation may be necessary if the spleen has been severely injured or in the treatment of the severe form of acholuric jaundice or auto-immune thrombocytopenic purpura. (See PURPURA.)

SPLENOMEGALY means enlargement of the spleen beyond its normal size.

SPLINTER HAEMORRHAGES are linear bleeds under the finger nails. Although they may result from injury they are a useful physical sign of infective endocarditis.

SPLINTS are supports for an injured or wounded part. They are most commonly employed in cases in which a bone is fractured, and consist then of some rigid substance designed to take the place of the broken bone in maintaining the shape of the limb, as well as to keep the broken ends at rest and in contact, and thus to ensure their union. Splints are most commonly made of wood either shaped to the limb or consisting merely of strips of wood about the width of the injured limb, and carefully padded with wool or similar soft material. Splints are also made of metal, poroplastic felt, leather, and cotton stiffened with plaster of Paris, as well as other materials. Splints may be improvized for first-aid out of walking-sticks, rifles, broom-handles, branches, folded-up newspapers, and in fact anything of suitable length and rigidity. (See FRACTURES.)

SPONDYLITIS is another name for arthritis of the spine. (See SPINE AND SPINAL CORD, DISEASES AND INJURIES OF.)

SPONDYLOLISTHESIS (see SPINE AND SPINAL CORD, DISEASES AND INJURIES OF).

SPONDYLOSIS (see SPINE AND SPINAL CORD, DISEASES AND INJURIES OF.)

SPONGIFORM ENCEPHALOPATHY: A disease of the neurological system caused by slow virus (q.v.) Spongy degeneration of the brain with progresive dementia occurs. Known examples of the disorder in humans are Creutzfeldt-Jakob disease and kuru. Among animals scrapie in sheep and bovine spongiform encephalopathy (BSE) (q.v.) are caused by slow viruses. They are believed not be be transferable to humans, but research on this aspect is continuing.

SPORADIC is the term applied to cases of disease occurring here and there, as opposed to epidemic outbreaks.

SPORE: Part of the life cycle of certain bacteria when the vegetative cell is encapsulated and metabolism falls to a low level. The spore is resistant to changes in the environment and, when these are unfavourable, the spore remains dormant; when they improve, it starts to grow. Certain dangerous bacteria, such as clostridium (q.v.), produce resistant ubiquitous spores so sterilization procedures need to be very effective.

SPORTS INJURIES, PREVENTION OF: There are four basic rules for the prevention of sports injuries. (1) Be fit for the sport or game. (2) Obey the rules, written and unwritten. (3) Wear the right clothes and shoes. (4) Use common sense. The first of these is obvious. In amplification of the others, Dr John Williams,

Medical Director of the Regional Sports Injuries Centre, Farnham Park Rehabilitation Centre, Slough, makes some cogent comments in his book, *Injury in Sport*.

'Obedience to the rules of the game (the spirit as well as the letter) is an essential component of injury prevention.' 'Reckless play is a not uncommon cause of injury.' 'It is the self-discipline of each individual player that finally determines whether sport will be safe or not. Since self-discipline is an essential component of sport, he who cannot discipline himself must be regarded as a menace on the sports field and if necessary permanently banned.'

Emphasis is laid on the importance of correct clothing and footwear. Clothing is often made of unsuitable material. Worn-out shoes and laces, jagged trouser buckles and sweat-rotted collars can all cause serious injury. The design of shoes may be faulty (e.g. the wrong siting of studs on football boots), or inappropriate (e.g. the same pair of shoes would not be suitable for running both on tartan track and asphalt road). A warning is given against advertisements that claim sports gear is in some way medically tested. Natural materials are better than man-made for clothes and footwear because of their absorbent and sweat evaporation qualities. When man-made fibres are worn, open weave is recommended.

All participants in sports should be immunized against tetanus (q.v.), and maintain this immunity by receiving regular booster injections every three years.

SPOTS BEFORE THE EYES can arise from a variety of causes including inflammation and bleeding in the eye, or preceding a retina detachment. They may also occur for a variety of totally harmless reasons.

SPOTTED FEVER (see MENINGITIS; EPIDEMIC; CEREBROSPINAL FEVER; TYPHUS FEVER).

SPRAINS are injuries in the neighbourhood of joints, consisting usually in tearing of a ligament with effusion of blood. (See JOINTS, DISEASES OF.)

SPRUE, or PSILOSIS, is a disease of uncertain origin, characterized by diarrhoea with the passage of large, fatty stools, anaemia, sore tongue, and loss of weight. The name was first given to the condition in 1879 by Sir Patrick Manson, and it was then considered to be a disease of tropical climates. Subsequent investigations have shown that a similar condition occurs in individuals who have never been in the tropics. To this latter condition the name of non-tropical sprue is usually given. The following description applies predominantly to the condition as it occurs in the tropics.

Causes: Many theories have been advanced concerning the cause of sprue, but the general consensus of opinion today is that it is due to an inborn error of metabolism characterized primarily by inability to absorb fats from the intestine. This explains the bulky, frothy stools due to excess of fat. Subsequently there is interference with the absorption of carbohydrate, vitamins and minerals. The poor absorption of vitamins is responsible for the anaemia and sore tongue, whilst the decreased absorption of calcium is responsible for the low level of calcium in the blood. One advantage of this theory is that it correlates three somewhat similar conditions: (1) tropical sprue; (2) non-tropical sprue; (3) coeliac disease (q.v.) which is a condition found in children. In all these the fundamental cause is the same. In children with coeliac disease the error of metabolism is so marked that the condition appears early in life. In adults the error is less marked and requires either some precipitating factor to provoke it, or else the normal ageing process. In the case of tropical sprue these precipitating factors are one or more of the following: an attack of dysentery; the strain of living in a hot, damp climate; dietetic indiscretions; the highly spiced diet so commonly eaten by Europeans in the tropics.

Tropical sprue is found chiefly in India, Burma, Malaysia, Indonesia and China. It also occurs in the Southern States of USA, the West Indies, and South America. It is more common in Europeans than in natives, and is more common in women than in men. As a rule it occurs after long residence in the tropics, and the onset is usually after the rains. There is quite often a preceding history of dysentery.

Symptoms: The onset may be gradual or rapid. Initially there are weakness, soreness of the tongue, difficulty in swallowing, indigestion, and diarrhoea. The diarrhoea is usually worst in the morning, and the stools are pale, bulky, and frothy. The appetite is usually poor. There is a marked degree of anaemia, usually of the macrocytic type: i.e. there is a high colour index. The tongue is smooth and red. Gastric acidity is low. Other characteristic findings are that the rise in the blood sugar level following the taking of sugar is less than normal, and there is an increase in the amount of fat in the stools. In untreated cases the patient steadily loses weight and becomes emaciated. Death is usually due to exhaustion and some intercurrent infection. The prognosis depends largely upon the stage at which treatment is begun.

Treatment: The essentials of treatment are rest in bed, a high-protein diet, and treatment of the anaemia and any other deficiency that may be present. It is usual to start the diet with skimmed milk and gradually add other items such as meat. Some authorities, on the other hand, recommend beginning with a diet consisting largely of beef. Whichever diet is used, the essential fact to be borne in mind is that the patient cannot tolerate fats, but that a high caloric intake is necessary to ensure that the patient is adequately nourished. This can best be done by a diet consisting predominantly of protein. For the anaemia folic acid and cyanocobalamin are required. Large doses of the vitamin B complex are also helpful: e.g.

Marmite. As the blood calcium level is also diminished, vitamins A and D should be given, and it is sometimes useful to supplement this by calcium lactate. As has already been pointed out, convalescence is often prolonged, resulting sometimes in marked depression on the part of the patient. Satisfactory results are seldom obtained unless the patient is sent home to a temperate climate. An individual who has had sprue should never return to residence in the tropics unless it is absolutely essential.

Non-tropical sprue or gluten enteropathy is due to a hypersensitivity to gluten and the treatment is a gluten-free diet.

SPUTUM means material spat out of the mouth. It may consist of saliva from the mouth, of mucous secretions from the throat or back of the nose, but is generally expectorated by coughing from the lower air passages. (See EXPECTORATION.)

SQUINT or STRABISMUS: A condition in which the visual axes of each eye are not directed simultaneously at the same fixation point (i.e. each eye is not pointing at the same object at the same time). Squints may be: (a) Paralytic, where one or more of the muscles, or their nerve supply is damaged; this type usually results in double vision. (b) Non-paralytic, where the muscles and nerves are normal. It is usually found in children. This type of squint can either result in poor vision, or occasionally may result from poor vision. Squints may be convergent (where one eye 'turns in') or divergent (one eye 'turns out'). Vertical squints can also occur but are less common. All squints should be seen by an eye specialist as soon as possible. Some squints can be corrected by exercises or spectacles; others require surgery.

STABS (see WOUNDS).

STAGHORN CALCULUS: A branched renal stone formed in the image of the collecting system of the kidney. It fills the calyces and pelvis and is commonly associated with an infection of the urine, particularly *Proteus vulgaris*. The calculus may lead to pyonephrosis and an abscess of the kidney.

STAMMERING is a disruption of the forward flow of speech. The individual knows what he wants to say but he temporarily loses his ability to execute linguistically formulated speech. Stammering is characterized by a silent or audible involuntary repetition/prolongation of an utterance, be it a sound, syllable or word. Sometimes it is accompanied by accessory behaviours, or speech-related struggle. Usually there are indications or the report of an accompanying emotional state, involving excitement, tension, fear or embarrassment.

Idiopathic stammering begins sometime between the onset of speech and puberty, mostly between 2 and 5 years of age. Acquired stammering at a later age due to brain damage is rare. The prevalence of stammering (the percentage of the population actually stammering at any point in time) is approximately 0·9 per cent. Three times as many boys as girls stammer. About 70 per cent of stammering children recover with little or no therapy. Stammerers have not been shown to demonstrate differences in personality from non-stammerers. There are, however, indications that at least some stammerers show minimal differences from fluent speakers in cerebral processing of verbal material.

There is a genetic predisposition towards stammering. The risk of stammering among first-degree relatives of stammerers is more than three times the population risk. In 77 per cent of identical twins either both stammer or both are fluent. Only 33 per cent of non-identical twins agree in this way. As there are identical twins who differ for stammering, environmental factors must be important for some stammerers. There are relatively large numbers of stammerers in highly competitive societies, where status and prestige are important and high standards of speech competence are valued.

Different treatments have been demonstrated to produce considerable benefit, their basic outline being similar. A long period of time is spent in training stammerers to speak in a different way (fluency-shaping techniques). This may include slowing down the rate of speech, gentle onset of utterance, continuous flow with correct juncturing, etc. When the targets have been achieved within the clinic a series of planned speech assignments outside the clinic is undertaken. In these assignments, and initially in everyday situations, the fluency-enchancing techniques have to be used conscientiously. Gradually speech is shaped towards normality requiring less and less effort. Therapy may also include some work on attitude change (i.e. helping the client to see himself as a fluent speaker) and possibly general communicative skills training.

STANNOSIS is the form of pneumoconiosis (q.v.) caused by the inhalation of stannous (tin) oxide, which occurs in tin ore mining.

STANOZOLOL (see ANABOLIC STEROIDS).

STAPES: The innermost of the small trio of bones in the middle ear. It is stirrup shaped and articulates with the incus and is linked to the oval window of the inner ear. (See EAR.)

STAPHYLOCOCCUS is a bacterium which under the microscope appears in small masses like bunches of grapes. It is one of the commonest infectious micro-organisms and is found, for example, in the pus discharged from boils (see MICROBIOLOGY).

STARCH is a substance belonging to that group of carbohydrates known as the amyloses. It is the form in which utilizable carbohydrate is stored in granules within the seeds and roots of many plants. It is converted into sugar when treated with heat in presence of a dilute acid. It is changed largely into dextrin when exposed to a considerable degree of dry heat, as in toasting bread; and a similar change into dextrin and malt-sugar takes place under the action of various ferments such as the ptyalin of the saliva. Starch forms a chief constituent of the carbohydrate foods (see DIET), and in the process of digestion the above-mentioned change takes place to prepare it for absorption. It is also slowly broken down in the process of cooking.

Starch is used externally to form a poultice for softening the skin in skin diseases. (See POULTICES.) It is also used as a constituent of dusting powders for application to chafed or irritable areas of the skin. (See CHAFING OF THE SKIN.) Starch enema is administered in inflammatory conditions of the bowel. (See ENEMA.)

STARVATION: Partial starvation, as a method of treatment, is used in certain diseases associated with previous excess of food, particularly obesity. (See OBESITY.) When a person is completely deprived of food for a time, not only is there great loss of weight but the chemical processes of the body are altered, and a poisoning effect is produced by the formation of acetone and other ketone bodies. In cases of slow starvation, the vitality of the tissues is reduced and they become more liable to tuberculosis and other diseases. (See also FASTING.)

STASIS is a term applied to stoppage of the flow of blood in the vessels or of the food materials down the intestinal canal. (For Blood Stasis, see CIRCULATION, DISORDERS OF.)

STATUS ASTHMATICUS: Repeated attacks of asthma, with no respite between the spasms, usually lasting for more than 24 hours. The patient is seriously distressed and, untreated, the condition may lead to death from respiratory failure and exhaustion. Corticosteroid treatment and other skilled medical care are urgently required.

STATUS EPILEPTICUS: Repeated epileptic fits with no return to consciousness between them. Breathing stops between each fit and the body is deprived of oxygen which causes damage to the brain. Urgent medical attention is required to control the condition or the patient may die.

STEATORRHOEA is any condition characterized by the passing of stools containing an excess of fat. (See MALABSORPTION SYNDROME.)

STENOSIS is a term applied to a condition of unnatural narrowing in any passage or orifice of the body. The word is specially used in connection with the four openings of the heart at which the valves are situated. (See HEART DISEASES.)

STENT: A surgical device used to assist the healing of an operative anastamosis – a joining up of two structures. A splint is left inside the lumen of a duct and this drains the contents.

STEREOGNOSIS means the faculty of recognizing the solidity of objects, and thus their nature, by handling them.

STEREOTAXIS is the procedure whereby precise localization in space is achieved. It is applied to that branch of surgery known as *stereotactic neurosurgery*, in which the surgeon is able to localize precisely those areas of the brain on which he wishes to operate.

STERILIZATION means either (1) the process of rendering various objects, such as those which come in contact with wounds, and various foods, free from microbes, or (2) the process of rendering a person incapable of producing children.

The manner of sterilizing bedding, furniture, and the like, after contact with a case of infectious disease, is given under DISINFECTION, whilst the sterilization of instruments, dressings, and skin surfaces, necessary before surgical procedures, is mentioned in the same article and also under ANTISEPTICS, ASEPSIS, and WOUNDS. For general purposes, one of the cheapest and most effective agents is boiling water or steam.
Use of sterilization: Milk is the chief article of food that calls for special sterilization. With regard to other foods, ordinary cooking has this for one of its chief objects.
Method of sterilization: One of the most effective modes is simply to boil the milk for a prolonged period in a covered pan; but this changes its taste considerably, and is therefore unsuitable for children and invalids, who tend to drink large amounts of milk.

Another method is to place the milk in a flask or bottle of which the neck is closed by a plug of cotton-wool, and set it in a pot of water, from the bottom of which it is separated by a triangle of wire or other means. The pot is placed on the stove and the water boiled for three-quarters of an hour, by which time the milk is sufficiently sterilized without appreciably affecting its taste. Many forms of sterilizer are on the market, but all depend upon this principle of having an inner vessel or set of bottles suspended within an outer pot containing water, which is boiled for three-quarters of an hour to one hour. Care must be taken that the milk is not uncovered, after being sterilized, until just before it is to be used.

Pasteurization is a slightly different method of treatment, which is sufficient to destroy the microbes that cause gastroenteritis, as well as those of many other diseases such as tuberculosis and typhoid fever, while preserving the natural state of the milk. (See PASTEURIZATION.)

Koch's method of sterilization is used in bacteriological investigation, where even the spores of bacteria must be destroyed. It is carried out by steaming the objects to be sterilized on three successive days. (See BACTERIOLOGY.)

BACTERIOLOGICAL STERILIZATION may be effected in many ways, and different methods are used in different cases, for it is evident that processes applicable to clothing or to a room may be quite unsuited for the sterilization of food.

SEXUAL STERILIZATION is being used to an increasing extent. In women it is performed by ligating, or cutting, and then tying the Fallopian tubes (q.v.), the tubes that carry the ovum from the ovary to the uterus. Alternatively the tubes may be sealed off by means of plastic and silicone clips or rings. It is usually performed through a small incision, or cut, in the lower abdominal wall. It has no effect on sexual or menstrual function, and, unlike the comparable operation in men, it is immediately effective. The sterilization is almost always permanent, but occasionally, for some unknown reason, the two cut ends of the Fallopian tubes reunite, and pregnancy is then again possible. Removal of the uterus and/or the ovaries also causes sterilization, but such procedures are only used when there is some special reason, such as the presence of a tumour.

The operation for sterilizing men is known as vasectomy (q.v.).

STERNUM is another name for the breastbone.

STEROID is the group name for compounds that resemble cholesterol chemically. The group includes the sex hormones, the hormones of the adrenal cortex, and bile acids.

STERTOR is a term applied to noisy breathing resembling snoring. It is due usually to flapping of the soft palate between a stream of air entering by the nose and one entering by the mouth. In ordinary snoring (q.v.) this results from the habit of sleeping with the mouth open, and in certain serious disorders it arises from paralysis of the soft palate. Some of these conditions affecting the nervous system and thus leading to paralysis of the soft palate are: apoplexy, suffocation, concussion of the brain, drunkenness, poisoning by opium or by chloroform. (For the means of distinguishing between these conditions see OPIUM POISONING.) In some of these paralytic conditions the snoring is very loud, and the noise is due then, not to flapping of the soft palate, but to lolling back of the tongue against the back of the throat as the patient lies on his back. In this case the breathing is at once relieved by pulling forward the lower jaw, by pulling the tongue out of the mouth, or by turning the patient upon one side, as is done, for example, in suffocation due to drowning.

Stertorous breathing is not to be confused with *sniffing* breathing produced by paralysis of the muscles that should hold the nostrils still and open; nor with *puffing* breathing due to paralysis of the muscles in the cheeks and lips; though all three conditions may be produced by the same causes. Nor must it be mistaken for *stridor*, or crowing breathing, due to spasmodic narrowing in the larynx; nor for the prolonged, noisy, *wheezing* breathing of asthma produced by narrowing of the bronchial tubes.

STETHOSCOPE is an instrument used for listening to the sounds produced by the action of the lungs, heart, and other internal organs. (See AUSCULTATION.)

STEVENS-JOHNSON SYNDROME: This is a form of erythema multiforme which is characterized by annular lesions which can develop into blisters. In addition to the skin lesions in this syndrome there is severe involvement of the eyes and the mucosa, giving rise to ulceration. It is commonly a hypersensitivity reaction to drugs particularly the sulphonamide group of antibiotics.

STIFFNESS is a condition which may be due to a change in the joints, ligaments, tendons, or muscles, or to the influence of the nervous system over the muscles of the part affected. Stiffness is associated with various forms of rheumatism. Stiffness of the neck muscles resulting in bending backward the head, and of the hamstring muscles, causing difficulty in straightening the lower limbs, is a sign of meningitis. Stiffness or spasticity also occurs in certain diseases of the central nervous system.

STIGMA means any spot or impression upon the skin. The term, stigmas of degeneration, is applied to physical defects that are found in mentally handicapped persons. (See MENTAL HANDICAP.)

STILBOESTROL is a synthetic oestrogen. Its physiological actions are closely similar to those of the natural ovarian hormone, and it has the great merit of being active when taken by mouth. An interesting property of stilboestrol is seen in the relief it affords when given to patients suffering from cancer of the prostate, inducing in some cases, it appears, regression of the primary tumour and of secondary deposits in bone. (See OESTROGEN.)

STILBOESTROL DIPHOSPHATE (see OESTROGEN).

STILET, or STILETTE, means the delicate probe or the wire used to clear a catheter or hollow needle.

STILLBIRTH: A stillborn child is 'any child which has issued forth from its mother after the twenty-eighth week of pregnancy and which did not at any time after being completely expelled from its mother, breathe or show any other sign of life'. In England, in 1990, the number of stillbirths was 3,068. (See PERINATAL MORTALITY.)

STILL'S DISEASE, or JUVENILE RHEUMATOID ARTHRITIS, is a disease of childhood first described by Sir Frederic Still (1868–1941). The characteristic of the disease is that the arthritis is usually symmetrical. It tends to start in the fingers, which become spindle-shaped due to the swelling of the affected joints. It then spreads to involve other joints, practically always in a symmetrical manner, including the wrists, elbows, knees and ankles. Occasionally, only one joint, such as the knee, may be involved initially. The onset may be abrupt, with high temperature, or gradual. The cervical spine is often involved, leading to stiffness of the neck, and some of these cases go on to ankylosing spondylitis (see SPINE AND SPINAL CORD, DISEASES AND INJURIES OF). As a result of the child's not moving the affected joints because of the pain this causes, there is marked wasting of the muscles. The heart is seldom involved, but there is often a characteristic rash. The age of onset is usually between 2 and 5 years, and the disease is marked by repeated recurrences. The disease is usally self-limiting, but tends to relapse and may persist for several years. Treatment is as for rheumatoid arthritis (q.v.) in the adult.

STIMULANTS are drugs and other agents employed to call forth special powers of the body or of individual organs in order to effect some special purpose or to offer resistance to some acute attack of disease. The use of stimulants presupposes a certain amount of reserve power on the part of the body or of the organ stimulated, which is lying dormant and requires an appropriate stimulus before it can be brought into action. In its broadest sense, the term stimulant includes all remedies which are not simply foods destined to supply the wear and tear of the body and to provide it with a store of energy-producing material. It also excludes remedies which have a sedative action upon the nervous system or other organs, and remedies which act directly upon the causes of disease without any reference to the body, such as antiseptics.

(For drugs which stimulate the intestines, see PURGATIVES; for those that stimulate the liver, see CHOLAGOGUES; for those that stimulate the kidneys, see DIURETICS.) Many substances, such as aromatics, spices, and bitters, stimulate the function of the stomach.

STINGS (see BITES AND STINGS).

STITCH is a popular name for a sharp pain in the side. It is generally due to cramp following unusually hard exertion (see CRAMP), but care must be taken that this trivial condition is not taken for pleurisy or for a fractured rib.

(For the stitches used to unite the edges of wounds, see WOUNDS.)

STOKES-ADAMS SYNDROME is a term applied to a condition in which slowness of the pulse is associated with attacks of unconsciousness, and which is due to a state of heart-block.

STOMA: A stoma refers to an opening constructed when the bowel has to be brought to the skin surface to convey gastrointestinal contents to the exterior. It is derived from the Greek word meaning mouth. In the United Kingdom there are about 100,000 patients with a colostomy, 10,000 with an ileostomy and some 2,000 with a urostomy in which the ureters are brought to the skin surface. They may be undertaken because of malignancy of the colon or rectum or as a result of inflammatory bowel diseases such as Crohn's disease. Urostomies usually take the form of an isolated loop of ilium into which the ureters have been implanted and which in its turn is brought to the skin's surface. This is undertaken because of bladder cancer or because of neurological diseases of the bladder. The stomas drain into appliances such as disposable plastic bags. Most of the modern appliances collect the effluent of the stoma without any leak or odour.

Patients with stomas often find explanatory booklets helpful. *Living with your Colostomy* and *Understanding Colostomy* are examples.

STOMACH: The stomach is a dilated portion of the alimentary canal, which in man has a shape somewhat resembling a pear. The larger end, known as the fundus, lies in the hollow of the left side of the diaphragm, and at one side of this is the opening from the gullet. The greater part of the stomach, into which the gullet opens, is known as the cardiac part, whilst the lower and narrower portion is known as the cardia, or cardiac orifice, and the pylorus. The stomach is slightly flattened from before backwards, and the two edges are known as the lesser curvature, which runs from one opening to the other direct, and the greater curvature, which sweeps round the fundus from the cardia to the pylorus.

Size and position: The stomach hangs freely suspended in the upper and left part of the abdomen, so that changes in position and shape take place readily according to the amount of food it contains. On the surface, the stomach corresponds to the ribs on the left side from about the fifth to the ninth, and extends below their protecting margin about halfway down to the navel, while the person is recumbent, and slightly below the navel when he stands up. The fundus lies immediately below the heart and base of the left lung, separated from them only by the diaphragm and their enveloping membranes. This explains the embarrassment of the heart's action and of breathing sometimes experienced by dyspeptics. The stomach is attached at the cardiac opening to the gullet, and at this point it is further secured to the diaphragm by a ligament. A broad band of peritoneum (small omentum) attaches the lesser curvature to the under surface of the liver, and a similar peritoneal fold unites its hinder surface to the spleen. The pyloric end, like the cardiac opening, is to a great extent fixed in position, but the greater curvature is quite freely movable.

The greatest length of the stomach from the fundus to the greater curvature near the pylorus is about 30 cm (12 inches), and the greatest breadth does not exceed 10 to 12·5 cm (4 to 5 inches). The capacity varies greatly in different people, but is usually about 1 to 1½ litres in adults. At birth its capacity is around 30 millilitres.

Structure: The stomach possesses four coats similar to those of the intestine. From within outwards, these are a lining of mucous membrane, a submucous layer, a muscular coat, and a peritoneal coat.

MUCOUS MEMBRANE lines the interior of the stomach and is of smooth, soft texture, though raised up into ridges when the stomach is empty. The surface can be seen with the naked eye to be thickly covered by minute pits into each of which several tube-shaped glands are found, on microscopic section, to open. The mucous membrane in fact consists almost en-tirely of these glands placed side by side, and supported by a small quantity of connective tissue and by fibres of unstriped muscle. The surface of the mucous membrane is composed of a single layer of columnar cells, and these also line the pits referred to. Each gland is composed of large cubical cells so arranged as to form a tube, open at the upper end where it meets the pit, and closed beneath. These cells secrete the gastric juice which exudes from all the minute tubes as digestion is proceeding. In the cardiac end of the stomach there are other larger cells in addition, mingled with those just described, and the large cells are supposed to secrete the acid of the gastric juice. Between the tubular glands lies some supporting connective tissue in which run numerous blood-capillaries and lymph-vessels.

SUBMUCOUS COAT is a loose connective tissue layer which joins the mucous coat to the muscular coat, and in which the large blood-vessels of the stomach run. The loose arrangement of its fibres allows the mucous membrane to glide freely over the muscular coat in the movements and variations in size of the stomach.

MUSCULAR COAT is of considerable thickness in the stomach, and is of great importance in varying the size of the organ according to the amount of food it contains, in making the peristaltic movements which mix the food with the digestive juice, and finally in expelling the softened food from the stomach into the small intestine. This coat consists of three layers: an outer one in which the fibres run lengthwise, a middle one where they are circular, and an inner layer in which they run obliquely across the stomach.

1 duodenum
2 pyloric sphincter
3 pylorus
4 pyloric canal
5 pyloric portion

6 greater curvature
7 cardiac portion
8 fundus
9 cardiac orifice
10 lesser curvature

The interior of the stomach.

PERITONEAL COAT is similar to the peritoneum covering the other organs of the abdomen. (See PERITONEUM.)

BLOOD-VESSELS: The stomach is abundantly supplied with blood from the coeliac trunk, a short, wide artery which comes directly from the aorta and also gives branches to the liver, pancreas, and spleen. There is a large arterial arch round either curvature, and from these two arches smaller branches run into the wall of the stomach and reach the submucous coat, from which minute branches are distributed to the other coats. The blood is collected by veins which ultimately return it to the portal vein.

NERVES: The stomach is richly supplied with nerves both from the brain and from the autonomic system. The tenth cranial nerve (vagus) of each side has a long course down the side of the gullet (hence its name: vagus or wanderer), and after giving branches to the larynx, heart, lungs, and other organs, terminates in the stomach, which has therefore important nervous connections with these vital organs. Other branches come from the solar (or coeliac) plexus of the sympathetic system. These nerves form a plexus in the submucous coat and another in the muscular coat, which exert a powerful influence over the secretions and movements of the organ, although these functions are, in the main, carried out automatically.

Functions of the stomach: The part played by the stomach in digestion consists in storing, warming, and softening the food, as well as partially digesting it, and then in passing it on in small quantities to the intestine, where the more important digestive processes that prepare it for absorption take place. The action of the gastric juice upon the food has been described under DIGESTION. The action of the muscular coat of the stomach is also very important. The movements, as seen by the aid of X-rays, consist of a series of waves, each of which takes about half a minute to pass along the stomach. These movements have also the effect of separating the more fluid parts from lumps still left in the later stages of digestion which are retained in the cardiac part of the stomach while the pylorus relaxes as each wave reaches it to allow some of the softened mass to pass through into the small intestine. This muscular movement takes place in health without causing any sensation, but in irritable conditions of the stomach, when digestion is not proceeding naturally, it may increase in force and give rise to irregular spasms which come and go, and which are attended by much pain. (See DYSPEPSIA.)

STOMACH, DISEASES OF: Only the more common and serious varieties of gastric disease can be considered here. The majority of them exhibit as their most marked and sometimes their only feature, the symptoms of dyspepsia. (See DYSPEPSIA.)

ACUTE GASTRITIS: **Causes**: Of these, the most important are: (1) Dietetic indiscretions: e.g. a large indigestible meal, or the excessive consumption of alcohol; (2) food poisoning; (3) infections: e.g. influenza, septicaemia; (4) toxins: e.g. uraemia; (5) the swallowing of poisons: e.g. acids, alkalis.

Symptoms: The chief change the stomach undergoes affects its mucous membrane, which is in a state of congestion, either throughout or in parts. The symptoms are those well known as characterizing an acute 'bilious attack', consisting in loss of appetite, sickness or nausea, and headache, frontal or occipital, often accompanied with giddiness and abdominal discomfort. An attack of this kind tends to subside in a few days, especially if the exciting cause is removed. Sometimes, however, the symptoms recur, in which case investigations, including possibly gastroscopy (q.v.), may be necessary.

Treatment: The offending cause must be removed and the patient must avoid alcohol and smoking. Antacids may help but, if there is any pain, aspirin must *not* be taken. Paracetamol may be used if the pain is troublesome but, if it is persistent, medical advice should be sought.

CHRONIC GASTRITIS may arise after repeated attacks of the acute form or may come on independently. It is of several types. The result of the chronic irritation of the gastric mucous membrane may be an excessively acid gastric juice, which gives rise to an acid dyspepsia. After a long period of irritation an atrophy of the secreting structures of the stomach may be produced, and there is then little or no secretion of gastric juice. In addition to this failure to secrete a proper gastric juice, the interior of the stomach becomes constantly coated with tough mucus, which further prevents digestion from proceeding normally.

Causes: Chronic gastritis is more common in women than men, and its incidence increases with age. A high proportion of its victims have a long-standing iron-deficiency anaemia. (See ANAEMIA.) Overeating and alcoholic excess are two common causes. It may be the result of some other disease such as cirrhosis of the liver or heart failure.

Symptoms: The symptoms are those of dyspepsia in an aggravated form (see DYSPEPSIA), of which loss of appetite, discomfort and pain after food, with distension and frequent vomiting, are the chief.

Treatment: This consists essentially of ensuring that the affected individual is having a bland diet of regular meals. The patient should obtain medical advice. Alcohol and smoking should be avoided.

ULCER OF THE STOMACH or GASTRIC ULCER, occurs quite commonly and can be serious. It occurs more often than is generally supposed, the result of necropsies showing that one person in every twenty or thereabout suffers from gastric ulcer at some period of life.

Causes: These are not fully understood, but the following points may be regarded as generally admitted: (1) gastric ulcer is more common in men than in women; (2) it becomes more frequent as age increases. Other factors include alteration in mucus production; duodenogastric reflux with bile damaging the gastric mucosa; the presence of the urease-producing bacterium, *Helicobacter pylori*; mucosal ischaemia; and damage to prostaglandins which help protect the mucosal cells. As the non-steroidal anti-inflammatory drugs are prostaglandin inhibitors, they predispose to the development of gastric ulcers. This ulcer is usually of small size (15 to 25 mm in diameter), of round or oval form, and tends to advance, not superficially, but to penetrate through the coats of the stomach. Its most usual site is upon the posterior wall towards the upper or lesser curvature of the stomach and near to the pyloric orifice. This is the point at which the mucous membrane is subjected to most friction by the food as it leaves the stomach. The ulcer may undergo a healing process at any stage, in which case it may leave but little trace of its existence. On the other hand, its scar may produce such an amount of contraction as to lead to narrowing of the pylorus, and later dilatation of the stomach. Also, perforation may take place, which, if not quickly operated upon, may be rapidly fatal, unless previously the stomach has become, as it may, adherent to another organ, by which the dangerous effects of this occurrence may be averted. It may also lead to severe bleeding, the condition known as haematemesis (q.v.). Usually there is only one ulcer, but sometimes there are more.

Symptoms: The symptoms to which this disease gives rise are sometimes indefinite and obscure, and in some cases the diagnosis has been first made by the sudden occurrence of a perforation. First among the symptoms is *pain*, which is usually worse before food. This pain is situated either in front, at the lower end of the breast-bone, or behind, about the middle of the back. It is often severe, and is usually accompanied with much tenderness to touch, and also with a sense of oppression and inability to wear tight clothing. Accompanying the pain there may be vomiting, particularly in more advanced cases. This tends in some measure to relieve the pain and discomfort, and in many instances the patient rather encourages this act. *Vomiting of blood* (haematemesis) occurs in about 25 per cent of cases and is most important diagnostically. Vomiting of blood, however, does not always indicate the presence of a gastric ulcer. Blood is also found mixed with the stools, rendering them dark and tarry-looking (melaena). There is usually constipation. X-ray examination may give little evidence of the presence of an acute ulcer, beyond showing that there is much irritation near the pyloric opening, with spasm in the rest of the stomach; but in chronic cases the deep ulcer often fills up with the barium that has been administered for the examination, and its outline can then be readily seen. Gastroscopy and gastric function tests are valuable investigations for determining whether or not an ulcer is present.

The course of a case of gastric ulcer is variable. In some instances it is acute, making rapid progress to a favourable or unfavourable termination. In others, however, the disease is chronic, lasting for months or years, and in those cases where the ulcers are multiple or of extensive size, incomplete healing may take place and relapses of the symptoms occur from time to time.

Although the majority of cases of gastric ulcer respond satisfactorily to a course of medical treatment, the relapse rate is high. This, however, has been reduced since the introduction of carbenoxolone and the histamine antagonists such as cimetidine and ranitidine in treatment. Further, as already noted, there is also the possiblity of three serious complications developing: (i) haemorrhage; (ii) perforation; (iii) obstruction of the pylorus as a result of contraction of the wall of the stomach produced by the ulcer.

Duodenal ulcer, in which a condition similar to gastric ulcer is found just beyond the pyloric opening, has symptoms like those of gastric ulcer, but is six to twelve times more common in males than females, and tends to occur at an earlier age. (See DUODENAL ULCER.)

Treatment: The mainstay of treatment is a derivative of liquorice known as carbenoxolone and the histamine receptor antagonists. This has largely replaced all other drugs. So effective is it that in many cases admission to hospital is no longer necessary. Attention to the diet, however, is still advisable. Alcohol should be taken in strict moderation and only with food – preferably in the form of light wines. Smoking should be given up.

When haemorrhage occurs, it is treated by complete rest in bed, morphine, and small two-hourly feeds of diluted milk for the first twenty-four hours. When much blood has been lost a transfusion may be necessary. In the event of perforation, treatment is by an immediate operation in which the peritoneal cavity is cleansed and the opening in the stomach wall stitched together.

Surgical treatment, usually in the form of removal of that part of the stomach containing the ulcer, is indicated: (i) in the presence of perforation of the ulcer; (ii) in the presence of severe pyloric obstruction; (iii) in the absence of satisfactory response to medical treatment.

CANCER OF THE STOMACH is more common in men than women. In 1986 there were over 10,500 cases of cancer of the stomach registered in England and Wales, of whom 6,500 were men. In all except the oldest age-groups its incidence has been falling in England and Wales over the last forty years. It occurs for the most part in persons at or after middle life, and is more common in men and in individuals belonging to blood group A. (See BLOOD GROUPS.)

The early symptoms of this disease are often vague. They are mostly those of dyspepsia, with more or less pain, discomfort, and vomiting, particularly after meals. The vomited material is often of coffee-ground appearance, due to admixture with blood, but copious haematemesis is less frequent than in cases of gastric ulcer. Treatment can usually be only palliative. In early cases an operation can sometimes be performed by which the disease is completely removed.

CONGENITAL PYLORIC STENOSIS is a congenital defect that occurs once in every 300 births. It is much more common in baby boys than baby girls, about 85 per cent of cases occurring in boys. It consists of marked hypertrophy, or enlargement of the muscles round the pylorus (q.v.): the opening from the stomach into the duodenum. The baby appears healthy at birth but within a fortnight he starts vomiting towards the end of his feed. The vomiting is described as projectile because the baby shoots the food out in one forceful volley. As the baby feeds, movements of the distended stomach can be seen moving across from left to right (*visible gastric peristalsis*), and the hypertrophied pylorus can be felt as a tumour or swelling. If surgical facilities are available operation is the recommended treatment. In mild cases, or if proper surgical facilities are not available, medical treatment with atropine methonitrate may be tried. If diagnosed and treated early, the results are excellent.

STOMACH TUBE is a soft rubber or plastic tube with rounded end, and usually about 75 cm (30 inches) in length, which is used for washing out the stomach when it contains some poisonous material, or when it is dilated and filled with fermenting food. (See WASHING OUT STOMACH.) A narrower tube, 90 cm (36 inches) in length, is used for the purpose of obtaining a sample of gastric juice for examination. (See also TEST MEAL.) Such a tube can also be allowed to pass out of the stomach into the duodenum so that the contents of the upper part of the small intestine are similarly obtained for analysis.

STOMATITIS means inflammation of the mouth. (See MOUTH, DISEASES OF.)

-STOMY is a suffix signifying formation of an opening in an organ by operation: e.g. colostomy (q.v.).

STONE (see CONCRETIONS; BLADDER, DISEASES OF; GALL-STONES).

STOOLS, or FAECES, consist of the remainder of the food after it has passed through the alimentary canal and been subjected to the action of the digestive juices, and after the nutritious parts have been absorbed by the intestinal mucous membrane. The stools also contain various other matters, such as pigment, derived from the bile, and large quantities of bacteria which are the main component of human stools. The stools are passed once daily by most people, but infants have several evacuations of the bowels in twenty-four hours. To some people the habit of opening the bowels only once or twice a week seems to be quite natural, though such cases are not common.

The *colour* of the stools is naturally of a dark brown, due to a pigment known as stercobilin, derived from the bile. This colour may be changed to green by the action of certain bacteria when decomposition is proceeding to a greater extent than usual in the bowels, and a deep green colour is also produced by some vegetables, such as spinach. White stools, having an appearance like that of clay or putty, are found in cases where the outlet of bile into the small intestine is stopped, and where jaundice is consequently present. When an excess of fat is taken in the food, as in the case of children fed on great quantities of cream, the digestive organs are unable to deal with it, and much of it is passed in the stools, giving the stools in these circumstances also a whitish colour. Black or slate-grey stools are produced when certain drugs are taken, as, for example, iron and bismuth; and a tarry blackness known as malaena is sometimes imparted to them when bleeding takes place from the stomach, the iron in the blood being acted upon by the sulphuretted hydrogen always present in the stools to produce the black sulphide of iron. Bright yellow stools are produced in diarrhoea, when the bile is passed almost unchanged, and a similar colour is caused by rhubarb, senna, and some other drugs. Mucus in the stools, whether in strings, or mixed with the food remnants, or in the form of membranes coating the hardened stools, is almost always a sign of irritation or inflammation in the mucous membrane low down in the bowel (colitis). Red blood in the stools signifies some diseased condition situated near the lower end of the bowel, such as an ulcer or piles. When the blood proceeds from a point higher up, such as an ulcer of the stomach, it is changed by the action of the digestive juices as already described.

Incontinence of the bowels, or inability to retain the stools, is found in several diseases of a prostrating nature in which the sphincter muscles, that naturally keep the bowel closed, relax. It is also a symptom of disease in, or injury to, the spinal cord.

Pain at stool is a characteristic symptom of a fissure at the anus or of inflamed piles, and in such cases is of a very sharp nature. Pain of a duller character associated with the movements of the bowels is often caused by inflammation in the other pelvic organs.

CONSTIPATION and DIARRHOEA are considered under separate headings.

STRABISMUS (see SQUINT).

STRANGULATION The constriction of a passage or tube in the body that blocks the blood flow and disturbs the working of the affected organ. It is usually caused by compression or twisting. Strangulation customarily occurs when part of the intestine (q.v.) herniates either inside the abdomen or outside as in an inguinal HERNIA (q.v.). If a section of the intestine twists this may strangulate and is known as a volvulus.

Strangulation of a person's neck either with a ligature or the hands obstructs the jugular veins in the neck preventing the normal outflow of blood from the brain and head. The trachea is also compressed, cutting off the supply of air to the lungs. The combination of these effects leads to hypoxia and damage to the brain. If not quickly relieved, unconsciousness and death follow. Strangulation may be deliberate or accidental – the latter being a particular hazard for children, for example, when playing with a rope. Removal of the constriction, artificial respiration, and medical attention are urgently necessary.

STRANGURY is a condition in which there is constant desire to pass water, accompanied by a straining sensation, though only a few drops can be voided. It is a symptom of inflammation situated in the kidneys, bladder or urinary passages.

STRAPPING means the application of strips of adhesive plaster, one overlapping the other, so as to cover a part and make pressure upon it. This method of treatment is used in cases of injury or disease when it is desired to keep a part at rest: for example, strapping may be applied to the chest in cases of pleurisy and fracture of the ribs. Also, it is often used to prevent the movement of joints which are sprained or otherwise injured.

STREPTOCOCCUS is a variety of bacterium which under the microscope has much the appearance of a string of beads. It is responsible for erysipelas and other virulent forms of inflammation. (See MICROBIOLOGY.)

STREPTOKINASE is an enzyme produced by certain streptococci, which has the property of removing blood clot and inflammatory material. It is now available on a commercial scale and is being used in the treatment of bruises and inflammatory conditions in order to facilitate the absorption of extravasated blood and inflammatory exudates. It is also being used to try to overcome the ill effects produced by the formation of clots (emboli or thrombi) in large blood-vessels.

STREPTOMYCIN is an anti-bacterial substance obtained from the soil mould, *Streptomyces griseus*. It was first isolated in 1944 by Dr Waksman in the United States of America. It was the first antibiotic to be effective against the tubercle bacillus.

Streptomycin has two disadvantages. The most important of these is the tendency of organisms to become resistant to it. This means that the administration of this antibiotic must be carefully supervized to ensure that correct dosage is being used. The other disadvantage is that streptomycin produces toxic effects, especially disturbance of the vestibular and hearing apparatus. This may result in deafness, giddiness, and tinnitus (q.v.). Whilst in many cases these toxic manifestations disappear when the antibiotic is withdrawn, they may be permanent. For this reason therefore streptomycin must always be used with special care.

STRESS FRACTURES are comparatively common in sportsmen. They tend to occur when an undue amount of exercise is taken: an amount of exercise which an individual is not capable of coping with in his (or her) state of training. The main initial feature is pain over the affected bone. This is usually insidious in onset, and worse at night and during and after exercise. It is accompanied by tenderness, and a lump may be felt over the affected site. X-ray evidence of them only appears after several weeks. Treatment consists of rest, some form of external support, and in the initial stage analgesics (q.v.) to deaden or kill the pain.

STRIAE ATROPHICAE is the term applied to atrophied strips of skin where this has been excessively stretched, as, for example, in pregnancy, when the greyish atrophied strips are known as STRIAE GRAVIDARUM.

STRICTURE means a narrowing in any of the natural passages of the body, such as the gullet, the bowel, or the urethra. It may be due to the development of some growth in the wall of the passage affected, or to pressure upon it by such a growth in some neighbouring organ, but in the majority of cases a stricture is the result of previous ulceration on the inner surface of the passage, followed by contraction of the scar. (See INTESTINE, DISEASES OF; URETHRA, DISEASES OF.)

STRIDOR is a noise associated with inspiration due to narrowing of the upper airway, in particular the larynx.

STROKE is sudden insensibility or bodily disablement connected with some diseased condition of the brain.
Causes: In subjects of heart disease, a clot may form in the cavities or on a valve of the heart, and being carried away by the blood-stream may lodge in a vessel of the brain so as to form a plug which prevents blood from reaching the part supplied by the vessel in question. The occurrence of this *embolism* is sudden and produces all the symptoms of stroke. When it occurs, the prospect of improvement is better than when the apoplectic symptoms are due to haemorrhage. In elderly people whose blood-vessels are extensively diseased and whose circulation is feeble, a type of stroke, of more gradual onset, may appear in consequence of the blood clotting in the interior of the vessels, this process being known as *thrombosis*.
The most important occasion of stroke is *haemorrhage* into the brain by the rupture of

blood-vessels. The blood-vessels of the brain, like those in other parts of the body, are liable to undergo degenerative changes after middle life. These changes affect the minute arteries as well as the larger vessels, rendering their texture fragile, and at the same time impairing their function in maintaining the healthy nutrition of the brain. Hence, in the immediate vicinity of the diseased blood-vessels the substance of the brain itself undergoes degeneration and becomes softened. The small vessels having thus lost the natural support of the surrounding tissues, and being here and there distended into aneurysms by disease, are liable to give way, and blood escapes into the brain. The haemorrhage may be slight in amount and in parts of the brain where its presence gives rise to little disturbance; but where a large blood-vessel has ruptured, and more especially where the blood has been extravasated in or around the important structures at the base of the brain, the result is a stroke or apoplexy, as described below, and death not infrequently follows within a short period. In favourable cases, in which a certain measure of recovery takes place, the effused blood undergoes gradual absorption, or becomes enveloped in a sort of capsule formed by the surrounding brain substance, and ceases to cause further disturbance. But even in such cases some degree of paralysis remains. Stroke in a young person is usually due to a subarachnoid haemorrhage resulting from the rupture of a congenital aneurysm.

Stroke is usually a disease of advanced life. A hereditary tendency is one of the predisposing causes of stroke. Important contributory factors are degenerative changes in the heart and blood-vessels and raised blood-pressure. With respect to the exciting causes of a stroke or apoplexy, it may be stated generally that whatever tends directly or indirectly to increase the tension within the cerebral blood-vessels may bring on an attack. Hence, such causes as severe exertion of body or mind, violent emotions, much stooping, and sudden shocks to the body, may precipitate the attack in a susceptible individual. Many cases in elderly people occur while some violent exertion is being made, such as hurrying to catch a train or during straining at stool.

Symptoms: Strokes vary both as regards their intensity, the particular symptoms shown, and the after-effects, but well-marked cases present the following symptoms. The person attacked becomes, more or less suddenly, deprived of consciousness and all power of voluntary motion. He lies as if in a deep sleep, with a flushed face, a slow pulse, stertorous breathing, accompanied with puffing of the cheeks during expiration, and with the pupils of the eyes insensible to light and contracted or unequal. This state in many respects resembles the coma of narcotic poisoning, and may sometimes be mistaken for alcoholic intoxication. The symptoms and history of the case, however, are usually sufficient to enable a correct diagnosis to be made.

The presence of complete paralysis down one or other side is a point which in general differentiates stroke from narcotic poisoning and alcoholic intoxication, the paralysis being demonstrable even during unconsciousness by lifting the limbs and noting the characteristic suddenness and helplessness with which those on the affected side fall when not supported. The fact that in either of the last-named conditions the person can generally be partially roused, while in stroke unconsciousness is complete, is also valuable. Assistance is also gained by observing the state of the pupils, which are usually unequal, whereas in narcotic poisoning they are usually much contracted, while in alcoholic intoxication they are widely dilated.

Death may occur within a few hours, or there may be a gradual return to consciousness, in which case it is usually found that the result of the attack remains in the form of paralysis of one side of the body (hemiplegia), while occasionally there may also be noticed some impairment of the mental powers, pointing to damage done to the brain. (See PARALYSIS; APHASIA.)

Stroke may occur without unconsciousness, a sudden paralysis of one side of the body being the only manifestation. Occasionally, when the haemorrhage takes place gently, the symptoms are gradually developed over a period of several hours (*ingravescent stroke*). Sometimes premonitory symptoms occur. Persistent headache of a dull throbbing character, a sense of fullness in the head, vomiting, giddiness, noises in the ears, slight confusion of mind, and numbness of a limb or of one side of the body are among the more important premonitory symptoms; and these may exist for a variable length of time before the attack comes on.

The effects of a stroke or apoplexy, as regards the paralysis which remains after the immediate attack is over, are described under *Hemiplegia* in the article on PARALYSIS.

Treatment: A knowledge of these facts is of the utmost importance in the treatment of stroke, as obviously much can be done in the way of warding off a stroke when it appears to threaten, and of preventing a recurrence in cases where there have been previous attacks. With respect to the treatment of stroke, little can be done during the state of unconsciousness, apart from skilled nursing. If the blood-pressure is very high, the administration of hypotensive drugs may be of value. (See ESSENTIAL HYPERTENSION.)

In the after-treatment of the resulting paralysis much may be done to prevent stiffness and to preserve the power of the muscles in the weakened limbs by physiotherapy, including exercises, massage and electrical treatment, and continuing reassurance. Advice for stroke victims may be obtained from the Stroke Association, CHSA House, Whitecross Street, London EC1Y 8JJ.

STROMA is the name applied to the tissue which forms the framework and covering of an organ.

STRONGYLOIDIASIS is the disease produced by *Strongyloides stercoralis*, a small nematode, which is found throughout the tropics, particularly in the Far East. It produces a characteristic itching skin rash, known as 'creeping eruption', as well as severe diarrhoea which, like hookworm, may lead to severe anaemia and prostration. The drug used in its treatment is thiabendazole.

STRYCHNINE is an alkaloid derived from *Strychnos nux-vomca*, the seeds of an East Indian tree, as well as from the seeds of several other closely allied trees and shrubs. It is a white crystalline body possessed of an intensely bitter taste, more bitter perhaps than that of any other substance, and it is not very soluble in water. It stimulates all parts of the nervous system, and was at one time widely used for this purpose. Strychnine poisoning is fortunately rare. It shows itself in convulsions, which come on very speedily after the person has taken the poison. The mental faculties remain unaffected, and the symptoms end in death or recovery within a few hours.
Treatment: The patient should be kept quiet. Artificial respiration may be necessary. At the earliest moment a benzodiazepine is injected intravenously in a large enough dose to stop the convulsions and put the patient to sleep.

STUPOR (see UNCONSCIOUSNESS).

STUTTERING (see STAMMERING).

STYE (see EYE, DISEASE AND INJURIES).

STYPTICS are applications which check bleeding, either by making the blood-vessels contract more firmly or by causing rapid clotting in the blood. Some possess both modes of action.
Varieties: Many substances have this action on account of their chemical or physical properties. Among them may be mentioned ice; hot water at 49 °C if brought directly in contact with the bleeding surface; perchloride of iron; acetate of lead and Goulard's water; nitrate of silver; sulphate of copper; sulphate of zinc; alum; tannin; hazeline; ergot; adrenaline; and Russell-viper venom.
Uses: The use of styptics is described under HAEMORRHAGE.

SUB- is a prefix signifying under, near, or moderately.

SUBACUTE: The description applied to a disease the duration of which lies between *acute* and *chronic*. An example is subacute endocarditis, a disorder that may not be diagnosed for several weeks or months, during which time it can severely damage valves in the heart.

SUBACUTE COMBINED DEGENERATION OF THE CORD is a degenerative condition of the spinal cord which most commonly occurs as a complication of pernicious anaemia. (See ANAEMIA.)

SUBACUTE SCLEROSING PANENCEPHALITIS is a rare complication of measles due to infection of the brain with the measles virus. It develops two to eighteen years after the onset of the measles, and is characterized by mental deterioration leading on to convulsions, coma and death. The annual incidence in Britain is about 1 per million of the childhood population. The risk of its developing is five to twenty times greater after measles than after measles vaccination.

SUBARACHNOID HAEMORRHAGE is a haemorrhage into the subarachnoid space. It is usually the result of rupture of an aneurysm on the circle of Willis (q.v.).

SUBARACHNOID SPACE is the space between the arachnoid and the pia mater, two of the membranes covering the brain (q.v.).

SUBCLAVIAN is the name applied to a large artery and vein which pass to the upper arm between the collar bone and the first rib.

SUBCLINICAL: A description of a disease that is suspected but which has not developed sufficiently or is too mild in form to produce clear signs and symptoms in an individual. Even so, damage may be caused to tissues and organs.

SUBCONSCIOUS is a state of being partially conscious, or the condition in which mental processes occur and outside objects and events are perceived with the mind nearly or quite unconscious of them. Such subconscious impressions or events may be forgotten at the time but may nevertheless exert a continued influence over the conscious mind, or may at a subsequent time come fully into consciousness. Much importance is attached to the influence of painful or unpleasant experiences which, though forgotten, continue to influence the mind, and these are held to be largely responsible for neurasthenic and similar states. This injurious influence is removed when the subconscious impressions come fully into consciousness and are then remembered and clearly seen in their relative importance.

SUBCUTANEOUS means anything pertaining to the loose cellular tissue beneath the skin: e.g. a subcutaneous injection. (See HYPODERMIC.)

SUBDURAL: Relating to the space between the strong outer layer of the meninges, the membrane which cover the brain, and the arachnoid, which is the middle layer of the meninges. A subdural haemorrhage occurs when bleeding takes place into this space. The trapped blood forms a large blood clot or haematoma within the skull and this causes pressure on the underlying brain. Bleeding may occur slowly as the result of disease or suddenly as the result of injury. Headaches, confusion, and drowsiness result, sometimes with paralysis. Medical attention is required urgently if a serious haematoma occurs soon after injury. (See BRAIN.)

SUBINVOLUTION is a term used to indicate that the womb has failed to undergo the usual involution, or decrease in size, which naturally takes place within one month after a child is born.

SUBJECTIVE is a term applied to symptoms, and sensations, perceived only by the affected individual. For example, numbness is a purely subjective sensation, whilst the jerk given by the leg on tapping the tendon of the knee is an objective sign.

SUBLIMATION is the conversion of a solid substance into a vapour and its recondensation. The term is also used in a mental sense for the process of converting instinctive sexual desires to new aims and objects devoid of sexual significance.

SUBLUXATION means a partial dislocation, and is a term sometimes applied to a sprain.

SUBMUCOSA: The layer of connective tissue that occurs under a mucous membrane – for example, in the intestinal wall.

SUBPHRENIC ABSCESS: An abcess that develops under the diaphragm, usually on the right side of the abdomen between the liver and the diaphragm. The cause may be an organ that has perforated – for instance, a peptic ulcer in the stomach or intestine. An abscess may also occur after an abdominal operation, usually when the bowel or stomach has been operated on. Antibiotics and sometimes surgery are the method of treatment.

SUCCUSSION is a method of examination by shaking the body of a patient in order to elicit splashing sounds, with a view to determining the presence of gas and fluid in a cavity such as the interior of the stomach or the pleural cavity.

SUCKLING (see INFANT FEEDING; BREASTS, DISEASES OF).

SUCRALFATE is a drug that is proving of value in the treatment of peptic ulcer (q.v.).

SUCROSE, or CANE SUGAR (see SUGAR).

SUCTION: The use of a reduction in pressure to clear away fluids or other material through a tube. Suction is used to remove blood from the site of a surgical operation. Suction is commonly necessary to remove secretions from the airways of newly born babies to help them breathe.

SUDDEN INFANT DEATH SYNDROME (SIDS): is a term applied to the unexpected death of an apparently healthy baby, usually during sleep. It is also known as Cot Death, and it is estimated that probably at least 1800 such deaths occur every year in Britain. Most babies who die in this way have been healthy, or only slightly unwell, the day before death. Death occurs silently and suddenly, the baby being found dead in his cot in the morning. Over half these deaths occur between the ages of 2 and 6 months, and boys are more affected than girls. They are more common in social classes III, IV and V (see SOCIAL CLASSES), and the incidence is highest in the winter. Most of the infants have been bottle fed.

The cause is still not really known and there may be no single cause. Prematurity and low birth weight may be factors. Smothering by a soft pillow may account for a few of the deaths, and a certain number are due to an infection of the lungs, such as broncho-penumonia or bronchitis, usually due to a virus. There is some evidence that these infants have an innate tendency to poor control of their breathing and are therefore likely to stop breathing should they have even a mild infection such as a cold. One possibility is that they may be associated with allergy to milk. Another is that they may be due to a sudden upset of the fluid balance of the baby as a result of bottle feeding. Yet another is that they may be associated with a deficiency of vitamin E. Smoking, drug addiction or anaemia in the mother may contribute to SIDS, but all that can really be said at the moment, however, is that the baby most likely to die in this way is one who is underweight when born, comes from a poor family, whose mother is young and already has several children, who has been bottle fed, has been unwell during the preceding fortnight and has signs of a cold in the head when put to bed. Bereaved parents can obtain help and advice from the Foundation for the Study of Infant Deaths, 35 Belgrave Square, London SW1X 8QB (071-235 0965).

SUDORIFICS are drugs and other agents which produce copious perspiration.

SUFFOCATION (see ASPHYXIA; CHOKING).

SUGAR is a substance containing carbon, hydrogen, and oxygen, and belonging therefore to the chemical group of carbohydrates. This group includes three subdivisions:

(1) Monosaccharides $(C_6H_{12}O_6)$
   e.g. Glucose, or dextrose, or grape sugar.
   Fructose, or laevulose, or fruit sugar.
   Galactose.
(2) Disaccharides $(C_{12}H_{22}O_{11})$
   e.g. Sucrose, or cane sugar, or beet sugar.
   Lactose or milk sugar.
   Maltose or malt sugar.
(3) Polysaccharides $(C_6H_{10}O_5)$
   e.g. Starch.
   Glycogen or animal starch.

Glucose, also known as grape sugar because it is found in various kinds of fruit, including grapes, is the form of sugar produced by the tissues and excreted in large amount by the kidneys in diabetes mellitus.

Sucrose is widely distributed through the vegetable kingdom, though it is specially plentiful in the juice of the sugar-cane, beetroot, and maple. When taken as a food, it is converted by the digestive juices into glucose before it is absorbed, this process being known as inversion. It is a valuable food, being utilized in the production of heat and energy, although it is also to a certain extent a tissue-builder so far as fat is concerned. It is to be avoided by people who tend to get fat as well as by diabetics.

Lactose is found in milk, and it is to the fermentation of this sugar and consequent production of lactic acid by certain bacteria that the souring of milk is due. The extent to which it is present in the milk of different animals is mentioned under INFANT FEEDING. It has little sweetening power compared with cane sugar, but it is used sometimes as a laxative.

Maltose is produced by the action of the ferment, diastase, upon the starch contained in barley, and also by the ferments of the saliva and pancreatic juice, and is still further changed by the intestinal ferments into glucose before it is absorbed.

Invert sugar is a natural mixture of dextrose and laevulose resulting from a chemical decomposition of cane sugar or of starch.

Starch is mentioned under a separate heading, and its use as a food under DIET and CEREAL.

The energy-producing value of sugars generally is taken as being, on the average, 4 Calories for each gram of sugar.

SUICIDE (see under MENTAL ILLNESS).

SULCUS is the term applied to any groove or furrow, but especially to a fissure of the brain.

SULFADOXINE is a long-acting sulphonamide (q.v.) with a range of action comparable to that of sulphamethoxypyridazine (q.v.). Along with pyrimethamine it is used in the prophylactic, or preventive, treatment of malaria. (See FANSIDAR.)

SULFAMETOPYRAZINE is a long-acting sulphonamide. Given in one weekly dose of 2 grams it is proving of value in preventing relapses during the winter in patients with chronic bronchitis.

SULINDAC is a drug of value in the treatment of rheumatic conditions. (See NON-STEROIDAL ANTI INFLAMMATORY DRUGS.)

SULPHACETAMIDE is one of the sulphonamides. Its main use today is in the form of eye drops of the sodium salt used locally in the treatment of infections of the eye.

SULPHADIAZINE is one of the sulphonamides. It is a highly active drug and in moderate dosage produces a high and persistent blood concentration. It is relatively non-toxic and is particularly useful in the treatment of meningitis.

SULPHADIMETHOXINE is one of the long-acting sulphonamides, only one dose of which is required daily.

SULPHADIMIDINE is comparable in activity to sulphadiazine, and has the advantage of being even more non-toxic and of producing higher blood concentrations.

SULPHAEMOGLOBIN is an abnormal pigment sometimes found in the blood as a result of the interaction of certain drugs derived from aniline, such as phenacetin and acetanilide.

SULPHAMETHOXAZOLE is one of the long-acting sulphonamides. It is related to sulphafurazole, has a duration of action of 12 hours, and is said to be particularly effective against streptococci.

SULPHANILAMIDE, or p-aminobenzene-sulphonamide, is a drug the discovery of which is one of the most important in medicine in the twentieth century. It was the first of the sulphonamide drugs. In 1935 the German chemist, Gerhard Domagk, announced the discovery of the effect of prontosil on streptococci. It was later found that this action was due to conversion in the body of prontosil into sulphanilamide, which acts by inhibiting the growth of various bacteria, especially the ubiquitous and dangerous *Streptococcus haemolyticus*. Although many other sulphonamides with various advantages have been subsequently introduced, sulphanilamide is still used to a certain extent. (See also SULPHONAMIDE.)

SULPHASALAZINE is a sulphonamide which is proving of value in the treatment of ulcerative colitis.

SULPHINPYRAZONE is a derivative of phenylbutazone which is proving of value in the treatment of gout.

SULPHONAMIDE: A drug having the sulphonamide grouping – SO_2NH_2. In 1935, Gerhard Domagk, a German chemist, announced the discovery of the effect of prontosil on streptococci. Subsequent work showed that this action was due to the conversion in the body of prontosil to sulphanilamide. The action of the sulphonamides is bacteriostatic and not bactericidal: i.e. they do not directly kill the bacteria but so interfere with their growth that they are unable to multiply. This action of the sulphonamides is now believed to be due to the similarity of their chemical structure to that of p-aminobenzoic acid. This latter substance is essential for the growth of many bacteria. If the bacteria are surrounded by a sulphonamide in greater concentration than p-aminobenzoic acid, then the bacteria take up the sulphonamide. This interferes with their development and they therefore never mature; nor are they able to reproduce themselves. Although the sulphonamides are being replaced to an increasing extent by penicillin, which is active against many of the same organisms, they are still a useful addition to our ability to control diseases due to bacterial infection.

SULPHONES are a group of drugs allied to the sulphonamides. They are used in the treatment of leprosy. The members of this group include dapsone.

SULPHONYLUREAS are sulphonamide derivatives which lower the blood sugar when they are given by mouth by enhancing the production of insulin. They are effective only when some residual pancreatic beta cell function is present. All may lead to a hypoglycaemia if given in overdose and this is particularly common when long-acting sulphonylureas are given to elderly patients. Tolbutamide was the first of the sulphonlyurea drugs. It has a short duration of action and is usually given twice daily. Chlorpropamide has a more prolonged action and only needs to be given once daily. Other oral hypoglycaemic agents of this family include glibenclamide, which has a duration of action intermediate between tolbutamide and chlorpropamide. Other sulphonlyureas include acetohexamide, glibornuride, Gliclazide, glipizide, gliquidone and tolazamide. Glymidine is a related compound with a similar action to the sulphonylureas. It is particularly useful in patients who are hypersensitive to sulphonylureas.

Sulphonylureas are best avoided in patients who are overweight as they tend to stimulate the appetite and aggravate obesity. They should be used with caution in patients with hepatic or renal disease. Side-effects are infrequent and usually not severe, the most common being epigastric discomfort with occasional nausea,

vomiting and anorexia. In about 10 per cent of patients chlorpropamide and tolbutamide may cause facial flushing after drinking alcohol (see DIABETES MELLITUS). Some patients are hypersensitive to oral hypoglycaemic agents and develop rashes which may progress to erythema multiforme and exfoliative dermatitis. These reactions usually appear in the first 6 to 8 weeks of treatment.

SULPHUR is a non-metallic element. Crude sulphur is obtained in volcanic districts, and from it sublimed sulphur is prepared by heating. In chemical combinations (sulphides and sulphates) sulphur has disinfectant and antiparasitic powers. When taken internally, the sulphides that are formed stimulate the action of the bowels, and, being excreted partly from the surface of the skin and mucous membranes of the air passages, they also stimulate these.
Uses: Sulphur is burned in order to produce sulphurous acid gas, which is used as a disinfectant. (See DISINFECTION.) Externally, sulphur ointment is an old remedy against the minute parasite that is responsible for the itch; and milk of sulphur is used in lotions for acne on the face. Sulphur is also used in baths for its stimulating action on the skin in cases of skin disease and rheumatism.

SULPHURIC ACID, or OIL OF VITRIOL, is, in its undiluted state, one of the most powerful of the mineral acids. It is a heavy, colourless liquid of oily consistence and is largely used in various manufacturing operations, so that poisoning by sulphuric acid is not uncommon. It chars any organic substance with which it is brought in contact, and acts as a violent corrosive poison. The treatment of sulphuric acid poisoning is that for corrosive poisons generally: e.g. to administer weak alkalis such as baking soda, whitening, magnesia, or soap in water, and to apply oil to the injured surfaces.
Uses: Dilute sulphuric acid, or aromatic sulphuric acid containing cinnamon and ginger, and commonly known as elixir of vitriol, is used in cases of diarrhoea for its astringent properties, in doses of 5 or 20 drops well diluted in water. A lemonade is also made, containing small quantities of sulphuric acid, for use by lead-workers; since it forms an insoluble sulphate with lead, and thus prevents absorption of any lead which may be accidentally swallowed at work.

SULPHUROUS ACID is a saturated solution of sulphur dioxide. It has an extremely pungent odour and strong disinfectant power.

SUMMER DIARRHOEA (see DIARRHOEA; INFANT FEEDING).

SUNBURN includes the various effects produced on the skin by the sun's rays. The effects produced on the skin by sunlight are predominantly due to the ultra-violet rays. They are more marked in fair-skinned than in dark-skinned people, and consist predominantly of darkening, or tanning, of the skin as a result of the production in the skin of a dark pigment known as melanin (q.v.), which protects the skin against the deleterious effects of continued exposure to ultra-violet rays. In addition there is thickening of the superficial layer of the skin (q.v.). This production of melanin is preceded by reddening of the skin due to dilatation of the blood-vessels of the skin, and it is this action on the unprotected white skin that is responsible for the painful manifestations of sunburn, using this word in the strict sense of the term. With substantial long-continued exposure to sunlight there is an increase in the risk of skin cancer. In northern Europe the sensitivity of the skin to sunshine decreases during the late spring and early summer, to increase again in the autumn. This is probably a result of increasing exposure to the sun inducing thickening of the superficial layers of the skin and increasing their content of melanin.

The first manifestation of sunburn, the reddening of the skin, begins to develop in a few hours. This persists for about two days, when it is gradually replaced by tanning or darkening of the skin which gradually develops in extent and depth, depending on how long the body is exposed to the sun's rays and the intensity of the sunlight. The effect of the sun in this respect is much diminished by cloud, and increased by snow. This latter effect is the result of reflection of the ultra-violet rays by the snow, and explains why particular care must be exercised when exposing oneself to the sun in snowy conditions, as on a skiing holiday. There is probably little extra risk of sunburn from exposure to the sun at sea as the surface of the sea does not reflect ultra-violet rays to any appreciable extent.

Symptoms: If the body is over-exposed to the sun, the initial reddening of the skin increases. The skin begins to itch and tingle, becomes swollen, and then blisters begin to form, with peeling of the skin. The speed with which these changes occur, and their extent, depend upon the individual susceptibility of the skin and also the degree and extent of exposure to the sun, but in severe caes the effects may be extensive enough to cause a general upset accompanied by fever.

Prevention: All these unpleasant effects of sunburn can be avoided by gradual exposure of the body to the sun. How gradual this should be depends on the susceptibility of the individual's skin to sunlight, and the intensity of the sun's rays. For the first few days such exposure should not exceed an hour or so, and initially only part of the body should be exposed. Those who are proposing to sunbathe in warm climates, as around the Mediterranean, would be well advised to 'get into training' by preliminary sunbathing in the garden at home. It is the parts of the body that are normally not exposed to the sun that are most susceptible to sunburn.

Other preventive measures include the sensible use of 'beach umbrellas', and other shades. Oiling of the skin is an ancient practice that has stood up well to the test of time. There is now a wide range of sunscreen preparations on the market, the active constituents of which include titanium dioxide and zinc oxide. Care, however, must be exercised in the choice of these, as there is by no means invariably a direct correlation between price and efficacy. A useful basic formula is 5 per cent para-aminobenzoic acid in 70 per cent ethanol. A more complicated prescription for those who are particularly sensitive to sunlight is 5 per cent para-aminobenzoic acid, 2·5 per cent amyl dimethylaminobenzoate, and 70 per cent ethanol. Another useful preparation is mexenone cream BPC (q.v.).

Treatment: Once sunburn, as opposed to suntan, has developed, the affected individual must keep in the shade. The itching and tingling of the skin may be relieved by applying calamine lotion or 2·5 per cent solution of coal tar. (See also MELANOMA.)

SUPER- is a prefix signifying above or implying excess.

SUPINATION means the turning of the forearm and hand so that the palm faces upwards.

SUPINE: Lying on the back, face upwards. or the position of the forearm where the hand lies face upwards.

SUPPOSITORY is a small conical mass made of oil of theobroma, to which white beeswax is sometimes added, or glycerin-jelly, and containing drugs intended for introduction into the rectum. This method of using drugs, which is more popular on the Continent than in the United Kingdom, may be chosen for various reasons. For example, the suppository, as in the case of soap or glycerin suppositories, may be used to produce an aperient action. Other suppositories, such as those of morphine, are used to quiet pain and check the action of the bowels. Others are used for the sake of their influence on neighbouring organs.

Method of use: The suppository is placed with its pointed end against the anus and with a firm but gentle screwing movement is pushed upwards. With the point of the forefinger, it must be pushed onwards for about 25 mm (1 inch), past the sphincter muscle, otherwise it will not be retained. It must be quickly introduced, as the material of which it is composed rapidly softens when brought into contact with the body. It may be retained in position by crossing the legs or lying on the side. To facilitate insertion it may be lubricated with a small amount of olive oil before insertion.

SUPPRESSION: (1) The stopping of any physiological activity. (2) A psychological defence mechanism by which an individual intentionally refuses to acknowledge an idea or memory that he finds distasteful or unpleasant. (3) A treatment that stops the visible signs of an illness or holds back its usual progress.

SUPPURATION means the process of pus formation. When pus forms on a raw surface the process is called ulceration, whilst a deep-seated collection of pus is known as an abscess. (For more detailed information, see ABSCESS; INFLAMMATION; PHAGOCYTOSIS; ULCER; WOUNDS.)

SUPRA- is a prefix signifying above or upon.

SUPRAPUBIC operation is one in which the abdomen is opened in its lower part, immediately above the pubic bones. (See LITHOTOMY.)

SUPRARENAL GLANDS, (see ADRENAL GLANDS).

SURAMIN is the *British Pharmacopoeia* name for a drug which has been much used, and with success, in the treatment of sleeping sickness (q.v.).

SURFACTANT is a surface-active agent lining the alveoli of the lungs, which plays an essential part in respiration (q.v.) by preventing the alveoli collapsing at the end of expiration. Absence, or lack, of surfactant is one of the factors responsible for hyaline membrane disease (q.v.), and it is now being used in the treatment of this condition by means of instillation into the trachea.

SURROGATE is a term applied in medicine to a substance used as a substitute for another.

SUSCEPTIBILITY: A reduced ability to combat an illness, usually an infection. The patient may be in poor general health or immunization or disease may have affected his defence mechanisms. For example, a person with AIDS (q.v.) is particularly susceptible to infection.

SUTURE is the name given either to the close union between two neighbouring bones of the skull, or to the series of stitches by which a wound is closed. (See WOUNDS.)

SWAB is a term applied to a small piece of gauze, lint, or similar material used for wiping out the mouth of a helpless patient or for drying out a wound. The term is also applied to a tuft of sterilized cotton-wool wrapped round a wire and enclosed in a sterile glass tube used for obtaining matter or membrane from the throat, from wounds, or the like, in order that this may be subjected to bacteriological examination.

SWAN-GANZ CATHETER is a flexible tube with a double lumen and a small balloon at its distal end. It is introduced into a vein in the arm and advanced until the end of the catheter is in the right atrium. The balloon is then inflated with air through one lumen and this enables the blood stream to propel the catheter through the right ventricle to the pulmonary artery. The balloon is deflated and the catheter can then record the pulmonary artery pressure. When the balloon is inflated the tip is isolated from the pulmonary artery and measures the left atrial pressure. These measurements are important in the management of patients with circulatory failure as under these circumstances the central venous pressure or the right atrial pressure is an unreliable guide to fluid replacement.

SWEAT (see PERSPIRATION).

SWEAT GLANDS (see SKIN).

SWEETBREAD is a popular term applied to several glands used for food, including the thymus gland of young animals (neck sweetbread), the pancreas (stomach sweetbread), and the testis.

SYCOSIS is a skin disease in which the hair follicles, especially of the chin, are inflamed, forming pustules round the hairs, surrounded by a swollen and reddened area of skin. The disease is directly due to infection of the hair follicles with staphylococcus or ringworm. The infection is generally attributed to a barber's utensils, and the condition is sometimes known as barber's itch, foul shave, or ringworm of the beard. (For treatment, see IMPETIGO; RINGWORM.)

SYMPATHETIC is a term applied to certain diseases or symptoms which arise in one part of the body in consequence of disease in some distant part. Inflammation may arise in one eye, in consequence of injury to the other, by the spread of organisms along the lymphatic channels connecting the two, and is then known as sympathetic inflammation. Pain also may be of a sympathetic nature. (See PAIN.)

SYMPATHETIC SYSTEM is part of the autonomic nervous system (q.v.). It consists of scattered collections of grey matter known as ganglia, united by an irregular network of nerve-fibres, those portions where the ganglia are placed most closely and the network of fibres is specially dense being known as plexuses. The chief part of the sympathetic system consists of two ganglionated cords that run through the neck, chest, and abdomen, lying close in front of the spine. (For further details, see NERVES.)

SYMPATHOMIMETIC DRUGS are those producing an effect comparable to those produced by stimulation of the sympathetic nervous system: e.g. adrenaline (q.v.).

SYMPHYSIS: An anatomical description of a joint in which two bones are connected by strong fibrous cartilage. One example is the joint between the two pubic bones in the front of the pelvis.

SYMPTOM is a term applied to any evidence of disease. The term, physical sign, is generally applied to evidence of disease of which the patient does not complain but which is elicited upon examination. For the symptoms indicative of the various diseases see under the headings of each disease.

SYN- is a prefix signifying union.

SYNAPSE is the term applied to the anatomical relation of one nerve-cell with another which is effected at various points by contact of their branching processes. The state of shrinkage or relaxation at these points (synapses) is supposed in some cases to determine the readiness with which a nervous impulse is transmitted from one part of the nervous system to another. Many drugs act upon the nervous system through their effect in closing or widening these junctions.

SYNCOPE, or fainting, is a loss of consciousness due to a fall in blood pressure. This may result because the cardiac output has become reduced or because the peripheral resistance provided by the arterioles has decreased. The simple faint or vaso-vagal attack is a result of a failure to maintain an adequate venous return of blood to the heart. This is likely to occur after prolonged periods of standing, particularly if one is standing still or if the climatic conditions are hot. It can also result from an unpleasant or painful experience. Pallor, sweating and a slow pulse are characteristic. Recovery is immediate when the venous return is restored by lying flat. Syncope can also result when the venous return to the heart is impaired as a result of a rise in intra-thoracic pressure. This may happen after prolonged vigorous coughing, the so-called cough syncope, or when elderly men with prostatic hypertrophy strain to empty their bladder. This is known as micturition syncope. Syncope is particularly likely to occur when the arterial blood pressure is unusually low. This may result from overtreatment of hypertension with drugs or it may be the result of diseases, such as Addison's disease, which are associated with low blood pressures. It is important that syncope is distinguished from epilepsy.

SYNDACTYLY is the condition which a child is born with, in which two or more fingers or toes are fused together to a varying extent. The condition is popularly known as webbed fingers or toes (q.v.).

SYNDROME is a term applied to a group of symptoms occurring together regularly and thus constituting a disease to which some particular name is given: e.g. *Cushing's Syndrome* comprising obesity, hypertension, purple striae and osteoporosis; *Korsakoff's Syndrome*, of loss of appreciation of time and place combined with talkativeness, forming signs of alcoholic delirium.

SYNECHIAE: Adhesions between the iris and adjacent structures, e.g. cornea, lens. They usually arise as a result of inflammation of the iris.

SYNERGIST: (1) A muscle that works in concert with an agonist muscle to perform a certain movement. (2) An agent, for example a drug, that acts with another to produce a result that is greater than adding together the separate effects of the two agents. Synergism in drug treatment may be beneficial as in the case of combined levodopa and selegiline, a selective monoamine oxidase inhibitor (q.v.), in the treatment of Parkinson's disease (q.v.). It may be potentially dangerous, however, as when monoamine oxidase inhibitors boost the effects of barbiturates (q.v.).

SYNOSTOSIS is the term applied to a union by bony material of adjacent bones normally separate.

SYNOVIAL MEMBRANE forms the lining of the soft parts that enclose the cavity of a joint. (See JOINTS.)

SYNOVITIS means inflammation of the membrane lining a joint. It is usually painful and accompanied by effusion of fluid within the synovial sac of the joint. It is found in acute rheumatism, various injuries and inflammations of joints, and in the chronic form in tuberculosis. (See JOINTS, DISEASES OF.)

SYNTHETIC is a term applied to substances produced by chemical processes in the laboratory or by artificial building up.

SYPHILIS is a contagious disease of slow development, which, at its start, shows a characteristic sore at the site of infection, later brings on constitutional effects resembling those of other infectious diseases, and at a still later period produces certain changes in the central nervous system, the arteries and elsewhere. Because, in the majority of cases the disease is acquired as a result of sexual intercourse with an infected individual, it is classed as one of the *venereal* diseases, or sexually transmitted diseases as they are now known. Syphilis affects only human beings, though it has been experimentally produced in anthropoid apes.

The disease seems to have first attracted public attention about or soon after the year 1494 in consequence of a severe and widespread outbreak among the French soldiers then occupied in the siege of Naples. An association with martial activity has persisted ever since. Thus it has been estimated that during the 1914–18 War a quarter of the armies in Europe were incapacitated by syphilis and gonorrhoea. For long it was known as the Neapolitan disease, French Pox, or Great Pox; and, in consequence probably of the licentiousness and the want of cleanliness that then prevailed, it spread in epidemic form. Later, it came to be called syphilis, the name being derived from that of the chief character in a Latin poem published by Fracastoro in 1530. It has been suggested that the disease existed in ancient times among the natives of America, and that the infection was brought to Europe by the followers of Columbus, but there are also grounds for supposing that the disease occurred among the Eastern races in ancient times, although it was most likely often confounded with leprosy and tuberculosis. Today, according to the World Health Organization, around 40 million new cases are notified annually in the world, and, according to many, this is an underestimate.

Causes: The causative organism is the *Treponema pallidum*, a long, thread-like wavy organism with pointed tapering ends. It is found in large numbers in the sores in the primary stage of the disease and in the skin lesions in the secondary stage.

The number of cases of syphilis reported in England in the year ending 30 June 1989, was around 1,400.

Syphilis may be *acquired* from people already suffering from the disease, or it may be *congenital*. The acquired form is usually got by sexual intercourse, but it may also result from kissing or from contact with a sore upon another person through some wound or abrasion. The epithelium covering the general surface of the skin seems to be an efficient protection, but the infective material apparently has the power of penetrating mucous membranes. Not only may the disease be spread as a venereal affection, but cups, spoons, towels, sponges, sheets, which have been used by the diseased, have been known to convey the contagion to others, although fortunately such inanimate articles appear to retain their infectiveness only for a short time. The acquired form of the disease is infectious from contact with sores, both in its primary and secondary stages; whilst infants suffering from the congenital form are also highly infectious. Accordingly any one frequently handling such an infant runs great risk of infection, although the mother may handle the babe with impunity (Colles' Law).

Symptoms: The *acquired form* of the disease is commonly divided into three stages – PRIMARY, SECONDARY, and TERTIARY, although in many cases the tertiary stage is wanting, whilst in others there is no dividing line between the secondary and tertiary symptoms. The disease presents great variations of intensity, being occasionally of a 'malignant' type, in which widespread ulceration speedily comes on and even causes death; and in other cases showing little more than a slight skin eruption. There are several laboratory tests for confirming the diagnosis.

The incubation period ranges from 10 to 90 days, though most frequently it occupies about four weeks. Then a small ulcer appears at the site of infection, which is accompanied by a typical cartilaginous hardness of the tissues immediately round and beneath it, and characterized by its resistance to all healing treatment. This, which is known as the PRIMARY SORE (or *chancre*), may be very much inflamed, or it may be so small and occasion so little trouble as to pass almost or quite unnoticed. A few days after this sore has appeared, the lymphatic glands in its neighbourhood, and later those all over the body, become swollen and hard. This condition lasts for several weeks as a rule, and then the sore slowly heals and the glands subside. After a variable period, usually about two months from the date of infection, the SECONDARY SYMPTOMS appear and resemble the symptoms of an ordinary fever in so far as they include rise of temperature and feverishness, loss of appetite, vague pains through the body, and a faint red rash seen best upon the front of the chest. The duration of this stage is largely dependent upon the efficiency with which it is treated.

In untreated or inadequately treated cases manifestations of the TERTIARY STAGE develop after the lapse of some months or years. These consist in the growth, here and there throughout the body, of masses of granulation tissue known as *gummas*. These gummas may appear as hard nodules in the skin, or form tumour-like masses in the muscles, or cause great thickening of bones, or they may develop in the brain and spinal cord, where their presence causes very serious symptoms. Gummas yield readily, as a rule, to appropriate treatment, and generally disappear speedily.

Still later effects are apt to follow, such as disease of the arteries, leading to aneurysm (see ARTERIES, DISEASES OF; ANEURYSM), to apoplexy, and to early mental failure (see MENTAL ILLNESS); also certain nervous diseases, of which tabes dorsalis and general paralysis are the chief.

The *congenital form* of syphilis, now rare, may affect the child before birth, leading then as a rule to miscarriage, or to a stillbirth if born at full time. Or he (or she) may show the first symptoms a few weeks after birth, the appearances then corresponding to the secondary manifestations of the acquired form.

Treatment: Any person who suffers from this disease forms a source of infection, and should take precautions not to spread it. Penicillin is the drug of choice in the treatment of syphilis in all its stages. Treatment must be instituted as soon as possible after infection is acquired;

(1) a full course of treatment is essential in every case, no matter how mild the disease may appear to be; (2) periodic blood examinations must be carried out on every patient for at least two years after he or she has been apparently cured.

SYRINGE is an instrument for injecting liquids into the body. Syringes vary considerably in shape and size according to the purpose for which they are used. (For the method of using a hypodermic syringe, see HYPODERMIC.)

SYRINGOMYELIA is a rare disease affecting the spinal cord, in which are found irregular cavities surrounded by an excessive amount of the connective tissue of the central nervous system. These cavities encroach upon the nerve tracts in the cord, producing especially loss of the sense of pain or of that for heat and cold in parts of the limbs, although the sensation of touch is retained. Another symptom sometimes present is wasting of certain muscles in the limbs. Changes affecting outlying parts like the fingers are also found. On account of their insensitiveness to pain, the fingers, for example, are often burnt or wounded, and troublesome ulcers, or loss of parts of the fingers, result. The condition of the spinal cord is probably present at birth, though the symptoms do not usually appear till young adulthood is reached. The disease is slowly progressive, though sudden exacerbations may occur after a cough, a sneeze, or sudden straining. Treatment consists simply in the maintenance of general good health.

SYRUP, formed of a mixture of sugar and water, is a fluid often used for the administration of drugs. It is employed partly on account of its pleasant taste, and largely also because it retards changes in drugs which deteriorate on exposure to the air.

SYSTEMIC: A description of something, for example, a drug, that affects the whole body and not just part of it.

SYSTOLE means the contraction of the heart, and alternates with the resting phase, known as diastole. The two occupy, respectively, about one-third and two-thirds of the cycle of heart action.

SYSTOLIC PRESSURE (see BLOOD PRESSURE).

T

TABES means, literally, a wasting disease, and is an old name applied to various diseases, such as tabes dorsalis and tuberculosis accompanied by enlargement of glands. At present the name

tabes dorsalis is used for locomotor ataxia and tabes mesenterica is used for tuberculosis affecting the glands in the abdomen: two diseases totally different in their nature and cause.

TABLET is the name given to a solid disc-like preparation made by compression and containing drugs mixed usually with sugar and other indifferent material. Tablets are widely used because of their convenience and accurate dosage. The word, 'tabloid', indicates a proprietary preparation.

TACHYCARDIA means a rapid pulse rate. (See HEART DISEASES.)

TACHYPNOEA means unusual quickness of breathing.

TACTILE: Perceptible to, pertaining to or related to the sense of touch.

TAENIASIS is the disease caused by taeniae, or tapeworms. Their shape is modified to present as large an absorbing surface as possible to the digested food passing down the intestine, so that they are flat, white and long (up to 12 metres [40 feet] in length), like a piece of tape, as their name implies. Each consists of a head, the size of a small pin's head, provided with suckers, and sometimes with hooklets, for adhesion to the bowel wall, and from this head segments are produced that gradually increase in size and develop ova the further they recede from the head. The mature segments at the extremity of the worm are crammed full of ova, and are constantly splitting off to be discharged in the stools. When these mature segments, or proglottides, are discharged, they fall upon the ground, and the ova they contain are afterwards conveyed either by food or drink into the stomach of an intermediate host, which may be a pig, ox or cattle, in the case of different parasites. The geographical distribution of different tapeworm infestation depends largely upon the eating habits of the inhabitants. Thus Taenia saginata, or the beef tapeworm, is found in beef-eating areas, especially in Europe and Mohammedan countries. Taenia solium, the pork tapeworm, is found most commonly in Germany and the Slav countries. Echinococcus granulosus is found where dogs are widely used, as in Iceland or sheep-rearing countries such as Australia, New Zealand and Argentina. When the ova reach the stomach of the intermediate host their capsule is dissolved, the embryos escape and find their way through the wall of stomach or intestine into the blood-vessels, by which they are carried to distant parts of the body. In the case of TAENIA SOLIUM the intermediate host is the pig, in the case of TAENIA SAGINATA it is cattle. In the muscles of these animals the embryos of the worm become encysted and remain so till they die, or till the animal's flesh happens to be eaten by the proper host, when they develop again into a new tapeworm in his intestine. The flesh of a pig thus infected shows plainly the encysted embryo (known as *Cysticercus cellulosae*), and is called measly pork. DIPHYLLOBOTHRIUM LATUM is seldom met with, except in the north of Europe and Asia, and the intermediate hosts are several varieties of fish. In the case of the tapeworm known as *Echinococcus granulosus*, relations are reversed, and man plays the rôle of intermediate host, the host of the mature tapeworm being the dog, from which the human being derives the embryo worm by allowing the dog to lick his hands and face, or to contaminate his food. Although the worm in the dog is very small (having only three segments, as a rule), the encysted form in man, known as a hydatid cyst, may reach a large size, situated in the liver, lungs, kidney or brain.

In the case of infestation with *Taenia saginata* there may be no symptoms or signs at all, and the 'host' only becomes aware that he is infested, when he sees the tapeworm, or rather part of it, in the stools. In the case of *Taenia solium*, the outlook is more serious because the eggs, when swallowed, are liable to migrate into the tissues of the body, as they do in the pig, and cause cysts. If these occur in the muscles they may cause little trouble but, if they occur in the brain, they can prove very serious.

Hydatid cysts often grow to a great size, budding off in their interior smaller cysts, which may have still smaller ones within them, the final contents of the smallest cysts being a salt, watery fluid and numerous heads of echinococci, each provided with a circle of hooks, and each capable, under proper conditions, of forming a new worm. The symptoms produced by a hydatid cyst depend mainly upon the effects of its size and consequent pressure. Very small cysts in the brain may produce serious results, like those of a tumour, whilst in the liver a cyst may grow to the size of a man's head before causing much trouble.

Treatment of tapeworm infestation consists of the administration of mepacrine, niclosamide or dichlorophen, followed by a purgative. Castor oil must not be used for this purpose. During treatment the stools must be carefully examined for the head of the tapeworm. Unless the head is passed in the stools, the worm will grow again. The treatment of hydatid cyst is surgical: i.e. the cyst must be removed by operation.

TALC is a soft mineral consisting of magnesium silicate. It is much used as an ingredient of dusting powders.

TALIPES is the technical name for club-foot (q.v.).

TALUS is the somewhat square-shaped bone which forms the lower part of the ankle-joint and unites the leg bones to the foot.

TAMPON: A plug or compressed gauze or cotton wool inserted into a wound or orifice to arrest haemorrhage. Also inserted into the vagina to absorb the flow of blood during menstruation.

TAMPONADE: The insertion of a tampon. It also may be used to describe the potentially life-threatening compression of the heart by the accumulation of fluid in the pericardial sac. This is characterized by tachycardia, pulsus paradoxus, low blood pressure, raised pressure in the jugular vein and abnormally quiet heart sounds.
Treatment consists of draining the fluid (which may be blood or an effusion) and treating the underlying cause.

TAMOXIFEN is a drug that is proving of value in the treatment of some cases of cancer of the breast.

TANNIN, or TANNIC ACID, is an uncrystallizable white or yellowish-white powder, which is soluble in water or glycerin. It is extracted from oak galls in large amount, but it is also present in almost all vegetable infusions. Tannic acid, acts as an astringent and also leads to rapid clotting of blood with which it is brought in contact.

TAPEWORM (see TAENIASIS).

TAPPING is the popular name for the withdrawal of oedema fluid from the cavities or the subcutaneous tissues of the body. (See ASPIRATION.)

TAR, or PIX LIQUIDA, is a thick, dark, oily substance obtained by the destructive distillation of several species of pine-tree. It is slightly soluble in water, more readily so in alcohol, oils, and strong alkaline solutions. Other tars of similar physical and medicinal properties are obtained from other woods, as well as from coal, shale, and peat. Tar is a substance of complex chemical composition, varying not only according to the source from which it is derived, but still more with the temperature at which it has been distilled. Generally speaking, wood-tar contains resin, creosote, and turpentine in considerable quantities, also benzol, carbolic acid, acetic acid, wood-spirit or methyl alcohol, methyl acetate, acetone, and wood-naphtha. The aniline dyes, many antipyretic bodies, saccharin, and various other medicinal substances and disinfectants are obtained indirectly from coal-tar.
Action: In consequence of the numerous medicinally active bodies it contains, tar exerts many marked effects upon the body. By reason of the creosote, carbolic acid, and methyl alcohol that it contains, it possesses an antiseptic and preservative power. Certain of its ingredients are of an irritating nature, and tar

therefore stimulates the action of any skin surface with which it is brought in contact, as well as the respiratory and other mucous membranes by which it is excreted after being taken internally.

Uses: Externally, tar is one of the most efficient preservatives of animal and vegetable tissues that we possess. For its germicidal action and stimulating properties it is used in chronic skin diseases, particularly psoriasis and dry eczema. To this end it is employed most commonly in the form of tar ointment. An alcoholic extract known as coal tar solution is also used to cleanse areas of skin affected by the disease.

TARGET CELL: Erythrocytes (q.v.) which are large and 'floppy' and have a ringed appearance, similar to that of a target, when stained and viewed under the microscope. This may occur with iron-deficiency anaemia, liver disease, a small spleen, haemoglobinopathies (disorders of haemoglobin) and thalassaemias (q.v.).

TARSAL: Of or pertaining to the tarsus (q.v.) of the foot and ankle – this comprises talus, calcaneus navicular, cuboid and three cuneiform bones – or eyelid.

TARSUS is the region of the instep with its seven bones, the chief of which are the talus supporting the leg-bones and the calcaneus or heel-bone, the others being the navicular, cuboid, and three cuneiform bones.

TARTAR is a concretion that forms on the teeth near the margin of the gum, consisting chiefly of phosphate of lime deposited from the saliva. Mixed with this are food particles, and in it flourish numberless bacteria. It is important that it should be prevented from forming by regular brushing of the teeth, or removal after it has formed by regular visits to the dentist, because it gives rise to wasting of the gums and loosening of the teeth.

TARTAR EMETIC is another name for antimony potassium tartrate, a drug used in the treatment of schistosomiasis. (See SCHISTOSOMIASIS.)

TASTE (see TONGUE).

TATTOOING has been a cult, or fashion, since the earliest days of history. Apart from the mixed motifs for its use, it has a definite therapeutic indication in matching the colour of skin grafts. It is performed by implanting particles of colour pigment into the deeper layer of the skin known as the corium (see SKIN). This is done by means of a needle or needles. The pigments commonly used are carbon for black, cinnabar (red mercuric sulphide) or cadmium salts for red, chrome salts for greens and yellows, cobalt for blue, ferric (iron) salts for

browns, pinks and yellows, and titanium for white. The main medical hazard of tattooing is infection, particularly of the liver, which may be fatal. The tattooed person may also become allergic to one of the pigments used, particularly cinnabar. Removal, which should be done by a plastic surgeon, always leaves a residual scar, and often needs to be followed by a skin graft. Removal is not allowed under the National Health Service unless there is some medical reason: for example, allergic reactions to it. Other methods of removal are by cryosurgery (q.v.), dermabrasion (q.v.) and salabrasion. These, too, must only be carried out under skilled medical supervision. Promising results are also being obtained from the use of laser (q.v.), a method that appears to produce less scarring than other methods, if it is carried out under expert medical supervision.

In order to reduce the health hazards, tattooists, along with acupuncturists, cosmetic skin-piercers and hair electrolysers, are required, under the Local Government (Miscellaneous Provisions) Act 1982, to register their premises with health and local authorities before starting business. The practitioners have to satisfy the authorities that adequate precautions have been taken to prevent the transmission of infections, such as hepatitis.

TAXIS is the method of pushing back, into the abdominal cavity, a loop of bowel which has passed through the wall in consequence of a rupture.

TEARS (see EYE).

TECHNETIUM-99: An isotope of the artificial element technetium. It emits gamma rays and is used as a tracer in building up a scintigraphic radioactive image of organs such as the brain.

TEETH are hard organs developed from the mucous membranes of the mouth and embedded in the jawbones. They are used to bite and grind food and to aid clarity of speech. In some animals the teeth may be modified in shape to enable them to be used as weapons.

Structure: Each tooth is composed of enamel, dentine, cement, pulp and periodontal membrane.

ENAMEL is the almost translucent material which covers the crown of a tooth. It is the most highly calcified material in the body, 96–97 per cent being composed of calcified salts. It is arranged from millions of long six-sided prisms set on end on the dentine. It is thickest over the biting surface of the tooth. With increasing age or the ingestion of abrasive foods the teeth may be worn away on the surface so that the dentine becomes visible. The outer sides of some teeth may be worn away by bad tooth-brushing technique.

DENTINE is a dense yellowish-white material from which the bulk and the basic shape of a tooth are formed. It is like ivory and it is harder

1 enamel   4 cement
2 dentine   5 dental periosteum
3 pulp cavity   6 bone of jaw

Vertical section through incisor tooth.

CEMENT or CEMENTUM is a thin bonelike material which covers the roots of teeth and helps hold the teeth in the bone. Fibres of the periodontal membrane are embedded in the cement and the bone. When the gums recede, part of the cement may be exposed and the cells die. Once this has happened, the periodontal membrane can no longer be attached to the tooth and, if sufficient cement is destroyed, the tooth support will be so weakened that the tooth will become loose.

PULP: This is the inner core of the tooth and is composed of a highly vascular, delicate fibrous tissue with many fine nerve fibres. The outer layer is formed by the odontoblasts which formed the dentine and are now dormant unless required to lay down a further thickness of dentine in response to a destructive stimulus at the outer edge of the dentine. The pulp is the tissue remaining after the tooth has been formed and may have helped in its eruption. The pulp is very sensitive to temperature variation and touch. If the pulp becomes exposed it will become infected and usually cannot overcome this. Root-canal treatment or extraction of the tooth may be necessary.

PERIODONTAL MEMBRANE: This is a layer of fibrous tissue arranged in groups of fibres which surround and support the root of a tooth in a bone socket. The fibres are interspersed with blood-vessels and nerves. Loss of the membrane leads to loss of the tooth. The membrane can release and re-attach the fibres to allow the tooth to move when it erupts or is being moved by orthodontic springs.

Arrangement and form: Teeth are present in most mammals and nearly all have two sets: a temporary or milk set followed by a permanent or adult set. In some animals, like the toothed whale, all the teeth are similar, but in man there are four different shapes: incisors, canines (eyeteeth), premolars (bicuspids), and molars. The incisors are chisel shaped and the canine is

than bone but softer than enamel. The crown of the tooth is covered by the hard protective enamel and the root is covered by a bonelike substance called cement. Dentine is formed from cells which produce cylinders of calcified material in the centre of which are tubules which contain protoplasmic processes which are extensions of the cells. These processes can transfer pain from the enamel to the sensitive pulp in the centre of the tooth. Dentine is formed from inorganic and organic matter. The composition is approximately 75 per cent inorganic salts and 25 per cent organic matter and water. Decay can erode dentine faster than enamel.

The permanent teeth of the right side.

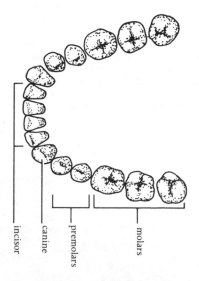

The permanent teeeth of the lower jaw.

enamel 1
dentine 2
pulp 3

Transverse section across the crown of a tooth.

pointed. Premolars have two cusps on the crown (one medial to the other) and molars have at least four cusps. They are arranged together in an arch in each jaw and the cusps of opposing teeth interdigitate. Some herbivores have no upper anterior teeth but use a pad of gum instead. As each arch is symmetrical, the teeth in an upper and lower quadrant can be used to identify the animal. In man the quadrants are the same, i.e. in the child there are two incisors, one canine and two molars (total teeth 20). In the adult there are two incisors, one canine, two premolars and three molars (total 32). This mixture of tooth form suggests that man is omnivorous. Anatomically the crown of the tooth has mesial and distal surfaces which touch the tooth next to it. The mesial surface is the one nearer to the centre line and the distal is the further away. The biting surface is called the incisal edge for the anterior teeth and the occlusal surface for the posteriors.

Development: The first stage in the formation of the teeth is the appearance of a downgrowth of epithelium into the underlying mesoderm. This is the dental lamina, and from it ten smaller swellings in each jaw appear. These become bell shaped and enclose a part of the mesoderm, the cells of which become specialized and are called the dental papillae. The epithelial cells produce enamel and the dental papilla forms the dentine, cement and pulp. At a fixed time the teeth start to erupt and a root is formed. Before the deciduous teeth erupt, the permanent teeth form, medial to them. In due course the deciduous roots resorb and the permanent teeth are then able to push the crowns out and erupt themselves. If this process is disturbed, the permanent teeth may be displaced and appear in an abnormal position or be impacted.

Eruption of teeth is in a definite order and at a fixed time, although there may be a few months leeway in either direction which is of no significance. Excessive delay is found in some congenital disorders such as cretinism. It may also be associated with local abnormalities of the jaws such as cysts, malformed teeth and supernumerary teeth.

The usual order of eruption of deciduous teeth is:

Middle incisors	6–8 months
Lateral incisors	8–10 ,,
First molars	12–16 ,,
Canines (eye-teeth)	16–20 ,,
Second molars	20–30 ,,

The usual order of eruption of permanent teeth is:

First molars	6–7 years
Middle incisors	6–8 ,,
Lateral incisors	7–9 ,,
Canines	9–12 ,,
First and second premolars	10–12 ,,
Second molars	11–13 ,,
Third molars (wisdom teeth)	17–21 ,,

TEETH, DISEASES OF: Teeth are important for appearance and speech and in the proper preparation of the food for its onward journey into the stomach. With modern foods biting and chewing are less important. Damage to the teeth can be painful.

TEETHING, or the process of eruption of the teeth, may be accompanied by symptoms which are particularly distressing in the child. There may be irritability, salivation, loss of sleep and a failure to feed. The child will tend to rub or touch the painful area. To a lesser extent this may also occur in the adult as the third molars try to erupt. Relief may be obtained in the child by allowing it to chew on a hard object such as a toy or rusk. If this is not sufficient, then various tinctures and pastes can be applied to the reddened area of gum. These remedies may contain salicylates or local anaesthetics.

TOOTHACHE is the pain felt when there is inflammation of the pulp or periodontal membrane of a tooth. It can vary in intensity and may be recurring. The commonest cause is caries when the cavity is close to the pulp. Once the pulp has become infected, this is likely to spread from the apex of the tooth into the bone to form an

permanent canine 1
permanent incisors 2
permanent incisors 3
permanent canine 4

10 premolars
9 first permanent molar
8 second permanent molar
7 second permanent molar
6 first permanent molar
5 premolars

Teeth of a six-year-old child. The permanent teeth are coloured black.

abscess (gumboil). A lesser but more long-lasting pain is felt when the dentine is unprotected. This can occur when the enamel is lost due to decay or trauma or because the gums have receded. This pain is often associated with temperature change or sweet foods. General debility makes a person more aware of minor discomforts. Expert dental advice should be sought early before the decay is extensive, even though the pain has disappeared temporarily. If a large cavity is accessible, temporary relief may be obtained by inserting a small piece of cotton wool soaked in one of the essential oils such as oil of cloves. A paste made from oil of cloves and zinc oxide powder is longer lasting but may make the pain more severe if the pulp is exposed and infected. Such a tooth requires root-canal therapy or extraction.

CARIES OF THE TEETH or dental decay is very common in the more affluent countries and is commonest in children and young adults. Increasing awareness of the causes has resulted in a considerable improvement in dental health, particularly in the last ten years. This has coincided with a rise in general health. Now 50 per cent of five-year-old children are caries free and of the others 10 per cent have half of the remaining carious cavities. Since the start of the National Health Service the emphasis has been on saving teeth. In south-east England, which has a high ratio of dentists for the population, less than 5 per cent of the people under 45 years have dentures. Now endentulous patients are mainly found among the elderly who had their teeth removed before 1948.

The precise cause of caries is still uncertain but the acidic theory is most widely held. Acid is produced by oral bacteria from dietary carbohydrates, particularly refined sugar, and this dissolves part of the enamel. The dentine is eroded more quickly as it is softer and the first time the person is aware of trouble is when the now hollow tooth collapses. Decay usually starts in a part of the tooth where cleaning is difficult, i.e. in the pits and fissures of the crown and between two teeth. The exposed smooth surfaces are usually protected as they are easily cleaned during normal eating and by brushing. Irregular and overcrowded teeth are more at risk from decay as they are difficult to clean. Primitive people who chew coarse foods rarely get caries. Fluoride in the drinking water at the rate of about 1 part per million is associated with a reduction in the caries rate. Prolonged severe disease in infancy is associated with poor calcification of the teeth, making them more vulnerable to decay. As the teeth are formed and partly calcified by the time of birth, the diet and health of the mother are also important to the teeth of the child. Pregnant mothers and children should have a good balanced diet with sufficient calcium and vitamin D. A fibrous diet will also aid cleansing of the teeth and stimulate the circulation in the teeth and jaws. The caries rate can be reduced by regular brushing with a fluoride toothpaste two or three times per day and certainly before going to sleep. This can be carried out with a brush and a tooth powder or

(Above) Natural crevices on healthy back teeth in which food collects. (Below) Front teeth of upper jaw showing places between teeth where food has collected and led to decay.

paste. Powders tend to be more abrasive and, if used too often and with too much force, can wear the teeth away. Confectionary should be avoided between meals. The provision of sweet or sugary juices in a pacifier or bottle to help an infant sleep will rapidly lead to the loss of the upper front teeth.

The dental health of children has improved greatly in the past fifteen years in most industrial countries. This appears to be due to a number of factors. Public awareness of the need to brush and clean the teeth has greatly increased. Toothpastes now contain additives which reduce the formation of plaque and fluoride will strengthen the enamel up to 50 per cent. Fluoride in the water, whether it occurs naturally or is added, is associated with a lower caries rate. Fluoride is also available in tablet form for children but probably the most common source of the ion is in toothpaste.

IRREGULARITY OF THE PERMANENT TEETH may be due to an abnormality in the growth of the jaws or to the early or late loss of the deciduous set. Most frequently it is due to an imbalance in the size of the teeth and the length of the jaws. Some improvement may take place with age but many will require the help of an orthodontist (specialist dentist) who can correct many mal-occlusions by removing a few teeth to allow him to move the others into a good position by means of springs and elastics on various appliances which are worn in the mouth.

LOOSENING OF THE TEETH may be due to an accident or inflammation of the gum. Teeth loosened by trauma may be replaced in the socket, even if knocked right out. If they are then splinted to the neighbouring teeth for a few weeks they may re-attach themselves to the bone. If the loosening is due to periodontal disease the prognosis is less favourable. The removal of any calculus and the use of some antiseptic mouthwashes will help.

DISCOLORATION of the teeth may be intrinsic or extrinsic, i.e. the stain may be in the calcified structure or stuck on to it. Intrinsic staining may be due to jaundice or the antibiotic tetracycline. Dark teeth are due to blood-breakdown products entering the dentinal tubules as a result of some trauma that has damaged the pulp. It may be possible to bleach such teeth but it usually needs to be repeated frequently. Extrinsic stain may be due to tea, coffee, tobacco, pan (a mixture of chuna and betel nuts wrapped in a leaf), iron-containing medicines or excess fluoride. Some of these can be removed by brushing with an abrasive paste but where the stain is within the tooth or the surface of the tooth is damaged, an artificial crown or veneer may be required.

GINGIVITIS or inflammation of the gums may occur as an acute or chronic condition. In the acute form it is often part of a general infection of the mouth and principally occurs in children or young adults and resolves after ten to fourteen days. The chronic form occurs later in life and tends to be progressive. There is moderate pain but the gums appear congested, bleed easily and may be ulcerated. Later calculus appears on the teeth. Eating may be difficult if the ulceration is extensive. Various micro-organisms may be found on the lesions including anaerobes. Treatment is initially supportive but the mouth should be kept as clean and moist as possible. Antiseptic mouthwashes may help and once the painful stage is past, the gums should be thoroughly cleaned and any calculus removed. In severe conditions an antibiotic may be required.

PERIODONTAL DISEASE is the spread of gingivitis to involve the periodontal membrane of the tooth and in its florid form used to be called pyorrhoea. In this, the membrane becomes damaged by the inflammatory process and a space or pocket is formed into which a probe can be easily passed. As the pocket becomes more extensive the tooth loosens. Although neglect hastens the process, the cause is still largely unknown. The production of calculus from plaque increases the trauma on the gingival margins and the injection of micro-organisms. The loss of the periodontal membrane also leads to the loss of supporting bone. Chronic inflammation soon occurs and is difficult to eradicate. The effect of chewing on mobile teeth is debatable but some shedding of bacteria into the bloodstream occurs and this may affect damaged organs such as heart valves after rheumatic fever. Acute flare-ups of the disease may occur when the patient is unwell and also during pregnancy. Pain is not a feature of the disease but there is often an unpleasant odour (halitosis). The gums bleed easily and there may be dyspepsia. Treatment is largely aimed at stabilizing the condition rather than curing it. This is done by meticulous care of the mouth and teeth and the removal of calculus. Where there is excess tissue, the edge of the gums can

be reshaped by surgical means, but attempts at replacing bone have only been partially successful.

DENTAL ABSCESS or ALVEOLAR ABSCESS is an infection that arises in or round a tooth and spreads to involve the bone. It may occur many years after a blow has killed the pulp of the tooth or more quickly after caries has reached the pulp. At first the pain may be mild and intermittent but eventually it will become severe and a swelling will develop in the gum over the apex of the tooth. The tooth may be sensitive to hot and cold at first, then will not respond but will feel extruded from the socket and be tender when touched. The swelling will enlarge until it feels like a bag of fluid, then may burst to discharge pus and will be more comfortable for a time. The discharge may become chronic. A radiograph of the tooth will show a round clear area at the apex of the tooth. Treatment may be by painting the gum with a mild counter-irritant such as a tincture of aconite and iodine in the early stages but later root-canal therapy or apicectomy may be required. If a swelling is present, it may need to be drained and antibiotics given. Where the tooth is beyond repair or of little use, then extraction may be preferable.

INJURIES TO TEETH are common. The more minor injuries include crazing and the loss of small chips of enamel, and the major ones include a broken root and avulsion of the entire tooth. A specialist dental opinion should be sought as soon as possible. The exposure of dentine will be painful for some weeks but can be easily treated by covering the tooth with a substance that does not easily conduct heat. Nail varnish or chewing gum will help for a few hours at least. When the pulp is exposed, it will almost certainly have to be removed before it becomes infected. A tooth that has been knocked out can be re-implanted if it is clean and replaced within a few hours. It will then require splinting in place for 4–6 weeks. Tinfoil can be used as a temporary splint. If the tooth was on the ground, then prevention of infection, including tetanus, will be necessary.

PREVENTION OF DENTAL DISEASE: As with other matters, prevention is better than cure. Children should be taught at an early age to keep their teeth and gums clean and to avoid refined sugars between meals. It is better to finish a meal with a drink of water rather than a sweetened drink. Sweetened drinks are particularly harmful just before going to sleep. Fluoride in some of its forms is useful in the reduction of dental caries and a vaccine now being developed may be useful. Overcrowding of the teeth, obvious maldevelopment of the jaw and persistent thumbsucking into the teens are all indications for seeking the advice of an orthodontist. Generally adults have less trouble with decay but more with periodontal disease and, as its onset is insidious, regular dental inspections are desirable. Dentures are also not without problem and should be checked at least every five years. If worn day and night, there is a risk of developing thrush under the denture and damaging the gum and mucous membrane.

TEETH GRINDING, or BRUXISM as it is technically known, is quite common in children during sleep, when it is of no significance unless really persistent. During the day it may be an attention-seeking device. There is no treatment for it and if ignored it will stop. It is more common and persistent in mentally retarded children.

In adults it is usually associated with stress or anxiety, but may be due to some local condition in the mouth such as an unsatisfactory filling. It may also be caused by certain drugs, including fenfluramine and levodopa. More rarely it may be due to brain disease. If not controlled, it produces excessive wear of the enamel covering of the teeth. Treatment consists of alleviation of any condition in the mouth and any anxiety and stress. It may be useful to wear a splint covering the teeth of one jaw at night.

TEETHING (see TEETH, DISEASES OF).

TEICHOPSIA: This refers to zigzag lines that patients with migraine often experience as an aura preceding an attack.

TELANGIECTASIS means an abnormal dilatation of arterioles and capillaries, forming sometimes a tumour or TELANGIOMA.

TEMAZEPAM is a relatively quick-acting hypnotic of short duration so that there is little or no 'hangover' the next morning. It is a derivative of diazepam. (See BENZODIAZEPINES.)

TEMPERAMENT is a term that includes those vague general peculiarities of mind and body that render some people more liable than others to be affected by particular diseases.

TEMPERATURE of the body is a subject of great importance. Animals are generally divided as regards their temperature into two classes: *cold-blooded animals*, including reptiles, amphibians, fish, and invertebrates generally, whose temperature varies to a great extent according to that of the surrounding medium; and *warm-blooded animals*, including mammals and birds, whose temperature remains almost constant, no matter how the surrounding temperature falls or rises. In warm-blooded animals, this constancy of body temperature is effected by a perpetual balancing of the various forces which produce heat and give off heat. The chief heat producer in the body is the oxidizing action that takes place on muscular contraction, and the chief cooling agents are the skin and lungs, which act by the exposure of the blood circulating in them to the air, and by the evaporation of moisture from their surfaces. The temperature of different warm-blooded animals varies considerably; in man it is somewhere between 36·7 and 37·2 °C (98 and 99 °F). It varies in different people but is generally stated to be about 37 °C (98·4 °F). Even in a given healthy individual the temperature is constantly changing, being lowest in the early morning and highest in the evening. The chief reason for this change is to be found probably in the variations as regards activity at different periods of the day. The temperature also varies in different parts of the body, that of the skin being about half a degree lower than that taken within the hollow organs of the body; and in stout people this difference between the surface and the interior is still more marked. In parts exposed to cold or provided with a feeble blood supply, such as paralysed limbs, the temperature may sink very low.

Temperature in disease: The maintenance of a nearly steady temperature is the result of a constant process of balancing between heat-production and heat-loss, controlled probably by a special centre in the nervous system. In disease, one or other of these processes may be impaired or the controlling mechanism may be thrown completely out of gear. The general temperature may rise as high as 43·3 °C (110 °F), or sink to 32·2 °C (90 °F) for a time; but the risk to life is great when it passes above 41 °C (106 °F) or below 35 °C (95 °F).

Fall of temperature may be due to many causes. Thus it generally accompanies great loss of blood, starvation, and the collapsed condition which sometimes results from severe attacks of fever, peritonitis, and other devitalizing acute diseases. Certain chronic diseases are generally accompanied by a subnormal temperature; of these, myxoedema is the most outstanding.

Rise of temperature is a characteristic of acute diseases, and of diseases due to microorganisms, the poisonous products of which lead to increased waste of the tissues. Injuries to the nervous system, even unpleasant sensations in children and nervous people, may have a similar effect. In people dying in a feverish condition, the temperature often rises very high immediately before death, owing probably to failure of the circulation and other conditions which diminish the body heat. Rapid rise of temperature in such a case is therefore an ominous sign.

Many diseases have a characteristic course of temperature, so that in hospital a glance at the temperature chart is often sufficient to acquaint a physician with the disease from which the patient is suffering. Thus pneumonia, enteric fever, measles, and malaria show, as a rule, quite recognizable temperature records.

High temperature in some diseases is a much less serious feature than in others. Thus in enteric fever or pneumonia 40·5 °C (105 °F) is an ordinary temperature, whilst in rheumatic fever and diphtheria the temperature generally ranges between 38·3 and 39·5 °C (101 and 103 °F), so that in these diseases a temperature of 40 °C (104 °F) gives cause for anxiety.

In most diseases the temperature gradually

abates as the patient recovers, but others, for example pneumonia and typhus fever, end rapidly by a *crisis* in which the temperature falls, perspiration breaks out, the pulse becomes slower, and the breathing quieter. The reason for the sudden change lies probably in the fact that in favourable cases, after the disease has lasted a certain time, the resisting power of the body becomes able fully to neutralize the poisons produced by the organisms of the disease. This crisis is often preceded by an increase of all the symptoms, including an epicritical rise of temperature.

Record of temperature: Temperature is generally measured by a thermometer. Those intended for clinical use possess a long, narrow bulb, an index registering from 35 to 43·3 °C (95 to 110 °F), and are made so that the column of mercury does not fall back into the bulb till it is shaken down.

There are two scales in common use: the Fahrenheit scale and the Centigrade or Celsius scale. (Hitherto, in Britain the term Centigrade has been preferred, but under the new International System of Units (SEE WEIGHTS AND MEASURES) the term Celsius is recommended.) The difference consists in this, that in the Centigrade scale the freezing-point of water is marked 0° and the boiling-point 100°, while in the Fahrenheit scale these are 32° and 212°, respectively. Accordingly 100 divisions on the Centigrade scale are equivalent to 180 divisions on the Fahrenheit scale, and 1 degree C equals 1·8 degrees F. To convert from degrees F to degrees C the following formula may be used:

$$n \text{ °F} = [(n - 32) \times \tfrac{5}{9}] \text{ C,}$$

and to convert from degrees C to degrees F the following:

$$n \text{ °C} = [(n \times \tfrac{9}{5}) + 32] \text{ F}$$

The Réaumur scale, in which the freezing-point is 0° and the boiling-point 80°, is also used in some countries, e.g. France, though not for scientific purposes.

As to the part of the body where the temperature is taken, the mouth is preferable, the bulb of the thermometer being placed beneath the tongue. The thermometer must be carefully washed with cold water before use, so that it does not convey infection, and care taken to ensure that the mercury is shaken down to below 35·5 °C (96 °F). The patient must be directed to keep the mouth shut but not to bite the thermometer with the teeth, and breathe through the nose. It is essential to ensure that the patient has not just had a hot drink. The thermometer must be kept in the mouth for at least three minutes. After use the thermometer must be thoroughly rinsed under running cold water and the mercury shaken down. When taken in the armpit the skin should be wiped dry, the bulb of the thermometer placed as high as possible, and the arm tightly folded across the chest. To obtain a correct reading, it is necessary to leave the thermometer in place for at least five minutes, because the skin surfaces do not at once represent the internal temperature of the body. Occasionally the temperature is taken by inserting the thermometer bulb about 5 cm (2 inches) into the rectum, a method which gives the most correct result of all, and is the most satisfactory in infants.

To keep a record, a piece of paper ruled with vertical lines to represent the periods at which the temperature is taken, and with horizontal lines corresponding to degrees, is used. A large dot is marked in the proper place each time the temperature is taken and the successive dots are afterwards joined by straight lines.

Treatment of high temperature is mentioned under ANTIPYRETICS; COLD, USES OF; FEVER.

TEMPLE is the side of the head above the line between the eye and ear. The term, temporal, is applied to the muscles, nerves, and artery of this region. The hair usually begins to turn grey first at the temples.

TEMPORAL: Referring or relating to the temporal region.

TEMPORAL ARTERITIS: Inflammation of the temporal artery. Also known as giant cell arteritis, it often affects other arteries too, mainly in the head. It predominantly affects the elderly. The artery becomes tender with reddening of the overlying skin. Headache and blindness may also occur. The diagnosis is confirmed by temporal artery biopsy, and treatment is with steroids.

TEMPORAL LOBE EPILEPSY: Epilepsy in which the abnormal cerebral activity originates in the temporal lobe of the brain. It is characterized by hallucinations of smell and sometimes of taste, hearing, or sight. There may be disturbances of memory, including déjà vu phenomena. Automatism (q.v.) may occur, but consciousness is seldom lost.

TENDERNESS is the term usually applied in medical nomenclature to pain experienced when a diseased part is handled, the term, pain, being reserved for unpleasant sensations felt apart from any manipulation.

TENDINITIS: Inflammation of a tendon. Usually caused by unusual or excessive physical activity, it may also be infective in origin or secondary to a connective tissue disorder. The pain and inflammation may be treated with non-steroidal anti-inflammatory drugs (q.v.), immobilization splinting and steroid injections. Repetitive strain injury, caused by constant use of a keyboard (typewriter, word processor or computer) is tendinitis occurring in the hands and arms.

TENDON, SINEW, or LEADER, is the cord that attaches the end of a muscle to the bone or other structure upon which the muscle acts when it contracts. Tendons are composed of bundles of white fibrous tissue arranged in a very dense manner, and are of great strength. Some are rounded, some flattened bands, whilst others are very short, the muscle-fibres being attached almost directly to the bone. Most tendons are surrounded by sheaths lined with membrane similar to the synovial membrane lining joint-cavities. In this sheath the tendon glides smoothly over surrounding parts. The fibres of a tendon pass into the substance of the bone and blend with the fibres composing it. One of the largest tendons in the body is the tendo Achilles, or tendo calcaneus as it is now known, which attaches the muscle of the calf to the calcaneus or heel-bone.

TENDON INJURIES are one of the hazards of sports. They usually result from indirect violence, or overuse, rather than direct violence. *Rupture* usually results from the sudden application of an unbalanced load. Thus complete rupture of the Achilles tendon is common in taking an awkward step backwards playing squash. There is sudden pain, the victim is often under the impression that he received a blow. This is accompanied by loss of function, and a gap may be felt in the tendon. *Partial rupture* is also accompanied by pain, but there is no breach of continuity or complete loss of function. Treatment of a complete rupture usually means surgical repair followed by immobilization of the tendon in plaster of Paris for six weeks. Partial rupture usually responds to physiotherapy and immobilization, but healing is slow.

TENDOVAGINITIS means inflammation of a tendon and of the sheath enveloping it.

TENESMUS is a term applied to a symptom of disease affecting the lower part of the large intestine, such as dysentery, piles, or tumour. It consists of a constant sense of weight about the lower bowel and desire to go to stool, coupled with straining at stool and the passage of little but mucus and perhaps some blood.

TENNIS ELBOW (see ELBOW).

TENO- is a prefix denoting some relation to a tendon.

TENOSYNOVITIS, or TENOSITIS, means inflammation of a tendon.

TENOTOMY means an operation in which one or more tendons are divided, usually with the object of remedying some deformity.

TENTORIUM is a wide process of dura mater forming a partition between the cerebrum and cerebellum and supporting the former.

TERATOGENESIS is the production of physical defects in the fetus. It is understandable that a drug may interfere with a mechanism that is essential for growth and result in arrested or distorted development of the fetus and yet cause no disturbance in adults, in whom these growth processes have ceased to be relevant. Thus the effect of a drug upon a fetus may differ qualitively as well as quantitively from its effect on the mother. The susceptibility of the embryo will depend on the stage of development it has reached when the drug is given. The age of early differentiation, that is from the beginning of the third week to the end of the tenth week of pregnancy is the time of greatest susceptibility. After this time the likelihood of congenital malformation resulting from drug treatment is less, although the death of the fetus can occur at any time as a result of drugs crossing the placenta or as a result of their effect on the placental circulation. The term teratogenesis has come into common usage since the thalidomide disaster.

Thalidomide was an effective non-barbiturate hypnotic which had passed stringent tests before being released for general use. In spite of this it produced a number of congenital defects, esecially of the limbs, in children born to mothers who had taken the drug while pregnant. As soon as this was discovered the drug was withdrawn from use. Subsequently the government set up a Committee of Drug Safety to try and ensure that there was no recurrence of such a distressing episode with subsequent drugs. Even the most stringent precautions, however, cannot ensure the complete elimination of this risk. Fortunately the risk is a remote one, but it is now realised that no drug should be given to a pregnant woman, particularly during the first few months of pregnancy, unless it is absolutely essential for her health or that of her unborn child. There is no satisfactory test on animals that will clear a drug of the possibility of producing congenital malformation in man. Indeed drugs such as aspirin, caffein, insulin and thyroxine cause fetal abnormalities in some animal species but there is no evidence that they do so in man. Furthermore, the problem must be kept in perspective and it should be appreciated that only 1 per cent of congenital malformations are the results of environmental factors, which include not only drugs but infections such as German measles and irradiation. The risk that any random pregnancy will end in some serious malformation is about 1 in 40. Of drugs in current use there is circumstantial evidence that the alkylating agents and antimetabolites used in the treatment of reticulosis and leukaemia are teratogenic. There is some evidence that oral hypoglycaemic agents and antihistamine agents may also be responsible for a few congenital malformations.

TERATOMA is a tumour that consists of partially developed embryonic tissues. The most common sites of this tumour are the ovary and the testicle.

TERBUTALINE is a drug that is proving of value in the treatment of asthma. It is given by injection under the skin or by inhalation. It is a beta adrenoreceptor agonist.

TERTIAN FEVER is the name applied to that type of malaria in which the fever reappears every other day. (See MALARIA.)

TESTICLE: The testes, or testicles, are the two male sexual glands. Each is developed in the corresponding loin, but before birth they descend through openings in the lower part of the front of the abdomen into a fold or pouch of skin known as the scrotum. This fold is strengthened by a layer of muscle fibres and fibrous tissues, and within it each testicle possesses a separate covering known as the tunica vaginalis. This tunic is a double layer of serous membrane similar in structure to the peritoneum or pleura, and it is derived from the peritoneum while the testicle is still within the abdomen. Occasion-ally, as the result of defective development, a more or less open channel of communication is left between the peritoneum and tunica vaginalis, and down this channel a hernia is liable to form in childhood or later. Throughout life, the openings in the abdominal wall remain, but each inguinal canal should be just large enough to allow the passage of one of the two spermatic cords, each of which is composed of the vas (or ductus) deferens, together with the blood-vessels, nerves, and lymphatics proceeding to the gland. Within the tunica vaginalis lies a dense fibrous coat known as the tunica albuginea, which affords protection to the gland. On microscopic examination, each testicle is found to consist of a series of minute tubes, from eight hundred to one thousand in number, supported by fibrous tissue in which the nerves and blood-vessels run, and lined by cells from which the spermatozoa are formed. Around 4·5 million spermatozoa are produced per gram of testicle per day. These tubes communicate with one another near the centre of the testicle, and are connected by a much convoluted tube, the epididymis, with the ductus, or vas deferens, which enters the abdomen, and passes on to the base of the bladder. This duct, after joining a reservoir known as the seminal vesicle, opens, close to the duct from the other side of the

1 urinary bladder	6 convoluted seminiferous tubule	11 prostatic follicle
2 prostrate utricle	7 canal of the epydidymus	12 ejaculatory duct
3 capsule of prostate	8 rete testis	13 seminal vesicle
4 urethra	9 efferent ductules	14 vas (ductus) deferens
5 penis	10 bulbo-urethral gland	15 ureter

Diagram of the male sex organs.

body, into that part of the urethra which is surrounded by the prostate gland. Owing to the convulutions of these ducts leading from the testicles to the urethra, and their indirect route, the passage from testicle to urethra is over 6 metres (20 feet) in length. In addition to producing spermotozoa, the testicle also forms an internal secretion which is responsible for the development of male characteristics. This hormone has been isolated and is known as testosterone.

TESTICLE, DISEASES OF: The pouch of skin, or scrotum, in which the testicles lie is liable to various general skin diseases, but particularly to eczema, which in many cases is often difficult to cure. Cancer of the skin in this region is specially common among chimney-sweeps, shale workers and cotton spinners, the result of chronic irritation by a carcinogenic agent in soot and paraffin products. Hernia, which in some cases passes into the scrotum, is treated under a special heading. (See HERNIA.) Sometimes, owing to defective development, the testicles are retained within the abdomen. HYDROCOELE is a local dropsy affecting one tunica vaginalis, and distending that side of the scrotum with fluid. (See HYDROCOELE.) VARICOCOELE is a condition in which the veins of the spermatic cord, especially on the left side, become unusually numerous and distended, the causes being much the same as those of varicose veins in other parts. The chief symptom is a dragging sensation in the testicle, which in some cases becomes at times very painful. This symptom is specially marked in warm weather and after exertion, the mass of veins at such a time becoming very distinct and resembling a 'bag of worms', though they empty quickly when the person lies down. Cold sponging of the part, careful regulation of the bowels, and the support of a suspensory net bandage afford all the treatment that is necessary in many cases; but an operation may sometimes be advisable. INFLAMMATION of an acute type (orchitis) may arise in people suffering from cystitis, stone in the bladder, and various forms of inflammation in the urinary organs, the most common cause of all being gonorrhoea. It may follow also upon some cases of mumps. The symptoms are intense pain and swelling with redness of the skin over the affected testicle; and the usual treatment consists of rest in bed, support of the scrotum with a suspensory bandage or wads of cotton-wool, the administration of analgesics (in some cases the pain may be so severe that morphine is necessary), and the administration of antibiotics if there is some definite causative micro-organism. In some cases the condition goes on to the formation of an abscess which bursts through the skin with immediate relief of pain. The condition is then treated as an abscess elsewhere. TORSION, or twisting or rotation, of the testes, or, strictly speaking, of the spermatic cord, is a relatively common occurrence in adolescent

and young adult males. It can occur during sleep, at rest, while playing games or doing hard physical work. About half the cases occur in the early hours of the morning during sleep. It is more liable to happen more often in the colder, than the warmer, months of the year. It makes itself felt by pain of varying severity – from slight to excruciating – either in the lower part of the abdomen or in the scrotum. In time the pain diminishes or disappears. The testes become hard and swollen. Treatment consists of immediate undoing of the torsion. If this is done within a few hours no harm ensues as a rule, but it should be followed within six hours by surgical operation to ensure that the torsion has been successfully undone and to fix the testes so that there should be no recurrence. TUBERCULOSIS occurs in the testicle occasionally, especially when some other organ, such as the bladder, is already the seat of the disease. It causes practically no pain, and is therefore often far advanced before it attracts attention. It responds well to chemotherapy with streptomycin, paraaminosaliylic acid and/or isoniazid. TUMOURS of the testes occur in around 600 males annually in Britain. They represent the second commonest form of malignant growth in young males. There are two types: seminomas and teratomas (q.v.). When adequately treated the survival rate for seminomas is 95 per cent, whilst that for teratomas is 50 per cent. INJURIES of the testicles are relatively rare. A severe blow may lead to shock and symptoms of severe collapse for a time, and may cause an effusion of blood into the tunica vaginalis. These symptoms are usually relieved by rest in bed.

TEST MEAL or gastric function test is a term originally applied to a meal given for the purpose of testing digestive function. The original gruel meal has been replaced by the injection of histamine (q.v.), which is a powerful stimulator of gastric juice, or pentagastin. After the stimulant has been injected, the digestive juices are withdrawn through a stomach tube (inserted through the nose and throat) and their volume and chemistry measured. A similar test is used to assess the working of the pancreas gland (q.v.).

TESTIS (see TESTICLE).

TESTOSTERONE is the name given to the male sex hormone secreted by the testes. It has also been prepared synthetically and has the formula $C_{19}H_{28}O_2$. In true eunuchoid conditions it has the power of restoring male sexual characteristics. (See ANDROGEN.)

TESTOSTERONE ENANTHATE (see ANDROGEN).

TESTOSTERONE PROPIONATE (see ANDROGEN).

TESTOSTERONE UNDECANOATE (see ANDROGEN).

TEST-TUBE is a tube of thin glass closed at one end, which is used for observing chemical reactions or for bacterial culture.

'TEST-TUBE BABY' (see EMBRYO TRANSFER).

TETANUS, or LOCKJAW, is a disorder of the nervous system, consisting in a greatly increased excitability of the spinal cord and manifesting itself by painful and lengthened spasm of the voluntary muscles throughout the body. The disease was well known in former wars, and Hippocrates (400 BC) refers to its rapidly fatal character.
Causes: The onset of the disease generally follows a wound, especially a deeply punctured, lacerated, or gunshot wound, usually appearing some 4 or 5 days after the wound has been inflicted, although it may be delayed for 3 or 4 weeks, by which time the wound is likely to be completely healed up. The presence in a wound of some foreign body, such as a splinter of wood or a portion of a bullet, seems to favour the onset of tetanus.

The direct cause of tetanus was discovered in 1889 by Kitasato, a Japanese observer, to be a bacillus: *Clostridium tetani*. This organism has a characteristic appearance, being long and bearing often at one end a large spore which gives to it a drumstick outline. It inhabits earth and dust, living especially a little distance below the surface in places where the manure of horses and cattle is collected. Hence it is found especially in the neighbourhood of stables, and is liable to infect wounds soiled with heavily manured earth. The bacillus develops a poison or toxin in the wound, and this, being absorbed, finds its way up the motor nerves to the spinal cord, which it renders excessively sensitive, so that its cells are excited by mild stimuli that under ordinary conditions would produce no reaction. After death, patients who have died of tetanus show very few lesions except congestion of the brain and spinal cord and degenerative changes in the cells of the latter.

In England and Wales, in 1974–78, there were 86 cases of tetanus, with 22 deaths, but fewer than 10 deaths a year occur now.
Symptoms: The onset of tetanus usually occurs within two days to three weeks of the wound responsible for the introduction of the infection. This is not necessarily an incubation period in the strict sense of the term because the causative organism may be dormant in the tissues of the body before producing toxin. The importance of this is that, whilst generally speaking, it is a fact that the longer the period between the wound and the onset of tetanus, the better the outlook, there are occasions when a delayed onset of the disease is acute and dangerous because a hitherto dormant strain of the organism has suddenly started to produce large amounts of toxin. The first signs of the disease usually show themselves as stiffness in the muscles near the wound, followed later, no matter where the wound is situated, by stiffness about the muscles of the jaw, causing difficulty in opening the mouth, which soon increases to *lockjaw* or trismus. This is accompanied by spasm in neighbouring muscles, and the drawn features and exposed teeth give to the countenance the peculiar expression known as *risus sardonicus*. The rigidity extends to the muscles of the neck, back, chest, abdomen, and extremities, and the body may assume a bent attitude, either backward (*opisthotonos*), forward (*emprosthotonos*), or laterally (*pleurosthotonos*). This general muscular rigidity, which at first is not constant but occasionally undergoes relaxation, is accompanied by frequently recurring convulsive seizures, which are readily excited by the slightest irritation, such as from a draught of cool air, a bright light, the closing of a door. In such attacks there is great suffering and the expression of the face is indicative of agony. The function of respiration may be seriously involved and asphyxia threaten or actually take place. The temperature sometimes rises to a high degree, and copious perspiration is also a constant symptom. These acute symptoms may subside after a few days and the patient gradually recover. On the other hand, the symptoms may increase in severity and death ensue either by asphyxia from prolonged spasm of the respiratory muscles, or exhaustion consequent on the violence of the symptoms, together with the absence of sleep. Throughout the whole course of the illness the mind is clear, and the patient waits with anxiety for the next convulsive attack. In milder cases the symptoms are less severe, the course more chronic, and recovery more common.

Tetanus sometimes occurs in new-born children, showing itself within a week of birth by obvious difficulty in the acts of sucking and swallowing, and, by the supervention of lockjaw, together with prolonged contraction of the muscles of the limbs and body, accompanied by convulsive seizures. *Local cases* of tetanus occur in which the muscles of a limb in the neighbourhood of the wound show spasms, but these do not become general, or they pass off after appearing to a slight extent. Such cases often show stiffness for several months.

The symptoms of strychnine poisoning bear a strong resemblance to those of tetanus, but in the former case they are more acute, less prolonged than the spasms of tetanus, come on after something has been swallowed, and end either in death or in recovery within a few hours. Hydrophobia (rabies), too, resembles tetanus in some respects.

The outcome depends upon various factors, including the virulence of the toxin, the age of the patient, his state of immunity and the availability of expert medical and nursing attention. If treated properly the prognosis is good, though those over 50 do less well.
Prevention: The outlook in tetanus has been entirely altered by the introduction of tetanus antitoxin and of tetanus toxoid. The latter

provides effective protection against the disease. Tetanus immunization is now an accepted part of the immunization programme for children in the United Kingdom. (See VACCINE.) Sportsmen using muddy playing fields are especially vulnerable and should have effective immunization, as should regular gardeners. Some authorities recommend booster injections of vaccine at intervals of ten years to maintain protection against the disease.

Whilst antitoxin is of primary value from the point of view of treatment, it is of prophylactic value if given immediately after an individual has received a wound which may be contaminated with the tetanus organism.

Treatment: Tetanus tends especially to follow wounds infected by stable refuse, by street dust, or by the deeper soil thrown up by shells on the battlefield. In all such cases, 1500 international units of antitoxin must be injected subcutaneously as soon as possible, unless it is definitely known that the individual has been completely immunized by a previous course of toxoid.

If the wound is only slight, all that may be required may be a dose of tetanus toxoid (0·5 ml) with or without an intramuscular injection of 1·2 mega units of benzathine penicillin. Other antibiotics active against *Cl. tetani* are benzylpenicillin, erythromycin and tetracycline, as is also metronidazole. In addition careful cleaning of the wound is required. An injection of 250 units of tetanus immunoglobulin (see IMMUNOGLOBULINS) provides immunity for four weeks.

TETANY is a condition characterized by spasm of muscle usually caused by a fall in the ionic calcium of the blood. This fall in ionic calcium results in hyperexcitability of the muscles, which are thus liable to go into spasm on the slightest stimulus. This is well demonstrated in two of the classical signs of the disease: *Chvostek's sign*, in which the muscles of the face contract when the cheek is tapped over the facial nerve as it emerges on the cheek; *Erb's sign*, in which muscles go into spasm in response to an electrical stimulus which normally causes only a contraction of the muscle. Tetany is most common in infants, in whom it may arise as a result of rickets, excessive vomiting, or certain forms of nephritis. It may also be due to lack of the active principle of the parathyroid glands. Overbreathing may also cause it. Treatment consists of the administration of calcium salts, and in severe cases this is done by giving calcium gluconate intravenously or intramuscularly. High doses of vitamin D are also required: calcitriol is the most active preparation.

TETRACYCLINES are a group of antibiotics which include chlorteracycline, oxytetracycline, tetracycline, demethylchlotetracycline, methacycline, lymecycline, minocycline, and clomocycline. Chlortetracycline, which is derived from *Streptomyces aureofaciens*, was the first to be discovered, followed by oxytetracycline which is derived from *Streptomyces rimosus*. Subsequently it was discovered that the active constituent of both these antibiotics was tetracycline, which can be prepared on a large scale by the catalytic hydrogenation of chlortetracycline. Methacycline, lymecycline, and clomocycline are subsequently discovered derivatives.

From the point of view of antibacterial activity, all the preparations are virtually identical, being active against both Gram-negative and Gram-positive bacteria, as well as certain rickettsiae (q.v.) and chlamydia including those causing Q fever, trachoma, psittacosis, and lymphogranuloma inguinale.

It is this wide range of activity, which has given them the name of broad-spectrum antibiotics, combined with the fact that they are given by mouth, that has made them such a useful contribution to the treatment of infective diseases. They must be used with discrimination in young children as they are liable to produce permanent discoloration of the teeth.

TETRALOGY OF FALLOT is the most common form of cyanotic congenital heart disease. The tetralogy consists of: (*a*) stenosis of the pulmonary valve; (*b*) a defect in the septum separating the two ventricles; (*c*) the aorta overrides both ventricles; (*d*) marked hypertrophy of the right ventricle.

THALAMUS is one of two masses of grey matter lying on either side of the third ventricle of the brain. It is an important relay and co-ordinating station for sensory impulses such as those for sight. (Plural: Thalami.)

THALASSAEMIA, also known as Cooley's anaemia, is a condition characterized by severe anaemia, due to the individual's having an abnormal form of haemoglobin in his blood. It is a genetically inherited disease which is widely spread across the Mediterranean through the Middle East and into the Far East. It has a particularly high incidence in Greece and in Italy.

THALIDOMIDE: A sedative and hypnotic drug now withdrawn from the market because it causes teratogenesis (q.v.). If taken during the first trimester of pregnancy it may cause an unusual limb deformity in the fetus known as phocomelia ('seal' of 'flipper' extremities).

THALLIUM: An element that is toxic to nerve and liver tissues. The radio-isotope thallium-201 is used as a tracer during special imaging studies of blood flow through the heart muscle in the diagnosis of myocardial ischaemia.

THECA: A sheathlike structure enclosing an organ or part.

THENAR EMINENCE is the projecting mass at the base of the thumb: what is popularly known as the ball of the thumb.

THEOPHYLLINE is an alkaloid similar to theobromine and occurs in small amounts in tea. It is a diuretic, usually administered in the form of theophylline and sodium acetate or of theophylline with ethylenediamine (aminophylline).

THERAPEUTICS is the general name applied to the science and art of healing.

THERAPY means the treatment of disease.

THERIAC means an antidote or substance given to neutralize poison. The name was specially given to Venice treacle, a celebrated mixture of 64 drugs prescribed in olden times as an antidote for poisons and a preventive of disease.

THERMO- is a prefix implying some relation to heat.

THERMOGRAPHY is a method of detecting cancer of the breast. It is based on the fact that abnormally hot areas of skin occur in an area of cancer. The process records such changes in temperature in a record known as a thermogram. Unfortunately, such hot areas of skin are caused by a number of other conditions. It is therefore a diagnostic method that can be used only as a rough screening procedure, but to this extent it is proving of some value in the early detection of cancer of the breast.

THERMOMETER SCALES (see TEMPERATURE).

THERMOPHORE is the name applied to a box or rubber bag filled with a mixture of glue, acetate of soda, chloride of soda, and sulphate of calcium. When it is placed in hot water for some time it has the property of retaining its heat for several hours and is used as a warm application.

THIABENDAZOLE is a drug that is proving of value in the treatment of various parasitic infections, including those due to guinea-worm and certain nematodes, as well as strongyloidiasis (q.v.).

THIAMINE is the *British Pharmacopoeia* name for vitamin B₁. Also known as ANEURINE, it is found in the husks of cereal grains. Its deficiency may be produced by too careful milling of rice in the East, or by a diet of white bread to the exclusion of brown bread and other cereal sources of this vitamin. The resulting disease is a form of neuritis with muscular weakness and heart failure, common in Japan and other parts of the East and known as beriberi (q.v.). Vitamin B₁ has been isolated in crystalline form, and a minute dose of this rapidly cures the symptoms of beriberi. The best sources of this vitamin are wholemeal flour, bacon, liver, egg-yolk, yeast and the pulses. The daily requirement is dependent, among other things, upon the total food intake, and has been estimated to be in the region of 0·5 mg of thiamine per 1000 Calories, increased during pregnancy to 2 mg daily as a minimum.

THIAZIDES (see BENZOTHIADIAZINES).

THIERSCH'S GRAFT is the term given to a method of skin-grafting in which strips of skin are shaved from a normal area and placed on the abnormal area to be grafted. (See SKIN-GRAFTING.)

THIGH is the portion of the lower limb above the knee. The thigh is supported by the femur or thigh-bone, the longest and strongest bone in the body. This fits by a rounded head at its upper end into the acetabulum, a hollow at the side of the pelvis, and at the lower end two large rounded condyles or knuckles rest upon the head of the tibia, and, along with the patella, or knee-cap, form the knee-joint. A large four-headed muscle, the quadriceps, forms most of the fleshy mass on the front and sides of the thigh and serves to straighten the leg in walking and to maintain the erect posture of the body in standing. At the back of the thigh, lie the hamstring muscles; and on the inner side the adductor muscles, attached above to the pelvis and below to the femur, pull the lower limb inwards. The large femoral vessels emerge from the abdomen in the middle of the groin, the vein lying to the inner side of the artery. These pass downwards with an inclination inwards deeply placed between the muscles, and at the knee they lie behind the joint. The great saphenous vein lies near the surface and can be seen towards the inner side of the thigh passing up to the groin, where it joins the femoral vein. The femoral nerve accompanies the large vessels and controls the muscles on the front and inner side of the thigh; while the sciatic nerve, about the thickness of a lead pencil, lies close to the back of the femur and supplies the muscles at the back of the thigh and muscles below the knee.

Deep wounds on the inner side of the thigh are dangerous by reason of the risk of damage to the large vessels. Pain in the back of the thigh is often due to inflammation of the sciatic nerve. (See SCIATICA.) The veins on the inner side of the thigh are specially liable to become dilated. (See VEINS, DISEASES OF.)

THIOPENTONE SODIUM is the *British Pharmacopoeia* name for a commonly used intravenous anaesthetic. Its main use is for inducing anaesthesia, which it does rapidly and painlessly.

THIORIDAZINE is a tranquillizer that is a useful anti-psychotic drug. (See NEUROLEPTICS.)

THIOTEPA is one of the alkylating agents that is proving of value in the treatment of certain forms of malignant disease, including cancer of the breast and ovary. (See CYTOTOXIC.)

THIOURACIL has the property of interfering with the synthesis of thyroxine in the thyroid gland. It was therefore introduced, with success, for the treatment of thyrotoxicosis, and is now widely used for this purpose, as the propyl salt. Thiouracil is used in one of two ways: (*a*) to control thyrotoxicosis, and for this purpose it usually needs to be taken for long periods; (*b*) as a preoperative measure in patients undergoing thyroid surgery.

THIRST, like appetite, is an instinctive craving for something necessary to the continuance of bodily activity. The sensation of thirst is generally referred to the back of the throat, because, when there is a deficiency of water in the system, the throat and mouth especially become parched by evaporation of moisture from their surface. The mere swallowing of water, however, is not sufficient to abolish thirst, as appears in cases where a fistulous opening into the gullet exists, through which the water escapes. Thirst is increased by heat, and is a constant symptom of fever; it is also present in diseases which remove a considerable amount of fluid from the system, such as diarrhoea, diabetes mellitus, and after great loss of blood by haemorrhage. A desire for water is also a feature of many conditions associated with great exhaustion.

THORACIC DUCT is the large lymph-vessel which collects the contents of the lymphatics proceeding from the lower limbs, the abdomen, the left arm, and left side of the chest, neck, and head. It is about the size of a goose quill, is provided with numerous valves, and opens into the veins at the left side of the neck. (See GLANDS; LYMPHATICS.)

THORACOCENTESIS means the withdrawal of fluid from the pleural cavity. (See ASPIRATION.)

THORACOPLASTY is the operation of removing a varying number of ribs so that the underlying lung collapses.

THORAX is another name for the chest.

THREADWORM (see ENTEROBIASIS).

THRESHOLD: The degree of stimulation, or electrical depolarization, necessary to produce an action potential in a nerve fibre (see NERVES). Stimulation below this level elicits no conducted impulse and supramaximal stimulation will elicit the same response as a threshold stimulus (see NERVES).

THRILL is a tremor or vibration felt on applying the hand to the surface of the body. It is felt particularly over the region of the heart in conditions in which the valve openings are narrowed or an aneurysm is present.

THROAT is, in popular language, a vague term applied indifferently to the region in front of the neck, to the larynx or organ of voice, and to the cavity at the back of the mouth. The last-mentioned use of the word, to denote the pharynx or cavity into which the nose, mouth, gullet, and larynx all open, is the correct one. (See PHARYNX. Information will also be found under LARYNX; NECK; TONSILS; NOSE.)

THROMBIN (see COAGULATION).

THROMBOANGIITIS OBLITERANS, also known as BUERGER'S DISEASE after the American surgeon who gave the first co-ordinated description of it in 1908, is an inflammatory disease involving the blood-vessels of the limbs, particularly the lower limbs. The cause is not known, but the use of tobacco is an important factor. It is almost entirely confined to men, and is more common in Jews than in Gentiles. Pain is the outstanding symptom, accompanied by pallor of the affected part. Sooner or later ulceration and gangrene tend to develop in the feet or hands. There is no specific treatment, but, if seen in the early stages, considerable relief may be given to the patient.

THROMBOCYTE (see PLATELETS).

THROMBOCYTOPENIA: A disorder in which the number of platelets (q.v.) in the blood is reduced. This predisposes to bruising and bleeding. It may be idiopathic (q.v.) but is also caused by malignant diseases (q.v.) (particularly haematilogical) and drugs. (See PLATELETS.)

THROMBOEMBOLISM: The formation of a thrombus (blood clot) in one part of the circulatory system from which a portion becomes detached and lodges in another blood vessel partially or completely obstructing the blood flow (an embolsim). Most commonly a thromous is formed in the veins of the leg and the embolism lodges in the pulmonary (lung) circulation.

THROMBOLYSIS: The breakdown of a blood clot by enzymic activity. Naturally occurring enzymes (q.v.) limit the enlargement of clots, and drugs – e.g. streptokinase – may be given to 'dissolve' clots – e.g., following a coronary thrombosis (q.v.).

THROMBOPHLEBITIS is the condition characterized by inflammation of the veins combined with clot formation. (See VEINS, DISEASES OF.)

THROMBOSIS means the formation of a blood-clot within the vessels or heart during life. The process of clotting within the body depends upon the same factors as in clotting of blood outside the body, involving the fibrinogen and lime salts circulating in the blood, as well as blood platelets. The indirect cause of thrombosis is usually some damage to the smooth lining of the blood-vessels brought about by inflammation, or the result of atheroma, a chronic disease of the vessel walls. The blood is also specially prone to clot in certain general conditions such as anaemia, the ill health of wasting diseases like cancer, and in consequence of the feeble circulation of old age.

Thrombosis may occur in the heart and terminate some chronic wasting disease; it often takes place in the vessels of the brain and thus causes stroke in people whose arteries are much diseased.

Thrombosis of a coronary artery of the heart is a very serious condition which affects, as a rule, middle-aged or elderly people. (See also ARTERIES, DISEASES OF; CLOT; COAGULATION; CORONARY THROMBOSIS; STROKE.)

THROMBOXANE is a substance produced in the blood platelets (see PLATELETS) which induces aggregation of platelets and thereby thrombosis (q.v.). It is also a vasoconstrictor (q.v.).

THROMBUS: A clot of blood. Usually describing the formation of a clot within a vessel obstructing the flow of blood, but it can also describe blood which has escaped from a damaged vessel and clotted in the surrounding tissue.

THRUSH is a type of inflammation affecting particularly the mouth of weakly children and causing a patchy white appearance on the lips, tongue, or palate. It is caused by the growth of a fungus on the surface of the mucous membrane. (See MOUTH, DISEASES OF.)

THUMB-SUCKING, or FINGER-SUCKING, is a universal and harmless habit in infancy. It is usually gradually given up during the preschool period, but quite often persists after school age especially if the child is tired, lonely or unhappy. In these cases the remedy is to deal with the cause. Threats should not be used to try to stop the habit.

THYMUS GLAND: The thymus gland was given its name by Galen in the second century AD because of its resemblance to a bunch of thyme flowers. It has two lobes and lies in the upper part of the chest. Each lobe is made up of a number of lobules divided into an outer portion, or cortex, and a central portion, or medulla. The cortex resembles lymphoid tissue and is made up of masses of small round cells called thymocytes. It is an area of intense lymphopoiesis and the rate of production of new cells is five times greater than that in lymph nodes and other lymphoid tissues. The medulla is more loosely cellular and consists of a stroma which contains far fewer lymphocytes than in the cortex but also contains epithelial cells and Hassall's corpuscles.

The thymus gland is now established as a vital part of the immunological system. Until 1960 the function of the thymus was completely unknown. Stem cells from the bone marrow come to the thymus where they develop into immunologically competent cells. They are then seeded out to the rest of the lymphoid tissue. There are two distinct populations of lymphocytes. One is dependent on the presence of the thymus (T lymphocytes) and the other is independent of the thymus (B lymphocytes). Both are concerned with immune responses. They differ in their distribution and in their life span. The thymus-dependent lymphocyte is a cell which in the absence of antigenic stimulation circulates through the blood, lymph nodes and back into the circulation again over a period of more than 10 years. It performs a policing role, awaiting recognition of foreign material which it is able to identify as such. It reacts by multiplication and transformation and these are the ingredients of the immune response. B lymphocytes are produced in the bone marrow and are concerned with the production of the circulating humoral antibodies.

The most common clinical disorder associated with abnormality of the thymus is myasthenia gravis (q.v.). Ten per cent of patients with myasthenia gravis will have a tumour of the thymus whilst the remainder will have inflammatory changes in the thymus called thymitis.

THYROID CARTILAGE is the largest cartilage in the larynx and forms the prominence of the Adam's apple in front of the neck. (See LARYNX.)

THYROID GLAND is a highly vascular organ situated in front of the neck. It consists of a narrow isthmus crossing the windpipe close to its upper end, and joining together two lateral lobes which run upwards, one on each side of the larynx. The gland is therefore shaped somewhat like a horseshoe, each lateral lobe being about 5 cm (2 inches) long and the isthmus about 12 mm (½ inch) wide, and it is firmly bound to the larynx. The weight of the thyroid gland is about 28·5 grams (1 ounce), but it is larger in females than in males, undergoes in many women a periodic increase at each time of menstruation, and often reaches an enormous size in the condition known as goitre (q.v.).

Minute structure: The gland is enveloped in a layer of fibrous tissue and possesses a rich blood supply. It is composed of multitudes of closed vesicles, each formed by a layer of cubical cells and containing a thick yellow fluid (colloid). Round the vesicles there is a dense network of capillary blood-vessels, whilst the finest lymphatic vessels communicate with the interior of these vesicles.

Function: The chief function of the thyroid gland is to produce a hormone rich in iodine. The main active ingredient of this hormone is thyroxine, and its probable mode of manufacture is:

This hormone, or secretion, which passes directly from the thyroid into the blood-stream, is de-iodinated in the body cells to triiodothyronine which exerts the physiological action of the thyroid hormone. The hormone is one of the most important in the body and controls the rate of metabolism. Thus, if it is deficient in children they fail to grow, a condition known as CRETINISM (q.v.). If the deficiency develops in adult life, the individual becomes obese, lethargic, and develops a coarse skin, a condition known as MYXOEDEMA (q.v.). Over-action of the thyroid, or HYPER-THYROIDISM, results in loss of weight, rapid heart action, and a highly strung nervous temperament.

The production of the thyroid hormone is controlled by a hormone of the pituitary gland – the thyrotrophic hormone.

THYROID GLAND, DISEASES OF (see CRETINISM; GOITRE; GRAVES' DISEASE; MYXOEDEMA).

THYROTOXIC ADENOMA is a variety of thyrotoxicosis in which one of the nodules of a multinodular goitre becomes autonomous and secretes excess thyroid hormone. The symptoms that result are similar to those of Graves' disease (q.v.), but there are minor differences. The first difference is that these autonomous adenomas tend to occur in long-standing nodular goitres so that the patients are older than those with Graves' disease. The symptoms of hyperthyroidism therefore tend to be more cardio-vascular, such as atrial fibrillation and heart failure. Exophthalmos and pre-tibial myxoedema do not occur as these are auto-immune manifestations of Graves' disease and toxic adenomas do not have an auto-immune basis.

Treatment: The first line of treatment is to render the patient euthyroid by treatment with antithyroid drugs. Then the nodule should be removed surgically or annihilated by radioactive iodine treatment.

THYROTOXICOSIS (see GRAVES' DISEASE).

THYROTROPHIN-RELEASING HORMONE: A hormone produced and released by the hypothalamus (q.v.) which stimulates the release of thyrotrophin-stimulating hormone (q.v.) by the pituitary gland (q.v.).

THYROTROPHIN-STIMULATING HORMONE (TSH): A hormone manufactured and released by the anterior part of the pituitary gland (q.v.) which stimulates the thyroid gland (q.v.) to manufacture and release thyroid hormones (thyroxine and tri-iodothyronine, qq.v.).

THYROXINE is a crystalline substance, containing iodine, isolated from the thyroid gland and possessing the properties of thyroid extract. It has also been synthesized. It is used in cases of defective function of the thyroid, such as cretinism, and myxoedema.

TIAPROFENIC ACID (see NON-STEROIDAL ANTI-INFLAMMATORY DRUGS).

TIBIA is the larger of the two bones in the leg. One surface of the tibia lies immediately beneath the skin in front and towards the inner side of the leg, forming the shin. Fractures of this bone are accordingly very liable to wound the skin and become compound. The thigh-bone rests upon the larger upper end of the tibia at the knee-joint, whilst below, the tibia and fibula together enter into the ankle-joint, the two bosses or malleoli at the ankle belonging, the inner to the tibia, the outer to the fibula.

TIC is the term applied to the habit spasm which forms a personal peculiarity in neurotic subjects. (See CRAMP.)

TICARCILLIN (see ANTIBIOTIC).

TIC DOULOUREUX is another name for facial, or trigeminal, neuralgia due to some affection of the fifth cranial nerve, and characterized by pain, situated somewhere about the temple, forehead, face, or jaw, and sometimes by spasm in the muscles of the affected region. (See TRIGEMINAL NEURALGIA.)

TICK is the general name given to a group of arachnid insects, some of which act as transmitters of diseases.

Ticks are blood-sucking arthropods which are responsible for transmitting a wide range of diseases to man, including Rocky Mountain spotted fever. African tick typhus and fièvre boutonneuse (see TYPHUS FEVER). Apart from being transmitters of disease, they cause intense itching and may cause quite severe lesions of the skin. The best repellents are dimethyl phthalate and diethyltoluamide. Once bitten, relief from the itching is obtained from the application of calamine lotion. Tick-bites are an occupational hazard of shepherds and game-keepers. (See BITES AND STINGS.)

TIMOLOL MALEATE is a beta-adrenoceptor-blocking drug which is proving of value in the treatment of angina pectoris, myocardial infarction, and hypertension. It is also used in the treatment of glaucoma. (See ADRENERGIC RECEPTORS.)

TINCTURE is an alcoholic solution, generally of some vegetable substance.

TINEA is the technical name for ringworm. (See RINGWORM.)

TINNITUS means a noise heard in the ear without any external cause. It is a frequent accompaniment of deafness.

Tinnitus is common, affecting about one in six adults at some time in their life. Only one-third of these consult a doctor and in less than one per cent does the tinnitus interfere with leading a normal life. The cause is damage to the auditory pathway and the most common part of the pathway to be damaged is the cochlea. It may be the result of drugs, particularly aspirin, chloroquine and quinine. Investigation is necessary to exclude any underlying cause but in most cases no cause can be found, and the management depends on relieving the effects of tinnitus on the patient because it is not usually possible to abolish the tinnitus altogether. Drugs such as carbamazepine, tocainide amide and mexiletine may help. The use of tinnitus maskers and hearing aids can suppress tinnitus by masking it with other sounds which the patient learns to listen to. Hearing aids suppress tinnitus by amplifying background noise.

Under the auspices of the Royal National Institute for the Deaf, the RNID Tinnitus Helpline has been established on 0345-090210. The service is open Monday to Friday, 10 a.m. to 3 p.m. Calls are charged at local rates. (See DEAFNESS; EAR, DISEASES OF; MENIÈRE'S DISEASE.)

TISSUES OF THE BODY are the simple elements from which the various parts and organs are found to be built. All the body originates from the union of a pair of cells but as growth proceeds the new cells produced from these form tissues of varying character and complexity. (See CELL.) It is customary to divide the tissues into five groups:

(1) Epithelial tissues, including the cells covering the skin, those lining the alimentary canal, those forming the secretions of internal organs. (See EPITHELIUM.)

(2) Connective tissues, including fibrous tissue, fat, bone, cartilage. (See these headings.)

(3) Muscular tissues (see MUSCLE).

(4) Nervous tissues (see NERVES).

(5) Wandering corpuscles of the blood and lymph (see BLOOD: LYMPH).

Many of the organs are formed of a single one of these tissues or of one with a very slight admixture of another, such as cartilage, or white fibrous tissue. Other parts of the body that are widely distributed are very simple in structure and consist of two or more simple tissues in varying proportion. Such are blood-vessels (see ARTERIES; VEINS), lymphatic vessels (see LYMPHATICS), lymphatic glands (see GLANDS), serous membranes (see SEROUS MEMBRANES), synovial membranes (see JOINTS), mucous membranes (see MUCOUS MEMBRANE), secreting glands (see GLANDS; SALIVARY GLANDS; THYROID GLAND) and skin (see SKIN).

The structure of the more complex organs of the body is dealt with under the heading of each organ.

TITRATION is a form of chemical analysis by means of standard solutions of known strength.

TITRE: The strength of a solution as determined by titration (q.v.). In medicine it is used to describe the amount of antibody (q.v.) present in a known volume of serum (q.v.).

TITUBATION means a staggering or reeling condition, especially due to disease of the spinal cord or cerebellum.

TNM CLASSIFICATION: A method of classifying cancers to determine how far they have spread. This helps doctors to determine the best course of treatment and the prognosis; it is useful in research. Originally defined by the American Joint Committee on Cancer, the T applies to the primary tumour, the N to any lymph node involvement and the M to any metastatic spread.

TOBACCO is the leaf of several species of Nicotiana, especially of the American plant *Nicotiana tabacum.*

The smoking of tobacco is the major public health hazard in Britain today. It causes a hundred thousand premature deaths per year in the United Kingdom alone. In addition to the deaths caused by cigarette smoking, it is also a major cause of disability and illness in the form of myocardial infarction, peripheral vascular disease, chronic obstructive airways disease and emphysema. Action on Smoking and Health (ASH) is a small charity founded by the Royal College of Physicians in 1971 that attempts to alert and inform the public to the dangers of smoking and to try to prevent the disability and death which it causes (see ASH).

Cigarette smoking is the major cause of chronic obstructive lung disease morbidity and 80 to 90 per cent of chronic obstructive lung disease in the United States is attributable to it. In 1982 the United States' Surgeon General stated that cigarette smoking was the major single cause of cancer mortality in the United States. Tobacco's contribution to all cancer deaths is estimated to be 30 per cent. Cigarette smoking is also the most important of the known modifiable risk factors for coronary heart disease.

Composition: In addition to vegetable fibre, tobacco leaves contain a large quantity of ash, the nature of this depending predominantly upon the minerals present in the ground where the tobacco plant has been grown. Of the organic constituents the brown fluid alkaloid known as nicotine is the most important. The nicotine content of different tobaccos varies, and the amount absorbed depends upon whether or not the smoker inhales.

Tobacco smoke also contains some sixteen substances capable of inducing cancer in experimental animals. One of the most important of these is benzpyrene, a strongly carcinogenic hydrocarbon. As this is present in coal-tar pitch, it is commonly referred to in this context as tar. Other constituents of tobacco smoke include pyridine, ammonia and carbon monoxide.

A very small amount of nicotine, such as that derived from a single cigarette, has a stimulating effect upon the mental and bodily powers.

In larger amount, the action is a depressant and narcotic one, which in habitual smokers is modified to a sedative.

The greatest hazard of smoking, however, is the fact that it is the major cause of lung cancer, coronary artery disease, peripheral vascular disease, chronic bronchitis and emphysema. It also has an adverse effect on the fetus when the pregnant mother smokes.

Another set of symptoms frequently arising in those who smoke is irritable cough and soreness of the throat. These symptoms pass off when smoking is discontinued. There is increasing evidence that passive smoking (inhaling smoke from someone else's cigarette) is also harmful. Children whose parents smoke are at increased risk of pneumonia and glue ear. There is growing pressure under health-and-safety-at-work legislation for employers to provide smoke-free working conditions for their staff.

The giving up of the smoking habit is largely a psychological problem, but there is some evidence that the use of nicotine chewing gum facilitates the process.

TOBRAMYCIN is an antibiotic related to gentamicin (q.v.) and with a similar range of activity. It is given by injection.

TOES (see CORNS AND BUNIONS; FOOT; NAILS).

TOLAZOMIDE (see SULPHONYLUREAS).

TOLBUTAMIDE is a sulphonamide derivative, or sulphonylurea, which lowers the level of the blood sugar in diabetes mellitus. As it is

rapidly excreted from the body, it has to be taken twice daily. Like chlorpropamide (q.v.), it may induce undue sensitivity to alcohol. (See also DIABETES MELLITUS, SULPHONYLUREAS.)

TOLERANCE: This occurs when the response to a particular amount of a drug or physiological messenger decreases (i.e. a larger dose must be given to produce the same response as before).

TOLMETIN (see NON-STEROIDAL ANTI-INFLAMMATORY DRUGS).

TOLNAFTATE is a preparation which in the form of a 1-per-cent solution, is proving useful as a local application in the treatment of certain forms of ringworm, particularly ringworm of the foot. It may also be applied as a powder or cream. It is used, too, in the treatment of tinea versicolor (see RINGWORM) and erythrasma (q.v.).

TOLUENE, or METHYLBENZENE, is a product of the distillation of coal tar widely used as a solvent in the manufacture of paint and rubber and plastic cements.

TOMOGRAPHY: A technique using X-rays or ultrasound to build up a focused image of a 'slice' through the body at a given level. By producing a series of such slices at different depths a three-dimensional image of the body structures can be built up (see X-RAYS).

-TOMY is a suffix indicating an operation by cutting.

TONGUE: The tongue is made up of several muscles, is richly supplied with blood-vessels and nerves, and is covered by highly specialized mucous membrane. It consists of a free part known as the tip, a body, and a hinder fixed part or root. The under surface lies upon the floor of the mouth, whilst the upper surface is curved from side to side, and still more from before backwards so as to adapt it to the roof of the mouth. At its root, the tongue is in contact with, and firmly united to, the upper edge of the larynx; so that in some persons who can depress the tongue readily the tip of the epiglottis may be seen projecting upwards at its hinder part.

Structure: The *substance* of the tongue consists almost entirely of muscles running in various directions. One runs along the upper surface and another along the lower surface from root to tip. Other fibres run vertically from the upper to the lower surface, whilst the chief bulk of the tongue is made up of muscle-fibres running from side to side. These various fibres are chiefly concerned in making changes in the shape of the tongue and moving it within the mouth. In addition to these, the tongue has numerous outside attachments; one muscle on

1 gustatory pore   3 sustentacular cell
2 stratified epithelium   4 gustatory cell with hairlet

Section showing taste buds. Magnified by 420.

each side unites it to the lower jaw-bone just behind the chin, and this muscle serves to protrude the tongue from the mouth; other muscles, which retract the tongue, attach it to the hyoid bone, the larynx, the palate, and the styloid process on the base of the skull.

The *mucous membrane* on the under surface of the tongue is very thin, so that the large blood-vessels on each side can easily be seen through it. In the middle line a fold of mucous membrane, the frenum, passes from the under surface to the floor of the mouth, and, when this frenum is attached too far forwards towards the tip of the tongue, the movements of the organ are impeded, and the condition is known as tongue-tie. On the upper surface or dorsum of the tongue the mucous membrane is thicker, and in its front two-thirds is studded with little projections of three kinds. The majority of these projections or *papillae* are of *conical* shape, and when the tongue becomes furred the apppearance is due to an unhealthy collection of epithelium upon them. Some of them end in long filaments, and are then known as *filiform* papillae. The roughness of the tongue in cats and other carnivorous animals is due to large backwardly directed conical papillae, which assist in cleaning the flesh off bones. On the tip, and towards the edges of the tongue, small red rounded *fungiform* papillae are seen, which act in all probability as end-organs for the sense of taste. On a line dividing the front two-thirds from the hinder one-third, and set in the shape of a V, is a row of seven to twelve large flat-topped *circumvallate* papillae, each placed in a corresponding depression and just visible, in most mouths, when the tongue is pressed firmly down with some flat instrument. These also act as end-organs for the nerves of taste. Each circumvallate papilla is surrounded by a trench, and upon both sides of the trench open numerous *taste-buds*. A taste-bud is shaped somewhat like a barrel, with an outer covering of flattened stave-like cells, enclosing a bundle of spindle-shaped cells which end in hairlike processes at the mouth of the bud, and are

connected at their deeply placed end with some filaments from the nerves of taste. These taste-buds are also found in the fungiform papillae, though in smaller numbers, and they are scattered over the throat, fauces, and palate; so that the popular expression 'a fine palate', as applied to the sense of taste, is quite correct.

No fewer than five *nerves* supply branches to each side of the tongue. These are the *lingual* branch of the 5th nerve, which is the nerve of ordinary sensation, to the front two-thirds of the tongue; the *chorda tympani* branch from the 7th nerve, which is supposed to be the nerve of taste, for a similar extent; the *glossopharyngeal* or 9th nerve, which conveys sensations both of touch and taste from the hinder third: the *superior laryngeal* branch of the 10th nerve, also sensory; and the *hypoglossal* or 12th nerve, which supplies the muscles of the tongue.

Functions: The chief uses of the tongue are of three kinds: (*a*) to push the food between the teeth for mastication, and then mould it into a bolus preparatory to swallowing; (*b*) as the organ of the sense of taste, and as an organ provided with a delicate sense of touch; and (*c*) to play a part in the production of speech. (See VOICE AND SPEECH.)

It is usual to classify any taste as:

1. Sweet   3. Bitter
2. Salt   4. Acid

since finer distinctions are largely dependent upon the sense of smell. The loss of keenness in taste brought about by a cold in the head, or even by holding the nose while swallowing, is well known. Sweet tastes seem to be best appreciated by the tip of the tongue, acids on its edges, and bitters at the back. It is possible, too, by chewing the leaves of an Indian plant, *Gymnaema sylvesive*, to do away with the power of tasting bitter and sweet substances, while the sensation for acids and salts remains, so that in all probability there are different nerve-fibres and end-organs for the different varieties of taste. Many tastes depend upon the ordinary sensations of the tongue, such as the constringent taste of tannin and the metallic taste of a weak galvanic current passed through the tongue. The sense of taste may be affected by certain drugs. Thus, penicillamine (q.v.) may reduce the sense of taste for sweet and salt, levodopa (q.v.) may induce a metallic or garlic-like taste, lithium (q.v.) may be accompanied by a rather vague unpleasant taste, captopril (q.v.) by a loss of the sense of taste, whilst metformin (q.v.) may cause a metallic taste.

Like other sensations, taste can be very highly educated for a time, as in tea-tasters and wine-tasters, but this special adaptation is lost after some years.

TONGUE, DISEASES OF (see MOUTH, DISEASES OF).

TONGUE, FURRING OF (see MOUTH, DISEASES OF).

TONICS are 'substances traditionally thought to give strength and vigour to the body, without producing sudden excitement or subsequent depression'. They are rarely prescribed nowadays.

TONSILLITIS is the inflammation of the tonsils.

ACUTE TONSILLITIS: It must never be forgotten that the infection is never entirely confined to the tonsils; there is always some involvement of the surrounding throat or pharynx. The converse is true in that many cases of 'sore throat' the tonsils are involved in the generalized inflammation of the throat.

Causes: The most common cause is the β-haemolytic streptococcus. Like most upper-respiratory-tract infections its highest incidence is in the winter months. It used to be an important precursor of rheumatic fever but early diagnosis and treatment have fortunately reduced the incidence of this disease in developed countries. Care should be taken to prevent the spread of infection in hospitals or institutions. Acute tonsillitis may also occur in infectious mononucleosis or glandular fever and, rarely, it may be the presenting feature of diphtheria. This disease is fortunately now extremely rare.

Symptoms: The onset is usually fairly sudden with pain on swallowing, fever and malaise. On examination, the tonsils are found to be enlarged, engorged and often covered with a varying amount of whitish or grey material. This material or exudate consists of purulent discharge from the tonsil. It may occur at scattered areas over the crypts of the tonsil when the condition is known as follicular tonsillitis, or it may be more extensive exudate covering practically the whole of the tonsil. This form of exudate occurs in simple streptococcal tonsillitis but may also occur in infectious mononucleosis (glandular fever). It is also a feature of diphtheria, although this condition is now extremely rare. The glands underneath the angle of the jaw are enlarged and tender. There may be pain in the ear on the affected side and, although this is usually referred pain, it may indicate spread up the Eustachian tube to the ear on that side. This is particularly so in children.

Occasionally an abscess develops around the affected tonsil, a peritonsillar abscess or quinsy. This abscess is formed by the collection of pus between the tonsil and the superior constrictor muscle of the pharynx. It usually comes on four to five days after the onset of tonsillitis and requires specialist treatment

Treatment: The drug of choice is still penicillin or erythromycin in penicillin-sensitive patients. Fluids should be encouraged and analgesia and antipyretic medication should also be prescribed.

In the past tonsillitis was often a precursor of rheumatic fever or of acute glomerular nephritis but this has fortunately become much less common, due to early recognition of tonsillitis and prompt treatment with the appropriate antibiotics. Improved socio-economic conditions have probably also contributed to the decreased incidence of these complications in developed countries.

Removal of tonsils is indicated: (*a*) when the tonsils and adenoids are permanently so enlarged as to interfere with breathing; in such cases the adenoids are removed as well as the tonsils; (*b*) when the individual is subject to recurrent attacks of acute tonsillitis which are causing significant debility, absence from school or work on a regular basis; (*c*) when there is evidence of a tumour of the tonsil.

TONSILS are two almond-shaped glands situated one on each side of the narrow fauces where the mouth joins the throat. Each has a structure resembling that of a lymphatic gland, and consists of an elevation of the mucous membrane presenting twelve to fifteen openings, which lead into pits or lacunae. The mucous covering is formed by the ordinary mucous membrane of the mouth, which also lines the pits; and the main substance of the gland is composed of loose connective tissue containing lymph corpuscles in its meshes, and packed here and there into denser nodules or follicles. The tonsils play an important rôle in the protective mechanism of the body against infection.

TOOTH, SUPERNUMERARY: Malformed extra teeth are frequently found, particularly in the upper incisor region. They often do not erupt but prevent the eruption of the permanent teeth.

TOOTHACHE (see TEETH, DISEASES OF).

TOPHUS is the name given to the concretions which form in connection with joints or tendon sheaths as the result of attacks of gout. At first the tophus is a soft mass, but later becomes quite hard. It is composed of biurate of soda. (See CONCRETIONS; GOUT.)

TOPICAL: Pertaining to drugs or other treatment applied locally to the area being treated – e.g. the skin, eye, etc.

TORPOR is a condition of bodily and mental inactivity, not amounting to sleep, but interfering greatly with the ordinary habits and pursuits. It is often found in people suffering from fever, and is a common symptom in aged people whose arteries are diseased. It may annoy young people after meals when they are the subjects of constipation or of dyspepsia, due to eating too much indigestible food.

TORSION means twisting. The term is applied to the process in which organs, or tumours, which are attached to the rest of the body by a narrow neck or pedicle, become twisted so as to narrow the blood-vessels or other structures in the pedicle. (See TESTICLES, DISEASES OF.)

Torsion is also the term applied to the twisting of the small arteries severed at an operation, by which bleeding from them is stopped.

TORTICOLLIS: This is shortness of the sternomastoid muscle on one side resulting in asymetry and limitation of movement of the neck. (See CRAMP; SPASMODIC TORTICOLLIS; WRY-NECK.)

TOUCH, according to the popular idea, is the fifth sense diffused all over the body, by which we become conscious of our surroundings otherwise than by the four special senses of hearing, seeing, tasting and smelling. But when this diffused sensitiveness is examined it is found to consist of a group of senses, several of which have special end-organs situated in the skin, muscles and elsewhere and special nerve-paths to convey their impressions to the brain. It is convenient, however, to adopt the popular view, and to consider all these under one heading. The cutaneous sense, then, is made up of the following:

Touch sense proper, by which we perceive a touch or stroke and estimate the size and shape of bodies with which we come in contact, but which we do not see.
Pressure sense, by which we judge the heaviness of weights laid upon the skin, or appreciate the hardness of objects by pressing against them.
Heat sense, by which we perceive that a body is warmer than the skin.
Cold sense, by which we perceive that a body touching the skin is cold.
Pain sense, by which we appreciate pricks, pinches and other painful impressions.

To these we may for convenience add:

Muscular sensitiveness, by which the painfulness of a squeeze is perceived. It is produced probably by direct pressure upon the nerve-fibres in the muscles.

Muscular sense, by which we test the weight of an object held in the hand, or gauge the amount of energy expended on an effort.
Sense of locality, by which we can, without looking, tell the position and attitude of any part of the body.
Common sensation, which is a vague term used to mean composite sensations produced by several of the foregoing, like tickling, or creeping, and the vague sense of well-being or the reverse that the mind receives from internal organs. (See the article on PAIN.)

The structure of the end-organs situated in the skin, which receive impressions from the outer world, and of the nerve-fibres which conduct these impressions to the central nervous system, have been described under NERVES.

Touch affects the Meissner's or touch corpuscles placed beneath the epidermis; as these differ in closeness in different parts of the skin, the delicacy of the sense of touch varies greatly. Thus the points of a pair of compasses can be felt as two on the tip of the tongue when separated by only 1 mm; on the tips of the fingers they must be separated to twice that distance, whilst on the arm or leg they cannot be felt as two points unless separated by over 25 mm, and on the back they must be separated by over 50 mm. On the parts covered by hair, the nerves ending round the roots of the hairs also take up impressions of touch.

Pressure is estimated probably through the same nerve-endings and nerves that have to do with touch, but it depends upon a difference in the sensations of parts pressed on and those of surrounding parts. Heat-sense, cold-sense and pain-sense all depend upon different nerve-endings in the skin; and thus, with care and delicate instruments like needles, bristles in holders and metal pencils through which hot or cold water can be made to circulate, the skin may be mapped out into a mosaic of little areas where the different kinds of impressions are registered. Whilst the tongue and finger-tips are the parts most sensitive to touch, they are comparatively insensitive to heat, and can easily bear temperatures which the cheek or elbow could not tolerate. The muscular sense, in all probability, depends on the sensory organs known as muscle-spindles, which are scattered through the substance of the muscles, and the sense of locality is dependent partly upon these and partly upon the nerves which end in tendons, ligaments and joints.

Disorders of the sense of touch occur in various diseases.

HYPERAESTHESIA is a condition in which there is excessive sensitiveness to any stimulus, such as touch. When this reaches the stage when a mere touch or gentle handling causes acute pain it is known as HYPERALGESIA. It is found in various diseases of the spinal cord immediately above the level of the disease, combined often with loss of sensation below the diseased part. It is also present in neuralgia, the skin of the neuralgic area becoming excessively tender to touch, heat or cold. Heightened sensibility to pain is seen sometimes in drunkards, who wince at a mere touch when not under the influence of alcohol. Heightened sensibility to temperature is a common symptom of neuritis. (See PAIN.)

ANAESTHESIA, or diminution of the sense of touch, causing often a feeling of numbness, is present in many diseases affecting the nerves of sensation or their continuations up the posterior part of the spinal cord. The condition of *dissociated analgesia*, in which a touch is quite well felt, though there is complete insensibility to pain, is present in the disease of the spinal cord known as syringomyelia, and affords a proof that the nerve-fibres for pain and those for touch are quite separate. In tabes dorsalis there is sometimes loss of the sense of touch on feet or arms; but in other cases of this disease there is no loss of the sense of touch, although there is a complete loss of the sense of locality in the lower limbs, thus proving that these two senses are quite distinct.

PARAESTHESIAE are peculiar forms of perverted sensation such as creeping, tingling, pricking or hot flushes.

TOURNIQUET is an instrument used for the temporary stoppage of the circulation in a limb, to control bleeding. There are various forms of tourniquet, the simplest being a tourniquet improvised from a band such as that made by a handkerchief folded cravat- wise, tied round the limb, and then twisted up by means of a rigid object passed beneath it. *Petit's tourniquet* has a linen strap passing over two pairs of brass rollers, which can be separated from one another by a screw, thus tightening the strap after it has been buckled round the limb. *Esmarch's tourniquet* consists of an elastic band which is wrapped with moderate tightness round the limb, and then prevented from unwrapping by tapes. It is the form generally used. (See HAEMORRHAGE.) A rubber tube knotted, or fixed with a clip, round the limb is also often used for

Two simple forms of tourniquet.

arresting the blood-flow. In applying a tourniquet for bleeding, it must be rendered sufficiently tight to stop the circulation completely. Otherwise if the veins only are compressed and the arteries still open, the bleeding is made worse. A tourniquet must not be left in position longer than is absolutely necessary; otherwise gangrene of the limb may result. It must be loosened cautiously after not more than 15 minutes. If bleeding has not stopped it is tightened again. This procedure must be repeated every 15 minutes.

TOW is a form of jute which is very hygroscopic, absorbing up to 25 per cent of moisture.

TOXAEMIA is a term applied to forms of blood-poisoning due to the absorption of bacterial products (toxins) formed at some local site of infection, such as abscesses. In other cases the toxaemia is due to defective action of some excretory organ, such as the kidney. As regards treatment, the most important consideration is to remove the source of infection.

Toxaemia of pregnancy is a term sometimes used to describe the two complications of pregnancy known as pre-eclampsia and eclampsia (q.v.).

TOXIC SHOCK SYNDROME is a syndrome, first described in 1978, characterized by high fever, diarrhoea, shock and an erythematous rash. It is frequently associated with the use of tampons, but has occasionally been reported in men. The disease is due to a staphylococcal toxin. The treatment consists of supportive measures to combat shock and eradication of the staphylococcus by antibiotics. A mortality rate of 10 per cent has been reported. The syndrome may recur.

TOXICOLOGY is the science dealing with poisons. (See POISONS.)

TOXINS are poisons produced by bacteria. (See IMMUNITY; IMMUNOLOGY; MICROBIOLOGY.) Toxins are usually soluble, easily destroyed by heat, sometimes of the nature of crystalline substances, and sometimes albumins. When injected into animals in carefully graduated doses, they bring about the formation of substances called antitoxins which neutralize the action of the toxin. These antitoxins are generally produced in excessive amount, and the serum of the animal when withdrawn can be used for conferring antitoxic powers upon other animals or human beings to neutralize the disease in question. The best known of these antitoxins are those of diphtheria and tetanus. Toxins are also found in many plants and in snake venom.

Some toxins are not set free by bacteria, but remain in the substance of the latter. They are known as endotoxins and are not capable of producing antitoxins.

TOXOCARIASIS is a disease acquired by swallowing the ova of a roundworm which lives in the intestine of cats (*Toxocara cati*) or dogs (*Toxocara canis*). In man, the small larval worms produced by these ova migrate to various parts of the body, including the retina of the eye, where they then die, and produce a small granuloma (q.v.) which in turn may produce allergic reactions. In the eye it may cause choroidretinitis. It is said that 2 per cent of apparently healthy people in Britain have been infected in this way. A course of treatment with diethylcarbamazine is said to kill the worm.

TOXOID is toxin (q.v.) which has been rendered non-toxic by certain chemicals, or by heat, or by being partly neutralized by antitoxin. The best-known example is diphtheria toxoid. (See IMMUNITY.)

TOXOPLASMOSIS is a disease which is due to infection with protozoa of the genus *Toxoplasma*. The infection may be acquired from eating raw or undercooked meat, from cats, or from gardening or playing in contaminated soil. It occurs in two forms: an acquired form and a congenital form. The acquired form may run such a benign course that it is not recognized, the patient scarcely feeling ill. In the congenital form the unborn child is infected by the mother. The congenital form, the incidence of which in the United Kingdom is 1 in 5000 pregnancies (1 in 2000 pregnancies in Scotland), may develop in one of two ways. The infant may either appear generally ill, or the brunt of the infection may fall on the nervous system causing hydrocephalus (q.v.), mental retardation, or loss of sight. In some cases the infection may be so severe that it kills the fetus, resulting in a miscarriage or stillbirth. In other cases the infection is so mild that it is missed until in later life the child begins to show signs of eye trouble. As the congenital form of the disease, which is most serious, seems to develop only if the mother acquires the infection during pregnancy, it would appear to be a wise precaution that pregnant women should avoid contact with cats and eating raw or undercooked meat foods.

TOY LIBRARIES: The National Toy Libraries Association, founded ten years ago to help handicapped children get suitable toys, now has links with over 500 toy libraries throughout the country. These libraries keep a wide range of toys that can either be played with at the Library or taken home. The range includes trucks for children to ride on, toys for babies, and others with an educational element. They also provide a convenient place for parents and child minders to meet, share common problems and seek advice if they want to. Further details can be obtained from: Play Matters National Toy Libraries Associations, 68 Churchway, London NW1 1LT (071-387 9592).

TRACE ELEMENTS are chemical elements that are distributed throughout the tissues of the body in very small amounts and are essential for the nutrition of the body. Nine such elements are now recognized: cobalt, copper, fluorine, iodine, iron, manganese, molybdenum, selenium and zinc.

TRACHEA is another name for the windpipe (q.v.). (See also AIR PASSAGES.)

TRACHEITIS means inflammation of the trachea. It may occur along with bronchitis, or independently, due to similar causes.

TRACHEOSTOMY, or TRACHEOTOMY, is the operation in which the windpipe is opened from the front of the neck, so that air may obtain direct entrance into the lower air passages. The opening is made through the second and third rings of the trachea (windpipe) (q.v.).
Reasons for operation: Conditions in which the opening of the larynx is narrowed are treated by the appropriate means but, should these fail, some form of airway intervention is necessary. In the majority of cases this would involve the insertion of an endotracheal tube, i.e. a tube is inserted either through the nose or mouth and down the pharynx through the larynx to bypass the obstruction, or by a tracheostomy. The majority of tracheostomies performed nowadays are for patients in intensive-therapy-unit situations. These patients require airway intervention for prolonged periods to facilitate artificial ventilation which is performed by means of a mechanical ventilator. The presence of a tube passing through the larynx for a prolonged period of time is associated with long-term damage to the larynx, and therefore any patients requiring prolonged intubation usually undergo a tracheostomy to prevent further damage to the larynx. Endotracheal intubation is also the preferred method of airway intervention for acute inflammatory disorders of the upper airway as opposed to tracheostomy. Tracheostomy in these cases is performed only in the emergency situation if facilities for endotracheal intubation are not available or if they are unsuccessful. Tracheostomy may also be performed for large tumours which obstruct the larynx until some form of treatment is instituted. Similarly it may be needed in conditions whereby the nerve supply to the larynx has been jeopardized impairing its protective function of the upper airway and its respiratory function.
Tracheostomy tubes: When the trachea has been opened it is necessary to introduce a tube in order to keep the opening from closing. The tubes are made either of hard rubber or more often of metal; and there is always an *outer tube* which is fixed in position by tapes passing round the neck, and an *inner tube* which slides freely out of and into the other, so that it may be removed at any time for cleansing, and is

readily coughed out should it happen to become blocked by mucus.

A dressing is generally applied between the edges of the outer tube and the wound to prevent trauma to the skin of the neck.

The inner tube must be removed and washed several times daily, and if at any time it gets blocked by coughed-up mucus, it must be instantly removed and wiped. The outer tube is not removed till one or two days have elapsed after the operation, and then it is replaced by a fresh tube carefully introduced.

After-treatment: When the operation has been performed for some permanent obstruction, the tube must be worn permanently; and the double metal tube is in such cases replaced after a short time by a soft rubber single one. When the operation has relieved some passing condition like diphtheria, the tube is left out now and then for a few hours, and finally, at the end of a week or so, is removed altogether, after which the wound quickly heals up.

TRACHOMA (see EYE, DISEASES AND INJURIES OF).

TRACTION: The application of a pulling force to the distal part of a fracture in order to allow the fracture to heal with the bone in correct alignment. There are many different methods for applying traction, usually involving weights and pulleys.

TRAINING (see DIET; EXERCISE).

TRANCE is a profound sleep from which a person cannot for a time be aroused, but which is not due to organic disease. The power of voluntary movement is lost, though sensibility and even consciousness may remain. It is usually due to hysteria, and may be induced by hypnotism. (See CATALEPSY; ECSTASY; and SLEEP.)

TRANEXAMIC ACID is a drug used in the control of bleeding. Its mode of action is similar to that of aminocaproic acid (q.v.).

TRANQUILLIZERS: A tranquillizer is a drug which induces a mental state free from agitation and anxiety, and renders the patient calm, serene and peaceful. Strictly speaking, tobacco, alcohol and the barbiturates might be included in this category, but the term 'tranquillizer' is usually restricted to certain new groups of drugs whose main action is the control of anxiety and psychomotor agitation without producing sleepiness, or clouding of consciousness. Among the more widely used drugs in this group are chlorpromazine, diazepam and chlordiazepoxide.

TRANSCUTANEOUS ELECTRICAL NERVE STIMULATION is a method of electrical stimulation that is being used for the relief of pain, including that of migraine, neuralgia and phantom limbs. Known as TENS, its mode of action appears to have some resemblance to that of acupuncture. Several controlled trials suggest that it provides at least a modicum of relief of pain after operations, thereby reducing the amount of analgesics that may be called for.

TRANSFUSION OF BLOOD is an old method of restoring a person believed to be dying by passing blood from another person into his veins. The practice was in vogue during the seventeenth century, and was performed either by bleeding a healthy person into a basin, and, by means of a syringe, injecting the blood into a cannula previously tied in one of the sick person's veins; or by uniting a vein in the healthy person with one in the sick person by means of two cannulae and a connecting tube, so that the blood passed directly from one to the other. In spite of all speed, the blood introduced by either of these methods was apt to clot; and the practice was adopted of whipping the blood with fine twigs, or straining it through muslin so as to remove its fibrin, and thus introduce merely the serum and blood corpuscles.

Apart from the difficulty caused by the tendency to clot, the major drawback to transfusion is that the corpuscles are liable to break up in the new circulation into which they are introduced; and the person into whom the new blood is transfused may suffer to a dangerous degree from symptoms such as nettle-rash, difficulty of breathing, purging, and signs of shock, whilst the immediate destruction of the red blood corpuscles leads to the passage of blood pigment in the urine and jaundice in some cases. A fatal result may quickly supervene.

To avoid this, it is necessary to find out that the blood of the donor is compatible with the blood already in the circulation of the recipient. (See BLOOD GROUPS.) Whenever possible, this should be done by people specially trained in the technique. In an emergency in a remote area, however, where such facilities are not available, compatibility of blood can be investigated by a relatively simple technique. A little blood is drawn from the recipient, and a drop of its serum mixed with a minute drop of blood from the donor, which has been allowed to drop into citrate of soda solution. If, in the course of a few minutes, the serum of the recipient causes clotting or breaking up of the donor's corpuscles, the two bloods are incompatible, and another donor of new blood must be chosen and similarly tested. Standard sera can also be obtained for testing the group to which the blood of the donor and that of the recipient belong.

Various methods of transfusion have been used at different times: such as by uniting a vessel in the donor with a vessel in the recipient by means of a short tube, while the two lie side by side; by withdrawing the blood into a syringe and then injecting it through a cannula into the recipient's vein; or by withdrawing the blood from the donor into a large glass vessel, coated with paraffin, which contains a small amount of citrate of soda solution intended to prevent clotting.

In Great Britain, however, all these methods have been given up since the inception, in 1946, of the National Blood Transfusion Service, which is responsible for the collection of blood from voluntary donors and for its storage in blood-banks throughout the country. In 1990 the service collected almost two million donations of blood which were screened for infectious agents that might transmit such diseases as syphilis, HIV or hepatitis. A standard transfusion bottle has been evolved, with special apparatus for the taking and the giving of blood. When such a set is used with the proper technique, the blood can be safely stored at a temperature of 2 to 6 °C for three weeks before use. In addition to whole blood, plasma or serum may be used for transfusion purposes. When stored in the dried form, human plasma and serum have proved to be valuable substitutes for whole blood. In the dried state human plasma is stable for five years provided it is stored at a moderate temperature (4·4 to 21·1 °C) and is not exposed to direct sunlight. It is reconstituted by adding pyrogen-free distilled water.

AUTOLOGOUS TRANSFUSION is the use of an individual's own blood, provided in advance, for transfusion during or after a surgical operation. This is a valuable procedure for operations that may require large transfusions or where a person has a rare blood group. Its use has increased because of the fear of AIDS.

EXCHANGE TRANSFUSION is the method of treatment in severe cases of haemolytic disease of the newborn (q.v.). It consists of replacing the whole of the baby's blood with Rh-negative blood of the correct blood group for the baby.

TRANSIENT ISCHAEMIC ATTACKS are episodes of transient ischaemia of some part of the cerebral hemispheres or the brain stem lasting anything from a few minutes to several hours and followed by complete recovery. By definition the ischaemic episode must be less than 24 hours. These episodes may be isolated or they may occur several times in a day. The cause is atheroma of the carotid or vertebral arteries and the embolization of platelets or cholesterol. These attacks present with strokes that rapidly recover.

TRANSLOCATION is the term used to describe an exchange of genetic material between chromosomes (q.v.). It is an important factor in the etiology, or causation, of certain congenital abnormalities such as, for example mongolism. It is one of the main abnormalities sought for in amnioscopy (q.v.).

TRANSPLANTATION of organs of the body has become a practical possibility within recent

years. The major outstanding problem is how to prevent the recipient's body from rejecting and destroying the transplanted organ. Such rejection of a foreign body is part of the normal protective mechanism of the body and is essential for the maintenance of the integrity of the body.

If the transplant comes from another person it is known as an *allotransplant*. If it comes from the patient himself – for example, a skin graft – it is known as an *autotransplant*. If it comes from an animal it is known as a *xenotransplant*.

Hitherto the major success has been achieved with transplantation of the kidney, and this has been most successful when the transplanted kidney has come from an identical twin. Less successful have been live transplants from other blood relatives, while least successful have been transplants from other live donors and cadaver donors. The results, however, are steadily improving. Thus the one-year functional survival of kidneys transplanted from unrelated cadaver donors has risen from around 50 per cent to over 80 per cent, and survival rates of 80 per cent after three years are not uncommon. For a well-matched transplant from a live related donor the survival rate after five years is around 90 per cent. And, of course, if a transplanted kidney fails to function, the patient can always be switched on to some form of dialysis (q.v.). In the United Kingdom the supply of cadaveric kidneys for transplantation is only about half that necessary to meet the demand, and around 3,000 people are awaiting transplants. Donor cards are now available in all general practitioners' surgeries and pharmacies but, of the millions of cards distributed since 1972, too few have been used. The reasons are complex but include the reluctance of the public and doctors to consider organ donation, poor organization for recovery of donor kidneys and worries about the diagnosis of death.

Drugs are now available that can depress the immune reactions of the recipient, which are responsible for the rejection of the transplanted organ. Notable among these is cyclosporin A. By these and other means, such as careful typing of the donor kidney, results are steadily improving. One of the more promising developments is the development of an anti-lymphocytic serum (ALS) which reduces the activity of the lymphocytes (q.v.), cells which play an important part in maintaining the integrity of the body against foreign bodies.

Other organs that have been transplanted are the heart, the lungs, the liver, bone marrow, and the cornea of the eye. With the exception of the last two of these, the results are not as satisfactory as in the case of kidney, but the results are improving. The one-year-survival rate in skilled hands is over 80 per cent, with many patients surviving for several years. Liver transplantation is now regularly carried out in specialist centres. It is estimated that in the United Kingdom approximately 200 patients a year between the ages of 15 and 55 would benefit from a liver transplant if an adequate number of donors were available. Over 100 liver transplants are carried out annually in the United Kingdom and one-year-survival rates of up to 80 per cent have been achieved.

A code of practice for procedures relating to the removal of organs for transplantation was produced in 1978 and this code has been revised in the light of further views expressed by the Conference of Medical Royal Colleges and Faculties of the United Kingdom on the Diagnosis of Brain Death. Under the Human Tissue Act 1961 only the person lawfully in possession of the body or his designate can authorize the removal of organs from a body. This authorization may be given orally. Patients who may become suitable donors after death are those who have suffered severe and irreversible brain damage. Such patients will be dependent on artificial ventilation. Patients with malignant disease or systemic infection and patients with renal disease, including chronic hypertension, are unsuitable. If a patient carries a signed donor card or has otherwise recorded his wishes there is no legal requirement to establish lack of objection on the part of relatives, although it is good practice to take account of the views of close relatives. If a relative objects, despite the known request by the patient, staff will need to judge, according to the circumstances of the case, whether it is wise to proceed with organ removal. If a patient who has died is not known to have requested that his organs be removed for transplantation after his death the designated person may only authorize the removal if, having made such reasonable enquiry as may be practical he has no reason to believe (a) that the deceased had expressed an objection to his body being so dealt with after his death, or (b) that the surviving spouse or any surviving relative of the deceased objects to the body being so dealt with. Staff will need to decide who is best qualified to approach the relatives. This should be someone with appropriate experience who is aware how much the relative already knows about the patient's condition. Relatives should not normally be approached before death has occurred but sometimes a relative approaches the hospital staff and suggests sometime in advance that the patient's kidneys might be used for transplantation after his death. The staff of hospitals and organ exchange organizations must respect the wishes of the donor, the recipient and their families with respect to anonymity.

Relatives who enquire should be told that some post-mortem treatment of the donor's body will be necessary if the organs are to be removed in good condition. It is ethical to maintain artificial ventilation and heart beat until removal of organs has been completed. This is essential in the case of heart and liver transplants and many doctors think it is desirable when removing kidneys.

TRANS-SEXUALISM is the psycho-sexual abnormality characterized by feelings of belonging to the gender opposite to that of the genitalia and the secondary sex characteristics.

Trans-sexuals or their families wanting help and guidance should contact the Gender Dysphoria Trust International, BM Box No. 7624, London WC1N 3XX (0323-641100) or the Partners' Group for Partners and Families of Trans-sexuals, BM Box No. 6093, London WC1N 3XX (0323-641100).

TRANSURETHRAL RESECTION: The use of a special cystoscope (q.v.) (a resectoscope) inserted through the urethra (q.v.) to resect the prostate gland (q.v.) or bladder tumours (see resection).

TRANSVERSE: An anatomical description of a line, plane or structure at right angles to the long axis of an organ or the body.

TRANSVESTITISM, or TRANSVESTISM, is the term given to a psycho-sexual abnormality in which there is a repetitive compulsion to dress in the clothes of the opposite sex to achieve orgasm.

TRANYLCYPROMINE (see ANTIDEPRESSANTS).

TRAUMA is the term used to indicate disorders due to wounds or injuries.

TRAVEL MEDICINE: Many countries have reciprocal health arrangements with Britain under which British visitors may receive emergency treatment free or at reduced cost. Information about these arrangements is available in leaflet SA40, available from any local DSS office. General and specific advice for travellers on such matters as immunizations needed can be obtained from their doctor, through travel agents or one of the high street travel 'health shops'. A useful source of information is the British Medical Association's *Well Away* booklet, available from major bookshops or through the BMJ Bookshop, BMA House, Tavistock Square, London WC1H 9TE.

The following centres specialize in medical advice for travellers going overseas:

Communicable Diseases (Scotland) Unit, Ruchill Hospital, Glasgow G20 9NB (041-946 7120).

Department of Infection and Tropical Diseases, East Birmingham Hospital, Bordesley Green East, Birmingham B9 5ST (021-766 6611).

Department of Health, Hannibal House, Elephant and Castle, London SE1 6TE (071-972 2000).

Travel Clinic, Hospital for Tropical Diseases, 4 St Pancras Way, London NW1 0PE (071-387 4411, fax: 071-383 0041).

Liverpool School of Tropical Medicine, Pembroke Place, Liverpool L3 5QA (051-708 9393).

Medical Advisory Services to Travellers Abroad, London School of Hygiene and Tropical Medicine, Keppel Street, London WC1E

7HT (071-927 2216, fax: 071-637 0248. For specific advice on malaria, contact the Malaria Reference Laboratory at the London School of Hygiene and Tropical Medicine (071-636 7929, 071-927 2435 and 071-927 2212 for taped advice and 071-636 8636 for particular queries).

TRAVEL SICKNESS is the sickness that is induced by any form of transport, whether by sea, air, motor-car or train. (See MOTION-SICKNESS.)
TRAVELLER'S DIARRHOEA is an all too common affliction of the traveller, which basks in a multiplicity of names: e.g. Aden gut, Aztec two step, Basra belly, Delhi belly, Gippy tummy, Hong Kong dog, Montezuma's revenge, Tokyo trots, turista. It is caused by a variety of micro-organisms, usually *E. coli*. Some people seem to be more prone to it than others, though for no good cause. Obvious preventive measures include the avoidance of salads, unpeeled fruit and ice cream, and never drinking unboiled or unbottled water. Two widely recommended preventive drugs are Streptotriad (one tablet twice daily for a week, and then one daily) and doxycycline (100 mg daily). Both are said to provide a satisfactory degree of protection, provided a fulminating infection is avoided, as long as taken.

TRAZODONE (see ANTIDEPRESSANTS).

TREMOR means a very fine kind of involuntary movement. Tremors may be seen in projecting parts like the hands, head and tongue, or they may involve muscles or even the individual fibres of a muscle here and there. They are of various grades of fineness. Very coarse tremors, which prevent a person from drinking a glass of water without spilling it, are found in multiple sclerosis and in chorea (see under these headings); somewhat finer tremors, which produce trembling of the hands or tongue when they are stretched out, are caused by alcoholism (see ALCOHOLISM, CHRONIC), by poisoning with other substances like lead, by Parkinsonism (q.v.), and by the weakness which follows some acute disease or characterizes old age; a fine tremor of the outstretched fingers is a characteristic of thyrotoxicosis (see GOITRE); very fine tremors, visible in the muscles of face or limbs, and known as fibrillary tremors, are present in general paralysis of the insane, and in progressive muscular atrophy or wasting palsy. Tremors may occur at rest and disappear on movement as in Parkinsonism, or they may occur only on movement (intention tremors) as in cerebellar disease.

TRENCH FEVER is an infectious disease caused by *Rickettsia quintana* which is transmitted by the body louse. Large epidemics occurred among troops on active service during the 1914–18 War. It recurred on a smaller scale in the 1939–45 War, and is endemic in Mexico.

TRENCH, or IMMERSION, **FOOT** is due to prolonged exposure of the feet to water, particularly cold water. Trench warfare is a common precipitating factor, and it was rampant during the 1914–18 War. Cases also occurred during the 1939–45 War, particularly during the slow winter advance up through Italy after the Anzio landings. Cases occurred, too, during the Falklands campaign. The less common form due to warm water immersion occurred with some frequency in the Vietnam war. It is characterized by painful swelling of the feet accompanied in due course by blistering and ulceration which, in severe, untreated cases, may go on to gangrene. In mild cases recovery may be complete in a month, but severe cases may drag on for a year.
Treatment: Drying of the feet overnight, where practicable, is the best method of prevention, accompanied by avoidance of constrictive clothing and tight boots, and of prolonged immobility. Frequent rest periods and daily changing of socks also help. The application of silicone grease once a day is another useful preventive measure. In the early stages treatment consists of rest in bed and warmth. In more severe cases treatment is as for infected tissues and ulceration. Analgesics (q.v.) are usually necessary to ease the pain. Technically, smoking should be forbidden, but the psychological effects in troops on active service may outweigh its advantages.

TRENDELENBERG POSITION: First described by Frederick Trendelenberg in 1881, this is a steep head-down tilt so that the patient's pelvis and legs lie above the heart. It is used to improve access and limit blood loss during surgery to the pelvis. It has been used to treat shocked patients, but, as the position increases pressure on the diaphragm and embarrasses breathing, raising the legs by themselves is better.

TREPHINING, or TREPANNING, is an operation in which a portion of the cranium is removed. Originally the operation was performed with an instrument resembling a carpenter's brace and known as the trephine or trepan, which removes a small circle of bone; but now this instrument is only used, as a rule, for making small openings, whilst, for wider operations, gouge forceps, circular saws driven by electric motor, or wire saws are employed in order to give greater ease and speed.
The operation is one requiring nicety of manipulation, but is neither difficult nor serious, and was one of the commonest major operations of antiquity. It is said, from the appearances presented by skulls found in old French burial mounds, to have been practised by prehistoric peoples; at all events Hippocrates describes fully the operation and the conditions that call for it, whilst Galen mentions two varieties of the instrument in common use. Both among the Greeks and Romans, and in the Middle Ages, resort seems to have been

made to trephining on very slight provocation for conditions traceable to the head.

At the present time, the conditions under which it may be thought advisable to trephine the skull are chiefly as follows. In cases of fracture, with splintering of the skull, the operation is performed to remove the fragments of bone and any foreign bodies, like a bullet, which may have entered, in order that the wound may be thoroughly cleansed. In compression of the brain with unconsciousness following an injury, the skull is trephined and any blood-clots removed, or torn vessels ligatured. When an abscess is present within the skull, the operation is called for in order to evacuate the pus. In certain forms of epilepsy, or in continued headache, when the symptoms point to a definite part of the brain being involved, the skull may be trephined over this area, so that any clot, scar, thickening of the bone or cyst, which is setting up the irritation, may be discovered and removed. For a cerebral tumour, trephining is often performed either with the view of removing the tumour, if possible, or at all events of relieving the great pressure within the skull caused by the growing mass.

TREPONEMA is the name of a genus of spirochaetal micro-organisms which consist of slender spirals and which progress by means of bending movements. *Treponema pallidum* (formerly called *Spirochaeta pallida*) is the causative organism of syphilis.

TRIAMCINOLONE is a corticosteroid (q.v.), which has a potency equivalent to that of prednisone, but is less likely to cause retention of sodium.

TRIAZOLAM (see BENZOTHIAZEPINES).

TRICHIASIS: A condition in which the eyelashes become ingrown.

TRICEPS: A muscle of the posterior upper arm which acts to extend the forearm. So named because it originates from three heads.

TRICHINOSIS, or TRICHINIASIS, is the name of a disease set up by eating diseased pork, in which the immature *Trichinella spiralis* is encysted. The full-grown female worm, which inhabits the intestine, is 3 mm in length, and the larvae, to whose movements the disease is due, are much smaller. The disease is acquired by eating raw or underdone pork from pigs that have been infected with the worm. When such a piece of meat is eaten, the embryos contained in it are set free, develop into full-grown trichinellae, and from each pair of these 1000 or more new embryos may arise in a few weeks. So soon as this new generation of embryos is produced they bore their way into the wall of the bowel, setting up sometimes severe irrita-

tion and diarrhoea, and thence wander all over the body, finally depositing themselves between the fibres of the voluntary muscles. During this migration, which lasts four or five weeks, they set up fever and pain in the limbs and muscles, often mistaken for rheumatism. Death may even result, but if the person survives to the end of four or five weeks, the trichinellae, which are now encysted in the muscles, give no further trouble.

Prevention is based on thorough inspection of meat in slaughter-houses, for even cooking, unless the meat is in slices, is not an efficient protection. Pigs should not be fed on unboiled garbage. Rats may be a source of sporadic outbreaks, as infected rats have been found near piggeries. The disease is now a rare one, thanks to sanitary inspection though it still occurs in these parts of the country, such as the Midlands, where raw sausage meat is considered a delicacy. The encysted trichinellae are just visible as fine white specks.

Treatment: In the early stages, tetrachlorocthylene, followed by a sharp purge, is of value. Recently, thiabendazole, which has proved of value in the treatment of affected pigs, has been used with promising results in human victims.

TRICHLOROETHYLENE, also known as TRILENE, is a volatile anaesthctic which has the advantages of being non-irritant and of inducing anaesthesia rapidly and pleasantly. It has been used mainly for inducing analgesia or light anaesthesia in obstetrics and dentistry. In an impure form it is used commercially in the dry-cleaning industry.

TRICHO- is a prefix denoting relation to hair.

TRICHOMONAS VAGINALIS is a protozoon normally present in the vagina of about 30 to 40 per cent of women. It sometimes becomes pathogenic and causes inflammation of the genital passages, with vaginal discharge. A man may become infected as a result of sexual intercourse with an infected woman and have a urethral discharge as a result; it may also cause prostatitis. Excellent results are being obtained from the use of metronidazole in its treatment. To obtain a satisfactory result it may be necessary to treat both partners.

TRICHOMONIASIS is the disease caused by infection with *Trichomonas vaginalis* (q.v.).

TRICHOPHYTON is the parasite that causes ringworm. (See RINGWORM.)

TRICHORRHOEA is the term applied to the falling-out of hair. It is usually due to some general disease such as scarlet fever or typhoid fever. When there is no obvious cause, such as this, treatment consists of attention to the general hygiene of the scalp. Vigorous massage is to be avoided.

TRICHOTILLOMANIA is the condition in which a person has an obsessional impulse to pull out his own hair.

TRICHURIASIS is a worldwide infection, particularly common in the tropics. It is caused by *Trichuris trichiura*, or whipworm, so called because of its shape, the rear end being stout and the front end hairlike, resembling the lash of a whip. The male measures 5 cm and the female 4 cm in length. Infection results from eating vegetables, or drinking water, polluted with the ova (eggs). These hatch out in the large intestine. The diagnosis is made by finding the eggs in the stools. The worms seldom cause any trouble unless they are present in large numbers when, especially in malnourished children, they may cause bleeding from the bowels, anaemia and prolapse of the rectum. The most effective drug at the moment is mebendazole: 100 mg twice daily for three days.

TRICUSPID VALVE is the valve, with three cusps or flaps, that guards the opening from the right atrium into the right ventricle of the heart. (See HEART.)

TRIFLUOPERAZINE (see NEUROLEPTICS).

TRIGEMINAL NERVE is the fifth cranial nerve. It consists of three divisions: (1) the ophthalmic nerve, which is purely sensory in function, being distributed mainly over the forehead and front part of the scalp; (2) the maxillary nerve, which is also sensory and distributed to the skin of the cheek, the mucous membrane of the mouth and throat, and the upper teeth; and (3) the mandibular nerve, which is the nerve of sensation to the lower part of the face, the tongue and the lower teeth, as well as being the motor nerve to the muscles concerned in chewing. The trigeminal nerve is of special interest, owing to its liability to neuralgia (q.v.), trigeminal neuralgia (q.v.), or tic douloureux as it is also known, being the most painful form known of neuralgia.

TRIGEMINAL NEURALGIA, or TIC DOULOUREUX, is one of the most severe forms of neuralgia. It affects the great nerve of sensation in the face (trigeminal nerve), and may occur in one or more of the three divisions in which the nerve is distributed. It is usually confined to one side. Women suffer, on the whole, more often than men, and they are usually over the age of 50. The attack is often precipitated by movements of the jaw, as in talking or eating, or by tactile stimuli such as a cold wind or washing the face. When the *first or upper division of the nerve* is involved, the pain is mostly felt in the forehead and side of the head. It is usually of an intensely sharp, cutting, or burning character, either constant or with exacerbations, and often periodic, returning at a certain hour each day while the attack continues. Occasionally the paroxysms are of extreme violence, and are brought on by the slightest provocation, such as a draught of cool air. The skin over the affected part is often red and swollen, and, even after the attack has abated, feels stiff and tender to the touch. As in all forms of neuralgia, there are certain localities where the pain is more intense, these painful points, as they are called, being for the most part in those places where the branches of the nerves emerge from bony canals or pierce the fascia to ramify in the skin. Hence, in this form, the greater severity of the pain above the eyebrow and along the side of the nose. There is also pain in the eyelid, redness of the eye and increased flow of tears. When the *second division of the nerve* is affected, the pain is chiefly in the cheek and upper jaw, the painful points being immediately below the lower eyelid, over the cheekbone and about the upper lip. This form is accompanied by pain of similar character to that affecting the first division; the pain often appears suddenly on slight provocation such as by taking a mouthful of hot or cold fluid. When *the third division of the nerve* suffers, the pain affects the lower jaw, and the chief painful points are in front of the ear and above the chin. Attacks of tic douloureux, extremely distressing as they are, may recur for years; and although, by depriving the sufferer of sleep and interfering with the taking of food, they may in some measure impair the health, they rarely appear to lead to any serious results. Nevertheless, the pain may be so intolerable as to make life a burden.

Treatment: The outlook in trigeminal neuralgia has been radically altered by the introduction of the drug carbamazepine, which is proving of outstanding value in relieving the pain of what is one of the most devastating of all forms of neuralgia. In view of its potential side-effects, it must only be taken under medical supervision. The introduction of this drug has radically cut down the need for killing the ganglion of the nerve, or its branches, by the injection of alcohol, electrocoagulation, percutaneous or radio frequency gangliolysis, or rhizotomy (q.v.).

TRIGGER FINGER, or SNAPPING FINGER, is the condition in which when the fingers are straightened on unclenching the fist one finger, usually the ring or middle finger, remains bent. The cause is obscure. In severe cases treatment consists of opening up the sheath surrounding the tendon of the affected finger. When confined to the thumb it is known as TRIGGER THUMB.

TRIGGER THUMB (see TRIGGER FINGER).

TRIGLYCERIDE: One of the basic chemical 'building blocks' from which fats are formed. A triglyceride molecules consists of three fatty-acid molecules which have chemically reacted with glycerol.

TRIGONE is the base of the bladder between the openings of the two ureters and of the urethra.

TRI-IODOTHYRONINE is the substance which exerts the physiological action of thyroid hormone. It is formed in the body cells by the de-iodination of thyroxine (tetra-iodothyronine) which is the active principle secreted by the thyroid gland. It has also been synthesized, and is now available for the treatment of myxoedema (q.v.). It is three times as potent as thyroxine. (See also THYROID GLAND.)

TRILENE (see TRICHLOROETHYLENE).

TRIMESTER: A period of three months. Normal human gestation is divided into three trimesters.

TRIMETHORIM is an anti-bacterial agent which is proving of value in the treatment of infections of the urinary tract. It is also a constituent of co-trimoxazole (q.v.).

TRIMIPRAMINE is a relatively weak antidepressant drug which also acts as a sedative. (See ANTIDEPRESSANTS.)

TRIMUSTINE is a nitrogen mustard derivative (q.v.) used in the treatment of certain forms of malignant disease. It is administered intravenously.

TRINITRIN (see GLYCERYL TRINITRATE).

TRIPLETS (see MULTIPLE BIRTHS).

TRISMUS is another name for lockjaw. (See TETANUS.)

TROCAR is an instrument provided with a sharp three-sided point fitted inside a tube or cannula, and used for puncturing cavities of the body in which fluid has collected.

TROCHANTER is the name given to two bony prominences at the upper end of the thigh-bone. The *greater trochanter* can be felt on the outer side of the thigh. The *lesser trochanter* is a small prominence on the inner side of this bone.

TROCHES is another name for lozenges. (See LOZENGES.)

TROCHLEAR NERVE is the fourth cranial nerve, which acts upon the superior oblique muscle of the eye.

TROPHIC is a term applied to the influence that nerves exert with regard to the healthiness and nourishment of the parts to which they run. When the nerves become diseased or injured, this influence is lost and the muscles waste, while the skin loses its healthy appearance and is liable to break down into ulcers. (See NERVOUS DISEASES; BED SORES.)

TROPHOBLAST is the outer layer of the fertilized ovum which attaches the ovum to the wall of the uterus (or womb) and supplies nutrition to the embryo.

TROPICAL DISEASES: This term includes some diseases that occur in temperate climates, but are more common or more severe in hot latitudes; as well as some that are found only in the tropics. (See ANCYLOSTOMIASIS; BERIBERI; BLACKWATER FEVER; CHOLERA; CLIMATE; DENGUE; DRACONTIASIS; DYSENTERY; ELEPHANTIASIS; FILARIASIS; HEAT-STROKE; LEISHMANIASIS; LEPROSY; LIVER DISEASES; MALARIA; ORIENTAL SORE; PLAGUE; PRICKLY HEAT; SCHISTOSOMIASIS; SLEEPING SICKNESS; STRONGLYLOIDIASIS; SUNBURN; YAWS; YELLOW FEVER.)

TRUNK: A major vessel or nerve from which lesser ones arise, or the main part of the body excluding the head, neck and limbs.

TRUSS is an instrument used to support a hernia; or to retain the protruding organ within the cavity from which it tends to pass. Every truss possesses a pad of some sort to cover the opening and a belt or spring to keep it in position.
    Before applying a truss the wearer must make certain that the hernia has been reduced. This may mean lying down before applying the truss. A truss will rarely control a hernia satisfactorily, and it should be considered as a temporary measure only until surgical correction is possible. In the past trusses have been supplied to patients considered too frail for surgery, but modern anaesthetic techniques means that most people can have their hernias surgically repaired.

TRYPANOSOMA is a genus of microscopic parasites, several of which are responsible for causing sleeping sickness and some allied diseases. (See SLEEPING SICKNESS.)

TRYPANOSOMIASIS (see SLEEPING SICKNESS.)

TRYPSIN is the chief protein ferment of the pancreatic secretion. It changes proteins into peptones and forms the main constituent of pancreatic extracts used for digestion of food. (See PANCREAS; PEPTONIZED FOOD.)

TSETSE FLY is an African fly of the genus *Glossina*. One or more of these is responsible for carrying the trypanosome which causes sleeping sickness and thus spreads the disease among cattle and from cattle to men.

TSUTSUGAMUSHI, or JAPANESE RIVER FEVER, is a disease of the typhus group. (See TYPHUS FEVER.)

TUBAL PREGNANCY: Implantation of the embryo in the fallopian tube (q.v.) rather than in the lining of the uterus (q.v.). The patient usually complains of pain between six and ten weeks' gestation and, if the fallopian tube is not removed, there may be rupture with potentially life-threatening haemorrhage (also known as ectopic pregnancy).

TUBERCLE is a term used in two distinct senses. As a descriptive term in anatomy, a *tubercle* means a small elevation or roughness upon a bone, such as the tubercles of the ribs. In the pathological sense, a *tubercle* is a small mass, barely visible to the naked eye, formed in some organ as the starting-point of tuberculosis. The name of *tubercle bacillus* was originally given to the micro-organism that causes this disease but this has now been changed to *Mycobacterium tuberculosis*. The term tubercular should strictly be applied to anything connected with or resembling tubercles or nodules, and the term *tuberculous* to anything pertaining to the disease tuberculosis.

When *Mycobacteria tuberculosis* have gained entrance to an organ, no matter whether inhaled, or whether absorbed from food and circulated through the lymphatics or blood-vessels, the following results ensue. The individual bacilli multiply, and around each group forms a minute tubercle, or granule, which is of a size almost invisible to the naked eye, and greyish in colour. These tubercles fuse together, and, at the same time, soften to a cheesy substance, so as to form yellow bodies about the size of pin-heads. Each grey tubercle, under the microscope, shows the appearance of a group of cells of medium size (epithelioid cells), surrounded by many smaller cells (connective tissue cells and white blood corpuscles), attracted to the spot as a result of the inflammation set up. Scattered between these cells lie the mycobacteria. Near the centre of the older tubercles there are often seen one or more large cells with many nuclei (giant cells). The larger yellow tubercles form a more or less structureless mass in the centre, but show numbers of the small grey tubercles round their edge. Thus the process spreads, the healthy tissue being broken down and giving place to the soft, cheesy mass, which, in the case of the lungs, finally bursts into a bronchial tube, is coughed up, and leaves a ragged cavity in its place. Another change, however, takes place at the same time, for, in consequence of the irritation set up by the tubercle, strands of fibrous tissue are built up round its edge, and, when the process is a very chronic one, these come to form a dense capsule for the tuberculous area, cutting it off from further advance on healthy tissue, and forming a natural cure.

TUBERCULIDE is the term given to any skin lesion which is the result of infection with the tubercle bacillus, or *Mycobacterium tuberculosis* as it is now known.

TUBERCULIN is the name originally given by Koch in 1890 to a preparation derived from the tubercle bacillus, or *Mycobacterium tuberculosis* as it is now known, and intended for the diagnosis or treatment of tuberculosis.
Varieties: *Old Tuberculin* (OT) is the heat-concentrated filtrate from a fluid medium on which the human or bovine type of *Mycobacterium tuberculosis* has been grown for six weeks or more. *Tuberculin Purified Protein Derivative* (Tuberculin PPD) is the active principle of Old Tuberculin, and is prepared from the fluid medium on which the *Mycobacterium tuberculosis* has been grown. It is supplied as a liquid, a powder, or as sterile tablets. The liquid contains 100,000 Units per millilitre, and the dry powder contains 30,000 Units per milligram. It is distributed in sterile containers sealed so as to exclude micro-organisms. It is more constant in composition and potency than Old Tuberculin.
Uses: The basis of the tuberculin reaction is that any person who has been infected with the *Mycobacterium tuberculosis* gives a reaction when a small amount of tuberculin is injected into the skin. A negative reaction means that either the individual has never been infected with the tubercle bacillus, or that the infection has been too recent to have allowed of sensitivity developing.

There are various methods of carrying out the test, of which the following are the most commonly used. The *Mantoux Test* is the most satisfactory of all and has the advantage that the size of the reaction is a guide to the severity of the tuberculous infection. It is performed by injecting the tuberculin into the skin on the forearm. The *Heaf Multiple Puncture Test* is reliable. It is carried out with the multiple puncture apparatus, or Heaf Gun. The *Vollmer Patch Test* using an impregnated filter paper, is useful in children because of the ease with which it can be carried out.

TUBERCULOSIS is the general name for the whole group of diseases associated with the presence of the *Mycobacterium tuberculosis*, of which pulmonary tuberculosis is the most important. (See MICROBIOLOGY.)

Tuberculosis not only affects the lungs, but may invade almost any organ, being seldom found, however, in the muscles or in tissues with few blood-vessels, like cartilage and sinews. The disease spreads usually by way of the lymphatic vessels. The severity of the disease varies considerably, according to the organ attacked – thus tuberculosis affecting the membranes of the brain and causing meningitis is a particularly dangerous disease, especially in infants and young children. Chronic inflammation of bones and white swelling of joints are manifestations of the disease, having less influence upon the general health. The enlargement of glands, most common in the neck, to which the name of scrofula was formerly given, because the swollen neck gives to the physiognomy a pig-like expression, is a well-known form of tuberculous disease. This form of the disease seems to have been much more widespread in former times, and was known also as 'king's evil', from the superstition that a touch of the royal hand conveyed a cure to the affected person. Many chronic abscesses are tuberculous in origin, arising from this affection in a bone, a gland, or the cellular tissue. The disfiguring skin disease known as lupus vulgaris is another of the manifestations of the disease. Other sites in which tuberculosis is apt to occur are the bowels and the genito- urinary tract: i.e. the kidneys, bladder and epididymis.

Consumption, or phthisis, is the name given, in popular language, to tuberculosis. It dates from the days when there was no effective treatment for tuberculosis, and the disease tended to be characterized by a rapid or gradual wasting away of the body. The term phthisis was usually restricted to that form of the disease in which the infection was restricted to the lungs: i.e. pulmonary tuberculosis.

The essential part of the disease, from which it receives its name of tuberculosis, is the formation in the substance of an organ of tubercles, fine granules of a size barely visible to the naked eye, these tubercles multiplying and changing in such a way as to lead finally to the destruction of the organ in which they are found.

Nature of the disease: Tuberculosis has been recognized as a disease from the earliest times. Hippocrates (460–375 BC) bestowed the name of phthisis upon the disease as it affects the lungs, and descriptions of the condition are found in the writings of classical authors. About AD 980 Haly Abbas of Baghdad, and again in 1779 Cullen, recognized the infectious nature of phthisis, but not till after the middle of the nineteenth century was it proved, by means of inoculating animals with tuberculous material from phthisical patients, that tuberculosis is really an infective disease, and that the tubercles result from an inflammatory process, due to some poison introduced with the diseased products. The nature of the poison was much disputed till 1882, when Koch announced the discovery of the tubercle bacillus, or *Mycobacterium tuberculosis* as it is now known, and so answered this important question.

The manner in which these bacilli gain access to the body is important. There are three possible channels:

(*a*) By INOCULATION: A person may prick himself with a knife contaminated by the sputum of a tuberculous patient, or may rub some of this material into a cut. Generally this results merely in a local skin disease, and it occurs only in doctors, nurses and others dealing with tuberculous patients, or in veterinary surgeons or others dealing with tuberculous animals.

(*b*) By INHALATION: The sputum and other discharges from tuberculous people swarm with bacilli. It has been calculated that a person suffering from a cavity in the lung may spit up 4,000,000,000 bacilli in the course of twenty-four hours, and each of these, when dried and blown about on dust, is potent for evil. Neither drying, nor freezing, nor putrefaction, nor the lapse of months destroys these bacilli, but direct sunlight is speedily fatal to them, so that dust which has lain for a short time in the open on a bright day becomes rapidly harmless. In rooms inhabited by tuberculous patients, and in hospital wards, the dust from the floor often contains *Mycobacterium tuberculosis*.

Probably almost all cases in which this disease primarily affects the lungs are due to inhalation of dust laden with the bacilli or inhalation of droplets coughed into the air by a tuberculous patient, whilst those cases in which the glands of the neck are first attacked arise by absorption of the bacilli through the tonsils.

(*c*) By INGESTION: It has long been known that tuberculosis, like other infectious diseases, can be conveyed by means of milk and other articles of food, and, acting upon this belief, sanitary authorities have enforced regulations designed to protect the public from the effects of consuming diseased meat and milk. In the case of meat there is practically no danger.

Tuberculosis is present throughout the world but it is especially prevalent in Asian countries where 60–80 per cent of children under 14 are infected. In England and Wales about 6,000 new cases of tuberculosis are notified annually. Mortality from the disease has fallen from 150 per 100,000 of the population at the turn of the century to 5 per 100,000 in the 1980s. The disease is more common in deprived urban areas, among elderly people and among immigrants from the Indian subcontinent. People suffering from immunodeficiency disorders – e.g. AIDS – diabetes mellitus and alcohol dependence are especially at risk of contracting tuberculosis.

A much larger number of the population suffer from early tuberculosis (it may be quite unsuspected) and recover. This is proved by the frequent presence on X-ray examination of old calcified tuberculous glands and by healed scars in the lungs found at post-mortem examination.

Causes: The direct cause of the disease is the *Mycobacterium tuberculosis*. (See BACTERIOLOGY.) But, in view of the fact that many people suffer from the disease in a mild degree and afterwards recover, and that many limited cases of tuberculosis in bones, skin and glands are successfully treated, it appears that there are other factors which determine whether a given case is serious or not, and whether it is likely to proceed towards recovery, if properly treated, or to end inevitably in death.

HEREDITY: There is probably a hereditary element in the predisposition to the disease. Over a long period those who are susceptible are gradually eliminated by the disease.

AGE is an important point. Young children are liable to tuberculosis affecting the bowels and the glands connected with them, and the meninges of the brain. At a slightly later age there is a greater tendency to that type of the disease formerly known as scrofula, the glands of the neck particularly being affected, and the greatest mortality from lung (or pulmonary) tuberculosis takes place after the age of 20.

Varieties: The forms of tuberculosis other than pulmonary tuberculosis, such as tuberculous disease of joints, bones and spine, meningitis, intestine, lupus, are considered under these headings. The lung disease may present in different ways.

Treatment: This falls very naturally into two classes: (*a*) preventive, and (*b*) remedial.

(*a*) PREVENTIVE TREATMENT: The problem of prevention is partly social and partly medical. Tuberculosis is commoner among the ill-fed and the badly housed. Abolition of overcrowding, provision of good homes, an adequate supply of protective foods and enough money to buy them have all gone a long way towards diminishing the incidence of tuberculosis. To a considerable extent, tuberculosis is a social disease. On the medical side, the problem is essentially to prevent uninfected susceptible people – especially children – from coming into contact with the infecting agent – the *Mycobacterium tuberculosis*. The great risk to the child is coming into contact with an adult who has the causative organism in his or her sputum. Every attempt must therefore be made to detect and treat all sufferers from tuberculosis.

Two of the most important preventive measures have been BCG vaccination (q.v.) and mass miniature radiography (q.v.).

(*b*) REMEDIAL TREATMENT: For all practical purposes this now consists of chemotherapy.

Chemotherapy: The outlook in tuberculosis was revolutionized by the introduction of effective antituberculous drugs. Since the isolation, in 1944, of streptomycin, the first chemotherapeutic substance to be of any value, several other drugs have been introduced. There are two important general aspects of chemotherapy. The first is that the *Mycobacterium tuberculosis* may become resistant to a drug given by itself. This can be prevented by using varying combinations of ethambutol, rifampicin and isoniazid, with streptomycin reserved for patients who fail to respond to these drugs. Most patients recover and suffer no recurrences; those who fail to respond – around 5 per cent – are usually the homeless and people who abuse alcohol and thus do not comply with treatment arrangements.

TUBEROSE SCLEROSIS, or EPILOIA, also sometimes known as TUBEROUS SCLEROSIS, is a hereditary disease due to a developmental abnormality of the brain. The prevalence is 1 in 50,000 of the population. It is characterized by mental retardation (usually from birth), epilepsy which usually starts before 2 years of age and multiple small nodules or tumours in the face which usually appear around puberty. Relatives of those with this condition can obtain help and guidance from the Tuberous Sclerosis Association of Great Britain, Little Barnsley Farm, Catshill, Bromsgrove, Worcestershire B61 0NQ (0527–71898).

TUBOCURARINE is the active constituent of curare (q.v.). It is a muscle relaxant (q.v.) which is widely used in anaesthesia.

TULARAEMIA is a disease of rodents such as rabbits and rats, caused by the bacillus, *Francisella tularense*, and spread either by flies or by direct inoculation, for example, into the hands of a person engaged in skinning rabbits. In man the disease takes the form of a slow fever lasting several weeks, with much malaise and depression, followed by considerable emaciation. It was first described in the district of Tulare in California, and is found widely spread in North America and in Europe, but not in Great Britain. Streptomycin, the tetracyclines and chloramphenicol, have proved effective in treatment.

TULLE GRAS: A dressing of gauze impregnated with soft paraffin to prevent it sticking to the wound.

TUMOUR means literally any swelling, but, by common consent, the term is held not to include passing swellings caused by acute inflammation, whilst the collections of diseased material arising in the course of chronic inflammation, like tuberculosis, syphilis, leprosy and glanders, sometimes are and sometimes are not classed as tumours, according to their size and appearance.

Varieties: Some are of an infective nature, as already stated; some arise undoubtedly as the result of injury; several contributing factors are mentioned under the heading of CANCER, but for the rest, the causes of tumours are really still undiscovered.

An old idea divides tumours into two great classes. On the one hand, some are *simple* or *benign*, growing slowly at one spot, pressing neighbouring parts aside but not invading them, not recurring after removal, and having little tendency to ulcerate; whilst others are *malignant*, spreading quickly from point to point, invading and destroying surrounding tissues, tending to recur after apparently complete removal, and being liable to ulcerate. This distinction is as old as the days of Hippocrates, who gave to gnawing tumours the name of carcinoma. Although in the majority of cases it is easy to decide whether a given tumour is of simple or malignant character, there is no sharp dividing line between the two kinds. Thus an expert sometimes has difficulty in stating from the microscopic characters of an *adenoma* (glandular tumour) growing in the breast or in the bowel, whether its progress will show a simple or malignant course. Again, *rodent ulcer*, a small ulcerating tumour situated generally on the face, may remain restricted to a single spot for twenty or thirty years, although it has the microscopic characters of a malignant tumour and finally spreads like one. Another fact connecting the two groups is that some simple tumours, persisting as such through middle life, are liable to assume a malignant character when old age is reached.

Formerly tumours were named according to some peculiarity of shape, colour, or the like. Thus a fungoid tumour was one resembling a mushroom, a polypus one which seemed to have one stalk with many feet, a mole was a dark hairy growth resembling the animal of that name, and sarcoma was originally the name given by Galen to a tumour of fleshy appearance. The use of the microscope, however, has brought about a more precise grouping, and tumours are now classed according to the tissues of which they are built, somewhat as follows:

(1) Simple tumours of normal tissue
(2) Hollow tumours or cysts, generally of simple nature
(3) Malignant tumours: (*a*) of imperfect cellular structure, resembling the cells of skin, mucous membrane, or secreting glands; (*b*) of imperfect connective tissue.

(1) SIMPLE TUMOURS OF NORMAL TISSUE: ADENOMA is a tumour growing from a gland and composed of gland-like tissue. These tumours are specially common in the breasts of young women; there may be several together, but usually they are easily removed.

ANGIOMA is a tumour formed by a mass of small blood-vessels or spaces in which blood circulates. These tumours may exist in internal organs, or on the skin, when they do not project much, and are known as naevi or 'mothers' marks'.

CHONDROMA is a tumour mainly formed of cartilage. These tumours develop especially on the fingers and toes.

FIBROMA is the name given to a tumour consisting mainly of fibrous tissue. Soft fibromas are often seen as wrinkled brownish tags upon the face or body.

LIPOMA means a tumour mainly composed of fat. Such tumours may be found in any part of the body, but they are especially common just beneath the skin. It is sometimes hard to distinguish such a tumour, which is very soft, from a chronic abscess; but the fatty tumour generally has a firm edge and can be seen to be attached at several points to the skin, which is puckered by these attachments.

MYOMA is a tumour composed largely of muscle fibres, usually unstriped muscle. These tumours are far more commonly found in the wall of the womb than in any other position, being known as fibroid tumours.

NEUROMA is a tumour growing upon a nerve, and therefore in many cases producing pain.

OSTEOMA is a tumour composed of bone. These are usually of small size and cause little trouble, except in so far as their position occasions discomfort.

PAPILLOMA is a tumour projecting from the surface of the skin or of a mucous membrane. It is composed of a core of fibrous tissue, which represents an overdevelopment of the papillae naturally found in these situations, covered by masses of cells. Warts are examples of papillomas on the skin (see WARTS), whilst soft papillomas sometimes develop in the bladder or bowel and cause much bleeding.

(2) HOLLOW TUMOURS are described under a special heading. (See CYSTS.)

(3) MALIGNANT TUMOURS of imperfect cellular structure resembling the cells of skin, mucous membranes or secreting glands, are known generally as CANCERS. This group and the following group are treated together under the heading of CANCER (q.v.). Many names are applied to cancers of different parts and according to their appearance. The name CARCINOMA is generally reserved at the present day for malignant epithelial tumours. EPITHELIOMA is a cancer springing from the skin surface, and ADENOCARCINOMA means one originating in glandular tissue. SCIRRHUS is a hard cancer in which much fibrous tissue has been developed; MEDULLARY or SOFT cancer is one in which the softer cellular element forms large masses; and COLLOID cancer is one in which a characteristic glue-like transformation takes place.

Malignant tumours of imperfect connective tissue are known as SARCOMAS; and, according to the shape of the embryonic cells, or the nature of attempts at the formation of connective tissues, these are subdivided as ROUND-CELLED, SPINDLE-CELLED, MELANOTIC, MYELOID.

Symptoms: The symptoms of a simple tumour are, as a rule, nothing beyond the presence of a swelling, and such accidental symptoms as those set up by its pressure upon neighbouring important organs, by the inconvenience of its size, its position, and the like. (For special symptoms of malignant tumours see CANCER.)

Treatment: The treatment of a tumour is, in general, its removal by operation. With regard to simple tumours, the advantage gained by removal may not be worth the inconvenience caused by an operation, and such tumours may be left alone. In particular cases the unsightliness of the tumour, the inconvenience of its size, or the tendency that some simple tumours have to become malignant may call for removal. If a tumour is malignant, or if there is any doubt as to its character, an operation should be performed at the earliest possible opportunity. For some surface tumours, and also for inoperable tumours in internal organs, the application of radiotherapy and X-rays has, in recent years, played a great part. (See RADIOTHERAPY; RADIUM; X-RAYS.) Chemotherapy is also playing in increasingly important part in treatment. (See CANCER.)

TURGOR: Being or becoming swollen or engorged.

TURNER'S SYNDROME is the condition of ovarian dysgenesis in which the gonad is represented by a ridge on the broad ligament in the normal position on the ovary. It is composed of connective tissue without follicles. The condition is due to a partial or complete lack of the second X chromosome, which appears to be necessary to maintain the ovary. As the patient is deficient in both ovaries the presenting complaint is amenorrhoea and absent development of the breasts and sexual hair. In the syndrome described by Turner these features of ovarian dysfunction were associated with shortness of stature, webbing of the neck and cubitus valgus and there was no impairment of intelligence. Although the development of the ovary is influenced to a varying degree most patients with this syndrome are of short stature and rarely reach a height of more than 155 cm (5 feet). A number of congenital defects additional to those originally described by Turner may be associated with the condition, and coarctation of the aorta, deafness and mental deficiency are well recognized.

Most women with this condition have only 45 instead of the normal 46 chromosomes and this is due to non-dysjunction of the sex chromosome occurring during meiosis. Their sex chromosome constitution is XO instead of XX. Patients with less severe forms of the syndrome may have a normal number of chromosomes but one of the X chromosomes is structurally abnormal and deficient in much of the genetic material.

TWINS (see MULTIPLE BIRTHS).

TYMPANIC MEMBRANE is the ear-drum, which separatees the external and middle ears. (See EAR.)

TYMPANITES means distension of the abdomen due to the presence of gas or air in the intestine or in the peritoneal cavity. The abdomen when struck with the fingers, gives under these conditions a drum-like (tympanitic) note.

TYMPANUM is another name for the middle ear. (See EAR.)

TYPHOID FEVER (see ENTERIC FEVERS).

TYPHUS FEVER is an infective disease of world-wide distribution, the manifestations of which vary in different localities. The causative organisms of all forms of typhus fever belong to the genus Rickettsia. These are organisms which are intermediate between bacteria and viruses in their properties and measure 0·5 micrometre or less in diameter.

LOUSE TYPHUS, in which the infecting Rickettsia is transmitted by the louse, is of world-wide distribution. More human deaths have been attributed to the louse via typhus, louse-borne relapsing fever and trench fever, than to any other insect with the exception of the malaria mosquito. Louse typhus includes Epidemic Typhus, Brill's Disease which is a recrudescent form of Epidemic Typhus, and Trench Fever (q.v.).

EPIDEMIC TYPHUS FEVER, also known as exanthematic typhus, classical typhus, and louse-borne typhus, is an acute infection of abrupt onset which, in the absence of treatment, persists for fourteen days. It is of world-wide distribution, but is largely confined today to parts of Africa. The causative organism is the *Rickettsia prowazeki*, so-called after Ricketts and Prowazek, two brilliant investigators of typhus, both of whom died of the disease. It is transmitted by the human louse, *Pediculus humanus*. The rickettsiae can survive in the dried faeces of lice for 60 days, and these infected faeces are probably the main source of infection of man.

Symptoms: The incubation period is usually 10 to 14 days. The onset is preceded by headache, pain in the back and limbs and rigors. On the third day the temperature rises suddenly, and the face and eyes become congested. At the same time the headache becomes more intense, and the patient is drowsy or delirious. Subsequently a characteristic rash appears on the abdomen and inner aspect of the arms, to spread over the chest, back and trunk. In cases which are not going to recover, death usually occurs from heart failure about the fourteenth day. In those who recover, the temperature falls by crisis about this time. In diagnosis the Weil-Felix reaction is helpful. The death-rate is variable, varying from nearly 100 per cent in epidemics among debilitated refugees to about 10 per cent.

FLEA TYPHUS, in which the infecting Rickettsia is transmitted by the flea, is represented by Murine Typhus.

MURINE TYPHUS FEVER, also known as flea typhus, is world-wide in its distribution and is found wherever individuals are crowded to-

Louse-borne	Flea-borne	Tick-borne	Mite borne
Epidemic typhus	Murine (endemic) typhus	Rocky Mountain spotted fever	Tsutsugamushi fever
Brill's disease		African tick typhus (Tick-bite fever)	(Scrub typhus)
Trench fever		Fièvre boutonneuse	Rickettsialpox

Classification of the typhus fevers.

gether in insanitary, rat-infested areas. Hence the old names of jail-fever and ship typhus. The causative organism, *Rickettsia mooseri*, which is closely related to *R. prowazeki*, is transmitted to man by the rat-flea, *Xenopsyalla cheopis*. The rat is the main reservoir of infection. Once man is infected, the human louse may act as a transmitter of the Rickettsia from man to man. This explains how the disease may become epidemic under insanitary, crowded conditions. As a rule, however, the disease is only acquired when man comes into close contact with infected rats.

Symptoms: These are similar to those of louse-borne typhus, but the disease is usually milder, and the mortality rate is very low (about 1·5 per cent).

TICK TYPHUS, in which the infecting Rickettsia is transmitted by ticks, occurs in various parts of the world. The three best-known conditions in this group are Rocky Mountain Spotted Fever, Fièvre Boutonneuse and Tick-bite Fever.

MITE TYPHUS, in which the infecting Rickettsia is transmitted by mites, includes scrub typhus, or tsutsugamushi disease, and rickettsialpox.

RICKETTSIALPOX is a mild disease caused by *Rickettsia akari*, which is transmitted to man from infected mice by the common mouse mite, *Allodermanyssus sanguineus*. It occurs in USA, West and South Africa and USSR.

Treatment: The general principles of treatment are the same in all forms of typhus, and can be divided into prophylactic and curative.

Prophylaxis consists of either avoidance of, or destruction of, the vector. In the case of louse typhus and flea typhus, the outlook has been revolutionized by the introduction of efficient insecticides such as DDT and Gammexane. The value of the former was well shown by its use after the Second World War. This resulted in almost complete freedom from the epidemics of typhus which ravaged Eastern Europe after the 1914–18 War being responsible for 30 million cases with a mortality of 10 per cent. Now only 10,000 to 20,000 cases occur a year, with around a few hundred deaths. Efficient rat control is another measure which reduces the risk of typhus very considerably. In areas such as Malaysia, where the mites are infected from a wide variety of rodents scattered over large areas, the wearing of protective clothing is the most practical method of prophylaxis.

Curative treatment was revolutionized by the introduction of chloramphenicol and the tetracyclines. These antibiotics altered the prognosis in typhus fever very considerably. Currently the most widely used is the long-acting tetracycline, doxycycline, one single oral dose of which is said to cure the disease.

TYROSINE: An amino acid (q.v.) important in the production of catecholamines, melanin and thyroxine (qq.v.).

U

ULCER means a breach on the surface of the skin or on the surface of the membrane lining any cavity within the body, which does not tend to heal quickly.

An ulcer consists of a floor or surface, which, in consequence of the loss of tissue, is usually depressed below the surrounding healthy surface, and an edge where the healthy tissues end. The floor of a healing ulcer is composed of granulations, which are small masses of cells engaged in forming connective tissue and richly supplied with capillary blood-vessels that give the ulcer a bright-red appearance; whilst the edge shows a blue line of growing epithelial cells, which are constantly spreading inwards. In the process of healing, the fibrous tissue formed by the granulations contracts and thus draws the edges of the ulcer together and gives a puckered appearance to the scar. If anything interferes with these natural processes, the ulcer is prevented from healing.

Varieties: VARICOSE ULCER generally comes on as the result of scratching the skin of a leg which has been rendered eczematous by the bad circulation. It will not heal so long as the patient walks about, and has a great tendency to develop into a callous ulcer.

INTERNAL ULCERS develop sometimes in the mouth (see MOUTH, DISEASES OF); in the stomach (see STOMACH, DISEASES OF); in the duodenum (see DUODENAL ULCER); in the bowels (see INTESTINE, DISEASES OF); and in other parts.

SYPHLITIC ULCERS have the characters of possessing a very abrupt edge, as if punched out, and of leaving behind after healing a brownish discoloured scar. TUBERCULOUS ULCERS may arise from the bursting of a tuberculous abscess under the skin; whilst the skin disease known as lupus vulgaris is a variety of tuberculous disease.

MALIGNANT ULCERS are developed when a cancer spreads so as to involve the skin. Such an ulcer has often a very offensive smell, requiring the use of deodorant substances.

TROPHIC ULCERS are apt to appear as the result of weakened nerve influence: e.g. the deep perforating ulcer on the sole of the foot in locomotor ataxia, or bed sores in people sick of some lingering disease. (See BED SORES.)

Causes: An ulcer may be set up by any cause which damages the surface of the body and prevents immediate healing. Naturally, any constitutional condition which diminishes the vitality or the healing power of the body acts in this way, and among these causes may be mentioned old age, general ill-health, scurvy, diabetes mellitus, gout, syphilis and tuberculosis, so that wounds produced in those suffering from any of these conditions are apt to form ulcers. Defective circulation in the direction either of a poor blood supply or of the stagnation which takes place in varicose veins is another important cause. Constant movement of any part on which there is a wound is quite

1 horny layer
2 Malpighian (growing) layer
3 tissue forming floor of ulcer

4 discharge on its surface
5 Malpighian layer growing
   over the edge of the ulcer

Vertical section through the edge of a simple ulcer. On the left is the
healthy surface, to the right is the bare ulcerated surface. Magnified by 21.

sufficient to delay its healing and produce an
ulcer.

Treatment: In treating an ulcer, three objects
must be kept in view: (1) to remove the cause
of ulceration; (2) to render the floor and edge
of the ulcer healthy so that healing may begin;
(3) to assist the healing process and ward off
any continuing source of irritation.

ULCERATIVE COLITIS (see COLITIS).

ULNA is the inner of the two bones in the
forearem. It is wide at its upper end, and its
olecranon process forms the point of the elbow.
In its lower part it is more fragile and is liable
to be broken by a fall upon the forearm while
something is grasped in the hand. Chipping off
of the olecranon process is a not uncommon
result of falls upon the elbow. (See FRACTURES.)

ULOGLOSSITIS means inflammation of the
gums and of the tongue.

ULTRAFILTRATION: Filtration carried out
under pressure. Blood undergoes ultrafiltration
in the kidneys to remove the waste products,
urea and surplus water that constitute urine.

ULTRASOUND or ULTRASONICS, relate to sound
in the frequency above 15 kilocycles per second:
that is, well above the upper frequency limit of
the human ear. These frequencies are now
being used to an increasing extent in medicine.
In diagnosis they are proving useful in obstetrics in assessing the stage of pregnancy and
detecting abnormality of the fetus, in the investigation of disease in the bladder, kidneys, liver,
ovaries and pancreas, and also in the diagnosis
of brain tumours. Their great advantage is that
they do not use ionizing radiation and can
therefore be used in the very young and in
pregnant patients without problems. They can
also be repeated without doing any harm to the
patient. Ultrasound is inexpensive, rapid and
versatile and scans can be performed in any
plane. It requires no contrast agent and the

running costs are low. Its reliability is dependent on the skill of the operator. It is replacing
isotope scanning in many situations, and also
radiography. Ultrasound of the liver can separate medical from surgical jaundice in approximately 97 per cent of patients. It is very
accurate in detecting and defining cystic lesions
of the liver but is less accurate with solid lesions
and yet will detect 85 per cent of secondary
deposits. This is less than CT scanning. It is
very accurate in detecting gall-stones and more
accurate than the oral cholecystogram. It is
useful as a screening test for pancreatic disease
and can differentiate carcinoma of the pancreas
from chronic pancreatitis with 85 per cent
accuracy.

It is the first investigation indicated in patients presenting with renal failure as it can
quickly determine the size and shape of the
kidney and whether there is any obstruction to
the ureter. It is very sensitive to the presence of
dilatation of the renal tract and it will detect
space-occupying lesions, differentiating cysts
and tumours. It can detect obstruction of the
ureter due to renal stones by showing dilatations of the collecting system and the presence
of the calculus. Adrenal tumours can be demonstrated by ultrasound though it is less accurate than CT scanning. Ultrasound is now the
first test for suspected aortic aneurysm and it
can also show the presence of clot and delineate
the true and false lumen. It is good at demonstrating sub-phrenic and sub-hepatic abscesses
and will show most intra-abdominal abscesses.
CT scanning is however better for the retroperitoneal region. It has a major application in
thyroid nodules as it can differentiate cystic
from solid lesions and show the multiple lesions
characteristic of the nodular goitre. It cannot
differentiate between a follicular adenoma and
a carcinoma as both these tumours are solid.
Ultrasound cannot demonstrate normal
parathyroid glands but it can identify adenomas
provided they are more than 6 mm in diameter.
Ultrasound can differentiate masses in the
scrotum into testicular and appendicular and it
can demonstrate impalpable testicular tumours.
This is important as 15 per cent of testicular
tumours metastasize whilst they are still impalpable.

Doppler is a new technique which shows the presence of vascular disease in the carotid and peripheral vessels as it can detect the reduced blood flow through narrowed vessels.

Ultrasound has particular applications in obstetrics. A fetus can be seen with ultrasound from the seventh week of pregnancy, and the fetal heart can be demonstrated at this stage. Multiple pregnancy can also be diagnosed at this time by the demonstration of more than one gestation sac containing a viable fetus. A routine obstetric scan is usually performed between the sixteenth and eighteenth week of pregnancy when the fetus is easily demonstrated and most photogenic. The fetus can be measured to assess the gestational age and the anatomy can also be checked. Gestational age, as determined from the last menstrual period, is often inaccurate. Ultrasound enables an objective definition of the expected date of delivery. In early pregnancy, from six to twelve weeks of gestation, the crown–rump length enables a prediction to be made to within five days. After the first trimester the bi-parietal diameter of the head is used. Intra-uterine growth retardation is much more reliably diagnosed by ultrasound than by clinical assessment. The site of the placenta can also be recorded and multiple pregnancies will be diagnosed at this stage. Foetal movements and even the heart beat can be seen. A second scan is often done between the thirty-second and thirty-fourth weeks to assess the position, size and growth rate of the baby. The resolution of equipment now available enables pre-natal diagnosis of a wide range of structural abnormalities to be diagnosed. Spina bifida, hydrocephalus and anencephaly are probably the most important but other anomalies such as multicystic kidney, achondroplasia and certain congenital cardiac anomalies can also be identified. Foetal gender can be determined from twenty weeks of gestation. Ultrasound is also useful as guidance for amniocentesis.

In gynaecology polycystic ovaries can readily be detected as well as fibroids and ovarian cysts. Ultrasound can monitor follicular growth when patients are being treated with infertility drugs. It is also useful in detecting ectopic pregnancies.

Ultrasonics are being used, too, in studying the flow of the blood. Among the interesting observations here is that blood flow in the carotid artery, the main artery carrying blood to the brain, is strongly influenced by extraneous stimuli, such as the telephone's ringing or someone's entering the room. They are also being used in the treatment of Menière's disease (q.v.) and of bruises and strains. In this field of physiotherapy, ultrasonic therapy is proving of particular value in the treatment of acute injuries of soft tissue. If in such cases it is used immediately after the injury, or as soon as possible thereafter, it is claimed, there is no question of delayed, chronic recovery. For this reason it is being widely used in the treatment of sports injuries. It acts by providing a form of micro-massage. (See MASSAGE.)

ULTRAVIOLET RAYS (see LIGHT TREATMENT).

UMBILICAL CORD: the fleshy tube containing two arteries and a vein through which the mother supplies the fetus with oxygen and nutrients. The cord, which is up to 60cm long, ceases to function after birth and is clamped and cut about 2·5cm from the infant's abdominal wall. The stump shrivels and falls off within two weeks, leaving a scar which forms the umbilicus.

UMBILICUS is the technical name for the navel.

UNCINATE FIT is a state in which a patient has a hallucination of smell or of taste; it may be a manifestation of epilepsy, or the result of a tumour pressing on that part of the brain concerned with the appreciation of smell and taste.

UNCONSCIOUSNESS is a condition depending usually on some disorder of the brain, and may be of various degrees.

Varieties: Sleep is a natural form of unconsciousness due to a resting condition of the brain (see SLEEP). When the brain remains irregularly active various peculiar forms of unconsciousness or of disturbed consciousness are apt to ensue, such as delirium, somnambulism, hypnotism, catalepsy, ecstasy. (See under these headings.) In syncope, or fainting, the brain ceases to act for a time in consequence of a bloodless state, brought on by feebleness of the heart's action. In the lesser forms of epilepsy (*petit mal*), the epileptic sometimes becomes unconscious of his surroundings, though able to perform such a simple act as to take off his clothing, or to run some distance, or even to attack another person.

STUPOR is the name given to a partial state of unconsciousness from which the person can be roused for a moment by some powerful stimulus such as a shout.

COMA means a condition of complete oblivion from which the individual cannot be aroused.

Causes: Fainting is due to deficient supply of blood to the brain. Among injuries to the brain, apoplexy, compression and concussion of the brain, and inflammation affecting the brain or its membranes are the chief causes of unconsciousness. Epilepsy is also a cause of passing unconsciousness, either accompanied by a fit, or, in the slighter forms, without any such seizure. Narcotic poisons also produce stupor. The poisons that accumulate in the blood during various diseases, such as glomerulonephritis and diabetes mellitus, may produce coma, that due to the latter disease being curable by insulin.

Treatment: The cause of unconsciousness must first of all be determined. Fainting brings with it its own cure, and little is necessary beyond leaving the unconscious person recumbent. (See FAINTING.) The means of distinguishing the effects of narcotic poisons from those of stroke are given under OPIUM, and this distinction is important, since in stroke the main requirement is absolute quiet, while in opium poisoning energetic treatment is necessary. Unconsciousness, due to compression of the brain resulting from severe injury to the head, may have to be treated by trephining the skull. The unconsciousness of uraemia due to glomerulonephritis is perhaps the form most liable to be mistaken or overlooked, but doubts as to this are set at rest by examination of the urine. In this case also prompt treatment is essential if life is to be saved. For the treatment of unconsciousness due to other causes, the special symptoms present will in general indicate the cause, and the treatment is given under other headings.

UNDECYLENIC ACID is a long chain fatty acid which is of value in the treatment of tinea pedis. (See RINGWORM.)

UNDULANT FEVER is another name for brucellosis (q.v.).

UNGUAL: An adjective relating to the finger nails or toe nails.

UNGUENTUM is the Latin name for ointment.

UNIT is the term applied to a quantity assumed as a standard for measurement. Thus, the *unit of insulin* is the specific activity contained in such an amount of the standard preparation as the Medical Research Council may from time to time indicate as the quantity exactly equivalent to the unit accepted for international use. The standard preparation consists of pure, dry, crystalline insulin. (See SI UNITS.)

URACHUS is a corded structure which extends from the bladder up to the navel, and represents the remains of the canal which in the fetus joins bladder with allantois.

URAEMIA describes the clinical state which arises from renal failure. It may be due to disease of the kidneys or it may be the result of pre-renal causes where a lack of circulating blood volume inadequately perfuses the kidneys. It may result from acute tubular necrosis and it may result from obstruction to the outflow of urine.

The word uraemia means excess urea in the blood, but the symptoms of renal failure are not due to the abnormal amounts of urea circulating but to the electrolyte disturbances and acidosis which are associated with impaired renal function. The acidosis results from a decrease in the ability to filter hydrogen ions from blood into the glomerular fluid and the reduced production of ammonia and phosphate means fewer ions capable of combining with the hydrogen ions so that the total acid elimination is diminished. The fall in glomerular filtration also leads to retention of sodium and water with resulting oedema, and to retention of potassium resulting in hyperkalaemia. The most important causes of uraemia are the primary renal diseases of chronic glomerular nephritis and chronic pyelonephritis. It may also result from malignant hypertension damaging the kidneys and amyloid disease destroying the kidneys. Analgesic abuse can cause tubular necrosis. Diabetes may cause a nephropathy and lead to uraemia as may myelomatosis and systemic lupus erythematosis. Polycystic kidneys and renal tuberculosis account for a small proportion of cases.

Symptoms: Uraemia is sometimes classed as *acute*, i.e. those cases in which the symptoms develop in a few hours or days, and *chronic*, including cases in which the symptoms are less marked and last over weeks, months, or years. There is, however, no dividing line between the two, for in the chronic variety, which may be said to consist of the symptoms of chronic glomerulonephritis, an acute attack is liable to come on at any time.

Headache in the front or back of the head, accompanied often by insomnia at night and drowsiness during the day, is one of the commonest symptoms, although it is apt to be attributed to some other cause. Unconsciousness of a profound type, which may be accompanied by convulsions resembling those of epilepsy, is the most outstanding feature of an acute attack and is a very dangerous condition.

Still another symptom, which often precedes an acute attack, is severe vomiting without apparent cause. The appetite is always poor, and the onset of diarrhoea is a serious sign.

Treatment: The treatment of the chronic type of uraemia includes all the measures which should be taken by a person suffering from chronic glomerulonephritis. An increasing number of these patients, especially the younger ones, are treated with dialysis and/or renal transplantation. (See KIDNEY, ARTIFICIAL; TRANSPLANTATION.)

URATES (see URIC ACID).

UREA, or CARBAMIDE, is a crystalline substance of the chemical formula $CO(NH_2)_2$, which is very soluble in water or alcohol. It is the chief waste product discharged from the body in the urine, being formed in the liver and carried to the kidneys in the blood. The amount varies considerably with the quantity and nature of the food taken, rising greatly upon an animal (protein) dietary. It also rises during the continuance of a fever. The average amount excreted daily, during health, on a mixed diet is about 33 to 35 grams.

Urea is administered for its diuretic action, and also as a test of kidney action, in doses of 5 to 15 grams. It is used, too, as a cream in the treatment of certain skin diseases, characterized by a dry skin, such as ichythyosis (q.v.).

Urea is rapidly changed, by a yeast-like micro-organism, into carbonate of ammonia; and to this chemical change the ammoniacal smell of badly kept latrines is due.

UREAPLASMA is a group of micro-organisms which plays a larger part in the causation of disease than was at one time suspected. One of them, *Ureaplasma urealyticum*, is now recognized as a cause of chronic prostatitis, nonspecific urethritis (see URETHRA, DISEASES OF.) and infertility.

URETER is the tube, about the thickness of a goose-quill, which on each side leads from the corresponding kidney down to the bladder. Each ureter begins above at the pelvis of its kidney and after a course of 25 to 30 cm (10 to 12 inches) through the loins and pelvis it opens by a narrow slit into the base of the bladder. The lower end pierces the wall of the bladder so obliquely (lying embedded in the wall for about 21 mm) that, though urine runs freely into the bladder, it is prevented from returning up the ureter as the bladder becomes distended.

URETHRA is the tube which leads from the bladder to the exterior, and by which the urine is voided. It is about 20 cm (8 inches) long in the male and 3·5 cm (1½ inches) long in the female.

URETHRA, DISEASES OF: The chief conditions which cause pain in the urethra, or interfere with the passage of urine, are urethritis or inflammation of the mucous lining, and stricture or narrowing of the tube.
URETHRITIS is often difficult to tell from inflammation of the bladder (cystitis), which, however, it may accompany and of which it is often the cause.
Causes: The most frequent cause of urethritis is gonorrhoea (q.v.), and this disease produces the most severe type of inflammation. Another common cause is the condition known as nonspecific urethritis (see NON-SPECIFIC GENITAL INFECTION). Like gonorrhoea, it is a venereal disease. Gout is another cause, producing its effects either owing to the repeated passage of irritating gravel with the urine, or to a highly acid state of this excretion. The damage caused by the passage of a rough stone from the bladder or of a catheter unskilfully introduced may also occasion a severe urethritis; and various drugs or articles of diet, such as alcohol or arsenic, may bring on an attack in those who are liable to suffer from it.
Symptoms: The symptoms consist chiefly in the constant oozing out of a small quantity of pus from the orifice of the urethra, a sense of scalding pain whenever urine is passed, increased redness of the mucous membrane as seen at the orifice, and tenderness along the course of the urethra. Subsequently, inflammation in neighbouring organs, e.g. the bladder, testicle, or even kidney, may be set up.
Treatment: This varies with the cause of the

inflammation, but in all cases the drinking of milk, water, and other bland fluids in large quantities is of advantage in order to flush out the urethra. The sulphonamide drugs and penicillin are highly effective in the treatment of gonorrhoea. The disease causing the inflammation requires special treatment according to its nature. (See also NON-SPECIFIC GENITAL INFECTION.)
STRICTURE is an abrupt narrowing of the tube at one or more places.
Varieties and causes: SPASMODIC or CONGESTIVE STRICTURE is a temporary condition which is not of much importance. It follows upon exposure to cold, excessive exercise like bicycling, alcoholic indulgence, and often upon operations near the urethra, such as that for piles. It prevents the passage of urine for a few hours or days. It is treated simply by a warm sitz-bath or warm fomentations to the fork, and, if necessary, the urine is drawn off by means of a soft or flexible catheter passed along the urethra and through the stricture.
ORGANIC STRICTURE is a much more serious condition. It is a scar, due to previous injury or ulceration of the mucous membrane, which, by contracting after the manner of all scars, produces narrowing of the urethral tube. This scar is almost always due to one or other of two conditions: severe laceration of the urethra as the result of injury, or long-continued chronic inflammation.
A stricture almost always occurs at one of two points: either just within the orifice of the urethra or in the fork, or crotch, where the urethra turns upwards as it enters the pelvis.
Symptoms: An organic stricture is of slow development, and gives rise at first to few symptoms beyond those of the urethritis, which causes it. As the stricture narrows, the stream of urine becomes smaller than natural, and there is straining and pain each time it is voided. Occasional attacks of spasmodic stricture are brought on by injudicious acts on the part of the person who already has an organic stricture; and this further narrowing of the tube causes complete stoppage of the urine for a time, accompanied by great pain, which results from distension of the bladder. After a stricture has lasted some years, unless it has been very carefully treated, and the person has led a well-ordered life, inflammation of the bladder almost certainly comes on, and the death of the patient may ultimately ensue from the spread of this inflammation upwards to the kidneys.
The existence, position, and calibre of a stricture are verified by the surgeon, who passes metal bougies of various sizes along the urethra.
Treatment: The diet should be simple and constipation must be prevented. By these means unnecessary irritation of the stricture is avoided, and thus spasmodic attacks with retention of the urine are warded off.
To check the gradual narrowing of the stricture some operative procedure is necessary, and, according to the situation and nature of the stricture, it is either *dilated* by means of

bougies passed along the urethra, or it is divided by a special instrument passed along the urethra (*internal urethrotomy*), or by an incision made through the fork (*external urethrotomy*). After-treatment, consisting in the passage of a bougie at regular intervals of some weeks or months, is necessary after any of these operations, in order to counteract the permanent tendency of the stricture to contract,

INJURIES TO THE URETHRA may follow a severe crush which has fractured the pelvis, or a fall astride of some object. The signs of this are the presence of blood in the urine, or inability to pass urine at all, after such an accident. The great risks are the occurrence of an abscess round the urethra, and the formation of a stricture at a later period.

URETHRITIS means inflammation of the urethra (q.v.).

URIC ACID is a crystalline substance, very slightly soluble in water, of chemical formula, $C_5N_4H_4O_3$. It is white in the pure state, but when found as a urinary deposit it is reddish-brown, presenting a supposed resemblance to cayenne pepper. The bi-urate of sodium and urate of ammonium occur in considerable amount in the urine during a feverish state or after great exertion, and produce, as the urine cools, a dense pink or yellow sediment. The average daily quantity of uric acid passed by human beings is 0·5 to 1 gram. In the urine of birds and reptiles uric acid is the chief nitrogenous constituent, taking the place of the urea excreted by human beings. Uric acid is formed in the liver and removed by the kidneys from the blood. The amount is increased in the following conditions: (*a*) Excessive consumption of meat, combined with sedentary habits. (*b*) Gout (see GOUT). (*c*) Diseases in which the white corpuscles of the blood are increased: e.g. leukaemia.

Owing to their insolubility, uric acid and the various urates often produce deposits in the urinary passages, which are known as urinary sand, gravel, or stones according to their size.

URINALYSIS: Analysis of the physical and chemical composition of urine (q.v.) to detect variations in the substances normally present and to identify abnormal constituents such as sugar, drugs, blood, or alcohol.

URINARY ORGANS form the system by which the urine is extracted from the blood, stored up, and from time to time discharged from the body. They comprise the two kidneys placed in the loins, two ureters leading from them to the bladder which is situated in the front of the pelvis, and the urethra which leads from the floor of the bladder out beneath the pubic bones to the exterior. (See BLADDERS; KIDNEYS; URETER; URETHRA.)

URINE is the excretion produced by the kidneys, and consists chiefly of waste substances resulting from the activity of the body, dissolved in water. The function of the kidneys consists almost entirely in selecting these substances from the blood; their actual formation takes place in the liver, muscles, etc. The urine and the perspiration are to a great extent interdependent; thus, in hot weather the amount of urine tends to decrease as more fluid is lost in perspiration, whilst the converse happens in cold weather. If the kidneys are acting vigorously the skin becomes very dry, whilst if there has been much perspiration, as in fevers, the urine is small in amount and highly concentrated. The amount of water lost from the body daily by perspiration is, in health, about half the amount passed as urine, and, though the sweat contains little of the waste material present in the urine, the glands of the skin can be made to take up the function of the kidneys to some extent when the latter organs are diseased. (See GLOMERULONEPHRITIS.) Many poisons taken into the body are excreted by way of the urine, e.g. morphine and strychnine, and so also are the germs of many diseases, e.g. those of typhoid fever.

Composition: About 96 per cent of the urine is water, the remaining 4 per cent being solids dissolved in it. Of the solids, far the most important is urea, of which there is, on an average, 25 grams in 1 litre. Common salt stands next in quantity, the average amount in 1 litre of urine being 9 grams. Phosphates and sulphates are also important constituents combined with potassium, sodium, calcium, and magnesium, whilst there is less than 1 gram each of uric acid, and ammonia, and just over 1 gram of creatinine.

Pigments are also present in the urine, and to them its colour is due. These pigments, the chief of which is urochrome, are derived indirectly from the colouring matter of the blood, and are produced also by the liver.

Amount: The amount of urine passed daily is about 1500 millilitres, subject to the variations mentioned above. A child, of course, passes much less than an adult; the average daily amount is: 430 ml at two years; 570 ml at four years; 850 ml at seven years; and 1140 ml at twelve years.

The amount of urine is *increased* in some diseases, of which diabetes is the chief. In other conditions it is *diminished*, notably in acute glomerulonephritis, in fevers and feverish states generally, and in heart failure.

COMPLETE STOPPAGE of the urine may occur for a time in the feverish conditions of children, or it may be due to acute glomerulonephritis, when the condition is a very serious one. When the stoppage is due to failure of the kidneys to secrete any urine, the condition is known as *suppression* or *anuria*. When the stoppage is due to such a cause as blockage of the ureters by stones or of the urethra by a stricture, although secretion by the kidneys still goes on, it is known as *retention*.

Colour: The tint of normal urine is generally

described as straw or amber coloured, but it may be considerably changed by various diseases or drugs.

PALLOR, giving the urine a watery appearance, is found in diabetes and in chronic glomerulonephritis, also in people who drink large quantities of water.

ORANGE OR RED COLOUR may appear when senna, beetroot or rhubarb has been taken; when blood is present the colour may be pink or bright red; urates cause a turbid red or yellow appearance.

SMOKY TINT, depriving the urine of transparency, is caused by small quantities of blood.

GREEN OR GREENISH-YELLOW urine is usually due to bile, or may be produced by taking santonin or quinine.

Odour: Healthy urine has a faint aromatic odour, but when it begins to decompose, an unpleasant ammoniacal smell is given off. Thus the presence of cystitis or of dribbling of the urine is betrayed by the odour of the patient's personal or bed clothes. Various items of diet may give a distinctive odour to the urine. Thus spinach may produce an acrid smell, mushrooms a fetid odour and truffles a stagnant smell. Cold meat containing preservatives may produce a smell that has been described as like boot polish. Many soups are fortified with glutamates and may give an ammoniacal smell, whilst garlic yields its characteristic odour to the urine as well as the breath.

Specific gravity of urine varies in health from 1015 to 1025 (distilled water being 1000). A urine of lower specific gravity suggests the presence of chronic glomerulonephritis, whilst a higher specific gravity may be due to diabetes mellitus, or to a feverish state.

Reaction: When the urine is tested with litmus paper the reaction is usually acid, and this is of importance, because the acid has an antiseptic action. This acidity is due, not to free acids, but to acid salts such as acid phosphate of sodium. In consequence of the secretion of acid from the blood into the gastric juice that is poured into the stomach shortly after meals, the urine may at such times become alkaline. In herbivorous animals and in vegetarians, owing to the great quantities of alkaline salts eaten in the diet, the urine is permanently alkaline.

Deposits: In healthy urine there is usually a fleecy deposit of mucus secreted by the mucous membrane of the urinary passages. A pink or yellow deposit, that settles as soon as the urine begins to cool, and that often leaves a stain upon the utensil in which the urine has stood, is due to urates. (See URIC ACID.) Uric acid is a rarer deposit, and, when present, falls in very scanty yellow or brownish, so-called 'cayenne-pepper' grains.

Abnormal substances: Many unusual substances taken into or formed in the body are got rid of in the urine, sometimes just as they have entered the body, in other cases considerably changed, e.g. drugs, and the poisons of various diseases. Further, various bacteria and parasites can be discovered in the urine in some diseases. Chemical or microscopical examination is necessary in order to reveal these, but there are six substances the detection of which is important in diagnosing diseases. These substances are (1) albumin; (2) blood; (3) sugar; (4) pus and tube-casts; (5) bile; (6) acetone. Strip tests, which merely involve the placing in urine of small specially impregnated strips of paper, are available for all of these, except pus and tube-casts.

URINE, EXCESS OF: The amount of urine passed in 24 hours is often markedly increased in diabetes mellitus, a fact which sometimes, without any other symptom, attracts the patient's attention. Any source of irritation or inflammation in the kidneys or bladder may also produce frequency, such as the formation of gravel or of a stone, tuberculosis of the kidney, inflammation of the bladder (cystitis), or enlargement of the prostate gland. The bladder, however, varies greatly in size in different individuals, and the necessity to pass water frequently may simply be a life-long personal peculiarity due to smallness of its capacity.

Increase in the urine at night may lead to wetting of the bed by children. (See NOCTURNAL ENURESIS.)

Treatment: Any increase in the amount of urine or the frequency with which it is passed calls for testing for the presence of sugar, albumin, gravel, pus, and the like. The treatment consists in that suited to any disease that may be discovered.

URINE, RETENTION OF: The term, retention, is applied to cases in which urine is duly secreted by the kidneys, but for some reason is retained in the bladder; while the more serious condition, in which the kidneys fail to produce urine, is known as suppression or anuria. (See URINE, amount.)

Causes: The urine may be retained either because the bladder is too weak to expel it, or because of some obstruction to the passage by which it should be voided. Weakness is a rare condition and is generally the result of some damage to the nervous system, this being one of the troublesome symptoms that follow an injury to the spinal cord; it is accompanied by dribbling away of the urine when the bladder becomes fully distended. A similar condition results from long-continued distension produced by some obstruction to the outflow.

Among the cases due to obstruction, some are acute and merely temporary, such as the difficulty of passing water that follows upon any operation near the bladder, e.g. one for piles, or that is apt to follow child-birth. In these cases the difficulty commonly is due to spasm, and does not persist more than a day or two. Among the more chronic cases of retention the commonest are those caused by enlargement of the prostate gland and consequent blockage of the outlet from the bladder; this condition is common in old men. In these the retention usually comes on gradually, and it is a common experience to find that the bladder never empties completely as it ought to do, but forms a sort of reservoir from which an overflow is discharged every few hours. The condition that leads to the most complete form of retention is a stricture or narrowing of the urethra due to the scar of previous injury or ulceration. (See URETHRA, DISEASES OF.) Similar blockage results also, in rare instances, from the pressure of some tumour upon the urethra, or the displacement of a neighbouring organ such as the womb in women.

Treatment: Cases in which retention is due to weakness of the bladder, in a chronic invalid, may be treated by the regular use of a soft rubber catheter, and this forms one of the most important duties in the nursing of such a case.

In any case of retention where the urine accumulates in and causes painful distension of the bladder, the condition may often be relieved by the sufferer's placing himself in a warm bath. This produces so much relaxation that the bladder often succeeds in emptying itself.

If relief is not gained by these means, the doctor may withdraw the urine by means of a catheter passed along the urethra. (See CATHETERS.) The instrument chosen varies according to the cause of the retention; thus, in cases due to weakness of the bladder or to moderate spasm at the outlet, a soft rubber catheter only is necessary. In cases of severer spasm, and in cases where the prostate gland is enlarged, a flexible instrument or a hard rubber catheter with a bend upon the point (known as a *coudé* catheter) is generally chosen; while, in cases of very narrow stricture, the surgeon may require to pass a rigid metal instrument. As a rule, great difficulty is experienced only in the last-named class of cases; and in them it may occasionally be necessary to tap the bladder above the pubis by means of a hollow needle.

URINOMETER or DENSIMETER, is a simple instrument designed for estimating the specific gravity of urine.

UROBILINOGEN: Urobilinogen is a chemical compound formed when bacteria in the intestine act on bilirubin (q.v.). Some is reabsorbed and returns to the liver and some is eliminated in the faeces.

URODYNAMICS: The measurement of the pressures within the bladder (q.v.) as well as the pressures of the urethral sphincter. The technique is useful in the investigation of patients with urinary incontinence. Special equipment is needed to carry out the procedure.

UROKINASE is an enzyme (q.v.) obtained from urine which dissolves blood clots. It is sometimes used in the treatment of pulmonary embolism (q.v.).

UROLOGY is that branch of medicine which treats of disorders and diseases of the kidneys, ureters, bladder, prostate, and urethra.

URSODEOXYCHOLIC ACID is a preparation used in the treatment of cholesterol gallstones (see GALL-BLADDER, DISEASES OF).

URTICARIA or NETTLE-RASH is a disorder of the skin characterized by an eruption resembling the effect produced by the sting of a nettle, namely, raised red or red-and-white patches, occurring in parts or over the whole of the surface of the body, and attended with great itching and irritation. It may be acute or chronic.

Causes: In some cases the attack appears to be connected with digestive derangements, or the taking of some foods particularly of a protein nature, such as various kinds of meat, fish, shell-fish, also occasionally from the use of certain drugs, such as penicillin. In some it is due to the injection of sera, or may follow the bite of an insect. In others it is due to exposure to cold – so-called cold urticaria – and occasionally may be the result of effort. There remains a considerable number of cases in which it is difficult to incriminate any one specific casual factor. The general consensus of opinion is that urticaria is an allergic reaction on the part of the affected individual to some substance to which he or she is hypersensitive. In other words, it comes into the same category as asthma and hay fever. In all three conditions the individual is allergic to some factor or factors, but the allergic response varies: in asthma it is the bronchioles of the lungs that are involved; in hay fever it is the mucous membrane of the nasopharynx, sinuses and eyes; whilst in urticaria it is the skin that gives the allergic response.

Symptoms: In severe cases there is at first considerable feverishness and constitutional disturbance, together with sickness and faintness, which either precede or accompany the appearance of the rash. The eruption may appear on any part of the body, but is most common on the face and trunk. In the former position is causes swelling and disfigurement while it lasts, and is apt to excite alarm in those unacquainted with its nature. The attack may pass off in a few hours, or may last for several days, the eruption continuing to come out insuccessive patches. The lesions are accompanied by severe itching. Occasionally a similar process takes place in the throat, and there is then considerable danger from blockage of the larynx. (See also ALLERGY.)

Treatment: The treatment of urticaria has been revolutionized by the introduction of the antihistamine drugs. There is now a large number of these, and it is necessary to find which particular preparation suits a particular individual. In addition, it is necessary to discover, if possible, the causative factor and to remove it. For instance, if an attack always follows the taking of a certain article of diet, this should be carefully noted and avoided in future.

UTERUS or WOMB, is a hollow organ suspended in the cavity of the pelvis. In shape, it is triangular from side to side, and flattened from before backwards. The lower angle is prolonged into a rounded neck (*cervix*), about 2·5 cm (1 inch) long, which communicates through a narrow opening or mouth (*os uteri*) with the vagina, the passage leading to the exterior of the body. In size, the normal uterus is only about 7·5 cm (3 inches) long, 5 cm (2 inches) in its greatest width, and 2·5 cm (1 inch) in thickness from front to back, while the walls are so thick that the cavity consists of a mere slit. It weighs 30 to 40 grams. During pregnancy, however, it enlarges to an enormous extent, and the walls increase still further in thickness. (See MUSCLE.) The cavity is lined by a thick, soft, mucous membrane, and the wall is chiefly composed of muscle fibres arranged in three layers. The outer surface, like that of other abdominal organs, is covered by a layer of peritoneum. The uterus has a copious supply of blood derived from the uterine and ovarian arteries. It has also many lymphatic vessels, and its nerves establish wide connections with other organs. (See PAIN.) The position of the uterus is in the centre of the pelvis, where it is suspended by several ligaments between the bladder in front and the rectum behind. On each side of the uterus are the broad ligaments passing outwards to the side of the pelvis, the utero-sacral ligament passing back to the sacral bone, the utero-vesical ligament passing forwards to the bladder, and the round ligament uniting the uterus to the front of the abdomen.

UTERUS, DISEASES OF: Among the most common symptoms are pain or irregularity in the menstrual functions, the presence of a white discharge (*leucorrhoea*), constant pain or sense of weakness in the back, and often the inability to bear children.

MALFORMATIONS sometimes occur and give rise to trouble in child-birth: for example, the uterus may be double, having a partition down the middle. The cervix may be long and furnished with a very narrow mouth.

DISPLACEMENTS are more common. The uterus is slung in the centre of the pelvic cavity, and has great freedom of movement up and down and from before backwards. It lies naturally with its long axis directed upwards and forwards between the bladder and rectum, but its position at any time varies considerably according to the state of distension of one or other of these organs. A flabby state of the muscular wall of the uterus, or a contraction of some of the ligaments that suspend it, may produce a bend upon the organ itself, or may permanently tilt it forwards or backwards. Bending forwards is known as *anteflexion*, tilting forwards is called *anteversion*, and the corresponding conditions towards the back are known as *retroflexion* and *retroversion*.

Downward displacement is known as *prolapse*, and in this condition the uterus slips bodily downwards in the space between the bladder and bowel, till, in bad cases, it may actually protrude from the vagina. The condition comes on in older women, usually those who are overweight and have in child-birth suffered laceration of the parts that should support the uterus. When the condition is slight it may be relieved by wearing a suitably shaped pessary, and in cases which are not relieved by this simple measure an operation (colporrhaphy), designed to repair the injury previously done, will often remedy the displacement.

INFLAMMATION is, perhaps, the commonest type of uterine disorder. It is of several forms, but the general term *endometritis* is applied to inflammation affecting the mucous membrane, *metritis* to the rarer condition in which the muscular substance is involved. This condition is often due to child-birth which has not passed off quite successfully; and it is still more often due to miscarriage. Inflammation spreading upwards from the vagina, and displacements of the uterus are other, though less common, causes. The usual treatment consists in rest, the employment of hot, antiseptic douches and other applications to the vagina. The sulphonamides or penicillin are given in severe cases. The interior of the uterus may be improved by the operation of curetting, which consists in scraping away the unhealthy mucous membrane with a special instrument, the curette.

TUMOURS of the uterus include fibroids and cancer.

FIBROID TUMOURS, or fibromyomas, are the most common form of tumour in any part of the body. They consist of masses of muscle fibres, similar to those of the uterus, and white fibrous tissue. They vary in size from that of a small seed to a mass weighing several pounds. The cause is not known, but they are much more common in women who have never borne children than in those with children. Whilst they may occur any time between puberty and the change of life, they are usually first recognized between the ages of 35 and 45. The symptoms depend upon the size and site of the tumour, and many fibroids give rise to no symptoms at all. The more important symptoms and signs are menstrual irregularity with of excessive loss of blood or excessive length of the period, sterility, frequency of micturition, and retention of urine. Pain is seldom a marked feature. Only those fibroids causing symptoms require treatment. If the symptoms are at all severe, operation is the treatment of choice.

CANCER OF THE UTERUS is one of the most common forms of cancer in women. It may occur in either the neck (or cervix) or the body of the uterus. Cancer of the cervix is more common than cancer of the body, and 95 per cent of cases occur in women who have borne children. Cancer of the body, on the other hand, is more common in unmarried women or women who have never borne children, and is rare before the menopause. The first sign is usually a blood-stained discharge. Treatment

1 peritoneum	6 clitoris	10 internal sphincter ani
2 uterus	7 labium minis	11 coccyx
3 bladder	8 labium majus	12 rectum
4 symphysis pubis	9 external sphincter ani	13 sacrum
5 urethra		

The female sex organs.

consists of radiotherapy or surgery or a combination of both. The earlier the cancer is detected and treated, the better the results. This is why it is so important that any woman over the age of 40 who has either excessive loss at the period, or irregular bleeding, should report at once to her doctor. In most cases there will be nothing serious to worry about, but if the bleeding should be due to cancer, then early diagnosis will permit of treatment being carried out at a stage when the expectation of cure is high. It is in the early diagnosis of cancer of the cervix, which tends to occur at an earlier age, that cervical cytology, as it is known, is so important. This consists of the simple procedure of taking a 'smear' of the cervix for examination in the laboratory. Such examination may reveal the presence of cancer long before it has produced any symptoms and signs, and treatment at this stage produces excellent results. It is recommended that a woman should have this procedure carried out every five years from the age of 30 to that of 70. In 1986, in England and Wales 7,800 cases of cancer of the uterus were reported: 3,800 involving the body, and over 4,000 the cervix.

UVEA is a term applied to the middle coat of the eye, including the iris, ciliary body and choroid.

UVEITIS: An inflammation of the uveal tract. *Iritis* is inflammation of the iris, *cyclitis* inflammation of the ciliary body and *choroiditis* inflammation of the choroid. The symptoms and signs vary according to which part of the uveal tract is involved and tend to be recurrent. The patient may experience varying degrees of discomfort or pain, with or without blurring of vision. The eye may be red or appear white. In many cases a cause is never found. Some known associations include various types of arthritis, some bowel diseases, virus illnesses, tuberculosis, syphilis, parasites and fungi. Treatment is with anti-inflammatory drops and occasionally tablets (e.g. steroid eye drops and tablets), plus drops to dilate the pupil.

UVULA is the small mass of muscle covered by mucous membrane that hangs down from the middle of the soft palate on its posterior aspect. Very rarely the structure is excessively long and may require trimming. Generally though its function is not certain and it seldom causes problems.

V

VACCINATION, from *vacca*, Latin for cow, means inoculation with the material of cowpox, performed to afford protection to the inoculated person against an attack of smallpox, or at all events with the view of diminishing the seriousness of, and averting a fatal result from, any such attack. This is the strict sense of the term, but it is used nowadays to describe the process of inoculating with any vaccine to obtain immunity, or protection, against the corresponding disease.

VACCINE is the name applied generally to a substance of the nature of dead or attenuated living infectious material introduced into the body with the object of increasing its power to resist or to get rid of a disease. (See also IMMUNITY.)

In cases where healthy people are inoculated with vaccine as a protection against a particular disease, this is done to produce antibodies which will confer immunity against a subsequent attack of the disease. (See IMMUNIZATION for programme of immunization during childhood.)

Vaccines may be divided into two classes: stock vaccines, prepared from micro-organisms known to cause a particular disease and kept in readiness for use against that disease; and autogenous vaccines, prepared from micro-organisms which are already in the patient's body and to which the disease is due. Vaccines intended to protect against the onset of disease are necessarily of the stock variety.

AUTOGENOUS VACCINES are prepared from the cultivation of bacteria found in the expectoration, the urine, the faeces, and in areas of inflammation such as boils. This type of vaccine was introduced by Wright about 1903.

ANTHRAX VACCINE was introduced by Pasteur about 1882 for the protection of sheep and cattle against this disease. A safe and effective vaccine for use in human beings has now been evolved.

BCG VACCINE is used to provide protection against tuberculosis. BCG vaccination is usually considered for five main groups of people:
(1) Schoolchildren: the routine programme in schools usually covers children aged between 10 and 14
(2) Students including those in teacher training colleges
(3) Children and new-born infants in families of Asian origin because of the high incidence of tuberculosis in this ethnic group
(4) Health service workers and others liable to infection at work
(5) Household contacts of people known to have active tuberculosis and new-born infants in households where there is a history of tuberculosis.
(See BCG VACCINE.)

CHOLERA VACCINE was introduced by Haffkine in India about 1894. Two injections are given at an interval of at least a week; this gives a varying degree of immunity for six months.

DIPHTHERIA VACCINE is available in several forms. (See DIPHTHERIA.) It is usually given along with tetanus and pertussis vaccine in what is known as Triple Vaccine. This is given in three doses: the first at the age of 3 or 6 months, the second six to eight weeks later, and the third six months later, with a booster dose at the age of 5 years.

HAY FEVER VACCINE is a vaccine prepared from the pollen of various grasses. It is used in gradually increasing doses for prevention of hay fever in those susceptible to this condition.

INFLUENZA VACCINE: a vaccine is now available for protection against influenza due to the influenza viruses A and B.

MEASLES, MUMPS AND RUBELLA VACCINES are given in combination early in the second year of life.

PERTUSSIS (WHOOPING-COUGH) VACCINE is prepared from *Bordetella pertussis*, and is usually given along with diphtheria and tetanus in what is known as Triple Vaccine. This is given in three doses: the first at the age of 2 to 6 months, the second and the third at four-week intervals, with a booster dose at 5 years.

PLAGUE VACCINE was introduced by Haffkine, and appears to give useful protection, but the duration of protection is relatively short: from two to twenty months. Two injections are given at an interval of 4 weeks. A reinforcing dose should be given annually to anyone exposed to the disease.

POLIOMYELITIS VACCINE gives a high degree of protection against the disease.

This is given in the form of attenuated Sabin vaccine which is taken by mouth – a few drops on a lump of sugar. Reinforcing doses of polio vaccine are recommended on school entry, on leaving school, and on travel abroad to countries where poliomyelitis is endemic.

RABIES VACCINE was introduced by Pasteur in 1885 for administration, during the long incubation period, to people bitten by a mad dog, in order to prevent the disease from developing.

RUBELLA VACCINE, usually given with mumps and measles vaccine in one dose, now provides protection against German measles. It also provides immunity for adolescent girls who have not had the disease in childhood and so ensures that they will not acquire the disease during any subsequent pregnancy, thus reducing the number of congenitally abnormal children whose abnormality is the result of their being infected with German measles via their mothers before they were born. The recommendation is that it should be given to all girls at the age of 10 to 14 years who have not had the vaccine in infancy, and to all women of child-bearing age shown on a blood test not to be immune – but not during pregnancy.

SMALLPOX VACCINE was the first introduced. As a result of the World Health Organization's (WHO) successful smallpox eradication campaign – it declared the disease eradicated in 1980 – there is now no medical justification for smallpox vaccination.

TETANUS VACCINE is given in two forms: (*a*) In the so-called Triple Vaccine, combined with diphtheria and pertussis (whooping-cough) vaccine. This is used for the routine immunization of children, the first dose being given at the age of 3 to 6 months, a second dose six to eight weeks later, and a third dose six months later. A booster dose of tetanus vaccine is recommended on leaving school, on entering higher education, or on starting employment. (*b*) By itself to adults who have not been immunized in childhood and who are particularly exposed to the risk of tetanus, such as soldiers and agricultural workers.

TYPHOID VACCINE was introduced by Wright and Semple for the protection of troops in the South African War and in India. TAB vaccine, containing *Salmonella typhi* (the causative organism of typhoid fever) and *Salmonella paratyphi* A and B (the organisms of paratyphoid fever) has now been replaced by Typhoid Monovalent Vaccine, containing only *S. typhi*. The change has been made because the monovalent vaccine is less likely to produce painful arms and general malaise and there is no evidence that the TAB vaccine gave any protection against paratyphoid fever. Two doses are given at an interval of four to six weeks, and give protection for one to three years.

YELLOW FEVER VACCINE is prepared from chick embryos injected with the living, attenuated strain (17D) of pantropic virus. Only one injection is required, and immunity persists for many years. Reinoculation, however, is desirable every ten years.

The hazards of vaccination, or immunization are minimal, compared with its benefits. Complications, however, do occur. A Vaccine Damage Payments Scheme has therefore been introduced. This provides for the payment of £10,000 tax free in respect of people who, since 5 July 1948 have suffered severe damage as a result of the following vaccinations which have taken place under routine public policy programmes: diphtheria, tetanus, whooping-cough, poliomyelitis, measles, German measles, tuberculosis (BCG), and smallpox (up to 31 July 1971).

VACCINIA is another term for cowpox, a disease in which vesicles form on the udders and teats, due to the same virus as is responsible for smallpox in man. It is also the term used to describe the reaction to smallpox vaccination.

VACUOLE: A space inside the cytoplasm of the cell. It is formed by a folding in of the cellular membrane when the cell ingests material from the outside – for example, when white blood cells attack bacteria.

VAGINA is the lower part of the female reproductive tract. It is a muscular passage leading from the labial entrance to the womb. It is lined with mucous membrane and receives the erect penis during sexual intercourse. The semen is ejaculated into the upper part of the vagina and from there the sperms must pass through the cervix and uterus to fertilize the ovum in the fallopian tube.

VAGINISMUS is spasmodic contraction of the opening of the vagina on attempted coitus. It is usually psychological in origin, due, for instance, to a neurotic temperament or to frigidity, but it may also be due to some local inflammatory condition.

VAGINITIS is inflammation of the vagina. (See LEUCORRHOEA.)

VAGOTOMY is the operation of cutting the fibres of the vagus nerve to the stomach. It is sometimes performed as part of the surgical treatment of duodenal ulcer, the aim being to reduce the flow or acidity of the gastric juice.

VAGUS, or PNEUMOGASTRIC, nerve is the tenth cranial nerve. Unlike the other cranial nerves, which are concerned with the special senses, or distributed to the skin and muscles of the head and neck, this nerve, as its names imply, strays downwards into the chest and abdomen, supplying branches to the throat, lungs, heart, stomach, and other abdominal organs. It contains motor, secretory, sensory, and vasodilator fibres.

VALGUS means literally knock-kneed, and is a bending inward at the knees (*genu valgum*), or at the ankle, as occurs in flat-foot (*pes valgus*).

VALVES are found in the heart, veins, and lymphatic vessels, for the purpose of maintaining the circulation of the blood and lymph always in one direction. (See HEART; LYMPH; VEINS.)

VALVULAR DISEASE (see HEART DISEASES).

VALVOTOMY: An operation that opens a stenosed heart valve and allows it to function properly again. Various techniques are used including a dilating instrument, a balloon or open-heart surgery.

VANCOMYCIN is an antibiotic derived from streptomyces, which is active against a wide range of Gram-positive organisms, including the staphylococcus.

VAN DEN BERGH TEST is one performed on a specimen of serum of the blood in cases of jaundice, to decide whether this is due to ordinary bile (immediate or direct reaction) or incompletely formed bile pigment (delayed or indirect reaction).

VAPORIZER: A device that turns water or a drug into a fine spray, thus enabling medicine to be taken by inhalation. It is used, for example, in the treatment of asthma.

VARICELLA is another name for chickenpox (q.v.).

VARICOCOELE means a condition in which the veins of the testicle are distended. (See TESTICLE, DISEASES OF.)

VARICOSE VEINS are veins that have become stretched and dilated. (See VEINS, DISEASES OF.)

VARIOLA is another name for smallpox (q.v.).

VARIX means an enlarged and tortuous vein.

VARUS, meaning bow-legged, is the term applied to a bulging condition at the hip (*coxa vara*), at the knee (*genu varum*), or at the ankle (*talipes varus*).

VAS is the Latin term for a vessel, especially a blood-vessel.

VASCULAR: Relating to the blood vessels.

VASCULITIS: Inflammation of the blood vessels. This may damage the lining of the vessels and cause narrowing or blockage, thus restricting blood flow. This, in turn, may harm or destroy the tissues supplied by the affected blood vessels. Vasculitis is probably caused by small particles called immune complexes, circulating in the blood, that adhere to the vessel walls and provoke inflammation. Normally these complexes are consumed by the white blood cells.

VASECTOMY is the surgical operation performed to render men sterile, or infertile. It consists of ligating, or tying, and then cutting the ductus, or vas, deferens (see TESTICLE). It is quite a simple operation carried out under local anaesthesia, through a small incision, or cut (or sometimes two) in the upper part of the scrotum. It has no effect on sexual drive or ejaculation, and does not cause impotency. It is not immediately effective, and several tests, spread over several months, must be carried out before it is safe to assume that sterility has been achieved. Although, in those who desire it, fertility can sometimes be restored by a further operation, to restore the continuity of the vas, this cannot be guaranteed, and only seems to occur in about one-fifth of those so operated on.

VASO-ACTIVE INTESTINAL PEPTIDE (VIP) was isolated in 1970. It stimulates the intestinal secretion of water and electrolytes, inhibits gastric secretion and promotes hyperglycaemia. It also has a secretin-like action on the pancreas, stimulating the production of pancreatic juice. It is secreted by the non-beta cells of the pancreas. Tumours of these cells, which are uncommon, provoke a watery diarrhoea syndrome or what is sometimes called pancreatic cholera.

VAS DEFERENS: A narrow tube that leads from each testis through the prostate gland to join a tube from the seminal vesicles to form the ejaculatory duct. Sperm and seminal fluid pass through this duct during ejaculation (see TESTICLE).

VASOCONSTRICTION: Narrowing of blood vessels which results in the blood flow to a particular part of the body's being reduced. Cold will cause vasoconstriction of the vessels under the skin thus reducing heat loss. Shock due to injury or loss of blood will also provoke vasoconstriction.

VASODILATORS are substances that cause dilatation of the blood-vessels. They may be drugs, such as amyl nitrite (q.v.), or natural substances in the body, such as kinins (q.v.).

VASOMOTOR NERVES are the small nerve fibres that lie upon the walls of blood-vessels and connect the muscle fibres of their middle coat with the nervous system. Through these nerves the blood-vessels are retained in a state of moderate contraction. There are vasodilator nerves, through which are transmitted impulses that dilate the vessels, and, in the case of the skin-vessels, produce the condition of blushing. There are also vasoconstrictor nerves which transmit impulses that constrict, or narrow, the blood-vessels, as occurs on exposure to cold. (See HYPOTHERMIA.) Various drugs produce dilatation or contraction of the blood-vessels and several of the substances produced by endocrine glands in the body have these effects: e.g. adrenaline (q.v.).

VASOPRESSIN is the fraction isolated from extract of the posterior pituitary lobe which stimulates intestinal activity, constricts blood-vessels, and inhibits the secretion of urine. It is also known as the antidiuretic hormone because of this last effect, and its only use in medicine is, on account of this effect, in the treatment of diabetes insipidus (q.v.). (See also PITUITARY BODY.)

VASOVAGAL ATTACK: The temporary loss of consciousness caused by an abrupt slowing of the heartbeat. This may happen following shock, acute pain, fear, or stress. A common cause of fainting in normal people, a vasovagal attack may be a consequence of overstimulation of the vagus nerve (q.v.) which is involved in the control of breathing and the circulation.

VEGANISM is a strict form of vegetarianism.

VEGETARIANISM means the principle of subsisting on a diet of vegetables which contains no meat. Such a diet may include milk, cheese and eggs, but there is a strict form of vegetarianism, known as veganism, the adherents of which will eat only vegetables and fruit.

VEGETATIONS are roughenings that appear upon the valves of the heart, usually as the result of acute rheumatism. They lead in time to narrowing of the openings from the cavities of the heart, or to imcompetence of the valves that close these openings. (See HEART DISEASES.)

VEGETATIVE SYSTEM is a term applied to that part of the nervous system which acts in an involuntary manner, to a large extent independently of the brain and spinal cord, and which regulates and connects movements and secretions of internal organs. It is also known as the autonomic nervous system. The term includes the sympathetic and parasympathetic nervous systems (q.v.).

VEINS are the vessels which carry blood to the heart after it has circulated through the tissues of the body. In general the veins lie alongside corresponding arteries that carry outwards to the tissues the blood which afterwards returns by the veins. The veins are, however, both more numerous and more capacious than the arteries, and, as a rule, there are two accompanying veins for each artery of moderate size. In addition to these deeply placed veins, there are superficial veins in the limbs, which can be readily seen in their distended state lying immediately beneath the skin.

Structure: A vein is of similar structure to an artery, consisting of three coats: outer of fibrous tissue, middle of muscular and elastic fibres, and inner composed of elastic membrane and flattened cells. Any vein has, however, a much thinner wall than its corresponding artery, especially as regards the middle coat. Most veins are provided with valves similar in structure to the valves of the heart, and consisting each of two segments or pouches, which lie flat against the wall of the vein as the blood passes in the proper direction, or which meet and close the passage whenever the blood tends to run backwards. The position of these valves can easily be seen upon the arm or leg by running the finger backwards along a large vein, when the distended vein shows a little swelling at each valve. The valves are most numerous in the veins of the lower limb, those in the arm stand next in point of numbers, whilst there are few valves in the veins of internal organs.

Chief veins: Four *pulmonary veins* open into the left atrium of the heart, two coming from each lung. Into the right atrium there open some small veins from the walls of the heart, and two great vessels, superior vena cava and inferior vena cava, that bring back blood from the body generally.

The *superior vena cava* brings the blood from the head, neck, and upper limbs. It is formed by the union of two *innominate veins*, each of which results from the junction, at the root of the neck, of the internal jugular vein, from the neck, and the subclavian vein, from the upper limb. The *internal jugular vein* receives the blood from within the skull and collects branches from the face and neck as it runs downwards alongside the carotid artery under cover of the thick sternocleidomastoid muscle. One of its most important branches is the *external jugular vein*, which runs beneath the skin from the angle of the jaw straight downwards to the middle of the collar-bone. This vessel can be readily seen when the veins of the neck are distended, and is liable to be opened in wounds of this region. The *subclavian vein* is the last section of the system of veins that accompany the arteries in the arm, each vein being named after its corresponding artery. The superficial veins of the arm are of special interest, because the large *basilic vein* that runs up the inner side of the upper arm is the vein usually opened in blood-letting. Its tributary, the median cubital vein, is used for punctures to get blood for various tests or in order to give intravenous injections. (See VENESECTION.)

The *inferior vena cava*, which lies to the right side and in front of the spinal column, starting at the junction of the two common iliac veins about the level of the navel, collects the blood from the lower limbs and abdomen. In the lower limbs and in the pelvis, the deeply placed veins correspond in name and in position to the arteries, while the surface veins of the lower limb empty their contents into the *small saphenous vein* on the back of the leg, and the *great saphenous vein* that runs from the instep up the inner side of the leg, knee, and thigh. These veins, and especially the great saphenous vein, are of special interest because of their liability to become distended or varicose. Within the abdomen, the inferior vena cava receives branches corresponding to several branches of the aorta, its largest branches being the *hepatic veins*, which return not only the blood that has reached the liver in the hepatic arteries, but also blood which comes from the digestive organs in the *portal vein* to undergo a second capillary circulation in the liver. (See PORTAL VEIN.)

It appears from what has been said that the blood circulating in the uppermost parts of the body is returned to the heart by the superior vena cava, that from below the diaphragm by the inferior vena cava. There are, however, several connections between these two great vessels, the most important being three *azygos veins* that lie upon the sides of the spinal column, the veins on the front of the abdomen, and some veins that emerge from the abdomen at the navel and connect the portal system with those of the inferior and superior vena cava. By these means the circulation is maintained even when one of these large vessels has been blocked by some disease within the chest or the abdomen.

VEINS, DISEASES OF: These vessels are subject to degenerative and inflammatory changes.

INFLAMMATION of a vein is a condition which is serious mainly on account of the clotting of the blood that usually takes place within the inflamed part (thrombosis), and the risk that such a clot may break up and portions be swept away by the circulation to lodge in other vessels (embolism). *Phlebitis*, or *thrombophlebitis*, is the name commonly applied to general inflammation of a vein, while the term *peri-phlebitis* is used when the inflammation is limited to the loose connective tissue immediately surrounding the vessel. Occasionally the inflammation is of a very acute character, the vein becoming filled with a clot containing bacteria, which are carried to distant parts of the body and there produce abscesses. This condition, known as pyaemia, is an extremely grave one. (See BLOOD-POISONING.) As a rule, however, phlebitis is of a more chronic type, running a course of three or four weeks and then improving under careful treatment.

Causes: Thrombophlebitis may occur as a result of local injury to the affected part, e.g. a bruise or a fracture, or it may be due to involvement of the vein from a neighbouring inflammatory or suppurative process. It not infrequently occurs in varicose veins. Most of the cases, however, occur following child-birth or an operation, and in these cases the main factor responsible for the condition is stagnation of the blood-flow through the veins, which is why physiotherapy and exercise for the legs are so important postoperatively. (See also WHITE LEG.) It may also occur in certain infectious diseases, particularly typhoid fever. In all these conditions the actual cause is probably one or more of three factors: (1) injury or inflammation of the lining endothelium of the vein; (2) slowing of the blood-stream in the vein; (3) some alteration in the blood which makes it more liable to clot.

Symptoms: In a typical case, the skin near the inflamed vein becomes red; the affected part becomes hot, and indeed the general temperature of the body may sometimes be raised; there is swelling both around the vein and of the part beyond it, so that, if a vein in the leg is inflamed, the foot is swollen; finally, considerable pain and tenderness to touch are experienced along the vein. When a clot forms in the vein, as it commonly does, the vessel can be felt as a hard line, and this blocked condition may persist for the rest of life, the vein being converted into a firm, fibrous cord; or a passage may be tunnelled through the clot after the inflammation has subsided in the course of three or four weeks.

Treatment: When the veins of the lower limbs are involved, the patient should rest in bed with the affected limb elevated and resting on pillows. Hot wet packs are applied to relieve the pain and to help to maintain an adequate circulation. If the pain is severe, sedatives may be required. Anticoagulants (q.v.) are necessary to prevent the clot's increasing in size and to reduce the risk of pulmonary embolism (q.v.). Within three days of going to bed, the patient should be encouraged to move the affected limb and foot, as this speeds the process of recovery. It is now recognized that prolonged rest in bed tends to delay recovery.

VARICOSE VEINS are veins that have become stretched and dilated out of proportion to the amount of blood they have to carry. There are three positions in which the veins have a special tendency to become varicose. These are the veins about the lower end of the bowel, producing the condition known as haemorrhoids or piles (see PILES); the veins of the testicle, producing varicocele (see TESTICLE, DISEASES OF); and the great saphenous vein, with its branches on the inner side of the leg, knee, and thigh. Further, small veins are apt to become varicose here and there on a mucous membrane that is the seat of chronic catarrh and congestion; these minute varicose veins are found especially on the mucous membranes of the throat and stomach, and may give rise, now and then, to haemorrhage, particularly in the case of alcoholics. Only the varicose veins of the limbs are considered here, the others having been dealt with elsewhere.

Causes: It is estimated that around two-thirds of adults in the United Kingdom have varicose veins. Undoubtedly some persons are more liable to the formation of varicose veins than others. The veins vary greatly in thickness in different persons and at different portions of the same vein, so that the formation of the vessel wall and the condition of surrounding parts have much to do with its dilatation. Occupations that necessitate long-continued standing, with little vigorous muscle exertion, not only throw a great strain upon the veins of the leg, but fail to provide the pumping action that muscular contractions exert in emptying the veins. Pregnancy is another common cause of varicose veins, though the condition tends to disappear after the child is born.

An important consideration is that, after a vein has begun to dilate, its walls become weaker and its valves useless. Thus the weight of the column of blood in the limb presses down with increasing force, the condition tends to worsen and to spread into neighbouring veins.

Symptoms: At first the only symptoms are heaviness and aching in the limbs accompanied sometimes by cramps. This is experienced either at night, after a long day's standing, or in the morning. After the condition becomes marked, there is often swelling of the feet, especially above the ankles, that quickly disappears when the patient lies down. Varicose veins that have lasted many years are liable to become inflamed, and to produce eczema and ulceration of the skin. (See ULCER.) Another risk attached to untreated varicose veins, particularly in older individuals, is that a blow on them may lead to severe haemorrhage.

Treatment: Palliative treatment is directed towards checking the deterioration of the veins and preventing ulceration, whilst the entire removal of the distended veins is known as radical treatment.

PALLIATIVE TREATMENT: In slight cases, it is often sufficient to avoid the use of tight stockings, to remedy constipation, to avoid standing as much as possible, and, in the evening, to sit with the feet elevated on a couch or chair. In more marked cases, some mechanical support for the superficial veins is necessary, in order to counteract the downward pressure of the blood in the great saphenous vein, whose valves have become useless. Elastic or crêpe bandage, elastic stockings or elastic bandages are probably the most satisfactory method of support. For some cases the one-way stretch bandage is satisfactory but most people prefer elastic stockings. For the treatment of varicose ulcers see ULCERS.

Successful results are sometimes obtained from the injection, into the veins of some irritating substance, such as sodium tetradecyl sulphate or sodium morrhuate. A clot forms at once in the vein, which later becomes solid. The veins must be firmly bandaged for the next few weeks. This treatment is practically painless.

RADICAL TREATMENT is adopted when the veins are excessively dilated, or when they are painful or unsightly. The most successful method consists in turning up a flap of skin on the inner side of the thigh or knee, ligaturing the vein in two places and removing the intervening dilated portions *en masse*. The wound heals quickly, and, in most cases, the cure is complete.

WOUNDS IN VEINS are not in general serious; for, although a considerable amount of dark blood flows steadily from that end of the vein more distant from the heart, it can be stopped by gentle pressure, and soon ceases of itself. When a varicose vein ruptures, as it may do if an ulcer is present, the condition is more serious, but bleeding can be checked easily by pressure above and below the wound, and by raising the limb.

VENA CAVA is the name applied to either of the two large vessels that open into the right atrium of the heart. (See VEINS.)

VENEPUNCTURE is the name applied to inserting a needle into a vein, usually for the purpose of injecting a drug or withdrawing blood for haematological or biochemical analysis.

VENEREAL DISEASES, SEXUALLY TRANSMITTED DISEASES as they are now officially known, are certain contagious maladies which are, as a rule, communicated from one person to another by sexual intercourse. They are also classified under the title of GENITO-URINARY MEDICINE. In 1989, there were 572,943 new cases registered in the clinics for these diseases in England. The commonest were non-specific infection (77,260) and gonorrhoea (19,761). The remaining cases included HIV/AIDS, syphilis (7,500), non-specific urethritis, chancroid (88), trichomoniasis (q.v.), candidiasis (see CANDIDA), scabies (q.v.), pediculosis pubis (see PEDICULOSIS), Reiter's disease (q.v.), condyloma (q.v.), and psychosexual problems. What might be described as the two 'classical' venereal diseases (syphilis and gonorrhoea), along with chancroid, account for less than 15 per cent of cases seen in these clinics today.

Among the means which have been proposed for reducing the incidence of these diseases are: education of the public; provision of means for immediate self-disinfection; early treatment; and compulsory treatment of all people found to be affected, the last measure almost necessarily implying notification of these diseases in the same manner as one of the ordinary infectious diseases. Such compulsory notification has never been favoured in Great Britain, though it is in force in certain European countries. For purposes of efficient treatment, clinics have been established under the aegis of the National Health Service in all the large towns in Great Britain.

There are over 200 such clinics, and they are playing an increasingly important role in an advisory and preventive capacity. The moral and ethical aspects of these diseases play a much more important part than in any other group of diseases and in the past have been either ignored or mishandled. This is one aspect of medicine in which health education in the widest sense is of paramount importance.

VENESECTION was a practice much in vogue for various ailments a century ago. Indeed, many people had themselves bled regularly for the purpose of avoiding the bad health consequent on over-eating and over-drinking. It came, in time, to be so much abused – many sick people undoubtedly having died, not of the original disease, but of the excessive bleeding practised for its cure – that it fell into almost complete disuse. Certain conditions are, however, benefited by withdrawing blood either from the affected part or from the general circulation. There are three chief methods of blood-letting.

VEIN PUNCTURE is employed when it is desired to obtain a small quantity of blood for analysis or the performance of various tests. For this purpose a hollow hypodermic needle is pushed into a vein, one of those at the bend of the elbow usually being chosen, while pressure by a band or by the fingers is exerted on the veins in the upper arm. If it is desired to obtain the serum of the blood, the blood is run off into a test tube and allowed to clot. If the blood is required for analysis, clotting may be prevented by adding to the tube, before the blood is drawn off, a few crystals of potassium oxalate or potassium citrate.

VENESECTION consists in the opening of a vein, usually, owing to its superficial position, one of the veins just above the bend of the elbow. After the desired amount has flowed out, a pad and tight bandage are used to stop the bleeding. This method was used in certain cases of acute heart failure, when life may depend upon quickly and temporarily relieving the strain on the heart. It is also used in the treatment of polycythaemia (q.v.).

CUPPING was at one time used either as dry-cupping to draw blood to the surface, or as wet-cupping to withdraw blood from a congested area. (See CUPPING.)

LEECHES were formerly used to draw blood. After they are removed, bleeding is generally free, and may be encouraged, if desired, by warm poultices. They are seldom used for this purpose at the present day.

VENOGRAPHY is the study of the veins, particularly by means of X-rays after the veins have been injected with a radio-opaque substance.

VENTILATION consists in the continuous dilution or removal, by pure fresh air, of the vitiated products from respiration, combustion, putrefaction of animal and vegetable material, and from industrial processes and trades. It includes the ventilation of houses, factories, buildings of every description, as well as of streets and sewers. Ventilation and warming must be considered together. A desirable atmosphere has been defined as 'cool rather than hot; dry rather than damp; and moving rather than still'.

Air-conditioning is increasingly used in hospitals, offices, hotels and other buildings to control the purity, temperature and humidity of the air. It filters out dust, smoke, pollen and smells as well as cooling or heating the air to provide a comfortable environment. Air-conditioning may reduce the risk of airborne infections or allergies and in hospitals the air in sterile units has been passed through special bacterial filters to reduce the risk of infection. Air-conditioning may, however, be the cause of certain disorders. Outbreaks of legionnaires' disease have been linked to faulty systems – perhaps improperly maintained. Other disorders such as humidifier fever and sick-building syndrome – headache, lassitude and irritability – are also attributed to air-conditioning.

AIR STERILIZATION: In order to reduce the risk of cross-infection, particularly in schools, dormitories, and offices, ultra-violet light has been used to kill pathogenic organisms. (See also HUMIDIFICATION.)

VENTILATION, ARTIFICIAL: The procedure, usually carried out in an operating theatre or intensive-care unit, in which a device called a ventilator takes over a person's breathing. This is done for someone who is unable to breathe normally. Damage to the respiratory centre of the brain as a result of head injury, disease of the brain, or an overdose of sedative or narcotic drugs may affect the respiratory centre. Chest injuries, disease of the lungs, nerve or muscle disorders or surgery of the chest or abdomen can also affect breathing and require the use of a ventilator to maintain normal breathing. (See ARTIFICIAL VENTILATION OF LUNGS.)

VENTILATOR: Machinery used to provide artificial ventilation. Also called respirator or life-support machine, it is an electric pump linked to a supply of air which it pumps into the patient through an endotracheal tube passed through the nose or mouth into the trachea. Sometimes the air is pumped straight into the trachea through an artificial hole called a tracheostomy (q.v.). During ventilation the patient's blood gases are closely monitored and other bodily activities such as pulse and heart pressure are regularly measured. Some patients need to be kept on a ventilator for several days or even weeks if their medical condition is serious. (See ARTIFICIAL VENTILATION OF LUNGS.)

VENTOUSE, or VACUUM EXTRACTOR, is used in obstetrics. It is based upon a suction-cup technique, whereby the baby is sucked out of the uterus instead of being drawn out by forceps.

VENTRAL means belonging to the belly.

VENTRICLE is the term applied to the two lower cavities of the heart (see HEART), and also to the cavities within the brain.

VENTRICULAR FIBRILLATION: a dangerous and rapid arrhythmia of the ventricle.

VENTRICULOGRAPHY is the process of taking an X-ray photograph of the brain after the fluid in the lateral ventricles of the brain has been replaced by air; in this way any alteration in the outline of the ventricles (e.g. from pressure by a tumour) can be detected.

VERAPAMIL is a drug used in the treatment of disordered rhythms of the heart and angina pectoris (q.v.), and is also proving of value in the treatment of high blood-pressure. (See CALCIUM-CHANNEL BLOCKERS.)

VERATRUM, also known as green hellebore, Indian poke, and poke root, is the root of *Veratrum viride*, a plant of the United States. It acts as a sedative and depressant of the heart and nervous system by virtue of veratrine and other alkaloids that it contains. Alkaloids obtained from it are used in the treatment of high blood-pressure. (See ESSENTIAL HYPERTENSION.)

VERBIGERATION means the insane repetition of meaningless words and sentences.

VERMICIDES, or VERMIFUGES, are substances that kill, or expel, parasitic worms from the intestines.

VERRUCA is the Latin term for a wart.

VERRUCOSE means covered with warts.

VERSION, or TURNING, is the name given to an operation in obstetrics which consists in turning the child in cases in which the lie of the child is abnormal.

VERTEBRA is one of the irregularly shaped bones that together form the vertebral column. (See SPINAL COLUMN.)

VERTIGO, or giddiness, is a condition in which the affected person loses the power of balancing himself, and has a false sensation as to his own movements or as to those of surrounding objects. The power of balancing depends upon sensations derived partly through the sense of touch, partly from the eyes, but mainly from the semicircular canals of the internal ear. In general, vertigo is due to some interference with this mechanism or with the centres in the cerebellum and cerebrum with which it is connected. Giddiness is apt to be associated with headache, nausea, and vomiting.
Causes: The simplest cause of vertigo is some mechanical disturbance of the body affecting the fluid in the internal ear; such as that produced by moving in a swing with the eyes shut, the motion of a boat causing sea-sickness, or a sudden fall. (See MOTION-SICKNESS.) The cause which produces a severe and sudden giddiness is Menière's disease (q.v.), a condition in which there is loss of function of the labyrinth of the inner ear. An acute labyrinthitis may result from viral infection and produce a severe vertigo lasting 2 to 5 days. Because it often occurs in epidemics it is often called epidemic vertigo. Vertigo is sometimes produced by the removal of wax from the ear, or even by syringing out the ear. (See EAR, DISEASES OF.) A third group of causes for vertigo is found in disorders of the stomach. Refractive errors in the eyes which have not received appropriate treatment by glasses, an overstrained nervous system, an attack of migraine, a mild attack of epilepsy, and gross diseases of the brain, such as tumours, form another set of causes acting more directly upon the central nervous system. Finally, giddiness may be due to some disorder of the circulation, e.g. bloodlessness of the brain produced by fainting, or by disease of the heart.
Treatment, while the attack lasts, consists in maintaining a recumbent posture, in a darkened, quiet room. Sedatives are the drugs which have most influence in diminishing giddiness when it is distressing. After the attack is over, careful examination is necessary in order to determine the cause, for upon this depends the appropriateness of treatment.

VESICAL is the term applied to structures connected with, or diseases of, the bladder. (See BLADDERS.)

VESICANTS are blistering agents. (See BLISTERS AND COUNTER-IRRITANTS.)

VESICLE means a small collection of fluid in the epidermis. The fluid in some cases consists of a drop of sweat collected at the mouth of a sweat-gland, but in general it is serum from the blood. The skin disease specially associated with the formation of vesicles is herpes; in this disease the vesicles usually burst and then scab over. Some infectious diseases show an eruption composed of vesicles: e.g. smallpox and chickenpox. When a large number of white corpuscles from the blood find their way into a vesicle, it becomes a pustule.
The term vesicle is also applied to minute sacs of normal structure, such as the air-vesicles in which the finest bronchial tubes end in the lungs.

VESICULAR BREATHING: Normal breath sounds heard in the lung by means of a stethoscope. These are soft regular sounds which become altered by disease and the changed characteristics may help the physician to diagnose a disease in the lung.

VESTIBULOCOCHLEAR NERVE is the eighth cranial nerve. It consists of two sets of fibres, which constitute two separate nerves. One is known as the vestibular nerve, which is the nerve of equilibration or balance. The other is known as the cochlear nerve, which is the nerve of hearing. Disturbance of the former causes giddiness, whilst disturbance of the latter causes deafness.

VESTIGIAL: An adjective referring to an organ which exists in a rudimentary form and whose function and structure have declined during the course of evolution. An example is the appendix.

VIBRATOR is an instrument used for vibratory massage in the mechanical treatment of disease. For its use see MASSAGE.

VIBRIO is a bacterium of curved shape, such as the vibrio of cholera.

VILLUS is the name given to one of the minute processes which are thickly planted upon the inner surface of the small intestine, giving it, to the naked eye, a velvety appearance, and greatly assisting absorption. (See DIGESTION, ABSORPTION AND ASSIMILATION; INTESTINE.)

VINBLASTINE is an alkaloid (q.v.) derived from the periwinkle plant (*Vinca rosea*) which is of value in the treatment of certain forms of malignant disease, particularly choriocarcinoma and Hodgkin's disease. (See CYTOTOXIC.)

VINCENT'S ANGINA is an ulcerative inflammation of the throat, often foul smelling, and caused by large, spindle-shaped bacilli and spirilla.

VINCRISTINE is an alkaloid derived from the common periwinkle which is proving of value in the palliative treatment of certain forms of malignant disease. (See CYTOTOXIC.)

VINEGAR (see ACETIC ACID.)

VINYL ETHER is an inhalational anaesthetic used in minor surgical procedures of short duration, and for the induction of anaesthesia (q.v.).

VIOMYCIN is an antibiotic which is active against the *Mycobacterium tuberculosis*, but less active than streptomycin or isoniazid.

VIRAEMIA: A condition occurring at various times in some viral infections in which the infecting virus is present in large amounts in the blood. In other virus infections the organisms are merely transported in the blood on their way to target tissues or organs.

VIRAL HAEMORRHAGIC FEVER or EBOLA VIRUS FEVER, is a highly fatal disease due to a virus related to that of Marburg disease (q.v.). Two large outbreaks of it were recorded in 1976 (one in the Sudan and one in Zaïre), with a mortality, respectively, of 50 and 80 per cent, and the disease reappeared in the Sudan in 1979. After an incubation period of 7 to 14 days, the onset is with headache of increasing severity and fever. This is followed by diarrhoea, extensive internal bleeding and vomiting. Death usually occurs on the eighth to ninth day. Infection is by person-to-person contact. Serum from patients convalescent from the disease is a useful source of antibodies to the virus.

VIRILISM is the term applied to the condition in which masculine characteristics develop in the female, and is commonly the result of an overactive suprarenal gland, or of a tumour of its cortex. It may also result from an androgen-secreting ovarian tumour and also from the polycystic ovary syndrome.

VIRULENCE: The power of a bacteria or virus to cause disease. Virulence can be measured by how many people the micro-organism infects, how quickly it spreads through the body, and how many people die from it.

VIRUS is the term applied to a group of infective agents which are so small that they are able to pass through the pores of collodion filters. They are responsible for some of the most important diseases affecting man: e.g. influenza, poliomyelitis, smallpox, and yellow fever. Some idea of their size may be obtained from the fact that the virus of influenza measures 80 nanometres, whereas the staphylococcus measures 1000 nanometres. (1 nanometre = one thousand-millionth of a metre.)

VISCERA is the general name given to the larger organs lying within the cavities of the chest and abdomen. The term 'viscus' is also applied individually to these organs.

VISION: Broadly speaking, vision is the ability to see.
PATHWAY OF LIGHT FROM THE EYE TO THE BRAIN: Light enters the eye by passing through the transparent cornea, then through the aqueous humour filling the anterior chamber. It then passes through the pupil, through the lens and the vitreous to reach the retina. In the retina the rod and cone photoreceptors detect light and relay messages in the form of electrochemical impulses through the various layers of the retina to the nerve fibres. The nerve fibres carry messages via the optic nerve, optic chiasm, optic tract, lateral geniculate body and finally the optic radiations to the visual cortex. Here in the visual cortex these messages are interpreted. It is therefore the visual cortex of the brain that 'sees'.
VISUAL ACUITY: Two points will not be seen as two unless they are separated by a minimum distance. This distance is such that the objects are so far apart that the lines joining them to the eye enclose between them (subtend) an angle of at least one minute of a degree. This amount of separation allows the images of the two points to fall on two separate cones (if the light from two points falls on one cone, the two points would be seen as a single point). There are many tests of visual acuity. One of the more common is the Snellen Test Type. This is made up of many letters of different size. Each letter is constructed in a specific manner so that the various components of the letter subtend an angle of one minute of one degree at the eye. Each letter when placed at specified distance from the patient subtends an angle of five minutes of a degree. Thus the top letter subtends an angle of 5 minutes when placed 60 metres from the eye, the lowest letter subtends the same angle when placed 4 metres away. By conventions the chart is placed 6 metres away from the patient. Someone able to see the lowest line at this distance has a visual acuity of

6/4. If they are only able to see the top letter they have 6/60 vision. 'Normal' vision is 6/6.

COLOUR VISION: 'White light' is made up of component colours. These can be separated by a prism, thereby producing a spectrum. The three cardinal colours are red, green, and blue. All other colours can be produced by a varying mixture of these three. Colour vision is a complex subject. The trichromat theory of colour vision suggests that there are three types of cones, each type sensitive to one of the cardinal colours. Colour perception is based on differential stimulation of these cone types. The opponent colour theory suggests that each cone type can generate signals of the opposite kind. Output from some cones can collaborate with the output from others or can inhibit the action of other cones. Colour perception results from these various complex interactions.

Defective colour vision may be hereditary or acquired and can occur in the presence of normal visual acuity. *Hereditary defective colour vision* is more common in men (7 per cent of males) than women (0·5 per cent of females). Men are affected, but women convey the abnormal gene to their children. It occurs because one or more of the photopigments of the retina are abnormal, or the cones are damaged. Red–green colour defect is the commonest. *Acquired defective colour vision* is the result of disease of the cones or their connections in the retina, optic nerve or brain, e.g. macular disease, optic neuritis. Colour vision can be impaired but not lost as a result of corneal opacification or cataract formation. *Tests of colour vision*: these include matching of coloured yarn, using specially designed numbers made of coloured dots surrounded by dots of confusing colour (e.g. Ishihara plates) and by means of coloured buttons which must be arranged in order of changing hue.

VISION, DISORDERS OF: The list of disorders resulting in poor or dim vision is huge. Disturbance of vision can result from an uncorrected refractive error, disease or injury of the cornea, iris, lens, vitreous, retina, choroid or sclera. It may also result from disease or injury to the structures comprising the visual pathway from the retina to the occipital cortex (see VISION, Pathway of light from the eye to the brain) and from lesions of the structures around the eye, e.g. swollen lids, drooping eyelids.

VISION, FIELD OF: When the eye looks at a specific point or object, that point is seen clearly. Other objects within a large area away from this fixation point can also be seen but less clearly. The area that can be seen around the fixation point, without moving the eye, is known as the field of vision. The extent of the field is limited inwards by the nose, above by the brow and below by the cheek. The visual field thus has its greatest extent outwards from the side of the head. The field of vision of each eye overlaps to a large extent so that objects in the centre and towards the inner part of each field are viewed by both eyes together. Because the eyes are set slightly apart, each eye sees objects in this overlapping part of the field slightly differently. It is because of this slight difference that objects can be perceived as three dimensional. Defects in the visual field (scotomas) can be produced by a variety of disorders. Certain of these produce specific field defects. For example, glaucoma, some types of brain damage and some toxins can produce specific defects in the visual field. This type of field defect may be very useful in diagnosing a particular disorder. The *blind spot* is that part of the visual field corresponding to the optic disc. There are no rods nor cones on the optic disc and therefore no light perception from this area. The blind spot can be found temporal (i.e. on the outer side) of the fixation point.

VISUAL ACUITY (see VISION).

VISUAL EVOKED RESPONSE: Stimulation of the retina with light causes changes in the electrical activity of the cerebral cortex. These changes can be measured from outside the skull and can give valuable information about the state of the visual pathway from the retinal ganglion cells to the occipital cortex. Not only can it determine that function is normal, it can also help to diagnose some causes of poor vision.

VITAL CAPACITY: The amount of air that can be forcibly exhaled from the lungs after a deep inspiration.

VITAMIN is a term applied to a group of 13 substances which exist in minute quantities in natural foods, and which are necessary to normal nutrition, especially in connection with growth and development. Some, A, D, E and K, are fat soluble and can be stored in the body. The remainder, C, B_{12} and other members of the B complex, are water soluble and are quickly excreted. Most vitamins have now been synthesized. When they are absent from the food, defective growth takes place in young animals and children, and in adults various diseases arise; whilst short of the production of actual disease, persistent deprivation of one or other vitamin is apt to lead to a state of lowered general health. Certain deficiencies in diet have long been known to be the cause of scurvy, beriberi, and rickets.

VITAMIN A is usually taken in more than ample quantity in the food, and is stored in the liver. It is developed originally by plants as a yellow colouring matter, carotene, for example in carrots, and it is also found in egg yolk, liver, milk, butter, and most green vegetables. When stored in the liver it is colourless and has a slight chemical difference from carotene. The two richest sources of this vitamin are halibut-liver oil and cod-liver oil. The daily requirement of vitamin A is in the region of 4000 international units. Children and pregnant women require relatively more than adults. Deficiency of vitamin A is responsible for serious inflammation of the eyes known as xerophthalmia, which is one of the chief causes of blindness in the developing world; also for night blindness, various skin eruptions, defective development of the teeth, and particularly for want of vitality in the tissues, which leads to localized inflammations. It is not destroyed by ordinary cooking processes.

Vitamin B complex

Vitamin B₁ (see THIAMINE).

Vitamin B₂ (see RIBOFLAVINE).

Vitamin B₃ (see PANTOTHENIC ACID).

Vitamin B₆ (see PYRIDOXINE).

Vitamin B₁₂ (see CYANOCOBALAMIN).

VITAMIN C is especially found in fresh fruits such as oranges, and also in fresh green vegetables, and to a smaller extent in milk, meat, and other fresh foods. Canned vegetables such as tomatoes also retain it if their reaction is acid. It is quickly destroyed by high temperature, by excess baking soda and other alkalis, and gradually by oxidation in process of keeping. Its deficiency leads to symptoms of scurvy (q.v.), including muscular weakness, haemorrhages under the skin, swelling and inflammation of the gums with loss of teeth, and serious damage to joints by haemorrhage; it occurs in people long deprived of fresh foods – sailors were once victims of this deficiency – and also in babies fed persistently on artificial foods. This vitamin has not only been obtained in a pure state, but has been manufactured in a crystalline form as ascorbic acid. The daily requirement of vitamin C (in terms of ascorbic acid) is 30 mg for adults and 60 mg for children. There is no convincing evidence that it is of any value in the treatment of disease other than vitamin deficiency.

VITAMIN D is of special importance for the growth of children, and its deficiency produces rickets (q.v.) with softening and irregular growth of bones, so that swollen joints, distorted limbs, deformities of the chest and similar malformations arise. It was formerly common in industrial conurbations but is rare now in developed countries. Osteomalacia (q.v.), a similar disease affecting the bones of adults, results from the same causes when lime salts are absorbed from the bones during pregnancy. It has long been known that cod-liver oil was the chief remedy for rickets, and for a time it was supposed that its anti-rachitic action depended upon vitamin A, but it is now known to be vitamin D. There are two forms of vitamin D. Vitamin D₂, also known as calciferol or ergocalciferol, is obtained from ergosterol, a waxy constituent of plants, by ultra-violet irradiation. Vitamin D₃, or cholecalciferol, is the natural form of the vitamin. It is produced by the ultra-violet irradiation of a sterol widely distributed in animal fats. This substance is also formed naturally in the fatty tissues of the body when the skin is exposed to the action of sunlight, or, when this is not available, to ultra-violet rays from an arc lamp. It can also be formed in food

such as milk when this is similarly exposed to light. Only a few foods contain vitamin D naturally, including cod-liver oil and other fish-liver oils (especially that from halibut liver), whilst egg yolk contains a smaller quantity; other fats and milk contain very small quantities. The mode of action of vitamin D is to aid the absorption of phosphorus and calcium from the food, increase their amount in the blood, and thus in the bones. In the case of this vitamin bad effects may follow over-dosage, or hypervitaminosis, because if too much calcium and phosphorus are maintained in the blood the bones and teeth become over-calcified, the arteries may become unduly hardened and calculi may be formed in the kidneys and other organs. The daily requirement for infants and nursing mothers is 400 to 800 international units, whilst for adults it is probably about 400 units. (See CALCIFEROL.)

VITAMIN E, TOCOPHEROL, has been known since 1923, when it was found that its absence in the case of rats caused failure to produce young. It is derived especially from the oil contained in seeds and in green leaves, and also is present in smaller amounts in other fresh fats. It can also be synthesized in the form of alpha-tocopherol. It is readily stored, like vitamin A, in the body, and thus is unlikely to be found wanting in human beings except in cases of very severe under-nutrition and in premature infants. It is possible, however, that miscarriages may occasionally be due to its deficiency.

VITAMIN K, also known as PHYTOMENADIONE, the anti-haemorrhagic vitamin, is essential for the proper clotting of blood. It has been given successfully in cases of bleeding in infants, and to patients with jaundice, who have a special tendency to bleeding. Bleeding in these conditions is thought to be due to deficiency of vitamin K. Synthetic chemical products with an identical physiological action have now been made. In the natural form it is widespread in nature, the main sources being spinach, leafy vegetables, tomatoes, and liver. The daily requirement of man is not known, but dietary deficiency rarely occurs, although people suffering from malabsorption disorders may become deficient.

VITAMIN P, CITRIN, or HESPERIDIN, present in citrus fruits, appears to be responsible for the resistance of the capillaries to pressure. If there is a deficiency of vitamin P in the diet the capillaries rupture easily, resulting, for example, in purpura.

Any person using a diet containing the protective foods, such as milk, eggs, butter, cheese, fat, fish, wholemeal bread, fresh vegetables and fruit, should obtain an ample supply of vitamins.

VITILIGO are patchy areas of depigmentation of the skin surrounded by areas of increased pigmentation. It is seen in many auto-immune diseases such as Graves' disease, chronic thyroiditis and Addison's disease and it is due to the auto- immune destruction of the melanin-secreting cells in the skin.

VITREOUS BODY is a semi-fluid, transparent substance which fills most of the globe of the eye behind the lens.

VIVISECTION: For over a century the medical profession has aimed at maintaining as high a standard as possible for vivisection. It was the medical profession led by Dr James Paget that was responsible for the passing of the Cruelty to Animals Act 1876, which aimed to eliminate cruelty. The infliction of pain was reduced to a minimum by the use of anaesthetics, and the licensing and surveillance of animal experiments was ensured.

Most experiments are carried out on specially bred mice and rats. Fewer than 1 per cent are done on cats, dogs, non-human primates, farm animals, frogs, fish and birds. Control on experiments have recently been strengthened. The great majority of animal experiments is done without anaesthesia because feeding experiments, taking blood, or giving injection, do not require anaesthetics in animals any more than in man. Universities in Britain are responsible for less than one-fifth of animal experiments; commercial concerns and government institutions are responsible for most of the rest. Tests on cosmetics account for under 1 per cent of all animal work, but are necessary because such materials are often applied with great frequency – and for a long time – to the skin of adults and infants.

A common argument is that animal research should be replaced by work on tissue culture. This is a method of research and investigation that is being increasingly used, but there is a limit to the extent to which infection, cancer, or drugs can be investigated on cultures of tissue cells. Other methods involving computerized or mathematical modelling of experiments are also being developed.

VOCAL CORDS (see LARYNGOSCOPE; LARYNX; VOICE AND SPEECH).

VOCAL RESONANCE: The air carrying the voice produced in the larynx passes through the throat, mouth and nose. The shape and size of these structures will influence the timbre of the voice, or vocal resonance. This will vary from person to person and even within an individual; i.e. with a cold.

VOICE AND SPEECH are two terms applied to the system of sounds which are produced in the upper air passages and in the mouth, and which form one of the means of communication between human beings.

Voice means the set of fundamental notes and tones produced by the larynx which are modified in various ways during their passage through the mouth so as to form speech or song. Speech differs from song in being less sustained and of smaller compass with regard to pitch, and in presenting sounds which have not a musical character.

VOICE is produced in the larynx of most animals. Voice production may be studied with the laryngoscope (q.v.), an instrument which enables the changes that take place in the larynx, when different notes are sounded, to be clearly seen.

Musical notes vary in three characters: loudness, pitch, and quality or timbre. The *loudness* of the voice depends upon the volume of air which is available for agitating the vocal cords, and therefore upon the size of the chest and the vigour with which its muscles can be made to act.

The *pitch* of the voice is determined by several things, the chief points being the size of the larynx; the degree of tenseness at which the vocal cords are, for the time being, maintained by the laryngeal muscles; the fact as to whether the cords vibrate as a whole or merely at their edges; and the shape which is given to the cavity of the larynx by movements of the arytenoid and epiglottic cartilages. In any given voice, the range of pitch seldom exceeds two and a half octaves, although the particular part of the musical scale that can be produced varies according as the voice is bass, tenor, contralto or soprano. Generally speaking, a large larynx with long vocal cords produces low notes, and hence men have a deeper voice than women. For the same reason the small larynx of childhood produces a shrill voice, whilst the rapid growth of the larynx at the time of puberty, and consequent uncertainty of muscular control over the vocal cords, produces the breaking of the voice that occurs in boys at this time. This is occurring at an earlier age. Thus fifty years ago, treble lines in cathedral choirs were made up of boys aged 11 to 16. Today choir schools are rarely catering for boys over 13, and voices are breaking as young as 12. Changes in the voice also occur at other ages as a result of the secondary action of the sex hormones. Thus, during menstruation there may be a slight decrease in the quality of the singing voice, affecting especially notes in the highest register, and there may be a lowering of pitch during pregnancy. At the menopause the entire vocal range for speaking and singing may be lowered, and with the onset of old age there tends to be increasing virilism of the voice.

The manner in which the muscles of the larynx act upon the cords allows the pitch to change at will. Thus if the thick part of each cord be held rigid and only the sharp free edge be allowed to vibrate, a high note is the result, and a still higher note is reached in men when only the front part of this free edge is allowed to move, as in the falsetto voice. On the other hand, by allowing a greater thickness of the cord to vibrate, the person loads the vibrating edge, and so produces a much deeper note.

The *timbre* of the voice is partly due to these differences in the larynx, but chiefly to peculiarities and to voluntary changes in shape of the mouth and other cavities associated with the air passages. These changes in shape are chiefly concerned with the alterations of the fundamental notes which produce speech.

It should be remembered, however, that, while the muscular arrangements of the larynx are chiefly concerned with the pitch of the voice, and the shape of the mouth with its modulation, the *loudness* is varied by the movements of the chest. The neglect of this fact is often responsible for the bad voice- production which leads to great straining of the throat, and is largely responsible for the throat affections of many of those who use the voice much.

There are certain peculiar forms of voice production. The *falsetto voice* has been already mentioned. *Whispering* is a form of speech in which voice is completely absent, the larynx being wide open and the sound produced entirely in the mouth. *Ventriloquism* is a form of speech in which the voice is produced by the indrawing of air, instead of in the usual way of expiration. Since it is always difficult to localize the source of sound, the ventriloquist can easily suggest to his audience a false place of origin for the unusual voice.

SPEECH consists of a series of rapid modifications of the voice, produced by changes in position of the palate, tongue, and lips.

DEFECTS OF SPEECH: The act of speech has a very elaborate controlling mechanism in the nervous system. Further, the power of speech is gained in early life by children hearing the sounds made by others and mimicking them, so that the centres for speech in the brain are intimately connected with those concerned in the sense of hearing.

MUTISM, or the entire absence of the power to speak, may be due to various causes, the most effectual being some mental deficiency which denies to the child sufficient intelligence to mimic the actions of those around him. In other cases the child seems to be quite intelligent, but, owing apparently to some defect in the nervous control of the voice and speech organs, or in these organs themselves, he is unable to make any sounds. A common cause of mutism is complete deafness present at birth, or caused by some ear diseases in early childhood. The child in this case cannot learn to speak, simply because he cannot hear, but, if properly educated, he can be taught to speak fluently and to understand what is said by watching the lips and throat of others. (See SPEECH DISORDERS.)

STAMMERING is a bad habit of speech due to want of co-ordination between the different parts of the speech mechanism. (See STAMMERING.)

Such minor peculiarities in speech as burrs and lisps are due to peculiarities in the action of the tongue or palate, whilst the deformities of tongue-tie and cleft-palate are accompanied by still greater defects of speech. When the nose is blocked by any condition, such as a cold in the head or polypus, the pronunciation of the resonants *m, n,* and *ng* is interfered with, these being heard as *b, d,* and *g,* respectively.

DYSPHASIA is a condition in which various forms of inability to speak, or to understand speech, come on, usually late in life, as the result of brain disease. (See DYSPHASIA.)

APHONIA, or loss of voice, causes speaking to be carried on in a whisper. It is usually either due to some disorder of the vocal cords, as in the laryngitis which may form part of a cold, or is a symptom of hysteria. It is generally of short duration. (See also DYSARTHRIA.)

VOLAR means something pertaining to the palm or sole.

VOLKMANN'S CONTRACTURE is the condition in which, as a result of too great a pressure from splint or bandage in the treatment of a broken arm, the flexor muscles of the forearm contract and thus obstruct free flow of blood in the veins; the muscles then swell and ultimately become fibrosed.

VOLUNTARY MUSCLE: Also known as skeletal muscle, this forms the muscles which are under a person's conscious control. Muscles that control walking, talking and swallowing are examples of those under such control (see INVOLUNTARY MUSCLE and MUSCLE).

VOLVULUS means an obstruction of the bowels produced by the twisting of a loop of bowel round itself. (See INTESTINE, DISEASES OF.)

VOMITING means the expulsion of the stomach contents through the mouth. When the effort of vomiting is made, but nothing is brought up, the process is known as retching. When vomiting occurs, the chief effort is made by the muscles of the abdominal wall and by the diaphragm contracting together and squeezing the stomach. The contraction of the stomach wall is no doubt also a factor, and an important step in the act consists in the opening at the right moment of the cardiac or upper orifice of the stomach. This concerted action of various muscles is brought about by a vomiting centre situated on the floor of the fourth ventricle in the brain.

Causes: Vomiting is brought about by some irritation of this nervous centre, but in the great majority of cases this is effected through sensations derived from the stomach itself. Thus, of the drugs which cause vomiting some act only after being absorbed into the blood and carried to the brain, although most are irritants to the mucous membrane of the stomach (see EMETICS); dyspepsia also acts thus, and lies at the root of most sick headaches; various diseases of the stomach, such as cancer, and ulcer, and food poisoning, act in a similar way. Irritation, not only of the nerves of the stomach, but also of those proceeding from other abdominal organs, produces vomiting; thus in obstruction of the bowels, peritonitis, gall-stone colic, renal colic, and even during pregnancy, vomiting is a prominent symptom.

Strong impressions of an unpleasant nature made upon the nerves of sense are apt to produce vomiting. Thus an offensive smell, a disagreeable sight, any interference with the balancing sense as in travel-sickness, irritation or even tickling of the throat, and the pain of an injury or operation are all likely to be attended by vomiting.

Direct disturbance of the brain itself is a cause: for example, a blow on the head, a cerebral tumour, a cerebral abscess, meningitis. Many cases of hysteria also show attacks of vomiting as one of their prominent symptoms.

Nausea and vomiting are common symptoms that may arise from local disease of the gastro-intestinal tract, but they are also associated with systemic illness and also with disturbances of labyrinthine function, such as motion sickness and acute labyrinthitis.

There are two centres in the brain concerned with vomiting. One is the chemo-receptor trigger zone. This centre is in contact with the blood and lies outside the blood-brain barrier. It is the site at which drugs such as apomorphine and toxins act. It is rich in dopamine receptors and hence dopamine antagonists are effective treatment for vomiting. The vomiting centre itself co-ordinates impulses received from the chemo-receptor trigger zone from the vestibular apparatus and the gastro-intestinal tract and also from higher centres in the cerebral cortex. The vomiting centre contains many cholinergic and histamine receptors and this is why anti-cholinergic drugs and anti-histamines are effective drugs in the control of vomiting.
CHARACTERS OF THE VOMIT: FOOD, more or less softened and made sour and bitter by digestion, constitutes the vomit in the simpler cases, such as those due, for example, to emetics and sea-sickness. It should be remembered that when milk is vomited up curdled, this indicates simply that the first step in its digestion has taken place, and it is a mistake to conclude, as is often done, that the curdling indicates some intolerance of the stomach for milk.
WATERY FLUID, brought up irrespective of meals, forms the vomitus in conditions where the vomiting is due to disturbances of the brain: e.g. brain tumours, and in certain other conditions such as the vomiting in the early months of pregnancy. When the vomiting continues for long, it tends to bring up mucus and bile also.
MUCUS, when vomited in considerable amount in strings, and especially when sour and brought up in the morning, is a sign of catarrh of the stomach, particularly that form associated with constant indulgence in alcohol.
BILE may be brought up by any long-continued attack of vomiting, after the contents of the stomach have been expelled and retching still continues: for example, in sea-sickness, or in migraine. Usually the bile is golden-yellow in colour; but sometimes it is grass-green.
FROTHY MATERIAL, with a yeasty smell, which divides into three distinct layers, froth on the surface, and a sediment of undigested food, with a layer of clearer fluid between, is characteristic of the vomit from a dilated stomach in which fermentative dyspepsia is taking place.
BLOOD may be red and brought up mixed with the food or in clots; but, much more often, it is vomited as a brown granular material, very much resembling 'coffee-grounds'. As a general rule, the vomiting of blood indicates some ulceration in the interior of the stomach, but the amount of blood is no guide to the size of the ulcer, because serious bleeding sometimes occurs from hardly perceptible erosions of the mucous membrane. Large quantities of blood are also occasionally brought up in chronic catarrh of the stomach (especially the alcoholic variety) which is accompanied by congestion.
Treatment: The cause of the vomiting must be sought and treatment directed towards this. If the vomiting is due to local disease in the gastro-intestinal tract the old-fashioned remedies of sodium bicarbonate and bismuth may be helpful, along with rest. If the vomiting is vestibular in origin and due, for example, to motion sickness, hyoscine or antihistamines are the drugs of choice, though the side effects of sedation, dry mouth and constipation may be troublesome.

Nausea and vomiting are a common feature of migraine. Metoclopramide is the drug of choice. This drug acts by encouraging gastric emptying and gastro-intestinal motility is altered by nausea and vomiting. Domperidone is also effective.

Vomiting is common in the post-operative period and this is due to the combined effects of morphine, analgesics, anaesthetic agents and the psychological stress of operation. Dopamine receptor antagonists such as metoclopramide are probably the drugs of choice.

Nausea and vomiting are common symptoms in pregnancy. Drugs are best avoided in this situation as they may damage the developing fetus. Simple measures, such as the taking of food before getting up in the morning and reassurance, are often all that is necessary. If drugs are required promethazine or metoclopramide are the drugs of choice as they appear to be free of teratogenic effects.

VON RECKLINGHAUSEN'S DISEASE: This description covers the inherited disease, multiple neurofibromatosis. About one new case occurs every 3,000 live births. The disease is characterized by tumours along the course of nerves which can be felt beneath the skin. Soft tumours may also develop beneath the skin. The condition may have other associated abnormalities such as scoliosis, decalcification of the bones due to overactivity of the parathyroid glands and fibrosis in the lungs. Surgery may be needed for cosmetic reasons or to relieve pressure on the nervous system.

VOYEURISM: The regular viewing of people who are naked or part naked or who are taking part in sexual intercourse. The voyeur's subjects are unaware that they are being watched. The voyeur, nearly always a man, usually becomes sexually excited and may induce orgasm by masturbation.

VULVA is the general term applied to the external female genitals.

VULVO-VAGINITIS is inflammation of the vulva and the vagina. It is more common in young girls than in adult women. It may be a manifestation of infection elsewhere in the body, or may indicate the presence of some infection in the vagina.

W

WALK (see GAIT).

WARFARIN is an anticoagulant which is active whether given by mouth, intramuscularly, intravenously or rectally. It is usually given by mouth, when its maximum effect occurs within about 36 hours. Its action passes off within 48 hours of cessation of treatment.

WARTS, or VERRUCAE, are small, solid growths, arising from the surface of the skin. They are due to a papovavirus infection of the skin. They are highly infectious, and it is estimated that 10 per cent of the population suffer from them. The infection is most likely to be spread in schools by hand-holding games, and among adolescents by walking barefoot on gymnasium floors and in swimming baths. COMMON WARTS develop on the skin of children and young people on the knuckles, on the backs of the hands and on the knees. Occasionally such warts come out in a crop. In structure, they consist of a bundle of fibres produced by overgrowth of the papillae in the true skin, each bundle enveloped by a cap of the horny cells that cover the surface of the epidermis, and the whole mass being surrounded by a ring of thickened epidermis. PLANE WARTS, which are flat-topped, are commonest on the face and the back of the hands. PLANTAR WARTS occur on the soles of the feet, most commonly in older children and adolescents. Epidemics are not uncommon in schools. SENILE WARTS are usually hard, wrinkled, and slightly raised areas of skin found in old people. SOFT WARTS, consisting of little tags of skin, are found especially upon the neck, chest, ears, or eyelids of people whose skin has been subjected for long to some irritation. HORNS are formed sometimes upon the face or hands, as the result of the drying up of the sebaceous material exuding from the skin that covers a wart, and, as the secretion goes on, these horns occasionally reach a length of some inches. TUBERCULOUS WARTS are developed sometimes as the result of a wound in the skin of the hands, especially of those who have come in contact with persons or animals suffering from

some form of tuberculosis: e.g. pathologists and butchers.

Treatment: There is much to be said for the old advice that the best way to manage warts is to let them manage themselves. Quite often they disappear spontaneously, which explains the large range of vaunted 'cures'. Warts can be treated with cryosurgery, electrocautery, curettage, laser treatment or by applying a preparation of salicylic acid or podophyllin.

WASHING (see DISINFECTION).

WASHING OUT OF THE STOMACH is performed for various reasons, particularly in order to remove poison that has been recently swallowed, before it shall have had time to act. Expert opinion today differs as to the value and safety of washing out the stomach in cases of poisoning. If it is done for this purpose, it should only be done by a doctor, nurse or experienced first-aider. The elementary rules are as follows:

(1) Place the head of the patient over the side of the bed so that the mouth and throat are at a lower level than the larynx and trachea.

(2) Use a wide-bore stomach tube (Jaques gauge 30) and lubricate it well with glycerin or some similar lubricant. In the adult 50 cm (20 inches) will reach the stomach. Make sure the tube is in the gullet (oesophagus) and not the trachea.

(3) For the first wash use 300 ml water, or olive oil if a tar oil derivative has been taken. Repeat this process, using 300-600 ml at a time, at least three or four times, saving all washings for analysis.

(4) If the patient is conscious, leave in the stomach 600 ml water containing 20 ml sodium or magnesium sulphate. If the patients is comatose, leave the stomach empty, and leave a nasogastric tube in place to keep the stomach empty. In the unconscious patient it is necessary to protect the airway with a cupped endotracheal tube.

Washing out is also employed to cleanse the stomach in cases in which the food tends to collect in the organ and to ferment. (See STOMACH TUBE.)

WASSERMANN REACTION is a test introduced for the diagnosis of syphilis by examination of the blood. It has now been largely supplanted by other more specific tests.

WASTING (see ATROPHY).

WASTING PALSY is a popular name for the disease more commonly known as progressive muscular atrophy. (See PARALYSIS.)

WATERBRASH, or PYROSIS, is a symptom of dyspepsia; during the course of digestion, the mouth fills with tasteless or sour fluid, which is generally saliva, but sometimes seems to be brought up from the stomach. At the same time, a burning pain is often felt at the pit of the stomach or in the chest. The condition is a symptom of excessive acidity of the stomach contents, due sometimes to an irritating diet, and often characteristic of a duodenal ulcer. (See DYSPEPSIA.)

WATER-HAMMER PULSE is a name given to the peculiarly sudden pulse that is associated with incompetence of the aortic valve of the heart, and suggests the philosophical toy after which it is named. (See PULSE.)

WATER ON THE BRAIN is a popular name for hydrocephalus and for meningitis. (See HYDROCEPHALUS; MENINGITIS.)

WAX is used in medicine as an ingredient of ointments, plasters, and suppositories. It is used either as yellow wax derived directly from honeycomb, or as white wax, which is the same substance bleached. It is also used in the form of paraffin wax to apply heat in the relief of rheumatic pains.

For wax in the ear, see EAR, DISEASES OF.

WEAKNESS (see ATROPHY; CACHEXIA; PARALYSIS; TONICS).

WEALS, or WHEALS, are raised white areas on the skin with reddened margins, which may result from sharp blows, or may be a symptom of nettle-rash.

WEANING (see INFANT FEEDING).

WEBBED FINGERS or TOES, or SYNDACTYLY, constitute a deformity sometimes present at birth, and liable to run in families. The web may be quite a thin structure, or the fingers may be closely united by solid tissue. In any case, separation is a matter of considerable difficulty, because, if the web is simply divided, it heals up as before. A special operation is necessary, consisting in turning back a flap of the web upon each of the united fingers, or some other device to produce healing in the new position.

WEBER'S TEST: A test with a tuning fork that is used to assess a person's deafness.

WEIGHT AND HEIGHT: The weight of a child at birth is about 3·2 to 3·6 kg (7 to 8 pounds) and the height 50 cm (20 inches). During the first six months the infant puts on weight at the rate of about 140 g (5 ounces) per week if no illness occurs, and during the second six months of life about 0·5 kg (1 pound) per month. At the age of one year he weighs from 8·2 to 10·9 kg (18 to 24 pounds). In the first year he increases

in height about 25 cm (10 inches), and measures almost 75 cm (30 inches) at one year old.

Age	Boys		Girls	
	Inches	Centi-metres	Inches	Centi-metres
Birth	20·0	50·9	19·5	49·5
2 weeks	20·3	51·7	20·1	51·0
3 months	23·7	60·2	23·2	58·8
6 months	26·2	66·7	25·6	65·0
9 months	28·0	71·2	27·4	69·6
1 year	29·6	75·1	29·1	73·9
2 years	34·0	86·4	33·7	85·5
3 years	37·8	95·9	36·9	93·8
4 years	40·6	103·0	40·0	101·6
5 years	43·1	109·5	42·9	108·9

Mean height of infants and young children. Thomson.

Age	Boys		Girls	
	Pounds	Kilo-grams	Pounds	Kilo-grams
Birth	7·5	3·4	7·3	3·3
2 weeks	7·5	3·4	7·3	3·3
3 months	12·9	5·8	12·0	5·5
6 months	17·4	7·9	16·4	7·4
9 months	20·4	9·2	19·2	8·7
1 year	22·8	10·3	21·7	9·8
2 years	27·0	12·2	25·7	11·6
3 years	31·5	14·3	30·4	13·8
4 years	35·6	16·2	34·5	15·7
5 years	40·2	18·3	39·4	17·9

Mean weight of infants and young children. Thomson.

In both boys and girls the growth in height amounts to 7·5 cm (3 inches) per year from the second to the fifth years. Boys continue to grow at the rate of 5 cm (2 inches) per year from the sixth to the fifteenth years, whilst girls continue to grow at this rate from the sixth to the eleventh years. In general, it may be said that the height is doubled at the end of five years, and trebled in the thirteenth or fourteenth year. After adolescence growth is more vigorous in boys, but girls attain their full height earlier than boys. Increase in height is greatest in the late spring and early summer, and least in the winter.

As a rule increase in height and increase in weight run parallel. At 2½ years the birth-weight has usually been increased fourfold, whilst at 5 years it has been increased fivefold. The general tendency of weight increase can be summarized as follows: (1) rapid increase in infancy and early childhood; (2) slow but constant increase from 3 to 12 years; (3) marked acceleration during puberty; (4) very slow increase to age of 25 or 30 years.

Charts relating height to age have been devised and give an indication of the normal rate of growth. The wide variation in normal children is immediately apparent on studying such charts. Deviations from the mean of this wide range are called percentiles. Centile or percentile charts describe the distribution of a characteristic in a population. They are obtained by measuring a specific characteristic in a large population of at least 1,000 of each sex at each age. For each age there will be a height, above and below which 50 per cent of the population lie and this is called the fiftieth centile. The fiftieth centile thus indicates the mean height at a particular age. Such tables are less reliable around the age of puberty because of variation in age of onset.

Minor variations from the mean do not warrant investigation but if the height of an individual falls below the third centile (3 per cent of normal children have a height that falls below the third centile) or above the ninety-seventh centile, investigation is required. Changes in the rate of growth are also important and skeletal proportions may provide useful information. There are many children who are normal but who are small in relation to their parents. The problem is merely growth delay. These children take longer to reach maturity and there is also a proportional delay in their skeletal maturation. The actual height must always be assessed in relation to maturity. The change in skeletal proportions is one manifestation of maturity but other features include the maturing of facial features with the growth of nose and jaw and dental development. Maturity of bone can readily be measured by the radiological bone age.

Failure to gain weight is of more significance. Whilst this may be due to some underlying disease, the commonest cause is a diet containing inadequate calories. Over the last six decades or so there has been quite a striking increase in the heights and weights of European children. Manufacturers of children's clothing, shoes and furniture have had to increase the size of their products. Growth is now completed at 20–21 years, compared with 25 at the turn of the century. This increase, and earlier maturation, it has been suggested, have been due to a combination of genetic mixing as a result of population movements, combined with the whole range of improvement in environmental hygiene, and not merely to better nutrition.

In the case of adults views have changed of recent years concerning 'ideal' weight. Life insurance statistics have shown that maximal

Weight in pounds

Height in inches	5 years	6 years	7 years	8 years	9 years	10 years	11 years	12 years	13 years	14 years
38	34	34								
39	35	35								
40	36	36								
41	38	38	38							
42	39	39	39	39						
43	41	41	41	41						
44	44	44	44	44						
45	46	46	46	46	46					
47	49	50	50	50	50	50				
48		52	53	53	53	53				
49		55	55	55	55	55	55			
50		57	58	58	58	58	58	58		
51			61	61	61	61	61	61		
52			63	64	64	64	64	64	64	
53			66	67	67	67	67	68	68	
54				70	70	70	70	71	71	72
55				72	72	73	73	74	74	74
56				75	76	77	77	77	78	78
57					79	80	81	81	82	83
58					83	84	84	85	85	86
59						87	88	89	89	90
60						91	92	92	93	94
61							95	96	97	99
62							100	101	102	103
63							105	106	107	108
64								109	111	113
65								114	117	118
66									119	122
67									124	128
68										134
69										137
70										143
71										148

Correlation of height, weight, and age in boys.
Bird T. Baldwin and Thomas D. Wood, from Bridges' *Dietetics for the Clinician.*
Courtesy of Lea & Febiger and Henry Kimpton.

Height		Small Frame	Medium Frame	Large Frame
Feet	Inches	Pounds	Pounds	Pounds
5	2	116–125	124–133	131–142
5	3	119–128	127–136	133–144
5	4	122–132	130–140	137–149
5	5	126–136	134–144	141–153
5	6	129–139	137–147	145–157
5	7	133–143	141–151	149–162
5	8	136–147	145–156	153–166
5	9	140–151	149–160	157–170
5	10	144–155	153–164	161–175
5	11	148–159	157–168	165–180
6	0	152–164	161–173	169–185
6	1	157–169	166–178	174–190
6	2	163–175	171–184	179–196
6	3	168–180	176–189	184–202

Ideal weights for men.

Weight in pounds with clothes. Height in feet and inches, with shoes on.
From Metropolital Life Insurance Company, as noted by Rynearson and Gastineau.

Height		Small Frame	Medium Frame	Large Frame
Feet	Inches	Pounds	Pounds	Pounds
4	11	104–111	110–118	117–127
5	0	105–113	112–120	119–129
5	1	107–115	114–122	121–131
5	2	110–118	117–125	124–135
5	3	113–121	120–128	127–138
5	4	116–125	124–132	131–142
5	5	119–128	127–135	133–145
5	6	123–132	130–140	138–150
5	7	126–136	134–144	142–154
5	8	129–139	137–147	145–158
5	9	133–143	141–151	149–162
5	10	136–147	145–155	152–166
5	11	139–150	148–158	155–169

Ideal weights for women.

Weight in pounds with clothes. Height in feet and inches, with shoes on.
From Metropolital Life Insurance Company, as noted by Rynearson and Gastineau.

life expectancy is obtained if the average weight at ages 25 to 30 years is maintained throughout the rest of life. These insurance statistics also suggest that it is of advantage to be slightly over average weight before the age of 30 years, to be of average weight after the age of 40, and to be under-weight from ages 30 to 40. In the past it has been usual, in assessing the significance of an adult's weight, to allow a 10 per cent range on either side of normal for variations in body build. A closer correlation has been found between thoracic and abdominal measurements and weight.

WEIGHTS AND MEASURES: It is over a hundred years since the metric system was legalized in Britain, but it was not until 1969 that it became illegal to use any system of weights and measures other than the metric system for dispensing prescriptions.

A rationalization of the metric system is now in operation, known as the International System of Units (SI). This has been described as 'a coherent system with seven basic units from which all other units are derived'. Among these derived units is that for force – the newton, the symbol for which is N. The new unit of pressure is the pascal, the symbol for which is Pa, while the universal unit for energy is the joule, symbolized by J. Some exceptions have had to be made for practical purposes. From the medical aspect, the most important of these is that the derived basic unit for volume, the metre cubed (m^3), is too clumsy. The litre (l) is therefore retained as an alternative, with its various submultiples such as millilitre (ml). To avoid the possible confusion arising from the use of the comma, and not a full stop, for the decimal point in continental Europe, it is recommended that in writing large numbers, groups of three figures are separated by a space, and not by a comma. Thus one-million-five-hundred-thousand is 1,500,000, or $1\cdot5 \times 10^6$.

WEIL'S DISEASE (see LEPTOSPIROSIS).

WERNICKE'S ENCEPHALOPATHY: Also called the Wernicke-Korsakoff syndrome, this uncommon disorder is characterized by mental

	Name of Unit	Unit Symbol
Length	Metre	m
Mass	Kilogram	kg
Time	Second	s
Electric current	Ampere	A
Thermodynamic temperature	Kelvin	°K
Luminous intensity	Candela	cd
Amount of substance	Mole	mol

Basic units of the International System of Units (SI).

Metric Measures of Weight

1 kilogram (kg)	=	1000·0 g	=	2·20 pounds (avoirdupois)
1 hectogram	=	100·0 g	=	3·53 ounces (avoirdupois)
1 dekagram	=	10·0 g	=	154·32 grains
	=	1·0 g	=	15·43 grains
1 decigram	=	0·1 g	=	1·54 grains
1 centigram (cg)	=	0·01 g	=	0·15 grain
1 milligram (mg)	=	0·001 g	=	0·015 grain
1 microgram (μg)	=	0·000001 g	=	0·00001 grain

Metric Measures of Capacity

1 litre (l) = 1000 millilitres = 35·196 Imperial fluid ounces
1 millilitre (ml) = 0·001 litre = 16·89 minims

N.B. - 1 millilitre is approximately equivalent to 1 cubic centimetre (cc).

Factors for Converting from One Scale to the Other

To convert grams into grains	× 15·432
„ grams into avoirdupois ounces	× 0·0353
„ kilograms into pounds	× 2·205
„ grains into grams	× 0·065
„ avoirdupois ounces into grams	× 28·35
„ troy ounces into grams	× 31·104
„ millilitres into Imperial fluid ounces	× 0·0352
„ litres into Imperial fluid ounces	× 35·2
„ fluid ounces into millilitres	× 28·42
„ pints into litres	× 0·568
„ metres into inches	× 39·37
„ inches into metres	× 0·0254

Approximate Value of Domestic Measures

Tumbler = 10 fluid ounces	Table-spoon (small) = ½ fluid ounce
Breakfast-cup = 8 „ „	Dessert-spoon = 120 minims
Tea-cup = 5 „ „	Tea-spoon = 60 minims
Wine-glass (large) = 2½ „ „	Drop (of water) = 1 minim

Note – When medicine is measured this should be done by means of a standardized measure, because domestic utentils vary greatly in size.

Multiple	Prefix	Symbol	Submultiple	Prefix	Symbol
10^1	deca	da	10^{-1}	deci	d
10^2	hecto	h	10^{-2}	centi	c
10^3	kilo	k	10^{-3}	milli	m
10^6	mega	M	10^{-6}	micro	μ
10^9	giga	G	10^{-9}	nano	n
10^{12}	tera	T	10^{-12}	pico	p

Prefixes for decimal multiples and submultiples in the International System of Units.

confusion or delirium that occurs in combination with an unsteady gait (q.v.), nystagmus (see EYE, DISEASE AND INJURIES), and paralysis of the eye muscles and eventually psychosis (q.v.). It is caused by a deficiency of vitamin B_1 (thiamine) which affects the brain and nervous system. It occurs in alcoholic individuals and in patients with persistent vomiting. As soon as the condition is diagnosed, it must be treated with large doses of thiamine. Unless the patient has developed symptoms of psychosis, the condition is usually reversible with treatment.

WERTHHEIM'S HYSTERECTOMY: A major operation done to remove cancer of the uterus or ovary. The ovaries, fallopian tubes, the uterus and its ligaments, the upper vagina, and the regional lymph nodes are all excised.

WET PACK is a method of treatment popular in some countries for the purpose of applying a moderate degree of cold or of heat, for some time, to a patient's skin.

WHEEZING is a popular name applied to the various sounds produced in the chest when the bronchial tubes are narrowed. It is applied particularly to the long-drawn breathing of asthma, and to the whistling or purring noises that accompany breathing in cases of bronchitis. (See ASTHMA; BRONCHITIS.)

WHIPWORM is a popular name for *Trichuris trichiura*. (See TRICHURIASIS.)

WHITE BLOOD CELL (see LEUCOCYTE).

WHITE HAIR: The greying or whitening of hair which takes place with age is due to a loss of its pigment, melanin (q.v.), and the collection of air bubbles in the shaft of the hair. There is no evidence that hair ever goes white overnight, whether in response to shock, strain or any other cause. Rapid whitening may occur patchily in a matter of days, but it is more often a matter of weeks or months. In the more rapid cases the cause is thought to be a form of alopecia areata (see BALDNESS), in which the dark hairs which fall out are replaced by white hairs. An alternative cause is vitiligo (q.v.). Certain drugs, including mephenesin and chloroquine (q.v.) may also cause whitening of the hair.

WHITE LEG is a fairly common and well-known condition in which a limb, usually one of the lower limbs, becomes enlarged, white, and painful.
Causes: Most commonly the condition occurs after child-birth; sometimes it occurs during convalescence from an acute febrile disease, especially typhoid fever or pneumonia. It is usually due to inflammation in, and blocking of, the veins of the limb, or may be caused by the spread of infection into the lymphatics of the limb from those within the pelvis, or to some morbid change in the blood causing it to clot.
Symptoms: The disease comes on during convalescence from one of the conditions mentioned above, beginning with slight feverishness and pain down the leg which is to be affected. The limb gradually swells, and in a few days may be greatly enlarged, hard, glossy, and of a strikingly white colour. The veins can generally be felt as solid lines down the inner side of the thigh, and the affected parts may be very tender to the touch. These symptoms persist for a week or so, but generally begin to subside within a fortnight from the onset, and about three-fourths of all cases recover completely in a few

weeks. In other cases, some degree of muscular weakness, swelling, or aching of the limb remains permanently, but the condition, though a serious one demanding most careful treatment, is seldom fatal.
Treatment consists chiefly of rest in bed with the affected limb supported on a pillow. Pain is relieved by laudanum fomentations or simply by wrapping the limb in cotton-wool. Anticoagulants such as heparin and dicoumarol are given to prevent the process spreading.

This is one of the conditions, however, in which it is now recognized that preventive measures can be most effective. These consist principally of not allowing patients to stay in bed longer than necessary, or of giving massage to the legs in cases which are confined to bed for long periods. (See also VEINS, DISEASES OF.)

WHITES (see LEUCORRHOEA).

WHITE SWELLING is a popular name applied to tuberculous disease of joints. (See JOINTS, DISEASES OF.)

WHITLOW is a popular term applied to all acute inflammations of the deep-seated tissues in the fingers, whether the structure affected is the root of the nail, the pulp of the finger-tip, the sheaths of the tendons that run along the back and front of the fingers, or the bone. Acute inflammation of the bones in the finger is rare, and in general a whitlow begins in the last part of one finger, being, when situated towards the back, a small abscess at the root of the nail, and, when starting in front, an abscess in the fat and fibrous tissue that compose the pulp of the finger. Suppuration may also begin in the sheath of the tendon, generally in front of the finger.

WHOOPING-COUGH, also known as HOOPING-COUGH, PERTUSSIS, and CHIN-COUGH, is an infectious disease of the mucous membrane lining the air passages, which manifests itself by frequently recurring attacks of convulsive coughing, followed by a peculiar, loud indrawing of the breath, and often by vomiting. It occurs mostly in children, and seldom more than once in a lifetime.
Causes: The cause of whooping-cough is a bacillus discovered by Bordet and Gengou in 1906 and found in the sputum. It is known as *Bordetela pertussis*. Although specially a disease of childhood, whooping-cough is by no means limited to that period, but may occur at any time of life, even to old age, should there have been no previous attack. It is most prevalent between the ages of 1 and 4, and is uncommon after 10. Whooping-cough can be a dangerous disease in infants, but is a much less serious malady in older children. It has been occasionally observed in newly born infants, and is more common in girls than in boys. Whooping-cough is infectious during any stage of its progress, but chiefly at its commence-

ment. It prevails mostly in the winter months, doubtless owing to the increasing predisposition to affections of the respiratory passages. In recent years the disease has tended to occur in cycles, with periods of increased prevalence occurring every three to four years. The incubation period is usually 7 to 10 days.

In an epidemic of whooping-cough, which extended from the last quarter of 1977 to mid-1979, 102,500 cases of whooping-cough were notified in the United Kingdom, with 36 deaths. This was the biggest outbreak since 1957 and its size was partly attributed to the fall in vaccination acceptance rates. In 1984 5,500 cases were notified in England and Wales.

Symptoms: Three stages of the disease are recognized: (1) the catarrhal, (2) the spasmodic, (3) the stage of decline.

The *first stage* is characterized by the usual symptoms of a catarrh, with sneezing, watering of the eyes, irritation of the throat, feverishness, and cough, but in general there is nothing in the symptoms to indicate that they are to develop into whooping-cough. There may be a slight rise of temperature to 37·2 to 37·7 °C (99 to 100 °F) in the first few days. The catarrhal stage usually lasts from ten to fourteen days.

The *second stage* is marked by the abatement of the catarrhal symptoms, but at the same time by increase in the cough, which now occurs in irregular paroxysms both by day and by night. Each paroxysm consists in a series of violent and rapid expiratory coughs, succeeded by a loud sonorous or crowing inspiration – the 'whoop'. The attacks are on the whole most severe at night. This stage of the disease usually lasts for two to four weeks, but it may be shorter or longer. It is during this time that complications are apt to arise which may become a source of danger greater even than the malady itself. The chief of these are inflammatory affections of the bronchial tubes and lungs, and convulsions, any of which may prove fatal. A milder complication is the formation of a small ulcer under the tongue from rubbing against the teeth in coughing. Hernia and prolapse of the rectum sometimes are produced by the strain of violent coughing.

When, however, the disease progresses favourably, as it usually does, it passes into the *third* or *terminal stage*, in which the cough becomes less frequent and generally loses in great measure its whooping character. The patient's general condition undergoes improvement, and the symptoms disappear in from one to three weeks. It is to be observed, however, that for a long period afterwards in any simple catarrh from which the patient suffers the cough often assumes a spasmodic character, which may suggest the erroneous notion that a relapse of the whooping-cough has occurred.

In severe cases it sometimes happens that the disease leaves behind it such structural changes in the lungs (eg. emphysema) as entail permanent shortness of breathing, or a liability to attacks of asthma. Occasionally the violence of the cough may rupture a blood-vessel in the eye, or in the brain with hemiplegia as a result.

Treatment: In mild cases, little is necessary beyond keeping the patient warm and carefully attending to the general health. The remedies applicable in the case of catarrh or the milder forms of bronchitis are of service here. In mild weather the patient may be in the open air. In the more severe forms, efforts have to be employed to modify the severity of the paroxysms. During convalescence, when the cough still continues to be troublesome, a change of air will often effect its removal.

Antibiotics, including tetracyclines, chloramphenicol, cephaloridine, erythromycin, and co-trimoxazole are of value, but it is not recommended that they should be used routinely. The main indications for their use are in young children and when there are complications.

A vaccine has been prepared which is effective as a prophylactic. This is given in the form of Triple Vaccine (Diphtheria, Tetanus, and Pertussis Vaccine) at the age of 3 or 6 months. A second dose is given six to eight weeks later, and a third dose six months later. It should not be given to a child with any disease or disorder of the central nervous system, to a child with a history of convulsions or to a child with a family history of convulsions. Administration should also be postponed in the case of a temporarily unwell child until he is well again.

WIDAL REACTION (see AGGLUTINATION).

WILMS' TUMOUR, or NEPHROBLASTOMA, is the commonest kidney tumour in infancy. It is a malignant tumour, which occurs in around 1 per 10,000 live births. The survival rate with modern treatment (removal of the kidney followed by radiotherapy and chemotherapy) is now around 80 per cent.

WILSON'S DISEASE or HEPATOLENTICULAR DEGENERATION, is a familial disease in which there is an increased accumulation of copper in the liver, brain, and other tissues including the kidneys. Its main manifestation is the development of tremor and rigidity, with difficulty in speech. In many cases there is improvement following the administration of dimercaprol, penicillamine, or trientine dihydrochloride; these substances cause an increased excretion of copper.

WINDPIPE is the popular name for the trachea, which extends from the larynx above to the point in the upper part of the chest where it divides into the two large bronchial tubes, one to each lung. It thus extends through the lower part of the neck and upper part of the chest, and is about 10 cm (4 inches) in length. It consists of a fibrous tube kept permanently open by about twenty strong horizontally placed hoops of cartilage, each of which forms about two-thirds of a circle, but is defective behind where the two ends are united by muscle-fibres. This fibro- cartilaginous tube is lined by a smooth mucous membrane, richly supplied with mucous glands and covered by a single layer of ciliated epithelium. (See also AIR PASSAGES.)

WINTER VOMITING DISEASE, or EPIDEMIC NAUSEA AND VOMITING, is a condition characterized by nausea, vomiting, diarrhoea and giddiness, which occurs during the winter. Outbreaks of it usually involve whole families or may affect communities like schools. It is due to parvoviruses. The incubation period is 24 to 48 hours, and attacks seldom persist for more than 72 hours.

WISDOM TOOTH is a popular name for the last molar tooth on either side of each jaw. These teeth are the last to appear and should develop in early adult life, but often they do not cut the gum till the age of 20 or 25 or indeed they may sometimes remain permanently impacted in the jaw-bone. This occurs in up to 25 per cent of individuals. The lower third molar is often impacted against the second because of the direction in which it erupts. (See TEETH.)

WITCH-HAZEL is a preparation of the bark, twigs, and dried leaves from *Hamamelis virginiana*, a plant of the United States possessed of strong astringent properties. It is used to check haemorrhages and excessive mucous discharges, and also for piles. The most commonly used preparation is the liquid extract, which is sometimes given internally and more often used in the strength of 4 ml to 85 ml of cold water, either as a lotion for bruises or as an enema for bleeding piles. Extract of hamamelis is employed as an application for varicose veins and ulcers; and ointments, known as hazeline snow and hazeline cream, are used as applications for irritable states of the skin.

WITHDRAWAL SYMPTOMS: Unpleasant physical and mental symptoms that occur when a person stops using a drug on which he or she are dependent. The symptoms include tremors, sweating, and vomiting which are reversed if further doses are given. Alcohol and hard drugs, such as morphine, heroin, and cocaine, are among the substances that induce dependence, and therefore withdrawal symptoms, when stopped. Amphetamines and nicotine are other examples.

WOLFFIAN DUCTS: The Wolffian ducts and the Mullerian ducts are separate sets of primordia that transiently co-exist in embryos of both sexes. In the male the Wolffian ducts give rise to the vas deferens, the seminal vesicles and the epididymis, while the Mullerian ducts disappear. In female embryos the Mullerian ducts grow and fuse in the midline to produce the Fallopian tubes, the uterus and the upper third of the vagina, whereas the Wolffian ducts regress. The former phase of development requires a functioning testis from which an inducer substance diffuses locally over the primordia to bring about the suppression of the Mullerian duct and the development of the Wolffian duct. In the absence of this substance development proceeds along female lines regardless of the genetic sex.

WOMB (see UTERUS).

WOMB MUSIC is the somewhat fanciful name given to the playing to crying babies of sounds comparable to those by which the unborn babe is surrounded in the womb, such as the beating of the mother's heart, the bowel sounds of the babe and the like. The claim is that the replaying of these brings back the 'peaceful music of the womb', to which they have become conditioned, and thus 'sings' them to sleep.

WOOL-SORTERS' DISEASE is another name for anthrax. (See ANTHRAX.)

WORD BLINDNESS is a condition in which, as the result of disease in the brain, a person becomes unable to associate their proper meanings with words, although he may be quite able to spell the letters. WORD DEAFNESS is an associated condition in which, though hearing remains perfect, the patient has lost the power of referring the names he hears to the articles they denote. (See DYSPHASIA.)

WORMS (see ASCARIASIS, ENTEROBIASIS, TAENIASIS).

WOUNDS: A wound is any breach suddenly produced in the tissues of the body by direct violence. An extensive injury of the deeper parts without corresponding injury of the surface is known as a bruise or contusion.
Varieties: Classified according to the immediate effect produced, four varieties are usually described as *incised, punctured, lacerated,* and *contused.*
INCISED WOUNDS are usually inflicted with some sharp instrument, and are clean cuts, in which the tissues are simply divided without any damage to parts around. The bleeding from such a wound is apt to be very free, but it can be readily controlled.
PUNCTURED WOUNDS, or stabs, are inflicted with a pointed instrument. These wounds are the most dangerous, partly because their depth involves the danger of wounding vital organs, partly because bleeding from a stab is hard to control, and largely on account of the difficulty of sterilization. The wound produced by the nickel-nosed bullet is a puncture, much less severe than the ugly lacerated wound caused by an expanding bullet, or by a ricochet, and, if no clothing has been carried in by the bullet, the wound is clean and usually heals at once.
LACERATED WOUNDS are those in which great

tearing takes place, such as injuries caused by machinery. The blood-vessels being torn and twisted, little bleeding is apt to result, and a limb may be torn completely away without great loss of blood. Such wounds are, however, specially liable to infection.

CONTUSED WOUNDS are those accompanied by much bruising of surrounding parts, as in the case of a blow from a cudgel or poker. In these wounds also there is little bleeding, but healing is slow on account of damage to the edges of the wound.

Any of these varieties may become infected by pus-forming germs and develop into a POISONED WOUND.

First-aid treatment: The first aim is to check any bleeding. This may be done by pressure upon the edges of the wound with a clean handkerchief, or, if the bleeding is serious, by putting the finger in the wound and pressing it upon the spot from which the blood is coming.

If medical attention is available within a few hours, it should not be interfered with further than is necessary to stop the bleeding and to cover the wound with a clean dry handkerchief or piece of lint. When expert assistance is not soon obtainable, one of the following procedures may be adopted. The bleeding being checked, the next step is to cleanse the wound and surrounding skin.

(*a*) *By painting freely with acriflavine, cetrimide, chlorhexidine or chloroxylenol* the wound and the surrounding skin, and covering with a piece of clean dry lint or strip dressing.

(*b*) *By washing with boiled water.*

The injured part should be fixed so that movement is prevented or minimized. A wounded hand or arm is fixed with a sling (see SLING), a wounded leg with a splint (see SPLINTS).

If the injury has caused severe shock, the patient must be treated for that. (See SHOCK.)

Healing of wounds: The reaction of the tissues to an injury is similar to that produced by any other irritation. If the wound has been accompanied by loss of tissue which has to be made good, or by death of a piece of tissue which has to be cast off as a slough, or by infection with bacteria which has to be overcome, the process of repair is tedious, and in some cases permanent damage is produced. The new tissue formed in the wound is mainly fibrous tissue, like that composing the supporting framework of the body.

Dangers of wounds: BLOOD-POISONING usually means that the germs themselves have entered the circulation, which is a grave occurrence and may be fatal. (See BLOOD-POISONING.)

ERYSIPELAS, TETANUS and GAS GANGRENE are conditions in which the germs, (or their toxins) responsible for these diseases enter the lymphatics and blood-stream and produce widespread effects. (See ERYSIPELAS; TETANUS; GANGRENE.)

HAEMORRHAGE: *Primary haemorrhage* means bleeding which occurs at the time of the injury. A large vein or artery may have been divided and may require to be tied. (See HAEMORRHAGE.) A wound of a large vessel like the femoral or the popliteal artery may cause death in a few minutes if untreated. *Reactionary haemorrhage* takes place sometimes from wounds which do not bleed much when they are first inflicted. The explanation is that the shock caused by the injury enfeebles the action of the heart, and, when the wounded person recovers from the shock in a few hours, the increased force of the heart's beating causes bleeding to recommence in the wound. *Secondary haemorrhage* occurs only in the case of poisoned wounds. The spread of the infection breaks down the blood-clot which has formed in the open end of a blood-vessel and allows the escape of blood. It is usually preceded by a slight oozing of blood, which serves to forewarn the medical attendant. This form of bleeding seldom occurs earlier than a week from the date of the injury.

SCALP WOUNDS usually heal well, but in deep scalp wounds there is a danger that suppuration may result and may pass within the skull. Again, a severe blow producing a scalp wound may cause fracture of the skull and concussion or compression of the brain. (See BRAIN, DISEASES AND INJURIES OF.)

CHEST WOUNDS: Stabs of the chest are serious chiefly because of the fatal bleeding likely to follow any wound of the heart or large vessels; a less serious danger attends wounds of the pleural cavity causing collapse of the lung or empyema.

ABDOMINAL WOUNDS: A penetrating wound of the abdomen, particularly when the bowel has been cut, is often fatal from the acute general peritonitis which it causes.

WRIST is the joint situated between the arm above and the hand below. The region of the wrist contains eight small carpal bones, arranged in two rows, each containing four bones. Those in the proximal row, that is the row nearest the forearm, are from the outside inwards when looking at the palm of the hand, the scaphoid, lunate, triquetrum, and pisiform. Those in the distal row, that is the row nearest the hand, are the trapezium, trapezoid, capitate and hamate. These intervene between the arm bones and the five metacarpal bones in the hand, and have the effect of diminishing jars communicated to the hand in virtue of a certain amount of sliding movement over one another, of which they are capable. These small bones are closely bound to one another by short, strong ligaments, and the wrist-joint is the union of the composite mass thus formed with the radius and ulna in the forearm. The wrist and the radius and ulna are united by strong outer and inner lateral ligaments, and by weaker ligaments before and behind, whilst the powerful tendons passing to the hand and fingers give it a great measure of strength.

The joint is capable of movement in all directions, and, on account of its shape and its numerous ligaments, is little liable to dislocation, although stretching or tearing of some of these ligaments is a common accident, constituting a sprain. (See JOINTS, DISEASES AND INJURIES OF.) Inflammation of the tendon-sheaths before and behind the wrist, causing the presence of fluid, also results occasionally from an injury, and produces a sense of weakness in the wrist. A fairly common condition is that known as a ganglion, in which an elastic swelling full of fluid develops on the back or front of the wrist in connection with the sheaths of the tendons. (See GANGLION.)

WRIST-DROP (see DROP WRIST).

WRITER'S CRAMP is a spasm which affects certain muscles when engaged in writing, and which may not occur when the same muscles are employed in other acts. Similar symptoms are observed in the case of musicians (guitar, clarinet and piano in particular), typists, word-processor and computer operators and artists.

WRY-NECK is a condition in which the head is twisted to one side. It may be caused by the contraction of a scar, such as that resulting from a burn or by paralysis of some of the muscles, but in the great majority of cases it is a spasmodic condition due to excessive tendency of certain muscles to contract. (See CRAMP; SPASMODIC TORTICOLLIS.)

X

XANTHELASMATA: These are yellow plaques of lipid deposited in the skin. They tend to occur in the eyelids. They are often associated with hyperlipidaemia.

XANTHOMATA: These are deposits of fatty tissue in tendon sheaths and over bony prominences such as knees, elbows and fingers. They are indicative of a state of hyperlipidaemia which may be a primary inherited disorder or secondary to such conditions as biliary cirrhosis, diabetes mellitus or nephrotic syndrome.

X CHROMOSOME: One of two sex chromosomes. Every normal female body cell has a pair of X chromosomes. Men have only one X chromosome and this is paired with a Y chromosome. The sex cells in men and women each have one X and one Y chromosome. Certain diseases are linked to the presence of an X chromosome: these include haemophilia (q.v.) (see GENES).

XENOGRAFT is a transplant from one animal to another of a different species. It is also known as a heterograft.

XERODERMA is a rough, dry condition of the skin accompanied by the copious formation of scales.

XERODERMA PIGMENTOSUM is a rare hereditary affection of the skin appearing first in early childhood. It is characterized by a dry skin which is heavily freckled and hypersensitive to sunlight.

XEROPHTHALMIA (see EYE, DISEASE AND INJURIES).

XEROSIS means abnormal dryness, especially of the eye.

XEROSTOMIA is the condition of dryness of the mouth due to lack of saliva. Its most extreme form occurs following radiotherapy of the mouth, and in the condition known as Sjögren's syndrome. No satisfactory substitute for natural saliva has been found though some find a methyl-cellulose substitute gives partial relief, as may a glycerin mouth-wash.

XIPHISTERNUM (see XIPHOID PROCESS.)

XIPHOID PROCESS or XIPHOID CARTILAGE: Also known as the xiphisternum, this is the small oval-shaped projection forming the lowest of the three parts of the sternum or breast bone.

X-RAYS (RÖNTGEN RAYS) were discovered in 1895 by Wilhelm Conrad Röntgen. Their use for diagnostic *imaging (radiology)* and for cancer therapy (see RADIOTHERAPY) is now an integral part of medicine. Many other forms of diagnostic imaging have been developed in recent years, sometimes also loosely called 'radiology'. Similarly the use of chemotherapeutic agents in cancer has led to the term *oncology* which may be applied to the treatment of cancer by both drugs and X-rays.

The rays are part of the electro-magnetic spectrum; their wavelengths are between 10^{-9} and 10^{-13} metres; in behaviour and energy they are identical to the gamma rays emitted by radioactive isotopes. Diagnostic X-rays are generated in an evacuated tube contining an anode and cathode. Electrons striking the anode cause emission of X-rays of varying energy; the energy is largely dependent on the potential difference (kilovoltage) between anode and cathode. The altered tissue penetration at different kilovoltages is used in radiographing different regions, for example in breast radiography (25–40 kV) or chest radiography (120–150 kV). Most diagnostic examinations use kilovoltages between 60 and 120. The energy of X-rays enbles them to pass through body tissues unless they make contact with the constituent atoms. Tissue attenuation varies with atomic structure, so that air-containing organs such as the lung offer little attenuation, while material such as bone, with abundant calcium, will absorb the majority of incident X-rays. This results in an emerging X-ray pattern which corresponds to the structures in the region examined.

The recording of the resulting images – *radiography* – is achieved in several ways, mostly depending on the use of materials which fluoresce in response to X-rays. Initially the use of such materials, mounted on card and examined in darkness, allowed brief study of bodily structures or events. Permanent images were on photographic glass plates. However photographic amulsions are relatively insensitive to X-rays so X-ray film is now also excited by light emitted by substances which fluoresce in response to X-rays. The film, usually doubly coated with emulsion to increase its responsiveness, is placed in a light-tight cassette. It is firmly compressed between screens faced with materials responsive to X-rays. Originally barium platino-cyanide and calcium tungstate were used; now more responsive materials – rare-earth compounds – such as zinc-cadmium sulphide are employed. The result has been a marked reduction in the X-ray dose needed for a given examination.

CONTRAST X-RAYS Many body organs are not shown by simple X-ray studies. This has led to the development of *contrast* materials which can be used to make particular organs or structures wholly or partly opaque to X-rays. Thus barium-sulphate preparations are largely used for examining the gastro-intestinal tract, i.e. barium swallow, barium meal, barium follow-through (or enteroclysis) and barium enema. Water-soluble iodine-containing contrast agents that ionize in solution have been developed for a range of other studies.

More recently a series of improved contrast molecules, chiefly non-ionizing, has been developed, with fewer side-effects. They can, for example, safely be introduced into the spinal theca for *myeloradiculography* – contrast X-rays of the spinal cord. Using these agents, it is possible to show many organs and structures mostly by direct introduction, e.g. via a catheter. In urography, however, contrast medium injected intravenously is excreted by the kidneys which are outlined, together with ureters and bladder. A number of other more specialized contrast agents exist, e.g. for cholecystography – radiological assessment of the gall bladder. The use of contrast and the attendant techniques has greatly widened the range of radiology.

IMAGE INTENSIFICATION The relative insensitivity of fluorescent materials when used for observation of moving organs – e.g. the oesophagus – has been overcome by the use of image intensification. A faint fluorographic image produced by X-rays leads to electron emission from a photo-cathode. By applying a high potential difference, the electrons are accelerated across an evacuated tube and are focused on to a small flourescent screen, giving a bright image. This is viewed by a TV camera and the image shown on a monitor and sometimes recorded on videotape or cine.

TOMOGRAPHY X-rays images are two-dimensional representations of three-dimensional objects. Tomography (Greek *tomos* – a slice) began with X-ray imaging produced by the linked movement of the X-ray tube and the cassette pivoting about a selected plane in the body: over- and underlying structures are blurred out, giving a more detailed image of a particular plane.

In 1975 Godfrey Hounsfield introduced *computerized tomography* (*CT*). This involves (i) movement of an X-ray tube around the patient, with a narrow fan beam of X-rays; (ii) the corresponding use of sensitive detectors on the opposite side of the patient; (iii) computer analysis of the detector readings at each point on the rotation, with calculation of relative tissue attenuation at each point in the cross-sectional plant. This invention has enormously increased the ability to discriminate tissue composition, even without the use of contrast.

The tomographic effect – imaging of a particular plane – is achieved in many of the newer forms of imaging – *ultrasount* (q.v.), magnetic resonance imaging (see NUCLEAR MAGNETIC RESONANCE) and some forms of nuclear medicine, in particular *positron emission tomography* (*PET*) (q.v.). An alternative term for the production of images of a given plane is *cross-sectional imaging*.

While the production of X-ray and other images has been largely the responsibility of radiographers, the interpretation has been principally carried out by specialist doctors called radiologists. In addition they, and interested clinicians, have developed a number of procedures, such as *arteriography* (see ANGLOGRAPHY), which involve manipulative access for imaging, e.g. selective coronary or renal arteriography.

The use of X-rays, ultrasound or computerized tomography to control the direction and position of needles has made possible quided biopsies, e.g. of pancreatic, pulmonary or bony lesions, and therapeutic procedures such as drainage of obstructed kidneys (percutaneous nephrostomy), or of abscesses. From these has grown a whole series of therapeutic procedures such as angioplasty (q.v.), stent insertion (q.v.) and renal-stone track formation. This field of *interventional radiology* has close affinities with minimally invasive surgery.

Radiotherapy, or treatment by X-rays: The two chief sources of the ionizing radiations used in radiotherapy are the gamma rays of radium (q.v.) and the penetrating X-rays generated by apparatus working at various voltages. For superficial lesions energies of around 40 kilovolts are used, but for deep-seated conditions, such as cancer of the internal organs, much higher voltages are required. X-ray machines are now in use which work at two million volts. Even higher voltages are now available through the development of the linear accelerator, which makes use of the frequency magnetron which is the basis of radar. The linear accelerator receives its name from the fact that it accelerates a beam of electrons down a straight tube, 3 metres in length, and in this process a voltage of eight million is attained. The use of these very high voltages has led to the development of a highly specialized technique which has been devised for the treatment of cancer and like diseases.

Like the photographic effect, the therapeutic effects were discovered almost accidentally. It was observed that prolonged exposures to the rays caused inflammation, and even ulceration of the skin, and further, that they caused loss of hair, and that they improved various diseased conditions. Repeated exposures, for example, of the hands of physicians using this method of treatment, have been observed to produce pigmentation of the skin, excessive growth of its horny layer, and even epithelioma. X-rays are particularly hurtful to the testes and ovaries of young people; and when these are exposed to the rays repeatedly, the genital glands must be covered by sheet-lead or some such protection, in case sterility should result. Too severe a reaction to the irritating effect of the rays upon the patient's skin at a single session must also be avoided. It is important to protect the surrounding areas, and this is done by the use of masks of sheet-lead, with a hole cut out over the affected area, and by enclosing the tube in a metal-lined box, with an opening opposite the affected spot. By these means, as well as by wearing lead-lined gloves, and by frequently anointing the skin with some simple ointment, people constantly applying the rays are effectually protected.

The greatest value of radiotherapy is in the treatment of malignant disease. In many cases it can be used for the treatment of malignant growths which are not accessible to surgery, whilst in others it is used in conjunction with surgery.

Leukaemia and other conditions, in which the spleen is enlarged, are often greatly benefited by exposure of the spleen or long bones to X-rays or radium. (See RADIOTHERAPY.)

In simple conditions, particularly superficial ones, X-rays have been used very successfully, but are being used less and less, in view of the increasing necessity to reduce to the absolute minimum the amount of irradiation to which people are exposed.

Y

YAWNING consists of an involuntary opening of the mouth, which is accompanied by marked dilatation of the pharynx, a characteristic distortion of the face and usually stretching of the limbs. The cause and function of yawning are quite obscure. It is classically regarded as a sign of drowsiness or boredom, but it not infrequently occurs following a severe haemorrhage, and it is also sometimes associated with indigestion.

YAWS, known also as FRAMBOESIA and PIAN, is a disease of the tropics, especially of Africa and the West Indies, affecting both white and black races. It consists in the appearance of small tumours covered with yellow crusts, scattered over the surface of the body.

Cause: The disease is directly contagious from person to person, and the infection is probably also carried by flies, and certainly by clothing and by the unclean huts of the natives. The direct cause is a spirochaete known as *Treponema pertenue*, and the occurrence of the disease in a person of unhealthy constitution, or one who is suffering from another disease, such as syphilis or tuberculosis, renders the attack much more serious.

Symptoms: The disease does not appear for a fortnight or more after infection, and during this time fever, malaise, pains, and itching of the skin may come on. It begins as a scaly eruption about the body and legs, in which small lumps form, and grow till they reach a size even of several centimetres in diameter. The surface of these is covered by a yellow crust of dried-up secretion, and in unhealthy people the tumours may break down and produce deep ulcers. After a duration of weeks or months the tumours gradually shrink and disappear.

Treatment: The outlook in yaws has been transformed by the introduction of penicillin, the effects of which are dramatic in this disease.

Y CHROMOSOME: One of two sex chromosomes that is present in every male body cell where it is paired with an X chromosome. The sex or germ cells in women as well as men contain one X and one Y chromosome (see GENES).

YEAST consists of the cells and spores of unicellular fungi belonging to the family of Saccharomycetaceae. The main species of yeast used in medicine is *Saccharomyces cerevisiae*, which is used in the fermentation industries, such as brewing. It is a rich source of the vitamin B complex (see VITAMIN), but its use has largely been given up since the various components of the vitamin B complex became available as separate entities.

YELLOW FEVER, also known as YELLOW JACK and VOMITO AMARILLI, is an acute disease of certain tropical localities, characterized by fever and jaundice.

Distribution: It is endemic in Africa from coast to coast south of the Sahara to Zambia. It also occurs in the northern part of South America and to a less extent today in Central America. In 1793 a very serious epidemic spread over the Northern United States, and, in Philadelphia alone, over 10 per cent of the population were swept off in the course of four months. Numerous other epidemics invaded the States in the end of the eighteenth and during the course of the nineteenth centuries, the last severe one taking place in 1878. In Europe the disease has from time to time invaded some of the Portuguese and Spanish ports, but it has never gained any permanent hold. When cases of yellow fever arrive at British or other northern European ports, no spread of the disease takes place. It is also unknown in the Far East.

Causes: The disease is due to a virus which is transmitted to man by the *Aedes aegypti* mosquito. Monkeys are an important reservoir of infection in areas where the disease is endemic. The virus is found in the blood of infected individuals during the first three or four days of the disease. The blood of a patient is directly infectious, and the deaths of three of the great investigators of the disease, Stokes, Noguchi, and Young, all of whom died of yellow fever, were probably due to direct contact with infected blood.

One attack gives more or less protection for life. Many adult natives in yellow fever areas therefore are protected against reinfection by having had the disease in childhood. In affected areas babies born to immune mothers are protected against the disease for several months.

Symptoms: Different cases vary greatly in severity, but the disease is apt to be especially serious during the prevalence of an epidemic, or when it affects people newly arrived from healthier parts. The incubation period is usually 3 to 5 days, but may be up to 10 days.

Three stages are usually described in a severe case. The *first stage* begins suddenly with headache, chill, pains in the back and limbs, and rise of temperature. The eyes are bloodshot. Vomiting also occurs, the tongue is furred, and the bowels are constipated. An important point is that the urine decreases in amount, and, if tested, is found to contain albumin, the result of inflammation of the kidneys. The degree in which these signs are present forms a valuable indication of the severity of the case and of the need for special treatment.

These symptoms last for about three days and then sometimes abate to some extent for a day and the patient appears better. This constitutes the *second stage*.

The *third stage* begins usually about the fourth day. The patient now becomes very weak and the black vomit comes on. This consists in bringing up constantly from the stomach a clear fluid containing black flakes formed of blood that has been acted upon by the gastric juice. Although this black vomit is regarded as an alarming sign, it is by no means an index that the patient is sure to die. Jaundice also appears with the third stage, and is the symptom to which the disease owes its name. Usually it amounts only to a pale yellow discoloration of the skin, but it may become mahogany brown in hue, and small haemorrhages under the skin and mucous membranes are also common. In fatal cases examined after death, the principal changes found are fatty degeneration of the liver, acute inflammation of the kidneys, and an inflamed and congested state of the stomach, which contains some of the black fluid mentioned above.

Treatment: PREVENTIVE TREATMENT is important, and consists of vaccination of everyone travelling to and from those parts of the world where the disease occurs. Such vaccination is compulsory, not only for the inhabitants of endemic zones and for travellers going to these areas, but, in addition, many countries outside endemic areas require that travellers who have come from, or have passed through, yellow fever areas shall have been vaccinated. The protection it gives comes on within ten days and is long-lasting, but it is wise for residents in yellow-fever areas to have it repeated every ten years. The sick must be kept for the first three days of illness in rooms protected by mosquito-netting, so that they may not infect mosquitoes which would pass on the disease to healthy people. The same general measures as in the case of malaria should be taken against mosquitoes.

CURATIVE TREATMENT must be directed towards checking symptoms as they arise. The patient must have plenty of water in small draughts, containing glucose, and flavoured with lime, orange, or grapefruit juice. Later on, the only food should be milk, thin soups, and similar liquid nourishment. The high temperature, which sometimes shows itself, is relieved by sponging or by the wet pack (q.v.).

YERSINIA is a genus of bacteria which includes the causative organism of plague, *Yersinia pestis*. (See PLAGUE.)

YOGHURT is sour milk curdled with one of the lactic-acid producing bacilli, such as *Lactobacillus acidophilus* or *Lactobacillus bulgaricus*. It contains all the protein, fat, calcium, and vitamins of the original milk, and is therefore a nutritious food, but there is no evidence that it has any unique beneficial properties of its own. In countries where standards of hygiene are low it has the advantage of having been sterilized by boiling and is therefore unlikely to be contaminated with dangerous micro-organisms.

YOHIMBINE is derived from the bark of *Pausinystalia yohimbie*, a West African tree. Once widely used as an aphrodisiac, an action for which there is no good evidence, it is now being used in the treatment of certain cases of postural hypotension and for the treatment of impotence. It is an alpha adrenoreceptor agonist.

YTTRIUM-90: An artificially produced isotope of the element Yttrium. The isotope is radioactive and emits beta rays which are utilized for the treatment of tumours.

Z

ZIDOVUDINE: An antiviral drug, with the trade name of Retrovir, used to treat AIDS and its related conditions, such as pneumocystis pneumonia. The drug slows down the growth of human immunodeficiency virus (HIV) but does not cure the disease. It may be given intravenously or by mouth. The drug, also called AZT, has been in use since 1987, and it works by blocking the enzyme that simulates HIV to grow and multiply. It may cause anaemia so regular blood tests are necessary.

ZINC is a metal, several salts of which are used in medicine for external application. It is essential for growth and development in animals and plants. The average human body contains a total of 1 to 2 grams, and most human diets contain 10 to 15 mg. In human beings, deficiency of zinc results in lack of growth, slow sexual development and anaemia. Deficiency is also associated with a skin disorder known as acrodermatitis enteropathica.

Uses: Zinc chloride is a powerful caustic and astringent which, combined with zinc sulphate, is used as an astringent mouth-wash. Zinc sulphate is also used in the form of eye-drops in the treatment of certain forms of conjunctivitis. (See EYE DISEASES AND INJURIES.)

Zinc oxide, zinc stearate, and zinc carbonate are made up in dusting powders, in ointments, in paste bandages or suspended in water as lotions for the astringent action they exert upon abraded surfaces of the skin. Zinc and castor oil ointment of the *British Pharmacopoeia* is a well-tried treatment for napkin rash.

Zinc undecenoate is used as an ointment and as a dusting- powder in the treatment of ringworm (q.v.).

ZOLLINGER-ELLISON SYNDROME: A rare disorder in which severe peptic ulcers recur in the stomach and duodenum (see DUODENAL ULCER; STOMACH, DISEASES OF). It is caused by a tumour in the pancreas that produces a hormone gastrin (q.v.) which stimulates the stomach and duodenum to produce excess acid and this causes ulceration. Treatment is by surgery.

ZONA and **ZOSTER** are two names for the eruption popularly known as shingles. (See HERPES ZOSTER.)

ZONULOLYSIS is the process whereby the zonule (see EYE) is dissolved by an enzyme (chymotrypsin) as part of intracapsular cataract surgery. Once the zonule has been dissolved the cataract can be lifted out of the eye (see CATARACT).

ZOONOSES are animal diseases which can be transmitted to man. There are over 150 infections of domestic and wild vertebrates which can be transmitted in this way, including bovine tuberculosis, brucellosis, hydatid cysts, ringworm, toxocariasis, toxoplasmosis, leptospirosis, listeriosis, and rabies. (See separate entries for details of these diseases.)

ZYGOMA, or ZYGOMATIC BONE, is the name given to a bridge of bone formed by the union of a process from the temporal bone with one from the malar bone. It lies in the region of the temple, gives attachment to the powerful masseter muscle which moves the lower jaw, and forms a protection to the side of the head.

ZYGOTE: This is the cell produced when an ovum is fertilized by a sperm. A zygote contains all the hereditary material for a new individual: half comes from the sperm and half from the ovum. After passing down the fallopian tube, when the zygote starts dividing, it becomes implanted in the uterus and develops into an embryo.

APPENDIX: BASIC FIRST AID

This appendix is designed to cover the basic principles involved in the immediate treatment of some common emergencies. It is not comprehensive, and anyone wishing to become proficient at first aid should attend a course run by a reputable organization such as the British Red Cross, 9 Grosvenor Crescent, London SW1X 7EJ (071-235 5454), St John Ambulance, 1 Grosvenor Crescent, London SW1X 7EF (071-235 5231, fax: 071-235 0796) and the St Andrew's Ambulance Association, Strachan House, 16 Torphichen Street, Edinburgh EH3 8JB (031-229 5419).

First-aid treatment in an emergency is intended:
- to preserve life and stop the victim's condition from deteriorating.
- to help recovery and save the victim from further harm.
- to make the casualty as comfortable as possible and reassure him/her and the family.
- to assess the events surrounding the illness or accident so that relevant facts can be given to a doctor, nurse or paramedical staff.

No ill or badly injured person should be moved without skilled assistance – especially if a neck or spinal injury is suspected – unless the individual's life is in immediate danger from the surroundings, for example, a fire. He or she should be kept warm; constricting clothing should be loosened; and a clear airway should be established, with any false teeth removed.

BLEEDING: This may occur from arteries, veins or capillary beds. The former is easily recognized as the blood tends to spurt from the wound at the same rate as the pulse. With the latter two types the blood tends to flow from the wound. Minor bleeding is usually treated in the home by the application of bandages, etc. However, the basic principles of treatment for major haemorrhages may be applied. Pressure should be applied to the bleeding point, via gauze or a clean piece of cloth if available, firmly enough to stop the flow of blood. With the pressure applied, the wound should be raised above the level of the heart. The patient should then be transferred to a place where medical care is available. If the loss of blood is severe enough for the victim to have become shocked, he or she should be laid flat with the legs raised, if possible.

BURNS: All but the most minor burns should be seen by a doctor as it is difficult to assess the severity of the burn immediately after it occurs. If the person or his or her clothing is actually on fire, then the first move must be to smother the flames by covering them with a blanket or coat, for example, and 'patting out' the flames without sustaining burns yourself. Many burns, however, are caused by hot liquids, hot gases, flashes from explosions or contact with a very hot object so that the person is not actually on fire. The treatment for all these burns is the same – to remove any clothing over the affected area, if possible, and to put the affected area under cold running water until the pain has stopped or the ambulance has arrived (the cold water should be applied for several minutes as cooling of the tissues, particularly the deeper layers of the skin, will limit the extent of the burn). The burn should be left exposed or covered with a piece of clean wet linen, e.g. a pillowcase, for the transfer to hospital. No lotions or potions should be applied to the burn until it has been seen by a doctor or a nurse.

CHOKING: Severe life-threatening choking occurs when a piece of food or a foreign object becomes lodged in the larynx or trachea (qq.v.) causing obstruction. The person may cough, gag, or wheeze and will become cyanosed (blue) as he or she fights to take a breath. Infants or small children should be held along the arm, head down, and several gentle blows with the flat of the hand should be delivered to the back between the shoulder blades. This will usually dislodge the foreign body. In older children or adults the Heimlich Manoeuvre should be employed. Stand behind the victim with your arms wrapped around the waist. Make a fist with one hand with the thumb placed at a point half way between the victim's navel and the bottom of the breastbone. Grasp the fist with your other hand and give a quick inward and upward thrust. This may be repeated several times if necessary. Alternatively, if the person is unconscious, he or she should be placed on the back, face up and the same thrust performed with the heel of the hand whilst kneeling astride the hips. If a choking person is alone, he or she can perform the manoeuvre by placing a fist in the correct position and delivering the thrust by pressing it against a firm surface.

CARDIAC/RESPIRATORY ARREST: The measures described here are basic life-support procedures – they can be performed if necessary without any equipment. Before commencing cardiopulmonary resuscitation on a person who has collapsed, it is essential to establish that it is required. Performing artificial ventilation and cardiac massage on a person who is breathing and whose heart is still beating can be dangerous. The person's chest and abdomen should be observed for respiratory movement and the pulse should be checked either at the neck or groin or by feeling directly over the heart.

The technique for simple resuscitation may be remembered by means of the mnemonic 'ABC (Airway, Breathing and Circulation)'. The aim of basic resuscitation is to maintain the flow of oxygenated blood to vital organs until the person's heartbeat and breathing can be restarted, if that is possible.

AIRWAY: If the airway is obstructed, no air can enter the lungs; therefore the mouth should be checked for foreign bodies, which can be removed by hooking them out with an index finger. False teeth should be removed. To prevent the tongue from obstructing breathing, the jaw should be pulled forward (using a finger behind the angle or the chin) and the head extended on the neck so that the person looks as if he or she is 'sniffing the morning air'. *Care must be taken if there is any suspicion of neck injury*.

BREATHING: If clearing the airway does not allow breathing to recommence, then artificial ventilation of the lungs must be started. Mouth-to-mouth ventilation, using the rescuer's expired air to inflate the victim's lungs, is probably the easiest and most satisfactory to use. The victim is positioned as described above. The rescuer uses one hand to obstruct the nose and steady the head and the other to pull the jaw forward and open the mouth. The rescuer then places his or her mouth completely over that of the victim and blows out so as to inflate the victim's lungs, starting with two slow breaths to reinflate the lungs. It is important to observe the victim's chest rise and fall normally before commencing the next breath. If the chest does not rise or there is marked resistance to the inflating breath, then the airway is probably obstructed and the head should be repositioned.

CIRCULATION: Ventilating the lungs without any blood's circulating will not provide oxygenated blood to vital organs. Therefore, if there is no pulse or heartbeat, cardiac massage should be started to produce this circulation. The person performing cardiac massage, who should preferably have been trained in the technique, should kneel beside the victim with the heel of one hand over the lower two-thirds of the breastbone and the other hand placed on top. Downward pressure is applied, keeping the arms straight with the elbows locked, so as to depress the breastbone 4–5 cm. Pressure is released slowly so that it takes the same time as compression. The rate of compressions should be 80 per minute. If there are two rescuers, then the person performing cardiac massage should stop after every five compressions to allow the other to perform one cycle of artificial ventilation. A lone rescuer should perform two breaths after every 15 compressions.

Once spontaneous ventilation and cardiac output have returned, the patient should be placed in the recovery, or coma, position. This consists of rolling the person on to his or her side, with the lower arm and leg straight and in line with the body. The upper arm and leg are flexed and brought forward to prevent the patient from rolling on to his or her front.

DROWNING: About 500 people die from drowning each year in Britain, and an unknown number survive a near drowning. About a fifth of drownings occur in salt water. Wet drowning (when water is aspirated into the lungs) occurs in 85 per cent of cases. The remaining 15 per cent develop laryngo-spasm so that, although they also die of asphyxia, no water enters the lungs.

There has been some controversy about what type of water carries the worst prognosis, but it is now thought that salt and fresh water are equally bad. The effect of salt water is to draw fluid into the alveoli from the vascular compartment with concomitant damage to the lung. This results in pulmonary oedema and hypoxia. Fresh water washes out pulmonary surfactant (causing pulmonary atelectasis and leading to hypoxia) and is absorbed into the vascular compartment causing volume overload and electrolyte disturbances. Both types may result in acidosis and circulatory collapse and may be complicated by hypothermia and trauma (which may have precipitated the drowning).

Treatment: Cardiopulmonary resuscitation (see CARDIAC/RESPIRATORY ARREST in this Appendix) should be started as soon as possible and the patient transferred to hospital. This should include people who recover consciousness fairly quickly as pulmonary oedema may develop over the next few hours. If the patient is hypothermic, resuscitation should continue until he or she has been warmed to normal body temperature. Patients may require admission to an intensive care unit for artificial ventilation, circulatory support, or correction of electrolyte imbalance or acidosis.

ELECTROCUTION: People may be electrocuted when they touch an object which is live so that a current passes through them to earth. A lightning strike has a similar effect. The severity of the outcome depends on the frequency and amplitude of the current which flows through them. Below 2mA there is only a feeling of strong paraesthesia, 15–100mA will produce muscular contraction in the muscles near the point of contact, which makes letting go of the object impossible, and 50mA–2A is the threshold for producing ventricular fibrillation (q.v.). [These thresholds are for the mains electricity supply, which in Britain has a frequency of 50Hz, a frequency that is particularly liable to induce ventricular fibrillation]. Thus electrocution can cause burns to the tissues at the sites where the current enters and leaves the body and may also induce ventricular fibrillation. If a person is seen being electrocuted, no attempt should be made to touch the victim until the power supply is turned off, as the helper may also be electrocuted. If the switch or mains supply cannot be found, then the victim should be knocked away from the power source using a non-conducting object such as wood. Burns should be treated as described above and, if the patient has developed ventricular fibrillation, then cardiopulmonary resuscitation should be started (see CARDIAC/RESPIRA-

TORY ARREST in this Appendix). Any person experiencing significant electrocution should be seen by a doctor.

FITS: A major fit or seizure is known as a Grand Mal convulsion and consists of two phases: the tonic phase when the person may let out a cry, falls to the ground and is observed to be rigid, and the clonic phase when he or she shakes. At the end of the fit there is usually a period of unconsciousness. The most important task in looking after people undergoing a fit is to prevent them from doing any damage to themselves. Any objects which might cause harm, particularly hot food and liquids, should be moved out of their way, but there is no need to try to move them unless they are in danger. At the end of the fit, when they are unconscious, they should be placed in the coma position.

POISONING: The number of substances with which people are poisoned, either deliberately or accidentally, is too great to list individually. This section will merely cover some basic principles to follow on discovering a person who has been poisoned.

If the person is unconscious, he or she should be nursed in the coma position [see CARDIAC/RESPIRATORY ARREST in this Appendix]. Vomiting should never be induced at home except under medical supervision. If corrosive substances have been ingested, then water or milk should be drunk to dilute the effects on the oesophagus and stomach, and any remaining on the skin should be washed away with copious volumes of water. The container from which the tablets or other substance came should be taken to hospital with the patient to help medical staff correctly identify the poison. Likewise if it is a plant, a leaf or berry should be taken to hospital. (See POISONS.)